Nelson Yuan-sheng Kiang

Veterinary Anesthesia

Veterinary Anesthesia

WILLIAM V. LUMB, D.V.M., M.S., Ph.D.
Charter Diplomate, American College of Veterinary Surgeons
Founding Diplomate, American College of Veterinary Anesthesiologists
Professor Emeritus of Clinical Sciences
College of Veterinary Medicine and Biomedical Sciences
Colorado State University
Fort Collins, Colorado

E. WYNN JONES, M.R.C.V.S., Ph.D.
Charter Diplomate, American College of Veterinary Surgeons
Founding Diplomate, American College of Veterinary Anesthesiologists
Vice Dean and Professor, College of Veterinary Medicine
Mississippi State University
Mississippi State, Mississippi
Professor Emeritus, College of Veterinary Medicine
Oklahoma State University
Stillwater, Oklahoma

Second Edition

Lea & Febiger *Philadelphia 1984*

Lea & Febiger
600 Washington Square
Philadelphia, PA 19106-4198
U.S.A.
215-922-1330

First Edition, 1973
Reprinted, 1977
Second Edition, 1984

Library of Congress Cataloging in Publication Data

Lumb, William V. (William Valjean), 1921–
Veterinary anesthesia.

Bibliography: p.
Includes index.
1. Anesthesia in veterinary surgery. I. Jones,
E. Wynn (Eric Wynn), 1924– . II. Title.
SF914.L82 1984 636.089'796 83–18736
ISBN 0–8121–0906–6

Although the authors and publisher have taken every precaution to assure that the dosages are accurate, they assume no responsibility for the use of these drugs or dosages under any circumstances.

PRINTED IN THE UNITED STATES OF AMERICA

Print number 3 2 1

To our families, who sacrificed many happy hours that this book could come to fruition.

Preface

Although all chapters have been revised, the general concepts of this edition remain unchanged from those of the first. The student is introduced to anesthetic principles, and those more experienced in anesthesiology will find it a comprehensive reference source. It will also benefit persons other than veterinarians who wish to anesthetize animals. Many older references have been deleted and over 500 new ones added.

The first edition was published at a time when the application of inhalation anesthesia was rapidly expanding; this edition comes at a time of resurgence of injectable anesthesia. Although advances in design of inhalation anesthetic equipment and the addition of new inhalants have dictated significant revision, it has been necessary to pay more attention to other methods of inducing anesthesia, especially those utilizing drug combinations and their application to domestic, laboratory, wild, and exotic species. The increasing number of narcotic and other preanesthetic agents in use has also required expansion of this section. Increasing sophistication of instrumentation and anesthetic-related care has also necessitated changes in relevant chapters. The Appendices, listing drug and equipment manufacturers, standard values, conversion tables, and commonly used symbols, have been retained and expanded.

Again, the authors are indebted to the many individuals who have assisted them in preparing this text. At Colorado State University, College of Veterinary Medicine and Biomedical Sciences, Dr. R. Bruce Heath consulted on most of the rough draft. Dr. Mollie Wright also read portions of the manuscript. Ms. Diane Perkins devoted many hours to development of the data on anesthetic deaths in the Veterinary Teaching Hospital. Mr. Alan Kilminster contributed his photographic expertise. At Mississippi State University, College of Veterinary Medicine, we thank Mr. Bruce Evans, Mrs. Ann Irby, Mrs. Minnie Williams, Mr. Robert Lucas, and Ms. Julia Heard for library and media assistance, and Mrs. Diane Sumner for secretarial help.

Dr. Richard W. Redding of the School of Veterinary Medicine, Auburn University, Auburn, Alabama, critiqued the chapter on the nervous system, for which we are appreciative.

Fort Collins, Colorado William V. Lumb
Mississippi State, Mississippi E. Wynn Jones

Contents

CHAPTER 1

An Outline of Animal Anesthesia

INTRODUCTION

Anesthesia provides freedom from pain and reflex response and, in general anesthesia, immobilization, relaxation, and unconsciousness. It is, indeed, one of the miracles of medicine, without which modern surgical techniques would have been impossible. The influence of improved anesthesia on the development of veterinary surgical techniques is well illustrated in equine surgery. During the last three decades, major developments have been made in equine inhalation anesthesia, with resulting advances in both orthopedic and abdominal surgical procedures. The advent of barbiturate anesthesia, a wide range of preanesthetic agents, and the use of fluorinated hydrocarbons have motivated the introduction of a variety of surgical procedures in smaller animals. In the last two decades, the use of muscle relaxants, sedatives, and tranquilizers has facilitated the restraint and therapy of wild and exotic animals.

HISTORY OF ANIMAL ANESTHESIA

The earliest recorded attempts to produce anesthesia appear to have been performed in humans. Apparently, its advantages for animal use were not recognized. The ancients used narcotics, alcohol, asphyxia, and even compression of the carotid arteries to alleviate pain during surgical intervention.

In 1540, Paracelsus produced ether and reported it to have a soporific effect on fowl. Despite this, no further progress was made until chemistry was developed and carbon dioxide and several other gases including oxygen were discovered. In 1800, Sir Humphrey Davy suggested that nitrous oxide might have anesthetic properties. Shortly thereafter, H. H. Hickman (1824) demonstrated, by animal experimentation, that the pain of a surgical operation could be alleviated by inhalation of carbon dioxide. Even so, it was not until 1842 that ether was used for human anesthesia.

Two years later, a dentist, Dr. Horace Wells (1844), discovered the general anesthetic properties of nitrous oxide. While this finding was neglected for several years, it was reintroduced in man in 1862.

In spite of animal experimentation to demonstrate the relief of pain by the inhalation of carbon dioxide (Hickman, 1824), general anesthesia was not introduced for veterinary surgery until after its use in man. Dr. C. P. Jackson (1853), a Boston physician, seems to have been the first to employ ether extensively in animals.

Although chloroform was discovered by Liebig in 1831, it was not until 1847 that it was used for general anesthesia in animals by Flourens and in man by Dr. J. Y. Simpson of Edinburgh, Scotland. With the introduction of chloroform as an anesthetic, reports began to appear in the veterinary literature of its use in animals.

Dadd (1854) routinely used general anesthesia in animals, and was the first in the United States to advocate humane treatment of animals and the application of scientific principles in veterinary practice.

In 1875, Ore published the first monograph on intravenous anesthesia using chloral hydrate and, three years later, Humbert described its use in the horse. Rectal anesthesia, attempted as early as 1847 by Pirogoff, was later employed in veterinary anesthesia largely for the administration of chloral hydrate. The intraperitoneal route of administration was first used in 1892 in France. Thus, the various routes for the administration of general anesthetics to animals were established by the end of the nineteenth century.

After the initial isolation of cocaine by Albert Niemann of Germany in 1860, Anrep, in 1878, suggested the possibility of using cocaine for local anesthesia. In 1884, Kolhler introduced cocaine for local anesthesia of the eye, and Halsted described nerve block anesthesia a year later. Its use was popularized in veterinary surgery by Sir Frederick Hobday, an English veterinarian. G. L. Corning, using cocaine, is credited with inducing spinal anesthesia in a dog in 1885. From his description, however, it would appear that he probably produced epidural anesthesia. In 1898, August Bier of Germany produced true spinal anesthesia in animals and then in himself and an assistant (Keys, 1942).

While the use of infiltration anesthesia was encouraged by Reclus in 1890, and Schleich in 1892, conduction anesthesia was introduced by Halsted and Hall in New York in 1884. These techniques became more popular with the introduction of substitutes for the toxic cocaine at the turn of the century. With these developments, it was possible for such workers as Cuille and Sendrail (1901) in France to induce subarachnoid anesthesia in horses, cattle, and dogs. While Cathelin (1901) reported epidural anesthesia in the dog, it remained for Retzgen, Benesch, and Brook to apply the techniques of epidural anesthesia to the larger animals in the 1920s. Although paralumbar anesthesia was introduced in man by Sellheim in 1909, it was not until the 1940s that Farquharson and Formston developed these techniques in cattle. Despite anesthetic developments in the latter half of the nineteenth century, and perhaps due to unfavorable results, general anesthesia was not readily adopted by the veterinary profession until well into the twentieth century. A heavy hand, without anesthesia, was the stock in trade of the average veterinarian.

In small domestic animals, ether and chloroform were commonly administered. However, general anesthesia in small domestic animals became more widely accepted after discovery of the barbiturates in the late 1920s and, in particular, with the development of pentobarbital sodium in 1930. Barbiturate anesthesia received an additional boost with introduction of the thiobarbiturates and particularly with thiopental sodium in 1934. Because of problems occurring during emergence from anesthesia, similar developments in large animal anesthesia awaited the introduction of such preanesthetic agents as the phenothiazine derivatives by Charpentier in France in 1950, the development of large animal anesthetic equipment, and the introduction of the fluorinated hydrocarbons by Raventos and others. Recently, fluorinated hydrocarbon anesthetics and combinations of tranquilizers, narcotic analgesics and dissociative agents have revolutionized veterinary anesthesia in both large and small animal practice.

In North America, development of veterinary anesthesia as a distinct discipline led to organization of the American Society of Veterinary Anesthesiology in 1970 and, in 1975, to establishment of the American College of Veterinary Anesthesiologists. The latter organization establishes criteria for and certifies specialty (diplomate) status in veterinary anesthesiology, under the auspices of the American Veterinary Medical Association. In the United States, numerous veterinary technician training programs have also developed, with a large component devoted to instruction in anesthesia.

Other groups around the world promoting veterinary anesthesia include the Association of Veterinary Anaesthetists of Great Britain and Ireland, and the International Congress of Veterinary Anaesthesia, the first meeting of which was held in Cambridge, England, in 1982.

For further information on the history of anesthesia, the reader is referred to Clark (1938), Smithcors (1957), and Lee (1959).

DEFINITIONS

The term "anesthesia," derived from the Greek *anaisthaesia*, meaning "insensibility," is used to denote loss of sensation to the whole or any part of the body. It is produced by agents that depress the activity of nervous tissue either locally or generally. From a pharmacologic point of view, there has been a significant redefinition of a general anesthetic (Heavner, 1983). Both central nervous stimulants and depressants can be useful general anesthetics (Winters et al., 1972). Several terms are used in describing anesthesia:

1. *Analgesia* refers to relief from pain.
2. *Tranquilization* is a state of behavioral change in which the patient is relaxed and unconcerned by his surroundings.
3. *Sedation* is a mild degree of central depression in which the patient is awake but calm.
4. *Narcosis* in man is defined as a drug-produced state of deep sleep accompanied by analgesia. In veterinary medicine, the narcotized patient is seldom asleep but is sedated and has decreased sensibility to pain.
5. *Hypnosis* is a condition of artificially induced sleep, or a trance resembling sleep, resulting from moderate depression of the central nervous system.
6. *Local anesthesia* is a loss of sensation in a limited body area.
7. *Regional anesthesia* is insensibility in a larger, though limited, body area.
8. *Basal anesthesia* is a light level of general anesthesia usually produced by preanesthetic agents. It serves as a basis for deeper anesthesia on administration of other agents.
9. *General anesthesia* is complete unconsciousness produced by controlled reversible intoxication of the central nervous system (CNS) in which there is lowered sensitivity to environmental stimuli and diminished response to such stimuli.
10. *Surgical anesthesia* is unconsciousness, accompanied by muscular relaxation to such a degree that surgery can be performed painlessly and without struggling on the part of the patient.
11. *Balanced anesthesia* is a state produced by a combination of drugs, which is characterized by unconsciousness, analgesia, and muscular relaxation.
12. *Dissociative anesthesia*, in contrast to balanced anesthesia, is produced by interruption of information flow from the unconscious to the conscious parts of the brain. This is in contrast to other agents that produce generalized depression of all brain centers. Dissociative agents stimulate some brain centers rather than depress them.

REASONS FOR ADMINISTRATION OF ANESTHETICS

Because anesthesia was first developed to alleviate pain and to provide relaxation for surgery, its use for other purposes is sometimes overlooked. These include restraint, transportation, various diagnostic and therapeutic procedures, behavior modification, euthanasia, and the humane slaughter of food animals.

TYPES OF ANESTHESIA

The diverse uses for anesthesia, the varying needs for analgesia, immobilization, and muscle relaxation, and the requirements peculiar to species, age, and disease state necessitate the use of a variety of agents by several methods. Anesthesia has therefore been classified according to method of administration of the drug employed.

1. *Inhalation*—anesthetic gases or vapors are inhaled.
2. *Intravascular*—anesthetic solution is administered by intravenous, intra-arterial, intracardiac, or intramedullary (bone marrow) injection.
3. *Other injectable routes*—anesthetic is ad-

ministered by intrathoracic, intraperitoneal, intramuscular, and subcutaneous injection.

4. *Oral or rectal*—liquid anesthetics may occasionally be administered per os or by enema.
5. *Local and conduction anesthesia*—anesthetic is applied topically, is injected locally into or around the surgical site (field block), or is injected around nerves supplying the specific site (conduction). In the latter instance, the injection may be perineural (nerve block), or into the epidural or subarachnoid space (spinal).
6. *Electronarcosis*—an electrical current is passed through the cerebrum.
7. *Transcutaneous electrical nerve stimulation (TENS, TNS, TES)*—local analgesia is produced by low-intensity, high-frequency electrical stimulation of the skin through surface electrodes.
8. *Hypnosis*—anesthesia is induced by placing the patient in a trance-like state.
9. *Acupuncture*—an ancient Oriental system of therapy utilizing long fine needles has been used more recently to induce anesthesia.
10. *Hypothermia*—body temperature is lowered, either locally or generally, to the level at which anesthesia occurs.

REFERENCES

Clark, A.J.: Aspects of the History of Anaesthetics. Br. Med. J., 2:1029, 1938.

Dadd, G.H.: *The Modern Horse Doctor*. J. P. Jewett and Company, Boston, 1854.

Heavner, J.E.: Veterinary Anesthesia Update. J.A.V.M.A., 182:30, 1983.

Jackson, C.T.: *Etherization of Animals*. Report of the Commissioner of Patents for the Year 1853. Beverly Tucker, Senate Printer. Washington, D.C., 1853, p. 59.

Keys, T.E.: The Development of Anesthesia. Anesthesiology, 3:11, 1942.

Lee, J.A.: *A Synopsis of Anaesthesia*, 4th ed. Williams & Wilkins, Baltimore, 1959.

Smithcors, J.E.: The Early Use of Anaesthesia in Veterinary Practice. Br. Vet. J., 113:284, 1957.

Stevenson, D.E.: The Evolution of Veterinary Anaesthesia. Br. Vet. J., 119:477, 1963.

Winters, W.D., Ferrer, A.T., and Guzman-Flores, C.: The Cataleptic State Induced by Ketamine: A Review of the Neuropharmacology of Anesthesia. Neuropharmacology, 11:303, 1972.

CHAPTER 2

General Considerations

INTRODUCTION

Anesthesia is, of necessity, a reversible process. Knowledge of the factors underlying production of anesthesia, and those that may modify it, is essential to success of the procedure. The dose of anesthetic and the techniques for its administration are based on the *average* animal. Because of the many phenomena that modify the effect of an anesthetic agent, however, it is unlikely that any given animal will be exactly "average."

Marked variations in response to a standard dose of anesthetic result from the interplay of many factors, especially those related to the metabolic activity of the animal and to the uptake and distribution of the anesthetic.

BIOLOGIC VARIATIONS

Since elimination of anesthetics depends especially on the metabolic processes of the animal, conditions affecting the metabolic rate exert a marked influence on anesthetic effect. Among these conditions are the following:

1. Relative Size. Small animals have a higher basal metabolic rate per unit of surface area than large animals; therefore, the smaller the animal, the larger the dose per unit of body weight necessary for anesthesia.

2. Physical Condition. Animals with large quantities of fat, which is a relatively inactive nonmetabolizing tissue, have a lower basal metabolic rate per unit of body weight and require less anesthetic than lean muscular animals in good condition. Greyhounds, an example of the latter, are notorious for their tendency toward excitability during induction and for a prolonged period of recovery (Knight, 1949).

Animals in poor condition also require less anesthetic. De Boer (1947) found that dogs kept on a low food intake resulting in weight losses of 10 to 20% showed a marked increase in duration of anesthesia following a single injection.

3. Age. In the newborn, the basal metabolic rate is low. It gradually increases to its highest point at the time of puberty through early adulthood and then gradually declines.

De Boer (1947) has shown that response to barbiturates varies in dogs of differing ages. Very young animals and older adult animals were found most sensitive, whereas dogs in the age range from 3 to 12 months were least sensitive. These age variations are also related to changes in liver enzyme activity (Kato and Takanaka, 1968). Changes of metabolism with age are not as clear-cut as originally thought. This reflects the fact that gross weight and surface area are not reliable measures of the active tissue mass of the body. In man, at least, data on fat-free body weight indicate little change between the young and aged adult (Keys, 1973).

4. Sex. The basal metabolic rate of males is approximately 7% higher than that of females. In the female, a rise occurs during pregnancy due to the metabolic activity of the fetuses. Conflicting evidence concerning sex differences in susceptibility to anesthetics has been presented.

The anesthetic used may be the determining factor.

Nicholas and Barron (1932) showed that definite sex variance existed in the susceptibility of rats to amobarbital anesthesia. Pregnant females were most susceptible, nonpregnant females less, and male rats least susceptible. Kennedy (1934) could find no sex variance in mice to hexobarbital anesthesia. Cameron (1938) has shown that normal females are less susceptible to pentobarbital sodium than spayed females. Female rats have been shown to be more sensitive to tubocurarine than males of a similar age (Green, 1979). Sex hormones may also cause differences in response to an anesthetic agent other than those resulting from the change in metabolic rate.

5. Genetic Differences. Genetic variation in dose response to anesthetics has been reported. A heritable difference in the ability of rabbits to hydrolyze atropine and cocaine (Stormont and Suzuki, 1970), genetic variations in response to pentobarbital in mice (Green, 1979), and strain sensitivity to nitrous oxide (Green, 1979) and to non-oxygen-dependent reductive biotransformation of halothane in rats (Gourlay et al., 1981) have all been reported. In a few people, plasma cholinesterase has been found to be completely absent or replaced by an inactive variant with resultant prolonged action of succinylcholine (Jenkins et al. 1967). Some breeds of swine are susceptible to malignant hyperthermia (Jones et al., 1972).

6. Activity and Biological Rhythms. The metabolic rate increases with activity; hence, active animals require relatively large doses of anesthetic agents. Mice have been shown to be most sensitive to pentobarbital at 7 A.M., a seasonal response to morphine has been recorded in the rabbit, and circadian rhythms have been shown to modify minimum alveolar concentrations for halothane and cyclopropane in rats by 5 to 10% (Green, 1979).

UPTAKE AND DISTRIBUTION OF ANESTHETICS

General anesthesia results from the action of an anesthetic upon the brain and spinal cord (see Chap. 4). The agent must, therefore, achieve access to the central nervous tissue.

Although Van Dyke and Chenoweth (1965) have demonstrated that significant quantities of some inhalation anesthetics are metabolized within the body, for practical purposes they are primarily exhaled. Small amounts are eliminated in feces and urine, or diffused through the skin and mucous membranes. Thus, providing respiration and circulation are maintained, inhalants are readily eliminated from the body. In contrast, injectable agents depend upon redistribution within the tissues, detoxification principally in the liver, and elimination via the kidneys. With these agents, the anesthetist has little control over the elimination process and, for this reason, they are considered to be more dangerous than the inhalant anesthetics.

Inhalation agents are, for the most part, nonreactive substances that can be absorbed, transported, and excreted from the body with little change. This suggests that they behave like inert gases, conforming to the general physical laws governing partial pressure, diffusion, and solubility in liquids. In general, this is true, though extremely soluble gases, those reacting with the solvent, or those undergoing ionization, do not follow Henry's law accurately. In the following description of the transport process, no distinction is made between gas and vapor.

Dalton's law states that the pressure of a mixture of gases is the sum of the partial pressures of the various gases. When a volatile liquid anesthetic agent is administered, it is vaporized into a carrier gas, usually oxygen. If an anesthetic gas is administered, it is diluted with oxygen. The partial pressure of anesthetic vapor or gas in the mixture can be controlled rather accurately by means of calibrated vaporizers or flowmeters. When the mixture is administered in a nonrebreathing system, the patient inhales a constant partial pressure of anesthetic, which is not modified by admixture with exhaled gases. In rebreathing systems, the partial pressure of the inhaled gas varies according to the volume of fresh gas flowing into the system. In actual practice, anesthesia is induced rapidly with a relatively high partial pressure of anesthetic and maintained with a lower partial pressure.

As the anesthetic mixture is inhaled, it passes through the upper airway and into the alveoli of the lungs. No blood-gas exchange occurs until the respiratory bronchioles and alveoli are reached. The anesthetic gas mixes by diffusion with the functional residual air of the lungs, and is thereby diluted. There is, therefore, a decrease in anesthetic partial pressure from inspired gas to alveolar gas. This decrease is the most important step between the source of the gas (the anesthesia machine) and the ultimate target (the brain).

Approximately 80% of the functional residual air is nitrogen. When a relatively impotent anesthetic agent such as nitrous oxide is used for anesthesia, it is important that the residual nitrogen be removed; otherwise, an anesthetic concentration of nitrous oxide cannot be achieved. By using a nonbreathing system, the residual air containing nitrogen is removed by "lung washout" in a few minutes and the alveolar concentration of nitrous oxide is thereby rapidly increased. Assuming a constant inspired concentration of the anesthetic, the rate of increase of alveolar concentration bears direct relation to the concentration inspired, and to the efficiency of delivery to the alveoli. The greater the alveolar ventilation, the more rapid the approach of the alveolar to the inspired concentration of gas or vapor. This approach of alveolar to inspired concentration ("washin") is adversely influenced by the residual volume of air (functional residual capacity—FRC) to be replaced. In fact, a useful constant to express "washin" time is the time required for flow (alveolar ventilation—V_A) through a container (FRC) to equal the capacity of the container. This happens to be the time required for 63% "washin" or "washout" of a new gas from the lungs, providing flow and gas concentration are constant and mixing is complete (Eger, 1974).

When nitrous oxide is administered, the relation of alveolar concentration (F_A) to the inspired concentration (F_I) is influenced by the concentration of nitrous oxide inspired. The higher the concentration (F_I), the less the effect. If, for instance, a lung is filled with 80% nitrous oxide in oxygen (80 volumes N_2O and 20 volumes O_2) and approximately half of the nitrous oxide is taken up into the blood, the concentration does not fall to 40%; 40 volumes remain in a total of 60 volumes (67%). As the uptake of nitrous oxide occurs, the lungs do not collapse, but instead draw in more gas to replace the gas taken up. This additional inspired volume may be quite significant in the early stages of nitrous oxide anesthesia, and further increases the alveolar N_2O concentration (Fig. 2–1). The increase in inspired ventilation and concentrating effect also accelerates the F_A/F_I rate of rise for a gas or vapor such as halothane given with nitrous oxide (the second gas effect) (Eger, 1979).

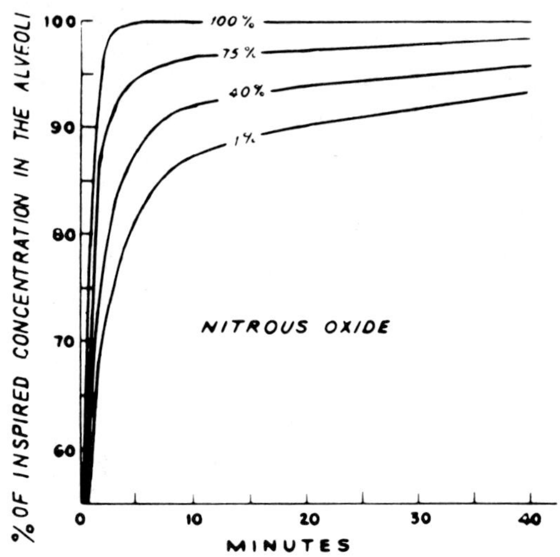

Figure 2–1. The concentration effect. This diagram illustrates that the higher the concentration of an anesthetic agent, the more rapidly the alveolar concentration approaches to that inspired. (From Wylie, W.D., and Churchill-Davidson, H.C.: *A Practice of Anaesthesia*, 2nd ed. Lloyd-Luke, Ltd., London, 1966.)

Factors that impede normal respiration delay "lung washout" and impair the ability of the anesthetist to achieve the necessary alveolar concentration of anesthetic. If the patient is heavily premedicated with an agent such as morphine or if mechanical dead space is increased, induction time is prolonged. Conversely, if alveolar ventilation is increased, induction may be quite rapid. Increased functional residual capacity, such as in emphysema, likewise delays production of desired alveolar concentrations of anesthetic, and thereby induction of anesthesia. These same factors have equal application to recovery from inhalation anesthesia.

As the gas enters the alveolus, it diffuses across the alveolar-capillary membrane, which is less than one micron thick and under normal circumstances presents little barrier to exchange of gas between the alveolus and the blood. Alveolar concentrations of anesthetic thus fail to rise as rapidly as predicted from a time constant derived from normal alveolar ventilation and FRC values (Eger, 1974). While ventilation delivers anesthetic to the alveolus, uptake by diffusion into the circulating blood removes anesthetic. The relation of delivery to uptake thus determines the alveolar concentration of anesthetic. Factors that determine anesthetic uptake are solubility (blood/gas partition coefficient) of the anesthetic, cardiac output, and the alveolar to mixed venous anesthetic partial pressure difference (Eger, 1974). On induction, a large concentration gradient exists owing to a high partial pressure of anesthetic gas within the alveolus and a low partial pressure within the pulmonary capillary. The body tissues remove nearly all anesthetic delivered in arterial blood and thereby markedly lower the partial pressure of venous blood. This gradient is responsible for the uptake of anesthetic gas from the alveolus to pulmonary capillary blood and, thus, via the left heart to the general circulation. Reduction of the area of alveolar membrane exposed to the anesthetic gas by exudate, transudate, atelectasis, emphysema, or by impaired permeability of the alveolar capillary membrane, as in pulmonary fibrosis, will impede diffusion and consequent uptake of anesthetic.

Blood from the right ventricle is pumped through the pulmonary capillary bed into the left atrium. Pulmonary capillary blood flow is dynamic and constantly changing. Arteriovenous shunts within the lungs may open, creating poorly perfused areas of lung tissue. Alveoli thus bypassed are considered physiologic dead space, since anesthetic uptake by the blood does not occur from them. Alternatively, pulmonary blood may perfuse alveoli which are not ventilated, due to atelectasis or other reasons, and gas uptake fails to occur. The mixed pulmonary venous blood entering the left heart is thus diluted with blood that has failed to take up anesthetic gas, due to bypass of the alveoli by shunting.

As pulmonary capillary blood passes the alveoli, it absorbs anesthetic gas, maintaining a low partial pressure on the capillary side of the alveolar membrane. By so doing, it lowers the partial pressure within the alveoli compared to that of the inhaled mixture. Other factors remaining constant, anesthetic solubility in blood determines the degree to which the pressure of gas within the alveoli is reduced. If the solubility is low, only small quantities will be removed per unit of time, and the pressure gradient between alveolus and blood will be low.

Anesthetic solubility may be expressed by several methods, but the partition (distribution) coefficient is the most general descriptive term (Eger and Larson, 1964). It is the ratio between anesthetic concentrations in each of two phases when equilibrium exists between these phases. For example, if tissue and blood concentrations are in equilibrium and there are 2 ml of anesthetic per ml of tissue and 1 ml of anesthetic per ml of blood, the tissue/blood partition coefficient is 2/1. When one expresses the partition coefficient, the numerator and denominator must be specified, i.e., blood/gas, tissue/gas, and tissue/blood. Solubility is usually expressed as per unit volume rather than as per unit weight (Table 2–1).

In Table 2–1, nitrous oxide has a blood/gas partition coefficient of 0.47 indicating that, at equilibrium, this amount is present in blood when one part is in the gaseous phase. Thus, nitrous oxide is relatively insoluble in blood compared to other agents listed in the table. Because of its relative insolubility in blood, an equilibrium is quickly established between inspired air, alveolar air, and pulmonary capillary blood. Since solubility in blood determines how much anesthetic is removed from the alveoli, the blood/gas solubility ratio is an indication of how rapidly the alveolar concentration rises toward the inspired concentration (Figs. 2–2, 2–3, 2–4, 2–5). Soluble agents such as methoxyflurane have high inspired air/alveolar air/

TABLE 2–1. Partition Coefficients at 37° C

		Tissue/Blood							
Anesthetic	*Blood/ Gas*	*Brain/(Grey)*	*Brain/ (White)*	*Liver*	*Kidney*	*Muscle*	*Fat*	*Lung*	*Oil/ Gas*
Cyclopropane	0.4 to 0.6	0.76*	1.5*	1.16*	0.62*	1.16*	12.9†		11.8
Nitrous oxide	0.47	1.06 (average grey and white)		0.80		1.15	2.3†	1.0	1.4
Fluroxene	1.37	1.43	1.43	1.37	1.05	2.3	23.0†		47.7
Isoflurane	1.41	2.6 (average grey and white)		2.5		4.0	45.0†		98
Enflurane	1.78	1.45 (average grey and white)		2.1		1.7	36.2†		98
Halothane	2.3	2.3	3.5	2.6	1.6	3.5	60		224
Divinyl ether	2.8	1.80	1.62	1.15	0.76	1.11	13.8†		58
Chloroform	8.4	1.38	2.39	1.98	1.22	1.89	30.8†		394
Diethyl ether	12.1	1.03	1.12	1.01	1.06	0.98	3.7†		65
Methoxyflurane	12.0	1.70	2.34	1.90	0.93	1.34	48.8†		970

*Assuming a blood/gas partition coefficient of 0.565.
†Estimated from the assumption that fat consists of 65% fat (oil) and 35% whole blood.
(Adapted from Eger, E. I., II.: *Anesthetic Uptake and Action*. Williams & Wilkins, Baltimore, 1974.)

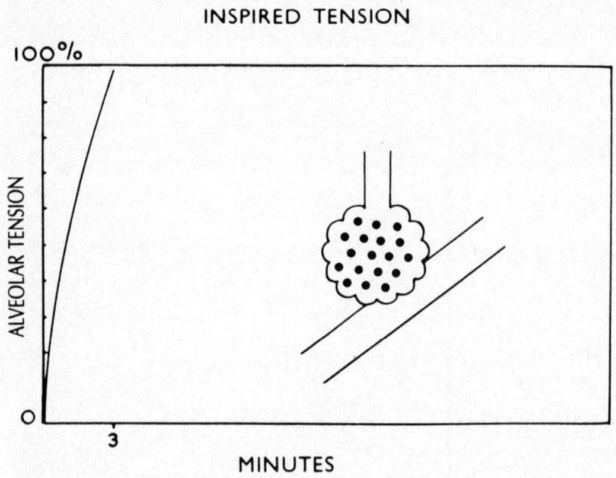

Figure 2–2. Alveolar tension curve of a gas that is totally insoluble in blood. (From Wylie, W.D., and Churchill-Davidson, H.C.: *A Practice of Anaesthesia,* 2nd ed. Lloyd-Luke, Ltd., London, 1966.)

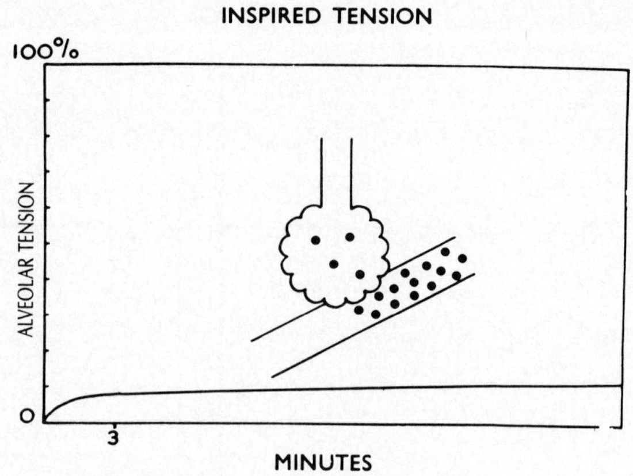

Figure 2–4. Alveolar tension curve of a gas that has a high solubility in blood, *i.e.,* ether. (From Wylie, W.D., and Churchill-Davidson, H.C.: *A Practice of Anaesthesia,* 2nd ed. Lloyd-Luke, Ltd., London, 1966.)

blood gradients, and the alveolar concentration rises slowly.

Tissue solubility determines the quantity of anesthetic removed from the peripheral circulation as it traverses the tissues, the amount removed being proportional to the tissue/blood partition coefficient. When this is high, tissue extraction of anesthetic from the blood is marked, venous blood returning to the alveoli contains little anesthetic agent, and a high alveolar/blood concentration gradient exists. The higher the tissue/blood coefficient, the longer the tissue will be able to extract anesthetic from blood or the longer it will take to saturate the tissue. Agents with high tissue/blood coefficients, therefore, require longer induction periods.

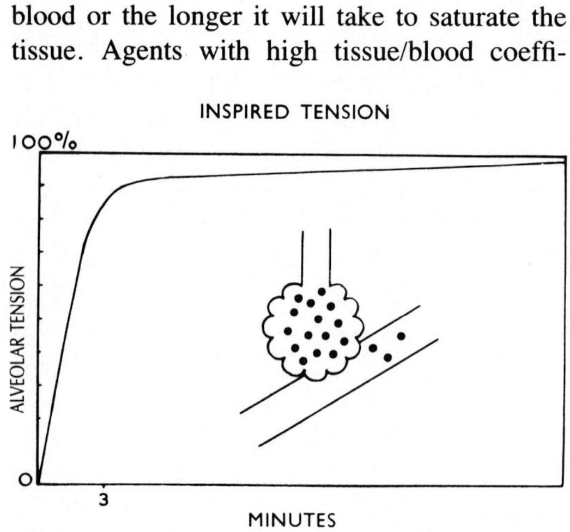

Figure 2–3. Alveolar tension curve of a gas that has a low solubility in blood, *i.e.,* nitrous oxide. (From Wylie, W.D., and Churchill-Davidson, H.C.: *A Practice of Anaesthesia,* 2nd ed. Lloyd-Luke, Ltd., London, 1966.)

Based on these facts, it is possible to determine from the blood/gas partition coefficient the relative speed with which induction can be accomplished. In general, anesthesia can be induced most rapidly with those gases having a low blood/gas partition coefficient. The partial pressure necessary for anesthesia must be maintained in the alveoli and pulmonary capillary blood. If alveolar anesthetic pressure is constantly lowered due to high blood solubility, neither the alveolar nor the arterial tension will be sufficient to produce anesthesia. To overcome this disadvantage during induction, the anesthesiologist supplies a higher inspired partial pressure of anesthetic than is required for maintenance of anesthesia.

Several factors affect anesthetic solubility. The solvent itself is of major importance, anesthetic agents being most soluble in lipids, less in proteins, and least in aqueous solutions. Electrolytes diminish solvent capacity. Fat is a better solvent than brain, and white matter of the brain is better than grey because of its higher lipid content. After a fatty meal, the blood/gas solubility for cyclopropane may rise as much as 20%. Anesthetic solubility increases in aqueous or oil media with decreasing temperature. Although variations in hematocrit, lipoid, protein, and electrolyte concentrations exert some effect

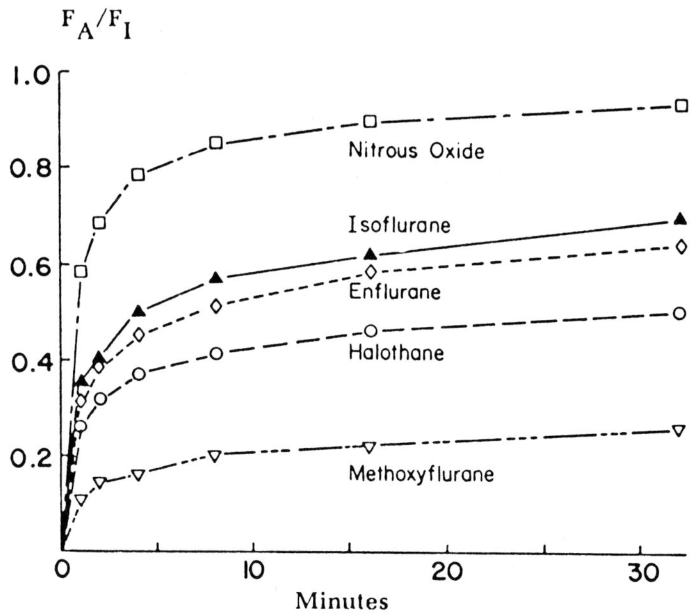

Figure 2–5. Volunteers breathed trace to subanesthetic concentrations of isoflurane or nitrous oxide, enflurane, halothane and methoxyflurane. Alveolar (F_A) and inspired (F_I) concentrations were measured by gas chromatography. The plot of the ratio of F_A/F_I expresses the rapidity with which the alveolar concentration approaches the concentration being inspired. It is most rapid with the least soluble anesthetic, nitrous oxide, and least rapid with the most soluble anesthetic, methoxyflurane. (From Eger, E.I., II: Isoflurane (Forane). A Compendium and Reference. Ohio Medical Products, Madison, Wisconsin, 1981.)

on anesthetic solubility, and thus on induction of anesthesia, changes in respiration and circulation are more important.

Tissue perfusion determines the amount of anesthetic presented to the various compartments of the body. In this respect, the body can be divided into four tissue groups: (1) vessel-rich group, (2) vessel-poor group, (3) muscle group, and (4) fat group. The vessel-rich group includes the brain, heart, kidney, hepatoportal system, and endocrine glands. The vessel-poor group contains bone, cartilage, tendons, and ligaments. The muscle group includes muscle and skin, and the fat group contains all adipose tissue. The vessel-rich group, muscle group, and fat group are the main determinants of uptake (Fig. 2–6). The vessel-rich group, which is perfused most thoroughly, dominates uptake during the first 5 to 15 minutes, after which the muscle group is dominant for 1 to 3 hours (Eger, 1974). The length of this period is determined by tissue solubility and a rising arterial gas tension. Fat, being poorly perfused, continues to absorb anesthetic agent after all other tissues have ceased, because of the high fat/blood coefficient of all anesthetics. The brain, heart, liver, and kidneys receive approximately 70% of the cardiac output, yet comprise only 7.3% of the total body weight (Table 2–2). Blood flow to the brain is estimated to be about 15% of the cardiac output and is much greater in shock; thus, it is not surprising that anesthesia can be quickly induced once an adequate arterial anesthetic partial pressure has been established. Increased blood flow to the muscles during fear and excitement may, on the other hand, delay anesthetic induction. Nervous tissue has little special affinity for anesthetics, its early saturation being due to intense perfusion.

There is an initial rapid uptake by organs of the vessel-rich group. This establishes anesthesia since the brain is one of these organs. Competition for the anesthetic by more poorly perfused tissue groups then develops. These groups become saturated slowly owing to poor blood supply. If the arterial tension is not held

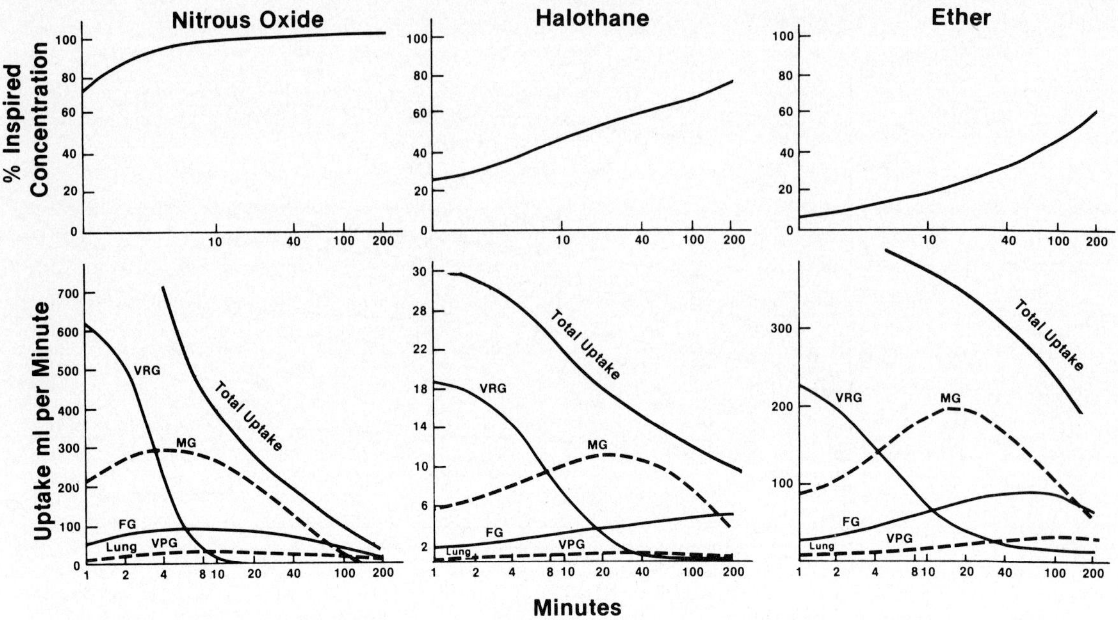

Figure 2–6. The three top graphs represent the approach of alveolar to inspired concentration, derived by analog computer. They are plotted on a logarithmic time scale. The inspired concentrations are 75% nitrous oxide, 1% halothane, and 10% ether.

The bottom graphs describe the uptake of gas by different tissue groups. The uppermost curve is total uptake. Uptake by various tissue groups is indicated by the lower curves. VPG = vessel-poor group; VRG = vessel-rich group; MG = muscle group; FG = fat group. Uptake by lung is of consequence in the first minute only. Uptake by the VPG (bone, cartilage, tendons, ligaments) is insignificant because of limited blood flow. The VRG (brain, heart, kidney, hepatoportal system, endocrines), MG (muscle and skin), and FG (fat) are the main determinants of uptake. The VRG dominates uptake during the first 5 to 10 minutes (longest in the case of halothane where the tissue/blood coefficient is highest). Following this, the MG is dominant for 70 to 170 minutes. The length of this period is determined by tissue solubility (muscle takes up halothane for a longer time than nitrous oxide) and by a rising arterial tension (the ether and halothane curves are similar, although halothane has a much larger muscle/blood coefficient than ether). Fat continues to take up agent after all other tissues have ceased doing so because of the high fat/blood coefficient of all anesthetics and because of the relatively low blood flow to this tissue. (From Eger, E.I., II, and Larson, C.P.: Anaesthetic Solubility in Blood and Tissues: Values and Significance. Br. J. Anaesth., 36:140, 1964.)

TABLE 2–2. Body Compartments Based on Tissue Perfusion

Group	*Region*	*Mass in Kg*	*% Cardiac Output*
Vessel Rich	Brain	1.4	14
	Liver (splanchnic)	2.6	28
	Heart	0.3	5
	Kidney	0.3	23
Intermediate	Muscle	31.0	16
	Skin	3.6	8
Fat	Adipose tissue	12.5	6
Vessel Poor	Residual tissue	11.3	Nil
Total	—	63.0	100

(From Bard, P.: Blood Supply of Special Regions. In *Medical Physiology,* 11th ed. Edited by P. Bard. The C.V Mosby Co., St. Louis, 1961. Data on adipose tissue and residual tissue have been added.)

constant by addition of more anesthetic to the system, there is, in addition to that lost by hepatic metabolism and renal excretion, a tendency for the concentration gradient to remove anesthetic from the brain to supply the less richly perfused tissue groups. Anesthesia will thus lighten. This redistribution effect continues for varying lengths of time depending upon the anesthetic agent employed. For this reason a so-called "steady state" of anesthesia requires a long period of administration to become established. Equilibration is finally reached when the inhaled, alveolar, arterial, venous, and tissue partial pressures become the same.

When anesthetic administration ceases, many of the same phenomena occur in reverse. The vaporizer is turned off and pure oxygen or air is inhaled by the patient. The anesthetic concentration of the alveolar air is reduced and, with each exhalation, anesthetic is removed from pulmonary blood. This output from venous blood to alveolar air is a function of solubility, cardiac output, and the venous to alveolar partial pressure difference. The balance between partial pressures in the alveolus and in the pulmonary capillary blood is now upset, a lower partial pressure existing within the alveolus. The concentration gradient is reversed between tissues, blood, alveolar air, and ambient air. The anesthetic gas flows from the area of high partial pressure in the tissues to the exterior. In contrast to induction, the ventilation-output relationship during recovery is not influenced by the concentration effect of nitrous oxide. Nonanesthetic gases are, however, affected by the rapid diffusion of nitrous oxide to the alveoli; alveolar oxygen may thus be so diluted that "diffusion hypoxia" results (Eger, 1974).

Adequate tissue perfusion and pulmonary ventilation are again essential for effective elimination of anesthetic. A reduced cardiac output or increased pulmonary ventilation permits a more rapid fall in alveolar anesthetic concentration. These changes in cardiopulmonary function may accelerate recovery from anesthesia with the more soluble agents; the concomitant increase in tissue "washout" time may delay recovery with relatively insoluble anesthetics. Increases in ventilation and circulation accelerate recovery, unless perfusion is increased to tissues of low perfusion such as muscle and fat (Eger, 1974). Fat, because of its affinity for anesthetic agents, is the last to lose its concentration. Slight traces of some agents may be found by gas chromatography in venous blood for as long as a week (Tevik et al., 1968).

Anesthetics and related drugs are commonly administered by intravenous injection and occasionally by intramuscular, intrathoracic, intraperitoneal, subcutaneous, and even oral or rectal routes. Intravenous administration bypasses the absorption phase of the drug with the consequences that onset and intensity of action are less variable, titration of dose according to response is facilitated, and the risk of toxicity lessens with progressive decline of drug concentration in the plasma (Hug, 1978).

As in inhalation anesthesia, the body may be considered to have multiple compartments (see Table 2–2) which are differentiated by blood supply and tissue-blood partition coefficient. After initial intravenous injection, mixing and dilution rapidly occur, and an initial blood plasma concentration of the drug is established. Blood plasma thus becomes the medium by which drug is delivered to and removed from its site of action. Factors affecting drug concentration and/or availability in the plasma also affect its concentration and availability at the site of action. Binding of drugs to plasma protein, in which form they cannot readily penetrate cellular membranes, and the removal of drugs by tissues that store, metabolize, and excrete them are all factors that lower the effective concentration of drugs at their site of action (Saidman, 1975; Hug, 1978). Binding is a reversible fusion of small molecules, such as barbiturates, with protein or other macromolecules, thereby limiting penetration of cellular membranes by molecular size, ionization, and limited lipid solubility. Protein binding varies with the nature of the drug, its concentration, and plasma pH and protein concentration. The fraction of bound ineffective drug increases with decreasing drug concentration and vice versa, and is modified by the presence of other drugs that compete for available binding sites. The rate of clearance of drug from the blood, its distribution to the tissues, and availability to produce its desired effects thus may all be modified by the drug concentration, the plasma pH and protein, the state of body hydration, and the presence of other drugs (Saidman, 1975).

After initial dilution within the vascular system, the drug is distributed to the various tissue compartments according to their perfusion, their capacity for the drug (volume of tissue × tissue-blood partition coefficient), and the partial pressure gradient of drug between blood and tissue. The vessel-rich group of tissues achieves equilibrium with the blood more quickly than do other tissue groups (Table 2–3). Although fat and muscle groups have similar tissue blood flows per unit of tissue, the higher solubility of most anesthetics (e.g., thiobarbiturates) in fat than in muscle accounts for the greater time to achieve equilibrium for fat than for muscle. Changes in tissue blood flow, solubility, and blood-tissue partial pressure gradients thus influence uptake and distribution of intravenous anesthetics. Since the plasma concentration of an intravenous anesthetic falls rapidly (Fig. 2–7), and its partial pressure is quickly exceeded by that in the vessel-rich tissues, anesthetic reenters the blood from these tissues to be redistributed to tissues having greater time constants. This redistribution reduces anesthetic concentration in the brain, anesthesia lightens, and anesthetic accumulates in muscle, fat, and vessel-poor tissues.

The ultimate effect of a general anesthetic is contingent upon its ability to cross the blood-brain barrier. This barrier, like the placenta, has permeability characteristics of cellular membranes and therefore limits the penetration of nonlipophilic, ionized, or protein-bound drugs. Penetration of these barriers is, in fact, so slow that little or no drug of the aforementioned types enters the brain or fetus after a single intravenous bolus dose. The barriers are not, however, absolute and slow penetration does occur, becoming significant when the level of drug is maintained over a prolonged period of time (Hug, 1978). The high lipid-solubility of thiopental relative to pentobarbital accounts for the rapid onset of and recovery from anesthesia induced by the former (Baggot, 1977).

Within moments of tissue uptake and redistribution, elimination of the drug begins. The circulation distributes it to vessel-rich organs able to biotransform and/or excrete it. The liver is the primary site of biotransformation while the kidney is primarily responsible for excretion. Other organs may occasionally be involved, such as in the elimination of morphine via the gastrointestinal tract (Hug, 1978). Biotransformation increases the rate of disappearance of the drug from active sites and converts most hypnotics and anesthetics from lipophilic nonpolar compounds to polar water-soluble derivatives capable of excretion by the kidneys. Without such conversion, elimination of lipophilic nonvolatile drugs is markedly prolonged due to reentry, after glomerular filtration, into

TABLE 2–3. Factors Influencing Rate of Tissue Equilibration of a Drug Such as Thiopental

Tissue	*Blood Flow (l/min)*	*Tissue Volume (l)*	*Thiopental Tissue-Blood Partition Coefficient*	*Capacity**	*Time Constant (min)†*
Vessel-rich group (VRG)	4.5	6	1.5	9	2
Muscle group (MG)	1.1	33	1.5	50	45
Fat group (FG)	.32	14.5	11.0	160	500
Vessel-poor group (VPG)	.075	12.5	1.5	19	250

*Tissue volume × tissue–blood partition coefficient.
†Capacity/blood flow.
(From Saidman, L.J.: Uptake and Distribution of Intravenous Agents: The Thiopental Model. Refresher Courses in Anesthesiology, 3: 141, 1975.)

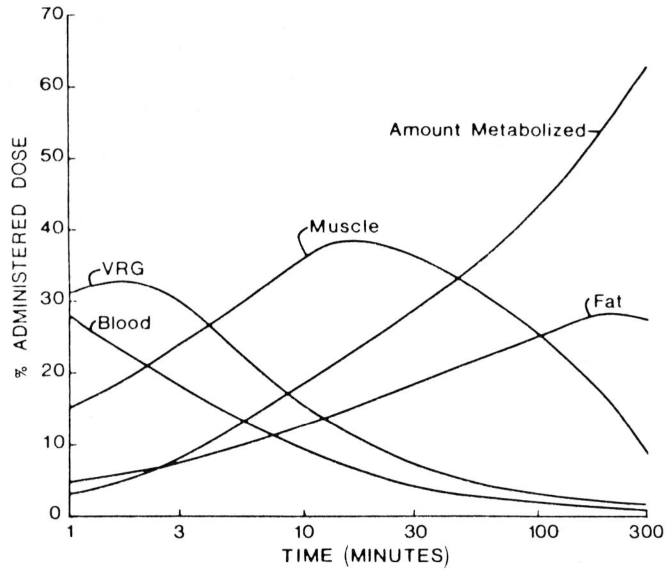

Figure 2–7. Following an intravenous bolus, the percent of thiopental remaining in blood rapidly decreases as drug moves from blood to body tissues. Time to attainment of peak tissue levels is a direct function of tissue capacity for barbiturate relative to blood flow. Thus, a larger capacity or smaller blood flow is related to a longer time to reach a peak tissue level. Initially, most thiopental is taken up by the VRG because of its high blood flow. Subsequently, drug is redistributed to muscle, and to a lesser extent to fat. Throughout this period, small but substantial amounts of thiopental are removed by the liver and metabolized. Unlike removal by the tissues, this removal is cumulative. Note that the rate of metabolism equals the early rate of removal by fat. The sum of this early removal by fat and metabolism is the same as the removal by muscle. (From Eger, E.I., II: *Anesthetic Uptake and Action*. Williams & Wilkins, Baltimore, 1974.)

the systemic circulation via the tubular epithelium. Although the metabolites resulting from biotransformation are usually less active, more toxic compounds may sometimes result (Brown, 1975). The rate of biotransformation is determined by the concentration of drug at the site of metabolism (e.g., plasma concentration and hepatic blood flow) and by the intrinsic rate of the process. The latter is determined by such factors as enzymic activity (see enzyme induction) and cofactor availability (e.g., genetics, presence of other drugs, nutrition, hypoxia) (Hug, 1978). Most drug metabolism follows first-order kinetics (a constant fraction is metabolized in a given period). In the event that the concentration exceeds the capacity of the biotransformation process, elimination assumes zero-order kinetics, a constant amount of drug is eliminated (Hug, 1978), and the pharmacologic effect is disproportionately prolonged with increasing or multiple doses (Baggot, 1977). Species variations in biotransformation may also be encountered, for example, lidocaine in man, dog, guinea pig, and rat, and glucuronide conjugation of drugs such as morphine, salicylic acid, and meprobamate in the cat.

Excretion subsequent to or independent of biotransformation is primarily a function of the kidney. Renal excretion is the principal process by which predominantly ionized drugs or those of limited lipid-solubility are eliminated (e.g., d-tubocurarine, gallamine triethiodide) (Baggot, 1977). The rate of excretion is determined by renal blood flow, glomerular filtration, and tubular secretion and reabsorption. Nonprotein-bound drug passes through the glomerulus. Other drugs and metabolites require the active transport processes of tubular secretion, which are sensitive to transport inhibitors and hypoxia. Reabsorption is efficient for those drugs (e.g., nonpolar lipophilic) able to penetrate cellular membranes, and is modified by pH and the rate of tubular urine flow (Hug, 1978). Intravenous agents used to produce or facilitate anesthesia such as barbiturates, narcotics, tranquilizers, and nondepolarizing relaxants are excreted primarily by the kidneys (Mazze, 1973; Eger, 1974). Although inhalant anesthetics are primarily eliminated by exhalation, their metabolites are excreted largely by the kidney.

FACTORS MODIFYING UPTAKE, DISTRIBUTION, AND ELIMINATION

It is thus apparent that many factors of common occurrence, such as rate of administration and concentration of anesthetic, physical status, muscular development, adiposity, respiratory and circulatory status, drug permeability coefficients, prior and/or concurrent drug administration, fear, recent feeding, and solubility of the anesthetic in bags and hoses may all modify the uptake, distribution, and elimination of anesthetics.

1. Concentration and Rate of Injection of the Anesthetic Agent. Concentration and rate of injection of a given dose affect anesthetic action, particularly with short-acting barbiturates. The more dilute the agent or slower the injection, the less effect produced (see Fig. 2–7).

2. Respiratory Function (see Chap. 6). Modification of effective ventilation, ventilation-perfusion ratios, and/or alveolar-capillary diffusion from any cause will influence both the uptake and elimination of inhalant drugs, more especially those of greater solubility. Commonly occurring examples include diaphragmatic hernia, pulmonary edema, pulmonary emphysema or atelectasis, and recumbency in large animals (Fig. 2–8).

Permeation of the blood-brain barrier by narcotics and narcotic antagonists is contingent upon partition coefficients, ionization, and protein binding, and is therefore influenced by hypocarbia and hypercarbia. Nishitateno et al. (1979) have indicated that during hypocarbia higher serum morphine concentrations, higher drug distribution in the lipid phase, and increased ratio of free base:acid salt of morphine facilitated penetration of morphine into the canine brain, in spite of decreased cerebral blood flow.

3. Circulatory Function (see Chap. 5). Variation in distribution of blood to the vessel-rich and vessel-poor tissues, to fat, to muscle, and to the alveoli themselves will modify the pattern of induction and recovery (see Fig. 2–8). In shock, the proportion of the cardiac output flowing to the brain is increased and the potential for redistribution is reduced. Due to reduced blood volume, dilution of the drug is also diminished, as is hepatic and renal blood flow. The reduction in blood volume diminishes both biotransformation and renal excretion. Induction is thus rapid, the dose required is reduced, and recovery is delayed. Even removal of 2% of the body weight in blood tremendously prolongs the recovery time from thiopental anesthesia in dogs (De Boer, 1947). It may thus be concluded that hemorrhage, such as might accompany a surgical procedure, will significantly increase sleeping time.

When fear, struggling, or fever occur, the decrease in circulation time may delay equilibration of anesthetic concentration between alveoli and pulmonary capillaries, muscle and skin blood flow is increased, induction of anesthesia is delayed, and more anesthetic is required. It is well-known that animals showing a period of excitement during induction of anesthesia always require more anesthetic. This causes a tendency toward overdosing with its attendant dangers. For this reason, preanesthetic sedation is recommended.

Hounds such as the whippet, greyhound, Afghan, borzoi, wolfhound, and saluki have a low fat-to-body mass ratio, a low muscle-to-body mass ratio, and consequent increased blood levels of unbound drug when anesthetized with barbiturate. Anesthesia is thus characterized by increased sleep times, stormy recoveries, and occasional fatalities. Thin-type muscled or emaciated patients may have similar characteristics (Rouse, 1978). The influence of some pathophysiologic states on anesthetic requirement is illustrated in Table 2–4.

4. Recent Feeding. According to Dukes (1947), a large meal of meat may increase the metabolic rate of dogs as much as 90% above the basal level (specific dynamic effect). Carbohydrate and fat also produce this elevation,

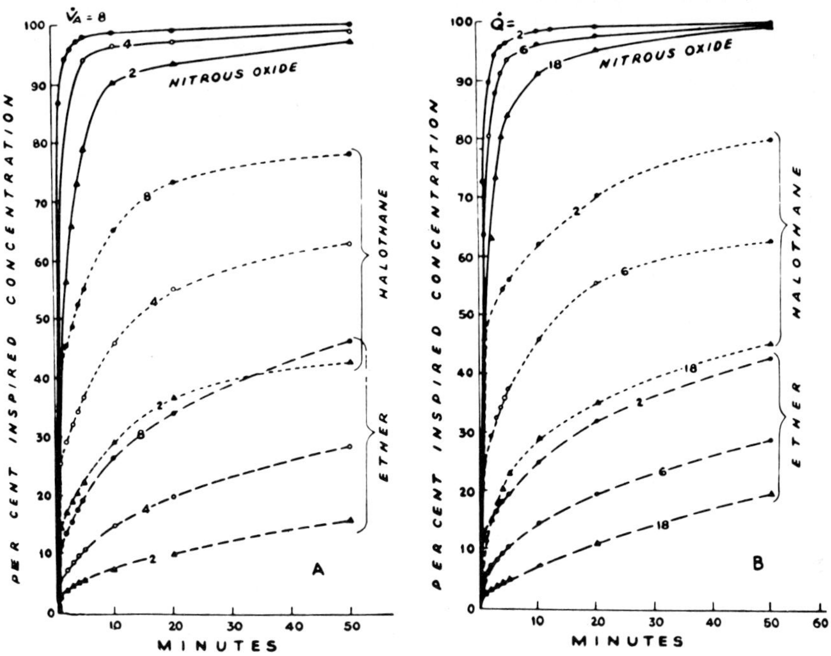

Figure 2–8. Effect of variations in cardiac output and ventilation on uptake and distribution of anesthetic agents. *(A)* Changes in alveolar concentration in relation to alteration of ventilation (2, 4, 8 liters per minute). *(B)* Effect of variations of cardiac output on alveolar concentration (2, 6, and 18 liters per minute). (From Wylie, W.D., and Churchill-Davidson, H.C.: *A Practice of Anaesthesia,* 2nd ed. Lloyd-Luke, Ltd., London, 1966.)

though to a lesser extent. It is usually 12 to 18 hours after the last meal before the basal metabolic rate is attained in carnivorous animals. In contrast, the bird is susceptible to starvation. A 6-hour preanesthetic fast may induce hypoglycemia and marked sensitivity to depressant drugs in small birds (Arnall, 1974). Certainly it is important to consider that starvation induces low plasma glucose, mobilized liver glycogen stores, and reduced circulating fatty acids, all of which may alter drug detoxification rates (Green, 1979).

In addition to altering the metabolic rate, feeding increases chylomicrons in the blood. It has been shown that thiobarbiturates localize in these and the duration of anesthesia is shortened (Anderson and Magee, 1956). Feeding also increases blood flow to the abdominal viscera and influences anesthetic distribution.

5. Uptake in Gas Spaces. With the excep-

TABLE 2–4. Pathophysiologic States That Change Anesthetic Requirement

State	*Anesthetic*	*MAC (% change)*	*Species*
Hypernatremia			Dogs
(Serum Na^+ 179 meq/L)	Halothane	↑ 43	Dogs
Hyperthermia (37° to 42° C)	Halothane	↑ 8° C	Dogs
Hypoxia (Pa_{O_2} 30 torr)	Halothane	↓ Progressively towards 0	Dogs
Hypercapnia (Pa_{CO_2} 95 to 245 torr)	Halothane	↓ Progressively to 0	Dogs
Hypocapnia (Pa_{CO_2} 10 torr)	Halothane	No change	Pregnant Ewes
Pregnancy	Halothane	↓ 25	Pregnant Ewes
Pregnancy	Methoxyflurane	↓ 32	Pregnant Ewes
Pregnancy	Isoflurane	↓ 40	Dogs
Hypotension (mean AP 40 to 50 torr)	Halothane	↓ 20	

(From Cullen, D.J.: Drugs and Anesthetic Depth. In *Drug Interactions in Anesthesia.* Edited by T.N. Smith, R.D. Miller, and A.N. Corbascio. Lea & Febiger, Philadelphia, 1981.)

tion of the gastrointestinal tract, nitrogen is the major gas constituent of closed internal body spaces. Owing to the high blood/gas partition coefficient of nitrous oxide relative to nitrogen and the gases of the intestinal tract, administration of nitrous oxide results in transfer of this gas to internal gas spaces of the body. Increased volume or pressure of the gases within these spaces may thus result. Volume increases occur in highly compliant spaces (e.g., intestinal, peritoneal, thoracic) and pressure changes in noncompliant spaces (e.g., sinuses, middle ear) (Eger, 1974). In intestinal loops of dogs anesthetized with halothane-oxygen and 75% nitrous oxide, the intestinal gas volume increased 1.8 times in 2 hours and 2.5 times in 4 hours. In experimental pneumothorax in dogs, the increase was more rapid; a 200 ml pneumothorax was doubled in 10 minutes, tripled in 45 minutes, and quadrupled in 2 hours. In pneumoencephalograms in dogs, the inhalation of 75% nitrous oxide increased cisternal pressure by 60 torr in 10 minutes (Eger, 1974). Use of nitrous oxide may thus be contraindicated in pneumothorax, pneumoencephalograms, intraocular surgery, and in intestinal obstructions requiring prolonged anesthesia.

6. Solubility of Inhalant Anesthetic in Rebreathing Bags and Hoses. The solubility of methoxyflurane and, to a lesser extent, halothane in rubber is such that uptake into the rubber of an anesthetic machine delays the rise and fall of anesthetic tension within the system (Fig. 2–9). Induction and recovery may thus be influenced.

7. Changes in Blood Constituents. Most noninhaled drugs are weak acids (barbiturates) or weak bases (narcotics, narcotic antagonists, muscle relaxants). Once the drug is injected, equilibrium between ionized and nonionized forms of drug depends on pH of the blood or tissues and the dissociation constant (pKa) of the drug. A difference in pH between tissue and blood may thus result in a drug concentration difference. Plasma acidosis, for instance, increases intracellular barbiturate, but decreases intracellular narcotic concentration (Saidman, 1975).

Drug availability at the site of action or of

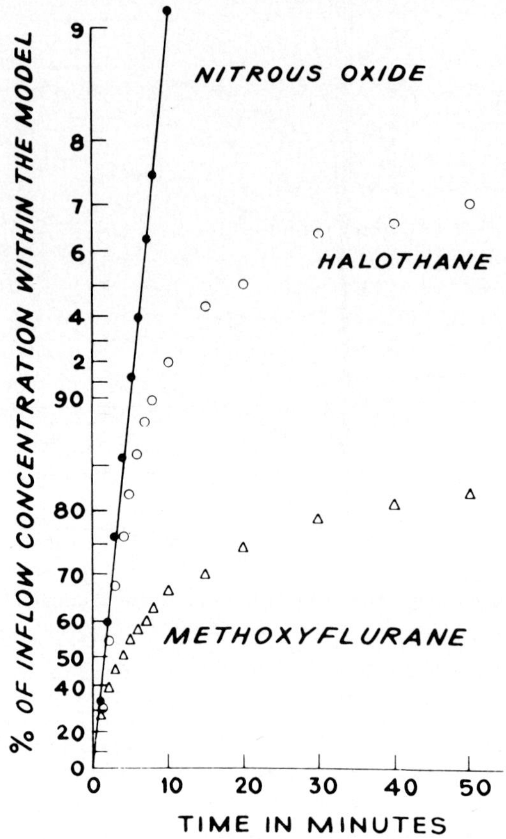

Figure 2–9. The effect of rubber solubility on the approach of tension of nitrous oxide (relatively insoluble), halothane (rubber/gas coefficient of 121), and methoxyflurane (rubber/gas coefficient of 724) toward that in the inflowing gas in a model anesthetic system. The model consisted of a double-ended 5-liter rubber bag, two corrugated rubber tubes identical to those commonly used in circle systems, and a Revel circulator. The components were arranged so that inflowing gas was rapidly distributed throughout the components. Inflow was matched by outflow such that the system neither became distended nor collapsed. The total system volume equaled 6.25 liters and inflow equaled 3 l/min in each of the experiments. Uptake of anesthetic by rubber opposes the rise of tension in the system. Since uptake is proportional to solubility, the rate of rise toward the inflowing concentration is most rapid with nitrous oxide, less so with halothane, and least with methoxyflurane. (From Eger, E. I., II, and Brandstater, B.: Solubility of Methoxyflurane in Rubber. Anesthesiology, 24:679, 1963.)

elimination is also modified by the degree of protein binding. Protein binding is diminished by uremia, by hypoproteinemia, and by administration of drugs competing for the binding sites. It may also be impaired by a change in pH, in the nature of the protein secondary to disease, or by dehydration. Such decreased binding may make more drug available for specific action with consequent apparent sensitivity to a normal dose (Saidman, 1975).

8. Preanesthetic Medication and Previous Administration of Drugs. Opioid analgesics lower the metabolic rate; atropine causes a slight rise. When they are administered in combination, however, the metabolic rate is decreased. Tranquilizers usually lower the metabolic rate.

It has been demonstrated repeatedly that administration of various drugs and pesticides will stimulate or inhibit hepatic microsomal drug-metabolizing enzymes (enzyme induction, enzyme inhibition). More than 200 drugs are recognized as enzyme inducers (Table 2–5). Maximal enhancement of enzyme levels occurs after approximately 5 days administration of the inducing agent; levels return to normal 48 to 72 hours after withdrawal of the enzyme inducer (Brown, 1975). The nature of the induction varies with the type of drug, its dose, age, thyroid function, and genetics (Brown, 1975; Baggot, 1977). Enzyme induction with accelerated biotransformation reduces the pharmacologic activity of drugs normally eliminated by biotransformation, such as certain barbiturates, tranquilizers, hypnotics, and anti-inflammatory agents. Since inhalation anesthetics also undergo biotransformation, their elimination is also influenced by enzyme induction. While this occurrence has little or no effect on the conduct of clinical anesthesia, it is of significance relative to viscerotoxicity. Methoxyflurane biotransformation may be modified quantitatively and qualitatively by enzyme induction to form nephrotoxic metabolites; chloroform hepatotoxicity is similarly induced by biotransformation. The potential for such toxicity in halothane anesthesia is enhanced by hypoxia. Toxicity associated with biotransformation is also enhanced by reduced liver antioxidants, such as glutathione or vitamin E. In all instances, toxicity of the organohalogens depends primarily on formation of reactive intermediates, especially those resulting from non-oxygen-dependent ("reductive") biotransformation (Brown, 1981), and is contingent upon the extent and type of biotransformation and the genetic, metabolic, and environmental drug pathways resulting from induction (Brown, 1979). The extent to which such induced metabolic effects influence clinical animal anesthesia is unknown.

Hepatic microsomal enzymes may also be inhibited with delay of biotransformation. Inhibitors include organophosphorus insecticides, pesticide synergists of the methylenedioxy phenyl type, guanidine, carbon tetrachloride, chloramphenicol, tetracyclines, and certain inhalation anesthetics (Brown, 1975; Baggot,

TABLE 2–5. Partial List of Drugs Capable of Producing Microsomal Enzyme Induction

Hypnotics	Antihistaminics
Barbiturates	Diphenhydramine (Benadryl)
Glutethimide (Doriden)	
Ethanol	Steroids
Chloral hydrate	Cortisone
	Prednisone
Tranquilizers	Norethynodrel (Enovid)
Chlorpromazine (Thorazine)	Methyltestosterone
Promazine (Sparine)	
Meprobamate (Equanil)	Anesthetics
Chlordiazepoxide (Librium)	Diethyl ether
	Halothane (Fluothane)
Anticonvulsants	
Diphenylhydantoin (Dilantin)	Insecticides
Methylphenylethylhydantoin (Mesantoin)	DDT
	Chlordane
	o,p′-DDD

(From Brown, B.B.: Enzymes of Biotransformation as Related to Anesthesia. ASA Refresher Courses in Anesthesiology, 3:27, 1975.)

1977). Inhibition is illustrated by prolonged plasma half-lives of barbiturates, narcotics, and local anesthetics during halothane anesthesia (Brown, 1975), and prolonged barbiturate anesthesia after prior or concurrent chloramphenicol medication (Teske and Carter, 1971).

Relevant drug interactions may also occur as a result of protein binding and interaction at receptor sites (Table 2–6).

Antibiotics are often administered prior to, during, or immediately after general anesthesia to prevent or treat bacterial infections associated with surgery. In many instances, little consideration is given to adverse responses that may occur from the interaction between antibiotics and drugs commonly used in the operating room (Adams et al., 1976). Although a variety of antibiotics have been shown to cause neuromuscular blockage, only the aminoglycoside group of antibiotics has been examined in detail (Pittinger and Adamson, 1972; Adams et al., 1974). Further information on antibiotic-anesthetic interactions is given in Chapter 5 and Chapter 14.

9. Concurrent Disease. The effect of disease on the metabolic rate usually varies with its duration. In the early febrile stage, the rate may be increased; however, as the disease progresses, toxemia may reduce it to low levels. Fever increases the metabolic rate in accordance with van't Hoff's law, which states that for each degree Fahrenheit the temperature rises, the metabolic rate is increased 7%. When animals suffer from toxemia or liver disease, the functions of this organ are impaired and the ability of the animal to detoxify anesthetics is depressed. Shock lowers the metabolic rate and, because of suppressed cardiovascular function, impairs uptake and distribution of anesthetic agents.

Hepatocellular disease causes reduced protein (primarily albumin) production with consequent limitation of protein binding, increased pharmacologically active drug, and unexpected sensitivity to such drugs as thiopental. Production of specific protein such as pseudocholinesterase may also be impaired with consequent increased

TABLE 2–6. Interactions at Tissue Receptor Sites

The following agents have neuromuscular blocking properties and may intensify effects of nondepolarizing neuromuscular blocking agents (tubocurarine, gallamine, dimethyl tubocurarine), or they may interact with each other.

Antibiotics	*General Anesthetics*
Bacitracin	Ether
Streptomycin, Dihydrostreptomycin	Halothane
Neomycin	Methoxyflurane
Kanamycin	
Gentamicin	*Other Agents*
Polymyxin B	Muscle relaxants
Oxytetracycline	Quinine
Lincomycin	Promethazine
Other tetracyclines	Magnesium sulfate
Colistimethate	Barbiturates
Paronomycin	Na citrate
Vancomycin	Organophosphorus insecticides

The following agents may intensify the neuromuscular blockade produced by succinylcholine.

Anticholinesterase agents
Magnesium sulfate

The following reactions occur at adrenergic receptor sites.

Drug 1	*Drug 2*	*Effect*
Epinephrine	Chloroform	Arrhythmias due to sensitization of the heart to catecholamines by drug 2
Levarterenol	Halothane	
Isoproterenol	Thiamylal	

(From Abbitt, L.E.: Drug Interactions. *In Drug Interactions, Incompatibilities and Adverse Reactions in Veterinary Practice.* Edited by L.E. Abbitt, L.E. Davis, S.D. Farey, and R.D. Scalley. Colorado State University, Fort Collins, Colorado, 1975.)

duration of action of succinylcholine. Hepatic disease may delay drug biotransformation due to enzyme inhibition or decreased hepatic blood flow (Stoelting, 1976). Some drugs and/or their metabolites (polar, molecular weight >300) are likely to be excreted in the bile in significant amounts (e.g., morphine, chloramphenicol, digitoxin) (Baggot, 1977). The doses of drugs contingent upon hepatic elimination must therefore be modified in the presence of hepatic disease.

Distribution and elimination of anesthetic and related drugs can also be impaired by renal disease with increased potential toxicity. Protein binding of organic acids with increased pharmacologic activity (sensitivity) is reduced in uremic patients; examples include pentobarbital, phenylbutazone, and cardiac glycosides. The increase of free drug fraction in plasma of patients with renal disease correlates with the degree of hypoalbuminemia (Baggot, 1977). Renal disease may also limit excretion and thereby prolong activity of muscle relaxants such as gallamine and pancuronium.

The degree by which renal disease influences drug protein binding, and, therefore, its activity and/or excretion, may be modified by fluid therapy (dilution, increased glomerular filtration) and by changes in plasma pH (see protein binding) (Eger, 1974).

Guinea pigs with vitamin C deficiency have been shown to be more susceptible to anesthesia as evidenced by earlier induction, deeper anesthesia, and slower recovery (Beyer et al., 1944).

Hyperthyroidism is accompanied by an elevated metabolic rate, whereas hypothyroidism is accompanied by lowering of the metabolic rate. Totally thyroidectomized dogs require small doses of anesthetic.

Leukemia in some forms increases the metabolic rate, as does severe pain (Adriani, 1958).

10. Ionizing Radiation and Anesthetic Effects. X-irradiation has been shown to affect (1) potency, onset, duration of action, and brain levels of barbiturate, and (2) activity of the hepatic microsomal enzyme system (Nair, 1969). A species sensitivity of the brain to radiation has also been identified. Earlier onset of drug action apparently results from radiation-induced modification of the blood-brain barrier. In adult animals, prolongation of drug action occurs which may be due to (1) sensitization with a region-specific increase in brain serotonin, and (2) partial inhibition of hepatic oxidase.

Prenatal irradiation produces impairment of the hepatic microsomal enzyme system in male rats. In young rats postnatally irradiated, a higher radiation dose is necessary to produce the same effect.

Saksonov and Kozlov (1968) have indicated that the anesthetic effect of barbiturates (barbital, hexobarbital, thiopental, pentobarbital) is decreased immediately after irradiation (1 to 3 hours). Later, as irradiation sickness develops (tenth to fifteenth day), an increased sensitivity develops.

CELLULAR EFFECTS AND TERATOGENICITY

Interest in mutagenic, carcinogenic, and teratogenic effects of anesthetics has increased significantly since an increase in spontaneous abortion of female anesthetists was noted in 1970 (Brown, 1977). It is assumed that this increased rate of abortion is due to chronic exposure to trace concentrations of anesthetics. Exposure to such anesthetic concentrations in the first trimester of pregnancy should be avoided. Exposure of rats to nitrous oxide on the ninth day of gestation has been shown to cause fetal resorption and skeletal and soft tissue anomalies. Others have also demonstrated that inhalation anesthetics are teratogenic in animals, especially the chick (Brown, 1977; Cullen, 1978). Corresponding teratogenesis in man has not been conclusively proved.

Epidemiologic studies have suggested an increased incidence of cancer among women, but not men, who work in operating rooms (Cullen, 1978). Commonly used anesthetics, with the exception of fluroxene, have not been shown to be potential carcinogens by in vitro tests. Both general and local anesthetics can inhibit cell division. Anesthetics also affect such immune phenomena as cellular adherence, phagocytosis, lymphocyte transformation, chemotaxis, and the killing of tumor cells (Duncan and Cullen, 1976) (see also Chap. 21).

PHYSICAL EXAMINATION

"For every mistake that is made for not knowing, a hundred are made for not looking."

—Anonymous

A thorough preanesthetic evaluation of the patient is essential for successful anesthesia and subsequent surgery. Every effort should be made to detect factors that may modify anesthetic action and safety. While such evaluation is important in all patients, it is especially important in the critically ill patient. In addition to body weight and vital signs, the following should be included:

1. History should include prior anesthetic history, previous and current health, pregnancy, exposure to drugs, and recent feeding. It is especially important to consider the status of cardiopulmonary function, the potential of acid base or electrolyte imbalance, the possibility of a full or distended stomach or of hepatic or renal disease, and the prior or concurrent administration of drugs (e.g., organophosphates, diuretics, digitalis preparations, anticonvulsants, corticosteroids, chloramphenicol, aminoglycoside antibiotics, sulfonamides, and barbiturates).
2. All body systems should be examined and any abnormalities identified. The latter will determine the extent to which additional examinations are necessary.
3. In all but extreme emergencies, routine hemograms, urinalysis, total protein, and blood chemistries to identify the status of kidney and liver function are essential.
4. Contingent upon the history and physical examination, additional examinations may include blood gases and pH, electrocardiography, clotting time and platelet counts, fecal and/or filarial examinations, and blood electrolyte determinations.
5. Roentgenographic and/or fluoroscopic examination may also be indicated, especially in animals susceptible to chronic respiratory infections, such as primates, calves, sheep, and rodents.

Following examination, the physical status of the patient should be classified and recorded so that accurate records are kept. (Table 2–7). This mental exercise forces the anesthetist to evaluate the patient's condition and proves valuable in proper selection of the agent to be used. Classification of physical status is an essential part of any anesthetic record system (see Chap. 23).

The preliminary physical examination should be done in the owner's presence, if possible, so that a prognosis can be given personally. This allows the client to ask questions and enables the veterinarian to allay any fears concerning management of the patient.

SELECTION OF THE ANESTHETIC AGENT

The ideal anesthetic agent is one that:

1. does not depend on detoxifying mechanisms within the body for its destruction and elimination;
2. permits rapid induction, quick alteration in depth of anesthesia, and rapid recovery;
3. does not depress respiratory and cardiac centers;
4. is not irritant to any tissue;
5. is inexpensive, stable, noninflammable, and nonexplosive; and
6. requires no special equipment for administration.

No agent available today possesses all of these qualities. Therefore, selection of an agent is a compromise based on appraisal of the situation. Factors to be considered include:

1. the patient's species, breed, and age;
2. physical status of the patient;
3. the time required for the surgical (or other) procedure, its type and severity, and the surgeon's skill;
4. familiarity with the proposed anesthetic technique; and
5. equipment and personnel available.

In general the veterinarian will have greatest

TABLE 2–7. Classification of Physical Status*

Category	Physical Status	Possible Examples of This Category
I	A normal healthy patient	No discernible disease; animals entered for ovariohysterectomy, ear trim, caudectomy, castration
II	A patient with mild systemic disease	Skin tumor, fracture without shock, uncomplicated hernia, cryptorchidectomy, localized infection, compensated cardiac disease
III	A patient with severe systemic disease	Fever, dehydration, anemia, cachexia, moderate hypovolemia
IV	A patient with severe systemic disease that is a constant threat to life	Uremia, toxemia, severe dehydration and hypovolemia, anemia, cardiac decompensation, emaciation, high fever
V	A moribund patient not expected to survive 24 hours with or without operation	Extreme shock and dehydration, terminal malignancy or infection, severe trauma

*This classification is the same as that adopted by the American Society of Anesthesiologists.

success with agents he has used most frequently and with which he is most familiar. The art of administration is developed only with experience; therefore, change from a familiar agent to a new one is usually accompanied by a temporary increase in the mortality rate. Clark (1938) speaking of anesthesia in man stated,

> "The outstanding fact is that thorough familiarity with a technique is equivalent at least to a 30 percent difference in efficiency. If a person has mastered a technique, it is not worth his while changing to a new and unfamiliar one unless the change promises some big advantage."

Often the length of time required to perform a surgical procedure and the amount of help available during this period dictate the anesthetic that is used. Generally, short procedures are done with short-lasting agents, such as thiobarbiturates or combinations utilizing dissociative, tranquilizing and/or narcotic agents. Although procedures of longer duration have utilized pentobarbital and/or chloral hydrate in the past, the established need for respiratory support in such procedures makes the use of inhalation equipment mandatory for safe anesthesia. Currently, where anesthesia of longer duration is required, inhalation or balanced anesthetic techniques are used.

Species differences may prevent the use of some drugs. For example, procaine is frequently lethal for parakeets and morphine can be excitatory for cats. On the other hand, most agents can be used interchangeably among species.

Anesthesia in the very young is attended with increased risk. This is due to size limitations, lower metabolic rate, limited muscular and adipose tissue in which anesthetic may be redistributed, and immature detoxification mechanisms. For this reason, the use of pentobarbital, and perhaps even thiobarbiturates, in the very young is contraindicated.

Aged animals are often poor anesthetic risks because of decreased stamina and the possibility of chronic heart, liver, or kidney disease which may be inapparent on casual examination. These animals, therefore, should not be given agents that are irritant to these body tissues or that require good liver and kidney function for their detoxification or elimination. The same is true of patients in a poor physical state due to febrile disease, since the liver and kidneys usually are somewhat affected, regardless of the location of the disease within the body.

General anesthesia is to be avoided, if at all possible, in animals with an elevated blood urea nitrogen. Local, regional, or epidural anesthesia should be used where possible. If general anesthesia must be used, the thiobarbiturates and inhalant anesthetics are preferred; pentobarbital should never be employed under these circumstances.

A cardiac murmur per se is not a contraindication for general anesthesia since surprisingly few animals with murmurs die from anesthesia *provided* they are compensated. However, they have less cardiac reserve and require more careful supervision during anesthesia. Dogs with heartworm infestation and congenital lesions of the heart and great vessels also fall in this category. Use of dissociative, narcotic-analgesic combinations in a balanced anesthetic technique is preferred in such instances.

Brachycephalic dogs, because of their pendulous soft palate and restricted respiratory passages, have difficulty in breathing even when awake. Under anesthesia, this difficulty is compounded and these animals often die because a patent airway is not maintained. Therefore, it is wise to use short-lasting agents with which the depth of anesthesia can be easily controlled so that a prolonged recovery period is avoided. Many small animal facilities are air-conditioned, and year-round surgery can be undertaken without considering the weather. During the summer months, in hospitals that are not air-conditioned, anesthesia may present a problem. This is particularly true of brachycephalic breeds. In hot, humid weather, it is sometimes better to delay surgery on these animals than to chance losing them through anesthesia and attendant struggling during the recovery period. There is a greater problem during anesthesia of larger animals when the use of a temperature controlled environment is often impossible.

In large animals such as horses and cattle, anesthetics should be selected to provide minimal recovery time and emergence struggling. Emergence struggling is usually more a problem in equine anesthesia, while general anesthesia in the ruminant is complicated by the hazards of rumen tympany, regurgitation, and aspiration. These latter complications make the use of regional anesthesia more desirable. In the event general anesthesia is used, endotracheal intubation is mandatory. In some instances, regional anesthesia in the standing position also presents the advantage that compression of abdominal viscera, as in a recumbent animal, is less likely to impede surgical intervention and respiratory and cardiovascular function.

As a group, the barbiturates are contraindicated for cesarean section because of the respiratory depression produced in the newborn. There is some indication that pentobarbital should not be used for any reason in pregnant animals if the effect on the fetuses is a consideration. Becker et al. (1958) have shown that administration of pentobarbital to pregnant guinea pigs on either the twenty-second, forty-second, or sixty-third day of gestation resulted in high mortality in the young. In addition, symptoms of neural damage were seen in the survivors. Thiobarbiturates can be used for cesarean section either alone or in combination with an inhalant, but a lower survival rate in the young may result. This is particularly true when the operation follows a prolonged labor.

A number of satisfactory anesthetic techniques are available for cesarean section including administration of inhalants, use of narcosis and balanced anesthesia or injection of local or regional anesthetics with or without sedation.

The anesthetic technique to be used should ultimately be selected after review of:

1. the factors likely to influence anesthesia;
2. the physical status of the animal;
3. the specific needs of the species; and
4. the specific needs of the case, including the relative requirements for sedation, immobilization, analgesia, relaxation, and safety.

PATIENT PREPARATION

Too often, operations are undertaken with inadequate preparation of the patient. Some foresight here is beneficial. With most types of general anesthesia, it is best to have the patient off feed for 12 hours previously. It should be recalled that some species are adversely affected by fasting. Pentobarbital sleeping time is prolonged in mice starved for 24 hours. Small birds may become hypoglycemic with but a few hours of starvation, and mobilization of glycogen stores may alter detoxification rates. The latter may be a factor in ruminants. In contrast, feeding in the dog increases the metabolic rate for up to 18 hours. Induction of anesthesia in an animal having a full stomach should be avoided if at all possible, because of the hazards of aspiration. Distension of the rumen in sheep has been shown to impair ventilation with consequent hypoxemia and hypercapnia (Ungerer et al., 1976). In the horse, a full stomach may rupture during induction and casting. Although limitation of food does not empty the ruminant stomach, the possibility of regurgitation is perhaps reduced if water is withheld for 12 hours prior to induction.

In most species, especially in the young and aged, water is usually offered up to the time that preanesthetic agents are given. It should be remembered that many old dogs suffer from nephritis. While these animals remain compensated under ideal conditions, the trauma of hospitalization, water deprivation, and anesthesia, even without surgery, may cause acute decompensation. To withhold water from these animals, even for short periods, may prove hazardous. In any case, it is good anesthetic practice to administer intravenous fluids during anesthesia to maintain adequate blood pressure, and urinary output, and to provide an available route for drug administration.

Systemic administration of antibiotics preoperatively is a helpful prophylactic measure if shock or contamination of the operative site is anticipated. Oral antibiotics have been shown to "sterilize" the bowel effectively and should be used prior to elective surgery of the gastrointestinal tract. The potential interaction of antibiotics with anesthetic or related drugs should receive careful consideration (see Table 2–6). In surgery of the colon, rectum, and anus, preoperative enemas administered a day or two prior to surgery will remove fecal material and facilitate manipulation. On the other hand, an enema just prior to surgery may complicate the situation, since feces will be fluid and the operative site may easily become contaminated.

Dehydrated animals should be treated with fluids and appropriate alimentation prior to operation; fluid therapy should be continued during operation. The delay occasioned by administration of fluids is more than compensated by the animal's increased ability to withstand the shock of anesthesia and surgical trauma. An attempt should be made to correlate the patient's electrolyte balance with the type of fluid that is administered. In hospitals where electrolyte balance studies are performed, exacting replacement therapy can be administered. Anemia and hypovolemia, as determined clinically and by hematologic determinations, should be corrected by administration of whole blood. Patients in shock without blood loss or in a state of nutritional deficiency will be benefited by administration of plasma or plasma expanders. Corticosteroids are indicated in aged or debilitated patients and those undergoing extensive surgery. Again, preanesthetic administration is more valuable than during operation.

Several conditions may severely restrict effective ventilation. These include pneumothorax, hemothorax, pyothorax, chylothorax, diaphragmatic hernia, and gastric or rumen distention. Affected animals are often in a marginal state of respiratory exchange. Respiratory support is indicated and intrapleural air or fluid should be removed by aspiration prior to induction, since the effective lung volume may be greatl reduced and severe respiratory embarrassment may otherwise result. While no attempt should be made to insert an endotracheal catheter in these patients prior to anesthesia, *this must be done immediately following induction*. Alternatively, a tracheotomy may be performed prior to induction. Many animals have been lost because the anesthetist was not prepared to carry out all phases of induction-intubation-controlled ventilation in one continuous operation.

In laboratory animals, especially rats, guinea pigs, mice, and rabbits, chronic respiratory disease may be endemic. In calves, sheep, and swine, lung lesions are common, and in primates tuberculosis may be encountered. Animals having such infections should receive specific therapy prior to anesthesia and, should resolution not occur, local or conduction anesthesia should be strongly considered.

Decompensated heart disease is a contraindication for general anesthesia, since fluid in the lungs reduces respiratory efficiency and the animal may have no cardiac reserve. If these animals must be anesthetized, an attempt at compensation through digitalization and diuresis should be made prior to anesthesia. If ascites is present, this fluid should be aspirated to reduce excessive pressure on the diaphragm.

In cases of hepatic or renal insufficiency, for instance in many bacterial and viral infections of mice, dogs, or primates, or in parasitism of calves, sheep, and rabbits, the mode of anesthetic elimination should receive strong consideration with inhalation anesthesia preferred. Under experimental conditions, animals with clinical or subclinical disease of any body system should be identified and rejected from the experiment.

Just prior to induction it is desirable to encourage defecation and/or urination by giving the animal access to a run or exercise pen. If this attempt is unsuccessful, catheterization or bladder compression may be necessary during surgical preparation.

Once the small animal is anesthetized, the bladder can be emptied by slow steady compression through the abdominal wall or by catheterization. An empty bladder is an advantage in abdominal surgery, particularly in the male, since urination may otherwise contaminate the operative field.

During anesthesia, the patient should, if possible, be restrained in a physiologic position. Compression of the chest, acute angulation of the neck, overextension or compression of limbs, and compression of the posterior vena cava by large viscera can all lead to serious difficulties. Complications include hypoventilation, nerve and/or muscle damage, and impaired venous return. The horse is especially susceptible to paralysis, resulting from excessive extension, abduction, or myodegeneration of the limbs. Such complications are more likely to occur when good relaxation is achieved, or blood pressure is depressed and recumbency is prolonged in a lateral position; such a position also adversely affects ventilation-perfusion ratios and thereby the efficiency of respiratory exchange. The inefficiency of respiratory exchange is even greater in the supine position (De Moor et al., 1974). Periodic change of position is therefore recommended (see Chap. 21).

Kilburn et al. (1960) have shown that tilting the canine patient alters the amount of respiratory gases that can be accommodated in the chest (functional residual capacity—FRC) by as much as 26%. Liu et al. (1969) found that, in dogs subjected to hemorrhage, tilting the animal head-up was detrimental, producing lowered blood pressure, hyperpnea, and depression of cardiac contractile force. When the animal was tilted head-down, no circulatory improvement occurred.

DeYoung and Lumb (1971) found that, in pentobarbital-anesthetized dogs lying on a horizontal table, sternal recumbency and left and right lateral recumbency positions consistently produced the least overall change in cardiopulmonary function. The supine position was the least physiologic of the level positions. Prone and supine head-down positions (60°) produced the greatest physiologic derangement.

In all species, the head should be extended to provide a free airway and to prevent kinking of the endotracheal tube. In ruminants, it is desirable to have the head tilted down to permit drainage of saliva. Downward tilting of the hindquarters and abdomen (below the thorax) with minimal compression of the abdomen will limit possible reflux of rumen contents. Precautions should also be taken to prevent accumulation of rumen gases during anesthesia. This may be done by passage of a large-bore stomach tube. During emergence from anesthesia, it is desirable to position the ruminant in sternal recumbency. When large species are restrained in recumbency, viscera, restraining ropes, and bands may restrict respiration or compress nerves or muscle groups severely. During restraint in dorsal recumbency, abdominal viscera may compress the large veins and restrict venous return. In all instances, thorough padding beneath the animal is mandatory.

REFERENCES

Adams, H.R., Goodman, F.R., and Weiss, G.B.: Alteration of Contractile Function and Calcium Ion Movements in Vascular Smooth Muscle by Gentamicin and Other Aminoglycoside Antibiotics. Antimicrob. Agents Chemother., 5:640, 1974.

Adams, H.R., Teske, R.H., and Mercer, H.D.: Anesthetic-Antibiotic Interrelationships. J.A.V.M.A., 168:409, 1976.

Adriani, J.: Anesthesia for Patients with Uncommon and Unusual Diseases. Anesth. Analg., 37:1, 1958.

Anderson, E.G., and Magee, D.F.: A Study of the Mechanism of the Effect of Dietary Fat in Decreasing Thiopental Sleeping Time. J. Pharmacol. Exp. Ther., 117:281, 1956.

Arnall, L.: Aspects of Anaesthesia in Cagebirds. In *Small Animal Anaesthesia*. Edited by O. Graham-Jones. Pergamon Press, Oxford, England, 1974.

Baggot, J.D.: *Principles of Drug Disposition in Domestic Animals*. W.B. Saunders Co., Philadelphia, 1977.

Becker, R.F., Flannagan, E., and King, J.E.: The Fate of Offspring from Mothers Receiving Sodium Pentobarbital before Delivery. A Study in the Guinea Pig. Neurology, 8:776, 1958.

Beyer, K.H., Stutzman, J.W., and Hafford, B.: The Relation of Vitamin C to Anesthesia. Surg. Gynecol. Obstet., 79:49, 1944.

Brown, B.R.: Anesthetic Hepatic Toxicity: A Scientific Problem? Annual Refresher Course Lectures, Lecture #106B. Am. Soc. Anesthes., 1979.

Brown, B.R.: Enzymes of Biotransformation as Related to Anesthesia. Refresher Courses in Anesthesiology, 3:27, 1975.

Brown, B.R.: Molecular Toxicity of Inhalation Anesthetics. Refresher Courses in Anesthesiology, 5:1, 1977.

Brown, B.R.: Pharmacogenetics and the Halothane Hepatitis Mystery. Anesthesiology, 55:93, 1981.

Cameron, G.R.: Some Recent Work on Barbiturates. Proc. R. Soc. Med., 32:309, 1938.

Clark, A.J.: Aspects of the History of Anaesthetics. Br. Med. J., 2:1029, 1938.

Cullen, B.F.: Cellular Effects and Toxicity of Anesthetics. Refresher Courses in Anesthesiology, 6:43, 1978.

De Boer, B.: Factors Affecting Pentothal Anesthesia in Dogs. Anesthesiology, 8:375, 1947.

De Moor, A., Desmet, P., and Verschooten, F.: Influence of Change of Body Position on Arterial Oxygenation and Acid-Base Status in the Horse in Lateral Recumbency. Zbl. Vet. Med. A., 21:525, 1974.

DeYoung, D.W., and Lumb, W.V.: Unpublished data, 1971.

Dukes, H.H.: *The Physiology of Domestic Animals*, 6th ed. Comstock Publishing Company, Ithaca, New York, 1947, p. 454.

Duncan, P.G., and Cullen, B.F.: Anesthesiology and Immunology. Anesthesiology, 45:552, 1976.

Eger, E.I., II: *Anesthetic Uptake and Action*. Williams & Wilkins, Baltimore, 1974.

Eger, E.I., II: Uptake and Distribution. Annual Refresher Course Lectures, Lecture #113. Am. Soc. Anesthes., 1979.

Eger, E.I., II, and Larson, C.P.: Anaesthetic Solubility in Blood and Tissues: Values and Significance. Br. J. Anaesth., 36:14, 1964.

Gourlay, G.K., Adams, J.F., Cousins, M.J., and Hall, P.: Genetic Differences in Reductive Metabolism and Hepatotoxicity of Halothane in Three Rat Strains. Anesthesiology, 55:96, 1981.

Green, C.J.: *Animal Anaesthesia*. Laboratory Animals Ltd., London, 1979.

Hug, C.C.: Pharmacokinetics of Anesthetics: Intravenous Drugs. Annual Refresher Course Lectures, Lecture #225A. Am. Soc. Anesthes., 1978.

Jenkins, J., Balinsky, D., and Patient, D.W.: Cholinesterase in Plasma: First Reported Absence in the Bantu; Half-Life Determination. Science, 156:1748, 1967.

Jones, E.W., Nelson, T.E., Anderson, I.L., Kerr, D.D., and Burnap, T.K.: Malignant Hyperthermia of Swine. Anesthesiology, 36:42, 1972.

Kato, R., and Takanaka, A.: Metabolism of Drugs in Old Rats. I. Activities of NADPH-linked Electron Transport and Drug Metabolizing Enzyme Systems in Liver Microsomes of Old Rats. Jpn. J. Pharmacol., 18:381, 1968.

Kennedy, W.P.: Sodium Salt of C-C-Cyclohexenylmethyl-N-Methyl Barbituric Acid (Evipan) Anaesthesia in Laboratory Animals. J. Pharmacol. Exp. Ther., 50:347, 1934.

Keys, A.: Age and the Basal Metabolism, Guidelines to Metabolic Therapy, Vol. 2. The Upjohn Company, Kalamazoo, Michigan, 1973.

Kilburn, K.H., McDonald, J., and Piccinni, F.P.: Effects of Ventilatory Pattern and Body Position on Lung Volume in Dogs. J. Appl. Physiol., 15:801, 1960.

Knight, G.C.: Barbiturate Anaesthesia in Small Animals. Proc. R. Soc. Med., 42:525, 1949.

Liu, C.T., Hoff, H.E., and Huggins, R.A.: Circulatory and Respiratory Responses to Postural Changes in the Hemorrhagic Dog. J. Appl. Physiol., 27:460, 1969.

Mazze, R.I.: Renal Toxicity of Anesthetics. Refresher Courses in Anesthesiology, 1:85, 1973.

Nair, V.: An Ontogenic Study of the Effects of Exposure to X-irradiation on the Pharmacology of Barbiturates. Chicago Med. School Quart., 28:9, 1969.

Nicholas, J.S., and Barron, D.H.: The Use of Sodium Amytal in the Production of Anesthesia in the Rat. J. Pharmacol. Exp. Ther., 46:125, 1932.

Nishitateno, K., Ngai, S.H., Finek, A.D., and Berkowits, B.A.: Pharmacokinetics of Morphine: Concentrations in the Serum and Brain of the Dog during Hyperventilation. Anesthesiology, 50:520, 1979.

Pittinger, C., and Adamson, R.: Antibiotic Blockade of Neuromuscular Function. Annu. Rev. Pharmacol., 12:169,1972.

Rouse, S.: Effects of Thiobarbiturate Anesthetics on Lean Dogs. Vet. Anesth., 5:22, 1978.

Saidman, L.J.: Uptake and Distribution of Intravenous Agents: The Thiopental Model. Refresher Courses in Anesthesiology, 3:141, 1975.

Saksonov, P.O., and Kozlov, V.A.: Features of the Pharmacological Action of Some Anaesthetic Drugs in Radiation Injury. Voennomed. Zh., 10:40, 1968.

Stoelting, R.K.: Estimation of Hepatic Function—Effects of Anesthetic Experience. Refresher Courses in Anesthesiology, 4:139, 1976.

Stormont, C., and Suzuki, Y.: Atropinesterase and Cocainesterase of Rabbit Serum: Localization of the Enzyme Activity in Isozymes. Science, 167:200, 1970.

Teske, R.H., and Carter, G.G.: Effect of Chloramphenicol on Pentobarbital-Induced Anesthesia in Dogs. J.A.V.M.A., 159:777, 1971.

Tevik, A., Nelson, A.W., and Lumb, W.V.: Chloroform and Halothane Anesthesia in Horses: Effect on Blood Electrolytes and Acid-Base Balance. Am. J. Vet. Res., 29:1791, 1968.

Ungerer, T., Orr, J.A., Bisgard, G.E., and Will, J.A.: Cardiopulmonary Effects of Mechanical Distension of the Rumen in Nonanesthetized Sheep. Am. J. Vet. Res., 37.807, 1976.

Van Dyke, R.A., and Chenoweth, M.B.: Metabolism of Volatile Anesthetics. Anesthesiology, 26:348, 1965.

CHAPTER 3

Facilities, Equipment, and Personnel

FACILITIES

Time and thought should be given to preparation of a place in the hospital for anesthetizing animals. All necessary items should be kept in supply and in a state of readiness. When anesthetic emergencies arise, there is no time to hunt for mislaid equipment.

The hospital area selected is, in some cases, the operating room itself. It is better, however, to have a separate "prep room" or place for preparing and inducing animals. This contributes to cleanliness in the operating room and leaves the surgeon undistracted. Regardless of the area used, it should be well lighted and equipped to facilitate examination, clipping, washing, and induction of anesthesia. A convenient method for storing clippers is to attach them to the wall or ceiling overhead, using a spring-activated reel.* This arrangement will pay for itself over a period of time since clippers usually break when dropped on the floor. A vacuum cleaner is useful to remove clipped hair from the patient and surroundings. A stainless steel sink with an overlying metal grid is effective for washing the surgical site and for expressing the bladder of small animals (Fig. 3–1). Alternatively, an examination or grooming table such as that illustrated in Figure 3–2, or an adjustable "V"-top operating table with central trough (Fig. 3–3), is also suitable when located adjacent to a sink with both hot and cold water.

*See Appendix A for manufacturer.

The preparation room should also have adequate storage space, a refrigerator, a source of oxygen, nitrous oxide, suction, and a scavenging system for waste gases. The gases and suction should preferably be piped from a central system. If gas cylinders are used, restraint for storage must be provided.

Preparation of large animals for anesthesia and surgery is commonly performed in the operating room itself. This is dictated both by economy of facilities and by the need in many cases for restraint and even anesthesia prior to all but the most simple procedures. Despite this, a preparation room for large animals is essential if thoroughly acceptable aseptic conditions are to be maintained. It can be a stall convenient to the operating room and may also serve as the recovery room, although this is not desirable. In addition to the operating room, the large animal preparation area should be readily accessible to other large animal holding space including a loading and unloading dock. The room or stall should be well lighted and may be equipped with both horse stocks and a cattle chute. The floor should be constructed to minimize slipping and to facilitate drainage and cleaning. As in the small animal preparation room, a sink, hot and cold water, clippers, a vacuum cleaner, oxygen, compressed air, suction, and a scavenging system should be pro-

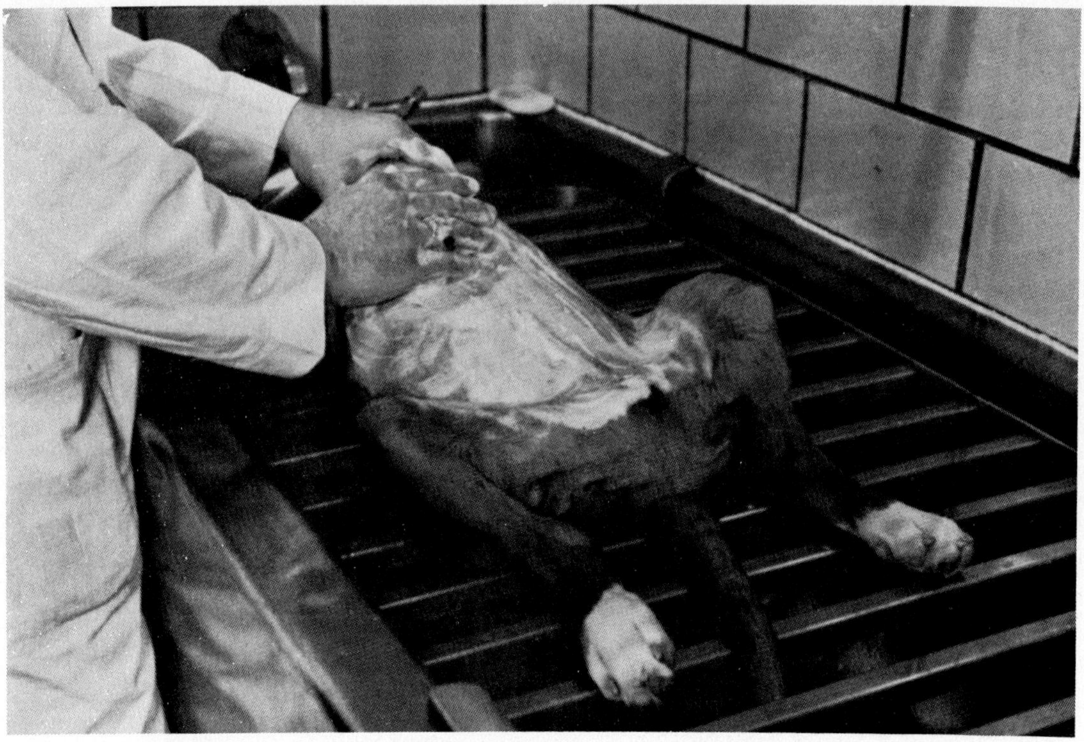

Figure 3–1. A sink with overlying metal grid for preoperative preparation of small animals. (From Leonard, E.P.: *Fundamentals of Small Animal Surgery.* W.B. Saunders Co., Philadelphia, 1968.)

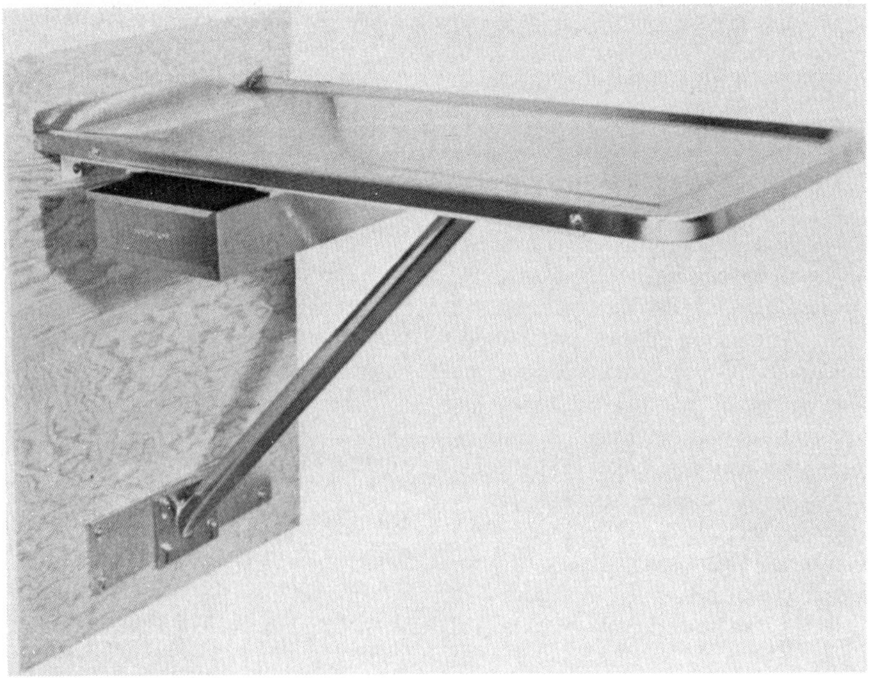

Figure 3–2. A table suitable for preparation, premedication, and induction of small animals. (Courtesy of Schroer Manufacturing Co., Kansas City, Missouri.)

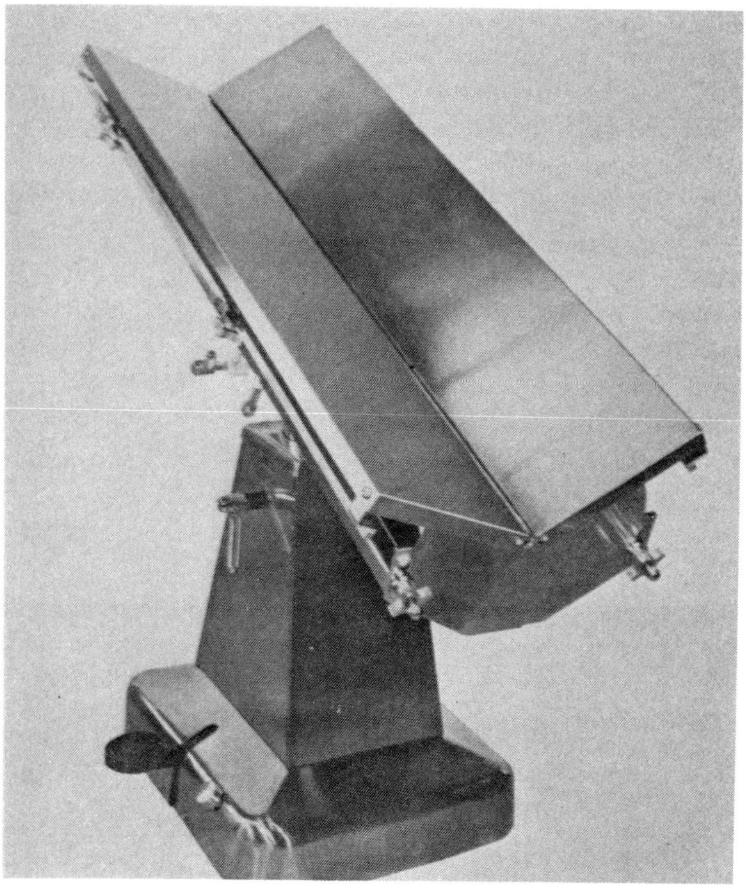

Figure 3–3. Adjustable "V"-top operating table. The top is constructed of two stainless steel panels either of which may be adjusted from horizontal to vertical. Adjustment may be made from either end of the table. A 3-inch wide stainless steel trough is located under the top at the center for collecting drainage from table. Top panels and trough lift off for easy cleaning. (Courtesy of Schroer Manufacturing Co., Kansas City, Missouri.)

vided. If the preparation room is to be used also as a recovery room, the floor and walls should be padded and it should be devoid of chute and stocks. An observation window that may be closed and an electric hoist or cart for moving the anesthetized animal should be installed. The room should be arranged to provide a quiet recovery, without light, and with minimal disturbance. Under such conditions, recovery is less likely to be complicated by struggling and excitement.

These facilities may comprise a suite of rooms or may be related functional areas in limited space. In any case, they should provide for an orderly flow of patients and personnel between animal holding space, preparation and induction areas, operating room or radiology, and recovery and/or intensive care. If the animal is induced with an inhalant anesthetic, it is preferable to transport the anesthetic machine with the animal. If this is not done, it will be necessary to equilibrate the gases in the new machine with those in the patient's respiratory tract.

Storage space, facilities for washing, cleaning, and, where appropriate, sterilizing anesthetic equipment are essential.

SUPPLIES AND EQUIPMENT FOR ANESTHESIA

The following supplies and equipment for anesthesia of animals are useful in the "prep," operating, and recovery rooms:

A. General

- Anesthetic machine with gas supply
- Masks of varying sizes
- Endotracheal tubes and connectors of varying sizes
- Syringes to inflate endotracheal catheter cuffs
- Forceps (rubber shod) to clamp endotracheal catheter cuff
- Laryngoscope with assorted blades, spare batteries, and bulbs
- Nonrebreathing valves
- Carbon-dioxide absorbent
- Rebreathing bags of assorted sizes
- Anesthetics, premedicants, and analeptics
- Antiseptics, sterile sponges, "prep" tray
- Cotton, gauze, adhesive tape
- Anesthetic jelly, topical and local anesthetic solutions
- Eye ointment
- Sterile syringes, hypodermic and spinal needles of assorted sizes
- Clippers with assorted heads
- Scissors
- Vascular catheters and sterile instruments, suture needles, and suture material for cut down
- Sterile gloves of assorted sizes
- Electrolyte solutions, plasma expanders, blood
- Fluid-administration sets
- Blood-collection and blood-administration sets
- Tourniquet
- Thermometer (rectal and/or telethermometer)
- Stethoscopes (chest and esophageal)
- Restraint ropes, straps, or thongs
- Heavy gauntleted leather gloves
- Small tool kit for minor adjustments (screwdrivers, wrench, Allen wrenches, pliers)
- Movable cabinet with lock to store smaller items listed above
- Infusion stand
- Stool for anesthetist
- Suction apparatus with catheters
- Kick buckets
- Adjustable examination and/or operating lights
- Cardiac defibrillator
- Cardiac-arrest and emergency kit
- Ventilator for assisted or controlled breathing
- Monitoring equipment (according to individual preferences)
- Equipment for blood gas and pH determinations
- Two- and three-way stopcocks

B. Small Animals

- Sandbags for positioning animal
- "V"-shaped trough for table top
- Anesthetist's screen
- Anesthetic chamber
- Small cart or stretcher on wheels and/or transporting cage
- Bathroom scale, self-registering
- Baby scales and/or balance and weights (metric system) for weighing birds and other small animals
- Bath towels and/or blankets
- Oxygen therapy cage

C. Large Animals

- Restraining ropes and hobbles
- Halters and headstalls
- Leg and tail bandages and cotton
- Tools for removing shoes and cleaning feet
- Pressure sprayer with soap and disinfectant dispenser
- Blankets
- Oral speculae
- Stomach tubes of assorted sizes
- Water mattress, padded hood or rubber pads for head, other body prominences, and limbs
- Rubber-covered bolsters or equivalent for positioning animal
- Movable cart and/or electric hoist for moving unconscious animal

Most of the aforementioned items are discussed in subsequent chapters.

Ideally, the anesthetized patient is placed in a relaxed, comfortable position. To prevent loss of body heat, a rubber pad beneath the animal is desirable (Fig. 3–4). Alternatively, an ab-

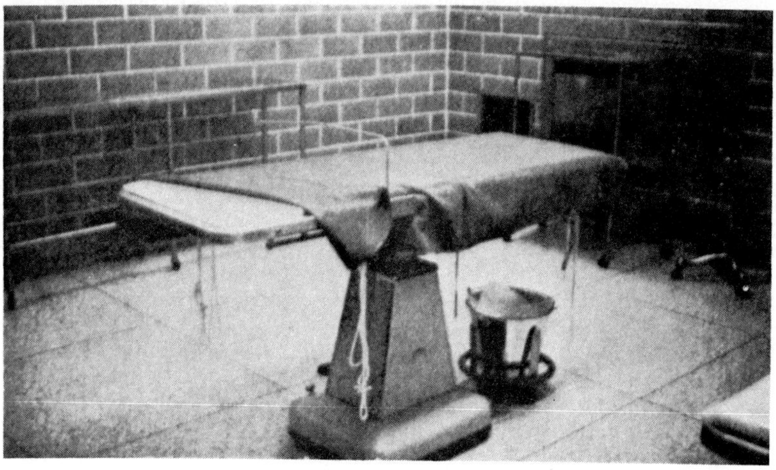

Figure 3–4. Insulating pad on operating table to prevent heat loss. The laundered cloth over the pad makes cleaning easy. Note anesthetist's shield to elevate drape and allow visualization of patient's head. (From General Anesthesia. Mod. Vet. Prac., *50*, 62, 1969.)

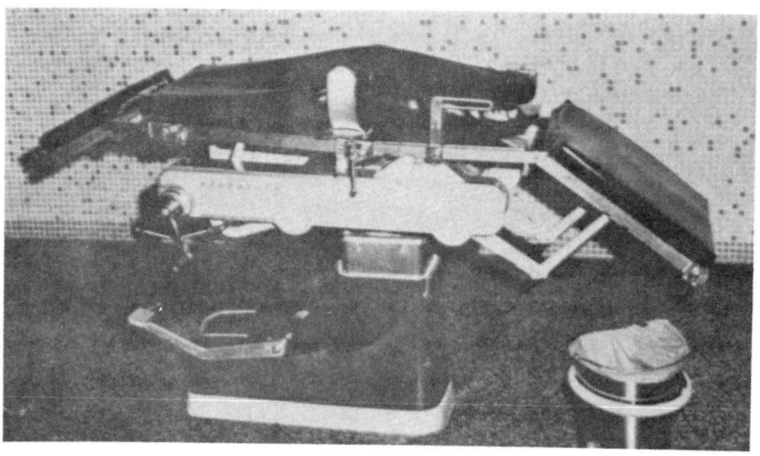

Figure 3–5. A human operating table* suitable for animal anesthesia and surgery. Note the body horns, pads, and flexion sites at head, mid- and foot sections.

sorbent paper cage liner or ordinary bath towels can be put beneath the small animal. The latter items also absorb fluids that drain onto the operating table.

Conventional small animal operating tables suitable for dogs, cats, primates, small ruminants, and swine are poorly designed for optimum positioning of the patient. Tables for humans are more flexible in that they are jointed and can be adjusted to requirements of the surgeon and comfort of the patient (Fig. 3–5). To overcome the shortcomings of inadequate table design, veterinarians use some additional aids, the least expensive of which is the sandbag. These can be fabricated in several sizes and shapes to fit the needs of various situations. The ordinary canvas-covered sandbag soon becomes bloodstained and unsightly; in addition, it continuously loses a small amount of sand. To correct these deficiencies, it can be sealed in a watertight plastic envelope that is easily cleaned (Fig. 3–6).

In many operations, stretching the patient's

*See Appendix A for manufacturer.

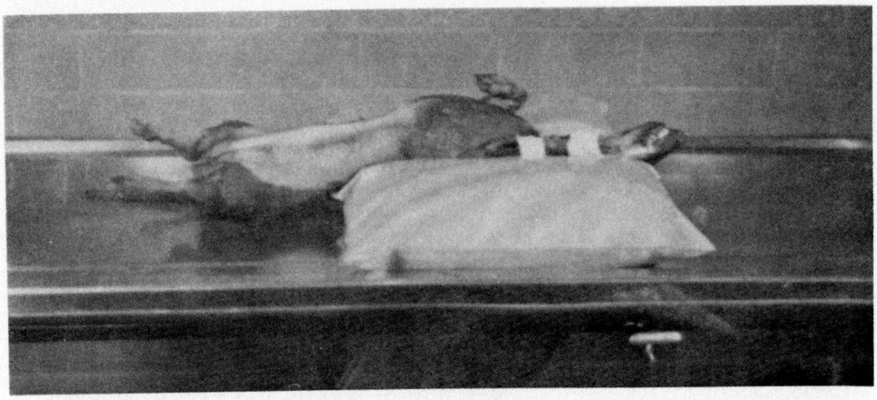

Figure 3–6. Plastic-covered sandbags hold the patient in position.

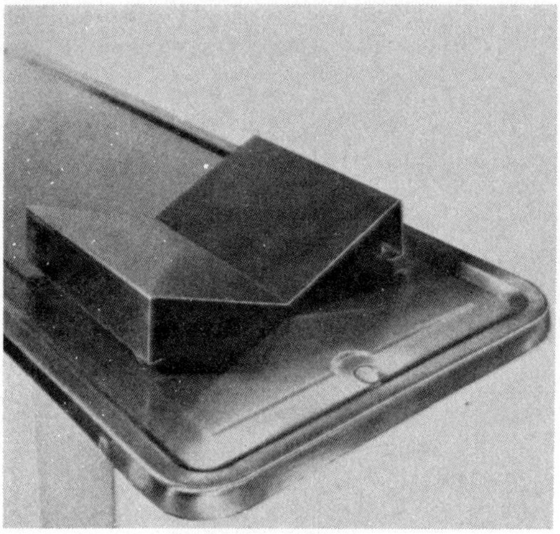

Figure 3–7. A portable metal trough to facilitate restraint in dorsal recumbency. (Courtesy of Schroer Manufacturing Co., Kansas City, Missouri.)

legs by tying them to the operating table with thongs may complicate the surgical procedure. When a flat-topped operating table is used, it is impossible to tie an anesthetized animal so that it will lie on its back and remain perfectly upright. This is true, despite the fact that this is a commonly used position especially in canine and feline operations. This problem may be overcome by the use of adjustable "V"-top tables or by the use of portable troughs of wood or metal placed on conventional tables (Fig. 3–7). Human operating tables are fitted with body horns that may be used to serve the same purpose (Fig. 3–5).

In larger animals, restraint, induction, and positioning during anesthesia present many physical problems. To overcome these, padded induction and recovery rooms and new types of operating tables have been developed (Fig. 3–8, A–F). Large animal operating tables should be padded and should have headrests and movable panels to facilitate access to the animal. Water-filled mattresses, inflated inner tubes, and movable pads are frequently used to protect the body, limbs, and head from undue pressure (see Chap. 21). Ability to lower the table to floor level or to tilt it to a vertical position facilitates restraint of the animal on the table either prior or subsequent to induction of anesthesia.

To assist positioning during anesthesia, tables may be tilted, an overhead hoist may be used, or trough-shaped operating tables may be employed (Figs. 3–8, 3–9, 3–10). When permanent facilities are not available, transportable large animal tables can be utilized (Fig. 3–9).

For operations in the standing position, use of a cattle chute or stocks is often indicated (Fig. 3–10). Chutes may be attached to a device that tilts the animal to a laterally recumbent position.

EQUIPMENT FOR RESTRAINT

In addition to the materials previously described, certain equipment is advantageous for handling wild and vicious animals. Included among these items are animal control poles, remote injection equipment, and squeeze cages.

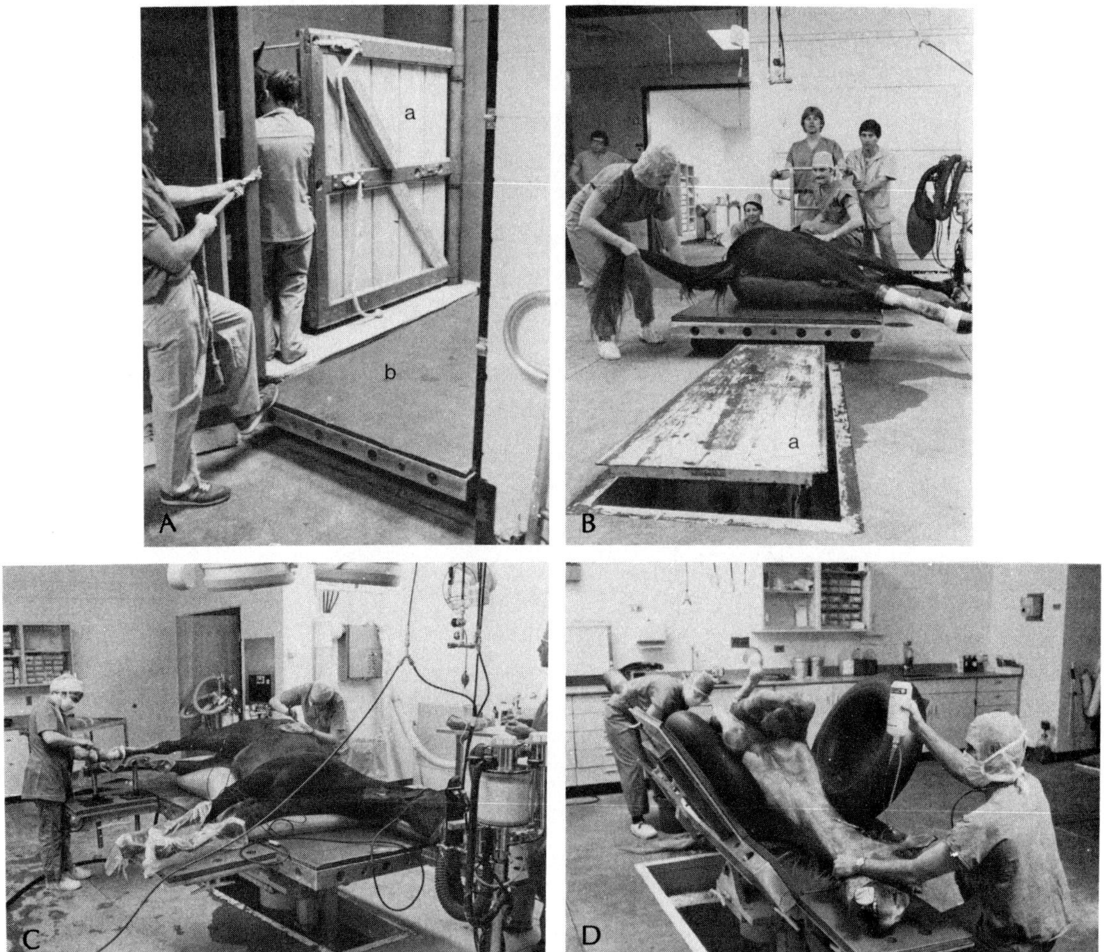

Figure 3–8. *A*, Large animal induction stall. Horse is confined behind swinging door (a). Anesthetic is administered in the jugular vein. As animal collapses, it is rolled onto operating table top (b). *B*, Horse is transported from induction stall to operating room on table top. Top slides onto hydraulic piston in floor (a). *C*, Table is elevated to proper position and horse is prepared for surgery. Note water-filled mattress under horse for extra padding. Limbs are inserted into plastic sleeves to reduce contamination from feet during surgery. *D*, Trough-type large animal table. Sides can be raised or lowered with hand cranks. Note inner tubes to protect horse's shoulders.

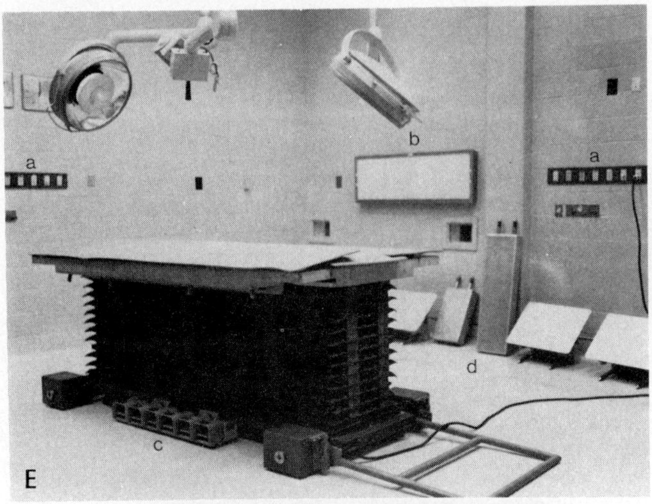

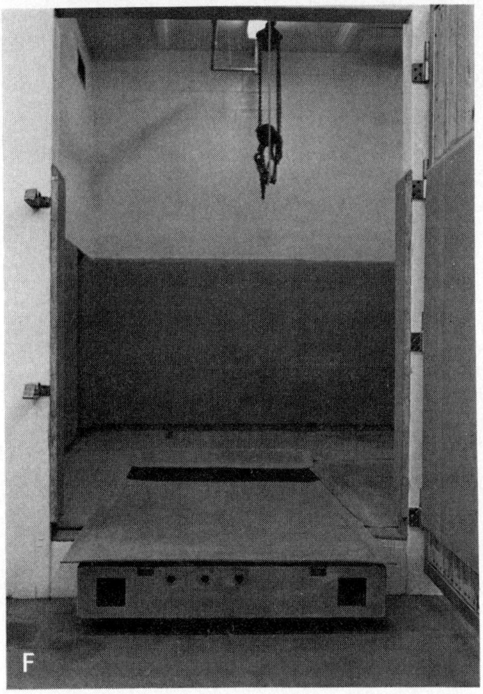

Figure 3–8 (Cont'd). *E*, Large animal operating room with wall-mounted medical gas, vacuum, and scavenging outlets *(a)*, and x-ray viewers *(b)*. The operating table is mobile; all four wheels will pivot. The foot-operated controls *(c)* for raising, lowering, and tilting the top can be seen at the bottom of the table. Panels *(d)* attach for positioning the head, body, and limbs. The electrically-controlled mechanism of the table is protected by an accordion-pleated shroud, extending from beneath the table to just above the foot controls. *F*, Padded recovery stall with ceiling hoist. Operating table top fits into floor.

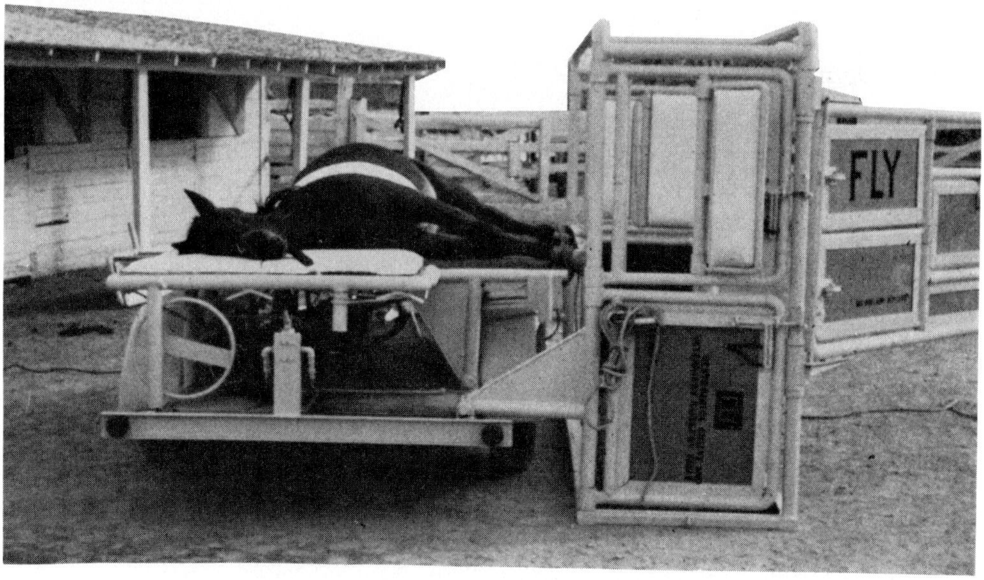

Figure 3–9. Transportable restraining chute and operating table. (Courtesy of Westwood Enterprise, Ovando, Montana.)

Animal Control Poles

To handle many species of wild or vicious animals, control poles are very useful. These generally consist of a long wooden or metal pole to which is attached a rope or steel cable, forming a noose which can be controlled by the operator from the opposite end (Fig. 3–11). In use, the animal's head or extremity is caught within the noose which is then tightened to hold the animal securely. Once the animal is caught, it usually is possible to inject a tranquilizer or anesthetic agent in order to facilitate handling. Caution must be employed in the amount of tension placed on the noose, since it is possible to asphyxiate animals with this device.

An excellent animal control pole* is available commercially, either in a standard length or with the ability to be extended up to 12 feet. An additional advantage of this pole over home-made types is that it has a quick release, allowing an animal to be freed immediately without the operator having to manipulate the noose.

Capture Equipment

In capture and restraint of wild animals, several devices are used. These include gunpowder- and carbon dioxide-powered rifles and pistols, crossbows, blowguns, and pole syringes* (Fig. 3–12). With them, it is possible to inject from 1 to 10 ml of any liquid into an animal for varying distances up to approximately 100 yards. The target area is usually the heavy muscles of the hip or neck.

According to Thomas (1961), who used a carbon-dioxide powered gun in a zoo practice, it seldom misfired or failed to inject the full quantity of drug. The range and accuracy varied somewhat and experience was necessary for best results. On cold days, with the ambient temperature between 20 and 40° F, it was difficult to make accurate shots over 30 yards unless the gun was prewarmed. On hot days, with the ambient temperature between 80 and 100° F, accurate shots could be made up to 50 yards.

Powder-propelled guns are more convenient and dependable. Both pistols and rifles require the same care and cleaning as other firearms.

Use of a crossbow and darts containing immobilizing agents has been reported by Pienaar et al. (1966). They stated that when used with a range finder, it has the advantages of being silent and more accurate than a carbon-dioxide powered gun.

*See Appendix A for manufacturers.

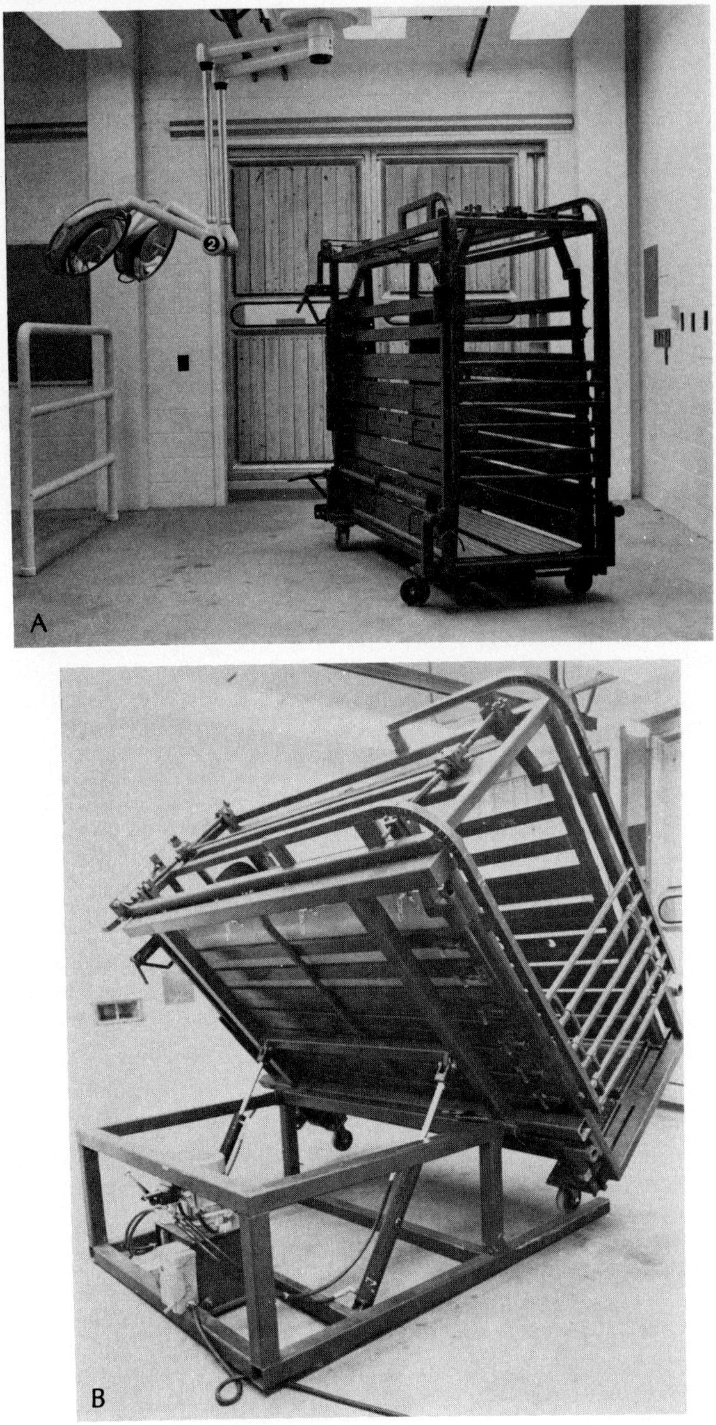

Figure 3–10. *A*, Bovine transporter for moving animals from receiving area to treatment and anesthesia induction. *B*, Transporter may be tilted to a horizontal position for surgery.

Figure 3–11. A commercially available animal control pole. (Courtesy of Ketch-All Company, San Diego, California.)

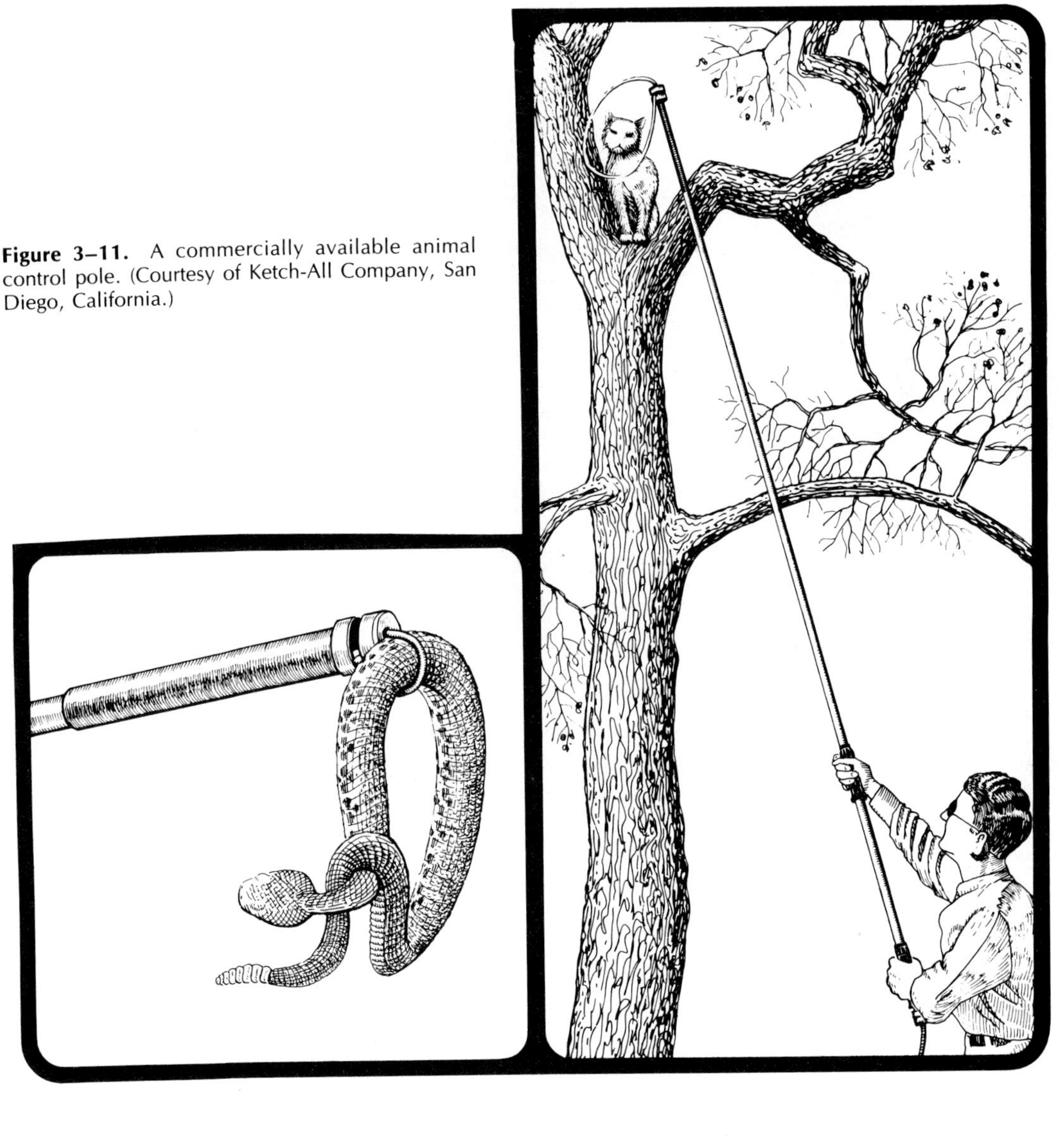

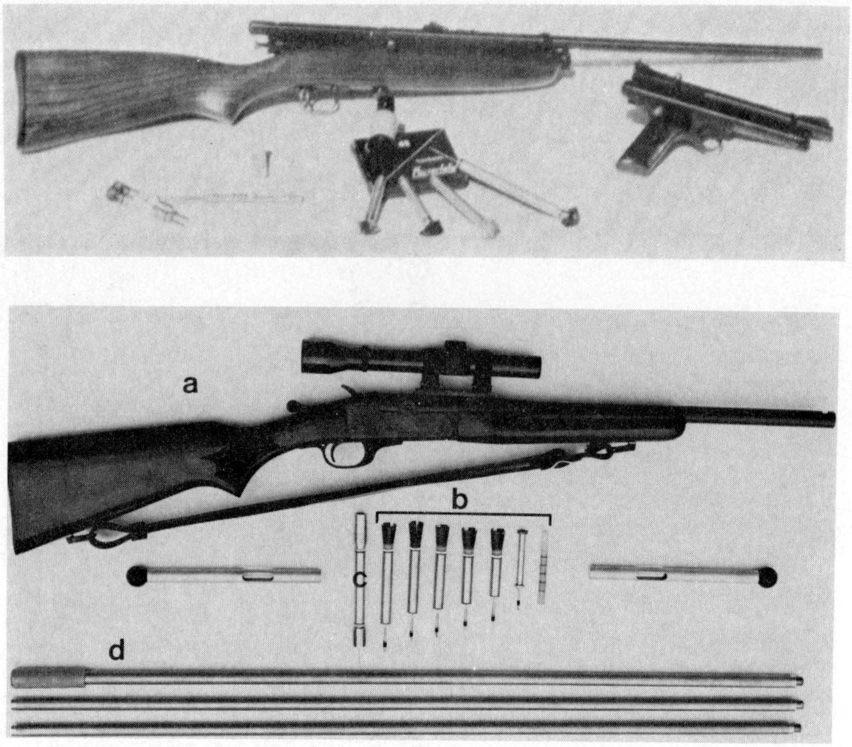

Figure 3–12. *A*, Palmer CO_2 powered short- and long-range syringe projectors with projectile syringes and loading equipment. (Courtesy of Palmer Chemical and Equipment Company, Inc., Atlanta, Georgia.) *B*, Remote injection equipment powered by .22 caliber gunpowder loads. Varirange syringe gun with telescopic sight (a) shoots syringes of various sizes (b). A pole syringe head (c) connects on the pole (d), which will extend to 9½ ft. (Courtesy of Gerwig Manufacturing Company, Ashland, Ohio.)

Haigh and Hopf (1976) have described how to make an inexpensive blowgun and darts from readily available materials. Blowguns are quiet and produce less trauma than gunpowder- or carbon dioxide-propelled capture guns; however, they do not have the range or penetrating power of the latter.

As emphasized by Sedgwick and Acosta (1969), many disastrous errors have been made by inexperienced individuals attempting to use capture equipment and immobilizing drugs. At best, these techniques lack precision. Many mechanical and physiologic variables affect drug administration, absorption, distribution, and elimination. The site and accuracy of injection, the mental state and general health of the animal, and climatic conditions all influence the effect produced. Most of the immobilizing drugs are potentially lethal for personnel and extreme caution should be employed in their use (see Chap. 21).

Use of a manual resuscitator and an endotracheal catheter will enable successful resuscitation of large animals immobilized under field conditions (Day et al., 1965). The Vetaspirator* is probably a more useful piece of equipment (Fig. 3–13).

Squeeze Cages

When zoo and other wild animals are to be anesthetized, the methods used vary with the species, their habitat, the degree of safety required, and the facilities available. The animal may be captured, treated, and released in its natural habitat; on the other hand, it may be necessary to premedicate or anesthetize it within its cage or in specially designed devices such as a squeeze cage* (Figs. 3–14, 3–15).

*See Appendix A for manufacturer.

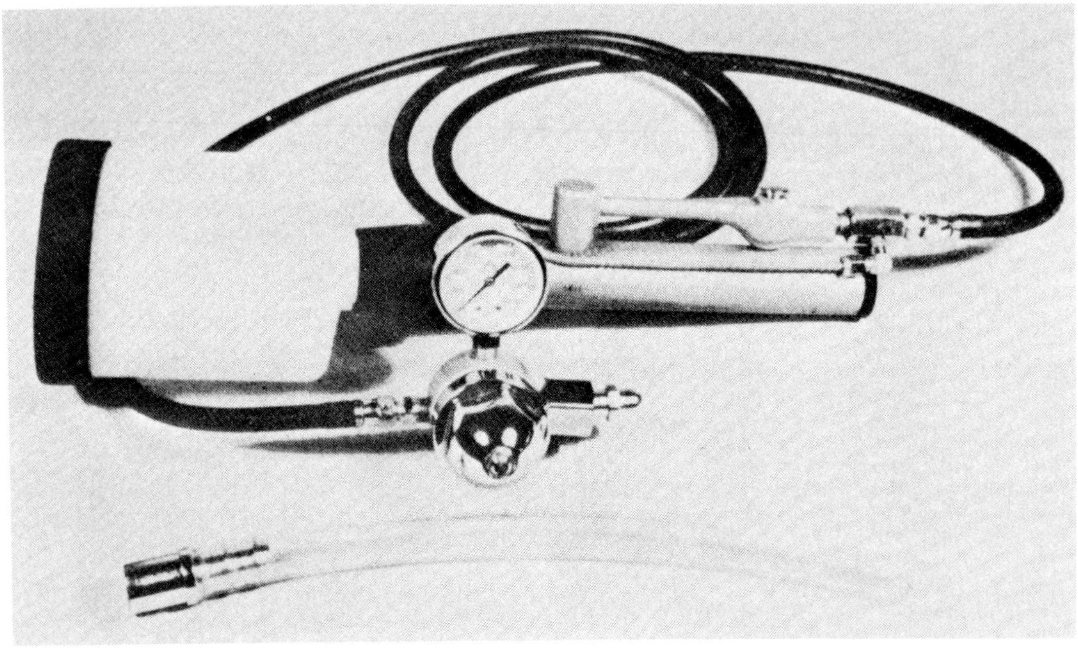

Figure 3–13. The Vetaspirator. This apparatus, when connected to a small oxygen tank, may be used for ventilatory assist, intermittent positive pressure ventilation, or aspiration of fluid and mucus from the respiratory passages and mouth.

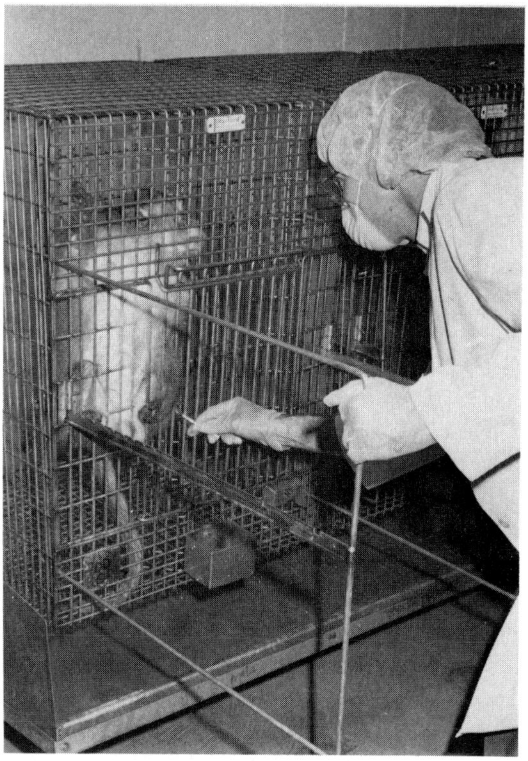

Figure 3–14. Primate squeeze cage. By pulling on handles, the operator brings a panel at the rear of cage forward, confining the animal against the bars at front. Injection can then be easily performed. Once this is accomplished, the handles are pushed to return the panel to its original position, thus freeing the animal. Note the protective clothing worn by the operator when working with primates. (Courtesy of the Department of Health and Human Services, National Institutes of Health, Bethesda, Maryland.)

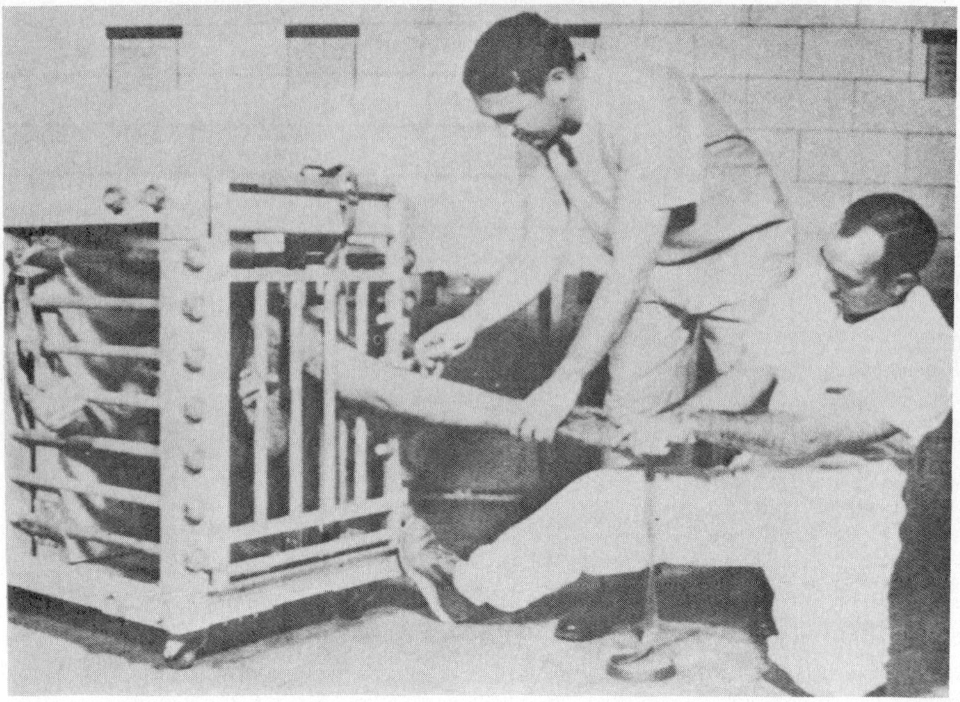

Figure 3–15. Administration of anesthetic agent to a chimpanzee by the intramuscular route. Both hands are restrained with straps. Intravenous administration can be accomplished via the cephalic vein in forearm. (From Day, P.W.: Anesthetic Technics for the Chimpanzee. Symposium Proceedings—Experimental Animal Anesthesiology, Brooks Air Force Base, Texas, p. 289, 1964.)

PERSONNEL

Well-trained lay personnel can do much to relieve the veterinarian from some of the more routine aspects of patient preparation and anesthesia. They are also invaluable for restraining and calming nervous animals prior to preanesthetic sedation. The ultimate responsibility for anesthesia rests with the veterinarian, but a lay assistant who does not have a working knowledge of these techniques is of little value other than to restrain the animal. For this reason, it is essential that the layman be taught the signs of anesthesia, and of anesthetic emergencies, and be able to initiate steps to cope with the latter. Among the techniques he should know are those of subcutaneous, intramuscular, and intravenous injection, endotracheal intubation, oxygen and blood administration, and cardiopulmonary resuscitation.

Considering the financial aspects of practice, a well-trained layman may be worth more to a veterinarian than a second colleague. A number of institutions currently conduct programs for training animal technicians.

REFERENCES

Day, G.T., Dyson, R.F., and Landeen, F.H.: A Portable Resuscitator for Use on Large Game Animals. J. Wildl. Man., 29:511, 1965.

Haigh, J.C., and Hopf, H.C.: The Blowgun in Veterinary Practice: Its Uses and Preparation. J.A.V.M.A., 169:881, 1976.

Pienaar, U.D., van Niekerk, J.W., Young, E., and van Wyk, P.: Neuroleptic Narcosis of Large Wild Herbivores in South African National Parks with the New Potent Morphine Analogues M–99 and M–183. J. S. Afr. Vet. Med., 37:277, 1966.

Sedgwick, C.J., and Acosta, A.L.: Capture Drugs. Mod. Vet. Pract., 50:32, 1969.

Thomas, W.D.: Chemical Immobilization of Wild Animals. J.A.V.M.A., 138:263, 1961.

CHAPTER 4

The Nervous System and Anesthesia

CENTRAL NERVOUS SYSTEM

Because anesthetics preferentially affect the nervous system, a general knowledge of its parts and functions is essential. Anatomically, the nervous system can be divided into central and peripheral divisions. The *central* division, comprised of the brain and spinal cord, contains all of the important nerve centers or nuclei. The *peripheral* division is composed of nerves and ganglia that supply the different organs and tissues.

Functionally, the nervous system can be divided into *somatic* and *autonomic* divisions. The former supplies the voluntary musculature while the latter innervates the viscera, blood vessels, and skin. Afferent fibers are found in both divisions. In anesthesia, one is concerned with both physiologic divisions, since obtunding of pain, relaxation of skeletal muscle, and maintenance of vital functions, such as cardiac output and respiration, are essential.

Brain

As the embryonic neural tube develops, the rostral part may be subdivided into five parts: the *telencephalon, diencephalon, mesencephalon, metencephalon,* and *myelencephalon* (Fig. 4–1, Table 4–1). Further development produces the cerebrum derived from the telencephalon. The brain stem, connecting the cerebrum and cerebellum, includes the entire diencephalon and mesencephalon, along with the ventral metencephalon and entire myelencephalon. The cerebellum is derived from the dorsal metencephalon.

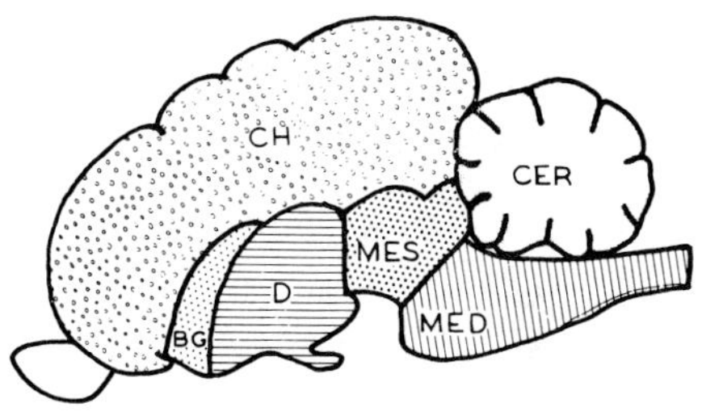

Figure 4–1. Schematic median section of the dog brain. CH, cerebral hemisphere; BG, basal ganglion; D, diencephalon; MES, mesencephalon; CER, cerebellum; MED, medulla oblongata. (From McGrath, J.T.: *Neurologic Examination of the Dog,* 2nd ed. Lea & Febiger, Philadelphia, 1960.)

Structurally, the cerebrum consists of an outer layer of gray matter containing nerve cell bodies

TABLE 4–1. Derivatives of the Primary Vesicles

Primary Vesicle	*Subdivision*	*Derivatives*	*Lumen*
Prosencephalon	Telencephalon	Cerebral cortex, corpus striatum, and rhinencephalon	Lateral ventricle and part of third ventricle
	Diencephalon	Thalamus and hypothalamus	Most of third ventricle
Mesencephalon	Mesencephalon	Collicular region and cerebral peduncles	Cerebral aqueduct
Rhombencephalon	Metencephalon	Pons and cerebellum	Fourth ventricle
	Myelencephalon	Medulla oblongata	Fourth ventricle and part of central canal
Remainder of neural tube		Spinal cord	Most of central canal

(From Gardner, E.: *Fundamentals of Neurology,* 5th ed. W. B. Saunders Co. Philadelphia, 1968.)

or neurons, and an inner core of white matter consisting mainly of myelinated nerve fibers. Centrally, at its base, are the basal nuclei.

The white matter of the cerebrum consists of corticocortical fibers and projection fibers. The corticocortical fibers connect different areas in the same hemisphere *(association fibers)* and in the opposite hemisphere *(commissural fibers).* Projection fibers originate or terminate in the cortex and connect it with the basal ganglia, brain stem, or spinal cord.

The diencephalon, or interbrain, is positioned between the cerebrum and midbrain. It contains the thalamus, which is concerned with sensory functions, and the hypothalamus, which is concerned with visceral functions.

The midbrain (mesencephalon) persists as such in the adult. It is formed in front by the two cerebral peduncles containing nerve tracts connecting the cerebrum with the brain stem and spinal cord.

The midbrain continues posteriorly into the pons which serves, in part, to connect the cerebral hemispheres and which also contains various nerve centers and tracts. Several pairs of cranial nerves connect to this structure: trigeminal (fifth), abducens (sixth), facial (seventh), and acoustic (eighth).

Behind the pons is the medulla oblongata and posterior to it is the spinal cord. In addition to nerve tracts, the medulla contains vital nerve centers that regulate respiration and circulation. Four pairs of cranial nerves connect to it: the glossopharyngeal (ninth), vagus (tenth), spinal accessory (eleventh), and hypoglossal (twelfth).

The cerebellum lies dorsal to the brain stem and is formed by two hemispheres separated by a central portion, the vermis. It is chiefly concerned with muscular coordination.

Reticular Activating System

Extending through the brain stem from the medulla anterior to the diencephalon is a meshwork of cells and fibers synapsing in all directions termed the *reticular activating system* (RAS). Ascending somatosensory fibers in the spinal cord (medial and lateral lemnisci) go directly over lateral pathways to the cerebral cortex and also synapse with cells in the RAS which, in turn, synapse diffusely with cortical cells (Fig. 4–2). Some impulses ascending through the dorsal columns also end in the RAS. Impulses ascending the cord directly to the cortex enable perception and sensory discrimination. Impulses through the RAS "activate" or "awaken" the cortex to receive perceptive and sensory impulses ascending the lateral pathways. When the RAS is blocked by injury or local or general anesthetics, perception does not occur despite the fact that the lateral pathways still function.

The RAS also facilitates the gamma efferent activity to skeletal muscle, which is responsible for muscle tone and enhanced skeletal reflexes. Anesthetics depress this gamma efferent activity and allow muscle relaxation.

The RAS is a multisynaptic structure, which

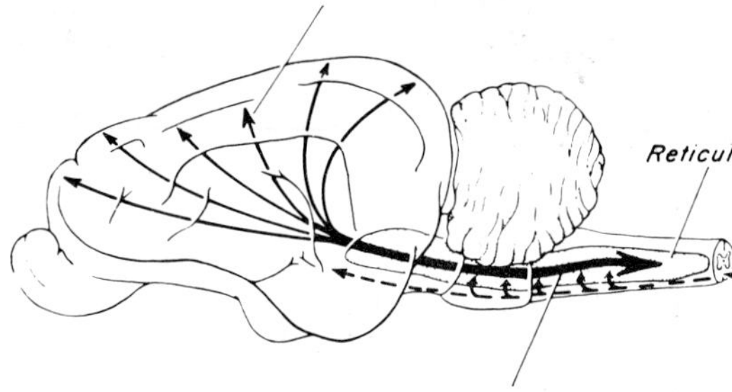

Figure 4–2. Ascending reticular activity results in an EEG and behavioral attention response. Descending reticular activity results in blockage of other sensory activity. (From Breazile, J.E., and Kitchell, R.L.: Pain Perception in Animals. Fed. Proc., 28:1379, 1969.)

probably accounts for its susceptibility to general anesthetics, since these agents block synaptic transmission better than nerve trunk conduction. Injection of a local anesthetic into the RAS produces general anesthesia, further substantiating the importance of this structure in controlling the overall degree of activity of the brain.

Cranial Nerves

Cranial nerves (Fig. 4–3) consist of 1) a peripheral portion, 2) a nuclear center in the brain stem (except olfactory and optic nerves), and 3) central connections with other parts of the brain. All twelve cranial nerves are paired.

Functionally, cranial nerves can be divided into those carrying impulses away from the brain *(efferent)*, those carrying impulses toward the brain *(afferent)*, and those performing both functions *(mixed)*:

Afferent Nerves

1. Olfactory
2. Optic
8. Acoustic

Efferent Nerves

3. Oculomotor } Motor to Eye Muscles
4. Trochlear }
6. Abducens }
11. Spinal Accessory
12. Hypoglossal

Mixed Nerves

5. Trigeminal
7. Facial
9. Glossopharyngeal
10. Vagus

Olfactory (Sensory). Cell bodies of the olfactory nerves are located in the olfactory nasal mucosa with their central processes passing through the cribriform plate to terminate in the olfactory bulbs.

Optic (Sensory). The optic nerves contain the central processes of the ganglion cells of the retina. Nerve fibers leave the eyeball as the optic nerve, and some decussate at the chiasm. They pass to the lateral geniculate bodies, then to the occipital cortex of the cerebrum. The optic nerve may be considered as a tract of the brain. Developmentally, it connects the retina, a derivative of the brain, and the diencephalon.

Oculomotor (Motor). The oculomotor nucleus is in the midbrain. It innervates the following muscles of the eye:

1. Dorsal } Recti
2. Medial }
3. Ventral }
4. Ventral oblique
5. Levator palpebrae superioris
6. Ciliary muscle
7. Sphincter pupillae

Trochlear (Motor). The trochlear nucleus is located in the midbrain. It innervates the dorsal oblique muscle of the eye.

Trigeminal (Motor and Sensory). The nucleus of the trigeminal nerve is in the medulla. In general, it is sensory to the skin of the muzzle and head, motor to the muscles of mastication. It has three main branches:

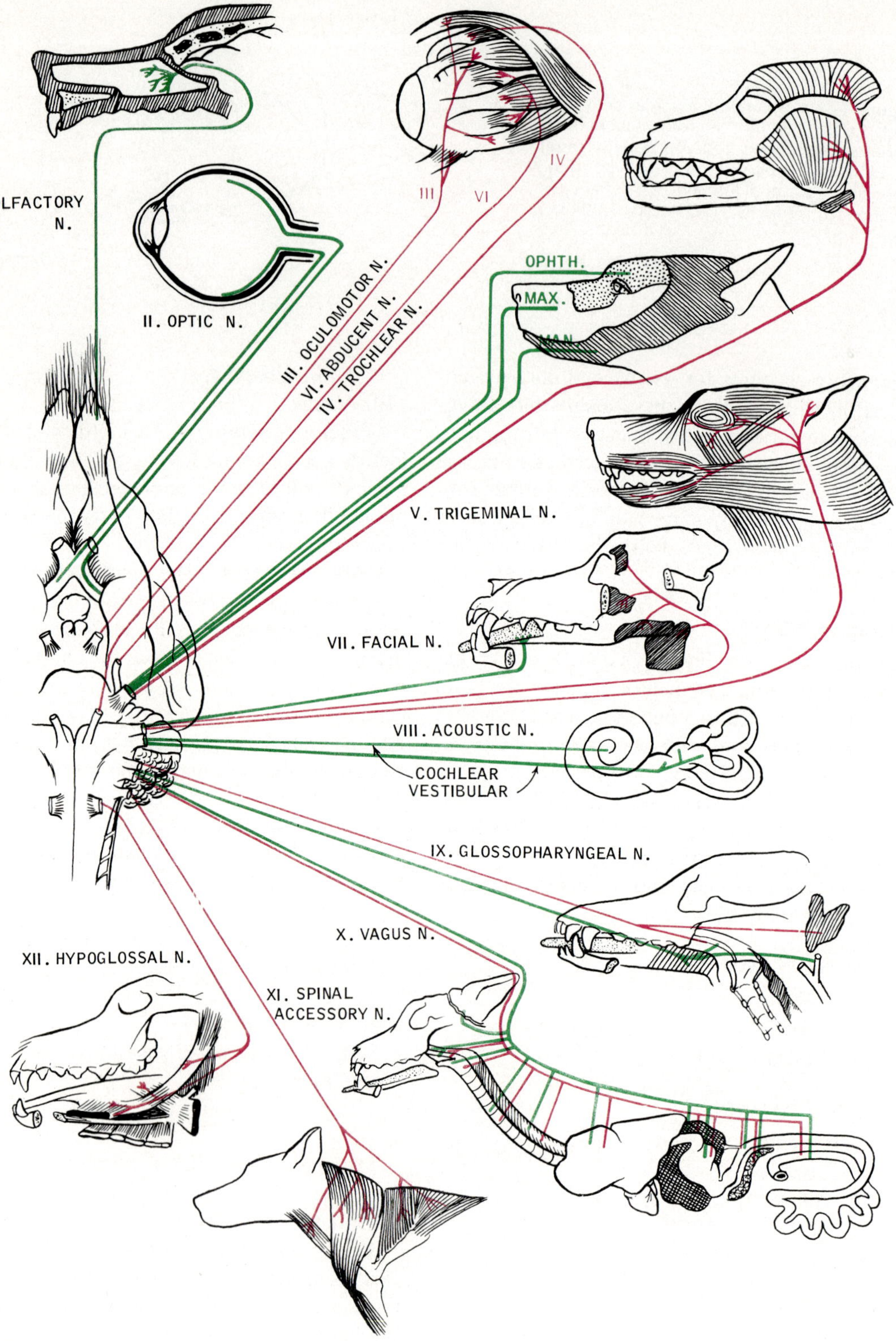

Figure 4–3. The origin and major distribution of the cranial nerves in the dog. (From Hoerlein, B.F.: *Canine Neurology, Diagnosis and Treatment,* 3rd ed. W.B. Saunders Co., Philadelphia, 1978.)

A. *Ophthalmic Branch (Sensory)*

1. Lachrymal
2. Frontal
3. Nasociliary

} Nerves

B. *Maxillary Branch (Sensory)*

1. Zygomatic
2. Sphenopalatine
3. Infraorbital

} Nerves

These two branches are sensory to the eyeball (corneal and palpebral reflexes), skin of the lower eyelid, mucous membrane of the nose, hard and soft palate, teeth of the upper jaw, and mucous membrane of the nasopharynx.

C. *Mandibular Branch (Motor and Sensory)*

1. Masseteric
2. Deep temporal
3. Buccinator
4. Pterygoid
5. Superficial temporal
6. Mandibular alveolar
7. Lingual

} Nerves

This branch supplies sensation to the lower part of face, side of the head, lower lip, ear, tongue, and lower teeth.

Motor fibers supply the muscles of mastication, tensor palati, and tensor tympani.

Masseteric
Temporal
Mylohyoideus
Anterior digastricus
Pterygoid

} Muscles

Abducens (Motor). The abducens nerve supplies the lateral rectus and retractor oculi muscles of the eye.

Facial (Motor and Sensory). The facial nerve is motor to all the skin muscles of the face, lips, nose, cheeks, ears, and ventral cutaneous muscles of the neck (muscles of expression). The facial nerve cells are located in the medulla.

Vestibulocochlear (Sensory). The acoustic nerve is composed of vestibular and cochlear portions. The former arises in the vestibular portion of the inner ear and is concerned with the sense of balance. Bipolar nerve cells of the latter are located in the spiral ganglion of the cochlea, transmit impulses from the hair cells of the cochlea centrally, and are concerned with the sense of hearing.

Glossopharyngeal (Motor and Sensory). The glossopharyngeal nerve is motor to the stylopharyngeus muscle and parotid and zygomatic salivary glands and sensory to the pharynx, tonsil, tongue, and carotid sinus.

Vagus (Motor and Sensory). The vagus is the longest cranial nerve, supplying organs and muscles of the neck, thorax, and abdomen. Preganglionic parasympathetic nerve fibers are supplied to the heart, visceral smooth muscle, and glands of the thorax and abdominal viscera. Motor innervation is also supplied to the pharynx and larynx. The sensory component transmits impulses centrally from the base of the tongue, pharynx, esophagus, stomach, intestines, larynx, trachea, bronchi, lungs, heart, and other viscera. Somatic afferent vagal fibers, following the facial nerve, supply sensation to the skin of the external ear canal.

Spinal Accessory (Motor). The spinal accessory nerve, as the name implies, has a dual origin from the medulla and from the cervical cord segments one to seven. The spinal root courses anteriorly, combines with the medullary roots and, subsequently, gives off some fibers to the vagus. It then passes posteriorly to supply muscles of the neck and shoulder.

Hypoglossal (Motor). The hypoglossal nerve supplies muscles of the pharynx, larynx, and intrinsic muscles of the tongue.

Spinal Cord

From the medulla, the spinal cord runs posteriorly in the vertebral canal. In domestic animals, it extends to the lumbosacral junction. It is surrounded by the meninges which support and protect it. From without inward, they are the dura mater, arachnoid, and pia mater. The spinal fluid is found in the subarachnoid space (Fig. 4–4).

Afferent fibers arriving at the cord through the dorsal nerve roots carry sensory impulses, which are conducted to motor reflex centers in the cord and to higher correlation centers in the brain. Efferent fibers, passing from the cord in the ventral nerve roots, transmit motor impulses from higher centers or reflex centers within the cord to muscles and glands. Ascending and descending tracts within the cord connect the

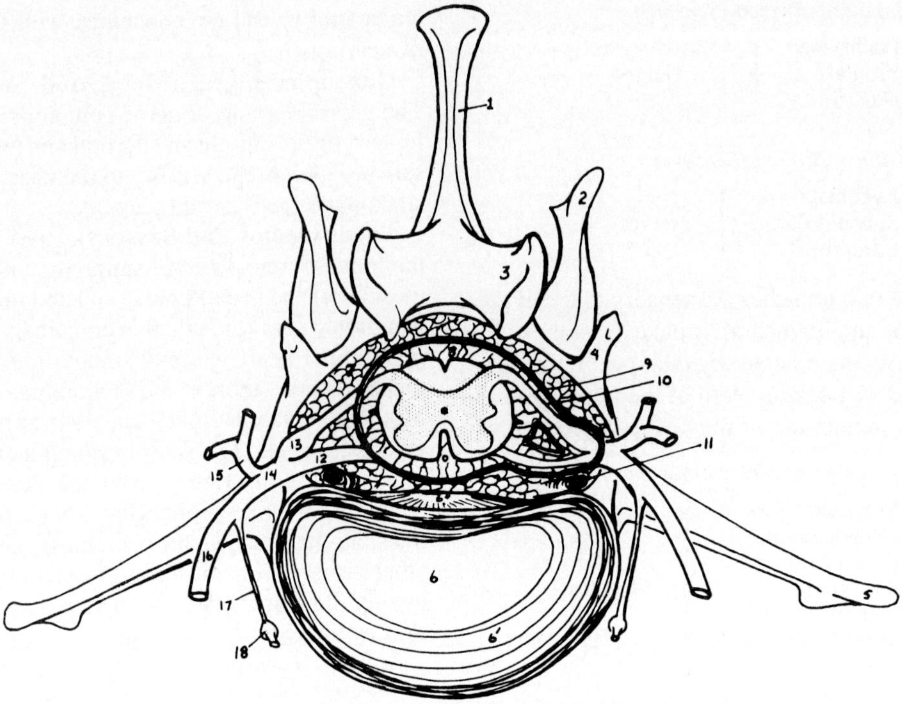

Figure 4–4. A cross section of the spine in the dog. (1) spinous process, (2) cranial articular process, (3) caudal articular process, (4) accessory process, (5) transverse process, (6) nucleus pulposus, (6′) fibrous ring or annulus fibrosus, (6″) dorsal longitudinal ligament, (7) epidural space, (8) subarachnoid space, (9) dura mater, (10) arachnoid, (11) longitudinal venous sinus, (12) ventral nerve root, (13) dorsal root ganglion, (14) spinal nerve, (15) dorsal branch of spinal nerve, (16) ventral branch of spinal nerve, (17) ramus communicans, (18) sympathetic trunk ganglion. (From Worthman, R.: *The Nerve of That Dog*. Washington State University, 1960.)

higher centers and the various cord segments with each other.

In cross section, the cord contains a central H-shaped area of gray matter composed of neurons and neuroglia along with their processes and some other fibers. Surrounding this area is an outer layer of white matter containing myelinated and nonmyelinated fibers supported by neuroglia. This outer white matter is divided into three major columns: dorsal, lateral, and ventral. Within these columns are ascending and descending tracts. For a more complete description in the dog, the reader is referred to Hoerlein (1978).

Cerebrospinal Fluid

The cerebrospinal fluid is found in both an internal (ventricular) system and an external (subarachnoid) system. The internal system consists of the paired lateral ventricles within the cerebellar hemispheres, the third ventricle medially between the thalamus and hypothalamus, and the fourth ventricle lying beneath the cerebellum and within the medulla. Cerebrospinal fluid is produced by the choroid plexus, a fringelike fold of pia mater found on the floor of both lateral ventricles and in the fourth ventricle, and also by the ependymal epithelium lining the ventricles (Milhorat, 1969). Fluid in the lateral ventricles empties into the third ventricle through the paired foramina of Monro. The third ventricle, in turn, empties into the fourth through the aqueduct of Sylvius. The central canal of the spinal cord is continuous with the fourth ventricle. The external or subarachnoid system overlies the brain and spinal cord. The bilateral foramina of Luschka allow fluid to pass between the ventricular and subarachnoid systems. In animals, phylogenetically below the ape, the foramen of Magendie is not found.

Cerebrospinal fluid is formed from the blood

by secretory and filtration processes and is absorbed into the blood by way of subdural venous sinuses and the spinal veins.

Because the skull forms an inelastic box, the brain-blood-cerebrospinal fluid relationship is a reciprocating one. A volume increase in any one component occurs at the expense of one or both of the other two. This phenomenon, first described by Monro (1783) and later modified by Kellie (1824), is termed the Monro-Kellie hypothesis or doctrine. It stresses that blood and cerebrospinal fluid are first to be moved. As the pressure of cerebrospinal fluid increases, it may reach the point that it inhibits blood flow to the brain.

In anesthesiology, hypotensive agents, osmotic diuretics, hypothermia, and hyperventilation may all be used to reduce intracranial pressure.

Increased cerebral or spinal fluid pressure produces a reflex increase in heart rate and blood pressure (Evans and Geddes, 1969). It has been hypothesized that the increase in cerebrospinal fluid pressure creates ischemia of neurons, and that this is the stimulus for increased sympathetic activity.

TABLE 4–2. Possible CNS Neuroregulators

Dopamine
Norepinephrine
Epinephrine
Tyramine
Octopamine
Phenylethylamine
Phenylethanolamine
Dimethoxyphenylethylamine (DMPEA)
Tetrahydroisoquinolines
Serotonin (5-hydroxytryptamine, 5-HT)
Melatonin
Tryptamine
Dimethyltryptamine (DMT)
5-Methoxytryptamine
5-Methoxydimethyltryptamine
5-Hydroxydimethyltryptamine (bufotenin)
Tryptolines
Acetylcholine
Histamine
γ-Aminobutyric acid (GABA)
γ-Hydroxybutyrate (GHB)
Glycine
Taurine
Purine
Aspartate
Glutamate
Prostaglandins
Corticosteroids
Estrogens
Testosterone
Thyroid hormone
Enkephalins
β-Endorphin
Substance P
Somatostatin
Angiotensin
Luteinizing hormone releasing hormone (LHRH)
Vasoactive intestinal polypeptide (VIP)
Adrenocorticotropic hormone (ACTH)
Thyroid releasing hormone (TRH)
Sleep factor delta

(From Barchas, J.D., Akil, H., Elliott, G.R., Holman, R.B., and Watson, S.J.: Behavioral Neurochemistry: Neuroregulators and Behavioral States. Science, 200:964, 1978. Copyright 1978 by the American Association for the Advancement of Science.)

NEUROREGULATORS

Neuroregulators play a key role in communication among nerve cells (Table 4–2). They may be subdivided into two groups: *neurotransmitters* convey information across synapses between adjacent cells; *neuromodulators* amplify or dampen neuronal activity. The latter can be released from within the brain or from other parts of the body to act on neurons distant from the release site (Barchas et al., 1978). In terms of anesthesia, many neuroregulators are known to be of great importance, whereas the significance of others may not be appreciated at this time.

OPIATE RECEPTORS AND ENDOGENOUS MORPHINE-LIKE SUBSTANCES

In 1973, several research groups demonstrated the existence of opioid receptors in the CNS that were not responsive to the known neurotransmitters (Pert and Snyder, 1973; Simon et al., 1973; Terenius, 1973). Concurrently, it was demonstrated by another group that focal electrical stimulation of the brain stem could relieve pain (Mayer et al., 1971). The marked similarity between the analgesia produced by stimulation and that produced by morphine, including the reversal by naloxone, led to the search for an endogenous ligand.

By 1974 Hughes reported evidence of an op-

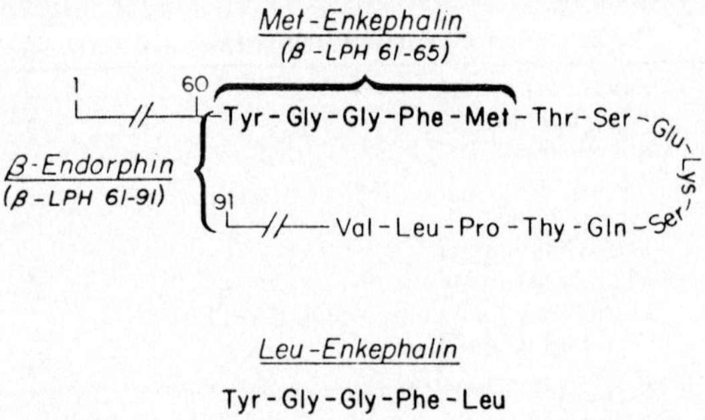

Figure 4–5. Endogenous opioids and their structural relationships to β-lipotropin. β-Lipotropin (β-LPH 1 to 91) is a pituitary hormone whose physiological functions remain to be established. Its carboxyl terminus (β-LPH 61 to 91) is an endogenous opioid called β-endorphin. The first five residues of β-endorphin (β-LPH 61 to 65) form another opioid peptide, methionine-enkephalin. A second pentapeptide with opiate-like properties, leucine-enkephalin, differs from the first only by substituting the leucine residue for the methionine residue. (From Barchas, J.D., Akel, H., Elliott, G.R., Holman, R.B., and Watson, S.J.: Behavioral Neurochemistry: Neuroregulators and Behavioral States. Science, 200, 964, 1978. Copyright 1978 by the American Association for the Advancement of Science.)

iate-like substance in brain extract and by 1975 had isolated two active pentapeptides. These differed only by a terminal amino group. They subsequently were termed methionine enkephalin (met-enkephalin) and leucine enkephalin (leu-enkephalin) since they were derived from the brain (Fig. 4–5). Hughes et al. (1975) noted that the peptide sequence for met-enkephalin corresponded to a portion of a larger pituitary hormone β-lipotropin (β-LPH). Teschemacher et al. (1975) reported that an endogenous opioid from the pituitary had a greater molecular weight than the enkephalins. Others (Li and Chung, 1976) found the substance, termed β-endorphin, corresponded to positions 61 to 91 of β-LPH, and still others (Bradbury et al., 1976) described its opiate properties. Guillemin et al. (1976) found another endogenous opioid with a fragment identical to 61 to 76 of β-LPH (α-endorphin). Today, it appears that at least three separate endogenous opioid neuronal systems are present in the brain: an enkephalin family with components similar to those found in the adrenal; a β-endorphin family, and a dynorphin family (Robbins et al., 1982).

Opiate receptors are specific sites on nerve cells which interact in a highly selective stereospecific fashion with opiate drugs (Pert and Snyder, 1973). These receptors are found only in nervous tissue and are most abundant in the brain stem (medulla and pons). The periaqueductal gray matter has a high receptor density. Other areas include the medial thalamus, solitary nuclei, area postrema, and anterior amygdala (Snyder, 1977). Receptors are also concentrated in the substantia gelatinosa of the spinal cord. Enkephalins appear to stimulate dopamine synthesis by acting on opioid receptors localized on dopamine nerve terminals (MacNichol et al., 1978). Others have shown that nonopiate receptor sites for β-endorphin are present within the body and have speculated upon the relationship between β-endorphin and stress (Hazum et al., 1979).

There is evidence that endorphins produce their analgesic effects by suppressing substance P (SP) release in the spinal cord. This peptide has a widespread distribution in nervous tissue, and is found in almost every division of the nervous system. High concentrations are found in the dorsal horn, and it has been shown that SP excites spinal cord nerve cells. Met-enkephalin blocks release of SP in isolated preparations of trigeminal nucleus. Some believe that prevention of SP release by enkephalin may be what closes the gate in the spinal cord pain transmission system. Descending neurons in the pain chain use the neurotransmitter serotonin. SP appears to excite neurons, whereas serotonin inhibits them (Marx, 1979).

Enkephalin analogs, which are longer-acting than natural enkephalins and are reversed by naloxone, have been synthesized (Pert and Pert, 1976; Chorev et al., 1979). It is probable that commercial preparations such as these will soon become available for therapy.

Narcotic analgesics have been shown to reduce the endogenous levels of brain monoamines and to increase their synthesis. Morphine produces dose-dependent increases in antinociception and accumulation of newly synthesized dopamine and norepinephrine in mouse brain. Stereospecific binding of morphine to opiate receptors in central nervous tissue triggers the chemical and physical responses involved in antinociceptive processes.

Chronic administration of moderate doses of morphine to rats increases the level of substance P (SP) within the spinal cord gray matter, particularly in areas classically associated with nociception. Vacca et al. (1980) reported that morphine may inhibit release of intraneuronal SP, and this mechanism could account for selective blockade by opiates of pain transmission in the dorsal horn.

Martin et al. (1976) first proposed that there are three types of receptors affected by morphine and nalorphine-like drugs. These they designated mu (μ), kappa (κ), and sigma (σ). Opioid-induced antinociception appears to be produced by μ and κ opioid receptor interactions, whereas opioid-induced hypermotility of animals is caused by μ and σ interactions (Iwamoto, 1981). The latter may be dependent upon CNS dopamine-containing systems.

PERIPHERAL NERVOUS SYSTEM

Spinal Nerves

Spinal nerves supply motor and sensory innervation to most of the body *(somatic nervous system),* with the exception of the head and viscera. They also form part of the autonomic nervous system which controls visceral functions. Spinal nerves vary in number depending on animal species. Anatomically, the spinal nerves are formed by a combination of dorsal and ventral spinal roots coming from the spinal cord. These join and leave the spinal canal through the intervertebral foramina. The dorsal root carries afferent fibers whose nuclei are in the dorsal root ganglion. The ventral roots contain efferent fibers.

The spinal cord is divided into segments for descriptive purposes, there being in the dog eight cervical, thirteen thoracic, seven lumbar, three sacral, and four or five coccygeal segments. The segmental distribution of the motor roots in the dog is set forth in Table 4–3.

After leaving the intervertebral foramen, each spinal nerve divides into dorsal and ventral branches. The dorsal branches generally supply the muscles and skin of the back, while the ventral branches supply the muscles and skin of the chest, abdomen, and extremities. Branches from several spinal nerves may combine to form major nerves (such as the sciatic) and plexuses (such as the brachial plexus) (Figs. 4–6, 4–7).

A *myotome* is the mass of musculature innervated from one ventral spinal nerve root (motor). It is derived from the somite of an embryonic segment and forms the skeletal musculature originating from that segment. Pelvic limb myotomes in the dog have been described by Fletcher (1970) (Table 4–4). The area supplied by a single dorsal nerve root (sensory) is called a *dermatome*. There is considerable overlap of areas supplied by adjacent roots. Knowledge of myotomes and dermatomes is essential for regional anesthesia of the thorax, abdomen, and limbs (see Fig. 16–12).

Branching off the spinal nerves in the thoracic and lumbar areas are *rami communicantes,* which connect the spinal nerves with a chain of ganglia lying lateral to the vertebral bodies, termed the vertebral sympathetic ganglia.

AUTONOMIC NERVOUS SYSTEM

The autonomic nervous system is often called the vegetative, visceral, or involuntary nervous system because its action requires no conscious control. In this respect, it contrasts with the somatic nervous system supplying the striated muscles. The hypothalamus is one of the major areas of the brain that controls the autonomic nervous system. The autonomic system can be further subdivided into the craniosacral or parasympathetic division and the thoracolumbar or sympathetic division (Fig. 4–8).

Parasympathetic System

Preganglionic fibers of the parasympathetic system arise in three areas: the midbrain (tectal outflow), the medulla (medullary outflow), and the sacral spinal cord (sacral outflow). These efferent fibers generally are long and synapse with one or two postganglionic fibers in a ganglion on or within the organ supplied. The tectal outflow originates in the Edinger-Westphal nucleus of the third (oculomotor) cranial nerve and synapses at the ciliary ganglion in the orbit to

TABLE 4–3. Segmental Distribution of Motor Roots in the Dog

C3–4–5	Distributed in segmental manner to most of the neck musculature.
C5	May send a branch to the phrenic nerve.
C6 (usually 7)	Phrenic nerves to the diaphragm.
C6–7–8, T1 (occasionally 2)	Brachial plexus to the forelimb.
T2–8	Intercostal nerves to the thorax.
T9–13	Nerves to the muscles of the ventral and lower lateral parts of the abdominal wall.
L1–2 (occasionally 3)	Nerves to the muscles of the caudolateral abdominal wall and the thigh in the region of the stifle.
L4–5–6–7, S1–2–3	Lumbosacral plexus to the hindlimb.
L4–5–6 (occasionally 3)	Femoral nerve to extensors of the stifle.
L5–6 (occasionally 4)	Obturator nerve, the abductor of the hip.
L6–7, S1	Sciatic nerve supplying all other muscles of the hindlimb.

(From McGrath, J.T.: *Neurologic Examination of the Dog,* 2nd ed. Lea & Febiger, Philadelphia, 1960.)

innervate the pupillary sphincter and ciliary muscles (Fig. 4–9). The medullary outflow is comprised of the parasympathetic components of the seventh (facial), ninth (glossopharyngeal), and tenth (vagus) cranial nerves. The facial nerve synapses at the submandibular ganglion to supply the submaxillary and sublingual glands, and at the pterygopalatine ganglion to innervate the lacrimal and nasal glands. The autonomic fibers of the glossopharyngeal nerve travel to the otic ganglion where they synapse to innervate the parotid and orbital salivary glands.

The vagus nerves contain approximately 80% of the parasympathetic nerve fibers in the body. The preganglionic fibers are long and synapse in small ganglia that lie directly on or in the viscera of the thorax and abdomen. Fibers are supplied to the heart, lungs, esophagus, stomach, small intestine, proximal colon, liver, gallbladder, pancreas, kidneys, and upper ureters. In the heart, they enter into intrinsic synapse in the muscle fiber. In the intestinal wall, they form the plexuses of Meissner and Auerbach. The vagus also carries afferent fibers, arising from the nodose ganglion, which produce visceral reflexes but apparently not pain.

The sacral outflow originates in the second, third, and fourth sacral segments of the spinal cord. Preganglionic fibers form the pelvic nerves *(nervi erigentes)* which synapse in ganglia near the bladder, distal colon, rectum, and sexual organs. The vagus and pelvic nerves thus provide secretory, vasodilator, and motor fibers for the thoracic, abdominal, and pelvic organs.

Autonomic nerve endings in the effector organ may terminate within cells or on the cell membrane. Smooth muscle cells may have protoplasmic bridges so that one stimulus causes many to react. No distinctive nerve ending exists comparable to the myoneural junction of somatic nerves.

Sympathetic System

The sympathetic nervous system arises from cells in the intermediolateral columns of the first thoracic to the fourth or fifth lumbar cord segments (canine). Their axons pass through the ventral spinal roots and synapse in sympathetic ganglia with postganglionic nerve cells.

There are three types of sympathetic ganglia: vertebral, prevertebral, and terminal. *Vertebral ganglia* are paired and lie in the lateral sympathetic chains paralleling the vertebral column. They are connected to each other by nerve trunks and to the spinal cord and spinal nerves by rami communicantes. White rami carry the preganglionic outflow from the spinal cord in myelinated fibers. These synapse with nonmyelinated fibers in the vertebral ganglia. The nonmyelinated fibers exit via the gray rami to join the spinal nerves supplying the blood vessels of skeletal muscle, the sweat glands, pilomotor muscles, and blood vessels of the skin.

Prevertebral ganglia are located in the abdomen and pelvis and consist mainly of the celiac, aorticorenal, and anterior and posterior mesenteric ganglia. The bladder and rectum are supplied by *terminal ganglia* located in close proximity to these organs.

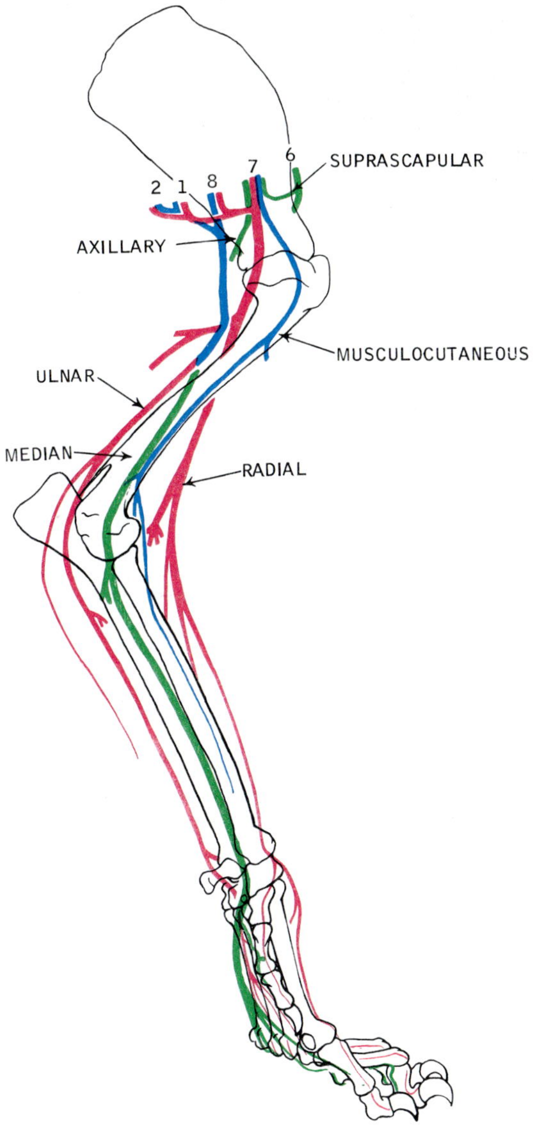

Figure 4–6. A medial view of the front limb of the dog illustrating the relative course and distribution of the major nerves to the leg. (From Hoerlein, B.F.: *Canine Neurology, Diagnosis and Treatment,* 3rd ed. W.B. Saunders Co., Philadelphia, 1978.)

Preganglionic fibers from the upper thorax form the cervical sympathetic chain and synapse with postganglionic fibers to form the sympathetic supply to the head and neck (sudomotor, pilomotor, vasomotor, secretory, and pupillodilator innervation). The upper thoracic chain supplies postganglionic fibers that form the cardiac, esophageal, and pulmonary plexuses. The splanchnic nerves are formed from preganglionic fibers which do not synapse until they reach the celiac ganglion. Postganglionic fibers from this and other prevertebral ganglia ramify widely to supply the abdominal viscera.

The adrenal medulla is unique in that it is embryologically, anatomically, and functionally homologous to the sympathetic ganglia. Chromaffin cells within the medulla originate from the neural crest and are innervated by preganglionic fibers.

In contrast to the parasympathetic system, preganglionic sympathetic fibers may synapse with many postganglionic nerve cells, thus being capable of producing massive sympathetic discharge.

The sympathetic and parasympathetic systems modulate each other and homeostasis is achieved through a balance between the two.

FUNCTION OF NEURONS

Axonal Conduction

Nerve impulses to skeletal muscles are electrical currents originating in the ventral horn cells of the spinal cord. They pass along the axon to the myoneural junction. From a pharmacologic standpoint, there is an important distinction between electrical *conduction* of a nerve impulse along an axon and chemical *transmission* of this signal across the neuromuscular junction. Local anesthetic agents block conduction, whereas a much larger group of drugs, including local anesthetics, alter transmission.

Using electrodes, it can be shown that the internal resting potential of an axon is approximately 70 millivolts (mv) negative to the exterior of the axon. This is termed the internal resting potential (RP) and is due to 1) a higher internal concentration of potassium and 2) selective permeability of the resting axonal membrane to potassium.

When a resting axon is stimulated electrically, a nerve action potential (NAP) is produced that will travel the full length of the neuron in either direction (Fig. 4–10). Most general anesthetics (ether, methoxyflurane, halothane,

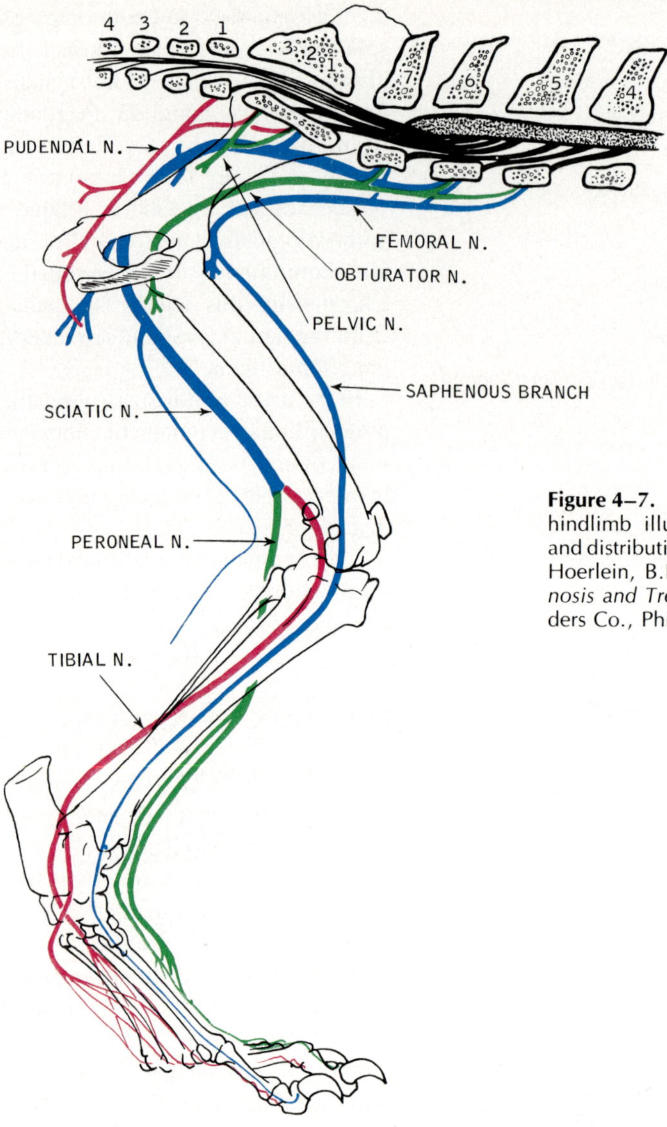

Figure 4–7. A medial view of the canine hindlimb illustrating the relative course and distribution of the major nerves. (From Hoerlein, B.F.: *Canine Neurology, Diagnosis and Treatment,* 3rd ed. W.B. Saunders Co., Philadelphia, 1978.)

and nitrous oxide) have little effect on nerve conduction velocity (deJong et al., 1966; deJong and Nace, 1967).

Chemical Transmission

The terminal axon connects with the sarcoplasm of the muscle fiber by the *terminal membrane*. Facing it is a second membrane, the *postjunctional membrane*. The two are separated by a space, the *subneural space*. The area where the nerve meets the muscle is termed the end-plate (Fig. 4–11).

The postjunctional membrane is preferentially permeable to sodium and potassium ions. The interior, facing the muscle, is negatively charged while the exterior, facing the nerve, is positively charged. This polarity is due to an excess of sodium ions outside and potassium ions inside. The electrostatic difference in potential between sides is approximately 90 mv.

When a nerve impulse reaches the end of the axon, it releases acetylcholine from its bound form in the synaptic vesicles. It is immediately adsorbed on the cholinergic receptors of the postjunctional membrane. This changes the configuration of proteins in the membrane and its

TABLE 4–4. Myotome Distribution in the Canine Pelvic Limb

Muscle	*Innervating Ventral Roots*	*Regional Nerve*
Sartorius	L4, L5, L6	Femoral
Rectus femoris	L4, L5, L6	Femoral
Vastus lateralis	L4, L5, L6	Femoral
Vastus intermedius	L4, L5, L6	Femoral
Vastus medialis	L4, L5, L6	Femoral
Capsularis coxae	L4, L5, L6	Femoral
Gracilis	L4, L5, L6	Obturator
Adductor magnus et brevis	L4, L5, L6	Obturator
Adductor longus	L4, L5, L6	Obturator
Pectineus	L4, L5, L6	Obturator
Tensor fasciae latae	L6, L7	Cranial gluteal
Middle gluteal	L6, L7	Cranial gluteal
Deep gluteal	L6, L7	Cranial gluteal
Superficial gluteal	L6, L7, S1	Caudal gluteal
Biceps femoris	L6, L7, S1	Sciatic
Abductor cruris caudalis	L6, L7, S1	Sciatic
Semitendinosus	L6, L7, S1	Sciatic
Semimembranosus	L6, L7, S1	Sciatic
Cranial tibial	L6, L7, S1	Peroneal
Long digital extensor	L6, L7, S1	Peroneal
Lateral digital extensor	L6, L7, S1	Peroneal
Fibularis longus	L6, L7, S1	Peroneal
Extensor hallucis longus	L6, L7, S1	Peroneal
Fibularis brevis	L6, L7, S1	Peroneal
Gastrocnemius	L6, L7, S1	Tibial
Superficial digital flexor	L6, L7, S1	Tibial
Deep digital flexor	L6, L7, S1	Tibial
Caudal tibial	L6, L7, S1	Tibial
Popliteus	L6, L7, S1	Tibial
Plantar muscles of pes	L7, S1	Tibial
Internal obturator	L7, S1, S2	Sciatic
Gemelli	L7, S1, S2	Sciatic
Quadratus femoris	L7, S1, S2	Sciatic
Bulbocavernosus	S1, S2	Pudendal
Ischiocavernosus	S1, S2	Pudendal
Coccygeus	S1, S2, S3	Sacral plexus
Levator ani	S2, S3	Sacral plexus
External anal sphincter	S2, S3	Caudal rectal

For each muscle, the myotome composition (determined by ventral root supply) is listed along with the regional nerve that supplies the muscle. The list is applicable to most dogs, i.e., dogs having median fixed plexuses. The external obturator, extensor digitorum brevis, and ischiourethalis muscles were not examined.

(From Fletcher, T. F.: Lumbosacral Plexus and Pelvic Limb Myotomes in the Dog. Am. J. Vet. Res., 31:35, 1970.)

permeability. Sodium migrates inward and potassium outward with decrease in negativity within the postjunctional membrane termed depolarization. From −90 to −45 mv nothing occurs. This range (−90 to −45) is termed the *end-plate potential* (EPP) (Fig. 4–12). Below −45 mv, electrical activity spreads to the muscle around the end-plate and is termed the *action potential* (AP). This reaches a positive value of up to +30 mv.

Depolarization requires 0.2 to 0.4 milliseconds. During this time, acetylcholine is hydrolyzed to acetic acid and choline by acetylcholine esterase present in the postjunctional membrane. As acetylcholine is hydrolyzed, the membrane permeability is restored to its normal state and the ions return to their respective sides *(repolarization)*. Muscle contraction is delayed 2 to 3 milliseconds; hence, repolarization is already complete when contraction occurs.

Acetic acid and choline recombine to form acetylcholine, through action of *cholineacetylase*. Acetylcholine is then adsorbed as a protein of one of the end-plate membranes.

When an impulse reaches a peripheral nerve ending, one of two chemical substances is released. Acetylcholine (ACH) is the chemical effector at: 1) all preganglionic autonomic end-

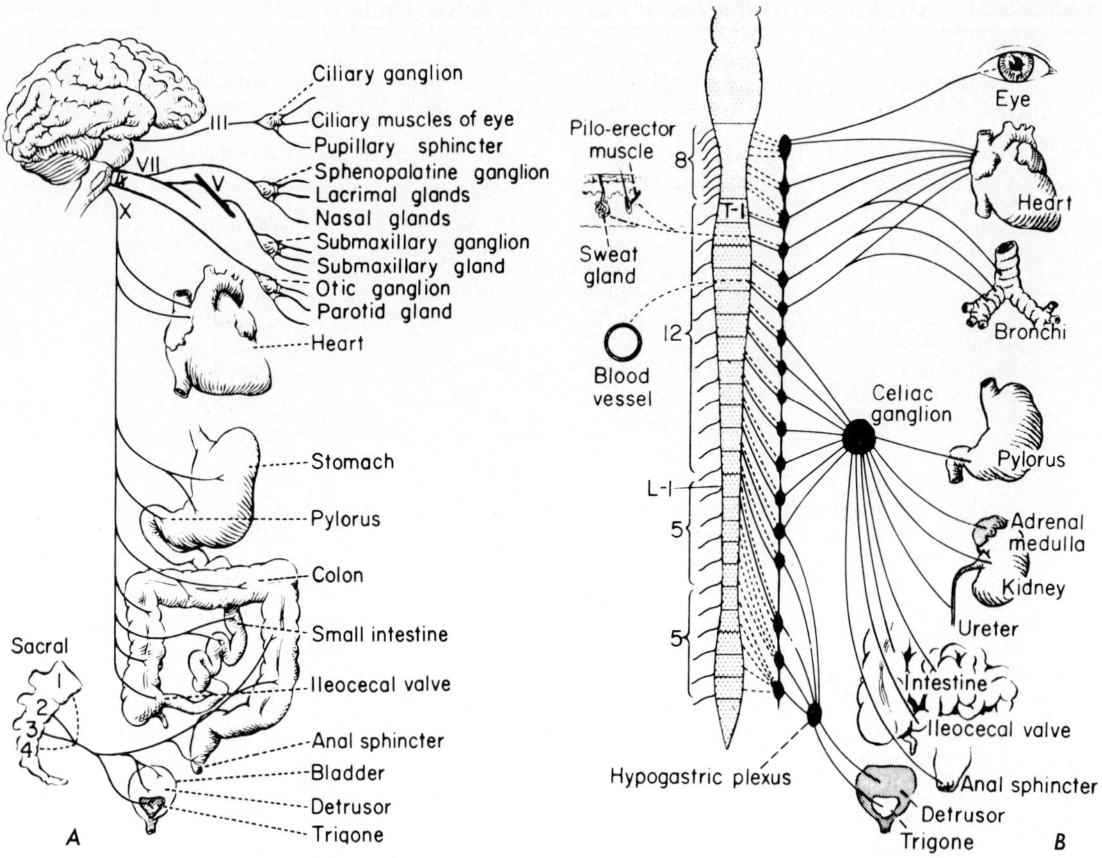

Figure 4–8. *A*, Parasympathetic nervous system. *B*, Sympathetic nervous system. (From Guyton, A.C.: *Textbook of Medical Physiology.* 6th ed. W.B. Saunders Co., Philadelphia, 1981.)

ings; 2) all postganglionic parasympathetic endings; 3) all motor nerve endings to skeletal muscle (somatic); 4) some central nervous system neurons; and 5) some postganglionic sympathetic fibers (sweat glands).

Norepinephrine (noradrenalin) is the effector at most postganglionic sympathetic endings. Small amounts of epinephrine may also be released here.

Many neurohumoral transmitters are active in the central nervous system. These include acetylcholine, norepinephrine, 5-hydroxytryptamine (5-HT or serotonin), γ-amino butyric acid (GABA), and others (see Table 4–2).

Synaptic and Parasympathetic Transmission

When a nerve impulse reaches the synapse, acetylcholine is released. It almost instantly crosses the synaptic cleft and unites with receptors on the postjunctional membrane causing a local increase in ionic permeability of the membrane (Fig. 4–13). Two types of permeability change may occur: 1) a generalized increase in permeability to all ions producing a depolarized membrane and an excitatory postsynaptic potential (EPSP), and 2) a selective increase in permeability only to small ions (K^+, Cl^-), resulting in stabilization of the membrane and an inhibitory postsynaptic potential (IPSP).

If an EPSP exceeds the threshold level, it initiates a nerve action potential (NAP) in a postsynaptic neuron or a muscle action potential (MAP) in skeletal or cardiac muscle. In smooth muscle, propagated impulses do not occur and a local contractile response is initiated; in glands, secretion results. An IPSP tends to op-

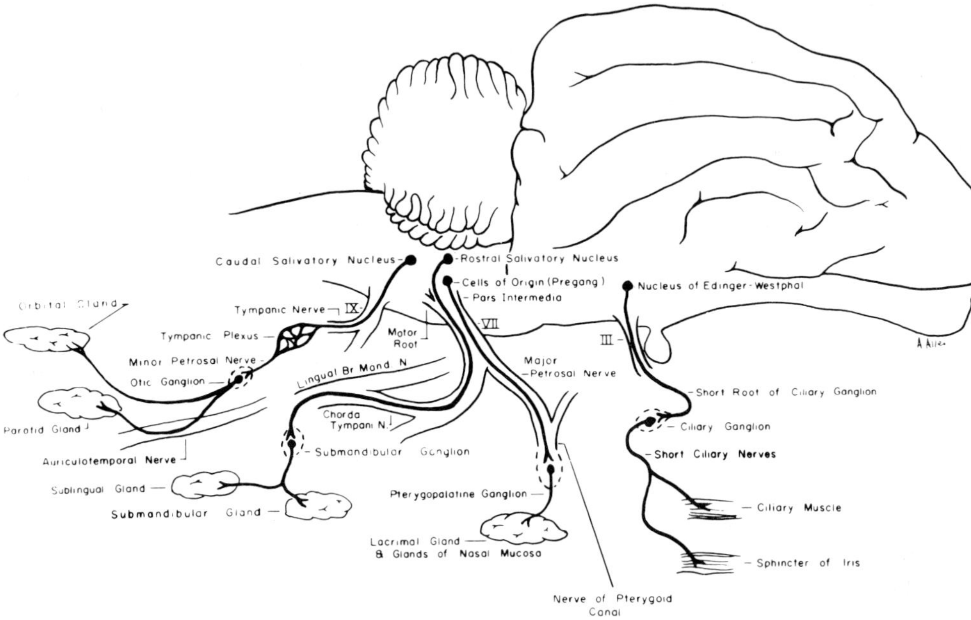

Figure 4–9. Routes of distribution of preganglionic and postganglionic parasympathetic fibers in the head region. (From Evans, H.E. and Christensen, G.C.: *Miller's Anatomy of the Dog*. W.B. Saunders Co., Philadelphia, 1979.)

pose an EPSP and the ultimate result is the algebraic sum of the reactions. Impulses can be transmitted across junctions at frequencies up to several hundred per second.

Nicoll and Iwamoto (1978) demonstrated that ganglionic transmission was approximately 20 times more sensitive to pentobarbital than was axonal conduction. The fast excitatory postsynaptic potential (EPSP) was approximately 10 times more sensitive to pentobarbital than were the slow potentials (slow EPSP and slow IPSP). Halothane, ether, chloral hydrate, chloralose, and phenobarbital also exerted some degree of selectivity toward the fast EPSP. Ethanol and urethan reduced all potentials indiscriminately.

Two cholinesterases are present in the body and are capable of hydrolyzing acetylcholine. Acetylcholine esterase (AChE), true, specific, "e"-type ChE, is found principally in neurons and at neuromuscular junctions, but also in erythrocytes, thrombocytes, and the placenta. It is responsible for terminating the action of acetylcholine by hydrolysis to acetic acid and choline. Practically all pharmacologic actions of anti-ChE agents are due to inhibition of AChE.

Butyrocholinesterase (BuChE, nonspecific, pseudo, plasma, or "s"-type ChE) occurs in glial cells of nervous tissue, in liver, plasma, and other organs. Its specific physiologic function is unknown, but it can hydrolyze ACh. Inhibition by drugs, however, produces no functional derangement.

Adrenergic Neurons

The catecholamines (dopamine, norepinephrine, and epinephrine) all function as neurotransmitters. They are synthesized by a series of enzymes (Fig. 4–14). The first step in the pathway is conversion of the amino acid tyrosine to L-DOPA. This reaction is followed by conversion of L-DOPA to dopamine, which is subsequently converted to norepinephrine (noradrenalin). In specific nuclei of the central nervous system and in the adrenal medulla, norepinephrine is further converted to form epinephrine (adrenalin). The catecholamines are taken up and stored within vesicles in sympathetic nerves and in the adrenal medulla (Fig. 4–15). They are released in response to nerve stimulation by a process of exocytosis, during

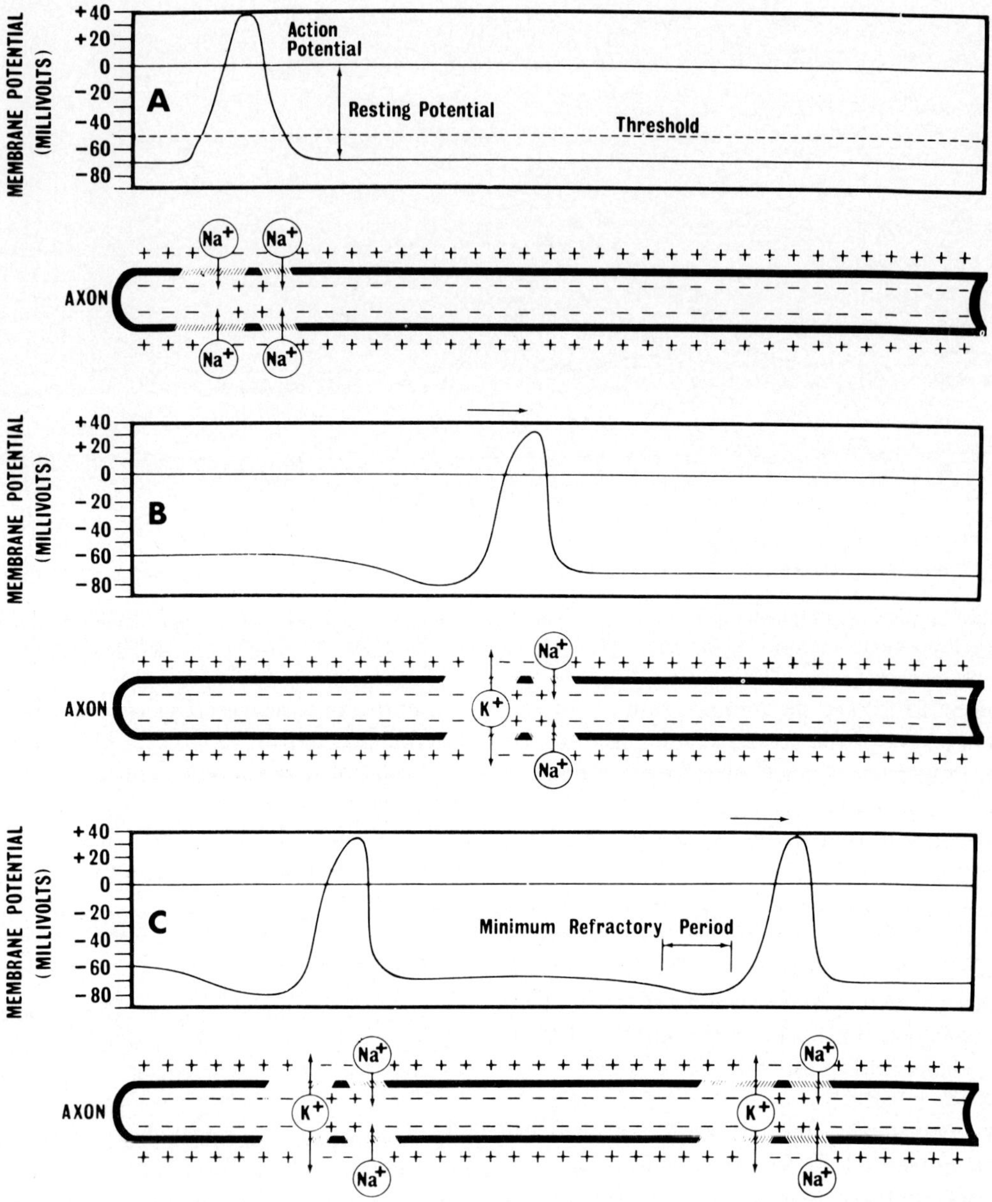

Figure 4–10. Schematic representation of nerve impulse. *A*, Depolarizing electrotonic effects result in sodium ions entering the axon. The resting potential is gradually altered until threshold is reached. At this time sodium ions enter the axon in great numbers, resulting in an action potential. *B* and *C*, Propagation of the nerve impulse is illustrated. Sodium ions enter the axon in advance of the nerve impulse, and potassium ions flow out after the impulse has passed. The outflow of potassium ions results in a brief refractory period. (Modified from Katz, 1961. From Miller, M.E., Christensen, G.C., and Evans, H.E.: *Anatomy of the Dog*. W.B. Saunders Co., Philadelphia, 1964.)

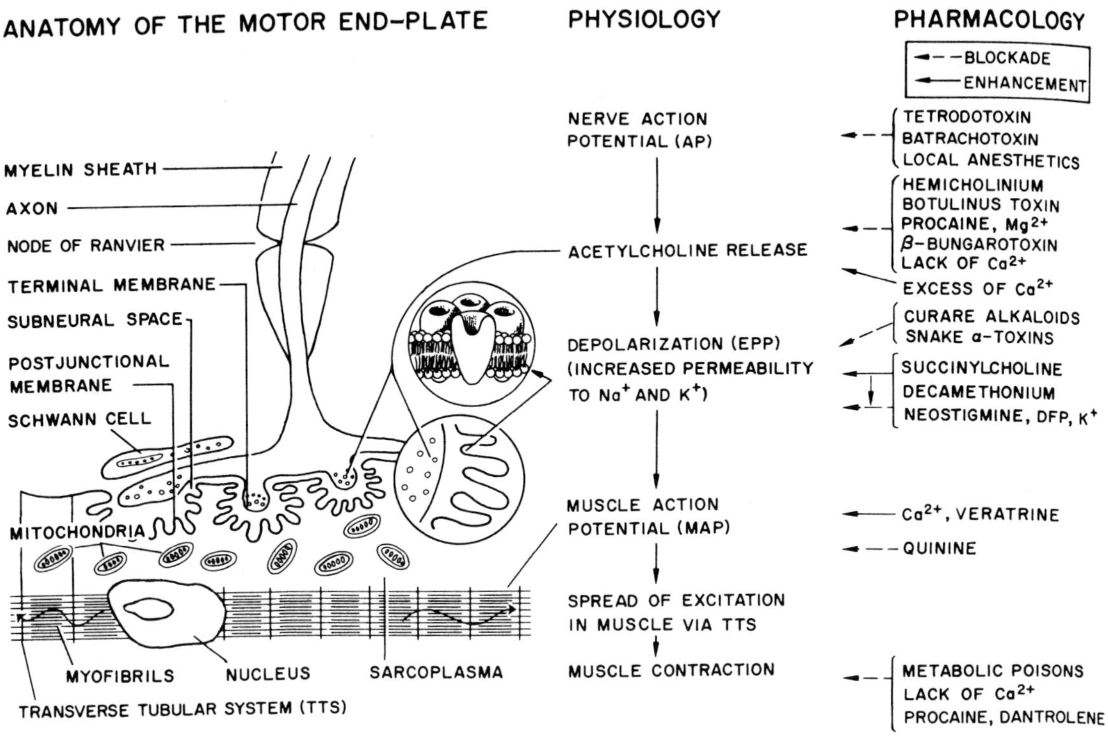

Figure 4–11. The anatomy of the motor end-plate and the sequence of events from the nerve action potential to the contraction of a muscle fiber. (From Gilman, A.G., Goodman, L.S. and Gilman, A. (Eds.): *The Pharmacological Basis of Therapeutics*, 6th ed. The Macmillan Co., New York, 1980.)

which the vesicle opens to the exterior of the cell and discharges its contents into the synaptic cleft. They cross the cleft and unite with adrenoreceptors on the effector cell to produce the appropriate response. The neurotransmitter actions of catecholamines are terminated principally by a process termed "uptake 1" (Fig. 4–16). A second uptake into non-neural cells has been designated "uptake 2." Neither of these processes is the same as the vesicular amine uptake that occurs within the neuron.

Generally, enzymatic degradation of catecholamines is not as important as neural membrane uptake in termination of neurotransmitter activity, although in some tissues metabolism of amines does play an important role. The two most important metabolic enzymes are catechol-O-methyltransferase (COMT) and monoamine oxidase (MAO). MAO is associated with mitochondria, whereas COMT is primarily a cytoplasmic enzyme.

Ahlquist (1948) first proposed that catecholamines produced their effects by interaction with cell surface receptors, which he termed alpha or beta adrenoceptors. He classified receptors on the basis of their ability to combine with the chemical structure of a series of adrenergic agonists. He further pointed out that neither the tissue site of the receptors nor the physiologic response (excitation or inhibition) was related to this recognition function. Thus, a drug may have entirely different actions from tissue to tissue, depending upon the type of receptor, and the biochemical change that occurs on binding of the receptor.

Ahliquist's original classification was expanded by Lands et al. (1967) who proposed that beta receptors could be subdivided into β_1 and β_2. β_1 receptors are found in the heart and control contractility and rate; in adipose tissue they control lipolysis. β_2 receptors mediate relaxation in smooth muscle, control lipolysis in

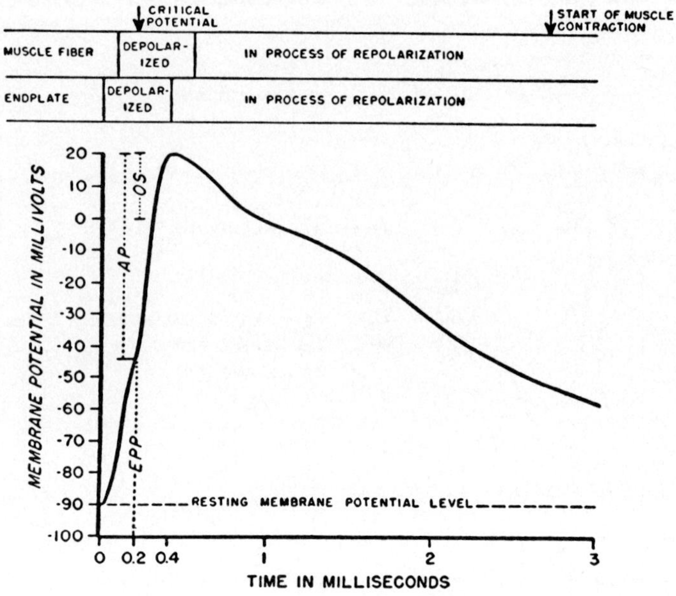

Figure 4–12. EPP, end-plate potential; AP, action potential; OS, overshoot. Owing to the release of acetylcholine by the nerve impulse at the end-plate at zero time, the end-plate potential is generated and in about 0.2 milliseconds the resting membrane potential of the end-plate (−90 millivolt decreases to −45 millivolts). When this critical level is reached, the potential change, from here on termed action potential, becomes propagated, within another 0.2 milliseconds overshoots and becomes electropositive (+15–20 millivolts). Within the next 2 to 3 milliseconds, the end-plate becomes repolarized and when the polarization process is almost complete, the contraction of the muscle fiber starts. (From Adriani, J.: *The Chemistry and Physics of Anesthesia,* 2nd ed. Charles C Thomas, Springfield, Illinois, 1962.)

skeletal muscle, and control glycolysis in the liver. At first it was believed that individual tissues contained only one of the β receptor subtypes. However, pharmacologic studies by Carlsson et al. (1972) demonstrated a mixture of β_1 and β_2 receptors in kitten, but not in rat hearts. Barnett et al. (1978) found a mixture of 25% β_1 and 75% β_2 receptors in rat lung, but in rat heart only β_1 receptors were found.

β_1 and β_2 receptors may be distinguished by their reactions with epinephrine and norepinephrine (Table 4–5). The action of catecholamines on cardiac β_1 adrenoceptors produces positive inotropic and chronotropic results. Vascular smooth muscle in some blood vessels and bronchial smooth muscle have β_2 receptors that produce vasodilatation or bronchodilation (Table 4–6).

Berthelsen and Pittinger (1977) demonstrated α_1 and α_2 receptors. Stimulation of α receptors located on the nerve terminal itself (presynaptic receptors) results in decreased exocytotic release of norepinephrine by the nerve (Fig. 4–17). The order of potencies for alpha adrenergic agonists and antagonists for presynaptic receptors is different from that for classic postsynaptic receptors. For this reason, receptors with pharmacologic properties of the postsynaptic receptor have been termed α_1, whereas those with properties of the presynaptic receptor have been designated α_2. There is evidence that α_2 receptors are also located postsynaptically in some vascular beds and in the brain. Thus, the classification is functional rather than anatomic.

Stimulation of a presynaptic β receptor increases exocytotic release of norepinephrine. It appears that the vascular presynaptic receptor may be β_2 in type, and thus more sensitive to circulating epinephrine than to norepinephrine released from nerves.

It is apparent that the adrenoreceptors play a large role in homeostasis throughout the sympathetic and central nervous systems.

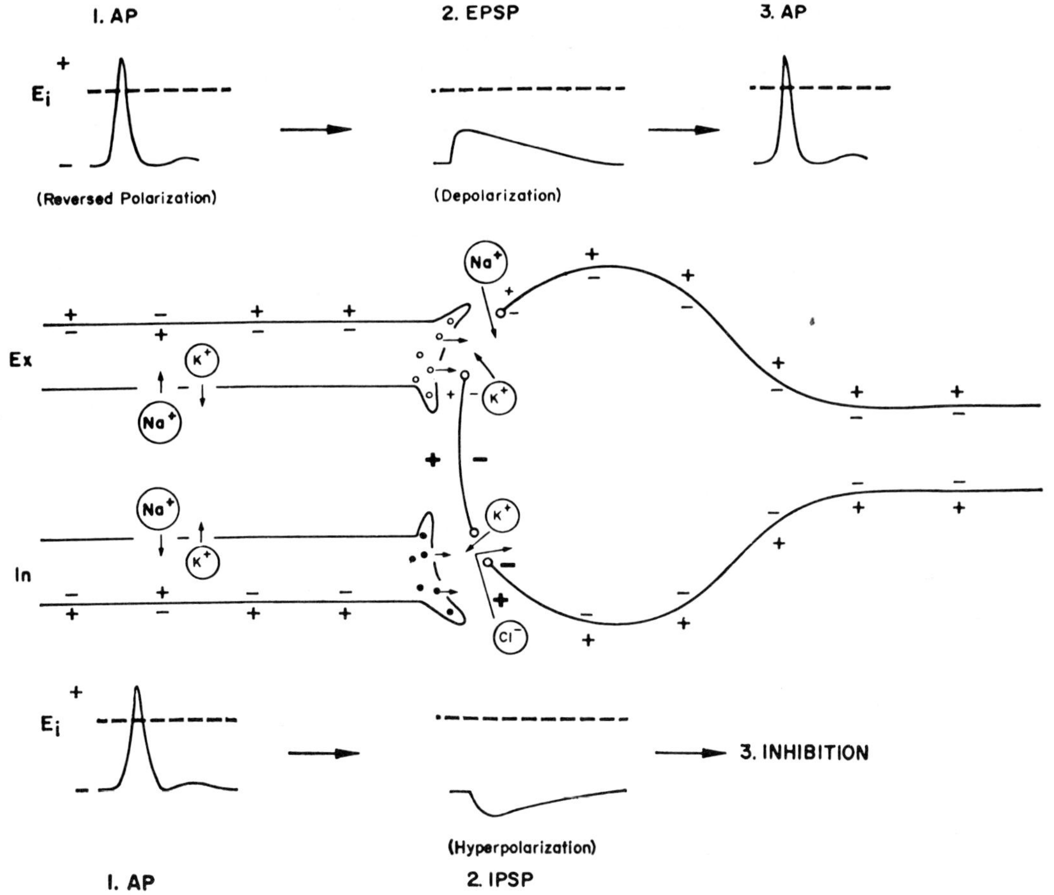

Figure 4–13. Steps involved in excitatory (Ex) and inhibitory (In) neurohumoral transmission. (1) The nerve action potential (NAP), consisting in a self-propagated *reversal* of negativity (the internal potential, E_i, goes from a negative value, through 0 potential, indicated by the broken line, to a positive value) of the axonal membrane, arrives at the presynaptic terminal and causes release of the excitatory (o) or inhibitory (•) transmitter. (2) Combination of the excitatory transmitter with postsynaptic receptors produces a localized depolarization, the excitatory postsynaptic potential (EPSP), through an increase in permeability to all ions (Na^+ and K^+ chiefly involved). The inhibitory transmitter causes a selective increase in permeability to the smaller ions (K^+ and Cl^- chiefly involved), resulting in a localized hyperpolarization, the inhibitory postsynaptic potential (IPSP). (3) The EPSP initiates a conducted NAP in the postsynaptic neuron; this can, however, be prevented by the hyperpolarization induced by a concurrent IPSP. The transmitter is dissipated by enzymatic destruction or by diffusion. (From Gilman, A.G., Goodman, L.S., and Gilman, A. (Eds.): *The Pharmacological Basis of Therapeutics,* 6th ed. The Macmillan Co., New York, 1980.)

PAIN RECEPTION

Relief of pain is the most compelling reason for anesthesia. Despite intensive research, the mechanism of pain is poorly understood and the term itself is not well defined. Discovery of opiate receptors, endorphins, and an increasing array of neuroregulators has broadened our knowledge of pain mechanisms.

Pain receptors are found throughout the body. Clinically, however, it is useful to classify pain into the following categories:

Superficial or cutaneous pain } Somatic pain
Deep pain (muscles, fascia, ligaments, joints, bones) } Somatic pain
Visceral pain
Referred pain
Psychogenic pain

Pain receptors in the tissues react to several stimuli. Whether pain is caused by direct receptor stimulation or release of a substance from the surrounding damaged tissue is unknown.

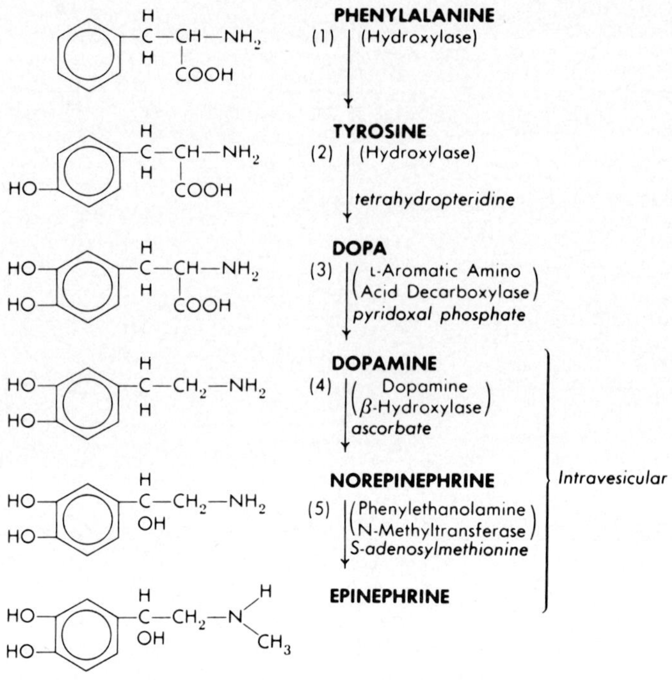

Figure 4–14. Steps in enzymatic synthesis of norepinephrine and epinephrine. (After Holtz et al., 1938; Blaschko, 1939; Gurin and Delluva, 1947; Levin et al., 1960.) (From Goodman, L.S., and Gilman, A.: *The Pharmacological Basis of Therapeutics*, 4th ed. The Macmillan Company, New York, 1970.)

Agents causing pain on injection include histamine, acetylcholine, angiotonin, serotonin, bradykinin, adenosine triphosphate, prostaglandins, endoperoxides, thromboxanes, substance P, and H^+ and K^+ ions, along with other less well-defined substances.

Impulses from painful stimuli travel centrally over both myelinated and nonmyelinated nerve fibers. In the epidermis and superficial dermis, pain impulses are conducted over A-delta and C fibers. Conduction is more rapid in the former (30 versus 1 meter/second), so that some impulses produced by a single stimulus reach the cerebral cortex more rapidly than others. The time interval in man may be so marked that a second or delayed pain may result (Table 4–7).

The cell bodies of nerves carrying pain impulses are in the dorsal root ganglia. The axons enter the spinal cord and branch diffusely, establishing reflex connections with motor neurons to skeletal muscle, and also synapsing in the dorsal horn. There are two classes of dorsal horn neurons: high-threshold and wide-dynamic range (Willis, 1980). High-threshold neurons do not respond to stimuli that activate mechanoreceptors, but do respond to stimuli activating nociceptors. In contrast, wide-dynamic-range cells are excited by mechanoreceptors as well as nociceptors, although they fire at highest rates when nociceptors are stimulated. These two types of neurons are in different locations within the spinal cord, and their receptive fields differ. High-threshold neurons are concentrated primarily in the marginal zone and adjacent substantia gelatinosa of the dorsal horn and have relatively circumscribed receptive fields.

Wide-dynamic-range neurons tend to be concentrated in the deeper layers of the dorsal horn. The receptive fields of these cells are generally larger than those of the other type of neuron and typically have a central sensitive zone surrounded by a less sensitive peripheral zone. Furthermore, they often receive a convergent input from deep or visceral receptors.

Wide-dynamic-range cells can signal pain intensity but are not likely to give good spatial

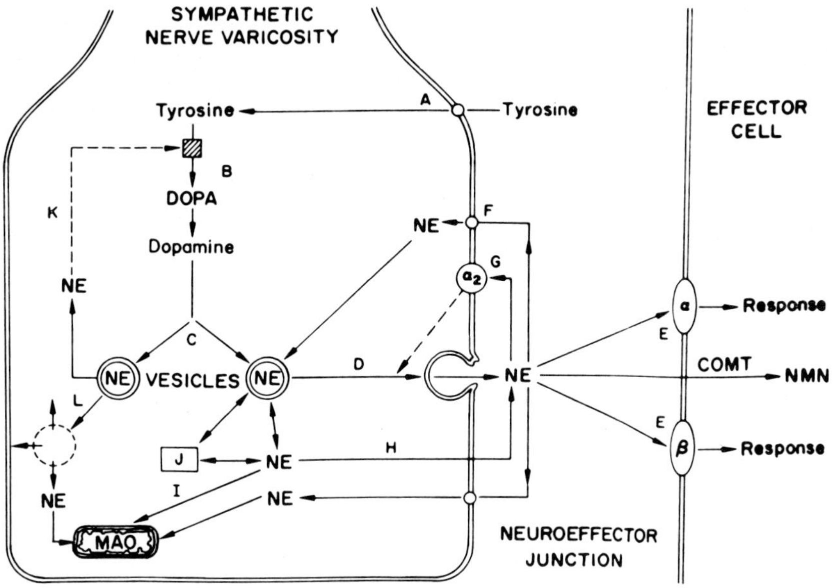

Figure 4–15. Proposed sites of action of drugs on the synthesis, action, and fate of norepinephrine at sympathetic neuroeffector junctions. The events proposed to occur in this model of a sympathetic neuroeffector junction are as follows. Tyrosine is transported actively into the axoplasm (A) and is converted to dopa and then to dopamine by cytoplasmic enzymes (B). Dopamine is transported into the vesicles of the varicosity, where the synthesis and the storage of norepinephrine (NE) take place (C). An action potential causes an influx of Ca^{2+} into the nerve terminal (not shown), with subsequent fusion of the vesicle with the plasma membrane and exocytosis of NE (D). The transmitter then activates α and β receptors in the membrane of the postsynaptic cell (E). NE that penetrates into these cells is probably rapidly inactivated by catechol-O-methyltransferase (COMT) to normetanephrine (NMN). The most important mechanism for termination of the action of NE in the junctional space is by active reuptake into the nerve and the storage vesicles. (F). Norepinephrine in the synaptic cleft can also activate presynaptic (α_2) receptors (G), the result of which is to inhibit further exocytotic release of norepinephrine (dashed line).

NE can also be displaced from storage vesicles by sympathomimetic amines such as tyramine, which gain access to the nerve terminal by active uptake as in F. A portion of this NE diffuses out of the nerve (H) to react with receptors. Another portion of the NE released in this manner, or by spontaneous diffusion, is deaminated by mitochondrial monoamine oxidase (MAO) (I). Observations that only a fraction of the total NE content is available for release by either nerve stimulation or tyramine indicate that pools of the transmitter are held in reserve (J).

The most important mechanism of regulation of NE synthesis involves the rate-limiting step, the hydroxylation of tyrosine. This regulation is complex but in part involves feedback inhibition by NE (K).

Sites of drug action in this scheme include: *(1)* Inhibition of MAO (e.g., by pargyline) or COMT (no pharmacologically significant example of inhibitor). *(2)* Inhibition of plasma membrane uptake mechanism for NE (F) by tricyclic antidepressants or cocaine, making more NE available for binding to receptors. *(3)* Inhibition of vesicular storage of NE by reserpine and, in part, by guanethidine (L). The NE thereby released is normally inactivated by MAO. Guanethidine and bretylium also block coupling of the action potential to the release of NE. *(4)* Displacement of NE by indirectly acting sympathomimetic amines (H). Exocytosis of vesicular contents does not occur. *(5)* Direct interaction with adrenergic receptors by agonists and antagonists (E, G).

Anatomical elements are not drawn to scale. Mitochondria are about 0.25 μm in diameter and 0.75 μm long; vesicles, 0.05 μm; a nerve varicosity, 2 to 10 μm; the junctional space, 0.1 μm. (From Gilman, A.G., Goodman, L.S., and Gilman, A. (Eds.): *The Pharmacological Basis of Therapeutics,* 6th ed. The Macmillan Co., New York, 1980.)

resolution of stimuli. On the other hand, they are well suited to explain the phenomenon of referred pain and pain radiation. High-threshold spinothalamic cells appear to signal stimulus location as well as intensity.

Afferent nociceptive neurons in the dorsal root release SP at their spinal terminals. These nociceptive inputs to the spinal cord activate tract cells that convey information to the thalamus and cerebral cortex in order to evoke the sensation of pain. In primates, including man, the spinothalamic tract is the main pathway responsible for transmission, with the neospinothalamic tract also participating. In

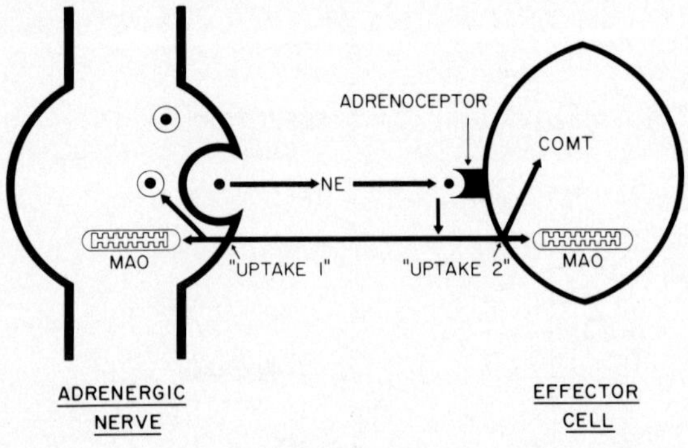

Figure 4–16. Release and fate of norepinephrine. Release of norepinephrine (NE) from an adrenergic nerve and its subsequent interaction with the adrenoceptor, uptake into the nerve terminal, uptake into other tissues, and metabolism are shown. MAO = monoamine oxidase; COMT = catechol-O-methyltransferase. (From Weinshilboum, R.M.: Antihypertensive Drugs that Alter Adrenergic Function. Mayo Clin. Proc., 55:390, 1980.)

other species, the spinocervical, spinoreticular, and spinotectal tracts may also carry afferent nociceptive signals.

Several spinal afferent systems thus participate in transmitting pain signals, but none is essential to it (King, 1979). The systems act in a nonspecific fashion carrying a variety of signals that are tactile, proprioceptive, or noxious. These systems interact with each other setting a bias that controls the final perception of a noxious stimulus. Present evidence indicates that exogenous opiates activate an efferent brain stem system that suppresses pain transmission at spinal levels. In contrast, the endogenous analgesia system appears to involve endorphin release at both brain stem and spinal levels. Serotonin (5HT) depletion prevents stimulation-produced analgesia and also opiate analgesia.

Nucleus raphe magnus (NRM) axons descend in the dorsolateral funiculus and terminate on dorsal horn neurons in lamina I (marginal layer) and deeper in the region of lamina V (Fig. 4–18). These neurons respond to noxious inputs and are strongly inhibited by NRM stimulation. Midbrain inputs to the NRM have been shown to come, in part, from the periaqueductal gray (PAG) and also from the gigantocellular reticular formation, which in the cat is a major receiving area for ascending pain transmission pathways. It is probable that the 5HT-containing terminals of the NRM synapse on enkephalin-containing interneurons of the dorsal horn, which in turn inhibit spinal neurons mediating pain sensations.

A major part of the PAG-induced analgesia appears to be mediated by a dorsolateral funiculus pathway that bypasses the NRM. A possible descending pathway is the ventromedial reticular formation of the medulla, which is a nonserotonergic cell group adjacent to the NRM. Thus, at least two pathways appear capable of producing analgesia. One, originating in the NRM, is serotonergic and has an enkephalin link. The other is neither serotonergic nor mediated by enkephalin. Its action is resistant to both naloxone and serotonin antagonists. When these pathways are activated in parallel by PAG stimulation, naloxone only partially reverses the analgesia resulting from stimulation of PAG.

Based on this information, Basbaum and Fields (1978) proposed the following hypothesis. A noxious stimulus activates pain transmission neurons (e.g., spinothalamic tract neurons in man). When the activity of these neurons reaches the appropriate level (pain threshold), pain is perceived. Activation of the transmission neurons turns on the pain-suppression system. The latter contains parallel modulating tracts, one naloxone-sensitive (presumably endorphin-mediated) and the other naloxone-insensitive. The pain suppression system thus feeds back and controls spinal and trigeminal nerve pain-transmission neurons. Enhancement of the descending portion of this loop, as occurs on administration of opiates or stimulation-produced analgesia, further reduces the intensity of pain perceived. Disruption of the loop by opiate

TABLE 4–5. Relative Potencies of Selected Agonists on α and β Adrenoceptors

Agonist	*α*	*β_1*	*β_2*
Isoproterenol	−	+	+
Epinephrine	+	+	+
Norepinephrine	+	+	−

(From Weinshilboum, R.M.: Antihypertensive Drugs that Alter Adrenergic Function. Mayo Clin. Proc., 55:390, 1980.)

TABLE 4–6. Responses of Effector Organs to Autonomic Nerve Impulses

Effector Organs	*Adrenergic Impulses*[1]		*Cholinergic Impulses*[1]
	Receptor Type	*Responses*[2]	*Responses*[2]
Eye			
Radial muscle, iris	α	Contraction (mydriasis) + +	———
Sphincter muscle, iris		———	Contraction (miosis) + + +
Ciliary muscle	β	Relaxation for far vision +	Contraction for near vision + + +
Heart			
S-A node	β_1	Increase in heart rate + +	Decrease in heart rate; vagal arrest + + +
Atria	β_1	Increase in contractility and conduction velocity + +	Decrease in contractility, and (usually) increase in conduction velocity + +
A-V node	β_1	Increase in automaticity and conduction velocity + +	Decrease in conduction velocity; A-V block + + +
His-Purkinje system	β_1	Increase in automaticity and conduction velocity + + +	Little effect
Ventricles	β_1	Increase in contractility, conduction velocity, automaticity, and rate of idioventricular pacemakers + + +	Slight decrease in contractility claimed by some
Arterioles			
Coronary	α,β_2	Constriction +; dilatation[3] + +	Dilatation ±
Skin and mucosa	α	Constriction + + +	Dilatation[4]
Skeletal muscle	α,β_2	Constriction + +; dilatation[3,5] + +	Dilatation[6] +
Cerebral	α	Constriction (slight)	Dilatation[4]
Pulmonary	α,β_2	Constriction +; dilatation[3]	Dilatation[4]
Abdominal viscera; renal	α,β_2	Constriction + + +; dilatation[5] +	———
Salivary glands	α	Constriction + + +	Dilatation + +
Veins (Systemic)	α,β_2	Constriction + +; dilatation + +	———
Lung			
Bronchial muscle	β_2	Relaxation +	Contraction + +
Bronchial glands	?	Inhibition (?)	Stimulation + + +
Stomach			
Motility and tone	α_2,β_2	Decrease (usually)[7] +	Increase + + +
Sphincters	α	Contraction (usually) +	Relaxation (usually) +
Secretion		Inhibition (?)	Stimulation + + +
Intestine			
Motility and tone	α_2,β_2	Decrease[7] +	Increase + + +
Sphincters	α	Contraction (usually) +	Relaxation (usually) +
Secretion		Inhibition (?)	Stimulation + +
Gallbladder and Ducts		Relaxation +	Contraction +
Kidney	β_2	Renin secretion + +	———
Urinary Bladder			
Detrusor	β	Relaxation (usually) +	Contraction + + +
Trigone and sphincter	α	Contraction + +	Relaxation + +
Ureter			
Motility and tone	α	Increase (usually)	Increase (?)
Uterus	α,β_2	Pregnant: contraction (α); nonpregnant: relaxation (β)	Variable[8]
Sex Organs, Male	α	Ejaculation + + +	Erection + + +
Skin			
Pilomotor muscles	α	Contraction + +	———
Sweat glands	α	Localized secretion[9] +	Generalized secretion + + +
Spleen Capsule	α,β_2	Contraction + + +; relaxation +	———
Adrenal Medulla		———	Secretion of epinephrine and norepinephrine
Liver	α,β_2	Glycogenolysis, gluconeogenesis[10] + + +	Glycogen synthesis +

TABLE 4–6. *Continued*

Effector Organs	*Adrenergic Impulses*[1]		*Cholinergic Impulses*[1]
	Receptor Type	*Responses*[2]	*Responses*[2]
Pancreas			
Acini	α	Decreased secretion +	Secretion + +
Islets (β cells)	α	Decreased secretion + + +	——
	β_2	Increased secretion +	——
Fat Cells	α,β_1	Lipolysis[10] + + +	——
Salivary Glands	α	Potassium and water secretion +	Potassium and water secretion + + +
	β	Amylase secretion +	
Lacrimal Glands		——	Secretion + + +
Nasopharyngeal Glands		——	Secretion + +
Pineal Gland	β	Melatonin synthesis	——

[1]A long dash signifies no known functional innervation.

[2]Responses are designated 1 + to 3 + to provide an approximate indication of the importance of adrenergic and cholinergic nerve activity in the control of the various organs and functions listed.

[3]Dilatation predominates *in situ* owing to metabolic autoregulatory phenomena.

[4]Cholinergic vasodilatation at these sites is of questionable physiologic significance.

[5]Over the usual concentration range of physiologically released, circulating epinephrine, β-receptor response (vasodilatation) predominates in blood vessels of skeletal muscle and liver; α-receptor response (vasoconstriction), in blood vessels of other abdominal viscera. The renal and mesenteric vessels also contain specific dopaminergic receptors, activation of which causes dilatation, but their physiologic significance has not been established.

[6]Sympathetic cholinergic system causes vasodilatation in skeletal muscle, but this is not involved in most physiological responses.

[7]It has been proposed that adrenergic fibers terminate at inhibitory β receptors on smooth muscle fibers, and at inhibitory α receptors on parasympathetic cholinergic (excitatory) ganglion cells of Auerbach's plexus.

[8]Depends on stage of menstrual cycle, amount of circulating estrogen and progesterone, and other factors.

[9]Palms of hands and some other sites ("adrenergic sweating").

[10]There is significant variation among species in the type of receptor that mediates certain metabolic responses.

(From Gilman, A.G., Goodman, L.S., and Gilman, A. (Eds.): *The Pharmacological Basis of Therapeutics*, 6th ed. The Macmillan Co., New York, 1980.)

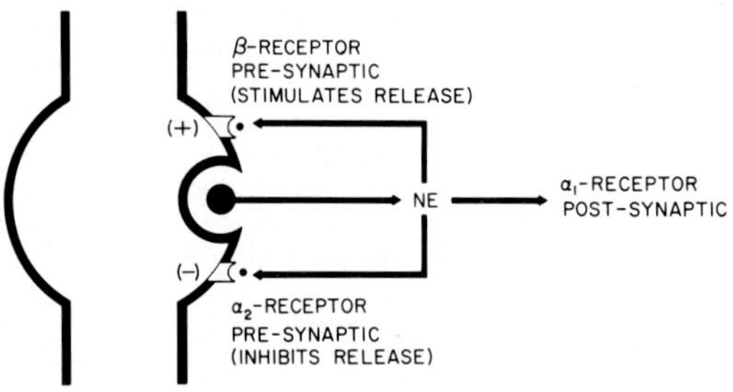

Figure 4–17. Presynaptic regulation of nonrepinephrine release by adrenoceptors. Regulation of release of norepinephrine from an adrenergic nerve terminal by presynaptic α and β adrenoceptors is shown. (From Weinshilboum, R.M.: Antihypertensive Drugs that Alter Adrenergic Function. Mayo Clin. Proc., 55:390, 1980.)

or 5HT antagonists increases the perceived intensity of the noxious stimulus.

This theory differs from that of Melzak and Wall (1965), which states that non-noxious inputs transmitted by large-diameter fibers activate the central control trigger. In contrast, Basbaum and Fields believe that negative feedback is due to noxious rather than innoxious stimuli and that these are critical for activation of descending modulation.

In animals, the fiber systems subserving pain perception are more diffuse than in man and are not as easily destroyed. Therefore, one should not assume that animals are not perceiving pain because man, in a similar situation, does not (Breazile and Kitchell, 1969).

Muscle relaxants such as curare may prevent movement when a noxious stimulus is applied, despite the fact that the animal has complete perception of the stimulus. Local anesthetics, on the other hand, block conduction in the peripheral nerves, preventing pain perception when a noxious stimulus is applied to the area supplied by these nerves.

Lewis et al. (1982) demonstrated that different patterns of foot shock in rats will activate opioid or nonopioid analgesia. They have also shown that release of adrenal medullary enkephalin-like peptides produces opioid (but not nonopioid) stress analgesia.

In lower animals, as in man, reaction to pain

TABLE 4–7. Classification of Nerve Fibers

		Terminology	*Fiber Diameter*	*Conduction Speed (meters/second)*
Myelinated somatic fibers	A	Alpha Beta Gamma Delta Epsilon	20μ ↓ (3–4μ) 2μ	120 ↓ (6–30)→pain fibers 5
Myelinated visceral fibers (preganglionic autonomic)	B		<3μ	3–15
Nonmyelinated somatic fibers	C		<2μ	0.5–2→pain fibers

(From Wylie, W.D., and Churchill-Davidson, H.C.: *A Practice of Anaesthesia.* Lloyd-Luke, Ltd., London, 1966, and Gasser, H.S.: Pain Producing Impulses in Peripheral Nerves. Assoc. Res. Nerv. Dis. Proc., 23:44, 1943.)

depends upon individual experience. Thompson and Melzack (1956) divided litters of Scottish terriers into two groups. One group led a normal life, while the other group was totally isolated from human or animal contacts. At 7 to 10 months of age, both groups of dogs were exposed to various stimuli, including painful ones. The normal dogs responded to pinpricks, electric shocks, and flame by quickly running to avoid the painful object, but retaining their composure. The isolated dogs, however, took much longer to learn to avoid the stimuli, and became disorganized and excited when the stimulating objects were in view. This indicates that pain avoidance is not an instinct, but is acquired in infancy.

THEORIES OF ANESTHESIA

Despite intensive studies for many years, the exact mechanism of anesthesia at the cellular or subcellular level has not been definitely established. Theories of anesthesia at the molecular and subcellular levels have been discussed by Kaufman (1977), Roth (1979), and Koblin and Eger (1979). They can generally be grouped as follows: 1) lipid theories; 2) aqueous-phase theories; 3) critical-volume theory; 4) protein conformational change theory; 5) microtubule theory; and 6) coacervate theory.

Anesthetic agents differ greatly in structure since they include hydrocarbons, alcohols, ethers, urethanes, sulfones, amides, steroids, and rare gases. It is impossible, except in a homologous series of substances, to show any relationship between anesthetic action and chemical constitution; therefore, many of the theories of narcosis have been based on physical properties of the anesthetics.

Because general anesthesia is produced by a wide range of compounds with no common chemical structure or activity, it must be a physical phenomenon working solely by forces acting between molecules. These electrostatic intermolecular forces (Van der Waals forces) are much weaker than the intermolecular chemical bonds between atoms and ions.

For many years it has been known that anesthetized animals can be awakened by an environment in which the pressure is increased. The physicochemical approach seeks correlations between anesthetic potency and physical properties of a series of anesthetics.

Meyer (1899) and Overton (1901) independently advanced what is now called the Meyer-Overton theory. It stated:

A. Anesthetic properties of substances are directly related to the partition coefficient of the substance in oil and water (Table 4–8). The higher the coefficient, the greater the anesthetic effect.

$$\text{Partition coefficient} = \frac{\text{solubility in oil}}{\text{solubility in water}}$$

B. All anesthetic substances must be both oil- and water-soluble.

C. Equivalent degrees of depression should be produced by equal molar concentrations (not equal amounts).

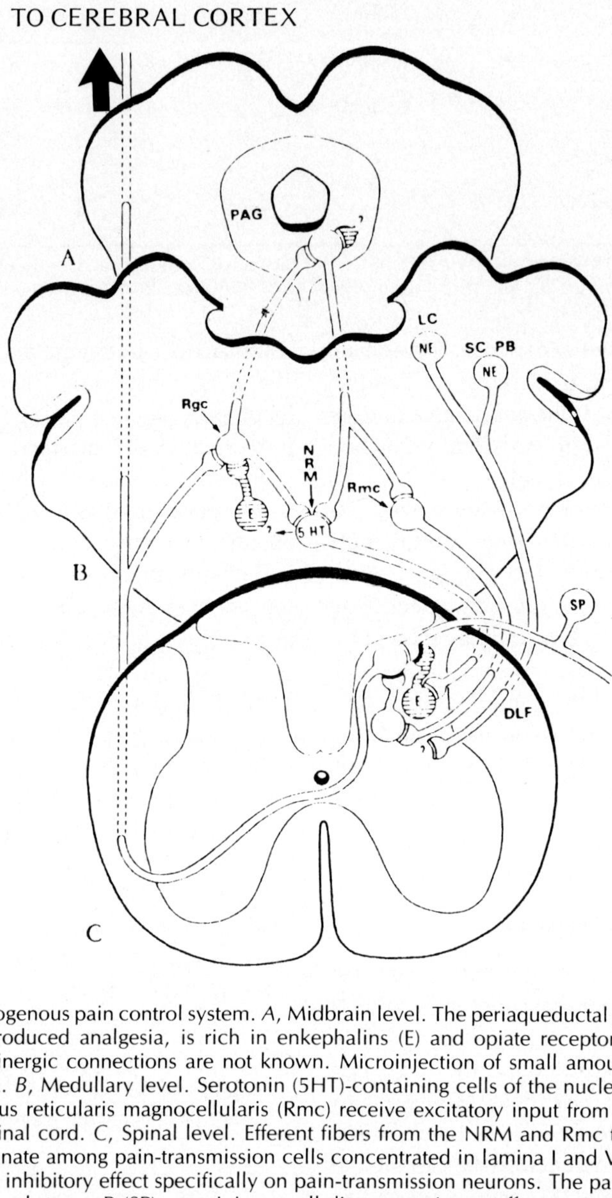

Figure 4–18. The endogenous pain control system. *A*, Midbrain level. The periaqueductal gray (PAG), an important locus for stimulation-produced analgesia, is rich in enkephalins (E) and opiate receptors, though the anatomic details of the enkephalinergic connections are not known. Microinjection of small amounts of opiates into PAG also produces analgesia. *B*, Medullary level. Serotonin (5HT)-containing cells of the nucleus raphe magnus (NRM) and the adjacent nucleus reticularis magnocellularis (Rmc) receive excitatory input from PAG and, in turn, send efferent fibers to the spinal cord. *C*, Spinal level. Efferent fibers from the NRM and Rmc travel in the dorsolateral funiculus (DLF) to terminate among pain-transmission cells concentrated in lamina I and V of the dorsal horn. The NRM and Rmc exert an inhibitory effect specifically on pain-transmission neurons. The pain-transmission neurons, which are activated by substance P (SP) containing small-diameter primary afferents, project to supraspinal sites and indirectly, via the nucleus reticularis gigantocellularis (Rgc), contact the cells of the descending analgesia system in the PAG and NRM, thus establishing a negative-feedback loop. Catecholamine-containing neurons of the locus ceruleus (LC) in the rat and subceruleus-parabrachialis (SC-PB) in the cat may also contribute to pain-modulating systems in the DLF. (NE = norepinephrine.) (From Basbaum, A.I., and Fields, H.L.: Endogenous Pain Control Mechanisms: Review and Hypothesis. Ann. Neurol., 4:451, 1978.)

TABLE 4–8. Narcotic Concentration, Partition Coefficient, and Molecular Concentration of Some Anesthetic Agents

Substance	*Narcotic Concentration in Volumes %*	*Oil/Water Partition Coefficient*	*Molecular Concentration in Lipoid*
Methane	370	0.54	0.08
Ethylene	80	1.3	0.04
Ether	5.8	31	0.07
Ethyl bromide	1.9	95	0.07
Chloroform	0.5	265	0.05

D. Depressants having a markedly changed partition coefficient with temperature changes should show corresponding changes in anesthetic potency at different temperatures. As an example, the partition coefficient of chloral hydrate decreases with cold. Tadpoles anesthetized in warm water awaken when cooled.

Objections to the Meyer-Overton theory are:

A. It is calculated with olive oil, which has no relationship to brain lipoids or plasma.

B. It does not apply to alkaloids or inorganic ions.

C. Many compounds with oil-water coefficient similar to powerful anesthetics possess no anesthetic power.

D. It is not a theory explaining narcosis but only a summary of factual observations.

Pauling (1961) and Miller (1961) independently proposed that the site of action of anesthetics lies in the aqueous phase of the CNS. Pauling proposed the formation of gas hydrates, which increased the impedance of the neural network or occluded pores in membranes. Hydrates also could impair the reactivity of enzymes by trapping protein polar groups. Miller theorized that anesthesia is caused by the ordering that simple solutes induce in nearby water molecules (''iceberg effect''). These ''icebergs'' were presumed to function in the same manner as Pauling's hydrates. Both theories suffer from lack of evidence.

Biophysical theories involve the site of anesthetic action and the site-anesthetic interaction. In 1954, Mullens proposed that anesthesia commences when a critical volume fraction of an inert substance is attained in membranes. He believed that anesthetics filled holes (free-volume) in membranes. Subsequent investigators have not supported free-volume theories, but the critical volume of anesthetic entering the membrane is thought to expand it rather than to fill holes (Fig. 4–19). Thus, sodium or potassium channels, acetylcholine receptors, or enzymes could be modified.

Allison and Nunn (1968) believed that general anesthesia results from reversible depolymerization of microtubules in nerve cells. The protein conformational change (PCC) theory proposes that anesthetics directly inactivate lipoproteins and that the site of anesthetic action is protein (Seeman, 1972).

In a spin-probe study of pressure, anesthetics, and membrane structure, Finch and Kiesow (1979) proposed that pressure and anesthetics alter the internal hydrophobic effects of cell membranes. They believed that anesthetics decrease membrane polarity by displacing water molecules in the membrane. This proposal differs from other hypotheses concerning the role of water in anesthetic effects on membrane structures, since it involves changes in membrane water penetration rather than water structure.

Ecanow et al. (1979) have stated that the cell membrane is a coacervate phase capable of undergoing subtle changes in structuring that correspond to different degrees of anesthesia. This allows the membrane to undergo a continuum of free energy changes from polar to nonpolar properties. The anesthetic state occupies one range on this continuum.

Today, the concept of anesthetic effect has changed from filling of free space to expansion and fluidization of the cell membrane. Evidence is clearly against the aqueous-phase theory of Pauling and Miller. The microtubule theory of

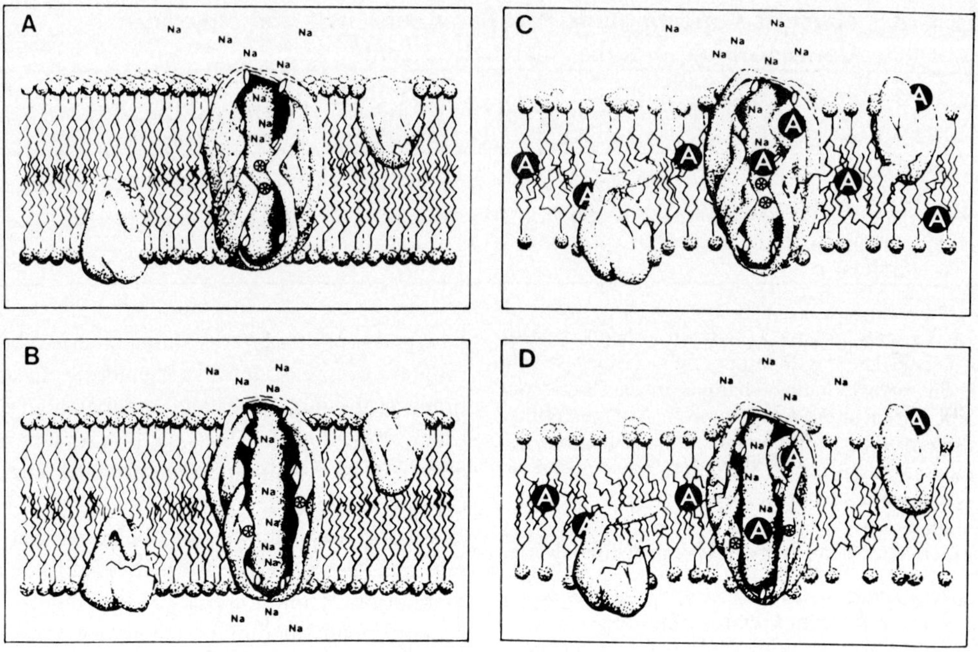

Figure 4–19. Anesthetic-membrane interactions: possible mechanisms of action. *A*, Membrane at rest. The membrane is composed of a phospholipid bilayer embedded with function protein (ionophore channel). The channel is "gated" by charged (⊗) or bulky constituents. *B*, A voltage-dependent conformational change of ionophore displaces the "gates," and creates an active (open) channel for ions (current) to flow. *C*, Anesthetic molecules bind to hydrophobic (and perhaps charged) sites within the membrane. Fluidization of bilayer and alteration of conformation of functional proteins result in an increase of membrane surface area (membrane expansion) with a decrease in membrane thickness. *D*, A sufficient voltage-dependent conformational change of ionophore to form an open channel cannot occur because of anesthetic-induced perturbation of bilayer and functional proteins. Anesthetic may also effectively block the channel. (From Roth S.H.: Physical Mechanisms of Anesthesia. Reproduced, with permission, from the Annual Review of Pharmacology and Toxicology, Volume 19. © 1979 by Annual Reviews, Inc.)

Allison and Nunn also has not accumulated supporting evidence.

Although the majority of investigators favor a lipid anesthetic site, the PCC theory remains viable. A hydrophobic protein site of action could cause many of the physical-chemical relationships that point toward the lipid phase.

Present evidence supports the assumption that the site of anesthetic action is on the cell membrane. It is believed that anesthetics act chiefly by depressing synaptic transmission. It has also been shown that several general anesthetics hyperpolarize CNS neurons, apparently because of an increase in potassium permeability (Nicoll and Madison, 1982). This is a nonsynaptic activity which, combined with synaptic depression, can result in decreased neuronal excitability and CNS unresponsiveness. However, the exact mechanism of anesthesia still remains an enigma.

Sites of Action of General Anesthetics

In the past, it was thought that the stages of anesthesia represented suppression of activity in the nervous system, starting first with the higher centers or those newest phylogenetically. Stage one (analgesia) was thought to be due to effect on the cerebral cortex; stage two (excitement), due to effect on the midbrain that had been released from cerebral control; and stage three (surgical anesthesia) was ascribed to progressive depression of the midbrain and spinal cord producing skeletal muscle relaxation. The assumption was made that the medulla, for some reason, was not depressed until the deepest stages of anesthesia were reached. Hence, stage four (toxic), involving respiratory and circulatory arrest, was due to medullary depression.

Larrabee and Posternak (1952) were able to demonstrate that pentobarbital, ether, chloroform, and chloretone depressed synaptic transmission in concentrations similar to those existing in the blood during surgical anesthesia, whereas higher concentrations were required to affect conduction along any type of axon. They concluded that this selective action of anesthetics on synapses was due either to a specific effect on synaptic transmission or to the relatively small "factor of safety" in transsynaptic excitation compared to axonal conduction.

The reticular activating system is a multisynaptic structure, which probably accounts for its susceptibility to anesthetics, since they block synaptic transmission better than nerve trunk conduction. Injection of local anesthetics into the RAS produces general anesthesia, thus supporting the theories that an intact RAS is necessary for conscious perception of impulses, and that the RAS is probably the most important site within the central nervous system for anesthetic action.

Melzack and Wall (1965) proposed that pain may be controlled by a presynaptic gating mechanism located in the dorsal horn of the spinal cord. Subsequently, it was demonstrated in cats by Wall (1967) that pentobarbital produced progressive "closure of the gate," which prevented cutaneous impulses from ascending to the brain. He postulated that cutaneous anesthesia was the result of a selective depression of impulse transmission across the first spinal synapse of the cutaneous sensory pathway located in the dorsal horn. This work was repeated by deJong and Wagman (1968), using halothane as the anesthetic agent. They suggested that the hypnotic action of anesthetics may be due to depression of synaptic transmission in the reticular substance, whereas the analgesic action may be due to depression of synaptic transmission in the dorsal horn.

Sites of Action of Local Anesthetics

Local anesthetic agents prevent passage of the nerve impulse in 1) sensory nerve endings, 2) ganglionic synapses, 3) myoneural junctions, and 4) nerve trunks. Clinically, the important sites of action are sensory nerve endings and nerve trunks. The smallest nerve fibers are paralyzed first because of the greater surface area per unit of volume. In mixed nerves, the sequence of anesthesia is autonomic, sensory, and motor. The order of anesthesia, as determined by loss of sensation and action potential, has been shown (Heinbecker et al., 1932, 1934) to be:

1. unmyelinated nerves (vasoconstriction and vasodilation);
2. smallest thinly myelinated nerves (temperature);
3. small thinly myelinated nerves (pain);
4. large thickly myelinated nerves (touch); and
5. largest thickly myelinated nerves (joint and pressure sense).

Return of sensation and action potential is in the reverse order.

In general, local anesthetics are acid salts of basic substances. The salt forms are water-soluble, whereas the substances themselves are water-insoluble or lipoid-soluble. Normal tissue fluids, which are slightly alkaline, hydrolyze the salt and liberate the base, which is then absorbed by nerve tissue.

The exact mechanism of action is still controversial, though it is probably a surface action. The free base that contains positively charged ions is strongly absorbed by the negatively charged nerve fibers and nerve endings. This, in turn, brings about a decrease in nerve membrane permeability or electrical conductivity.

Sax and Pletcher (1969) have suggested that local anesthetics form a hydrogen-bonded complex with a receptor in the nerve cell membrane. All commonly used local anesthetics possess at least one polar group capable of participating as the donor in a hydrogen bond. They indicate that any chemical group on the lipoprotein membrane capable of accepting a hydrogen bond is a potential binding site for local anesthetics. The acetylcholine receptor is one such possible site of action. In this fashion, acetylcholine would be blocked from the active site, and transmission would be inhibited.

REFERENCES

Ahlquist, R.P.: A Study in the Adrenotropic Receptors. Am. J. Physiol., 15:586, 1948.

Allison, A.C., and Nunn, J.F.: Effects of General Anaesthetics on Microtubules. A Possible Mechanism of Anaesthesia. Lancet, 2:1326, 1968.

Barchas, J.D., Akil, H., Elliott, G.R., Holman, R.B., and Watson, S.J.: Behavioral Neurochemistry: Neuroregulators and Behavioral States. Science, 200:964, 1978.

Barnett, D.B., Rugg, E.L., and Nahorski, S.R.: Direct Evidence of Two Types of β-Adrenoceptor Binding Sites in Lung Tissue. Nature, 273:166,1978.

Basbaum, A.I., and Fields, H.L.: Endogenous Pain Control Mechanisms: Review and Hypothesis. Ann. Neurol., 4:451, 1978.

Berthelsen, S., and Pettinger, W.A.: A Functional Basis for Classification of α-Adrenergic Receptors. Life Sci., 21:595, 1977.

Bradbury, A.F., Seldberg, W.F., Smyth, D.G., and Snell, C.R.: Lipotropin C-Fragment: An Endogenous Peptide with Potent Analgesic Activity. In *Opiates and Endogenous Opioid Peptides*. Edited by H. W. Kosterlitz. Elsevier/North Holland Biomedical Press, Amsterdam, 1976.

Breazile, J.E., and Kitchell, R.L.: Pain Perception in Animals. Fed. Proc., 28:1379, 1969.

Carlsson, E., Ablad, B., Brandstrom, A., and Carlson, B.: Differentiated Blockade of the Chronotropic Effects of Various Adrenergic Stimuli in the Cat Heart. Life Sci., 11:953, 1972.

Chorev, M., Shavitz, R., Goodman, M., Minick, S., and Guillemin, R.: Partially Modified Retro-Inverso-Enkephalinamides: Topochemical Long-Acting Analogs In Vitro and In Vivo. Science, 204:1210, 1979.

deJong, R.H., Hershey, W.N., and Wagman, I.H.: Nerve Conduction Velocity during Hypothermia in Man. Anesthesiology, 27:805, 1966.

deJong, R.H., and Nace, R.A.: Nerve Impulse Conduction and Cutaneous Receptor Responses during General Anesthesia. Anesthesiology, 28:851, 1967.

deJong, R.H., and Wagman, I.H.: Block of Afferent Impulses in the Dorsal Horn of Monkey. A Possible Mechanism of Anesthesia. Exp. Neurol., 20:352, 1968.

Ecanow, B., Gold, B.H., and Ecanow, C.S.: Unified Theory of Anesthesia. J. Pharm. Sci., 68:4, 1979.

Evans, A.F., and Geddes, L.A.: Vasomotor Response to Increased Cerebrospinal Fluid Pressure in the Spinal Animal. Cardiovascular Res. Ctr. Bull., Baylor College of Medicine, 7:100, 1969.

Finch, E.D., and Kiesow, L.A.: Pressure, Anesthetics, and Membrane Structure: A Spin-Probe Study. Undersea Biomed. Res., 6:41, 1979.

Fletcher, T.F.: Lumbosacral Plexus and Pelvic Limb Myotomes in the Dog. Am. J. Vet. Res., 31:35, 1970.

Guillemin, R., Ling, N., and Burgus, R.: Biochimie: Endorphines, Peptides, d'Origine Hypothalamique et Neurohypophysaire a Activite Morphinomimetique. Isolement et Structure Moleculaire de l'α-Endorphine. C. R. Acad. Sc. Paris, 282:783, 1976.

Hazum, E., Chang, K., and Cuatrecasas, P.: Specific Nonopiate Receptors for β-Endorphin. Science, 205:1033, 1979.

Heinbecker, P., Bishop, G.H., and O'Leary, J.: Allocation of Function to Specific Fiber Types in Peripheral Nerves. Proc. Soc. Exp. Biol. Med., 30:304, 1932.

Heinbecker, P., Bishop, G.H., and O'Leary, J.: Analysis of Sensation in Terms of the Nerve Impulse. Arch. Neurol. Psychiat., 31, 34, 1934.

Hoerlein, B.F.: *Canine Neurology: Diagnosis and Treatment,* 3rd ed. W. B. Saunders Co., Philadelphia, 1978.

Hughes, J.: Isolation of an Endogenous Compound from the Brain with Pharmacological Properties Similar to Morphine. Brain Res., 88:295, 1975.

Hughes, J., Smith, T.W., Kosterlitz, H.W., Fothergill, L.A., Morgan, B.A., and Morris, H.R.: Identification of Two Related Pentapeptides from the Brain with Potent Opiate Agonist Activity. Nature (London), 258:577, 1975.

Iwamoto, E.T.: Locomotor Activity and Antinociception after Putative Mu, Kappa and Sigma Opioid Receptor Agonists in the Rat: Influence of Dopaminergic Agonists and Antagonists. J. Pharmacol. Exp. Ther., 217:451, 1981.

Kaufman, R.D.: Biophysical Mechnisms of Anesthetic Action: Historical Perspective and Review of Current Concepts. Anesthesiology, 46:49, 1977.

King, R.B.: Principles of Pain Management. A Short Review. J. Neurosurg., 50:554, 1979.

Koblin, D.D., and Eger, E.I., II: Theories of Narcosis. N. Engl. J. Med., 301:1222, 1979.

Lands, A.M., Arnold, A., McAuliff, J.B., Luduena, F.P., and Brown, T.G.: Differentiation of Receptor Systems Activated by Sympathomimetic Amines. Nature, 214:597, 1967.

Larrabee, M.G., and Posternak, J.M.: Selection Action of Anesthetics on Synapses and Axons in Mammalian Sympathetic Ganglia. J. Neurophysiol., 15:91, 1952.

Lewis, J.W., Tordoff, M.G., Sherman, J.E., and Liebskind, J.C.: Adrenal Medullary Enkephalin-Like Peptides May Mediate Opioid Stress Analgesia. Science, 217:557, 1982.

Li, H.L., and Chung, D.: Isolation and Structure of an Unknown Untriakontapeptide with Opiate Activity from Camel Pituitary Glands. Proc. Natl. Acad. Sci. U.S.A., 73:1145, 1976.

MacNichol, E.E., Jr., Kunz, Y.W., Levine, J.S., Harosi, F.I., and Collins, B.A.: Stimulation of Dopamine Synthesis in Caudate Nucleus by Intrastriatal Enkephalins and Antagonism by Naloxone. Science, 200:552, 1978.

Martin, W.R., Eades, C.G., Thompson, J.A., Huppler, R.E., and Gilbert, T.E.: The Effects of Morphine and Nalorphine-like Drugs in the Non-Dependent and Morphine-Dependent Chronic Spinal Dog. J. Pharmacol. Exp. Ther., 197:517, 1976.

Marx, J.L.: Brain Peptides: Is Substance P a Transmitter of Pain Signals? Science, 205:886, 1979.

Mayer, D.T., Wolfe, T.L., Akil, H., Carder, B., and Liebeskind, J.C.: Analgesia from Electrical Stimulation of the Brain Stem of the Rat. Science, 174:1351, 1971.

Melzack, R., and Wall, P.D.: Pain Mechanisms: A New Theory. Science, 150:971, 1965.

Milhorat, T.H.: Choroid Plexus and Cerebrospinal Fluid Production. Science, 166:1514, 1969.

Miller, S.L.: A Theory of Gaseous Anesthetics. Proc. Natl. Acad. Sci., 47:515, 1961.

Mullins, L.J.: Some Physical Mechanisms in Narcosis. Chem. Rev., 54:289, 1954.

Nicoll, R.A., and Iwamoto, E.T.: Action of Pentobarbital

on Sympathetic Ganglion Cells. J. Neurophysiol., 41:977, 1978.
Nicoll, R.A., and Madison, D.V.: General Anesthetics Hyperpolarize Neurons in the Vertebrate Central Nervous System. Science, 217:1055, 1982.
Pauling, L.: A Molecular Theory of General Anesthesia. Science, 134:3471, 1961.
Pert, C.B., and Pert, A.: (D-Ala^2)-Met-Enkephalinamide: A Potent, Long-Lasting Synthetic Pentapeptide Analgesic. Science, 194:330, 1976.
Pert, C.B., and Snyder, S.H.: Opiate Receptor: Demonstration in Nervous Tissue. Science. 179:1011, 1973.
Robbins, K.C., Devare, S.G., Reddy, E.P., and Aaronson, S.A.: Comparison of the Distribution of Dynorphin Systems and Enkephalin Systems in Brain. Science, 218:1134, 1982.
Roth, S.H.: Physical Mechanisms of Anesthesia. Annu. Rev. Pharmacol. Toxicol., 19:159, 1979.
Sax, M., and Pletcher, J.: Local Anesthetics: Significance of Hydrogen Bonding in Mechanism of Action. Science, 166:1546, 1969.
Seeman, P.: The Membrane Actions of Anesthetics and Tranquilizers. Pharmacol. Rev., 24:583, 1972.
Simon, E.J., Hiller, J.M., and Edelman, I.: Stereospecific Binding of the Potent Narcotic Analgesic [^{3}H] Etorphine to Rat-Brain Homogenate. Proc. Natl. Acad. Sci., 70:1947, 1973.
Snyder, S.H.: Opiate Receptors in the Brain. N. Engl. J. Med., 296:266, 1977.
Terenius, L.: Characteristics of the "Receptor" for Narcotic Analgesics in Synaptic Plasma Membrane Fraction from Rat Brain. J. Pharmacol. Toxicol., 33:377, 1973.
Teschemacher, H., Opheim, K.E., Cox, B.M., and Goldstein, A.: A Peptide-like Substance from Pituitary that Acts like Morphine. Life Sci., 16:1771, 1975.
Thompson, W.F., and Melzack, R.: Early Environment. Sci. Am., 194:38, 1956.
Vacca, L.L., Abrahams, S.J., and Naftchi, E.N.: Effect of Morphine on Substance P Neurons in Rat Spinal Cord: A Preliminary Study. Brain Res., 182:229, 1980.
Wall, P.D.: The Mechanisms of General Anesthesia. Anesthesiology, 28:46, 1967.
Willis, W.D.: Neurophysiology of Nociception and Pain in the Spinal Cord. In *Pain*. Edited by J.J. Bonica. Raven Press, New York, 1980.

CHAPTER 5

The Cardiovascular System and Anesthesia

GENERAL FUNCTIONS

The functions of the cardiovascular system are to carry oxygen and nutrients to the tissues, remove wastes and, in general, maintain the homeostasis of the cellular environment. To conduct these functions, blood must be pumped by the heart through the lungs and then distributed to all areas of the body. Distribution and return are accomplished by the arteries, capillaries, and veins. Proper function of these organs is essential for tissue metabolism and, during general anesthesia, for the delivery and removal of anesthetics to and from the central nervous system.

THE HEART

For practical considerations, only four-chambered hearts are considered here, although it should be emphasized that hearts in many lower vertebrates may contain fewer than four chambers.

Anatomically, the heart can be divided into right and left sides, each composed of an atrium and a ventricle. Physiologically, it comprises a low-pressure side (right) and a high-pressure side (left). Electrically, it can be divided into atria insulated from ventricles.

Blood enters the right atrium from the venae cavae (superior and inferior), passes into the right ventricle, and is pumped via the pulmonary artery through the lungs, at which time exchange of oxygen and carbon dioxide with the alveolar air occurs (Fig. 5–1). Blood returns from the lungs via the pulmonary veins to enter the left atrium, from which it passes to the left ventricle and is pumped into the aorta for distribution to the body.

Four rings of dense connective tissue form a fibrous "skeleton" for the heart. The atria, ventricles, valves, and arterial trunks are attached to this skeleton, which also serves to insulate the atria from the ventricles. Contraction of the ventricular walls furnishes the major source of energy for the circulation of blood. Because the left ventricle performs more work, the musculature of its wall is thicker than that of the right ventricle.

Four sets of valves control blood flow within the heart. The aortic and pulmonary valves are similar, each consisting of three cusps. The atrioventricular valves, interposed between the atria and ventricles, are termed tricuspid on the right and mitral on the left. The tricuspid has three cusps, whereas the mitral has only two. Chordae tendineae connect the valves to papillary muscles within the ventricles.

The muscles of the ventricles can be divided

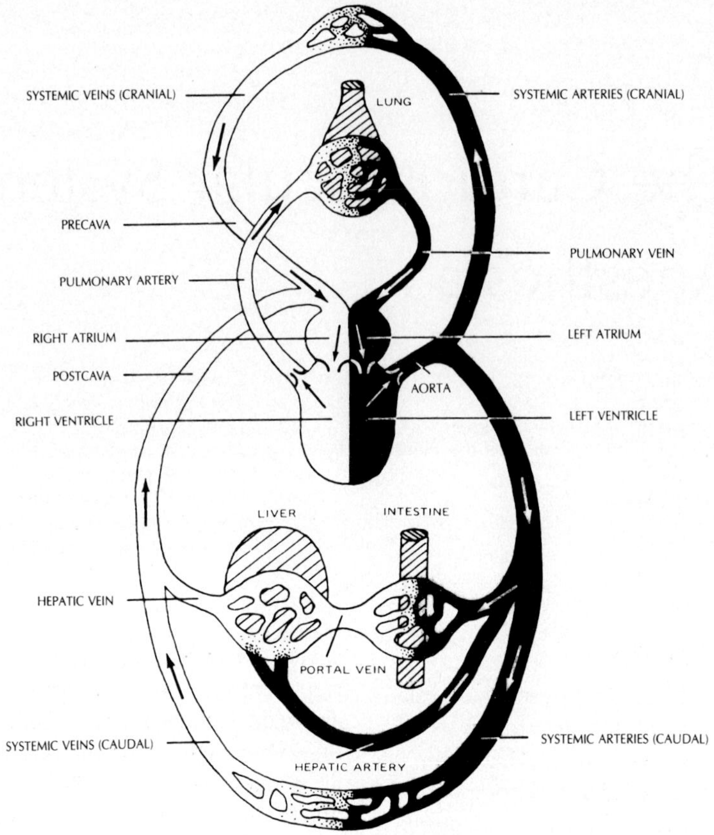

Figure 5–1. Schematic representation of the circulatory system. (From Anonymous: Mod. Vet. Pract., 50:68, 1969.)

into two groups: spiral muscles and the deeper constrictor muscles. Histologically, heart muscle is a syncytium. Functionally, the heart muscles must contract simultaneously. This is accomplished through the conduction system and the syncytial nature of the muscle fibers, excitation spreading from one muscle fiber to another in a coordinated fashion.

PHYSIOLOGY OF CARDIAC MUSCLE

Rhythmic beating of the heart is caused by a complex series of biochemical events. The basic contractile unit of a heart muscle cell is the sarcomere, composed of interdigitating protein filaments, actin (thin filament), and myosin (thick filament) (Fig. 5–2). Muscle shortening occurs when the actin and myosin filaments are activated. Activation is regulated by a protein assembly unit, composed of tropomyosin and troponin associated with actin molecules. In diastole, tropomyosin prevents the interaction of actin and myosin, perhaps by blocking myosin-interacting sites on actin filaments. Systole is initiated when tropomyosin moves from its blocking position, allowing cross linkages to form between projections of myosin and exposed sites on actin. As cross bridges form, the projecting heads of myosin filaments pull sets of thin filaments toward each other, the thick and thin filaments move laterally in relation to one another, and contraction occurs. Diastole is initiated when tropomyosin returns to its blocking position. Ionized calcium (Ca^{++}) in the vicinity of the troponin unit of the contractile apparatus is the immediate and obligate modulator of the relaxation-contraction cycle (Fuchs et al., 1970).

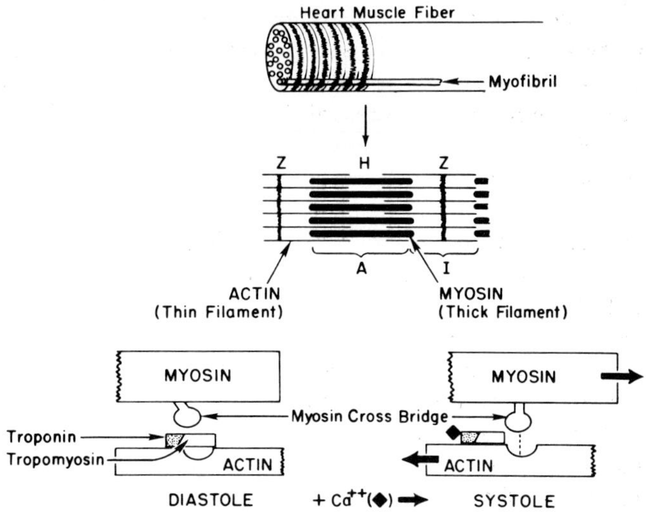

Figure 5–2. Structural arrangement of actin and myosin filaments in the contractile apparatus of cardiac muscle. Interaction of calcium with troponin results in the removal of tropomyosin from its diastolic blocking position on actin, allowing activation and muscle contraction. (From Parker, J.L., and Adams, R.H.: Drugs and the Heart Muscle. J.A.V.M.A., 171:78, 1977.)

Entry of Ca^{++} into the myocardial cell and the resulting intracellular Ca^{++}-dependent events with each heartbeat are initiated by bioelectrical events at the cell membrane. These are represented by the cardiac action potential (Fig. 5–3).

The diastolic (resting) membrane potential in heart cells is about −90 mV intracellularly, due primarily to selective permeability of the cell membrane to electrolytes and also to active ion transport. This results in asymmetric distribution of charged ions across the cell membrane. The membrane momentarily loses its selective permeability characteristics when the cell is stimulated above a threshold, and the resulting change in ion distribution can be recorded as an action potential. The ventricular action potential is composed of two basic components, depolarization and repolarization, which can be further divided into five phases. The rapid upstroke, phase 0, is similar to the depolarization spike seen in skeletal muscle and neurons, representing a rapid influx of Na^{+} into the cell. As the permeability characteristics of the cell membrane are quickly reestablished, rapid (phase 1) and delayed (phase 3) repolarization occur, restoring the membrane potential to its diastolic level (phase 4). Efflux of K^{+} is the primary determinant of late repolarization. Phase 0 and phase 3 of a single cell action potential can be temporally related to the QRS complex (depolarization) and the T wave (repolarization) of

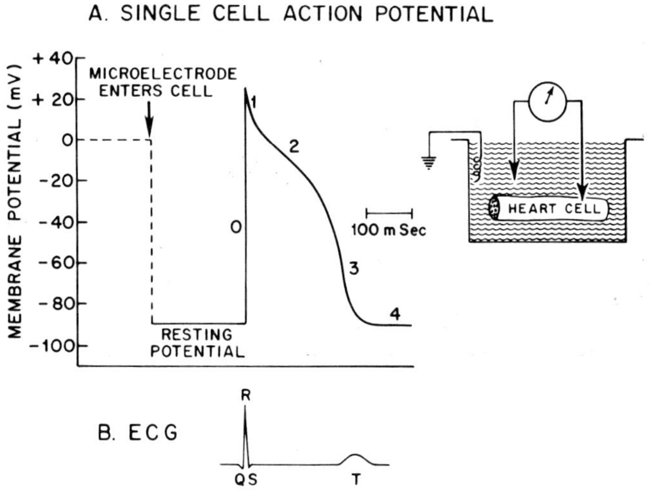

Figure 5–3. *A,* Cardiac action potential recorded from a single myocardial cell. The phases listed are: 0, rapid depolarization upstroke; 1, rapid repolarization; 2, plateau; 3, delayed repolarization; and 4, diastolic potential. The plateau phase (2) is thought to be the slow current representing electrogenic entry of Ca^{++} into the cell. *B,* Cardiac electrocardiogram (ECG) of the ventricle correlating with the respective phases above. (From Parker, J.L., and Adams, R.H.: Drugs and the Heart Muscle. J.A.V.M.A., 171:78, 1977.)

the electrocardiogram. The plateau or phase 2 is characteristic of cardiac muscle and represents a slow, inward current carried by Ca^{++} through membrane channels or pores, distinct from those participating in the rapid upstroke phase of the action potential. The plateau phase caused by the Ca^{++} is believed to be the link in heart muscle that couples membrane excitation with activation of the contractile apparatus. A portion of the contractile-dependent Ca^{++} in heart muscle is in rapid equilibrium with extracellular Ca^{++} and is probably derived from superficial binding sites on the cell membrane.

Activation of the contractile mechanism begins with movement of the action potential impulse along the sarcolemma of the muscle fiber and into its intricate microinvaginations known as the transverse tubular system (T-tubules, Fig. 5–4). Muscle contraction follows the onset of depolarization in about one-fiftieth of a second and is due to an immediate increase in intracellular Ca^{++}. Although many aspects of the processes involved in excitation-contraction coupling are unknown, there is no question that the supply of superficial membrane-bound Ca^{++} must be adequate for heart muscle contraction to occur. During repolarization, Ca^{++} is sequestered by the sarcoplasmic reticulum which stores it with greater affinity than troponin.

There is a net influx of Na^+ and Ca^{++} and reflux of K^+ with each action potential. Membrane-bound enzymes act as pumps to relocate ions and to prevent their improper accumulation. A Na^+-K^+ activated adenosine-triphosphatase (ATPase) pump propels Na^+ out of the cell and K^+ into the cell against their respective concentration gradients. Excess intracellular Ca^{++} is removed from the cell by pumps in the sarcoplasmic reticula which are close to the sarcolemma.

The mechanisms of action of various cardiac drugs can be described in relation to positive or negative inotropic effects on the contractile strength of the heart (Sperelakis and Schneider, 1976). Adrenergic or sympathomimetic amines, such as epinephrine, norepinephrine, and isoproterenol, have potent positive inotropic activity, causing an increase in heart rate and force of myocardial contraction. Left ventricular pressure is increased. The rate of ventricular pressure increase is accelerated, and this in turn causes increased stroke volume and cardiac output. These contractile changes are primarily effects on mechanical function and do not depend on the tachycardia induced, or on venous return, afterload, or other variables. The excitatory effect of the catecholamines is mediated initially by stimulation of the cardiac beta-adrenergic receptors (β_1). Cardiac β-receptor stimulation activates adenylate cyclase, a membrane-bound

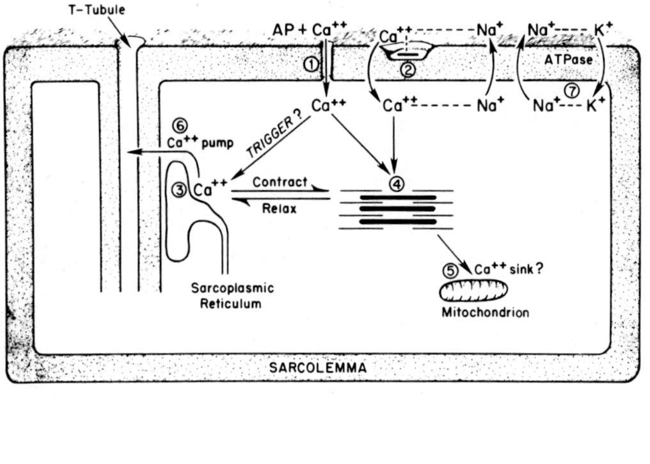

Figure 5–4. Schematic representation of cellular ion movements controlling excitation-contraction coupling in heart muscle. An action potential (AP) instigates the inward movement of Ca^{++} through "Ca^{++} pores"(1), or from superficial stores of Ca^{++} at the sarcolemmal membrane (2), or both. Inward-moving calcium may trigger the release of additional Ca^{++} from intracellular storage sites of the sarcoplasmic reticulum (3). These Ca^{++} sources and perhaps that resulting from Na^+–Ca^{++} exchanges across the sarcolemma (2) activate the contractile proteins (4). Relaxation occurs as calcium is sequestered at storage sites of sarcoplasmic reticulum (3) and perhaps mitochondria (5). Ca^{++} is pumped out of the cell (6). Altered sodium-pump activity (7) may also affect sodium concentrations available for Na^+–Ca^{++} exchange. (From Parker, J.L., and Adams, R.H.: Drugs and the Heart Muscle. J.A.V.M.A., 171:78, 1977.)

enzyme that catalyzes conversion of ATP to the cyclic nucleotide, adenosine 3′,5′-monophosphate (AMP). Cyclic AMP has been shown to possess positive inotropic activity and to act as a "second messenger" that translates β-receptor occupancy into the contractile response (Fig. 5–5). A relationship has been shown among β-receptor stimulation, adenylate cyclase activation, increased intracellular cyclic AMP concentration, and increased systolic Ca^{++} influx by way of the slow Ca^{++} channels of the sarcolemma. The augmented systolic Ca^{++} influx makes more Ca^{++} available for activation of the contractile proteins and an increase in contractility results. Glucagon and histamine can also increase cyclic AMP concentrations by stimulating the adenylate cyclase system. Phosphodiesterase inhibitors (methylxanthines) increase cyclic AMP concentrations through inhibition of the phosphodiesterase enzyme-mediated metabolism of cyclic AMP to its inotropically inactive metabolite cyclic 5′ AMP. Cardioactive prostaglandins may also increase cyclic AMP availability. Another cyclic nucleotide, cyclic guanosine monophosphate (GMP) has been found to decrease contractile force and may be involved in negative inotropic action of certain cardioactive drugs.

Pentobarbital has been shown to decrease binding and availability of Ca^{++} at superficial membrane sites in the heart cells (Naylor and Szeto, 1972). Halothane not only affects superficial membrane events, but may also affect intracellular Ca^{++}-dependent inotropic processes (Price, 1974). The magnitude of the cardiodepressive actions of anesthetics is more pronounced during pathologic cardiovascular states. Furthermore, hazardous interactions of anesthetics with other therapeutic but potentially cardiodepressive drugs may occur through mutual inhibition of Ca^{++}-dependent processes (Adams et al., 1976).

It is not surprising that changes in concentrations of circulating cations have important influences on cardiac function. Alterations in Ca^{++}, Na^{+}, K^{+}, H^{+}, and Mg^{++} concentrations in the fluid bathing myocardial cells produce direct effects. Cardiac contractile strength increases rapidly following an increase in extracellular Ca^{++}, apparently owing to increased movement of Ca^{++} down the transmembrane concentration gradient, and to increased sequestration and release of Ca^{++} intracellularly. Decreased contractile strength occurs following reductions in extracellular Ca^{++}. Rapid infusion of blood preserved with acid-citrate-dextrose (ACD) solution lowers Ca^{++} in dogs and man and depresses myocardial function (Denlinger and Nahrwold, 1976). K^{+} excess induces almost immediate decrease in contractile strength, whereas small decreases cause relatively substantial increases in strength. K^{+} deficiency enhances the toxicity of cardiac glycosides and conversely K^{+} is sometimes of therapeutic value

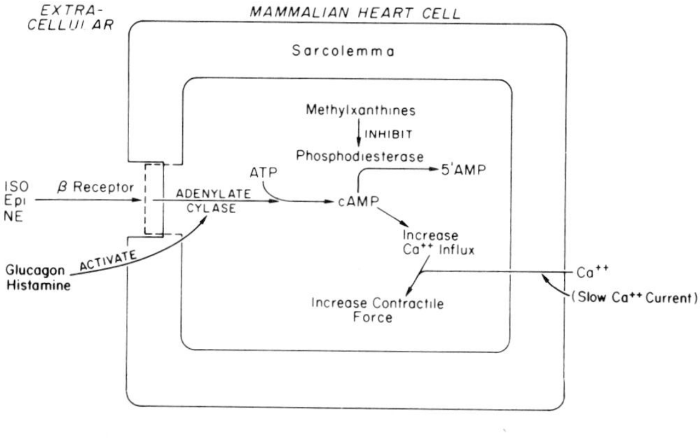

Figure 5–5. Proposed mechanism for the modulation of cardiac contractile force by agents that alter intracellular cyclic 3′,5′adenosine monophosphate (cAMP) concentrations. Catecholamines, glucagon, and histamine increase cAMP concentrations by activation of adenylate cyclase, whereas phosphodiesterase inhibitors such as methylxanthines (e.g., caffeine, theophylline) increase cAMP concentration by reducing enzymatic destruction of the nucleotide. In turn, increased cAMP concentrations increase contractile force by promoting influx of calcium through the slow Ca^{++} channel and probably by other mechanisms not shown. (ISO = isoproterenol; Epi = epinephrine; NE = norepinephrine) (From Parker, J.L., and Adams, R.H.: Drugs and the Heart Muscle. J.A.V.M.A., 171:78, 1977.)

in control of cardiac manifestations of digitalis intoxication. Thiazide diuretics may induce serum electrolyte abnormalities, such as hypokalemia and hyponatremia due to increased excretion of these ions.

Increases in H^+ concentration have direct negative inotropic effects on isolated heart muscle. The direct effect of H^+ has not been fully determined, although inhibition of the binding of Ca^{++} to troponin, altered binding of Ca^{++} to sarcoplasmic reticulum, and displacement of sarcolemmal bound Ca^{++} may be involved. Intracellular myocardial acidosis appears to be the critical factor, suggesting that metabolic or respiratory acidosis associated with certain disease conditions and drug administration may be involved in the myocardial depression observed (Sperelakis and Schneider, 1976). Alterations of plasma osmolarity, such as occur with dehydration or administration of hyper- or hypo-osmolar fluids, may indirectly induce alterations in myocardial electrolyte concentrations and may modify cardiac function.

THE CONDUCTION SYSTEM OF THE HEART

The sinoatrial (S–A) node is a small mass of specialized tissue in the right atrial wall near the entrance of the anterior vena cava (Fig. 5–6). It is the normal pacemaker of the heart, spontaneously originating electrical impulses that travel throughout the atria. It receives nerve impulses from the sympathetic and parasympathetic nervous systems. Vagal (parasympathetic) fibers release acetylcholine, which slows impulse formation, and sympathetic fibers release norepinephrine, which increases impulse formation. Epinephrine secreted into the blood by the adrenal medulla may also greatly accelerate the pacemaker. Under normal conditions, vagal influence predominates in most mammals. The S–A node remains the pacemaker as long as it produces impulses at a rate faster than any other region of the myocardium, and as long as these pass through atrial muscle to the ventricles. Anesthesia frequently produces disturbances in the normal control of the heart by the S–A node.

Once an impulse is generated in the S–A node, it spreads rapidly in all directions through the atrial muscle syncytium (Fig. 5–7). As it reaches the interatrial septum, it contacts the atrioventricular (A–V) node, another specialized conducting tissue mass. After a short delay, the impulse is conducted along the bundle of His, through the insulating fibrous "skeleton," and into the upper margin of the interventricular septum where the bundle divides into right and left branches. These descend on either side of

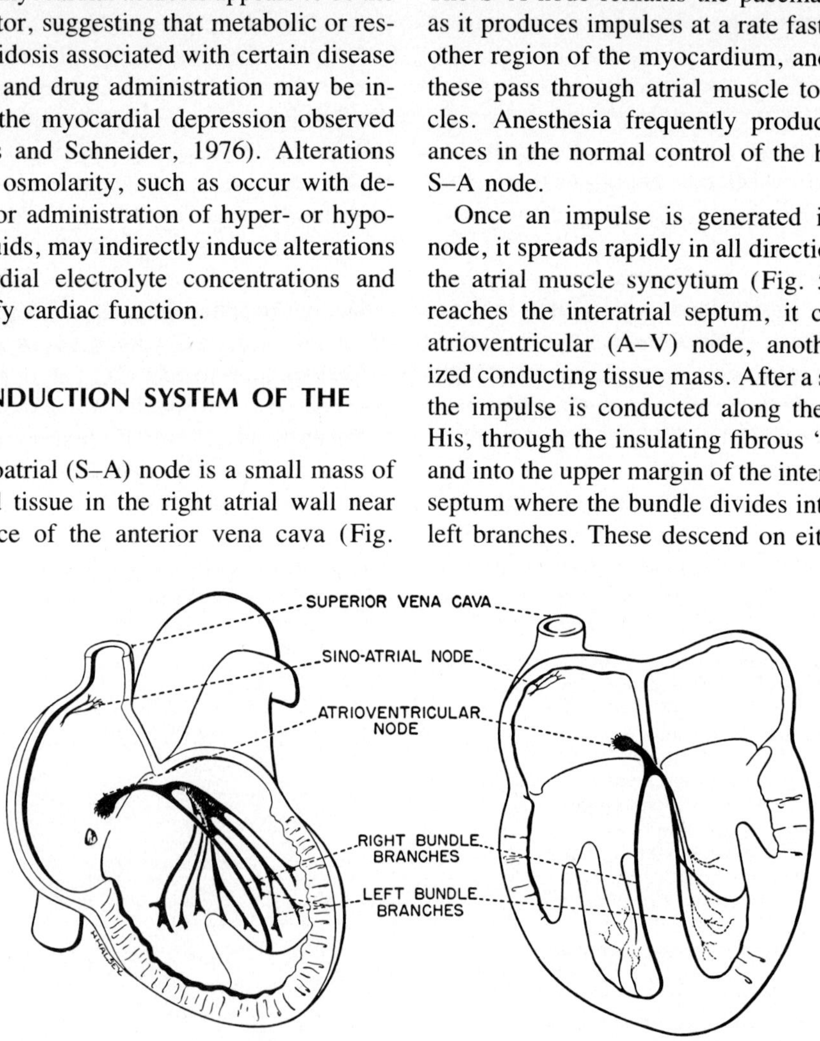

Figure 5–6. The sinoatrial (SA) node is the normal pacemaker of the heart. No specialized conduction system has been described in the atria. The atrioventricular (A–V) node, common bundle, and bundle branches conduct the wave of excitation from the atrium to the ventricular myocardium. (From Rushmer, R.F.: *Cardiovascular Dynamics*, 4th Ed. W.B. Saunders Co., Philadelphia, 1976.)

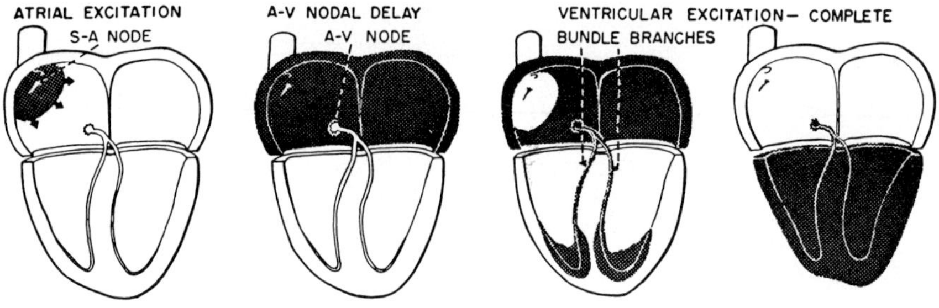

Figure 5–7. Sequence of cardiac excitation. Excitation of the heart is normally initiated by an impulse that is generated by the S–A node and that spreads rapidly in all directions through the atrial musculature. After a slight delay at the A–V node, impulses are conducted by the Purkinje system into the ventricles, where a wave of excitation spreads from the endocardial surfaces through the ventricular musculature. (From Rushmer, R.F.: *Cardiovascular Dynamics,* 4th ed. W.B. Saunders Co., Philadelphia, 1976.)

the septum to ramify into Purkinje's fibers, which spread over the inner surface of the respective ventricles.

On leaving the A–V node, the impulse travels the bundle and its branches rapidly and penetrates the ventricles to produce an almost simultaneous contraction of the ventricular walls. An abnormal sequence of ventricular contraction results either if waves of contraction originate at unusual sites in the heart wall, or if conduction is impaired in His's bundle or Purkinje's network.

The sinoatrial node, atrioventricular node, His's atrioventricular bundle, and Purkinje's fibers have been studied in several species of animals. The histologic characteristics of the conduction system differ widely in the hearts of reptiles, birds, and mammals. S–A and A–V nodes can be identified in most mammals, but are poorly defined in hearts of reptiles and birds (Truex and Smythe, 1965).

THE CARDIAC CYCLE

Clinically, there are only two phases in the cardiac cycle: the phase of ventricular muscle contraction termed *systole*, and a resting phase or phase of ventricular relaxation termed *diastole* (Fig. 5–8). The atria also undergo systole and diastole, atrial systole occurring during ventricular diastole and vice versa; however, the phase of the cardiac cycle is determined by the action of the ventricles and not of the atria.

CONTROL MECHANISMS

Several factors control the heart rate. As previously described, the S–A node is the normal pacemaker. It, in turn, is influenced by nerve impulses passing through vagal and sympathetic fibers. Both sets of fibers have their origin in the base of the medulla in a poorly localized site termed the "cardioregulatory center." Vagal fibers are carried in the vagus nerve to the heart (Fig. 5–9). Sympathetic fibers descend the spinal cord to T1, T2, T3 (this varies with species), course to the lateral sympathetic chain, and ascend to the stellate ganglion from which they pass to the heart in the cardiac nerves. The two sets of fibers are mutually antagonistic in their actions on the S–A node. In addition, the sympathetic and parasympathetic medullary centers are mutually antagonistic. Gross innervation of the heart in the dog, cat, pig, and horse has been described by McKibben and Getty (1968a, 1968b, 1969a, 1969b).

Afferent nerves converge on the medullary cardioregulatory center and continuously modify its activity (Fig. 5–10). These originate from the cerebral cortex, the carotid and aortic bodies, and the visceral and somatic body areas. Their input is moderated by the cardioregulatory center and is expressed as impulses transmitted to the heart via vagal and sympathetic fibers.

At the bifurcation of the carotid artery into internal and external branches is a dilatation of the internal carotid, the *carotid sinus*. Nerve endings sensitive to stretch are located in this

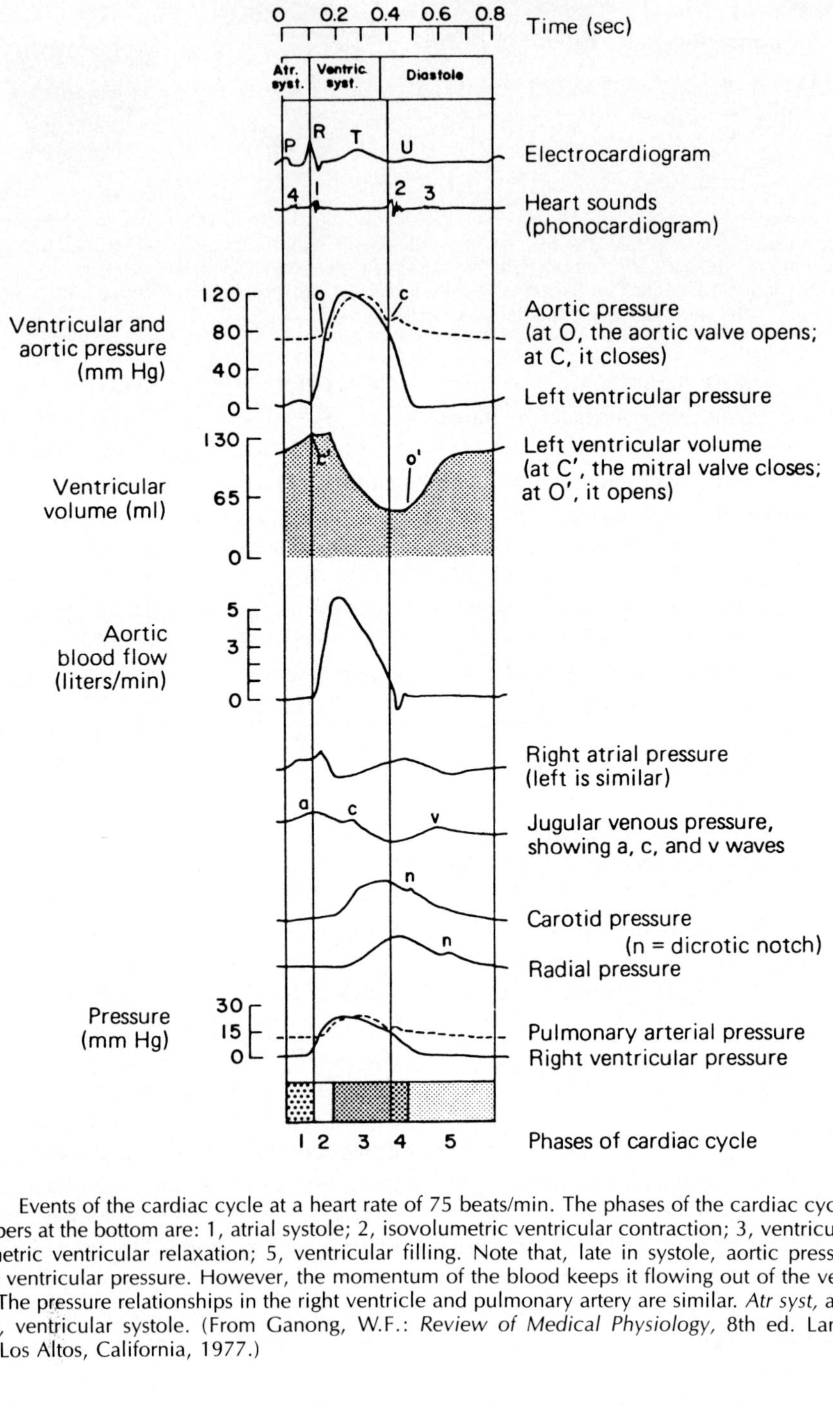

Figure 5–8. Events of the cardiac cycle at a heart rate of 75 beats/min. The phases of the cardiac cycle identified by the numbers at the bottom are: 1, atrial systole; 2, isovolumetric ventricular contraction; 3, ventricular ejection; 4, isovolumetric ventricular relaxation; 5, ventricular filling. Note that, late in systole, aortic pressure actually exceeds left ventricular pressure. However, the momentum of the blood keeps it flowing out of the ventricle for a short time. The pressure relationships in the right ventricle and pulmonary artery are similar. *Atr syst,* atrial systole. *Ventric syst,* ventricular systole. (From Ganong, W.F.: *Review of Medical Physiology,* 8th ed. Lange Medical Publishers, Los Altos, California, 1977.)

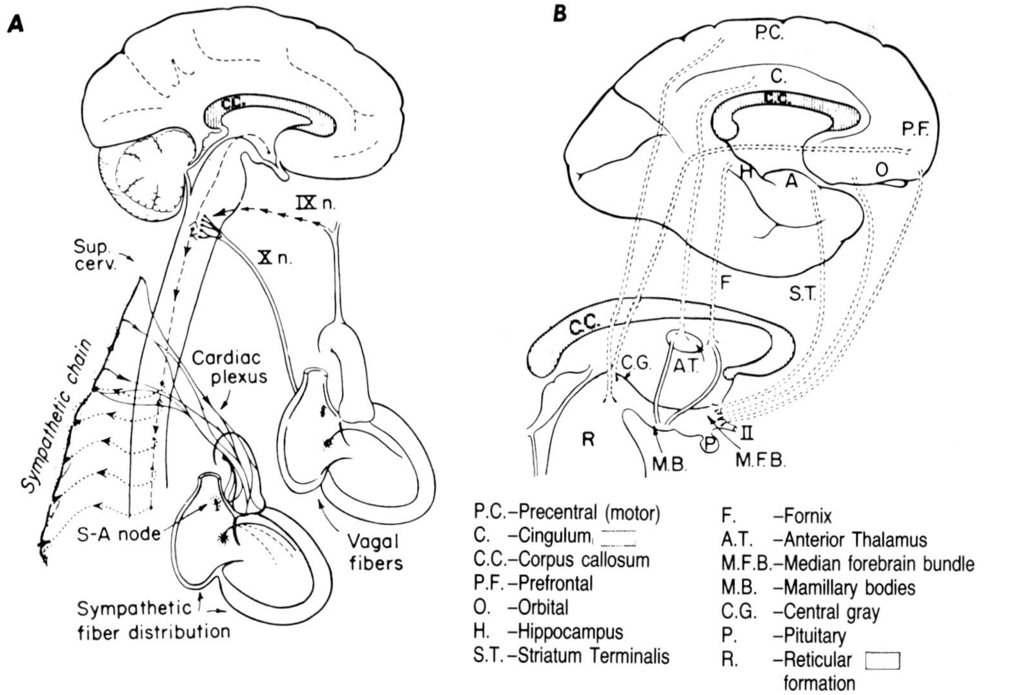

Figure 5–9. Neural control of the heart in man. *A,* The vagus nerve endings are concentrated in the region of the sinus node and atrioventricular node and are more diffusely distributed over the atrium. They do not extend to the ventricular myocardium. Sympathetic fibers from T_1–T_5 are distributed to all parts of the atrium and ventricles. Impulses traveling along the vagus and sympathetic nerves to the heart come from the medulla or the diencephalon. *B,* Neural pathways from many parts of the brain converge on the diencephalic region to influence autonomic outflow to the heart and other visceral structures. (From Rushmer, R.F.: *Cardiovascular Dynamics,* 4th ed. W.B. Saunders Co., Philadelphia, 1976.)

area and, when the vessel dilates due to pressure, they communicate this fact to the central cardioregulatory center via the glossopharyngeal (ninth) nerve. Other stretch-sensitive fibers are located in the aortic arch and transmit impulses centrally via the vagus (tenth) nerve.

An increase in arterial pressure increases the rate of discharge from these pressoreceptors (baroreceptors) and stimulates the cardioregulatory center to slow the heart both by vagal stimulation and by sympathetic inhibition. Simultaneously, the vasoconstrictor center is inhibited and peripheral resistance is decreased by inhibition of sympathetic vasoconstrictor outflow.

Less widely appreciated is the fact that there are sensory nerve endings in the atria and ventricles of the heart and lungs, which exert a tonic inhibitory influence on the vasomotor centers (Thames, 1980). These endings are particularly sensitive to changes in cardiac volume, and thus to changes in blood volume. They exert a tonic inhibitory effect on secretion of renin and release of vasopressin which are important in salt and water homeostasis and in blood pressure regulation (Fig. 5–11). They also participate to a smaller degree in the sympathetic outflow to muscle.

Studies indicate a reciprocal relationship between the magnitude of carotid input and the response to vagal block. Thus, there is an important interaction between carotid and cardiopulmonary receptors.

Clinical use can be made of two reflexes during tachycardia. Pressure on the skin over the carotid sinus (carotid sinus reflex) will produce bradycardia. Pressure on the eyeball at the lateral canthus (oculocardiac reflex) will also slow the heart.

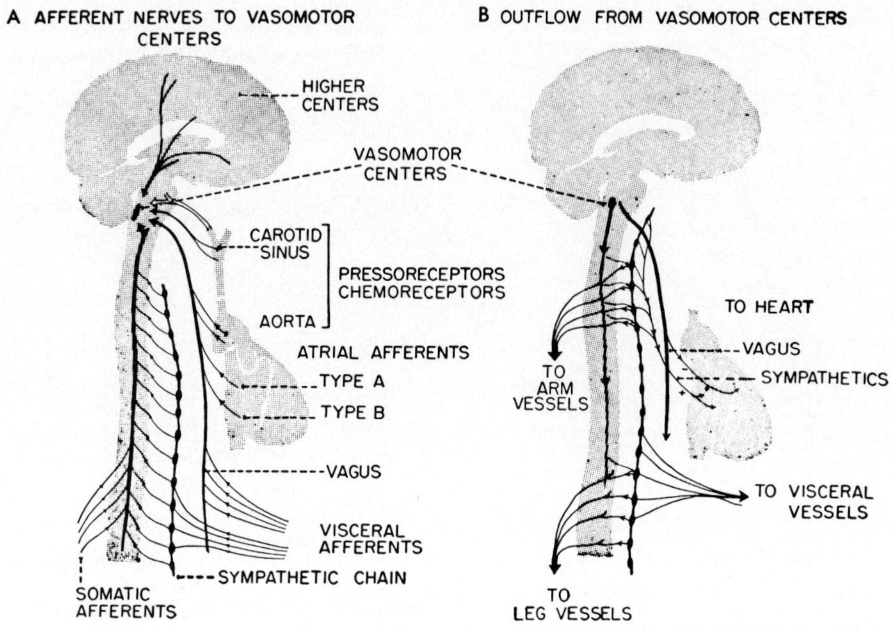

Figure 5–10. Neural mechanisms for peripheral vascular control. *A*, The vasomotor centers in the medulla receive afferent impulses originating from many different areas in the body, including the higher centers of the nervous system, pressoreceptors from the heart and great vessels, afferent nerves from the viscera, and somatic pain afferents. *B*, Impulses discharged from the vasomotor centers descend the spinal cord and influence cell bodies in the intermediolateral cell column which in turn initiate sympathetic nerve impulses conducted to the blood vessels in all parts of the body. (From Rushmer, R.F.: *Cardiovascular Dynamics,* 4th ed. W.B. Saunders Co., Philadelphia, 1976.)

HEMODYNAMIC DETERMINANTS OF CARDIAC FUNCTION

Various hemodynamic determinants and their mathematical relationships have been used to define cardiac contractile force (Muir, 1977). These include: 1) initial fiber length from which the myocardium begins to contract (preload); 2) the force of contraction independent of loading (contractility); 3) intraventricular systolic tension at semilunar valve opening (afterload); and 4) heart rate. The first two are influenced primarily by intrinsic mechanisms, and all are greatly influenced by the autonomic nervous system. In cardiac dysrhythmias, a fifth determinant, dyssynergia, becomes important because ventricular contraction follows an abnormal sequence.

In attempting to assess myocardial contractility, researchers have developed several mathematical indices of cardiac function. Measurement of intracavitary ventricular pressure during isovolumetric contraction (dp/dt max) was an early index (Fig. 5–12). To minimize the effect of pre- and afterload, normalization of the first derivative of left ventricular pressure (dp/dt max) to the simultaneous absolute isovolumetric pressure and an elasticity constant (K) were developed (dp/dt/Kp max). Plotted values for dp/dt/Kp max versus left ventricular pressure at each moment during contraction can be extrapolated to zero pressure (V max) to furnish another load-independent index of myocardial function.

The most common invasive technique for quantitating ventricular function is measurement of cardiac output. Cardiac output can be plotted against central venous pressure or left ventricular end-diastolic pressure as shown in Figure 5–13. Cardiac output is dependent on preload, contractility, afterload, heart valve function, and ventricular synergy.

CARDIAC RESERVE

The normal heart in a resting animal is functioning at one-fourth to one-third of its capacity.

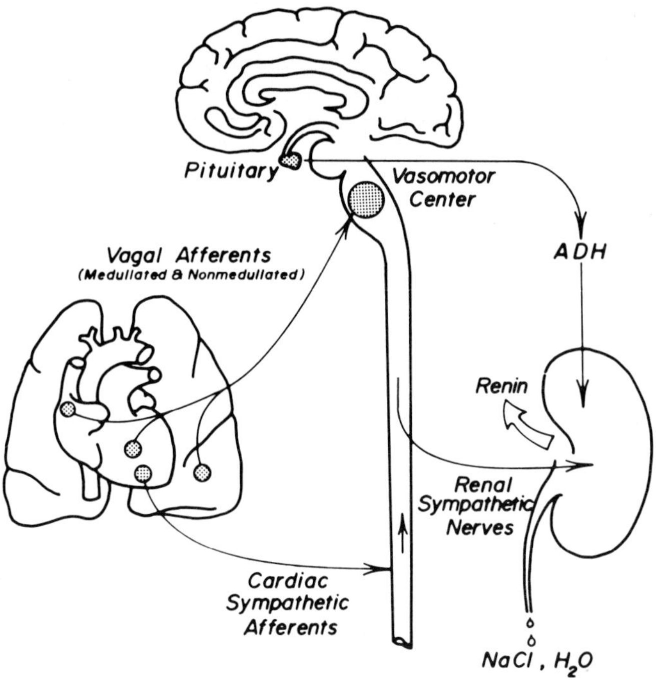

Figure 5–11. Cardiopulmonary-renal reflex effects thought to be mediated by receptors with vagal and sympathetic afferents. (From Thames, M.D.: Contribution of Cardiopulmonary Baroreceptors to the Control of the Kidney. Fed. Proc., 37:1209, 1978.)

The difference between the work capability at rest and that during maximum physical exertion is termed the *cardiac reserve*.

The amount of exercise that can be performed over a prolonged period is limited by the ability of the cardiovascular system to deliver oxygen to the tissues, since oxygen is the essential substance stored in smallest quantity in tissues in relation to its utilization rate. The amount of oxygen available to the tissues is limited by the cardiac output and the amount of oxygen that can be extracted from each unit of blood (arterial-venous oxygen difference).

As exercise increases the need for tissue oxygenation, an increase in cardiac output occurs through increased heart rate and venous return. Simultaneously, the tissues extract more oxygen from the blood and the A–V oxygen difference increases. In a normal subject, a 100% increase in oxygen consumption necessitates only a 70% increase in cardiac output; the remainder is obtained by increased oxygen extraction by the tissues. Oxygen extraction from coronary artery blood is almost complete; therefore, increase in cardiac function is almost totally dependent on increased coronary blood flow.

As the heart rate increases, the cardiac output increases up to a point. When the heart rate exceeds the ability of the ventricles to fill during diastole, cardiac output falls. The maximal effective heart rate varies with species. In man, it is about 2½ times the resting value or 170 to180 beats/min, whereas in birds, it is several hundred times a minute. Tachycardia also interferes with coronary blood flow, thus reducing the efficiency of the myocardium.

In heart disease and other stress situations such as anesthesia and shock, the cardiac reserve may be markedly reduced (see Fig. 5–13).

THE PERIPHERAL VASCULAR SYSTEM

There are two peripheral vascular systems: the general systemic system and the pulmonary system. The general systemic system is supplied by blood under high pressure from the left ventricle (Fig. 5–14). The pulmonary system, by

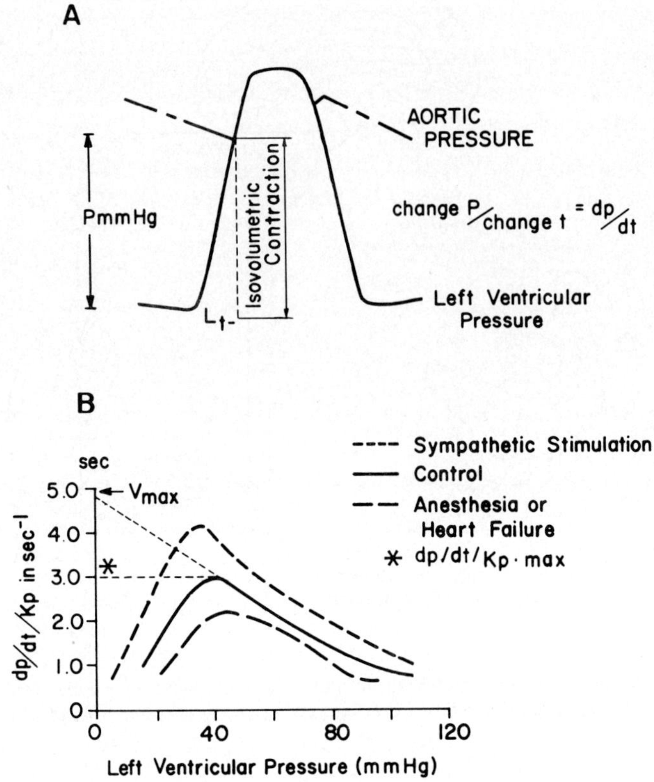

Figure 5–12. *A*, Relationship between pressure changes during isovolumetric contraction and time (dp/dt). P = Pressure; t = time. *B*, Effect of sympathetic stimulation and anesthesia on 2 indices of cardiac contractility (dp/dt/Kp max and V max). P = Pressure; t = time. (From Muir, W.W.: Anesthesia and the Heart. J.A.V.M.A., 171:92, 1977.)

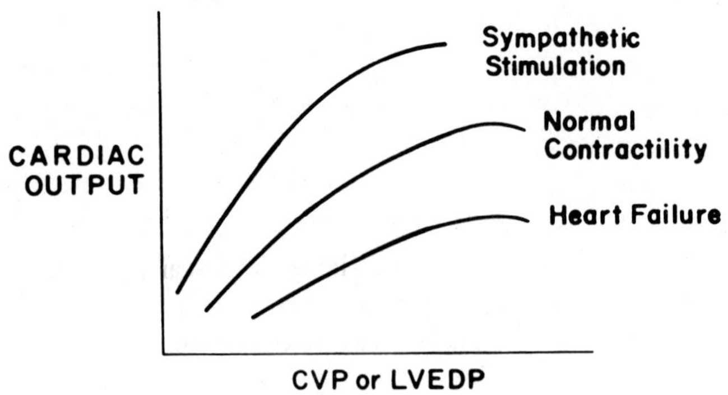

Figure 5–13. Effect of sympathetic stimulation and heart failure on the ventricular function curve. During heart failure, relatively large increases in central venous pressure (CVP) or left ventricular end diastolic pressure (LVEDP) result in only small increases in cardiac output. (From Muir, W.W.: Anesthesia and the Heart. J.A.V.M.A., 171:92, 1977.)

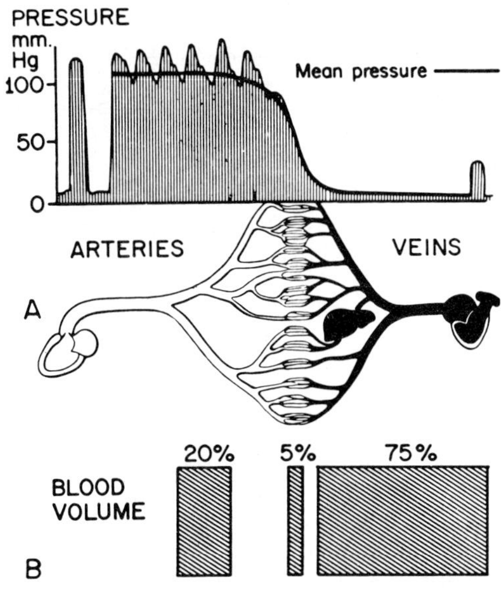

Figure 5–14. Pressures and volumes of blood in the systemic circulation. *A*, The pressures in the arterial system are elevated and pulsatile. The mean arterial pressure declines gradually as blood flows through the main branches of the arterial tree. In the small vessels, the pressure head diminishes rapidly and the fluctuations are damped out because of the high resistance to flow. In the major veins, the pressure gradient is again shallow. *B*, The volume of blood in the arteries is relatively fixed at about 20% of the total. The veins contain about 75% of the systemic blood volume but can alter their capacity over a wide range. (From Rushmer, R.F.: *Cardiovascular Dynamics*, 4th ed. W.B. Saunders Co., Philadelphia, 1976.)

contrast, is a low-pressure system (Fig. 5–15). The work performed by the right ventricle is significantly less than that of the left, the pulmonary artery pressure being only about one-fifth of that in the systemic circulation. The following discussion will center on the systemic vascular system rather than on the pulmonary system.

Blood pressure in the arterial tree is maintained by cardiac output and peripheral vascular resistance* (Fig. 5–16). The latter is created by tonic contraction of the arterioles and precapillary sphincters. Therefore, the arterial side of the circulation is termed the *resistance system* and the vessels are *resistance vessels*.

A seldom appreciated fact is that the venous side of the circulation contains 70 to 80% of the total blood volume (Wiedeman, 1963) (Fig. 5–14, Table 5–1). For this reason, and because they dilate easily, veins are termed *capacitance vessels* and the venous system is termed the *capacitance system*. In shock, the venous system may dilate and sequester as much as 20 times the amount of blood contained on the arterial side of the circulation.

In cat muscle, intense vasoconstrictor fiber stimulation produces a luminal reduction of roughly 35% in the average resistance vessel, in contrast to a 25% reduction in the average capacitance vessel. Constrictor fiber control in resistance vessels can increase resistance up to seven times that of "basal tone." In capacitance vessels, mobilization of up to 40% of the total blood volume at "basal tone" can be achieved. The constrictor responses produced by circulating adrenal medullary hormones are weak, producing roughly 25% of the reaction produced by sympathetic stimulation (Mellander, 1960).

FLOW DISTRIBUTION

Blood leaving the heart enters the aorta and is distributed by the great vessels to the various body areas. Extensive bifurcation occurs in the tissues. The arteries divide into arterioles and, finally, capillaries. Little change in blood pressure or exchange of oxygen occurs until the capillaries are reached. Capillaries permeate every body tissue and are rarely more than 0.1 mm from any cell. Many materials readily diffuse through the capillary walls to supply adjacent cells and, conversely, cellular wastes easily gain access to the capillaries for removal. Tissues with high metabolic rates (e.g., brain, viscera) have dense capillary beds for ready diffusion of essential metabolites, whereas tissues with lower requirements (e.g., fat, bone) are less well supplied (Table 5–2).

Two types of capillaries have been described, arteriovenous (A–V) or "thoroughfare" capillaries and "true" or secondary capillaries. Blood flows continuously through A–V capil-

*Peripheral vascular resistance may be calculated from the formula

$$PVR = \frac{\text{Mean Arterial Pressure}}{\text{Mean Cardiac Output}}$$

and expressed as arbitrary peripheral vascular resistance units (PRU) or as dynes (sec)(cm^{-5}).

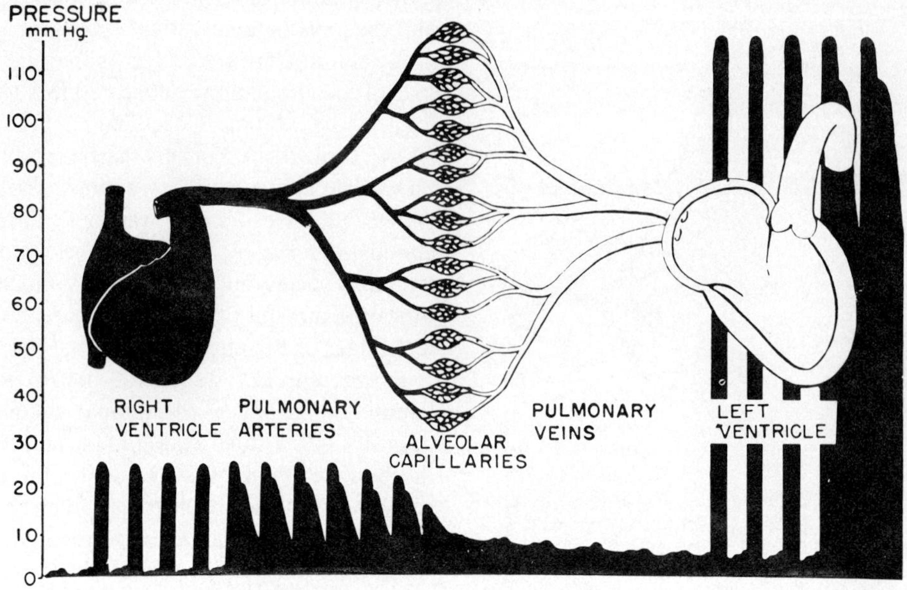

Figure 5–15. Pressures in the pulmonary vascular system. Since the pulmonary arterial system offers slight resistance to blood flow, the pressure difference between pulmonary artery and left atrium amounts to only 4 to 6 mm Hg. The low-pressure head drives the same volume of blood through the pulmonary circuit as flows through the systemic circulation with a gradient of approximately 90 mm Hg. (From Rushmer, R.F.: *Cardiovascular Dynamics,* 4th ed. W.B. Saunders Co., Philadelphia, 1976.)

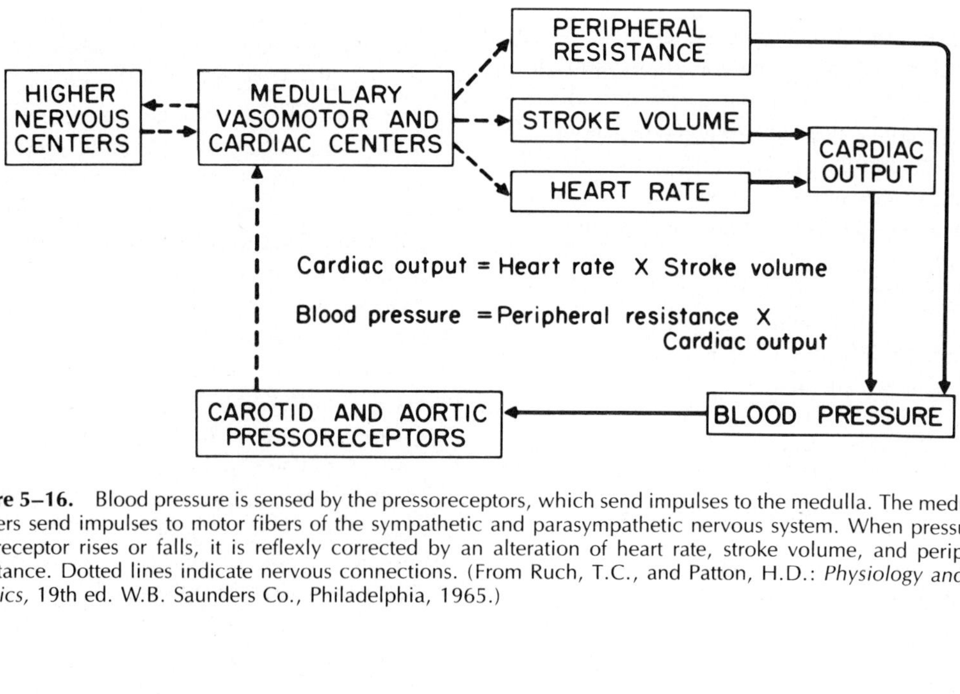

Figure 5–16. Blood pressure is sensed by the pressoreceptors, which send impulses to the medulla. The medullary centers send impulses to motor fibers of the sympathetic and parasympathetic nervous system. When pressure at the receptor rises or falls, it is reflexly corrected by an alteration of heart rate, stroke volume, and peripheral resistance. Dotted lines indicate nervous connections. (From Ruch, T.C., and Patton, H.D.: *Physiology and Biophysics,* 19th ed. W.B. Saunders Co., Philadelphia, 1965.)

TABLE 5–1. Geometry of Mesenteric Vascular Bed of the Dog

Kind of Vessel	*Diameter (Mm)*	*No.*	*Total Cross-sectional Area (Cm²)*	*Length (Cm)*	*Total Volume (Cm³)*	
Aorta	10	1	0.8	40	30	
Large arteries	3	40	3.0	20	60	
Main artery branches	1	600	5.0	10	50	
Terminal branches	0.6	1,800	5.0	1	25	
Arterioles	0.02	40,000,000	125	0.2	25	
Capillaries	0.008	1,200,000,000	600	0.1	60	
Venules	0.03	80,000,000	570	0.2	110	
Terminal veins	1.5	1,800	30	1	30	740
Main venous branches	2.4	600	27	10	270	
Large veins	6.0	40	11	20	220	
Vena cava	12.5	1	1.2	40	50	
					930	

(From Burton, A.C.: *Physiology and Biophysics of the Circulation.* Year Book Medical Publishers, Inc., Chicago, 1965.)

TABLE 5–2. Comparison of Organ Blood Flow (expressed in ml/min/100 g of tissue)

Organ	*Baboon*	*Dog*	*Man*
Heart	138.74	133	84
Lungs (bronchial)	71.8	145	
Lungs (pulmonary)	570.4	927	433
Liver (HA)	49.87	45	25
Liver (PV)	74.89	80	80
Liver (total)	124.76	120	109
Spleen	102.91	60	
Stomach	39.26	40	
Gut	30.51	60	
Pancreas	109.61	100	
Thyroid	50.66	184	550
Adrenals	108.61	217	590
Kidneys	448.09	426	420
Skin	3.91	7	12
Carcass	5.25	5	3

HA = Hepatic artery
PV = Portal vein

(From Fife, W.P.: *Cardiac Output and Regional Blood Flow in the Anesthetized Baboon.* SAM-TR-66-50. U.S. Air Force School of Aerospace Medicine, 1966.)

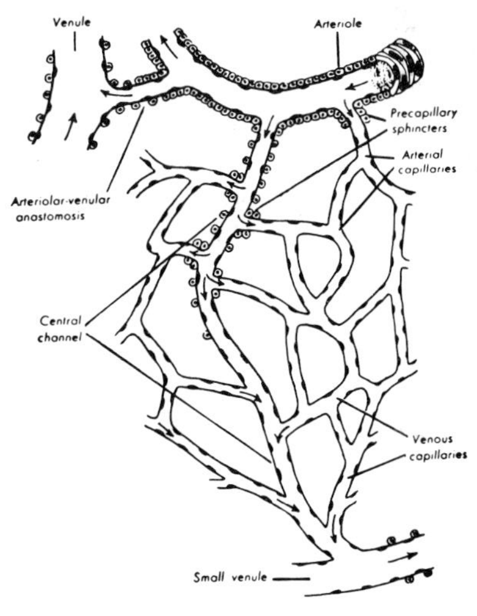

Figure 5–17. Bifurcation of the vascular system with diagrammatic capillary bed. Arrows indicate direction of blood flow. Muscle cells (highly diagrammatic) are shown surrounding arteriole, less densely around venule, and scattered along the proximal part of a through channel. They are present at the point of origin of the true capillaries. An arteriovenous (A–V) anastomosis, or by-pass, is also shown. (From Copenhaver: In *Bailey's Textbook of Histology,* 17th ed. Williams & Wilkins, Baltimore, 1978.)

laries, the amount being controlled by sphincters in the arteriole and along the capillary wall. "True" capillaries, which branch from the A–V capillaries, are controlled by precapillary sphincters located where they branch from the A–V capillaries. These capillaries have no muscle in their walls and flow is intermittent, being controlled by the precapillary sphincter. A continuously changing pattern of flow is produced by this type of system in response to tissue need and pressure gradients (Fig. 5–17).

Arteriovenous anastomoses are present in virtually every tissue and are capable of diverting blood directly from resistance to capacitance vessels without passing through a capillary bed (Prinzmetal et al., 1948). These are of significance, particularly in the lungs where gaseous exchange is thus circumvented. In shock, opening of A–V shunts deprives tissues of capillary perfusion.

Mellander and Lewis (1963) found that changes in the reactivity of the vascular bed of cat muscle varied with the various sections of vessel. The precapillary sphincter was most sensitive to reduction in regional blood flow, losing its constrictor response to sympathetic vasoconstrictor nerve stimulation and to norepinephrine injection. The next most sensitive were the precapillary resistance vessels. Thus, when regional blood flow was reduced, inflow to the capillary bed became unrestricted.

The postcapillary and capacitance vessels were most resistant to low flow abolition of vasoconstrictor response.

Some implications that may be derived are that:

1. In early shock, vasoconstrictors may be of benefit (a) by increasing the precapillary-to-postcapillary resistance ratio, thus enhancing movement of extravascular fluid into the circulation and (b) by constricting the capacitance vessels, thus increasing venous return to the heart.
2. As shock deepens, vasoconstrictors may have their greatest effect on postcapillary sphincters, increasing fluid loss into the tissues.
3. Use of sympatholytic agents in deepening shock blocks postcapillary vasoconstriction, thus preventing escape of fluid into the tissues. These agents also block neurogenic vasoconstriction of the capacitance vessels leading to pooling of blood. This is more than counter-balanced by prevention of fluid loss due to outward filtration produced by postcapillary constriction.

CHEMICAL MEDIATORS

Because catecholamines can produce either of two effects on vascular smooth muscle, Ahlquist (1948) proposed that two types of receptors exist in smooth muscle: *alpha* and *beta* (Fig. 5–18, Table 4–6). Norepinephrine acts principally on alpha receptors, whereas epinephrine acts on both, but mainly on alpha receptors. Circulating catecholamines, epinephrine and norepinephrine, are thought to play a minor role in normal peripheral vascular control.

Several substances have been proposed as being the cause of vasodilatation in the normal subject. Among these are carbon dioxide, histamine, serotonin, and prostacyclin (PGI_2). Reactive hyperemia is believed to be due to adenosine leaving the cells.

Prostaglandins (PG) exert an action on systemic arterial and venous vessels, pulmonary vascular bed, heart, carotid sinuses, and autonomic and central nervous systems involved in control of the cardiovascular system. The effects vary according to the PG and the animal species involved. Prostaglandins bind to cellular membrane receptors, increasing intracellular levels of cyclic nucleotides (cAMP, cGMP) and altering intracellular calcium pools. A dynamic balance of PG activities appears to exist, producing cardiovascular homeostasis (Jacobsen, 1983). The two most prominent PGs in this balance appear to be prostacyclin (PGI_2) and thromboxane (TXA_2). Prostacyclin, released by the pulmonary and other vascular endothelium, is a potent vasodilator and inhibitor of intravascular platelet aggregation. Thromboxane is produced by platelets and strongly stimulates vasoconstriction and platelet aggregation.

Prostaglandins play an important role in regulation of pre- and postsynaptic release of catecholamines from adrenergic nerve endings and the adrenal medulla. In the rat, PGE_2, PGI_2, and PGF_2 produce cardiac acceleration. PGE_2 and PGI_2 are potent antagonists of the increased heart rate and blood pressure caused by spinal cord stimulation and catecholamine release. This is a postsynaptic effect on the peripheral vessels and cardiac muscle (Feuerstein and Kopin, 1981).

VENOUS REGULATION

The venous system has been estimated to contain 70 to 80% of the total blood volume. Venomotor control is performed by both nervous and humoral factors. Sympathetic constrictor fi-

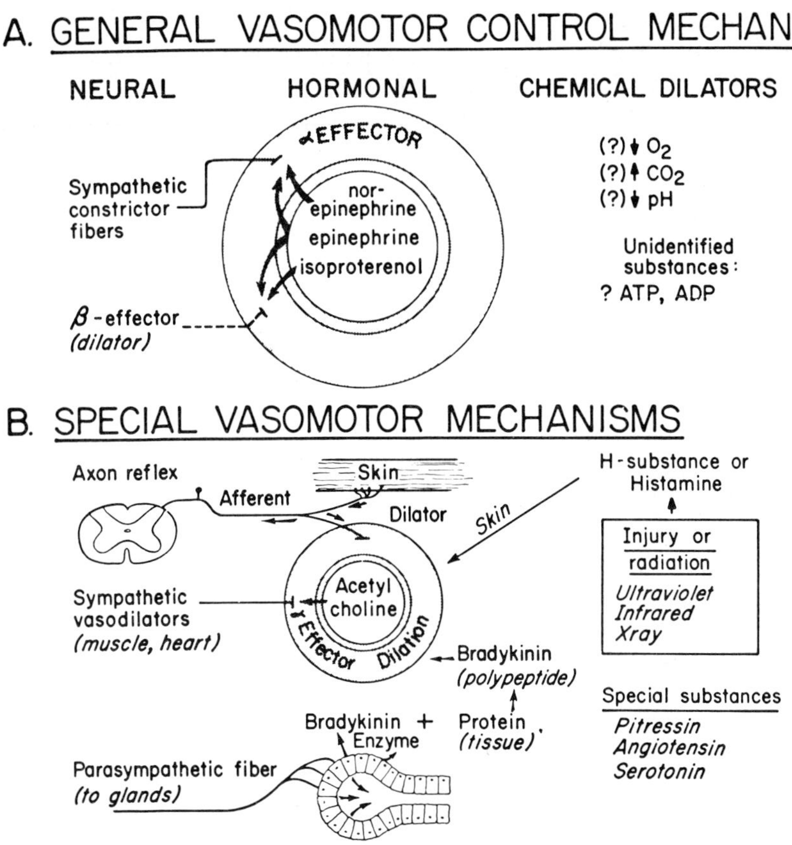

Figure 5–18. Vasomotor control. *A*, Vasoconstriction or vasodilation can be produced in various tissues by means of many neural, hormonal, and chemical mechanisms. Sympathetic fibers and circulating norepinephrine and *l*-epinephrine are widely believed to act at specific sites (α effectors). The β effectors are not innervated. The chemical dilators are proposed mechanisms for explaining vasodilation following temporary occlusion of blood supply to a vascular bed (reactive hyperemia). *B*, The special vasomotor mechanisms are found prominently in the skin, although the sympathetic vasodilators (muscle and heart) and the postulated bradykinin mechanism affect glands. No definite role in normal vascular regulation has been assigned to the special constrictor substances, vasopressin (Pitressin), angiotensin, serotonin. (From Rushmer, R.F.: *Cardiovascular Dynamics,* 4th ed. W.B. Saunders Co., Philadelphia, 1976.)

bers have been demonstrated to supply large superficial veins.

Carbon dioxide has been shown to dilate veins by direct local action. Decreased oxygen tension produces venoconstriction, whereas increased oxygen tension causes dilatation.

In canine veins, Ishikawa et al. (1980) demonstrated regional differences in contraction with vasoactive substances. Veins of the body wall and extremities were sensitive to norepinephrine and to 5-hydroxytryptamine (5-HT), whereas the pulmonary, portal, and mesenteric veins were highly sensitive to histamine. The renal veins were contracted by 5-HT. In general, the contraction values for norepinephrine and 5-HT were considerably higher than those for acetylcholine and histamine.

Venous return from the systemic veins is increased during inspiration by more negative intrathoracic pressure. Conversely, increase in portal vein flow and liver volume occurs during expiration. When the diaphragm is paralyzed, preventing mechanical compression of the liver, splanchnic and systemic venous flows occur together, producing wider variations in the volume of the thoracic vena cava. Normal respiration thus seems to prevent wide fluctuations in the volume of the central venous reservoir and to provide a more constant venous supply to the heart (Moreno et al., 1967).

Venous contraction is controlled at least in part by the carotid sinus mechanism. Decreased perfusion pressure in the sinus stimulates afferent impulses from the medullary vasomotor center, stimulating alpha receptors in the veins. As a consequence, the smooth muscles of the veins contract, forcing blood from the capacitance system. The action is reciprocal, increased carotid sinus pressure causing relaxation of the vein walls (Dow and Fry, 1968).

Blood flow in veins is also affected by the efficiency of the heart, arteriolar tone, muscular activity, valves, thoracic pressure, and gravity.

Increasing arterial resistance lowers venous return to the heart; however, as shown in Figure 5–19, for a given increase in venous resistance, the venous return decreases approximately eight times as much as with a similar increase in arterial resistance. This is due to the ability of veins to dilate with little increase in pressure (capacitance), in contrast to the arterial system.

VASCULAR CONTROL IN SPECIFIC TISSUES

Rushmer (1976) has pointed out that concise descriptions of peripheral vascular control are impossible owing to lack of knowledge and the complexity of the system. In addition to pressor and depressor areas of the medulla, diencephalic centers also exist which integrate reactions involving the vascular system, such as thirst, hunger, water balance, and temperature control. Impinging on these hypothalamic centers are multiple impulses from other areas of the brain.

The peripheral vasculature is controlled by several factors. Arterioles are supplied with nerve fibers from the sympathetic system. Stimulation of these fibers releases norepinephrine at the nerve endings causing the arteriolar muscle to contract, narrowing or closing the lumen of the vessel.

Stimulation of parasympathetic nerves supplying certain glands may cause an intense vasodilatation. It has been shown that this may be due to release of bradykinin into the interstitial spaces.

The cerebral blood flow is probably the most stable in the body as far as vasomotor influences are concerned. Carbon dioxide increases cerebral blood flow, but rarely elevates it twofold. Reduced oxygen tension also dilates cerebral blood vessels. Blood flow is not uniform throughout the central nervous system, varying

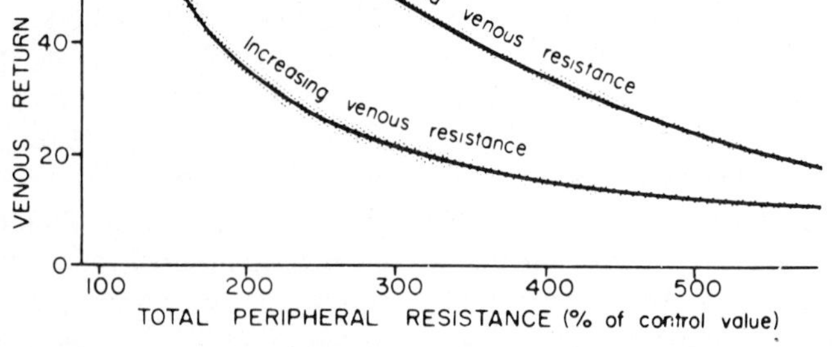

Figure 5–19. Effect on venous return of increasing the total peripheral resistance when the resistance is increased in three different ways: (1) by injecting microspheres into the arteries to increase arterial resistance, (2) by constricting the inflow veins to the heart, and (3) by combining these two procedures. (From Guyton, A.C.: Venous Return. Am. J. Physiol., 196:1008, 1959.)

from 0.14 ml/g in spinal white matter to 1.8 ml/g in the inferior colliculus.

The pulmonary vascular bed is also rather unresponsive to normal vascular control. Pulmonary resistance is low, and can become even lower to allow two to three times the flow with little increase in pressure gradient. Hypoxia apparently induces some vasoconstriction, tending to shunt blood from inactive lung parenchyma to areas where gases can be exchanged.

The pulmonary bed serves as an overflow reservoir for the extrathoracic capacitance vessels and also as a reservoir to allow the left ventricle to adjust to sudden changes in venous return. The right heart acts much as a sluice gate separating systemic veins from the pulmonary circulation. Mean pressures in the central veins and pulmonary artery rise and fall together.

The liver is served by two vascular systems: the portal vein carrying about four-fifths of the inflow and the hepatic artery carrying the remainder. Sympathetic nerve stimulation and norepinephrine cause constriction of both the portal and hepatic systems. A significant feature in the canine liver is the presence of "throttling veins." These are sublobular veins containing sphincters that, when closed, produce hepatic venous pooling (Arey, 1941).

The spleen can be contracted by stimulation of the splenic nerve, greatly increasing the vascular resistance and forcing blood cells into the systemic circulation. Norepinephrine is said to cause increased resistance, whereas epinephrine empties the cells into the general circulation. Cholinergic substances produce dilatation.

Norepinephrine and epinephrine cause vasoconstriction of the renal vessels. Temporary clamping of these vessels produces a reactive hyperemia due to unknown vasodilator substances. Above 70 mm Hg, blood flow through the kidney shows little change, despite increases in arterial pressure, because of an autoregulatory mechanism.

The gastrointestinal tract is profusely supplied with splanchnic nerves that also control the splanchnic vascular bed. Alpha receptors in these vessels respond to norepinephrine by vasoconstriction. Dilatation occurs following isoproterenol injection. The autonomic nerves act only on the alpha receptors. A slight dilatation occurs with acetylcholine administration, suggesting that gamma receptors may be present. Inhalation of 5 to 15% carbon dioxide has been shown to cause vasodilation.

The heart is supplied by coronary arteries and drained by coronary veins. The major portion of coronary blood flow occurs during diastole because the pumping action of the heart actually impedes coronary artery flow. Increase in myocardial contraction, such as occurs when catecholamines are given, increases myocardial work while simultaneously impeding coronary flow.

The direct effects of epinephrine, norepinephrine, and acetylcholine on the coronary arteries are equivocal. Carbon dioxide and pH changes also appear to have little effect, though low oxygen tension in coronary blood causes dilatation.

Skeletal muscle has a double sympathetic innervation. The constrictor fibers activate alpha receptors while a second fiber type causes vasodilatation through cholinergic gamma receptors. Beta receptors, which react only to circulating catecholamines, are also present, but their role is obscure. The vascular bed in muscle also reacts to vasodilator substances released by exercise.

The most complex control system is in the skin where a myriad of effects have been described. Nervous control is predominantly sympathetic vasoconstrictor. No vasodilator fibers are known to exist, but unidentified vasodilator substance are known to occur. Changing oxygen and carbon-dioxide tensions do not seem to produce vasomotor changes. Heat and cold, on the other hand, produce marked vasodilatation or vasoconstriction.

In summary, it may be said that blood flow, oxygen consumption, and vasomotor control vary in the vascular beds of various tissues. Circulating hormones, epinephrine, norepinephrine, and acetylcholine appear to have little activity under normal circumstances. The role of vasodilator substances developed in hypoxic tissues has not been well defined.

CARDIOVASCULAR EFFECTS OF GENERAL ANESTHESIA

> ". . . no general anesthetic is known which, when present in anesthetic concentration, fails to depress contractility in mammalian hearts."
>
> —Price, 1961

TABLE 5–3. The Effect of pH Changes on the Function of the Dog Heart-Lung Preparation

Control pH	*Study pH*	*% Decrease in Function*	*How pH Change Produced*
7.33	6.96	77	CO_2
7.37	7.18	54	CO_2
7.54	7.38	38	CO_2
7.76	7.22	45	HCl
7.65	6.99	55	CO_2
7.60	7.37	48	HCl

(From Price, H.L., and Helrich, M.: The Effect of Cyclopropane, Diethyl Ether, Nitrous Oxide, Thiopental, and Hydrogen Ion Concentration on the Myocardial Function of the Dog Heart-Lung Preparation. J. Pharmacol. Exp. Ther., 115:206, 1955.)

Knowledge of the probable cardiovascular responses to a given drug or combination of drugs during anesthesia is of great importance to the anesthesiologist. Anesthetics, through direct effects on the myocardium, affect conductivity and contractility, producing changes in cardiac rate, rhythm, and output. Peripherally, these agents have direct action upon the arterioles, capillaries, and venules.

Changes in cardiovascular function during anesthesia may be due to factors other than the direct effect of anesthetic drugs on the heart or vasculature. The two most important of these are changes in ventilation and autonomic nervous system activity. At surgical levels, almost all anesthetic agents depress ventilation and produce hypoxia and hypercapnia, either of which, if not corrected, will alter cardiac function (Table 5–3). Although the changes in heart rate are variable, severe hypoxia will produce a deep depression of myocardial contraction. An increase in blood pressure, related to the release of catecholamines, commonly occurs during the early phase of hypercapnia and, at the same time, increased carbon dioxide depresses myocardial contraction and adds to the cardiac depression produced by hypoxia and drugs. In studies on humans, Theye et al. (1966) found that hypocapnia during ether or halothane anesthesia decreased cardiac output, probably through altered sympathetic nervous system activity.

As carbon dioxide is eliminated during recovery from anesthesia, the effect is similar to withdrawal of a vasopressor, and hypotension may occur. Selection of an anesthetic agent thus must take into consideration its effect upon blood pressure, cardiac output, cardiac rate, and related responses in other body systems. Anesthetic agents act upon the vasomotor center, as well as on the cardioaccelerator and cardioinhibitor centers of the central nervous system. They also act upon the respiratory centers, thereby indirectly producing cardiovascular changes.

The relative potency of various anesthetic agents in causing depression of cardiac reflexes is (from most to least depressant): volatile agents (chloroform, ether, halothane) > oxybarbiturates > cyclopropane > thiopental-nitrous oxide > chloralose (Price, 1961). Kohli et al. (1966) studied the influence of anesthetics and blood pressure on the functional refractory period (FRP) of spinal vagotomized dogs. The FRP may be defined as the minimum interval between two consecutive ventricular impulses propagated from the atrium. They found the FRP was prolonged in the following order: thiopental > pentobarbital > halothane or ether > cyclopropane. They postulated that anesthetic sensitization of the heart to epinephrine is not related to depression of A–V conduction.

The pure effect of an anesthetic agent may be altered by preanesthetic agents, since the latter also tend to change normal physiologic conditions. It has been shown that when narcotics are used, the S–A and A–V nodes and the bundle of His may be affected. This knowledge is important because certain of the general anesthetic agents commonly used also have direct action upon these structures.

Use of a laryngoscope, insertion of an endotracheal tube, and inflation of endotracheal tube cuffs produce an effect upon the cardiovascular system that must be recognized as a part of anesthesia. Surgical manipulation of the thoracic and abdominal viscera, irritation of the respiratory tract, and stimulation of the vagus nerve cause a marked response by the myocardium. These actions may produce both atrial and ventricular extrasystoles, delayed conduction time, and slowing or even arrest of the heart. Irritation of the nasal mucosa with gases also can reflexly cause cardiac arrest.

Although many investigators have reported the effects of individual anesthetic agents on the heart, it is often difficult to maintain or reproduce the same condition clinically in a patient at any given time. These variable results might well be expected since there are many influencing factors that cannot be controlled, such as age, sex, general physical condition, and species variation.

ANESTHETIC AGENTS AND THE HEART

Virtually all clinically useful general anesthetics produce direct depression of myocardial contractility (Table 5–4). Some cause minimal net depressant actions, owing to reflex sympathetic nervous system stimulation (indirect effect) which counteracts the depression. Ketamine or low doses of morphine can produce positive inotropic effects; diethyl ether and cyclopropane also have sympathetic stimulatory activity. Other inhalation anesthetics produce

TABLE 5–4. Effects of Anesthetic Drugs on Determinants of Cardiac Function

A. Direct Effects

Preload	Contractility	Afterload	Heart Rate
↓	↓	↓	↓

B. Indirect Effects*

PRELOAD	*Increased* 1. Barbiturates 2. Inhalation anesthetics	*Decreased* 1. Butyrophenones 2. Phenothiazines 3. Narcotics 4. Benzodiazepines 5. Xylazine	*Unchanged* 1. Belladona derivatives 2. Dissociative agents 3. Nitrous oxide 4. Muscle relaxants
CONTRACTILITY	*Increased* 1. Dissociative agents 2. Morphine (low doses)	*Decreased* 1. Butyrophenones 2. Phenothiazines 3. Narcotics 4. Barbiturates 5. Inhalation anesthetics 6. Nitrous oxide	*Unchanged* 1. Belladona derivatives 2. Benzodiazepines 3. Xylazine 4. Phenothiazines (?) 5. Muscle relaxants
AFTERLOAD	*Increased* 1. Dissociative agents 2. Nitrous oxide	*Decreased* 1. Butyrophenones 2. Phenothiazines 3. Narcotics 4. Benzodiazepines 5. Xylazine 6. Barbiturates 7. Inhalation anesthetics	*Unchanged* 1. Belladona derivatives 2. Muscle relaxants
HEART RATE	*Increased* 1. Belladona derivatives 2. Butyrophenones 3. Phenothiazines 4. Barbiturates 5. Dissociative agents 6. Nitrous oxide 7. Inhalation anesthetics	*Decreased* 1. Narcotics 2. Xylazine	*Unchanged* 1. Benzodiazepines 2. Muscle relaxants (?)

↓ = Depressant effect.
*Indirect effects are modulated primarily by the amount of autonomic nervous system activity.
(From Muir, W.W.: Anesthesia and the Heart. J.A.V.M.A., 171:92, 1977.)

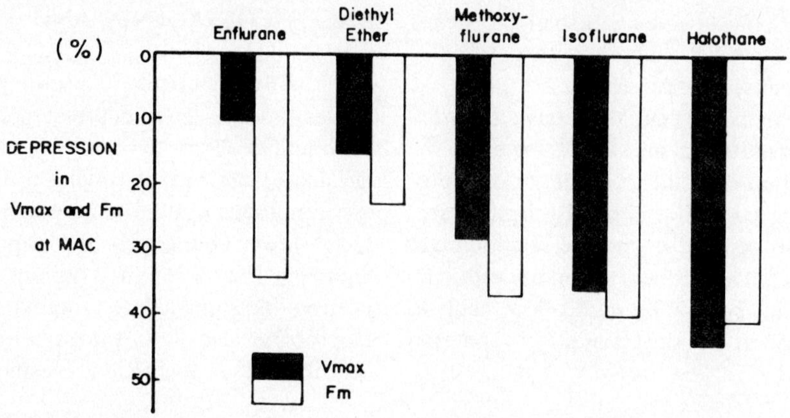

Figure 5–20. The mean maximal velocity of shortening (Vmax) and mean maximal developed force (Fm) in isolated cat papillary muscle at 32° C are depressed about 40% by 1 MAC isoflurane, halothane, or methoxyflurane. Enflurane and diethyl ether show less depression. (From Kemmotsu, O., Hashimoto, Y., and Shimasato, S.: Inotropic Effects of Isoflurane on Mechanics of Contraction in Isolated Cat Papillary Muscles from Normal and Failing Hearts. Anesthesiology, 39:470, 1973.)

dose-related decreases in ventricular contractility (Fig. 5–20). In light planes of anesthesia, this effect is minimal owing to some degree of sympathetic activity. With most inhalation agents given at low concentrations, cardiac output is maintained in spite of decreased contractility and arterial blood pressure (afterload) by increasing heart rate. All anesthetics can potentially depress the myocardium severely in high doses, or if the physiologic status of the patient is impaired. Neuromuscular blocking agents and local anesthetics have minimal effects on cardiac function in normal dosages (Fig. 5–21).

Heart rate, intramyocardial systolic-developed tension, and cardiac contractility are factors determining myocardial oxygen demands. Myocardial oxygen demand and oxygen delivery are closely interdependent. Coronary blood flow (oxygen delivery) correlates closely with arterial blood pressure (afterload). The latter also influences the tension that must be developed by the ventricle (oxygen demand). The normal heart matches oxygen delivery to oxygen demand, providing that near-normal cardiac rates and blood pressures are maintained. If, however, oxygen demand increases because of hypertrophy, dilatation, or tachycardia, or if oxygen delivery is decreased due to hypoxia or hypotension, the delicate balance is disrupted. Anesthetic depression of myocardial function is generally considered undesirable. However, if depression is accompanied by a reduction in

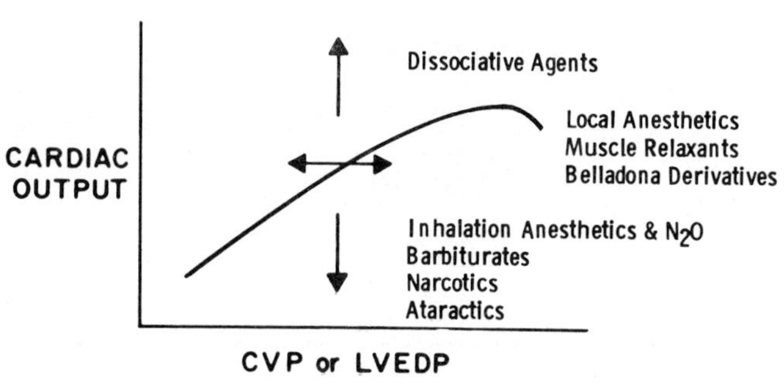

Figure 5–21. Effects of anesthetic drugs on the ventricular function curve in the clinically normal dog with intact reflex responses. CVP = Central venous pressure; LVEDP = left ventricular end diastolic pressure. (From Muir, W.W.: Anesthesia and the Heart. J.A.V.M.A., 171:92, 1977.)

cardiac work and an even greater reduction in myocardial oxygen demand, this effect might be beneficial. As an example, halothane decreases arterial blood pressure, thus decreasing afterload, myocardial systolic tension, and oxygen demand (Table 5–5). If pronounced hypotension develops, decreased coronary blood flow and decreased oxygen delivery result. If arterial blood pressure and coronary blood flow are maintained, however, potential benefit may result if reduced myocardial oxygen demand equals or is less than oxygen delivery. For example, the negative inotropic effects of fentanyl and halothane have been shown to reduce cardiac oxygen demand more than the corresponding decrease in oxygen delivery. Table 5–6 lists the effects of some agents on myocardial oxygen consumption.

There are two mechanisms by which anesthetics can depress cardiac energy sources: 1) interference with oxygen delivery and 2) depression of oxidative and glycolytic phosphorylation. Energy in the form of adenosine triphosphate and creatinine phosphate appears to be reduced by general anesthesia. There is no evidence to indicate a direct depressant effect of anesthetics on the contractile proteins of the myocardium. At high concentrations, anesthetics can irreversibly uncouple oxidative phosphorylation or cause reversible, partial inhibition of myocardial mitochondrial activity. This could affect nonesterified free fatty acid oxidation, which under normal conditions is the major energy source of the heart. This, in turn, could cause a dependence on glycolytic pathways that are also affected by anesthetics. A relative insulin insufficiency has been demonstrated and has been proposed to be the cause of decreased myocardial glucose extraction during inhalation anesthesia, resulting in a negative inotropic effect.

It has also been proposed that anesthetics interfere with myocardial Ca^{++} metabolism. The cardiac action potential correlates closely with electrolyte shifts across the cardiac cell membrane. Anesthetics may interfere with these

TABLE 5–5. Cardiovascular Effects of Four Anesthetic Agents in Miniature Swine* (Percent Change from Preanesthesia Control Values)

Agent	*Halothane*	*Methoxyflurane*	*Pentobarbital Na*	*Thiamylal Na*
Cardiac Output (ml/min)	−50	−39	−41	−38
Stroke Volume (ml)	−50	−48	−45	−41
Stroke Work (mm Hg L)	−69	−66	−40	−20
Mean Arterial Pressure (mm Hg)	−41	−29	+8	+34
Heart Rate (beats/min)	0	+20	+8	+9
Peripheral Vascular Resistance (mm Hg/L/min)	+14	+21	+86	+122
Hematocrit (%)	−22	−14	−17	−16

*Mean values from 8 measurements at 15-minute intervals.
(From Sawyer, D.C., Lumb, W.V., and Stone, H.L.: Cardiovascular Effects of Halothane, Methoxyflurane, Pentobarbital, and Thiamylal. J. Appl. Physiol., 30:36, 1971.)

TABLE 5–6. Effects of Anesthetic or Preanesthetic Drugs on MVO_2

Increased or Unchanged	*Decreased*
1. Diethyl ether	1. Enflurane
2. Cyclopropane	2. Halothane
3. Nitrous oxide	3. Methoxyflurane
4. Dissociative agents	4. Fluroxene
	5. Barbiturates
	6. Narcotics
	7. Ataractics

$M\dot{V}O_2$ = Myocardial O_2 consumption.
(From Muir, W.W.: Anesthesia and the Heart. J.A.V.M.A., 171:92, 1977.)

electrolyte alterations and Ca^{++} transcellular transport, resulting in a negative inotropic effect.

The many drugs used in anesthesia vary widely in their ability to produce dysrhythmias. With adequate oxygenation, most dysrhythmias are caused by autonomic nervous system imbalance. Disease states may also produce or exacerbate cardiac dysrhythmias.

For further information, the reader should consult the respective sections on individual anesthetic agents.

Several antibiotics have been shown to cause cardiovascular depression in anesthetized patients and to alter the cardiovascular effects of other unrelated drugs. The aminoglycosides interfere with uptake of Ca^{++} at superficial membrane-binding sites in vascular smooth muscle (Adams et al., 1974). As a result, contractile responses to norepinephrine, angiotensin II, serotonin, potassium chloride, and Ca^{++} are inhibited. Injection of Ca^{++} was found to antagonize the renal vasodilatory effects of streptomycin (Wolf and Wigton, 1971). Intravenous administration of Ca^{++} antagonizes the hypotensive effects of streptomycin during pentobarbital anesthesia in dogs (Pandey et al., 1964). It has been proposed that aminoglycosides cause a negative inotropic effect, by disrupting Ca^{++} transport in the excitation-contraction coupling process in heart cells (Fig. 5–22).

In experiments with isolated heart muscle, Ca^{++} completely overcame the myocardial depressant effects of gentamicin; however, norepinephrine only partially antagonized these. During pentobarbital anesthesia, isoproterenol and norepinephrine transiently antagonized the cardiovascular depression from neomycin, whereas Ca^{++} caused a sustained antagonism of the depression produced by neomycin and gentamicin (Adams et al., 1976).

By altering Ca^{++}-dependent functions, the

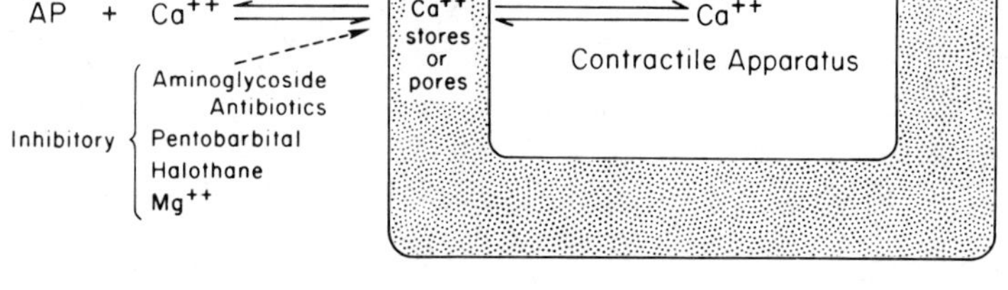

Figure 5–22. Schematic representation of excitation-contraction coupling in mammalian heart cell. An action potential (AP) instigates the inward movement of Ca^{++} through "Ca^{++} pores" or from superficial "stores" of Ca^{++} at the sarcolemmal membrane. Inward moving Ca^{++} activates the contractile mechanism or triggers the release of Ca^{++} from intracellular sites. The drugs listed are believed to exert at least part of their positive (facilitory) or negative (inhibitory) inotropic effects by altering Ca^{++} movements at the cell membrane. Solid lines denote physiologic pathways; dashed lines represent proposed sites of drug actions. (From Adams, H.R., Teske, R.H., and Mercer, H.D.: Anesthetic-Antibiotic Interrelationships. J.A.V.M.A., 168:409, 1976.)

aminoglycoside antibiotics act synergistically with anesthetics, resulting in accentuated cardiovascular depression.

REFERENCES

Adams, H.R., Goodman, F.R., and Weiss, G.B.: Alteration of Contractile Function and Calcium Ion Movements in Vascular Smooth Muscle by Gentamicin and Other Aminoglycoside Antibiotics. Antimicrob. Agents Chemother., 5:640, 1974.

Adams, H.R., Teske, R.H., and Mercer, H.D.: Anesthetic-Antibiotic Interrelationships. J.A.V.M.A., 168:409, 1976.

Ahlquist, R.P.: A Study of the Adrenotropic Receptors. Am. J. Physiol., 15:586, 1948.

Arey, L.B.: Throttling Veins in the Livers of Certain Mammals. Anat. Rec., 81:21, 1941.

Denlinger, J.K., and Nahrwold, M.L.: Cardiac Failure Associated with Hypocalcemia. Anesth. Analg., 55:34, 1976.

Dow, R.W., and Fry, W.J.: Regulation of Venous Capacity: The Carotid Sinus Mechanism. Surgery, 64:346, 1968.

Feuerstein, G., and Kopin, I.J.: Effect of PGD_2, PGE_2, PGF_2 and PGI_2 on Blood Pressure, Heart Rate and Plasma Catecholamine Responses to Spinal Cord Stimulation in the Rat. Prostaglandin, 212:189, 1981.

Fuchs, F., Reddy, Y., and Briggs, N.F.: The Interaction of Cations with the Calcium-binding Site of Troponin. Biochem. Biophys. Acta, 221:407, 1970.

Ishikawa, N., Ishikawa, T., and Shigei, T.: Possible Embryogenetical Differences of the Dog Venous System in Sensitivity to Vasoactive Substances. Jpn. J. Pharmacol., 30:807, 1980.

Jacobsen, D.C.: Prostaglandins and Cardiovascular Disease—A Review. Surgery, 93:564, 1983.

Kohli, J.D., Tuttle, R.R., Dresel, P.E., and Innes, I.R.: Influence of Anesthetics and of Arterial Blood Pressure on the Functional Refractory Period of Artrioventricular Conduction. J. Pharmacol. Exp. Ther., 153:505, 1966.

McKibben, J.S., and Getty, R.: A Comparative Morphologic Study of the Cardiac Innervation in Domestic Animals, I: Canine. Am. J. Anat., 122:533, 1968.

McKibben, J.S., and Getty, R.: A Comparative Morphologic Study of the Cardiac Innervation in Domestic Animals, II: Feline. Am. J. Anat., 122:545, 1968.

McKibben, J.S., and Getty, R.: Innervation of Heart of Domesticated Animals: Horse. Am. J. Vet. Res., 30:193, 1969.

McKibben, J.S., and Getty R.: Innervation of Heart of Domesticated Animals: Pig. Am. J. Vet. Res., 30:779, 1969.

Mellander, S.: Comparative Studies on the Adrenergic Neuro-hormonal Control of Resistance and Capacitance Blood Vessels in the Cat. Acta Physiol. Scand., 50:5, 1960.

Mellander, S., and Lewis, D.H.: Effect of Hemorrhagic Shock on the Reactivity of Resistance and Capacitance Vessels and on Capillary Filtration Transfer in Cat Skeletal Muscle. Circ. Res., 13:105, 1963.

Moreno, A.H., Burchell, A.R., van der Woud, R., and Burke, J.H.: Respiratory Regulation of Splanchnic and Systemic Venous Return. Am. J. Physiol., 213:455, 1967.

Muir, W.W.: Anesthesia and the Heart. J.A.V.M.A., 171:92, 1977.

Naylor, W.G., and Szeto, J.: Effect of Sodium Pentobarbital on Calcium in Mammalian Heart Muscle. Am. J. Physiol., 222:339, 1972.

Pandey, K., Kumar, S., and Badola, P.R.: Neuromuscular Blocking and Hypotensive Effects of Streptomycin and Their Reversal. Br. J. Anaesth., 36:19, 1964.

Price, H.L.: Calcium Reverses Myocardial Depression Caused by Halothane. Anesthesiology, 41:576, 1974.

Price, H.L.: Circulatory Actions of General Anesthetic Agents and the Homeostatic Roles of Epinephrine and Norepinephrine in Man. Clin. Pharmacol. Ther., 2:163, 1961.

Prinzmetal, M., Ornitz, E.M., Simkin, B., and Bergman, H.C.: Arterio-venous Anastomoses in Liver, Spleen, and Lungs. Am. J. Physiol., 152:48, 1948.

Rushmer, R.F.: Cardiovascular Dynamics, 4th ed. W.B. Saunders Co., Philadelphia, 1976.

Sperelakis, N., and Schneider, J.A.: A Metabolic Control Mechanism for Calcium Ion Influx That May Protect the Ventricular Myocardial Cell. Am. J. Cardiol., 37:1079, 1976.

Thames, M.D.: Reflex Control of the Circulation. Annual Refresher Course Lectures, American Society Anesthesiologists Annual Meeting, 1980.

Theye, R.A., Milde, J.H., and Michenfelder, J.D.: Effect of Hypocapnia on Cardiac Output During Anesthesia. Anesthesiology, 27:778, 1966.

Truex, R.C., and Smythe, M.O.: Comparative Morphology of the Cardiac Conduction Tissue in Animals. Ann. N.Y. Acad. Sci., 127:19, 1965.

Wiedeman, M.P.: Dimensions of Blood Vessels from Distributing Artery to Collecting Vein. Circ. Res., 12:375, 1963.

Wolf, G.L., and Wigton, R.S.: Vasodilation Induced by Streptomycin in the Perfused Canine Kidney. Arch. Int. Pharmacodyn. Ther., 194:285, 1971.

CHAPTER 6

Physiology of Respiration

INTRODUCTION

Respiration is the transfer of gases between living organisms and their environment. In mammals, respiration entails the absorption of oxygen and the excretion of carbon dioxide. The mechanisms by which these gases are transported to and from the cell are likewise utilized for the passage of anesthetics. This transport of gases and anesthetics requires both effective respiratory and cardiovascular function. The latter is discussed in Chapter 5. It is axiomatic that safe, effective anesthesia must not impair the gaseous and metabolic environment of the cell and, therefore, the transport systems associated with the maintenance of this environment. Despite such a prerequisite for safe anesthesia, most anesthetics currently in use do suppress respiratory and cardiovascular functions—functions that are already impaired in many animals requiring anesthesia. It is thus essential that the anesthesiologist comprehend both respiratory and cardiovascular physiology.

DEFINITIONS

Pulmonary ventilation is accomplished by expansion and contraction of the lungs. Several terms are used to describe the various types of breathing that may be observed.

1. *Eupnea* is ordinary quiet breathing.
2. *Dyspnea* is labored breathing.
3. *Tachypnea* is increased respiratory rate.
4. *Hyperpnea* is fast and/or deep respiration, indicating "overrespiration."
5. *Polypnea* is a rapid, shallow, panting type of respiration.
6. *Bradypnea* is slow regular respiration.
7. *Hypopnea* is slow and/or shallow breathing indicating "underrespiration."
8. *Apnea* is transient cessation of breathing.
9. *Cheyne-Stokes respirations* increase in rate and depth and then become slower followed by a brief period of apnea.
10. *Biot's respirations* are sequences of several gasps, apnea, and several deep gasps.
11. *Kussmaul's respirations* are regular deep respirations without pause.
12. *Apneustic respiration* is long gasping inspirations with several subsequent ineffective exhalations.

To describe the events of pulmonary ventilation, air in the lungs has been subdivided into four different *volumes* and four different *capacities* (Fig. 6–1).

1. *Tidal volume* (V_T) is the volume of air inspired or expired in one respiration.
2. *Inspiratory reserve volume (IRV)* is the volume of air that can be inspired over and above the normal tidal volume.

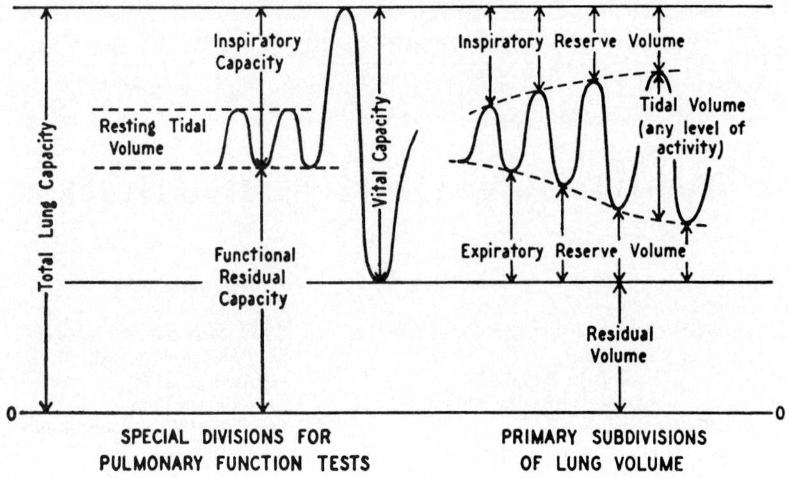

Figure 6–1. Lung volumes and capacities. (From: Standardization of Definitions and Symbols in Respiratory Physiology. Fed. Proc., 9:602, 1950.)

3. *Expiratory reserve volume (ERV)* is the amount of air that can be expired by forceful expiration after a normal tidal expiration.
4. *Residual volume (RV)* is the air remaining in the lungs after the most forceful expiration.

Another term frequently used is the *minute respiratory volume* or *minute volume*. This is equal to the tidal volume times the respiratory rate.

Occasionally, it is desirable to consider two or more of the aforementioned volumes together. Such combinations are termed *pulmonary capacities*.

1. *Inspiratory capacity (IC)* is the tidal volume plus the inspiratory reserve volume. This is the amount of air that can be inhaled starting after a normal expiration and distending the lungs to the maximum amount.
2. *Functional residual capacity (FRC)* is the expiratory reserve volume plus the residual volume. This is the amount of air remaining in the lungs after a normal expiration. Values for the dog are illustrated in Table 6–1.
3. *Vital capacity (VC)* is the inspiratory reserve volume plus the tidal volume plus the expiratory reserve volume. This is the maximum amount of air that can be expelled from the lungs after first filling them to their maximum extent.
4. *Total lung capacity (TLC)* is the inspiratory reserve volume plus the tidal volume plus the expiratory reserve volume plus the residual volume, or the maximum volume to which the lungs can be expanded with the greatest possible inspiratory effort.

The important factor in pulmonary ventilation is the rate at which *alveolar* air is renewed by atmospheric air. This is not equal to the minute respiratory volume because a large portion of inspired air is used to fill the respiratory passages, rather than the alveoli, and no significant gaseous exchange occurs in this air. Air that fills the respiratory passages, the nose, pharynx, trachea, and bronchi, is termed *dead space air.* On inspiration, new air must displace that in the dead space before it reaches the alveoli. The volume of air entering the alveoli with each breath is equal to the tidal volume (V_T) minus the dead space volume (V_D).

Dead space has been further divided into anatomic and physiologic divisions. Anatomic dead space is the volume of all spaces of the respiratory system except the alveoli. If alveoli

TABLE 6–1. Functional Residual Capacity (FRC) of the Dog as Reported by Several Investigators, Using Different Methods of Measurements

Investigator	*Breed*	*Method*	*Anesthetized*	*Position*	*FRC (ml/kg ± S.D.)*
Dubin and Westcott	Beagle	Open circuit	No	Standing	34.8 ± 6.6
Kleinman, et al.	Mongrel	Closed circuit	Yes	Supine	38.7 ± 7.5
Harvey and Schilling	Mongrel	Pressure volume	Yes	Not specified	30.7 ± 2.6
Simmons and Hemingway	Mongrel	Open circuit	Yes	Supine	24.9 ± 5.4
Simmons and Hemingway	Mongrel	"Direct"	Yes	Supine	31.2 ± 4.1
Cook, et al.	Mongrel	Pressure volume	Yes	Prone	32.9 ± 8.3

(From Dubin, S., and Westcott, R.J.: Functional Residual Capacity of Normal Unanesthetized Beagle Dogs. Am. J. Vet. Res., 30:2027, 1969.)

for some reason are nonfunctional, or if pulmonary blood flow to some alveoli is low, then these too may be considered dead space. Thus, physiologic dead space includes not only the anatomic dead space, but any alveolar dead space that may be present. In a normal animal, the anatomic and physiologic dead space are essentially the same but, in pulmonary disease, the physiologic dead space may be several times larger.

RESPIRATORY CHARACTERISTICS OF VARIOUS SPECIES

Data concerning respiration of several species are listed in Table 6–2 and Figure 6–2. Stahl (1967) has correlated respiratory variables on the basis of log-log relationships (allometry) in animals varying in size from the rat to man. He suggests that prediction formulas probably cover animals from mice to steers and possibly all mammals (Table 6–3).

The higher metabolic rate of smaller species is reflected in a relatively high oxygen requirement (Table 6–4).

Anesthesia lowers the metabolic rate and oxygen consumption. Tanaka et al. (1961) found that thiopental-anesthetized dogs had a mean oxygen uptake of 10.45 ml/kg/min. When cooled to 30° C, this was reduced to 6.25 ml/kg/min.

Farhi et al. (1957) measured intrapleural pressure in anesthetized dogs and found that, at the peak of inspiration, negative pressure was as much as −14.3 cm H_2O. At any given point within the pleural cavity, pressures did not vary more than 1 cm.

CONTROL OF RESPIRATION

With the aid of the circulation, respiration regulates the oxygen, carbon dioxide, and hydrogen ion environment of the cell. Respiratory function is controlled by central respiratory centers, central and peripheral chemoreceptors, pulmonary reflexes, and certain other reflexes. This complex control system produces a combination of respiratory frequency and depth which is best suited for optimum ventilation with minimal effort (Comroe, 1974).

Central respiratory centers (Fig. 6–3) are the pneumotaxic center in the upper pons, the apneustic center in the lower pons, hydrogen ion receptors in the upper and lateral medulla, and the medullary respiratory center in the lower medulla. The medullary center includes both inspiratory and expiratory centers and, as might be expected, is the most primitive. Acting alone, this center initiates and maintains a gasping, arrhythmic inspiratory-expiratory sequence. The apneustic center, when uncontrolled, is responsible for prolonged inspiratory movements that are normally modified by the pneumotaxic center and by various vagal reflexes. Thus, with the aid of the various stimuli that they receive, the central respiratory centers are able to induce a normal respiratory pattern (Comroe, 1974).

Variations in oxygen, carbon dioxide, and hydrogen ion concentrations are detected by both peripherally and centrally located chemoreceptors, and the information is transmitted to the

TABLE 6–2. Respiratory Rate, Tidal and Minute Volumes: Vertebrates
(Values, unless otherwise specified, are for the resting state)

Animal	*Body Weight kg*	*Condition*	*Respiratory Rate breaths/min*	*Tidal Volume[1] ml*	*Minute Volume L/min*
		MAMMALS			
Beaver *(Castor canadensis)*	18		16		
Cat *(Felis catus)*	3.7 (2.3–5.7)		30 (24–42)	34 (20–42)	0.96 (0.86–1.09)
Cattle *(Bos taurus)*	144–514	Lying	30–35	1400–3400	46–104
	144–514	Standing	27–32	1500–4200	49–114
Dog *(Canis familiaris)*[2]	30.5		16 (11–18)	432	6.1 (5.1–7.4)
	28.6		17 (11–21)	302	5.3 (4.9–5.4)
	19.1		22 (13–37)	251	5.5 (4.5–6.4)
	16.4		13 (12–16)	296	4.1 (3.3–4.9)
Giraffe *(Giraffa sp.)*		Standing	31.8 (17–58)	3404 (3090–3508)	
Goat *(Capra hircus)*			19	310	5.7
Guinea pig *(Cavia cobaya)*	0.466 (0.274–0.941)		90 (69–104)	1.8 (1.0–3.9)	0.16 (0.10–0.38)
Hamster *(Mesocricetus auratus)*	0.092 (0.065–0.134)		74 (33–127)	0.8 (0.42–1.2)	0.06 (0.033–0.083)
Horse *(Equus caballus)*	486 ± 3.5		10.0 ± 1.2	7500 ± 370	200 ± 24.6
Marmot *(Marmota marmota)*	2.13	Awake[3]	8.0	22	0.174
		Hibernating[4]	0.68	13 (11.3–14.8)	0.0089
Monkey *(Macaca rhesus)*	2.68 (2.05–3.08)		40 (31–52)	21 (9.8–29)	0.86 (0.31–1.41)
Mouse *(Mus musculus)*	0.02 (0.012–0.026)		163 (84–230)	0.15 (0.09–0.23)	0.024 (0.011–0.036)

Porpoise *(Tursiops truncatus)*[5]	170		1.1 (0.9–1.93)	9000 (8000–10,000)	9.7 (9.0–10.4)
Rat, cotton *(Sigmodon hispidus)*	0.77		94.5 (75–115)	0.35 (0.24–0.70)	0.04 (0.023–0.071)
white *(Rattus norvegicus)*	0.113 (0.063–0.152)		85.5 (66–114)	0.86 (0.60–1.25)	0.073 (0.05–0.101)
Seal *(Phoca vitulina)*[6]	27.5		9 (6–12)		3.97
Sheep *(Ovis ories)*	59.9 (46.6–74.0)	Rectal temperature 39.69 (39.30–40.13)°	20 (15.7–23.6)	362 (287–455)	7.10 (5.95–7.69)
Sloth *(Cholepus hoffmanni)*	4.5		13		0.844 (0.78–0.96)
(Bradypus griseus)	3.1		6.2 (4.5–8.0)		0.485 (0.33–0.73)
		BIRDS			
Canary			108 (96–120)		
Chicken *(Gallus domesticus)*, ♂	4.2		17 ± 1	46 ± 2	0.777 ± 0.039
♀	3.4		27 ± 2	31 ± 2	0.766 ± 0.044
Duck (*Anas* sp.), ♂		Standing	42	30 (35–38)	
♀		Supine	110		
Goose (*Anser* sp.), ♂			20		
♀			40		
Pigeon *(Columbia livia)*		Standing	(25–30)	4.7 (4.5–5.2)	
		Supine	(25–30)		
Turkey *(Meleagris gallapavo)*, ♂			2.8		
		REPTILE			
Turtle *(Malaclemys terrapin centrata)*[7]	0.65–0.72		3.7	14	0.051

[1]Air inspired or expired in one respiration. [2]Measurements made after 30-minute rest in hammock, at 24° C; values corrected to BTPS conditions. [3]Rectal temperature = 37.8° C. [4]Rectal temperature = 5–6° C. [5]Captive animal. [6]Cheyne-Stokes respiration. [7]Ambient temperature 24–29° C. (Modified from Gleysteen, J.J., and Stroud, R.C.: In: *Respiration and Circulation*. Federation of American Societies for Experimental Biology, Bethesda, Maryland, 1971.)

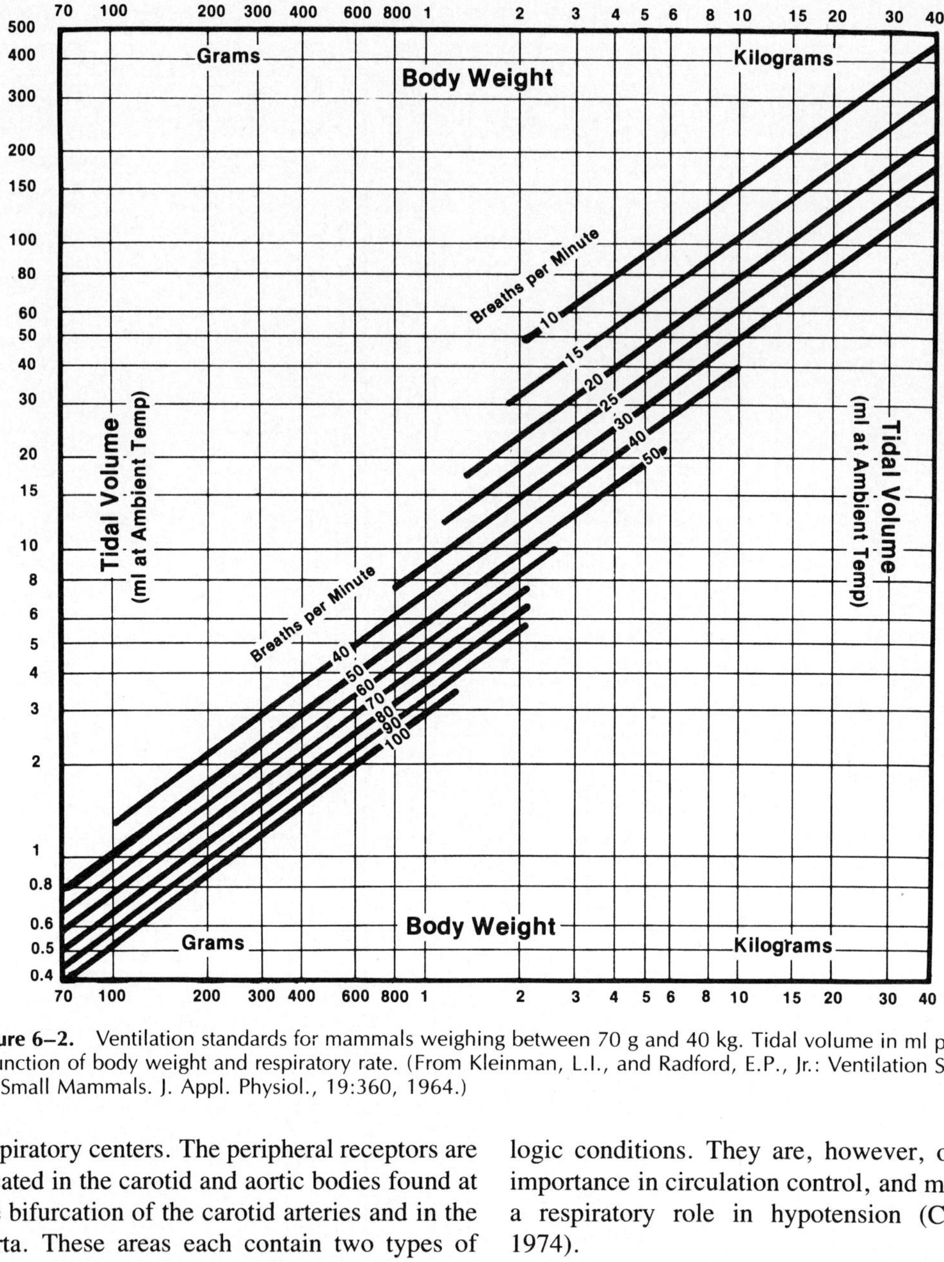

Figure 6–2. Ventilation standards for mammals weighing between 70 g and 40 kg. Tidal volume in ml plotted as a function of body weight and respiratory rate. (From Kleinman, L.I., and Radford, E.P., Jr.: Ventilation Standards for Small Mammals. J. Appl. Physiol., 19:360, 1964.)

respiratory centers. The peripheral receptors are located in the carotid and aortic bodies found at the bifurcation of the carotid arteries and in the aorta. These areas each contain two types of receptors: one type (pressoreceptor or baroreceptor) responds to pressure, the other (chemoreceptor) responds to chemical stimulation. Pressoreceptors are situated in the wall of the carotid sinus and the aortic arch; stimulation with consequent depression of respiration results from an increase in pulse pressure, pulse frequency, or mean pulse pressure. In mammals, the pressoreceptors do not appear to serve any respiratory function under normal physiologic conditions. They are, however, of great importance in circulation control, and may play a respiratory role in hypotension (Comroe, 1974).

The peripheral chemoreceptors are stimulated by a low partial pressure of oxygen rather than by a low oxygen content of the blood. The acute ventilatory response to hypoxia is mediated solely by these receptors, the stimulation of which becomes obvious upon breathing 18% oxygen or when the Pa_{O_2} becomes 70 mm Hg or less. These same chemoreceptors are sensitive to increased arterial partial pressures of carbon dioxide, probably via a decline in hydrogen

TABLE 6–3. Predicted and Observed Basal Values of Respiratory Variables in Common Mammals*

Animal	*TLC*	*FRC*	*V_T*	*V_D*	*f*	*$\dot{V}_E$*	*C_L*	*R*	*D_{LCO}*	*W_{BR}*
RAT										
Predicted	7–17	3–7	1.0–2.7	0.38–1.2	45–105	0.07–0.18	0.31–0.64	38–93	0.02–0.07	217–470
Reported	8–11	1–2	1.5–1.8		97–115	0.16–0.24	0.3–0.6	71–119		250–1,000
CAT										
Predicted	130–300	58–160	16–44	5–15	22–52	0.6–1.6	5–12	6–14	0.5–1.5	1,500–3,900
Reported	130–260	66–145	25–34	5–16	26–30	0.3–1.0	5–15	8–20	0.7–1.2	1,300–2,900
DOG										
Predicted	550–1,400	270–800	69–192	17–67	15–37	1,800–4,900	25–54	2.1–5.6	2.4–7.7	4,500–12,000
Reported	900–1,000	250–600	140–260	70–100	18–26	2,000–6,000	30–75	0.6–3.7	1.7–10	2,200–9,500
MAN										
Predicted	2,700–7,300	1,500–4,700	330–970	67–330	10–25	6,000–17,000	130–290	0.7–2.0	13–47	15,000–44,000
Reported	5,000–6,000	2,400–3,700	400–500	150	11–22	6,000–7,000	125–200	0.9–1.9	17–50	30,000–50,000

The reported range is usually the total range from one or more references. *Predicted values for 0.25-kg rat, 3.7-kg cat, 15.0-kg dog, 70.0-kg man, shown with estimated 1 standard error limits based both on slope and intercept values. TLÇ = total lung capacity (ml); FRC = functional residual capacity (ml); V_T = tidal volume (ml); V_D = dead space (ml); f = frequency of respiration (min); V_E = minute volume (ml/min); C_L = lung compliance (ml/cm H_2O); R = flow resistance (cm H_2O/(liters/sec)); D_{LCO} = diffusing capacity CO (ml/mm Hg per min); W_{BR} = power of breathing (g-cm/min).

(From Stahl, W.R.: Scaling of Respiratory Variables in Mammals. J. Appl. Physiol., 22:453, 1967.)

TABLE 6–4. Oxygen Consumption: Vertebrates

Species (Synonym)	No. and Sex	Body Weight g	Temperature, °C		O_2 Consumption $ml \cdot g^{-1} \cdot hr^{-1}$
			Body	Ambient	
PRIMATES					
Homo sapiens Caucasians	6♂	71,500	....	....	0.210
	♀	60,000	....	....	0.198
Macaca mulatta[1]	11	3,200	....	....	0.43
Pan troglodytes[1]	22	38,000	....	20–29	0.249
Papio ursinus	17	16,400	37	27	0.304
Saguinus geoffroyi	1	225	....	~27	1.04
Saimiri sciureus[1]	....	840	....	....	0.83
ARTIODACTYLA					
Bos taurus, Hereford[1]	♂[2]	700,000	....	....	0.11
	♀	500,000	....	....	0.114
Holstein[1]	♀	500,000	....	....	0.125
Shorthorn	♀[3]	380,000	39.0	18	0.160
Camelus dromedarius[1]	4	407,000	38.1	....	0.099
Capra sp.	....	36,000	....	....	0.193
Jamnapuri	26	26,600	....	....	0.272
Odocoileus virginianus	4	51,200	....	−7 to +24.7	0.226
Ovis aries[1]	5	51,500	....	....	0.256
Dorset[4]	♂	70,000	....	....	0.179
	♀	60,000	....	....	0.164
Sus scrofa	♂	250,000	....	....	0.130
	♀	250,000	....	....	0.121
PERISSODACTYLA					
Equus asinus	♀	190,000	37.2	20	0.204
		165,000	37.0	20	0.204
E. caballus[1]	....	703,000	....	....	0.145
Percheron[4]	♂[2]	650,000	....	....	0.110
	♀	675,000	....	....	0.125
CARNIVORA					
Canis familiaris[1]	3	9,700	38	25.4	0.342
Bull terrier	9	23,600	37.8	....	0.319
Mixed breed	59	13,900	....	18–24	0.327
	31	12,400	....	18–24	0.342
	14	20,800	39	....	0.359
	5	16,300	39	....	0.363
Felis catus[2]	....	3,000	....	....	0.44
Mustela vison	3	700	....	25	0.738
RODENTIA					
Cavia porcellus[1]	....	500	38.5	32	0.78
Chinchilla laniger[1]	....	402	....	....	0.68
Mus musculus	47	35.7	....	32	1.59
Rattus norvegicus[1]	40	545	37.5	28	0.84
LAGOMORPHA					
Oryctolagus cuniculus[1]	20	1,520	38.4–41.0	28	0.470
AVES					
Gallus domesticus (Chicken)	....	....	....	....	497
PISCES					
Carassius auratus (Goldfish)	....	....	....	20	85[4]*
Cyprinus carpio (Carp)	....	....	....	19.5	100*
Salmo trutta (Brown trout)	....	....	....	15	226*

*Values are cubic millimeters oxygen per gram fresh weight per hour for adult animals.
[1]Domestic animals. [2]Castrate. [3]Heifer. [4]Composite of data
(Abstracted from Altman, P.L., and Dittmer, D.S. (Eds.): *Biology Data Book*. Federation of American Societies for Experimental Biology, Washington, D.C., 1972.)

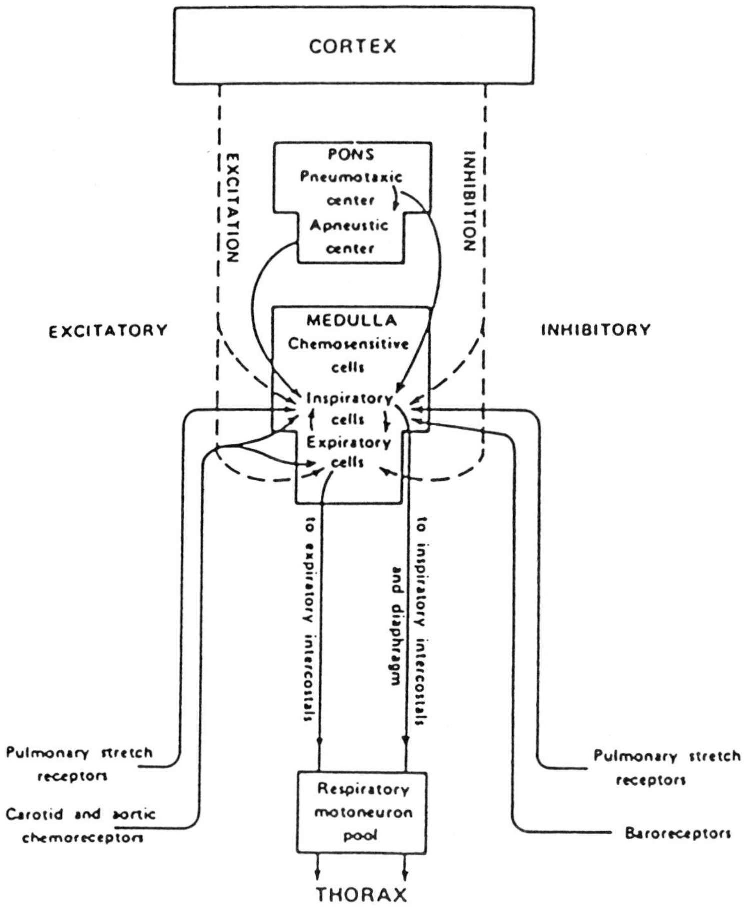

Figure 6–3. Schematic representation of the respiratory centers and the important connections. (From Lambertsen, C.J.: Neural Control of Respiration. In *Medical Physiology,* 14th ed. Edited by V.B. Mountcastle. The C.V. Mosby Co., St. Louis, 1980.)

ion concentration. The response to hypoxia is accentuated by a concurrent increase in $PaCO_2$ (Fig. 6–4). The greater ventilatory response to respiratory acidosis, in contrast to that which occurs from metabolic acidosis, results from response of the central chemoreceptors (Pavlin, 1976). Stimuli from peripheral chemoreceptors are transmitted to the respiratory center and thence to the respiratory apparatus.

Central chemoreceptors respond, as do the peripheral, to changes in the hydrogen ion concentration of their environment. Their location and sensitivity to hydrogen ions enable them to guard the environment of the cerebrospinal fluid (CSF). In contrast to the peripheral receptors, central chemoreceptors are not responsive to changes in oxygen tension, but do play a primary role in the total response to $PaCO_2$. Denervation of the peripheral chemoreceptors only reduces the respiratory response to CO_2 by 15% or less.

Most ions cross the blood-brain barrier slowly. Hydrogen and bicarbonate ions penetrate this barrier less readily than does carbon dioxide, which readily crosses. Because the CSF lacks a buffering system, the elevation of hydrogen ion concentration induced by CO_2 transfer is much greater than that of the blood. A time lapse is necessary, however, for these changes to occur in the CSF; the response of central receptors is therefore slower than their peripheral counterparts. Selective permeability

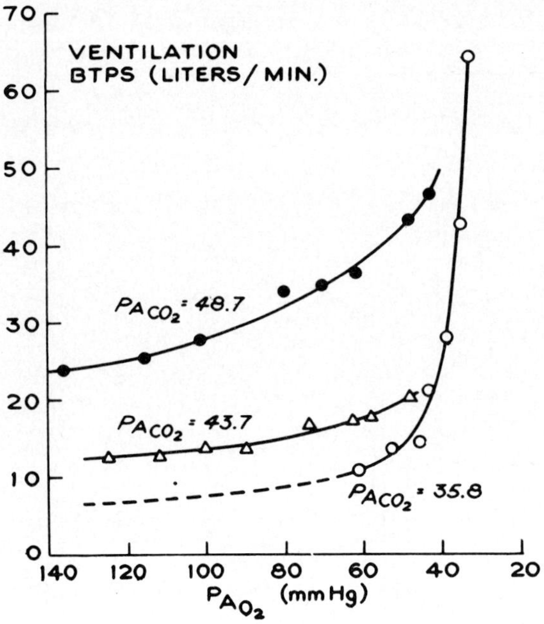

Figure 6–4. Increase in ventilation due to hypoxia associated with low and high levels of CO_2. Alveolar P_{CO_2} (P_{ACO_2}) was maintained close to 35.8 mm Hg *(bottom curve)*, 43.7 mm Hg *(middle curve)* and 48.7 mm Hg *(top curve)* in a subject given low O_2 mixtures to breathe. The two upper curves start *(left)* at higher levels because of the effect of higher CO_2 tensions. The slope of the upper curve becomes steeper than that of the lower ones because of interaction between the low O_2 and high CO_2 stimuli. Volume of ventilation corrected to BTPS; this = gas at body temperature, ambient pressure, saturated with water vapor. (Reproduced with permission from Comroe, J.H., Jr.: *Physiology of Respiration: An Introductory Text.* Copyright © 1965 by Year Book Medical Publishers, Inc., Chicago.)

of the blood-brain barrier to carbon dioxide explains the greater ventilatory response to increased carbon dioxide (respiratory acidosis) than to metabolic acidosis. In fact, hypocapnia resulting from stimulation of peripheral chemoreceptors by metabolic acidosis creates a central alkalosis and depresses respiratory drive.

Because the blood-brain barrier is not totally impermeable to hydrogen and bicarbonate ions, compensatory regulation across this barrier does occur in a matter of hours in the presence of sustained arterial acid-base disorders. In chronic hyperventilation due to hypoxia with ensuing CSF changes, there is an initial hypocapnic alkalosis of both blood and CSF. This is followed by a decrease in CSF bicarbonate with little apparent compensation in the plasma. Similar changes can be induced by hyperventilation under anesthesia. In dogs so hyperventilated, CSF bicarbonate concentration decreased after 2 hours and continued to decrease, although plasma bicarbonate remained unchanged. If, after several hours, hyperventilation ceases, the patient continues to hyperventilate despite arterial gas tensions indicative of respiratory alkalosis. This is because the CSF still has a low bicarbonate with a consequent central stimulus to maintain hyperventilation (Pavlin, 1976).

Although peripheral chemoreceptors are not essential for the characteristic respiratory response to carbon dioxide, they are important in the response to relatively large increases in Pa_{CO_2}. They facilitate the maintenance of ventilation when central carbon dioxide receptors are depressed, as by anesthesia and hypoxia. Peripheral chemoreceptors continue to function even after the death of other tissues, and under such circumstances are stimulated by decreased oxygen pressure rather than by changes in carbon dioxide and hydrogen ion concentration. Thus, they serve as a last line of defense against respiratory failure, and are even responsible for the last gasps of dying animals.

Most anesthetic and narcotic agents are respiratory depressants. They influence respiratory responses to carbon dioxide, and thereby the resting pulmonary artery CO_2 tension, the apneic threshold, and the ventilatory response to inspired CO_2 and to reduced tensions of inspired oxygen. In general, anesthetic agents elevate resting Pa_{CO_2} in a dose-related fashion, the respiratory system normally being set to maintain a Pa_{CO_2} between 38 and 43 mm Hg at sea level. The halogenated anesthetics, such as isoflurane, enflurane, and halothane, all elevate resting Pa_{CO_2}.

The apneic threshold refers to the $PaCO_2$ at which an anesthetized patient hyperventilated to the point of apnea will resume spontaneous ventilation. An increase in this threshold is an index of ventilatory depression. As ventilation becomes depressed in terms of an elevated resting Pa_{CO_2}, the apneic threshold is elevated an equivalent amount (Pavlin, 1976). The respiration of anesthetized patients can therefore be assisted

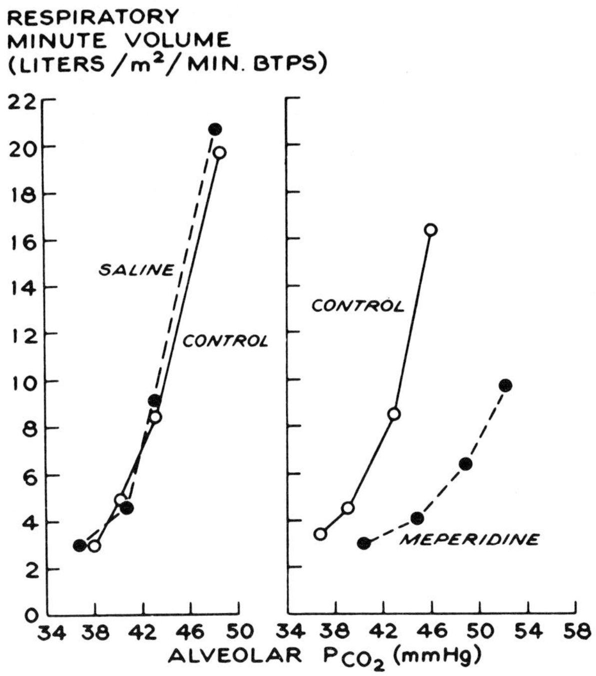

Figure 6–5. The CO_2 response curve. As the alveolar P_{CO_2} rises, the respiratory minute volume increases *(left)*. Saline injection has no effect on the curve. Narcotics, such as meperidine, and many anesthetics cause the curve to shift down and to the right, indicating a reduced response to CO_2 *(right)*. (Reproduced with permission from Comroe, J.H., Jr.: *Physiology of Respiration: An Introductory Text*. Copyright © 1965 by Year Book Medical Publishers, Inc., Chicago.)

to 5 to 9 mm Hg below the Pa_{CO_2} developed during spontaneous breathing. Apneic thresholds are then reached and controlled ventilation is required.

If minute ventilation is recorded in response to increasing inspired CO_2 concentrations, a CO_2 response curve is obtained. The slope of this response curve is linear; it is increased by progressive hypoxia, and is decreased by increasing concentrations of inhalation anesthetics. Cyclopropane and ether are least depressant, fluroxene and methoxyflurane are intermediate, and halothane, isoflurane, enflurane, and nitrous oxide depress the response most (Pavlin, 1976). Narcotic agents also increase resting Pa_{CO_2} values and decrease the slope of the CO_2 response curve (Fig. 6–5). During operation, afferent stimuli from the surgical field tend to overcome such respiratory depression. These stimuli cease after surgery, and respiration during recovery frequently becomes depressed.

Changes in ventilatory response to decreasing arterial oxygen tensions tend to follow a hyperbolic curve, in contrast to the linear response to CO_2. A response is first evident when the Pa_{O_2} falls below 100 mm Hg and increases sharply as Pa_{O_2} values fall to 60 mm Hg or less. Significant depression of this curve has been demonstrated in halothane, morphine, and barbiturate anesthesia.

Clinically, it is important to appreciate that respiration of hypoxic patients may be unresponsive to carbon dioxide and driven only by oxygen want. When this occurs, administration of oxygen relieves the hypoxia but eliminates the mechanism responsible for stimulation of the respiratory center. Prolonged, even fatal apnea may thus result if the central respiratory centers have been sufficiently depressed. In any case, respiratory depression continues until the Pa_{CO_2} rises to a threshold level sufficient to stimulate the respiratory reflexes or until the central depressant effects wear off.

In addition to stimuli originating in the central nervous system and the peripheral chemoreceptors, there are numerous pulmonary stimuli which modify respiration and which are initiated by three major classes of lung receptor: the pulmonary inflation-deflation receptors, the irritant receptors, and the type J receptors (Berger et al., 1977). The Hering-Breuer (inflation-deflation) receptors are thought to be within the airway smooth muscle; Miserocchi et al. (1973) found that the greatest concentration of stretch receptors occurred in the hilar portions of the airways in dogs. The inflation reflex is activated by pulmonary distension and sustained by continued inflation of the lungs. The primary effect via the vagal nerves is increased expiratory time; other effects are bronchodilation, tachycardia, and vasoconstriction (Berger et al., 1977). The threshold for their activation varies with age and species and is lowered by general anesthesia (Comroe, 1974; Berger et al., 1977). The reflex discharge is suppressed by elevated carbon dioxide concentrations, a response similar to that found in avian pulmonary receptors (Berger et al., 1977). Deflation of the lungs causes tachypnea, but it is uncertain whether this is due to lack of stimulation of the inflation receptors, to specific receptors, or to a response of irritant on "J" receptors (Comroe, 1974).

Irritant receptors were initially called rapidly adapting stretch receptors. They are presumed to lie between airway epithelial cells. Excitation results from such irritants as ether or ammonia, from particulate matter, and from histamine. Effects include cough, hyperpnea, and bronchoconstriction (Berger et al., 1977).

Juxtapulmonary-capillary ("J") receptors are supposedly located in the wall of the pulmonary capillary. They are believed, but not proved, to respond to pulmonary congestion. In the cat they are activated by hyperinflation of the lung (Berger et al., 1977).

The upper airways also possess receptors. Mechanical stimulation of the nose in anesthetized animals causes apnea, bradycardia, and sneezing. Similar stimulation of the epipharynx initiates a sniff or aspiration reflex, as well as bronchodilation and hypertension. Mechanical stimulation or irritation of receptors in the larynx and trachea induces coughing, slow deep breathing, apnea, bronchoconstriction, and hypertension (Berger et al., 1977).

Reflexes from the carotid sinuses and aortic arch also modify the respiratory pattern. Arterial hypotension induces hyperpnea, while hypertension depresses breathing. Certain chemoreceptors in the pulmonary and coronary circulations may induce bradycardia, hypotension, and apnea. The dog, for instance, has such receptors in the epicardium of the left ventricle. These chemoreceptors are not activated by chemical changes that normally occur in the body but may, depending upon the animal species, be activated by drugs such as veratrine, nicotine, serotonin, ATP, and some antihistamines (Comroe, 1974). It has been suggested that such reflexes may be activated by rapid intravenous injections (Comroe, 1974).

In horses under barbiturate anesthesia, when respiration is irregular and prolonged periods of apnea may occur, slight manual compression of the chest will often initiate a respiratory response. This may be due to stimulation of Hering-Breuer receptors.

In emergencies, advantage has been taken of the fact that certain afferent stimuli tend to produce reflex respiratory movements. Among these stimuli are dilation of the anal sphincter, traction on the tongue, and alternate immersion in hot and cold water. In cats, the point of a curved hemostat can be pressed on the hard palate and, with continuing pressure, slid posteriorly onto the soft palate to evoke a reflex respiration. A bilateral respiratory reflex initiated by light pressure on a localized area of the thoracic wall has been described in dogs and rabbits by Whitehead and Draper (1947). The area is approximately 1½ inches in diameter and is located at the point where the scalenus and rectus abdominis muscles and their aponeurotic tendons are in apposition. Pressure on this area produces smooth, normal respirations that are largely diaphragmatic. Although the reflex may become fatigued, its sensitivity returns rapidly. It is abolished by severe hypoxia, shock, and deep anesthetic depression. Compared with anal stretching and tongue traction, however, this is the last reflex to disappear with deepening anesthesia. Such procedures do not replace the need for assisted or controlled respiration when respiratory depression persists for more than a brief interval.

In some species, such as the dog, an increase in body temperature not only increases respiration but causes panting. This is induced by the hypothalamic thermoregulatory center and controlled by a panting center closely related to the pneumotaxic center (Guyton, 1981).

MECHANICAL FACTORS IN BREATHING

Now that the mechanisms by which alternating inspiration and expiration are controlled have been discussed, it is appropriate to consider transport of gases to and from the lungs. This depends on a pressure gradient between the atmosphere and the alveoli, on the resistance to flow between these two regions, and on the resistance of the lungs to distension. During inspiration, there is active muscular effort, a result of which is enlargement of the pleural cavity.

The intrapleural pressure is thereby reduced to a subatmospheric value, and a pressure gradient is established. In contrast to inspiration, expiration is normally passive and depends on the return of the chest and lungs to a resting position. Intrapleural pressure and, consequently, alveolar pressure are elevated, and the pressure gradient is reversed. Fluctuating pressure gradients between the atmosphere and the alveoli thus cause air to flow in and out of the lungs.

The ease with which air moves through the airways is contingent not only upon the driving pressure, but also upon airway resistance. According to the Hagen-Poiseuille law, gas flow through a tube is proportional to the pressure gradient across the tube, the fourth power of the diameter of the tube, and inversely to the viscosity of the liquid:

$$\text{pressure loss} = \text{constant} \times \text{viscosity} \times \frac{\text{length of tube}}{(\text{diameter})^4} \times \text{flow rate}$$

the constant depends on the units used and is 6.94×10^{-2}, if flow is expressed in liters per minute, pressure loss in millimeters of water, length and internal diameter in centimeters, and viscosity in terms relative to that of water (Macintosh et al., 1963). These relationships are true only if the gas particles or molecules move parallel to the tube (laminar flow). If the walls of the tube in which the gas is flowing are irregular or the critical flow rate of the gas is exceeded, the flow becomes disorderly (turbulent flow). The critical flow rate varies directly as the internal diameter of the tube and is modified by the ratio of the viscosity of the gas to its density.

The significance of a transition from laminar to turbulent flow is illustrated by the fact that, at rates approximating critical flow, the pressure loss increases by about 50% if the flow becomes turbulent (Macintosh et al., 1963). Airway resistance during respiration can be minimized by an airway that is as wide as possible, and in which sudden alterations in direction or diameter are avoided. (The hazards of increased airway resistance to expiration and inspiration are discussed in Chapter 7.)

The pressure across the airway can be measured by the difference between the pressure at the mouth and that recorded within the esophagus. Only 80% of the intraesophageal pressure is used, the remaining 20% in healthy individuals being considered to result from pulmonary tissue resistance (Comroe, 1974). It should be noted that a vertical gravity-related pleural pressure gradient also plays a role in intrapulmonary gas distribution (Rehder et al., 1975).

Airway resistance increases with the rate of respiration and with narrowing of the airway by contraction of the bronchiolar muscles. Constriction of bronchiolar smooth muscles, by stimulation of the vagal constrictor fibers, hypoxia, increased arterial P_{CO_2}, cold, emboli in certain parts of the pulmonary circulation, and by chemical irritation, not only increases airway resistance, but also decreases anatomic dead space. Locally elevated blood P_{CO_2} may cause bronchial constriction only in that part of the lung whose pulmonary blood flow is reduced, thereby limiting ventilation of alveoli not supplied with blood. This may be the mechanism by which there is proper matching of air supply and of mixed venous blood to the alveoli (Comroe, 1974).

Airway resistance is also increased by disease of the bronchioles, by foreign bodies, by collapse or kinking due to loss of normal support, and by parasympathomimetic drugs.

To inflate the lungs, it is necessary to apply force. The greater the force applied, the greater the pulmonary distension and, consequently, tidal volume. The relationship of the distending pressure to the resulting increase in volume serves as a measure of the elasticity or distensibility of the lungs. The volume change in liters in relation to a centimeter of water increase in pressure is termed *compliance* of the lungs. Since this may vary with the volume of the lung at the time of measurement, it is desirable to know the lung volume at the time. Compliance divided by lung volume is called specific compliance (Comroe, 1974). If compliance is increased, the lung is more distensible. Alternatively, if it is decreased, the lung is more rigid.

Lung compliance plus thoracic compliance equals total compliance.

Since the lungs consist of many bubble-like alveoli that are lined with a mucous-like substance, it is to be expected that resistance of the lungs to distension results from surface tension. The alveoli are lined by a surface-active complex lipoprotein, termed surfactant, which is first formed by alveolar cells relatively late in fetal life (Comroe, 1974). In bubbles, surface tension increases as the bubble size decreases. In alveoli, the surface tension is high when the lungs are inflated and low when they are deflated, thereby tending to prevent collapse of small alveoli and overinflation of large alveoli. In the absence of surfactant, collapse of the lungs may occur, as in congestive collapse, after prolonged inhalation of 100% oxygen, or in the neonatal respiratory distress syndrome. Production of surfactant is enhanced by administration of corticosteroids, and it is depleted by air pollution, infection, high and low tidal volumes, and overventilation of the lungs (Comroe, 1974; Rehder et al, 1975; Polgar and Weng, 1979).

Inflation and deflation of the lungs are dependent not only upon compliance of the lungs themselves, but also upon resistance of the thorax to movement. Since the lungs and thoracic cage tend to adhere to each other, these two structures act in unison. Because the thorax enlarges slightly in the resting state, the recoil of the thorax opposes that of the lung. Thoracic compliance can be measured by subtracting pulmonary compliance from the combined compliance of the lungs and thoracic wall (Comroe, 1974). When anesthetized and unanesthetized paralyzed patients were compared, reduced compliance of the respiratory system was reported during anesthesia. Reduced compliance of the lung during anesthesia has been attributed to atelectasis and is reversible by hyperinflation (Rehder et al., 1975). Alterations in the mechanical properties of the lung and chest wall in general anesthesia reduce FRC in recumbent positions (Rehder et al., 1975). Lai et al., (1979), studying dogs anesthetized with thiopental, were unable to detect any significant effect upon lung volumes, static pressure-volume curves of the chest or lung, or static compliance of the lung or chest wall. During halothane anesthesia, however, there was a significant reduction in FRC and mean lung compliance and an increase in mean chest wall and total system compliance in dogs in a supine position. (Southorn et al., 1980).

GASEOUS EXCHANGE ACROSS THE ALVEOLAR-CAPILLARY MEMBRANE

Having reached the pulmonary alveoli, inhaled gases must traverse the alveolar-capillary membrane to enter the blood; during exhalation, exchange in the reverse direction is likewise necessary. Gases passing between the alveolar lumen and capillary blood do so by diffusion, moving from places of high partial pressure to those of a lower partial pressure. At identical partial pressures, the rate of diffusion of gases depends on the size of their molecules and is inversely proportional to the square roots of their molecular weights (Graham's law) (Macintosh et al., 1963). Since a molecule of oxygen is smaller than one of carbon dioxide, the former diffuses faster. When diffusion occurs across a gas-fluid interface as in the alveolar-capillary membrane, the rate of diffusion of the gas is also directly proportional to the solubility of the gas in the liquid. Since carbon dioxide is more soluble in water than oxygen, it diffuses more rapidly across the alveolar membrane despite its larger molecule (Macintosh et al., 1963).

Provided flow of air to and from the alveoli and of blood through the pulmonary capillaries is optimal, and the characteristics of the intervening tissues remain normal, alveolar-capillary gaseous exchange is satisfactory. It is, therefore, readily apparent that there are three basic causes for impaired exchange of gases between the alveoli and pulmonary capillaries (Fig. 6–6): 1) abnormal alveolar-capillary membrane with impaired diffusion; 2) bypass of the pulmonary capillary circulation; and 3) failure to match functional pulmonary alveoli and capillaries. To be transported in the red blood cell, the gas must pass through surfactant, alveolar epithelial and capillary endothelial membranes, plasma, and the red cell membrane.

The pathway may be increased by thickening

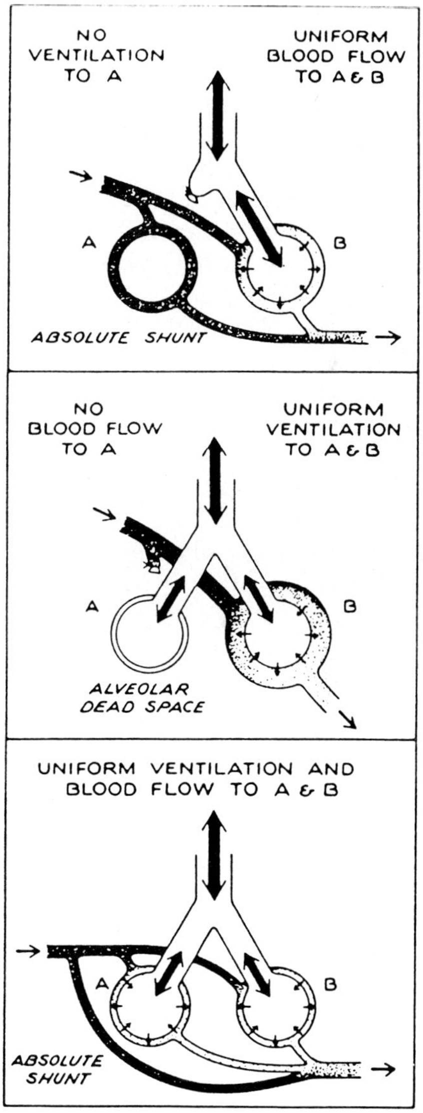

Figure 6–6. Uneven ventilation and pulmonary blood flow. The alveoli, where rapid gas exchange occurs, are represented by rounded areas. Leading into these are tubes depicting the conducting airways of anatomic dead space in which no effective gas exchange occurs. *Arrows* entering the alveoli show distribution of total inspired gas *(large arrow)* to various alveoli. *Small arrows* crossing alveolar walls show the process of diffusion of O_2 out of the alveoli into the blood and of CO_2 from the blood into the alveoli. The *shaded channel* surrounding the alveoli represents pulmonary blood flow. It enters the capillary bed as mixed venous blood *(dark)* and emerges as arterialized blood *(light)*. Top, lung *A* has no ventilation but normal blood flow, while lung *B* has normal ventilation and blood flow. Center, lung *A* has normal ventilation but no blood flow, while lung *B* has normal ventilation and increased blood flow. Bottom, a shunt of venous to arterial blood completely bypasses the lung. (Reproduced with permission from Comroe, J.H., Jr.: *Physiology of Respiration*, 2nd ed. Copyright © 1974 by Year Book Medical Publishers, Inc., Chicago.)

of alveolar and capillary membranes, by separation of these membranes by fluid, exudate, and cellular infiltration, and by capillary distension.

Just as gases must enter and leave the lungs from the atmosphere and must traverse the alveolar-capillary membrane, so their passage to and from the lungs via the pulmonary circulation is equally essential. The characteristics of blood flow through the alveolar capillaries are, therefore, as important as the exchange of air to and from the alveoli. Since blood flow through the capillaries is pulsatile, this allows more time for gas exchange, providing, of course, that cardiac stroke volume does not exceed the volume of the capillary bed. Should this happen, some blood passes directly through the capillaries and does not receive the benefit of the momentary pause between each pulse for gas exchange. Such a relationship can perhaps be compared to the carbon dioxide absorber in the circle-type anesthetic machine, in which it is necessary for the capacity of the absorber to be at least equal to the tidal volume of the patient. Not only does pulmonary flow vary with the heartbeat, it is also influenced by inflation and deflation of the lungs. Pulmonary blood flow is restricted by increased vascular resistance due to local hypoxia, a mechanism that may provide for shunting blood from poorly ventilated alveoli. This mechanism has, however, been shown to be inhibited by anesthetics in cats, and may contribute to greater alveolar/arterial Po_2 gradients observed during anesthesia (Nunn and Hulands, 1973). A decrease in pH has a similar effect (Comroe, 1974). Variations in pulmonary capillary blood flow are also caused by an open chest, varying degrees of vascular occlusion, venous-to-arterial shunts, cardiovascular disturbances (such as shock or cardiac failure), lesions (such as pulmonary necrosis and fibrosis), and by gravity.

Nonuniform ventilation, with failure to match functional alveoli and capillaries, is caused by variations in local compliance, airway resistance, airway closure following reduction of functional residual capacity (Nunn and Hulands, 1973; Gilmour et al., 1976), uneven transpulmonary pressure such as during thoracic operations, and by nonuniform expansion of the chest. Lack of ventilation of one part of the lung results in a mixture of oxygenated and poorly oxygenated blood and cannot be compensated for to any great extent by hyperventilation of the remainder as far as oxygen uptake is concerned. Hyperventilation can, however, compensate for lack of elimination of carbon dioxide in unventilated portions of the lungs providing the respiratory centers, muscles, thorax, and lungs are fully responsive to the elevated $Paco_2$. This difference between oxygen and carbon dioxide is due to their respective dissociation curves. When venous blood from pulmonary arteries passes into the pulmonary capillaries prior to the oxygen exchange, it is about 60% saturated with oxygen; after passing through normally ventilated lungs, it becomes approximately 97% saturated. Since saturation is already almost complete and since oxygen is relatively insoluble in plasma, additional ventilation or even addition of oxygen to the inspired gas is unlikely to cause any marked increase in saturation.

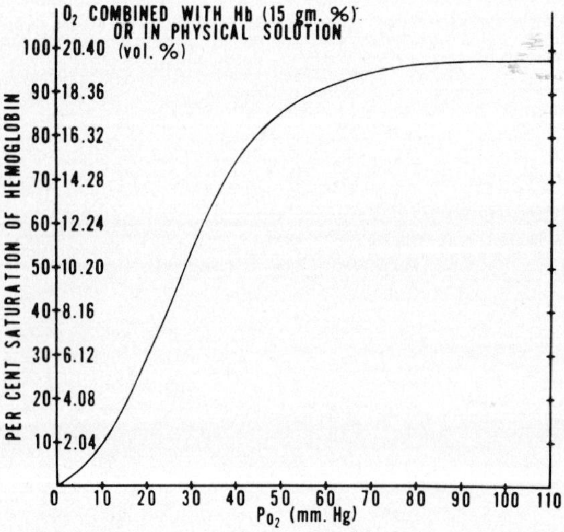

Figure 6–7. Oxygen-hemoglobin dissociation curve of dog blood at pH 7.40. The percentage HbO_2 and O_2 content change little when the Po_2 changes from 100 mm Hg (normal Po_2) to 60 mm Hg as may occur during cardiopulmonary dysfunction or disease. (From Gillespie, J.R., and Martin, D.B.: Long-Term Oxygen Cage Therapy for Hypoxemic Dogs. J.A.V.M.A., 156:717, 1970.)

This inability of blood to accept additional

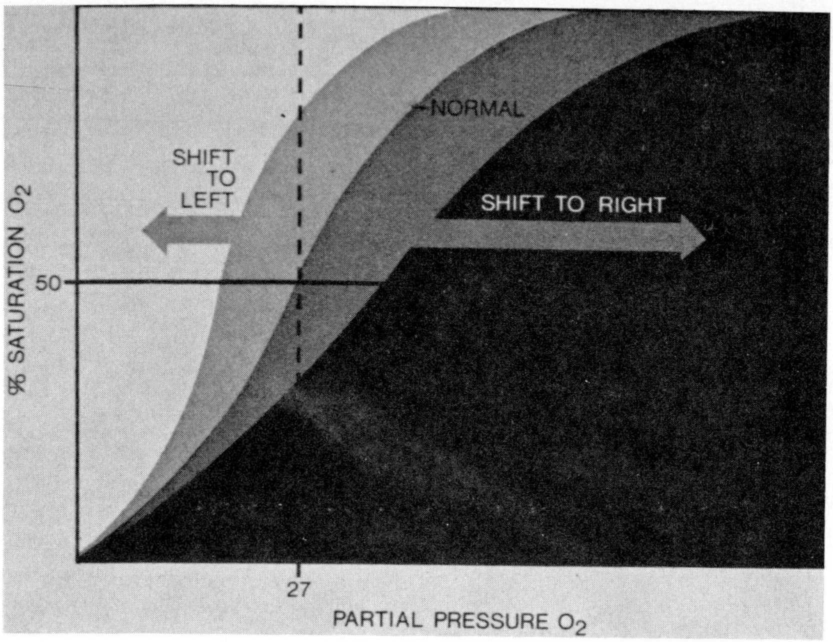

Figure 6–8. Hemoglobin affinity for oxygen. Increased oxygen affinity *(shift to the left)* means there will be a higher oxygen content at any given PO_2. Conversely, decreased oxygen affinity *(shift to the right)* means there will be a lower oxygen content at any given PO_2. A shift to the left is the result of alkalemia (decreased H^+), hypothermia (cold), hypocarbia (decreased PCO_2), and decreased 2,3-diphosphoglycerate. A shift to the right is the result of acidemia (increased H^+), hyperthermia (fever), hypercarbia (increased PCO_2), and increased 2,3-DPG. (Reproduced with permission from Shapiro, B.A., Harrison, R.A., and Walton, J.R.: *Clinical Application of Blood Gases*, 3rd ed. Copyright © 1982 by Year Book Medical Publishers, Inc., Chicago.)

oxygen is due to the nature of the hemoglobin dissociation curve (Fig. 6–7). At oxygen tensions similar to those of venous blood, hemoglobin is already 75% saturated (Fig. 6–8). Additional increments in the partial pressure of oxygen induce diminishing increases in the percent saturation of hemoglobin and the dissociation curve gradually flattens. Unlike the oxygen dissociation curve, that for carbon dioxide is more linear and the degree to which *hypocapnea* can be induced is limited only by the amount of hyperventilation.

When blood circulates through nonventilated lungs, this has the same effect as a venous-to-arterial shunt (see Fig. 6–6). In the event that this shunt is complete (absolute), even pure oxygen in the inspired gas will not increase the percent saturation of pulmonary venous blood to normal. If the shunt is only partial, or if the absolute shunt in relation to the total perfused area is relatively small, oxygen saturation of hemoglobin may increase to maximum. A maximal PO_2 value will not be achieved, however, because dissolved oxygen will not be increased to a maximum (Comroe, 1974).

If the reverse should occur—in other words, normal alveolar ventilation with inadequate alveolar blood flow (see Fig. 6–6)—circulation to the remainder of the lung would be increased. That part which is ventilated but which has an impaired blood supply constitutes dead space (alveolar dead space). In this instance, the alveolar gas remains as inspired air that moves back into the trachea on exhalation, and exhaled air assumes more of the characteristics of inspired air. At the same time, the remaining functional pulmonary surfaces are required to oxygenate a greater amount of blood. Compensation by hyperventilation thus becomes necessary. In the case of $PaCO_2$, complete or partial compensation for uneven ventilation occurs due to increased ventilation induced by hypercapnea, hypoxia, or both (Comroe, 1974).

Impaired gaseous exchange due to a combination of the aforementioned factors is well illustrated in anesthetized horses in supine and lateral recumbency. Under these circumstances, Gillespie et al. (1969) and DeMoor et al. (1974) have reported large differences between alveolar oxygen tension and arterial oxygen tension. During the anesthetic period, the estimated pulmonary shunt flow to total blood flow ratio was 14% when the thorax was open, and 11% when it was closed. This effect on oxygen uptake is especially apparent in the supine position in heavy and old animals; when the animal is breathing atmospheric air, a low Pa_{O_2} has been found (DeMoor et al., 1974). This large alveolar-arterial O_2 gradient is believed to result from 1) maldistribution of perfusion due to gravity, 2) hypoventilation of the dependent lung, 3) development of atelectasis, especially in the down lung, and 4) decrease in cardiac output. A reduction in the volume of the lowermost lung of the laterally recumbent horse has been suggested as a result of radiographic studies of ponies (McDonell et al., 1979). Recommendations have therefore included turning the animal from side to side during prolonged recumbency and administering supplemental oxygen during recovery (DeMoor et al., 1974).

It has been suggested that arteriovenous anastomoses open during halothane anesthesia and thereby contribute to the alveolar-arterial P_{O_2} difference. Studies during halothane anesthesia of dogs have not supported this premise (Pavlin et al., 1980).

The ventilation-perfusion ratio expresses the relationship of ventilation and blood flow in the lungs. If the alveolar ventilation per minute relative to the pulmonary-capillary blood flow per minute is greater than 0.8, ventilation is excessive and alveolar dead space is inferred. On the other hand, if the relationship is less than 0.8, venous-to-arterial shunt characteristics occur (Comroe, 1974). Lack of uniformity or failure of blood flow and ventilation to match causes respiratory inefficiency, although compensatory mechanisms to prevent this have been described. For instance, if the pressure of oxygen in an alveolus is low, this tends to induce constriction of the arterioles to this alveolus, with resulting reduction in blood supply. Low alveolar carbon dioxide, on the other hand, constricts bronchioles and reduces ventilation to the alveolus, thereby diverting air to more adequately diffused alveoli (Comroe, 1974). Various methods are available to detect uneven ventilation and perfusion. The single-breath carbon dioxide test is one; more recently, radioactive gases have been used and their distribution plotted by means of a surface-scanning procedure.

TABLE 6–5. Composition of Respiratory Gases in Man

Gas	*Inspired Air (%)*	*Expired Air (%)*	*Alveolar Air (%)*
O_2	20.95	16.1	14.0
CO_2	0.04	4.5	5.6
N_2*	79.0	79.2	80.0

*There is no change in the absolute concentration of N_2. The change in percent occurs because more oxygen is used than carbon dioxide produced.

OXYGEN TRANSPORT IN THE BLOOD

Under normal conditions, oxygen is taken into the pulmonary alveoli, and carbon dioxide is removed from them at a rate that is sufficient to maintain the composition of alveolar air at a relatively constant concentration. The composition of respiratory gases in man is set forth in Table 6–5. At body temperature, alveolar air is saturated with water vapor, which has a pressure at 37° C of 48 mm Hg. If the pressure in the alveolus is 760 mm Hg, then the pressure due to dry air is 760 − 48 = 712 mm Hg. Knowing the composition of alveolar air, one can calculate the pressure of each gas in the alveolus.

Pressure of Respiratory Gases in the Alveolus

$$O_2 = (760 - 48) \times 0.14 = 100 \text{ mm Hg}$$
$$CO_2 = (760 - 48) \times 0.056 = 40 \text{ mm Hg}$$
$$N_2 = (760 - 48) \times 0.80 = 570 \text{ mm Hg}$$

Oxygen pressure in the lungs at sea level is approximately 100 mm Hg at 38° C. Under these conditions, 100 ml of plasma will hold 0.31 ml of oxygen in physical solution. Whole blood, under the same conditions, will hold 20 ml of oxygen or about 60 times as much as plasma. Carbon dioxide is similarly held by blood. Thus, it is apparent that oxygen and carbon dioxide in blood are transported largely in chemical combination, since both are carried by blood in much greater quantities than would occur if simple absorption took place.

In the lung, gas exchange occurs across the alveolar membrane and the capillary membrane. The total distance across which exchange takes place is less than 1 micron; therefore, it occurs rapidly. Equilibrium *almost* develops between blood in the lungs and air in the alveolus, and the Po_2 in the blood almost equals the Po_2 in the alveolus. At complete saturation, each gram of hemoglobin combines with 1.36 ml of oxygen. This is the total carrying capacity of hemoglobin, or four oxygen molecules combined with each hemoglobin molecule. The ability of hemoglobin to combine with oxygen depends on the partial pressure of oxygen in the surrounding environment. The degree to which it will become saturated at various oxygen partial pressures varies considerably (see Figs. 6–7, 6–8). It is adjusted so that, even when ventilation is inefficient or the supply of oxygen is sparse as at higher altitudes, the degree of saturation still approaches 100%. For instance, although it is probably not fully saturated until it is exposed to a Po_2 of 250 mm Hg, it is still over 92% saturated when the oxygen partial pressure is only 70 mm Hg.

Although there is relatively little change in saturation between 70 and 250 mm Hg partial pressure of oxygen, a marked change occurs between 10 and 40 mm Hg, a partial pressure characteristic of actively metabolizing tissues. Thus, as hemoglobin is exposed to tissues having partial pressures of oxygen within this range, it must yield its oxygen to the tissues. The lower the Po_2 of these tissues, the greater the amount of oxygen that hemoglobin must give up. The degree to which hemoglobin gives up its oxygen is influenced by the environmental pH, Pco_2, and temperature (see Fig. 6–8)—all mechanisms that protect the metabolizing cell. As the pH decreases and the Pco_2 and local temperature increase, at any given Po_2 value, especially in the range of 10 to 40 mm Hg, hemoglobin carries less oxygen and must give it up to the surrounding environment. It is also interesting to note that nature has adapted for the relatively lower oxygen environment of the fetus, since fetal hemoglobin carries a greater percentage of oxygen at a low partial pressure.

Certain enzyme systems aid dissociation of oxygen from hemoglobin, the most completely studied being the enzyme system producing 2,3-diphosphoglycerate (2,3-DPG). This system enhances dissociation of oxygen from hemoglobin by competing with oxygen for the binding site. Lowered levels of enzyme increase the affinity of hemoglobin for oxygen, and thus act as if the curve is shifted to the left (see Fig. 6–8). The oxygen tension at which 50% saturation of hemoglobin is achieved (P50) is used to measure affinity of hemoglobin for oxygen. Reduced P50 occurs in septic patients and in carbon monoxide poisoning. The reverse has been encountered in chronic anemia (Shapiro et al., 1977). Since tissues require a given volume of oxygen per unit of time, the hemoglobin concentration of blood also has a significant influence upon oxygen delivery to the tissues.

Although an increase in the partial pressure of alveolar oxygen above normal results in only a small increase in that carried by hemoglobin, plasma carries oxygen in an amount directly proportional to the partial pressure of oxygen in the alveoli. At normal atmospheric pressure, when the animal is breathing air at 38° C, 0.3 ml of oxygen is carried in solution in 100 ml of blood. If pure oxygen is administered, the partial pressure of oxygen in the alveoli is raised from 100 to almost 700 mm Hg. Plasma oxygen is thus elevated almost seven times, that is, from 0.3 to 2.1 ml per 100 ml of blood. The result is an increase of about 10% in oxygen carried by the blood. This is of some importance since oxygen transfers from blood to tissues by diffusion, and the process occurs at a rate proportional to the difference in oxygen tension between plasma and body tissues.

A common misconception is that oxygenation of a patient can be improved by increasing the *pressure* at which oxygen is administered. Except in hyperbaric chambers, improved oxygenation of the patient is not obtained by increasing the pressure of the gas mixture, but by increasing the *proportion* of oxygen in the mixture. At a positive pressure exceeding 40 mm Hg, the capillary circulation in the lungs is inhibited;

therefore, it is not practical to administer oxygen at a pressure exceeding this figure.

The partial pressure of oxygen in various body areas is:

Inspired air = 160 mm Hg
Alveolar air = 100 mm Hg
Arterial blood = 90–95 mm Hg
Interstitial fluid = 30 mm Hg
Intracellular fluid = 10 mm Hg
Venous blood = 40 mm Hg

Little oxygen is lost in large blood vessels. A continuous pressure gradient is present from the alveolus to the tissue cell.

Oxygen has a weak covalent link with hemoglobin. Four factors influence oxygen uptake: 1) change in pH due to carbon dioxide, 2) specific effect of carbon dioxide, 3) temperature, and 4) effect of salts and enzymes (see Fig. 6–8).

Decreasing the carbon dioxide tension in blood raises the pH and causes hemoglobin to bind more oxygen; when the carbon dioxide tension increases, the oxygen dissociation curve shifts to the right. Carbon dioxide reacts with hemoglobin to form carbaminohemoglobin, which has much less affinity for oxygen than does hemoglobin. Thus, it exerts a specific effect also.

Increased temperature favors dissociation of oxyhemoglobin. As metabolic rates increase, there is increased heat in the tissue which, in turn, makes more oxygen available.

The salt or electrolyte concentration of blood has been shown to affect oxygenation, although the mechanism of action is obscure. Ordinarily, variations in electrolyte concentration of blood have little effect on oxygen transport.

Several factors increase the availability of oxygen in tissues when needed:

1. *Increased circulation*. Up to three times as much blood may flow through the tissues.
2. *Increased respiratory rate*. The carbon dioxide tension of the blood regulates the respiratory center.
3. *Increased deoxygenation of a given volume of blood*. This may be due to: *a)* lowered oxygen tension in the cells, *b)* increased temperature with increased dissociation, and *c)* metabolic products, such as carbon dioxide and lactic acid, which are acidic. All of these favor local vasodilation with the consequent benefit of increased supply of oxygen in instances of increased tissue metabolism.

These factors combine to make up to ten times as much oxygen available to tissues as would be available in the resting state. The rate of muscular activity is not limited by oxygen supply since muscle can incur an oxygen deficit.

CARBON DIOXIDE TRANSPORT AND THE CHLORIDE SHIFT

Carbon dioxide is an end product of glucose oxidation. During severe exercise, the production of carbon dioxide is increased enormously. In the tissues, carbon dioxide reacts with water to form carbonic acid. Because of the blood buffer systems, transport of carbon dioxide to the lungs for excretion is effected with little change in blood pH. The importance of the lungs in excreting this volatile acid is illustrated by the fact that, in man, the kidneys eliminate 40 to 80 mEq per day, while the lungs eliminate 13,000 mEq per day (Comroe, 1974).

$$CO_2 + H_2O \underset{\text{Anhydrase}}{\overset{\text{Carbonic}}{\rightleftarrows}} H_2CO_3 \leftrightarrows H^+ + HCO_3^-$$

Under ordinary circumstances, the pH of venous blood is only 0.01 to 0.03 lower than that of arterial blood. A carbon dioxide pressure gradient, opposite to that of oxygen, exists from the tissues to the atmospheric air:

Tissues = 50 mm Hg (during exercise may be higher)
Venous blood = 46 mm Hg
Alveolar air = 40 mm Hg
Expired air = 32 mm Hg
Atmospheric air = 0.3 mm Hg
Arterial blood = 40 mm Hg (equilibrium with alveolar air)

Some carbon dioxide is carried dissolved in the plasma. This is divided into: 1) H_2CO_3, and 2) carbon dioxide in simple solution. These are referred to as *carbonic acid*. The amount of carbon dioxide transported as carbonic acid is about 10% of the total and is found in the plasma.

The greater portion of carbon dioxide transport is as *bicarbonate*. This may occur: 1) in plasma through buffering action with plasma protein (this accounts for 5% of carbon dioxide transport), or 2) by formation in the red blood cell through the chloride shift (this accounts for the largest amount). The excellent buffering capacity of hemoglobin allows greater changes in hydrogen ion content to occur during this process with minimal change in pH (Shapiro et al., 1977).

As blood passes to the venous side of the vascular system, carbon dioxide is absorbed and diffuses into the red blood cell (Fig. 6–9). Here it is converted to carbonic acid. Reduced hemoglobin, a weaker acid, gives up its alkali, chiefly potassium, to carbonic acid. As bicarbonate is thus formed and accumulates in the erythrocyte, the ionic equilibrium between cell and plasma is upset. The corpuscular membrane is impermeable to potassium, but bicarbonate diffuses through into the plasma. Chloride ions, in turn, shift into the cell to restore ionic equilibrium and balance the potassium. The chloride shift enables carbon dioxide to be carried without any change in blood pH and is the main method of transport.

A third method by which carbon dioxide is carried is in the form of carbamino compound. Amino acids and aliphatic amines combine with carbon dioxide to form unstable carbamino compound. Hemoglobin is the main protein acting in this manner, though many can do so. The efficiency of this reaction is greater with Hb than with HbO_2. Thus, as HbO_2 dissociates, its capacity to carry CO_2 increases (Comroe, 1974).

The mechanisms of carbon dioxide and oxygen transport are integrated in the blood in at least three ways.

1. The acidity of carbonic acid produced in the tissues favors release of oxygen without a change in oxygen tension. The release of carbon dioxide in the lungs favors oxygen uptake.
2. Release of oxygen favors carbon dioxide uptake and vice versa in the carbamino mechanism. Upon the release of oxygen, hemoglobin becomes a weaker acid and is more capable of accepting hydrogen ions thereby facilitating its buffering effect (Shapiro et al., 1977).
3. The two acid forms of the hemoglobin molecule favor dissociation by shifting from one form to the other. Oxygen uptake favors carbon dioxide loss and vice versa.

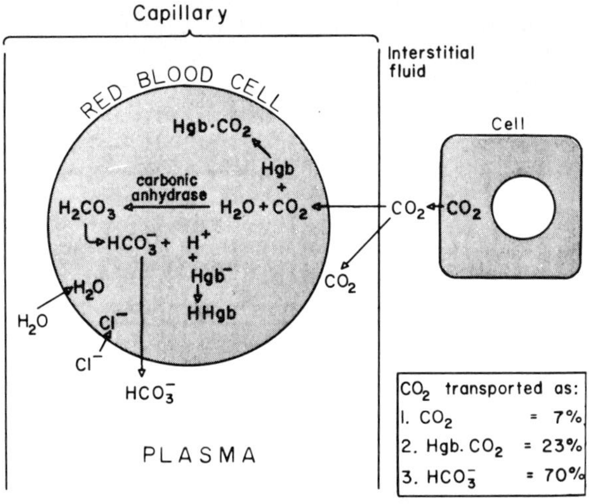

Figure 6–9. Transport of carbon dioxide in the blood. (From Guyton, A.C.: *Textbook of Medical Physiology*, 6th ed. W.B. Saunders Co., Philadelphia, 1981.)

Just as the amount of oxygen transported by the blood depends on the partial pressure of oxygen to which the blood is exposed, so is carbon dioxide transport likewise affected; however, the carbon dioxide dissociation curve is more or less linear, as previously mentioned. Thus, hyper- and hypoventilation have marked effects on the carbon dioxide content of the tissues in contrast to that of oxygen. For instance, doubling the ventilation halves the alveolar P_{CO_2}; halving the alveolar ventilation doubles the alveolar P_{CO_2}.

ACID-BASE BALANCE

In normal animals, the blood pH is 7.4 ± 0.05. If the pH rises above 7.45, the condition is termed *alkalosis;* below 7.35, it is termed *acidosis* (Fig. 6–10). Normal metabolic processes continuously produce acidic substances such as lactic acid, sulfuric acid from protein metabolism, and carbon dioxide. Some alkaline substances are also being added, though to a lesser extent. The pH of the blood is kept constant through three mechanisms: blood buffers, respiration, and the kidneys.

Pathologic changes in metabolism almost always result in acidosis. The pH shift during prolonged surgery with poor lung ventilation may result in values below 7.

The state of acid-base balance within the body depends primarily upon the relative quantities of carbonic acid and base bicarbonate in the extracellular fluid. Carbonic acid is the major blood acid and is formed from CO_2. It is volatile and controlled directly by ventilation. The remainder are nonvolatile fixed acids and are controlled predominantly by renal excretion. Blood base is primarily bicarbonate. It is produced with the aid of carbonic anhydrase in the kidney, with concurrent buffering and excretion of hydrogen ions and the addition of bicarbonate ions to the blood. By this mechanism, the kidney assumes a significant role in acid-base balance. Normally, carbonic acid and base bicarbonate are present in a ratio of 1 to 20 respectively. If this ratio is altered, there is a deviation in pH of the body fluids and a state of acidosis or

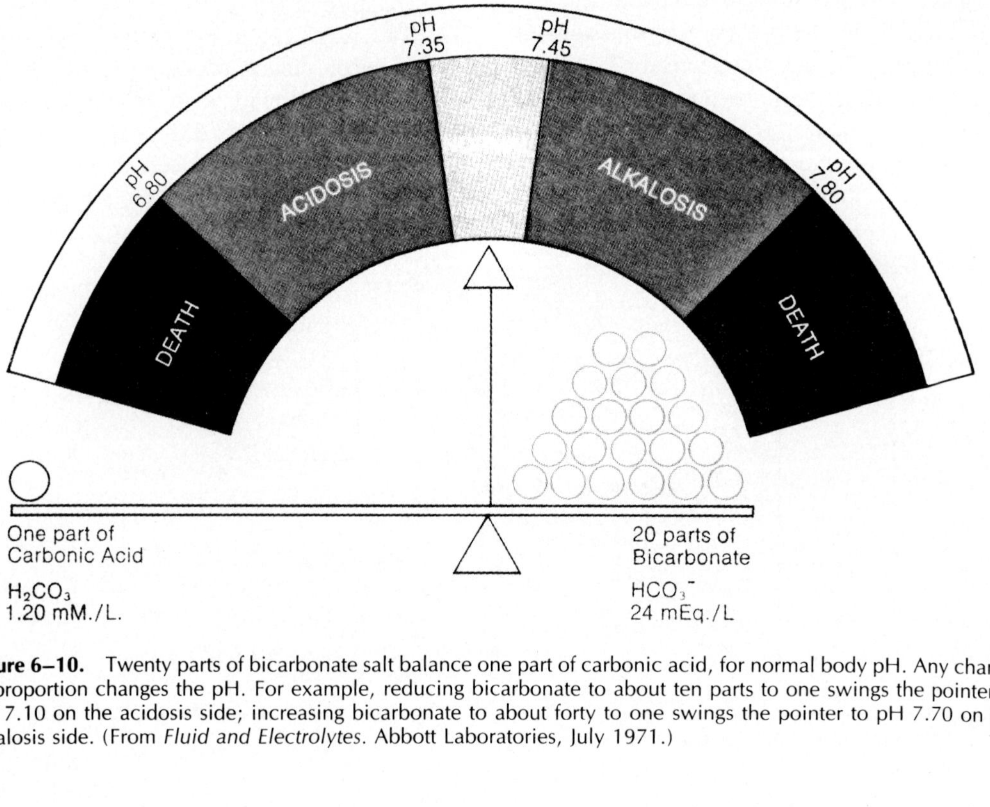

Figure 6–10. Twenty parts of bicarbonate salt balance one part of carbonic acid, for normal body pH. Any change in proportion changes the pH. For example, reducing bicarbonate to about ten parts to one swings the pointer to pH 7.10 on the acidosis side; increasing bicarbonate to about forty to one swings the pointer to pH 7.70 on the alkalosis side. (From *Fluid and Electrolytes.* Abbott Laboratories, July 1971.)

alkalosis exists. Other buffer systems within the body play only a minor role in regulation of acid-base balance.

Two general types of acid-base imbalances may occur. Metabolic disturbances affect *bicarbonate*, whereas respiratory disturbances affect *carbonic acid*.

Metabolic Disturbances
- Bicarbonate deficit—acidosis
- Bicarbonate excess—alkalosis

Respiratory Disturbances
- Carbonic acid deficit—alkalosis
- Carbonic acid excess—acidosis

Metabolic acidosis may be caused by diarrhea with loss of sodium bicarbonate in the feces, renal insufficiency with retention of organic acid ions, ketosis with production and accumulation of ketonic acids in the tissues (as occurs with diabetes mellitus or starvation), administration of acidic drugs, or severe infectious disease with production of ketone bodies. The body attempts to compensate for bicarbonate deficit by increased respiratory activity to remove carbon dioxide, and through conservation of bicarbonate ions and excretion of hydrogen ions in the urine.

Metabolic alkalosis may occur as a result of excessive acid loss through vomiting, or through potassium loss such as might occur with overdoses of adrenal corticoids. To correct the imbalance, breathing is slow and shallow. In addition, the kidneys excrete bicarbonate ions and retain hydrogen ions.

Respiratory acidosis results from hypoventilation with retention of carbon dioxide. Increased PCO_2 causes an elevation of plasma hydrogen ion concentration. An excess carbon dioxide tension in the blood is termed *hypercapnia* or *hypercarbia*. The kidney compensates by conserving bicarbonate ions and excreting hydrogen ions in the urine. Compensation therefore occurs over a period of time. A high $Paco_2$ accompanied by acidemia is indicative of acute ventilatory failure. The presence of partial or complete compensation for the excessive hydrogen ion concentration is indicative of subacute or chronic ventilatory failure. Because basic cellular processes are very susceptible to sudden pH changes, the severity of acidemia relative to $Paco_2$ levels is an important prognostic indicator (Shapiro et al., 1977).

Respiratory alkalosis occurs with hyperventilation and resultant loss of carbon dioxide. A deficient carbon dioxide tension in the blood is termed *hypocapnia* or *hypocarbia*. The kidneys compensate by excreting bicarbonate ions and retaining hydrogen ions. Chronic alveolar hyperventilation (respiratory alkalosis) is thus characterized by decreased $Paco_2$ with a normal or near-normal arterial pH (Shapiro et al., 1977).

It should be emphasized that both respiratory and metabolic aberrations in acid-base balance can occur simultaneously. For methods of monitoring acid-base status, see Chapter 19.

HYPOXIA

The term *anoxia* literally means without oxygen. Through common usage, it has come to mean inability of tissues to receive or utilize an adequate amount of oxygen. Since a literal anoxia seldom if ever exists, the word *hypoxia*, indicating a state of decreased oxygen availability or diminished utilization of oxygen by tissues (impaired tissue respiration), is a preferable term. Blood hypoxia refers to an insufficient content of oxygen in the blood; hypoxemia is defined as a relative deficiency of oxygen tension in the arterial blood. In assessment of tissue oxygenation, hypoxemia is defined as Pao_2 less than 80 mm Hg (Shapiro et al., 1977).

Saklad (1953) has classified hypoxia into seven categories in contrast to the four conventional types of anoxia. This classification achieves a better etiologic designation (Tables 6–6, 6–7).

Atmospheric hypoxia is due to reduction in available oxygen in the inhaled atmosphere. This could result from high altitude, dilution with inert gases such as anesthetic gases, or confinement in unventilated areas, such as an airtight box.

Tidal hypoxia is the result of decreased oxygen uptake because of decreased respiratory

TABLE 6–6. Classification of Oxygen Want

*Types of Anoxia**	*Types of Hypoxia†*
1. Anoxic	1. Atmospheric
	2. Tidal
	3. Alveolar
2. Anemic	4. Hemoglobic
3. Stagnant	5. Stagnant
4. Histotoxic	6. Histotoxic
	7. Demand

*Conventional classification
†Saklad, 1953

exchange. Disease, drugs (anesthetic agents are an example), respiratory obstruction, or altered respiratory dynamics (such as convulsions) are causes.

Alveolar hypoxia is produced by a decrease in number or efficiency of the functioning alveoli such as occurs with pneumonia, emphysema, atelectasis, pleural effusion, intrapulmonary exudates, or shunt effect (pulmonary perfusion in excess of ventilation).

Hemoglobic hypoxia is due to reduction in hemoglobin content of the blood, or reduction in available hemoglobin as in carbon monoxide poisoning.

Stagnant hypoxia is the result of poor circulation.

Histotoxic hypoxia results from inability of cells to utilize oxygen properly and may be produced by alcohol, anesthetics, cyanide, or carbon monoxide.

Demand hypoxia is caused by metabolic conditions in which body requirements for oxygen are elevated above normal, such as hyperthyroidism, hyperpyrexia, or blood dyscrasia.

Susceptibility of dogs to oxygen want varies greatly (Davis, 1949). Dogs are better able to withstand hypoxia than cats because of their greater ability to increase ventilatory volume through response to chemoreceptor stimulation (Stacy and Whitehorn, 1947). Resistance to hypoxia is greater in young animals than in adults. Survival of tissues under hypoxic conditions varies considerably.

BODY RESPONSE TO HYPOXIA

Hypoxia produces a fall in body temperature, probably as a homeostatic reaction that tends to protect the animal. (Traumatic shock is also accompanied by reduction in oxygen consumption.) The time of appearance and degree of response to hypoxia vary greatly in individual patients and are dependent to a large extent upon their condition. Animals with cardiovascular or respiratory disease often develop hypoxia under conditions that ordinarily would not affect a normal animal. These patients lack ability to compensate by circulatory and respiratory adjustment.

Stimulation of the chemoreceptors by low oxygen tension induces increased alveolar ventilation and also plays a significant part in initi-

TABLE 6–7. Oxygen Capacity, Content, Tension, and Arteriovenous Difference in Various Forms of Hypoxia

		Arterial Oxygen		*Venous Oxygen*		
Hypoxia	*Oxygen Capacity*	*Content*	*Tension*	*Content*	*Tension*	*A–V Difference*
Atmospheric	Normal	Decreased	Decreased	Decreased	Decreased	Decreased
Tidal	Normal	Decreased	Decreased	Decreased	Decreased	Decreased
Alveolar	Normal	Decreased	Decreased	Decreased	Decreased	Decreased
Hemoglobic						
Carbon Monoxide	Decreased	Decreased	Normal	Decreased	Decreased	Decreased
Hemorrhage	Decreased	Decreased	Normal	Decreased	Decreased	Decreased
Stagnant	Normal	Normal	Normal	Decreased	Decreased	Decreased
Histotoxic	Normal	Normal	Normal	Increased	Increased	Decreased
Demand	Normal	Normal	Normal	Decreased	Decreased	Increased

(From Saklad, M.: *Inhalation Therapy and Resuscitation.* Charles C Thomas, Springfield, Illinois, 1953.)

ating cardiac responses. Ultimately, the work of large increases in ventilation with concomitant increased oxygen consumption negate any gain in available oxygen (Shapiro et al., 1977).

The immediate circulatory responses to lack of oxygen are dilation of the coronary and cerebral vessels, elevation of the pulse rate, and increase in cardiac output. In the pulmonary circuit, pulmonary arterial pressure likewise increases as a result of alveolar hypoxia in all animal species tested (Orr et al., 1977). In conditions of oxygen deficiency, three mechanisms tend to protect the heart: 1) decreased tonicity of the coronary vessels, 2) increased coronary circulation due to greater diversion of the cardiac output, and 3) decrease in cardiac work.

Capillaries are extremely vulnerable to hypoxia, the endothelium being easily injured with resultant relaxation and dilation. They thus become packed with stagnant red blood cells and their walls become progressively permeable to fluid and plasma proteins.

Drinker (1925) has pointed out that capillaries in different parts of the body vary in their resistance to hypoxia, and the endothelium of pulmonary capillaries is least resistant to low oxygen tensions. This results in fluid accumulation in the alveolar wall, further obstructing exchange of oxygen and carbon dioxide in the lungs.

The early response to hypoxia is an increased efficiency of the cardiovascular system. Continued lack of oxygen, however, produces a fall in blood pressure, pulse rate, and cardiac output. Fatal hypoxia in dogs almost invariably results in ventricular standstill rather than fibrillation (Harris, 1946).

The liver parenchyma is quite sensitive to hypoxia, more so than kidney and muscle, and a decrease in hepatic function results. Lack of oxygen caused by ligation of the hepatic artery produces a lethal bacterial necrosis in dogs. Recently it has become apparent that impaired hepatic perfusion with resulting altered biotransformation contributes to the toxicity of certain of the inhaled anesthetics. The kidney can tolerate lack of oxygen for approximately 2 hours (Hamilton et al., 1948). Renal disease being absent, urinary output reflects renal blood flow so that urinary output is a useful indicator of renal perfusion status (Shapiro et al., 1977).

Rats exposed to low oxygen tension for long periods of time have necrosis and hemorrhage in the adrenal glands. Lewis et al. (1942) have shown that if adrenalectomized animals are given adrenocortical hormone, they withstand oxygen deficit to a greater degree.

Several chemical changes take place in the blood during hypoxia. Overventilation with blowoff of carbon dioxide may cause alkalosis, particularly if the kidneys do not compensate by excretion of bicarbonate. In extreme hypoxia, acidosis will result, owing to incomplete combustion of carbohydrates resulting in lactic acid formation, and also to decreased respiratory efficiency with carbon dioxide retention (Fig. 6–11).

Lack of oxygen has been shown to produce hyperglycemia with glycosuria. This is probably mediated by the effect of hypoxia on the central nervous system and is associated with increased output of epinephrine.

When cell metabolism is reduced by lack of oxygen, there is a short period of stimulation followed by paralysis and, finally, cell death. During the paralytic stage, the intracellular electrolytic changes that occur continue to affect the cell even though hypoxia may have ceased. These consist of a loss of intracellular potassium and a rise in intracellular sodium. The latter causes retention of water in the cell or intracellular edema. This edema disrupts normal cell function after the hypoxic insult has been withdrawn, and may be so severe that the cell becomes distended and finally ruptures, producing irreversible cellular changes. Intracellular edema probably does not occur until the hypoxic insult has finished and does not reach its maximum effect for 6 to 8 hours. In terms of the central nervous system, this may be manifested clinically by return of the patient to consciousness followed by drowsiness and confusion that persist for another 24 hours.

SYMPTOMS OF HYPOXIA

Symptoms of acute oxygen insufficiency include increased respiratory rate, rise in systolic

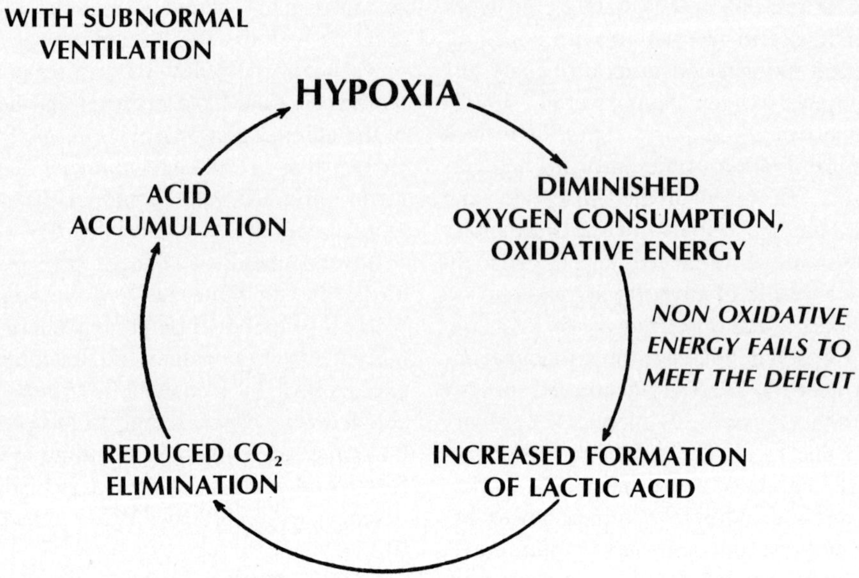

Figure 6–11. The tendency toward acidosis due to subnormal ventilation. (From Saklad, M.: *Inhalation Therapy and Resuscitation*. Charles C Thomas, Springfield, Illinois, 1953.)

blood pressure, elevated pulse rate, nausea and vomiting, dilated pupils, muscular incoordination, and twitching followed by convulsions. Cyanosis is not a reliable sign of the extent of hypoxia. Cyanosis is caused by reduced hemoglobin in the capillary blood, and a minimum of 5 g for each 100 ml of blood is required to make a visible color change. In anemic animals, color changes may not occur until arterial oxygen saturation has fallen to as low as 55%. In very anemic animals, cyanosis may never become evident even though the animal dies from hypoxia. Cyanosis is not a prominent characteristic of shock because there is marked capillary constriction.

Because the brain is the organ most sensitive to oxygen deficit, the main characteristic of a hypoxic state is unconsciousness. The severity of the insult determines the depth of unconsciousness but, as far as the central nervous system is concerned, it is impossible to determine what form of hypoxia has caused the insult. Following *severe* hypoxia, all reflexes are absent in the early stages except for the light reflex. Later, the reflexes may become exaggerated. Usually, there is a state of vasoconstriction with a fall in blood pressure and increased heart rate, indicating diminished cardiac output. When extensive damage occurs to the vasomotor center, the systolic blood pressure falls to shock levels. Swann (1953) has shown that irreversible cerebral damage occurs in unanesthetized hypoxic dogs approximately 1 minute following circulatory failure or when the blood pressure falls below 55 mm Hg. With mild hypoxia, mental confusion is transitory and recovery may occur after several days of unconsciousness. If a decerebrate state exists for more than 72 hours, complete recovery does not occur, and the patient usually dies within 1 to 6 weeks. Hyperpyrexia may develop terminally with temperatures as high as 110° F.

HYPERVENTILATION

Hyperventilation may be induced mechanically or may result from three general pathophysiologic states: hypoxemia sufficient to stimulate peripheral chemoreceptors, metabolic acidosis with stimulation of chemoreceptors, and abnormal stimulation of ventilatory centers (Shapiro et al., 1977). Anesthetized patients that are hyperventilated with oxygen-rich mixtures cease to breathe spontaneously; their color remains good, and as soon as blood carbon dioxide is allowed to accumulate, breathing resumes. Concurrent with the alveolar hyperventilation (respiratory alkalosis) are an increase in blood pH, a decrease in Pa_{CO_2} and, in the event of compensation, reduced bicarbonate and base excess.

Biddulph et al. (1960) hyperventilated dogs with a respirator for 1 hour and reported the arterial blood pH was 7.65. Kanter (1961), in a similar experiment, could find no change in glomerular filtration rate, renal plasma flow, hematocrit, rectal temperature, heart rate, or total solids in the plasma. In the latter experiment, hyperventilation was conducted for 3 hours and the arterial blood pH reached 7.63.

Garcia et al. (1971), when hyperventilating anesthetized dogs to a Pa_{CO_2} of 15 mm Hg, reported an increase of blood lactate and pyruvate within 10 to 15 minutes. This increase persisted for a 2- to 3-hour period and subsequently declined despite continued hypocapnia. An increase in anesthetic depth as a result of alkalosis can probably be explained by an alteration of protein binding of injected drugs, by increased anesthetic uptake and alveolar concentration, by reduction of reticular action, and by reduced reflex input responses (Smith, 1976).

OXYGEN TOXICITY

Despite reports by Bert in 1847 and Smith in 1899 (cited by Winter, 1974), the hazards of oxygen toxicity have largely been ignored until recently. There is now, however, no doubt that this is a serious hazard. It has been shown to be a function of both the Pa_{O_2} and the duration of exposure.

Inhalation of 100% oxygen eliminates nitrogen from the lungs in a few minutes and from the rest of the tissues at a slower rate. As might be expected, there is some respiratory depression due to diminished stimulation of carotid and aortic chemoreceptors, with resultant carbon dioxide retention. Since increased oxygen saturation of hemoglobin reduces available reduced hemoglobin, the transport of carbon dioxide is also impaired. Some stimulation of respiration may ultimately result from irritation of respiratory mucous membranes. Modification of chemoreflexes also induces a decreased pulse rate and a reduced cardiac output. Direct stimulation by oxygen constricts most blood vessels (Lee and Atkinson, 1968).

Continuous exposure to oxygen concentrations in excess of 60 to 70% for 24 hours or longer induces signs of oxygen toxicity due to irritation of the respiratory tract, pulmonary congestion, and pulmonary edema, with or without hyaline membrane formation (Balentine, 1966). Similar lesions have been encountered subsequent to exposure to hyperbaric oxygen. Pneumonitis has been induced in laboratory animals exposed to high oxygen tensions for prolonged periods. Since this has been observed also in germfree animals, it is believed to be a direct toxic effect (Balentine, 1966).

Survival times of animals breathing 0.9 to 1.0 atmospheres of 100% oxygen are variable. Guinea pigs live 49 to 118 hours, dogs 55 to 119 hours, and rabbits 82.7 ± 24.7 hours. Primates appear to have a greater tolerance, and poikilotherms (frogs, turtles, snakes) appear resistant (Winter, 1974). Clinical signs become apparent only during the last quarter of the exposure period. In one study, the respiratory rate fell, tidal volume increased, and a marked reduction in arterial oxygen saturation occurred. Death was seemingly due to hypoxia (Smith et al., 1963). In similar studies in rats, Kistler et al. (1967) reported progressive changes in the alveolar blood-gas barrier commencing 24 hours after the onset of exposure to 100% O_2. There was a progressive increase in the pulmonary interstitial space due to edema and hemorrhage, so that the thickness of the blood-gas barrier doubled by 72 hours. Inhalation of 80 to 100% oxygen has likewise been shown to be fatal to 1- to 2-week-old lambs in 2 to 4 days. Artificial ventilation did not seem to modify the effect, and there was no significant alteration in pulmonary surfactant (deLemos et al., 1969).

There is a biphasic response to oxygen inhalation in primates. Initially, there is exudation with pulmonary capillary destruction, hemorrhage, and alveolar type I cell disintegration. This is followed by a reparative phase with alveolar type II cell and fibroblast proliferation, septal thickening, capillary hyperplasia, and progressive fibrosis (Winter, 1974). A consistent finding in both man and animals has been decreased compliance and vital capacity. In rabbits, decreased mucus transport, inhibition of ciliary function, and depressed alveolar macrophage function have been reported (Winter, 1974).

In premature human infants, inhalation of oxygen concentrations greater than 40% causes retrolental fibroplasia. Necrosis of the visual cell layer of the retina of rabbits and degeneration of the axons in the ganglion cell layer of the canine retina have also been observed (Balentine, 1966). Convulsions result from exposure to hyperbaric oxygen (5 atmospheres). The incidence of these appears to be related to high cerebral P_{CO_2} values (Bennet, 1966).

EFFECTS OF EXCESS CARBON DIOXIDE

Carbon dioxide was discovered by Joseph Priestley about 1770, and its anesthetic properties first noted by Hickman in 1824. The latter demonstrated on dogs that the pain of surgery could be abolished by inhalation of this gas; however, strange as it may seem, it was not until 1929 that the anesthetic properties of carbon dioxide were confirmed by Leake and Waters.

Carbon dioxide is the normal physiologic respiratory stimulant and is found in a concentration of 0.25% in air. Its administration has been recommended: 1) for replacement therapy, 2) for its effect on respiration, 3) for its effect on circulation, and 4) for mental conditions in man. As far as replacement therapy is concerned in conditions encountered clinically, carbon dioxide is already retained and further administration is probably detrimental. Although carbon dioxide is a powerful respiratory stimulant under normal circumstances, in hypoxia its action becomes reversed and administration may produce respiratory depression.

Many methods for oxygen administration are confined extensions of the respiratory tract resulting in considerable dead space, which is a significant hazard in small species and pediatric patients. This tends to cause carbon dioxide accumulation in the patient because of insufficient elimination. Five percent carbon dioxide can be tolerated by a patient. Higher concentrations produce a rise in pulse rate and systolic blood pressure, increased depth of respiration (often with little increase in rate), and muscular twitching followed by convulsions. The color of the mucous membranes may be good. Concentrations of 20 to 30% are subanesthetic, 30 to 40% are anesthetic, and over 40% may be fatal (Fig. 6–12).

When illustrated graphically, ventilatory response to carbon dioxide excess is nearly a straight line. The normal response is accentuated by hypoxia and catecholamine stimulation. With all anesthetic agents studied (except perhaps ketamine), there is a dose-related decrease in slope (response to CO_2) with increase in depth. During light to moderate halothane anesthesia, pulmonary artery pressure rises with increasing Pa_{CO_2} values. Airway resistance is also increased with elevated Pa_{CO_2} values. Increased anesthetic depth due to halogenated agents with elevated Pa_{CO_2} increases the propensity for epinephrine-induced arrhythmias in dogs. With hyperventilation, alkalosis, and consequent hypokalemia, digitalis effects increase. During anesthesia, cardiac output is affected by CO_2 in a linear manner, blood pressure rises, and peripheral resistance is lowered slightly. Increased anesthetic depth alters this response and may cause hypotension. With halothane and hypocapnia, cardiac output may decrease rapidly. Cerebral blood flow increases with hypercapnia and decreases with hypocapnia. Increased CO_2 stimulates the sympathetic nervous system with increases in epinephrine, norepinephrine, and 17-hydroxy-ketosteroids. Hypercapnia also decreases resting muscle blood flow and neuromuscular transmission, and facilitates and prolongs tubocurarine effects (Smith, 1976).

Biddulph et al. (1960) have shown that dogs anesthetized with thiopental and respired with a mixture of 30% carbon dioxide and 70% oxygen had a mean blood pH of 6.78 after 1 hour. Miller et al. (1950) found that alveolar carbon dioxide concentrations above 15% depress adrenal function in the dog as evidenced by absence of an eosinopenia following injection of

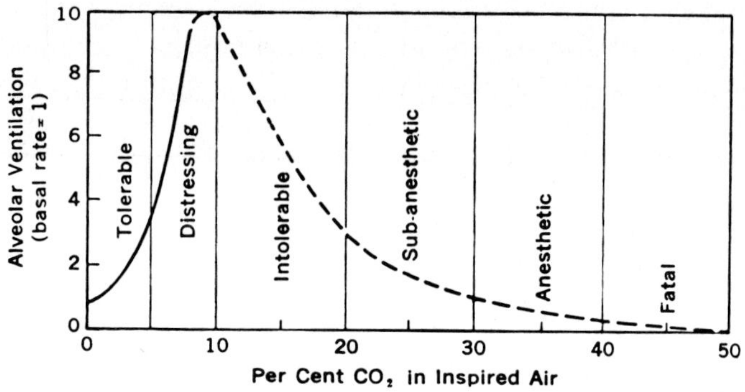

Figure 6–12. Effect on alveolar ventilation of breathing carbon dioxide in the inspired air. (From data of Gray, J.S.: *Pulmonary Ventilation and Its Physiological Regulation.* Charles C Thomas, Springfield, Illinois, 1950.)

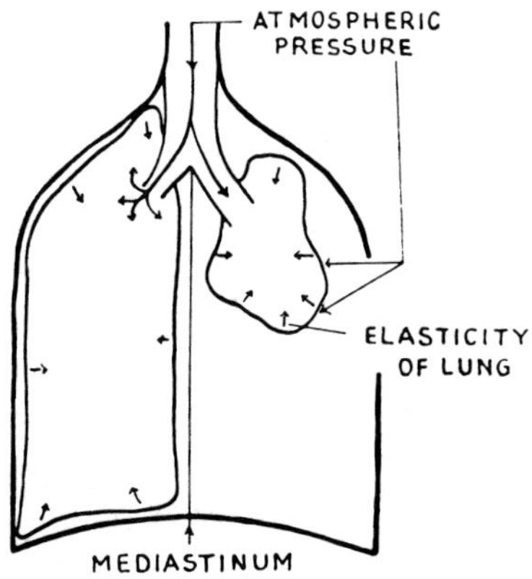

Figure 6–13. Forces responsible for collapse of lung when chest wall is opened. (From Hall, L.W.: *Wright's Veterinary Anaesthesia and Analgesia,* 7th ed. Baillière Tindall, London, 1971.)

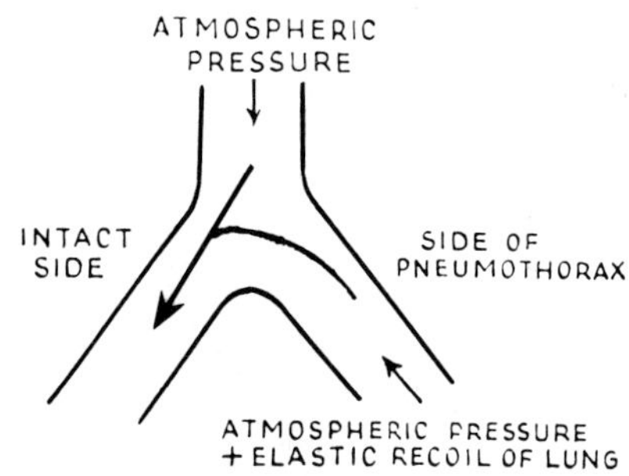

Figure 6–14. Forces responsible for "pendulum air" transfer from lung to lung in open penumothorax. (From Hall, L.W.: *Wright's Veterinary Anaesthesia and Analgesia,* 7th ed. Baillière Tindall, London, 1971.)

epinephrine. Dogs given a mixture of 30% carbon dioxide and 70% oxygen exhibited a decreased tolerance to thiopental and pentobarbital; in some dogs that subsequently survived, the blood pH reached 6.61.

A high incidence of cardiac malformations can be produced in rats by exposing the mother to carbon dioxide during pregnancy (Haring, 1960). A gas mixture containing 6% carbon dioxide, 20% oxygen, and 74% nitrogen was found to produce ventricular septal defects, with or without other cardiac abnormalities. For this reason, particular care should be exercised to prevent development of high carbon dioxide levels in pregnant animals.

PNEUMOTHORAX

When air enters the pleural cavity, the condition known as pneumothorax is produced. Pneumothorax is divided into two types depending upon the cause. In *open* pneumothorax, a penetrating wound exists between the pleural cavity and the body surface; in *closed* (tension or valvular) pneumothorax, air enters the pleural cavity through rupture of the lung. In the latter, it is assumed that a tissue check-valve closes during exhalation, trapping air in the pleural cavity. The extent and severity of the actions that occur from pneumothorax depend upon the size of the opening and the amount of air gaining access to the cavity.

Three events occur in open pneumothorax:

1. The lung on the affected side collapses (Fig. 6–13). The collapsed lung acts as a

venous-arterial shunt, since blood passing through the lung is returned unoxygenated to the left side of the heart and reduces cardiac efficiency.

2. The mediastinum, which forms a fragile barrier between the two halves of the chest cavity, shifts toward the side away from the opening. This causes partial collapse of the other lung. As respiratory movements continue, the mediastinum is drawn toward the closed side of the chest during inspiration and, on expiration, is forced toward the opening. The action further reduces the effective respiratory volume of the remaining lung.
3. When an open pneumothorax is created, the animal continues to breathe, but the exposed lung, instead of moving in the conventional manner, becomes smaller on inspiration and larger on expiration. This movement is termed "paradoxical respiration." On inspiration, air pressure in the main bronchus of the exposed lung exceeds that in the trachea, since the pressure is a combination of the elastic recoil of the lung plus the atmospheric pressure (Fig. 6–14). Air drawn into the intact lung comes first from the collapsed lung and then from the exterior, the collapsed lung becoming smaller on inspiration and enlarging on expiration. Consequently, an animal with open pneumothorax has considerable "pendulum air," which transfers from lung to lung and is ineffective in respiratory exchange.

When a thoracotomy is performed, air enters the lungs through the trachea and the pleural cavity through the wound. The amount of air entering the chest by each route depends on the relationship between the cross-sectional area of the trachea and that of the thoracotomy opening (Wright and Hall, 1961). In the dog and cat, the mediastinum is flexible and thin, and changes of intrapleural pressure on one side are immediately communicated to the other. Open thoracotomy in these animals is thus essentially bilateral. The size of the opening determines the length of time the animal can survive without artificial ventilation. With a small aperture, respiration may continue for a long period before asphyxia results.

REFERENCES

Balentine, J.D.: Pathologic Effects of Exposure to High Oxygen Tensions: Review. N. Engl. J. Med., 275:1038, 1966.

Bennet, P.B.: Hyperbaric Oxygen and the Signifiance of Increased Cerebral Oxygen and CO_2 Tension. In: *A Symposium on Oxygen Measurements in Blood and Tissues and Their Significance*. Edited by J.P. Payne, and D.W. Hill. Churchill, London, 1966.

Berger, A.J., Mitchell, R.A., and Severinghaus, J.W.: Regulation of Respiration. N. Engl. J. Med., 297:92, 1977.

Biddulph, C., Hof, H., Clancy, R., and Brown, E.B., Jr.: Plasma and Tissue Electrolyte Changes Produced in Dogs by Hypercapnia, Hypocapnia, and Hypoxia. Publication 60–83, School of Aviation Medicine, U.S. Air Force Aerospace Medical Center, Brooks Air Force Base, Texas, 1960.

Comroe, J.H., Jr.: *Physiology of Respiration: An Introductory Text*, 2nd ed. Year Book Medical Publishers, Inc., Chicago, 1974.

Davis, H.A.: *Shock and Allied Forms of Failure of the Circulation*. Grune & Stratton, New York, 1949.

deLemos, R., Wolfsdorf, J., Nachman, R., Block, A.J., Leiby, G., Wilkinson, H.A., Allen, T., Haller, A., Morgan, W., and Avery, M.E.: Lung Injury from Oxygen in Lambs. Anesthesiology, 30:609, 1969.

DeMoor, A.,, Desmet, P., and Verschooten, F.: Influence of Change of Body Position on Arterial Oxygenation and Acid-Base Status in the Horse in Lateral Recumbency, Anaesthetized with Halothane and Efficiency of Postanaesthetic Oxygen Administration. Zbl. Vet. Med. A, 21:525, 1974.

Drinker, C.K.: The Efficiency of the Oxygen-Carbon Dioxide Treatment of Carbon Monoxide Poisoning. J. Indust. Hyg., 7:539, 1925.

Farhi, L., Otis, A.B., and Proctor, D.F.: Measurement of Intrapleural Pressure at Different Points in the Chest of the Dog. J. Appl. Physiol., 10:15, 1957.

Garcia, A.C., Lai, Y.L., Attebery, B.A., and Brown, E.B., Jr.: Lactate and Pyruvate Accumulation During Hypocapnia. Respir. Physiol., 12:371, 1971.

Gillespie, J.R., Tyler, W.S., and Hall, L.W.: Cardiopulmonary Dysfunction in Anesthetized Laterally Recumbent Horses. Am. J. Vet. Res., 30:61, 1969.

Gilmour, I., Burnham, M., and Craig, D.B.: Closing Capacity Measurement During General Anesthesia. Anesthesiology, 45:477, 1976.

Guyton, A.C.: *Textbook of Medical Physiology*, 6th ed. W.B. Saunders Company, Philadelphia, 1981.

Hamilton, T.B., Phillips, R.A., and Hiller, A.: Duration of Renal Ischemia Required to Produce Uremia. Am. J. Physiol., 152:517, 1948.

Haring, O.M.: Cardiac Malformations in Rats Induced by Exposure of the Mother to Carbon Dioxide during Pregnancy. Circ. Res., 8:1218, 1960.

Harris, A.S.: Ventricular Fibrillation and Standstill in Coronary Occlusion. Fed. Proc., 5:41, 1946.

Kanter, G.S.: The Effect of Hyperventilation on Glomercular Filtration and Renal Plasma Flow. Publication

61–48, School of Aviation Medicine, U.S. Air Force Aerospace Medical Center, Brooks Air Force Base, Texas, 1961.

Kistler, G.S., Caldwell, P.R.B., and Weibel, E.R.: Development of Fine Structural Damage to Alveolar and Capillary Lining Cells in Oxygen Poisoned Rat Lungs. J. Cell Biol., 33:605, 1967.

Lai, Y.L., Rodarte, J.R., and Hyatt, R.E.: Respiratory Mechanics in Recumbent Dogs Anesthetized with Thiopental Sodium. J. Appl. Physiol., 46:716, 1979.

Lee, J.A., and Atkinson, R.S.: *A Synopsis of Anesthesia,* 6th ed. Williams & Wilkins, Baltimore, 1968.

Lewis, R.A., Thorn, G.W., Koepf, G.F., and Dorrance, S.S.: The Role of the Adrenal Cortex in Acute Anoxia. J. Clin. Invest., 21:33, 1942.

Macintosh, R., Mushin, W.W., and Epstein, H.G.: *Physics for the Anaesthetist,* 3rd ed. Blackwell Scientific Publications, Oxford and Edinburgh, 1963.

McDonell, W.N., Hall, L.W., and Jeffeott, L.B.: Radiographic Evidence of Impaired Pulmonary Function in Laterally Recumbent Anaesthetized Horses. Equine Vet. J., 11:24, 1979.

Miller, F.A., Hemingway, A., Nier, A.O., Knight, R.T., Brown, E.B., Jr., and Varco, R.L.: The Development of, and Certain Clinical Applications for, a Portable Mass Spectrometer. J. Thorac. Surg., 20:714, 1950.

Miseroccchi, G., Mortola, J., and Sant'Ambrgio, G.: Localization of Pulmonary Stretch Receptors in the Airways of the Dog. J. Physiol., 235:775, 1973.

Nunn, J.F., and Hulands, G.H.: Gas Exchange During Anaesthesia. Proc. R. Soc. Med., 66:980, 1973.

Orr, J.A., Ungerer, T., Bisgard, G.E., and Will, J.A.: Hemodynamic Effects of Acute Hypoxia and Minute Amounts of Endotoxin in Awake Swine. Am. J. Vet. Res., 38:1753, 1977.

Pavlin, E.G.: Chemical Control of Ventilation. Refresher Course in Anesthesiology, 4:63, 1976.

Pavlin, D.J., Ferens, J., Allen, D.R., and Cheney, F.W.: Pulmonary Arteriovenous Shunts during Halothane Anaesthesia in Dogs. Br. J. Anaesth., 52:763, 1980.

Polgar, G., and Weng, T.R.: The Functional Development of the Respiratory System from the Period of Gestation to Adulthood. Am. Rev. Respir. Dis., 120:625, 1979.

Rehder, K., Sessler, A.D., and Marsh, H.M.: General Anesthesia and the Lung. Am. Rev. Respir. Dis., 112:541, 1975.

Saklad, M.: *Inhalation Therapy and Resuscitation.* Charles C Thomas, Springfield, Illinois, 1953.

Shapiro, B.A., Harrison, R.A., and Walton, J.R.: *Clinical Application of Blood Gases,* 2nd ed. Year Book Medical Publishers Inc., Chicago, 1977.

Smith, C.W., Lehan, P.H., and Monks, J.J.: Cardiopulmonary Manifestations with High O_2 Tensions at Atmospheric Pressure. J. Appl. Physiol., 18:849, 1963.

Smith, T.C.: Carbon Dioxide and Anesthesia: Respiratory, Circulatory, and Metabolic Effects. Refresher Courses in Anesthesiology, 4:125, 1976.

Southorn, P., Rehder, K., and Hyatt, R.E.: Halothane Anesthesia and Respiratory Mechanics in Dogs Lying Supine. J. Appl. Physiol., 49:300, 1980.

Stacy, R.W., and Whitehorn, W.V.: The Comparative Susceptibility of Cats and Dogs to Anoxia. Fed. Proc., 6:210, 1947.

Stahl. W.R.: Scaling of Respiratory Variables in Mammals. J. Appl. Physiol., 22:453, 1967.

Swann, H.G.: The Principles of Resuscitation. Anesthesiology, 14:126, 1953.

Tanaka, R., Fujimori, M., and Virtue, R.W.: Oxygen Utilization by Dogs after Administration of Potassium Perchlorate during Hypothermia, and at a Pressure of 2 Atmospheres. Anesthesiology, 22:20, 1961.

Whitehead, R.W., and Draper, W.B.: A Respiratory Reflex Originating from the Thoracic Wall of the Dog. Anesthesiology, 8:159, 1947.

Winter, P.M.: Pulmonary Oxygen Toxicity. Refresher Courses in Anesthesiology, 2:163, 1974.

Wright, J.G., and Hall, L.W.: *Veterinary Anaesthesia and Analgesia,* 5th ed. Williams & Wilkins, Baltimore, 1961.

CHAPTER 7

Oxygen Administration and Artificial Respiration

Safe anesthetic induction, maintenance, and recovery require effective pulmonary and cardiovascular function. This implies the transfer of sufficient oxygen to and carbon dioxide from the pulmonary alveoli, and adequate circulation through both pulmonary capillaries and those of other vital organs. Since pulmonary ventilation may be depressed by drugs, disease, equipment, or by the procedure planned, assisted or controlled ventilation with concomitant gas transport and exchange may be advantageous, or even mandatory, during anesthesia or supportive therapy.

OXYGEN ADMINISTRATION

Determining Oxygen Cylinder Content

A rule of thumb for determining the number of liters of oxygen in commercial cylinders is to multiply the pressure by 3. The length of time a cylinder will last can be estimated by multiplying the pressure times 3 and dividing by the flow in liters per minute.

Example:
Cylinder pressure 350 pounds and flow 6 liters per minute,
$350 \times 2 \div 6 = 175$ minutes

Table 7–1 shows the approximate hours of service in standard 244 cubic feet cylinders of oxygen.

Regulators

When one is using gases from large cylinders, it is necessary that they be reduced to safe pressures. This is accomplished by means of a regulator that may be of one, two, or three stages. The regulator facilitates control and stabilization of the gas flow and provides pressures low enough to allow the controlled release of gas over a relatively narrow range of flow rates (e.g., 1 to 15 liters per minute) and to be compatible with the use of rubber tubing. Single-stage regulators reduce tank pressure to approximately 60 psi in a single step; two- and three-stage regulators reduce tank pressure to intermediate pressures and to 50 to 60 psi in the final stage, following which the gas is metered through a flowmeter (Fig. 7–1). Single-stage regulators may be preset to deliver gas at no more than 50 psi or they may be adjustable. An adjustable regulator has a threaded hand control on its face; this control can be opened to permit a wide range of flow while limiting the output pressure to 50 psi. The amount of gas going to

TABLE 7–1. Approximate Remaining Hours of Service in Standard 244 Cubic Feet Cylinders of U.S.P. Oxygen

	Full Cylinder	*Contents at Diminishing Gauge Pressure*		
Rate of flow in L per min	*244 cu ft 2,200 lbs 6,900 L*	*183 cu ft 1,650 lbs 5,175 L*	*122 cu ft 1,110 lbs 3,450 L*	*61 cu ft 550 lbs 1,725 L*
4	28¾ hrs	21½ hrs	14¼ hrs	7½ hrs
6	19 hrs	12¼ hrs	9½ hrs	4¾ hrs
8	14¼ hrs	10¼ hrs	7¼ hrs	3½ hrs
10	11½ hrs	8½ hrs	5¾ hrs	2¾ hrs
12	9½ hrs	7¼ hrs	4¾ hrs	2¼ hrs
14	8 hrs	6 hrs	4 hrs	2 hrs
16	7 hrs	5¼ hrs	3½ hrs	1¾ hrs

Examples—Full cylinder, at 2,200 lbs pressure, flowing at a rate of 4 liters should last 28¾ hours. A cylinder with 1,100 lbs pressure flowing at a rate of 6 liters per minute should last 9½ hours.
(Courtesy of Ohio Chemical & Surgical Equipment Company, Madison, Wisconsin.)

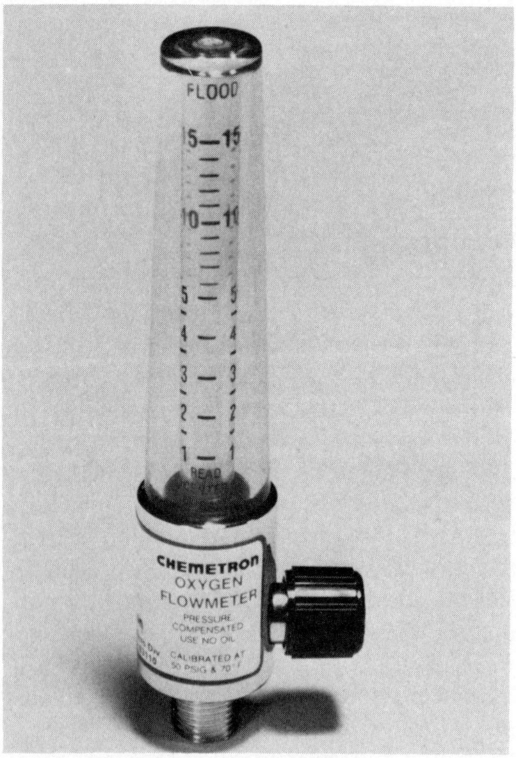

Figure 7–1. Dual-scale, Thorpe-type flow tube. The expanded scale reads from 0 to 5 LPM, while the 5 to 15 LPM scale is for general use. The "Flood" position delivers a minimum of 65 LPM. (Courtesy of Chemetron Medical Division, Allied Healthcare Products, Inc., St. Louis, Missouri.)

the patient from a single-stage regulator is metered by a Thorpe-tube flowmeter, the gas from an adjustable regulator via a Bourdon flowmeter (Fig. 7–2). The latter is a low-pressure device that meters the gas leaving the regulator with a scale that converts pressure to flow rate. A multiple-stage regulator may be provided with either Bourdon or Thorpe-tube flowmeters.

One-stage-regulators present certain hazards and disadvantages. If the valve on an oxygen tank provided with a single-stage regulator is opened rapidly and the regulator valve is also open, the regulator may shatter. Single-stage regulators do not maintain oxygen pressure as cylinder pressure drops, so frequent adjustments are necessary to produce a uniform delivery of oxygen. With multiple-stage regulators, oxygen flow is maintained at a uniform rate until the cylinder is almost exhausted.

After a regulator is attached to the cylinder, the liter-flow mechanism should be turned to the "off" position before the cylinder valve is opened. The cylinder valve should be opened slowly, since oxygen should never be permitted to enter a regulator suddenly. One asset of a piped hospital gas system is that pressure is reduced at a central location. Gas is thus at its working pressure at the various outlets.

The Air Injector Valve

If oxygen at concentrations lower than 100% is desired, an air injector valve can be attached to the regulator (Fig. 7–3). Oxygen entering this apparatus from the regulator passes into a cham-

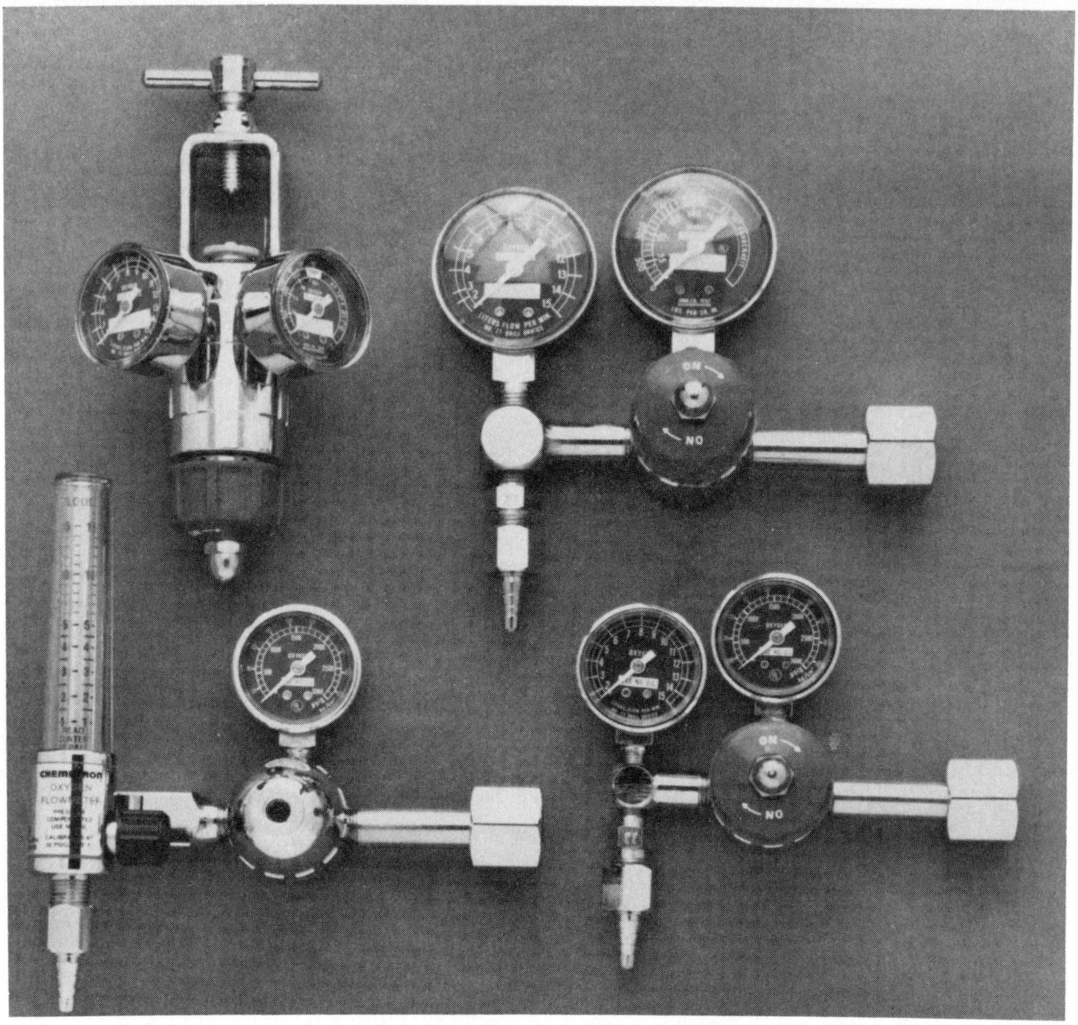

Figure 7–2. *A*, Single-stage adjustable regulator with Bourdon gauge for small cylinders. *B*, Single-stage adjustable regulator with Bourdon gauge for large cylinders. *C*, Single-stage preset regulator with Thorpe-type flowmeter for large cylinders. *D*, Small compact single-stage adjustable regulator with Bourdon gauge. (Courtesy of Chemetron Medical Division, Allied Healthcare Products, Inc., St. Louis, Missouri.)

ber through a narrow orifice. This creates a negative pressure and draws air into the chamber via entrainment ports. The oxygen-air mixture is then forced out the bottom. The volume of air aspirated into the chamber depends upon the size of the entrainment port. Diluters based on this principle are usually provided with a sequence of different sized ports, which are calibrated to provide specific concentrations of oxygen at given flow rates. Mixing devices of this type are not reliable in the presence of fluctuating downstream resistance.

Safety Precautions with Oxygen

At high pressures, the oxidizing powers of oxygen are greatly enhanced. Fats, oils, and paints may oxidize with explosive force, producing so-called *flash-flames* or *oxygen-fires*.

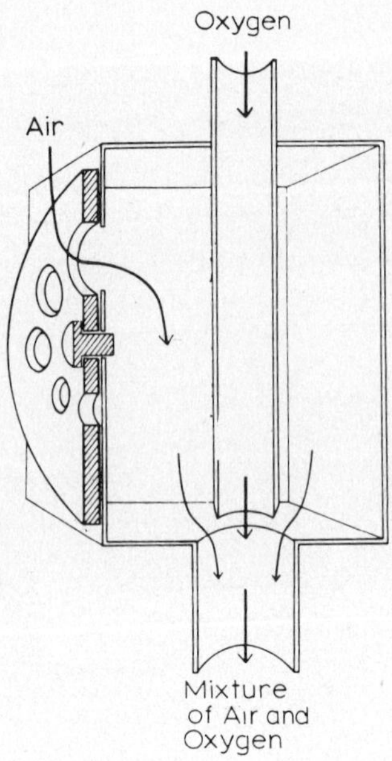

Figure 7–3. Cutaway of air injector valve for mixing room air and oxygen. The Venturi principle is used in its operation.

For this reason, grease or oils should never be used around oxygen cylinders and equipment. Smoking must be prohibited in areas where oxygen is used. Since oxygen supports combustion, all possible sources of fire should be eliminated. Candles, open flames, electrical devices such as heating pads or fans, x-ray equipment, and electrocautery machines are dangerous sources of combustion.

Oxygen cylinders should be stored so they cannot tip over; otherwise, in falling, the cylinder valve may be opened or broken. In this event, the cylinder can become jet-propelled in the same manner as a rocket. A handcart with safety chain should be used in transporting cylinders. If stored against a wall, a safety chain should be installed to hold the cylinder upright. Hazards and precautions associated with the use of compressed gases have been reviewed by Webb and Warren (1982).

Permanent Oxygen Supply

In building new hospitals, planners should consider permanent installation of an oxygen pipeline system (Fig. 7–4). Advantages of such an arrangement include: 1) ability to buy oxygen in larger tanks with increased economy, 2) removal of unsightly tanks from the operating room and other areas, 3) ability to use oxygen in several areas of the hospital without duplication of equipment, 4) an increased inclination to use oxygen when indicated because of availability and ease in administration, and 5) reduction of gas pressure at a central location.*

Methods of Oxygen Administration

Methods for delivery of controlled gas concentrations fall into two categories: nonrebreathing and rebreathing systems (see Chap. 11). In the former, exhaled gases have little or no contact with those inhaled. Exhaled carbon dioxide is therefore not a problem, but gas flows must be adequate to satisfy the needs of respiratory minute volume and of peak inspiratory flows. The latter is usually accomplished by provision of an inspiratory reservoir in which fresh gas accumulates during nondemand periods of the respiratory cycle. As a further safeguard, these systems have a one-way valve by which room air enters the system when inspiratory demands are not met. A nonrebreathing system that totally satisfies ventilatory needs is called a high-flow system. If environmental air is required, the system is considered a low-flow system. Rebreathing systems require a carbon dioxide absorber, and are usually used for administration of inhalant anesthetics, but may occasionally be used for therapy.

Oxygen therapy is generally administered by nonrebreathing systems. High-flow systems usually incorporate an entrainment (Venturi) device to add environmental air in static proportion to oxygen flows, and thus can provide oxygen concentrations from 24 to 100% (see Fig. 7–3). Nebulizers may also utilize the Venturi principle and provide 30 to 100% oxygen concentrations (Shapiro et al., 1979). Such high-flow systems, if properly applied, provide a constant controlled inspired concentration of oxygen (FIO_2) with the potential for control of temperature and

*A brochure entitled "Standard for Nonflammable Medical Gas Systems, NFPA 56-1983" is available from the National Fire Protection Association, Inc., Batterymarch Park, Quincy, Massachusetts, 02269. It sets forth requirements for construction and testing of oxygen and other nonflammable medical gas systems.

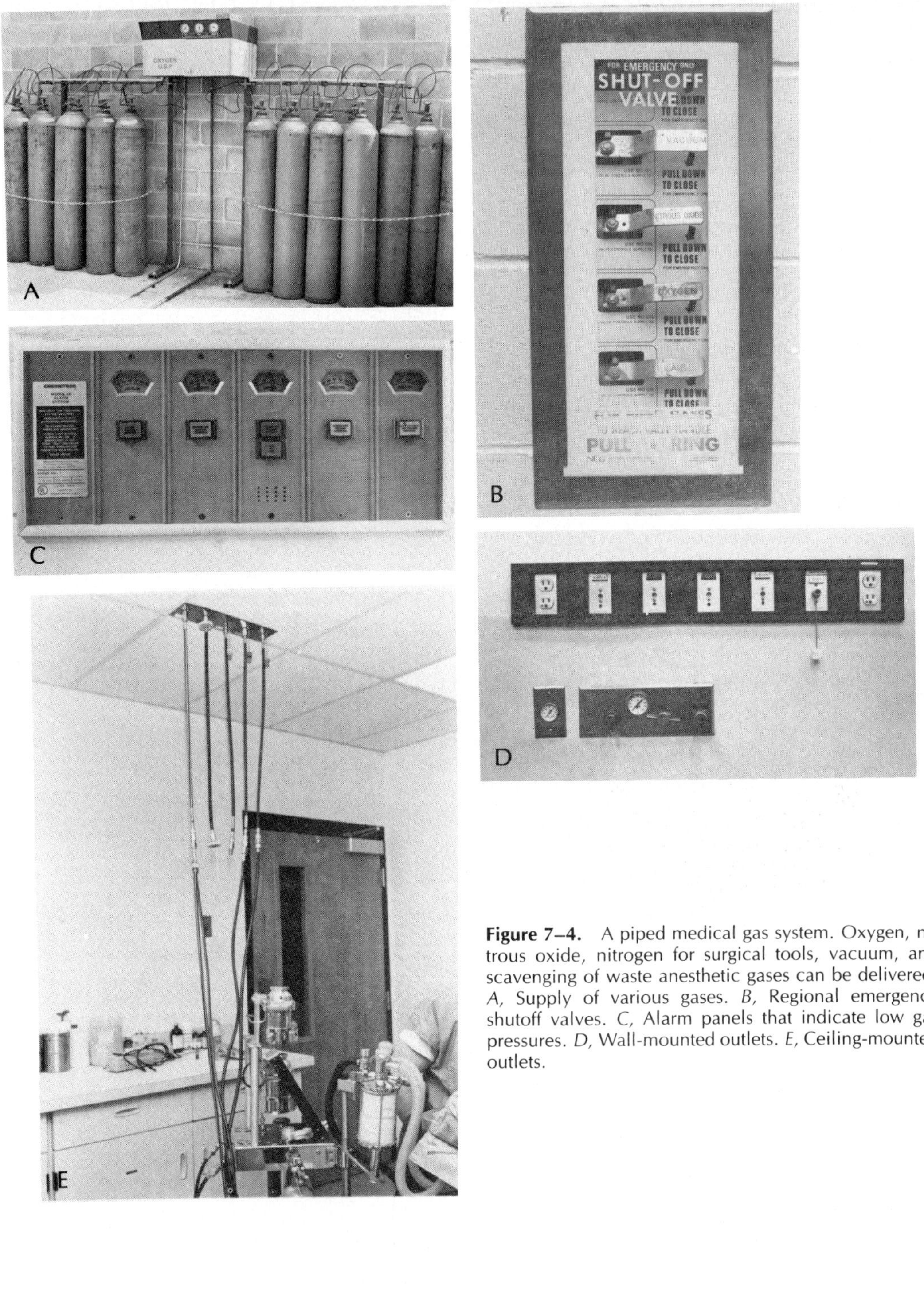

Figure 7–4. A piped medical gas system. Oxygen, nitrous oxide, nitrogen for surgical tools, vacuum, and scavenging of waste anesthetic gases can be delivered. *A,* Supply of various gases. *B,* Regional emergency shutoff valves. *C,* Alarm panels that indicate low gas pressures. *D,* Wall-mounted outlets. *E,* Ceiling-mounted outlets.

humidity. Low-flow systems require the use of environmental air to provide part of each tidal volume; oxygen concentrations from 21 to 90% can be administered in this way. These systems thus depend upon a reservoir of oxygen (directly from a tank, or indirectly via bag) and its dilution with air. In the event that oxygen flows directly into the upper airways, these constitute an anatomic reservoir that is replenished with oxygen during each respiratory pause.

Oxygen can be administered to animals by the following means:

1. Tent or chamber
2. Nasal catheter
3. Face mask or endotracheal catheter (diffusion respiration, nonrebreathing valve, respirator [ventilator], or gas machine)
4. Hyperbaric chamber

The simplest equipment is relatively inexpensive and proves lifesaving in emergencies. In any case, ready availability of oxygen during anesthetic procedures, for intensive care, and for other inhalation therapy is essential.

Tents or Chambers

A simple and traditional method for administration of oxygen to man is with an oxygen tent. The canopy of the tent covers the head of the patient's bed, and cooled oxygen is pumped into it. The closest approach to this method in veterinary practice has been the use of a transparent plastic bag into which the whole animal or its head is placed. This has not proved satisfactory for use with small animals because of the restraint problem. With small animals, oxygen chambers are therefore preferred. The use of either tents or chambers for large animals is unsatisfactory because restraint is difficult and the chamber is of such a size that attainment of efficacious concentrations is expensive, slow, and difficult.

Structurally, chambers are usually of two types: 1) a box or aquarium-like chamber with a fitted top or side door or 2) a hospital cage with solid walls, the door of which has been altered to make it airtight and to which have been attached the necessary fittings (Fig. 7–5).

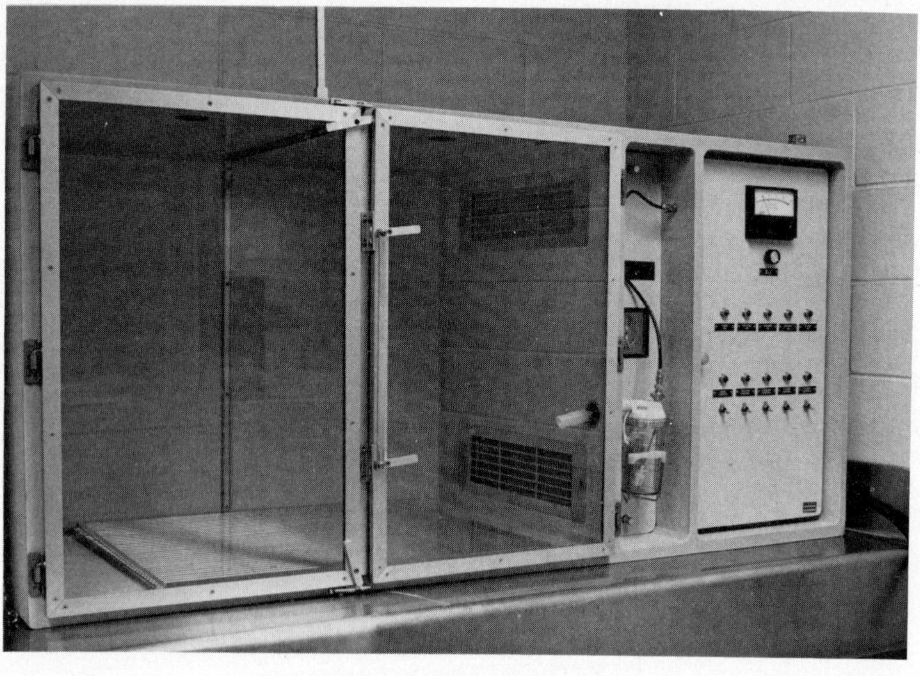

Figure 7–5. Temperature-controlled oxygen therapy cage for small animals. A similar model for birds also has controlled humidity.

Plastic chambers manufactured for the maintenance of germfree animals are also satisfactory as therapy chambers. Equipment for proper use of chambers should include a thermometer, a gauge for determining relative humidity, a flowmeter, and an oxygen analyzer.

Tents or chambers may be operated as modified open or as modified closed systems (Gillespie, 1972). The modified open system comprises a leaking reservoir supplied by a high flow of oxygen, thereby flushing out residual air, accumulations of carbon dioxide, and excessively humid gases. Often modified open chambers are built so that oxygen enters at the top, is cooled by passing over ice in a container, and then settles to the patient. Water, produced by the melting ice, is drained to the exterior to prevent a rise in chamber humidity. Warm carbon dioxide rises to the top of the chamber and escapes through vents. In other chambers, humidity and temperature are controlled automatically. The oxygen content should be tested at least three times a day with an oximeter because flow into the chamber is not necessarily an indication of oxygen concentration.

Relative humidity within the chamber should be maintained between 40 and 60% in most instances. The carbon dioxide content should not be more than 1.2%. Maintaining a minimum flow of 6 to 8 liters of oxygen per minute with a concentration of 50% prevents harmful accumulations of carbon dioxide from developing, even in the absence of soda lime.

A thermometer should be used to determine chamber temperature. Oxygen chambers that are not equipped to cool and dry the air may be detrimental to the patient and even cause death by heat stroke.

In the presence of fever, metabolism is increased, and oxygen requirements are thereby increased. When an animal with fever is placed in a chamber, the oxygen flow should be increased to 10 liters per minute, flooding the cage, cooling the ambient temperature, and thereby lowering the animal's temperature.

If desired, a nebulizer can be inserted in the oxygen line and various solutions, such as antibiotics, antifoaming agents, and bronchodilators, can be vaporized into the oxygen chamber.

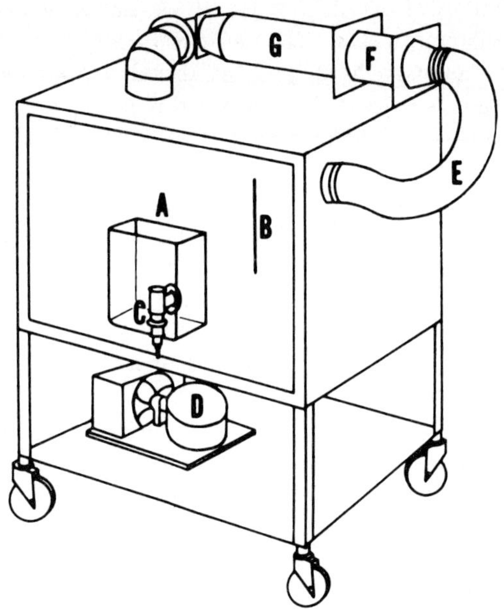

Figure 7–6. Modified Gourley O_2 cage. Heavy Plexiglas door, sealed tightly to the cage (A); thermometer within cage (B); port for putting O_2 into cage (C); refrigeration compressor (D); 4-inch flexible hose for carrying gas out of cage (E); CO_2-absorbent canister (F); and housing for condensing and cooling coils from refrigeration compressor leading to circulating fan and gas inlet pipe on top of cage (G). (From Gillespie, J.R., and Martin, D.B.: Long-term Oxygen Cage Therapy for Hypoxemic Dogs. J.A.V.M.A., 156:717, 1970.)

The modified closed system utilizes a gastight cage, a low flow of oxygen, and carbon dioxide absorption. Temperature and humidity are controlled automatically. Gillespie and Martin (1970) recommended a modified Gourley small animal cage for dogs with hypoxemia. It was modified by addition of cooling and condensing coils, a CO_2 absorber, and a circulating fan (Fig. 7–6). Oxygen therapy may also be administered with the aid of a human pediatric incubator that has similar environmental controls. No matter which system is used, the animal should not be handled more than 3 or 4 times daily owing to disruption of the environment within the chamber.

Nasal Catheter

For continuous administration of oxygen to small animals that are severely depressed, a nasal catheter of small gauge polyethylene (PE

200) or of soft flexible rubber or plastic tubing is quite effective. The catheter is held against the animal's head, and the distance from the external nares to the pharynx marked on the catheter with adhesive tape. An anesthetic jelly is applied to the catheter, which is then inserted along the floor of the nasal passage as far as the mark. Adhesive tape is applied around the catheter and to the nose to hold the catheter in position. Oxygen is then regulated to flow to the patient at the desired rate. Because of the drying effect of oxygen, it should first be passed through a humidifier.

Oxygen may be similarly administered to large animals. To keep the nasal tube in position, use of a self-retaining catheter or a cuffed canine endotracheal catheter is advantageous.

Face Mask

Administration of oxygen by means of a mask is effective during anesthesia and for short periods during emergencies; however, unless the animal is quite depressed or is anesthetized, it probably will resist the mask and reduce its effectiveness. To minimize mechanical dead space and improve effective ventilation, the mask should be as small as practical, and provision for exhalation should be as close to the external nares as possible. Masks are also satisfactory for oxygen therapy in horses of placid temperament. Modified plastic buckets or plastic bags have been used for this purpose.

Endotracheal Intubation

Endotracheal intubation is used for one or more of the following purposes:

1. to maintain an open airway while the patient is under anesthesia, to prevent aspiration of secretions or regurgitated stomach contents, especially in the ruminant, and to improve effective ventilation by reducing the dead space of the upper airway;
2. to provide a means for administration of inhalation anesthetics, aerosols, and/or oxygen; and
3. to facilitate assisted or controlled ventilation.

Endotracheal tubes should be smooth, easily cleaned and sterilized, and sufficiently rigid to resist kinking and compression. They may or may not have inflatable cuffs and may be curved or straight. Endotracheal tubes for use in small animals vary in size from 4 to 15 mm inside diameter (12 to 44 French*). In adult cattle and horses, tubes up to 35 mm in outside diameter are necessary. Endotracheal tubes are made of rubber or plastic (Fig. 7–7). Conductive materials should be used when employing explosive anesthetics. Tube length should equal the distance from the external nares to the midcervical region. A tube that is too long may be inadvertently inserted into one of the bronchi, thereby occluding the other. Extension of the tube unnecessarily beyond the external nares increases the mechanical dead space. A simple tube is sufficient, provided maintenance of an airway is all that is desired, and can be made from rubber or plastic tubing of various diameters. Plastic (Tygon†) tubing is suitable for making large animal endotracheal tubes. A smooth, rounded bevel should be produced on the end of the tube to be inserted into the trachea. Potential trauma to the larynx and trachea is thereby minimized. It is important to appreciate that the use of thin-walled tubing predisposes to kinking and occlusion of the lumen.

Intubation Procedure

If the trachea is to be completely occluded except for the catheter lumen, an inflatable cuff is attached to the catheter. Cuffs are not available for tubes smaller than 4 mm, and probably should not be used on those smaller than 5 mm in diameter. The most suitable cuffs have a signal balloon on the opposite end of the inflation tube. When the catheter is inserted in the trachea, the degree of inflation of the hidden cuff can be determined by observation of the balloon. Overinflation may occlude the tube lumen, or may cause pressure necrosis of the tracheal mucosa.

Cuffs that have a large volume, high compliance, a large surface area of contact, and that do not distort either the tube or the tracheal

*See Appendix B for comparison of French, Davol, and Magill catheter sizes.

†See Appendix A.

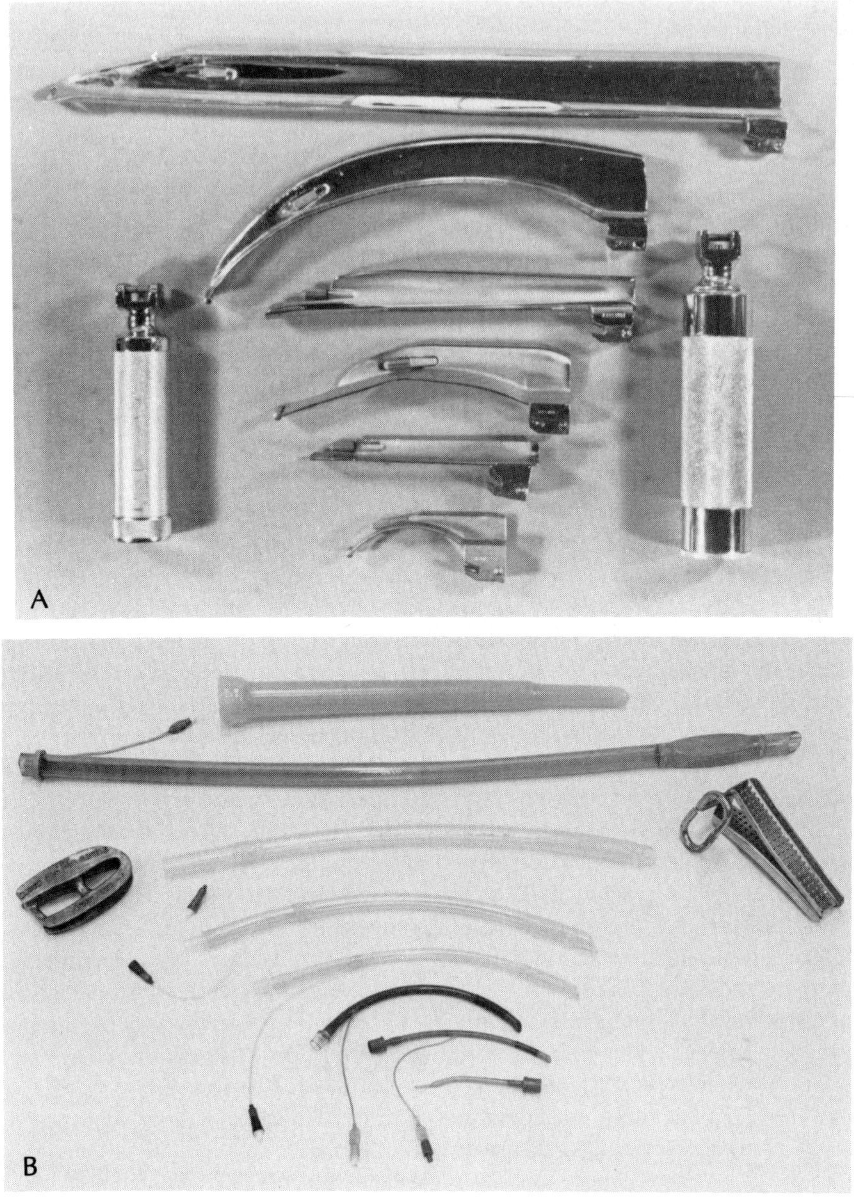

Figure 7–7. A variety of large- and small-animal laryngoscopes *(A)*, and endotracheal tubes *(B)* ranging from a Cole tube for large animals at the top to a Cole tube for cats at the bottom. The speculum on the left (Drinkwater) is used for intubation of cattle and that on the right (Bayer's wedge) for horses.

anatomy are preferred. Long tubes should be shortened to reduce dead space.

Pedersoli and Krista (1979) studied the effects of five different commercially available endotracheal tubes on the tracheas of dogs anesthetized for two hours with methoxyflurane. Lateral tracheal wall pressure (LWP) and measurements of the inside and outside diameters of the trachea were made. The cuffed endotracheal tubes commonly used in dogs produced excessively high LWP. Significant changes were observed in the tracheal epithelium and cilia, varying from loss of cilia to loss of tracheal epithelium thickness.

An inexpensive and effective technique for

making new cuffs has been described by Wycoff (1947). The inflation tubing, blunted needle, and signal balloon are salvaged from leaking cuffs. These are then inserted into new cuffs made from Penrose drain tubing. With practice, cuffs can be easily and simply constructed at a fraction of their commercial cost.

If hemostats are used in clamping an inflation tube to keep the cuff distended, they tend to cut the tube. This can be prevented by using self-sealing adapters, by wrapping the hemostat blades with adhesive tape, or by using rubber-shod tongue forceps.

If the tubes are to be connected to ventilators or anesthetic machines, plastic or metal catheter connectors are required. The largest connector that can be inserted into the catheter should be used to avoid restriction of the airway. When small catheters are used, the connector should be fitted *around* the tube rather than within the lumen, since the latter method severely constricts the lumen. Sudden constriction or sharp angulation of the lumen of the adapter or tube markedly increases airway resistance.

Following use, the endotracheal catheter should be washed thoroughly to remove respiratory secretions and anesthetic jelly from the lumen and exterior. It should then be cold sterilized in a suitable solution. Care should be taken to see that antiseptic solutions do not enter the inflation tube since leakage within the patient could irritate the respiratory mucosa.

When one is choosing an endotracheal catheter, the largest diameter that can be introduced through the larynx without force should be selected. Those having a diameter considerably smaller than the natural airway increase airway resistance, impair gaseous exchange, including uptake and elimination of inhalant anesthetics, and require increased respiratory effort by the patient. Increased negative pressure associated with the latter may result in pulmonary edema. It is good practice to have at hand a catheter thought to be the correct size and also one larger and one smaller. This ensures that the correct size will be available.

When an endotracheal catheter is to be used, *patency should be assured and the cuff should be checked by inflating it prior to the time the animal is anesthetized*. The cuff and tip of the tube are lubricated with a minimal amount of water-soluble jelly, preferably one containing an anesthetic. Use of an anesthetic jelly tends to prevent trauma and irritation to the larynx and trachea which otherwise cause postintubation cough.

Prior to intubation, pharyngeal and laryngeal reflexes should be obtunded sufficiently by anesthesia to prevent reflex cardiac arrhythmias, apnea, laryngospasm, and coughing. If laryngeal reflexes hinder intubation, force should not be used; instead, anesthetic depth should be increased or a topical anesthetic or muscle relaxant administered.

Endotracheal catheters can be inserted by visualization, by palpation of the glottis, by blind intubation, or by passage over a previously inserted stomach tube or catheter. The latter is especially helpful in rabbits and guinea pigs. Because the sight method depends upon a light source and favorable position of the animal, many individuals prefer the touch or palpation method in dogs. The palpation procedure is also used in larger ruminants, whereas in small ruminants and swine, laryngoscopy is desirable. Blind intubation is easily accomplished in the horse, but less readily in ruminants. In domestic cats, intubation is by direct visualization. A laryngoscope aids visualization of the larynx and facilitates placement of the endotracheal tube in some species. A Miller 0 neonatal laryngoscope is especially helpful in rabbits and guinea pigs. Alternatively, a canine otoscope may be used.

Intubation in Dogs (Tube 5 to 15 mm ID). Once anesthesia has been induced and the jaw muscles have relaxed, the tongue is grasped between the thumb and fingers of the left hand and pulled anteriorly. This brings the larynx into the pharynx for a short distance. The index finger of the left hand is extended to depress the epiglottis, and the tip of the catheter is guided along the finger into the laryngeal opening. The epiglottis and arytenoid cartilages are landmarks for this procedure. When the catheter is properly inserted, the arytenoid cartilages can always be felt making an inverted ''V'' (Λ) over it. It should be emphasized that *the catheter must be placed in this position*. If it is pushed into the animal's pharynx, in the hope that it will enter the larynx, it *always* enters the esophagus instead.

Should visual intubation be preferred, this is accomplished with the dog in lateral or sternal recumbency, the head extended upon the neck, and the tongue pulled well forward. The mouth is held wide open with the thumb and second finger of the left hand. The tip of the epiglottis is located (it may be necessary to deflect the soft palate to do this) and depressed by the tip of the endotracheal tube, which is subsequently advanced into the trachea. Trauma to the larynx during intubation, either by excessive digital manipulation or by application of forceps to the epiglottis, should be avoided because edema may result. The presence of the tube in the trachea should be confirmed by digital palpation, direct observation when possible, or by detection of rhythmic exhalation from the lumen of the tube. Holding the open end of the catheter to one's ear should never be used as a test of its position as it is not reliable.

The catheter should be inserted so that the cuff is just beyond the larynx. No advantage is achieved by inserting it further. If inserted too far, one bronchus will be intubated and the other occluded, in which event the lung on the occluded side will be inadequately ventilated or even collapse. In breeds that are not brachycephalic, the endotracheal catheter is fixed to the upper jaw by passing tape around the catheter and the bridge of the nose twice. In brachycephalics, the lower jaw is used. An alternate method is to fasten the catheter by means of a heavy rubber band looped about the patient's jaw. If a simple airway is all that is desired, the cuff need not be inflated. Occasionally, if the anesthesia is light, or inflation of the cuff is excessive, momentary reflex apnea may occur. In any case, the cuff should never be inflated more than necessary to prevent loss of gas around the tube. Resistance to withdrawal and palpation of the pilot bulb are useful guidelines. If mechanical ventilation is to be employed, the cuff is inflated, the inflation tube is sealed, and the intubation procedure is complete (Fig. 7–8).

In cases of oropharyngeal surgery or of orthopedic surgery of the facial region, the endotracheal tube may be inserted via a pharyngotomy or tracheotomy incision. The former is

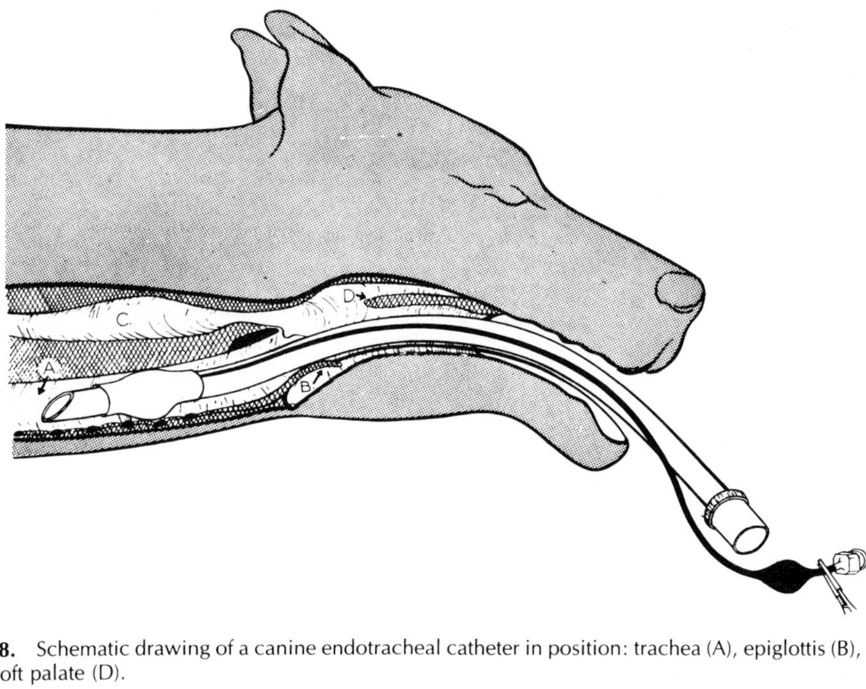

Figure 7–8. Schematic drawing of a canine endotracheal catheter in position: trachea (A), epiglottis (B), esophagus (C), and soft palate (D).

preferable due to less aftercare and fewer complications (Hartsfield et al., 1977). When these procedures are completed, *patency of the airway should be confirmed* by detecting the flow of air to and from the end of the tube.

Following surgery, the catheter should be left in position until the animal shows signs of recovery as evidenced by return of the swallowing reflex. If it is removed prematurely, reinsertion will be difficult if the animal is beginning to regain upper airway reflexes. Prior to removal, the clamp holding air within the cuff should be loosened. Tape fixing the catheter in position is then cut and the catheter carefully removed, taking care to see that the animal does not chew it.

Intubation in Domestic Cats (Tube 1.5 to 8.5 mm ID). After the tongue is pulled forward, intubation is performed by direct vision. A 3.5- to 6-mm Cole tube is usually satisfactory for the adult cat. In kittens, it may be necessary to use a Cole pediatric tube (1.5 to 3.5 mm diameter), appropriate plastic tubing, or a modified urethral catheter. In the use of small-diameter tubes, endotracheal tube adapters should fit *around* the tube unless a soft pliable catheter or Cole tube is used. The main problem encountered when intubating cats is the extreme sensitivity to largyngeal spasm, especially when vagotonic agents such as barbiturates have been used for induction. Under such circumstances, it is essential that the plane of anesthesia be deep or that the laryngeal reflexes be obtunded by administration of a muscle relaxant (succinylcholine chloride, 0.5 mg/lb body weight) or by use of a topical anesthetic or 4% lidocaine hydrochloride solution.

Preferably the anesthetic is sprayed from a small syringe and fine-gauge needle. It also may be applied with a cotton applicator. It should be kept in mind that 10 mg/kg of lidocaine hydrochloride is strongly epileptogenic and produces excitement and convulsions in the cat when given intravenously (Acheson et al., 1956).

Intubation in Ruminants (Tube 10 to 35 mm OD). Induction of general anesthesia in ruminants is especially hazardous because of possible aspiration of accumulated saliva and regurgitated stomach contents. Suppression of salivation by the intravenous administration of 0.02 mg/lb body weight of atropine sulfate may thus be indicated. Atropine, however, is considered by some to be contraindicated in ruminants since their copious secretions become viscid and contribute to airway obstruction (Hall, 1971). Intubation with a cuffed endotracheal tube or a Cole tube as soon as possible during the induction period is mandatory. Fortunately, with the possible exception of the goat, laryngeal reflexes permit intubation in a light plane of anesthesia. In fact, in certain instances, it is possible to intubate tranquilized cattle. In adult cattle, the mouth is held open by a wedge-shaped speculum (a Drinkwater gag* [Fig. 7–7] is preferred), the tongue is pulled forward, the head is extended upon the neck, and the lubricated end of the tube is guided into the larynx by passage of the hand into the pharynx. In the event that the size of the oral cavity makes this difficult, a stomach tube may be passed per os into the trachea. This tube is used as a guide over which the endotracheal tube is threaded. When the endotracheal tube reaches the larynx, some resistance usually is encountered. Occasionally, this resistance prevents passage of the tube into the larynx. It can often be overcome by rotation of the endotracheal tube or, alternatively, by use of a smaller tube. When the endotracheal tube is inserted, the guide tube is removed and the cuff inflated. The speculum remains in situ to prevent damage to the tube.

Visual intubation can be performed with the aid of a large animal laryngoscope.* This is used to insert a stomach tube or other such guides into the trachea. The laryngoscope is then removed, and the endotracheal tube is passed over the guide. With the head extended and the head and neck straight, blind intubation is also possible. Lateral deviation of the neck should be avoided. The tube with concavity dorsad is inserted as far as the pharynx, rotated 180° to engage the laryngeal orifice and gently advanced. Assistance may be required by manipulation of the larynx externally.

In smaller ruminants (calves, sheep, and goats), intubation is most readily performed vis-

*See Appendix A.

ually by means of a laryngoscope. Preferably, the animal should be in either lateral or dorsal recumbency. Sheep may be placed in an upright sitting position. The tongue is pulled forward, and the laryngoscope blade is passed over and pressed down on the base of the tongue. The laryngeal orifice is thus visualized, and the endotracheal tube inserted. Should a laryngoscope not be at hand, it is possible to intubate blindly. The mouth is held open, the tongue is drawn forward, and the head extended. The tube is passed as far as the pharynx with the concavity of the tube dorsad. After reaching the pharynx, it is rotated 180° and gently guided into the larynx by gripping the latter externally. Intubation is facilitated by rotating the tube gently back and forth as it is passed into the larynx. Any lateral deviation of the head should be avoided.

Intubation in Horses (Tube 14 to 30 mm OD). This is accomplished easily by blind intubation. A Bayer's wedge (Fig. 7–7) or an equivalent speculum, inserted between the upper and lower molars, will keep the mouth open and protect the endotracheal catheter. The horse should be in lateral recumbency, the head and neck extended, and the tongue pulled forward. The tube, its concavity toward the hard palate, is passed orally into the pharynx, at which time it is rotated 180° and advanced into the larynx during inspiration. Difficulties are most frequently encountered when the tube deviates from the midline or when the head and neck are not sufficiently extended. Intubation with smaller, more flexible tubes can be performed through the inferior nasal meatus.

Intubation in Swine (Tube 5 to 15 mm OD). Endotracheal intubation in swine is more difficult. Laryngeal spasm is easily induced, the larynx is set at an angle to the trachea, and the tube often may enter the middle ventricle of the larynx (Fig. 7–9). The head and neck should be fully extended, with the animal in dorsal or lateral recumbency. The mouth is held open with a speculum, and the animal is intubated visually by means of a laryngoscope with a 250-mm blade. Once the tube is introduced into the lumen of the larynx, passage into the trachea requires slight flexion of the head on the neck or rotation of the tube through 180°.

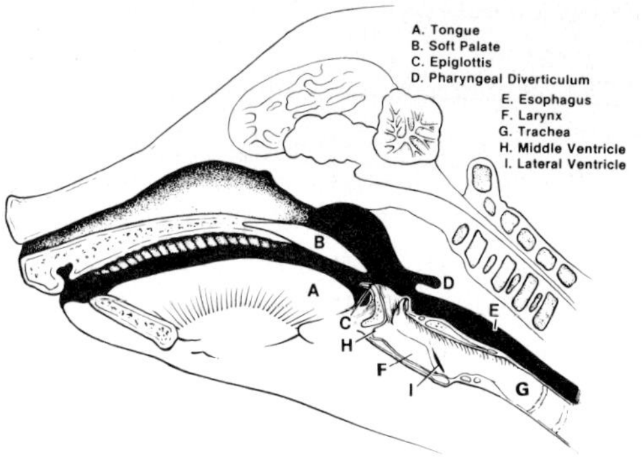

Figure 7–9. Sagittal section of pig's head. Curved endotracheal catheters will not pass area near I, unless rotated so that curve is ventral. Once past this area, the tube is rotated 180° so that the curve is dorsal.

Whatever the species, the advantages of endotracheal intubation far outweigh the disadvantages. Advantages of an endotracheal catheter are:

1. It assures a patent airway.
2. It prevents aspiration of vomitus, blood, or secretions if an inflated cuff is used.
3. It facilitates administration of oxygen and inhalant anesthetics.
4. Respiration can be easily controlled, permitting open chest surgery.
5. There is decreased respiratory effort.
6. Dead space is minimized, increasing efficiency over a closed system with a mask or cone.

Unfavorable complications and sequelae that may occur from endotracheal intubation are:

1. laryngitis and tracheitis due to trauma;
2. overinflation of the cuff with ischemia and subsequent mucosal necrosis;
3. aspiration or deglutition of the catheter;
4. massive atelectasis if the catheter is inserted too far;
5. reflex arrhythmias, coughing, apnea, bronchospasm, and laryngospasm; and
6. kinking, collapse of the tube, or rupture of the cuff.

Oxygen Therapy

The most beneficial results from oxygen therapy are in anoxic anoxia, in which the blood oxygen tension is decreased. Benefits are limited in anemic and stagnant anoxia because little increase in oxygen saturation results, although the amount of oxygen dissolved in the plasma is increased. There is probably little advantage to be gained from oxygen therapy in cases of histotoxic anoxia.

Administration of oxygen is necessary only to a degree sufficient to maintain normal arterial oxygen tensions (80 to 120 mm Hg) or hemoglobin saturation of 90% or more. If the character of the hemoglobin dissociation curve is recalled, it will be realized that Po_2 values above this range induce little change in oxyhemoglobin saturation. Below 80 mm Po_2, a small decrease significantly reduces the percentage saturation of hemoglobin with oxygen.

Administration of oxygen is advantageous in acute pulmonary disease, cardiac failure, trauma of the chest, shock, and severe hemorrhage (Atkinson et al., 1977).

The anesthesiologist also commonly encounters hypoxemia due to regional areas of uneven ventilation of the lung (ventilation/perfusion inequality), and to absolute shunting of venous (pulmonary artery) blood that mixes with saturated blood. The latter is refractory to oxygen therapy. The effect of such intrapulmonary shunting upon the Pao_2 is also directly related to the degree of desaturation of the venous blood that is shunted. Decreased venous oxygen content results from increased metabolic activity of the tissues, from reduced tissue blood flow per unit of time due to decreased cardiac output, and from lowered Pao_2, which is often secondary to existing hypoxemia or to anemia.

Breathing fractions of inspired oxygen (FIO_2) greater than that in air (21%) increases alveolar oxygen tensions, may decrease the ventilatory work necessary to maintain a given alveolar oxygen tension (PAO_2), and may decrease the myocardial work necessary to maintain a given Pao_2 (Shapiro et al., 1979).

Inhalation of 100% oxygen eliminates nitrogen rapidly from the lungs and more slowly from the tissues. This fact has been utilized to reduce pneumothorax, emphysema, and gaseous distension of the gut. Rapid absorption of oxygen from alveoli may, however, lead to atelectasis when nitrogen has been largely removed from the alveoli. Oxygen therapy is also indicated in carbon monoxide poisoning and in instances of severe hyperthermia.

When one is administering 100% oxygen, it is important to appreciate that it makes less reduced hemoglobin available for transport of carbon dioxide. It initially depresses respiration slightly owing to removal of chemoreceptor stimulation, but later causes some stimulation owing to its effect on the mucosa of the respiratory tract. The chemoreceptor effect also decreases pulse rate and cardiac output (Atkinson et al., 1977). Oxygen therapy may also induce hypoventilation, respiratory arrest, or even coma in cases in which the hypoxia is chronic. In such cases, it is believed that the patient has become tolerant to the concomitant hypercapnia and that reflex stimulation results primarily from the lack of oxygen. Administration of oxygen eliminates this stimulus with consequent suppression of chemoreflexes.

Humidification

Methods employed for administration of oxygen often bypass the upper airway, thereby inducing water and heat loss, drying of the airways, and thickening of secretions. Ciliary function and respiratory defense mechanisms are impaired, resulting in retained secretions, blocked airways, and infection. This loss of water with consequent drying may be prevented by the use of a bubbler jar or humidifier, or a nebulizer. Vaporization provided by the bubbler jar is limited and of value only for administration via mask or nasal catheter (Dripps et al., 1967). Once the gas mixture is warmed from room to body temperature, additional water vapor is required to achieve 100% relative humidity. To satisfy such requirements, humidifiers maintained at approximately body temperature may be used. More frequently, in-line pneumatic or ultrasonic nebulizers are used. These emit a spray of water particles, most of which vary from 0.001 to 5 microns in size.

Ultrasonic nebulizers emit more uniform particles of a size (0.8 to 1 micron) least likely to fall out in the delivery tubes or upper airways (Dripps et al., 1967). Unlike the pneumatic nebulizer, the ultrasonic nebulizer cannot be used to deliver drug aerosols. The output of the ultrasonic nebulizer is so great that prolonged use may be hazardous because of the introduction of large quantities of water into the patient's lungs. A simple method requiring no special equipment is to drip water at the rate of 1 to 4 drops per minute into a nasal catheter through which oxygen is being administered.

Aerosol Therapy

The site of deposition of inhaled liquid droplets is contingent upon the droplet size. Most effective deposition occurs with droplets of 0.5 to 1.5 microns in diameter (Dripps et al., 1967). Droplets of 8 microns in diameter predominate in the bronchioles, of 15 microns in the bronchi, and of 40 or more microns in the upper airway (Modell, 1968). In addition to humidification, bronchodilators, detergents and wetting agents, antifoaming agents, mucolytic agents, enzymes, antibiotics, and steroids may be administered in this manner. Although such drugs are commonly used in human medicine, some doubts exist regarding the merits of many aerosols over simple humidification. Ethyl alcohol (20 to 30%) in water has been found to be effective, however, in severe pulmonary edema (Modell, 1968).

Hyperbaric Oxygen

At 3 atmospheres of ambient pressure, sufficient oxygen is dissolved in the blood to supply tissue needs, hemoglobin thus being unnecessary for oxygen transport (Boerema et al., 1959). This improved oxygen transport is, however, achieved at a cost to carbon dioxide transport owing to the lack of desaturated hemoglobin in the venous blood. The resulting rise in venous and tissue P_{CO_2} thus increases pulmonary ventilation with a consequent fall in arterial P_{CO_2}. This latter change may be responsible for cerebral vasoconstriction during hyperbaric oxygen therapy. Pulmonary vascular resistance is also increased by such therapy.

The potential for supplying additional oxygen to tissues, especially in cases of stagnant and anemic hypoxia, has caused this technique to be applied to such syndromes as hemorrhagic shock, carbon monoxide poisoning, coronary and cerebral ischemia, and traumatic ischemia of the extremities (Hall, 1968). The use of high-pressure oxygen may facilitate cardiac surgery by reducing the necessity for extracorporeal circulation (Bernhard et al., 1963), and by permitting the substitution of saline for blood during perfusion. Hyperbaric oxygen therapy has also been shown to be beneficial in the early stages of anaerobic infections (Hall, 1968) and may improve results from radiation therapy for malignant disease (Atkinson et al., 1977).

Because of the dangers of oxygen toxicity, dysbarism, and fire, as well as the necessity for special chambers, the application of hyperbaric oxygen therapy has been limited.

ASSISTED AND CONTROLLED RESPIRATION

The optimal respiratory pattern consists of a regular rhythm with normal rate and depth, thereby providing normal ventilation. Observation of the excursion of the chest is a simple measure of the degree of ventilation. The efficiency of ventilation may also be roughly assessed on the basis of color of the mucous membranes when oxygen is not being administered, degree of capillary oozing, heart rate, and gas flow required to maintain inflation of the reservoir bag in a nonrebreathing system, or it may be determined by a ventilation meter or spirometer. These means of assessing ventilation have some marked inadequacies. For example, cyanosis does not become evident in the anemic animal until there is severe hypoxia, and it is difficult to assess the efficiency of carbon dioxide elimination unless the arterial P_{CO_2} is determined.

When ventilation is inadequate, respiration should be *assisted* or *controlled*. In assisted respiration, ventilation is enhanced by assistance during spontaneous breathing. In controlled respiration, the normal respiratory mechanisms are inactive, and the anesthesiologist assumes control of breathing. Once pulmonary ventilation is controlled, assessment of adequate volume exchange becomes even more difficult. Ventilation should, however, be sufficient to maintain normal tissue oxygenation and removal of carbon dioxide. Unless laboratory facilities for blood or end-tidal gas monitoring are available, sufficiency can be determined only by observation for chest excursion and for signs of hypoxia and hypercapnia, which can be grossly inaccurate. Hypoxia is indicated by cyanosis and by compensatory circulatory changes that take place in an effort to maintain a supply of blood to the brain. These include a rise in blood pressure and pulse rate and subsequent sharp and progressive fall (Mushin et al., 1969). Despite controlled breathing, hypoxia may result from the use of a pressure-cycled ventilator, arising from change of compliance, the presence of secretions, changes in posture, the use of retractors, or other limitations of the vital capacity. Unlike oxygenation, which results from a volume exchange that is not especially critical, the clearance of carbon dioxide is directly related to the efficiency of ventilation. Accumulation of carbon dioxide induces hypertension, increased bleeding at the surgical site, increase in salivary and bronchial secretions, cerebral congestion, and increased predisposition to cardiac arrhythmias and arrest (Atkinson et al., 1977).

Assisted or controlled respiration is required for emergencies, open chest surgery, during the administration of muscle relaxants, and whenever ventilation is suppressed. In general, the earlier controlled respiration is commenced, the better; delay in initiating adequate ventilation decreases the chances of ultimate survival and recovery. During assisted or controlled breathing, tidal exchange should be maintained at values equal to or above normal (10 to 15 ml/kg body weight).

Ventilation may be assisted or controlled by methods using pressure changes on the chest wall, abdomen, or diaphragm, or through the airway, and by electrical stimulation. Manual compression of the chest may be used for brief periods, but is generally unsatisfactory. Most methods of resuscitation utilize pressure changes within the airway. When pressure is applied to the airway, it is necessary to consider the hazards that may result.

The fluctuating subatmospheric intrapleural pressures (Fig. 7–10) that occur during normal respiration not only move air in and out of the alveoli, but also assist venous return and diastolic filling of the heart-thoracic pump mechanism (Gerst, 1961; Rochford, 1959). In the event of an elevated mean airway pressure, this pressure change is transmitted to the pleural cavity, and venous return and cardiac output are impaired. Studies (Morgan et al., 1966) of intermittent positive-pressure breathing (IPPB) in lightly anesthetized dogs revealed that cardiac output (Fig. 7–11) and stroke volume decreased as the airway pressure increased (peak airway pressures from 10 to 30 cm of water). At the same time, venous return was inhibited by increased airway pressure. The adverse effects of increasing airway pressure were accentuated by increasing the inspiratory to expiratory ratio (1:2 to 1:1 to 2:1). Under normal conditions, however, venous return is reestabished by compensatory vasoconstriction. Should this be impaired by disease, hypovolemia, or even anesthesia, an elevated airway pressure may cause additional embarrassment to cardiac output (Gerst, 1961). Airway pressure is raised by prolonged pressure inhalation, by increased inspiratory to expiratory (I:E) ratio, and by obstruction of exhalation (Hunter, 1962). If the chest is closed, ventilator-produced subatmospheric pressure during exhalation contributes to a normal mean airway pressure and thereby assists venous return and cardiac filling (Fig. 7–12). Unfortunately, application of a negative pressure to the airway often induces a decrease in arterial Po_2 probably due to closure of small airways and associated air trapping (Grenvik et al., 1977). The benefits of subatmospheric pressure are, of course, inapplicable when the chest is opened. During controlled ventilation and positive-pressure inflation of the lungs, the heart is compressed somewhat by the inflated lungs, and its output may suffer. The higher the peak pressure and the longer its duration of action, the greater are the cardiac tamponade and reduction of cardiac output (Mushin et al., 1969). Since the pulmonary circulation is a low-pressure circuit, this

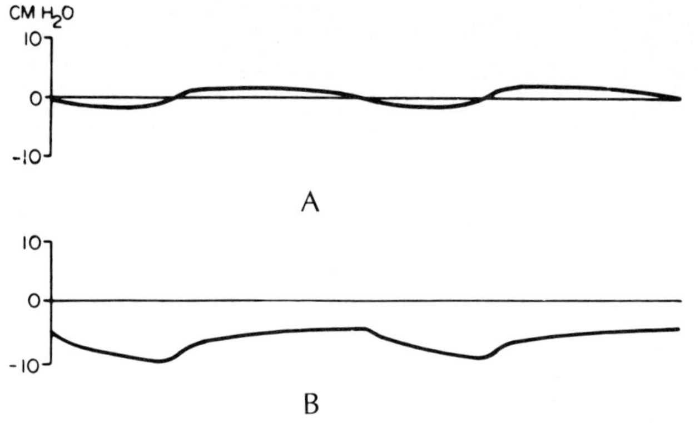

Figure 7–10. *A,* The calculated changes in pressure in the alveoli of a conscious patient breathing spontaneously. Tidal volume = 800 ml; compliance of lungs and thorax = 0.1 liter/cm H_2O; compliance of lungs alone = 0.2 liter/cm H_2O; airway resistance = 2 cm H_2O/liter/sec); respiratory frequency = 15/min. *B,* The calculated changes in intrapleural pressure in the same circumstances as shown in *A.* (From Mushin, W. W., Rendell-Baker, L., Thompson, P.W., and Mapleson, W.W.: *Automatic Ventilation of the Lungs,* 2nd ed. F.A. Davis Co., Philadelphia, 1969.)

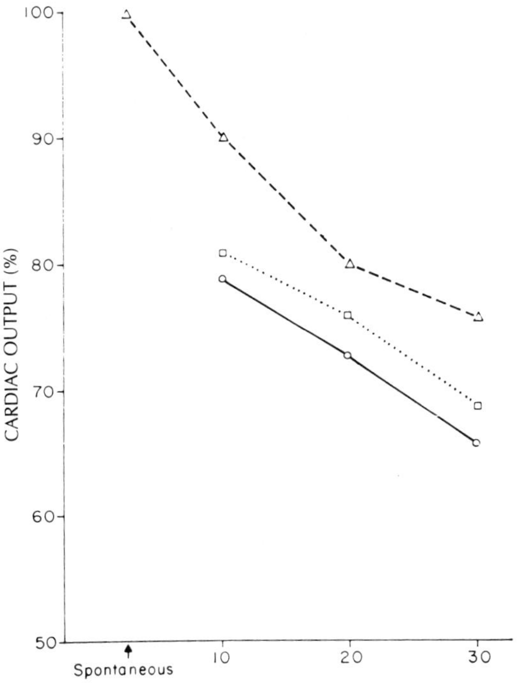

Figure 7–11. Effect of increasing airway pressure and inspiratory/expiratory ratio on cardiac output (average of 12 experiments). Dashed line, triangles indicate values at I:E ratio 1:2, dotted lines, squares at 1:1; and solid line, circles at 2:1. (From Morgan, B.C., Martin, W.E., Hornbein, T.F., Crawford, E.W., and Guntheroth, W.G.: Hemodynamic Effects of Intermittent Positive Pressure Respiration. Anesthesiology, 27:584, 1966.)

likewise is easily suppressed by increased intrapulmonary pressures with an added burden on the right ventricle. In patients with an open chest, the thoracic pump mechanism no longer operates; tamponade, unless from surgical interference, is less likely, and impaired pulmonary circulation by high airway pressure may be of considerable significance. With the advent of the use of continuous positive pressure breathing in contrast to intermittent positive pressure breathing, it has been recognized that changes are also induced in other organs. There is a redistribution of renal blood flow away from the outer cortex with decreased sodium excretion, urine output, and creatinine clearance and an increase in plasma antidiuretic hormone (ADH) (Baratz et al., 1971; Hall et al., 1974). In the liver there is increased portal venous pressure and decreased portal blood-flow (Johnson and Hedley-White, 1975). Positive end-expiratory pressure may increase intracranial pressure (ICP) secondary to increased intrathoracic and systemic venous pressure or may decrease it owing to a decrease in systemic arterial pressure (Fairley, 1978).

During positive-pressure inflation of the lungs, maintenance of a low mean airway pressure with an adequate I:E ratio is, therefore, desirable unless there are indications for continuous positive-pressure breathing. A low mean airway pressure can be accomplished by a brief period of rapid inflation and a period of expiration long enough to allow return to normal atmospheric pressure in the trachea. An I:E ratio of approximately 1:2 is suitable for intermittent positive pressure (Hunter, 1962). If a negative

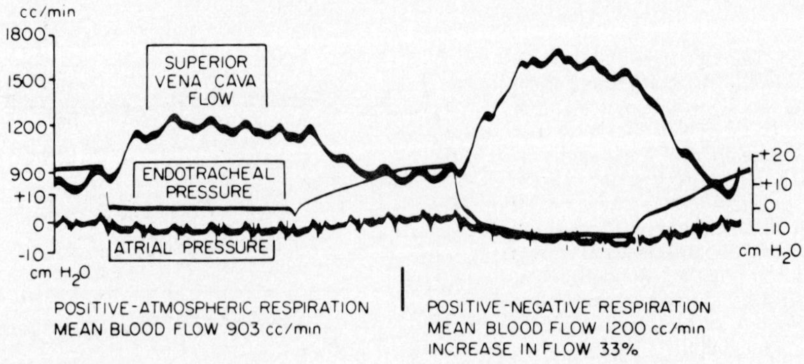

Figure 7–12. Effect of a negative-pressure phase in increasing the venous return to the heart. The tracing is from a dog. Substitution of negative pressure during the expiratory phase, instead of atmospheric, increased blood flow in the superior vena cava by 33%. (From Mushin, W.W., Rendell-Baker, L., Thompson, P.W., and Mapleson, W.W.: *Automatic Ventilation of the Lungs,* 2nd ed. F.A. Davis Co., Philadelphia, 1969.)

pressure exhalation phase is used, an I:E ratio of 1:1 or 1:1.5 is probably adequate (Mushin et al., 1969). The influence of inflation/deflation characteristics on the mean airway pressure is illustrated in Figure 7–13 A–E.

Hyperventilation of a duration likely to occur in anesthesia is generally not considered hazardous, although elimination of carbon dioxide below the threshold value required for respiratory stimulation is associated with postventilation apnea, reduced cardiac output, and reduced cerebral blood flow (Rochford, 1959; Sugioka et al., 1962; Sullivan et al., 1967). This reduced blood flow may be useful during intracranial surgery, although it generally is undesirable and may be detrimental to the metabolism of ischemic brain. To avoid hypercapnia, the degree of ventilation should err on the side of hyperventilation unless P_{CO_2} monitoring is available, in which case eucapnia is preferred. Hypercapnia with increased catecholamine release, a depressant action on vascular smooth muscle, and increased cardiac output may be undetected when oxygen-rich gas mixtures are used. Since hyperventilation decreases arterial CO_2 tension, return to normal tension is contingent upon a period of hypoventilation (Dejours, 1966). If, during this period of hypoventilation, the animal breathes air, the arterial oxygen tension falls to a low level that does not return to normal for nearly 1 hour (Fig. 7–14). This postventilation hypoxia can be prevented by use of oxgyen-enriched mixtures (Fig. 7–15) (Sullivan et al., 1967).

Overinflation causes such pulmonary damage as emphysema, pneumothorax, and pneumoperitoneum. Instances have also been reported in which interstitial pulmonary gas gained access to pulmonary veins and to the pericardial sac (Grenvik et al., 1977). Rupture in experimental animals is usually into the mediastinum with passage of air into the cervical region. Pressures above 30 cm of water are possibly harmful; pressures of 40 to 80 cm of water are required to rupture unsupported mammalian lungs. Higher pressures (80 to 90 cm of water) do occur during coughing. Damage resulting from overinflation is more likely to occur when the chest is open and the lungs are unsupported. The maximum safe pressure in the intact mammal is probably about 70 cm of water (Mushin et al., 1969). Just as high pressures may be harmful, so excessive subatmospheric pressures also may damage the lungs. Negative pressures greater than 10 cm of water are reported to cause pulmonary damage in the dog, especially when the chest is closed (Waltz et al., 1954). During thoracotomy, low negative pressures cause a predisposition to atelectasis and consequent lowered pulmonary compliance. An occasional increase in inflation pressure is therefore necessary to overcome this. Negative pressures may also cause a "check-valve" or "trapping" mechanism, especially in diseased lungs with weak small airways, in which case these airways

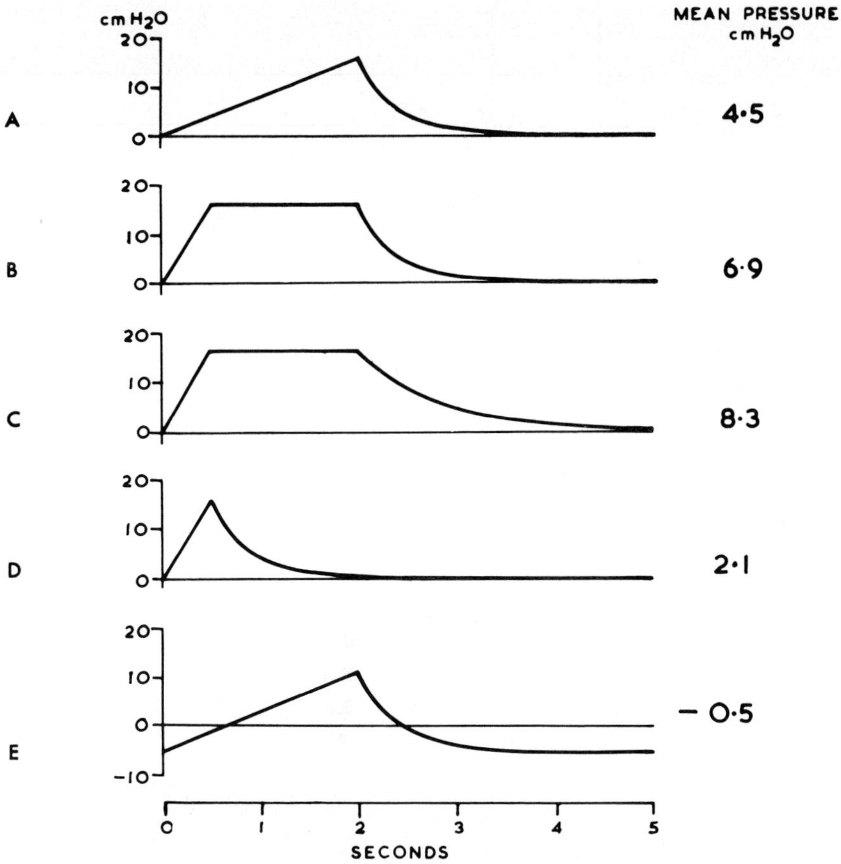

Figure 7–13. Diagrams illustrating the meaning of the term "mean pressure in the lungs" during artificial ventilation. In each case the total respiratory cycle lasts 5 seconds; the tidal volume is 800 ml, and the compliance is 0.05 liter/cm H_2O. Hence the pressure range is 16 cm H_2O. The airway resistance is taken as 6 cm H_2O/(liter/sec). However, possible changes in other variables produce a wide range of mean pressures. *A,* Inflation is slow (flow of inflating gas is 24 liters/min). Expiration is "free." The resistance of the apparatus is taken as 2 cm. H_2O/(liter.sec.). The mean pressure is 4.5 cm H_2O. *B,* Inflation is rapid (flow of inflating gas is 96 liters/min) at the beginning of the inspiratory phase. The lungs are then held inflated for some time so that the inspiratory phase lasts for 2 seconds, as in *A*. Expiration is again "free." The mean pressure is 6.9 cm H_2O. *C,* The inspiratory phase follows the same course as in *B,* but expiration is impeded by an apparatus resistance of 10 cm H_2O/(liter/sec). The mean pressure is 8.3 cm H_2O. *D,* Inflation is rapid (flow of inflating gas is 96 liters/min) and is followed immediately by the "free" expiration. The mean pressure is 2.1 cm H_2O. *E,* Inflation is slow (flow of inflating gas is 24 liters/min) and again occupies 2 seconds. During the expiratory phase a steady negative pressure (−5 cm. H_2O) is introduced. Expiration is "free." The mean pressure is −0.5 cm H_2O. (From Mushin, W.W., Rendell-Baker, L., Thompson, P.W., and Mapleson, W.W.: *Automatic Ventilation of the Lungs*. 2nd ed. F.A. Davis Co., Philadelphia, 1969.)

tend to collapse and exhalation is impaired (Mushin et al., 1969).

During the past decade, the needs of human neonatal and adult ventilatory support have spawned several modifications. Intermittent mandatory ventilation (IMV) was initially developed for weaning from mechanical ventilation. It permits unassisted, unrestricted, spontaneous respiration interspaced periodically with mechanical breaths ("sighs") and may avoid the respiratory alkalosis commonly associated with other forms of mechanical ventilation when it is properly utilized (Downs and Modell, 1977). Subsequently, it has become apparent that this also provides a primary form of ventilatory support. Most ventilators incorporate this mode.

To keep unstable air spaces open during ex-

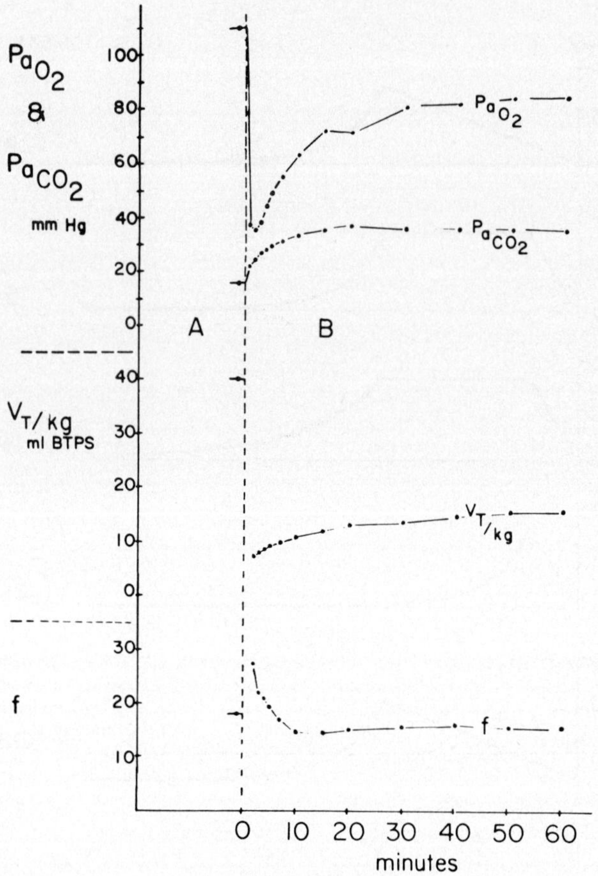

Figure 7–14. Ventilatory response of the dog to posthyperventilation blood gas tensions. Period A represents steady hyperventilation with air for 60 min. Period B represents mechanical ventilation discontinued, allowing spontaneous return of breathing. (From Sullivan, S.F., Patterson, R.W., and Papper, E.M.: Posthyperventilation Hypoxia. J. Appl. Physiol., 22:431, 1967.)

piration, thereby increasing the functional residual capacity (FRC), and to improve oxygenation in the respiratory distress syndrome and in pulmonary edema, a system by which a positive end-expiratory pressure (PEEP) is maintained has been developed. This technique was originally initiated to avoid the need to administer potentially toxic concentrations of inspired oxygen. It is generally considered applicable when PaO_2 is less than 70 mm Hg with an inspired concentration of oxygen 50% ($FIO_2 = 0.5$), or when venous admixture is greater than 10 to 15%. The minimal pressure necessary is utilized since PEEP impedes venous return and at higher levels increases pulmonary vascular resistance. When levels >15 mm Hg are utilized, pulmonary vascular resistance and reduced cardiac output may be offset by intentionally increased blood volume and by inotropic agents (Fairley, 1978).

Modifications of PEEP, continuous positive airway pressure (CPAP), and expiratory positive airway pressure (EPAP) are used during spontaneous ventilation, in conjunction with IMV or via a T-piece system (see next section). Both are used to maintain lung distension; the distinction between them is during inspiration. Positive airway pressure from a distended reservoir bag or demand valve is maintained throughout inspiration in CPAP. With EPAP inspiration is solely dependent upon the efforts of the patient. The work of breathing is thus less with CPAP.

Recently, interest has developed in high-fre-

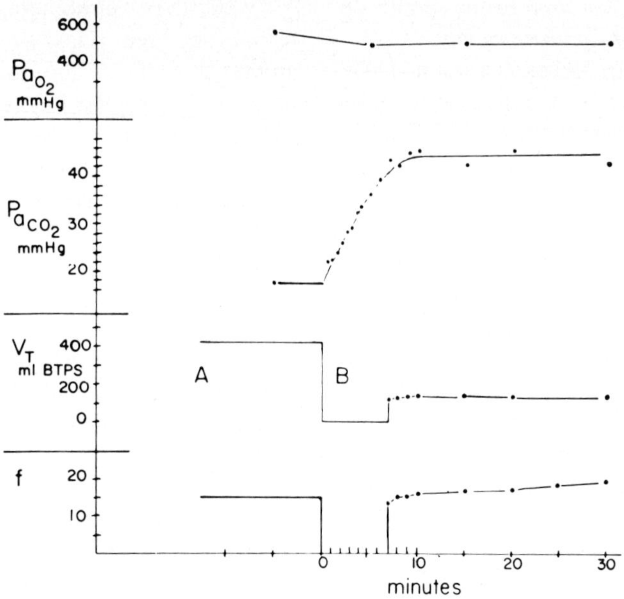

Figure 7–15. Effect of O_2 breathing on ventilation and blood gas tensions of the dog following hyperventilation. Period A, hyperventilation with O_2 for 60 min. Period B, mechanical ventilation discontinued, allowing spontaneous return of breathing. (From Sullivan, S.F., Patterson, R.W., and Papper, E.M.: Posthyperventilation Hypoxia. J. Appl. Physiol., 22:431, 1967.)

quency ventilation. The tidal volume is less than dead space, mean airway and peak inflation pressures are reduced, and there is less compromise of cardiovascular function and danger of barotrauma. Oxygenation and elimination of carbon dioxide are nevertheless adequate. Three basic forms are recognized: high-frequency positive pressure ventilation (HFPPV), high-frequency jet ventilation (HFJV), and high-frequency oscillation (HFO). Original investigators utilized HFPPV with frequencies greater than 60/minute; rates as high as 900/minute have now been utilized. High-frequency jet ventilation employs a Venturi mechanism by which gas is delivered through a small catheter (14- to 16-gauge) with entrainment of additional gas to supplement tidal volume and humidification. Rates are usually greater than 80/minute. High frequencies necessitate accurate control of the inspiratory time. Such times are as low as 0.01 seconds and are optimally 20 to 30% of the entire cycle.

High-frequency oscillation (HFO) involves a "to and fro" movement of the same volume of air in and out of the airway. Methods, such as an in-line CO_2 absorber or a bypass circuit, are required for elimination of carbon dioxide. Best results have been obtained at frequencies greater than 900/minute.

The mechanism by which these methods achieve adequate oxygenation and ventilation and their specific application have yet to be elucidated (Gallagher, 1981).

Diffusion Respiration

Provision of oxygen can be achieved for brief periods by diffusion respiration, providing the airway is patent and the circulation efficient. The phenomenon of diffusion respiration was first described in the dog by Draper and Whitehead (1944). *Diffusion respiration* may be defined as exchange of oxygen and carbon dioxide between the atmosphere and lung alveoli without respiratory movements. This phenomenon was first noted during resuscitation of dogs from respiratory arrest produced by thiopental. It was found that artificial respiration could be suspended for a period of up to one-half hour, if there was a high oxygen concentration in the respiratory tract and if a tube in the mouth delivered 10 liters of oxygen per minute.

Three conditions are necessary for this phenomenon to be successful: 1) replacement of the nitrogen in the respiratory tract and in the atmosphere at the glottis by oxygen, 2) an adequate circulation, and 3) a patent airway.

Diffusion respiration produces a fall in blood pressure and oxygen content of arterial and venous blood with a progressive rise in carbon dioxide content. Concurrently, the pH of arterial and venous blood falls (to 6.72 and 6.84 respectively at 45 minutes). Urine production in dogs during diffusion respiration ceases within a few minutes after arrest of breathing, with either thiopental or muscle relaxants (Kopecky et al., 1952; Irwin et al., 1957) (Fig. 7–16).

Practical application of this phenomenon has been made in hypoxia of small animals by insertion of an endotracheal catheter and flow of 5 to 10 liters per minute of oxygen into the respiratory tree. Gas flows from the lungs around the tube to the atmosphere. This temporarily relieves the oxygen want, whether the patient is breathing or not, and is often lifesaving. The technique is now more commonly used when terminating controlled ventilation, especially when hyperventilation has occurred or the animal's response to CO_2 has been depressed.

T-Tube

By a slight modification, the diffusion respiration system can be adapted to achieve intermittent, manually operated, positive-pressure ventilation.

The simplest apparatus consists of an oxygen cylinder or source of air fitted with a reduction valve and flowmeter, a length of tubing leading to a T-piece, and a cuffed endotracheal catheter (Fig. 7–17; see also Ayres T-tube, Chap. 11).

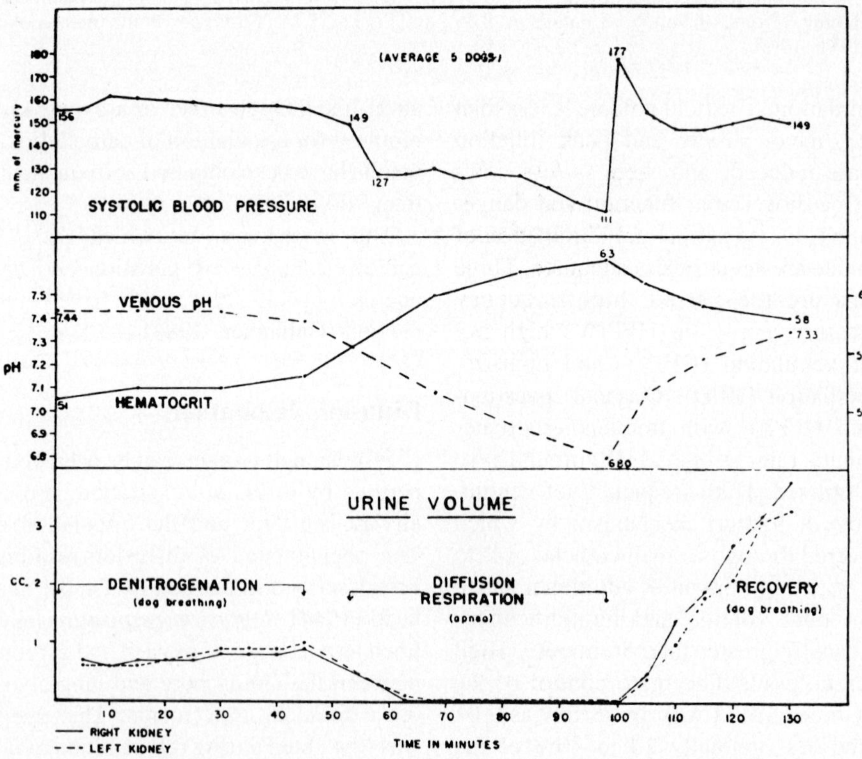

Figure 7–16. Average changes in blood pressure, venous pH, hematocrit, and urine volume in 5 dogs during diffusion respiration. Renal innervation intact on both sides. No intravenous fluid given. (From Kopecky, F.A., Rayburn, C.J., Whitehead, R.W., and Draper, W.B.: A Study of Anuria Occurring during Apnea under Diffusion Respiration. Am. J. Physiol., 168:131, 1952.)

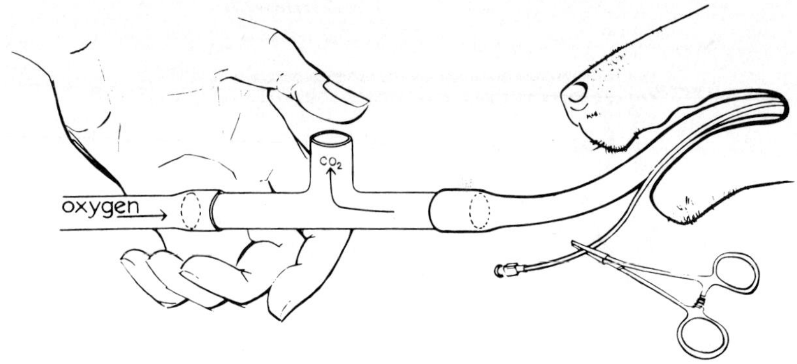

Figure 7–17. Oxygen administration with a T-tube. Positive pressure is produced by intermittently closing the tube with the thumb. Carbon dioxide is exhaled when the thumb is removed.

The diameter of the T-piece and of the exhalation orifice should be at least as large as that of the endotracheal tube. The endotracheal catheter is connected to one arm of the T, the oxygen supply to the other, and the third arm is left open. To avoid excessive mechanical dead space, this orifice should be close to the endotracheal tube. To conserve gases and to avoid rebreathing, the expiratory limb should have a capacity greater than the tidal volume, and the gas flow should be 1.5 to 2.0 times the minute volume.

Positive-pressure inflation is achieved by intermittent occlusion of the orifice to the atmosphere, the duration of which, together with the gas flow rate, determines respiratory rate and depth. An open-ended bag may be attached to the end of the expiratory limb to facilitate controlled or assisted ventilation. For emergency purposes in the horse, a T-piece is unnecessary; oxygen is insufflated directly into the pharynx or trachea via a nasopharyngeal or endotracheal tube, and the nostrils are intermittently occluded. The degree of excursion of the thorax or lungs should be carefully observed to avoid overinflation and consequent permanent pulmonary damage. The duration of exhalation, which occurs by elastic recoil of the chest and lungs, should be at least twice that of the inspiratory phase. Occasional positive-pressure breaths should be used to assure adequate ventilation and to overcome potential atelectasis during spontaneous ventilation.

Although the technique has been used predominantly in small animals, it has also been used in larger animals and is, in fact, limited only by the available gas flow, the tube size, and the physical endurance of the anesthetist. The technique has been modified in small animals for the administration of inhalant anesthetics (see Chap. 11).

Nonrebreathing Systems

Inclusion of a reservoir bag between the oxygen supply and the T-tube of the previous system minimizes the loss of oxygen, which is stored in the bag during each exhalation. Inspired gases are supplied from the reservoir bag, which should be connected to the endotracheal tube (or mask) by an airway larger than the diameter of the animal's trachea. Corrugated hose is usually used. The reservoir bag should be eight to ten times the tidal volume of the animal and should not be so large as to preclude easy determination of the ventilatory excursion. The minimal flow of gas now required must equal only the minute volume rather than the peak inspiratory flow. Replacement of the T-tube with an exhalation valve provides a system incorporating the basic principles of the Magill system (Fig. 7–18; see also Chap. 11). Rebreathing of exhaled gases is possible but minimized by a gas flow exceeding the respiratory minute volume. Modifications of the system to minimize dead space include use of the Norman Elbow and the Bain Circuit (Fig. 7–19). Controlled or assisted ventilation can be readily accomplished by these systems. Manual or auto-

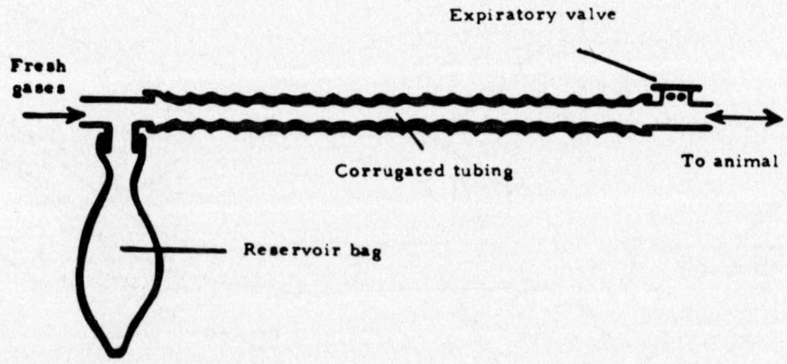

Figure 7–18. Magill attachment. During inhalation, the expiratory valve is closed and fresh gases flow from the corrugated tubing and reservoir bag to the patient. During exhalation, fresh gases flow into the reservoir bag and corrugated tubing while exhaled gases pass out through the expiratory valve. If the fresh gas flow does not exceed respiratory minute volume, significant amounts of exhaled gases pass into the corrugated tubing and rebreathing occurs. (From Hall, L.W.: *Wright's Veterinary Anaesthesia and Analgesia,* 7th ed. Baillière Tindall, London, 1971.)

matic techniques may be used. When a Bain Circuit and a pressure-limited ventilator were used, fresh gas flows (FGF) of 80 to 100 ml/kg/minute were generally satisfactory in dogs. When tidal volumes of 20 ml/kg at a rate of 20 per minute were used, 90 and 100 ml/kg FGF tended to induce hypocapnea. The latter FGF was generally satisfactory when the respirations were reduced to 10 to 12 per minute or were spontaneous (Manley and McDonell, 1979).

To assure separation of inspired and expired gases, a nonrebreathing valve is often incor-

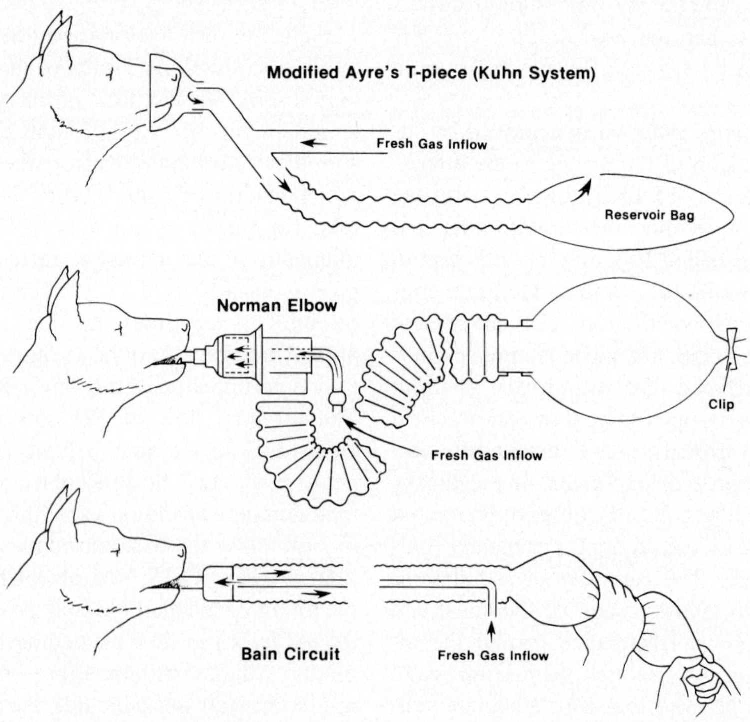

Figure 7–19. Examples of T-tube modifications. The Norman Elbow and Bain Circuit minimize dead space by having the fresh gas inflow at the endotracheal tube entrance to wash out exhaled gases. (Modified from Muir, W.W.: *An Outline of Veterinary Anesthesia*. Ohio State University, Columbus, Ohio, 1981.)

porated in the system in place of the T-tube or expiratory valve. The nonrebreathing valve obviates the possibility of carbon dioxide buildup, providing the dead space of the valve is small and it is situated as close to the patient as possible. Such valves can be used for either spontaneous or controlled breathing.

Several types of nonrebreathing valves, originally designed for infant anesthesia, can be employed. Among these are the Stephen-Slater, Digby-Leigh, Fink, and Ruben valves (Figs. 7–20, 7–21). Nonrebreathing valves should have negligible resistance at normal respiratory flow rates, a low intrinsic dead space, and minimal reflux. The valves should not stick when wet, and the complete unit should be compact, light, and easily cleaned and serviced (Sykes, 1959).

Digby-Leigh or Ruben valves are commonly used in simple nonrebreathing systems. During spontaneous or passive exhalation, a valve opens to allow flow of the exhaled gases to the atmosphere; at the same time, the pressure of these exhaled gases closes a valve guarding the orifice to the oxygen tubing and reservoir bag. Oxygen, which is flowing continuously, thus accumulates within the bag. If respiration is spontaneous, a negative pressure is generated within the airway during inspiration, closing the exhalation valve and opening the valve over the orifice of the oxygen tubing and/or reservoir bag. Oxygen thus flows from the reservoir bag and is inhaled. Should inspiration be controlled, the bag is compressed and a positive pressure is induced in the bag, opening the valve to the patient. Loss of gases to the atmosphere is prevented automatically by the Digby-Leigh and Ruben valves. During assisted or controlled breathing with this equipment, the gas flow should be sufficient to keep the reservoir bag half to two-thirds full.

Available nonrebreathing valves are designed for human use and are therefore suitable only for small animals and immature larger species.

Nonrebreathing System with Self-Inflating Bag

Assisted or controlled ventilation with the nonrebreathing systems described so far necessitates a gas supply. If, however, the reservoir bag is replaced with a self-inflating bag, an oxygen supply is unnecessary unless supplementary oxygen is required. The Hope resuscitator is such a device. It consists of a rubber self-inflating bag, a nonrebreathing valve, and a close-fitting mask (Fig. 7–22). When the bag is squeezed, air is forced into the patient and, on release, exhaled gases are vented into the room. A connection on the device enables administration of oxygen if desired, and an endotracheal catheter can be substituted for the mask.

Several similar devices are commercially available.

Ventilators

Although manual techniques are simple and satisfactory, the desirability of freeing the anesthesiologist from manual operation, coupled with limited availability of assistance, has established a need for mechanically controlled ventilators (Jones, 1964). These may be flow or pressure generators that are time-pressure-, volume-, or patient-cycled. These fundamental characteristics may differ during inhalation and exhalation.

Ventilators have also been classified as 1) controllers that operate independently of the patient's inspiratory effort, 2) assistors that augment inspiration of the spontaneously breathing patient, and 3) assistor-controllers that may act as either assistor or controller (Hedley-Whyte, 1968).

A flow generator determines the gas flow and volume delivered, without regard in most cases to the pressure pattern obtained. A pressure generator dictates the pressure pattern, while the resulting flow and minute volume are determined by the physical characteristics of the lung ventilated (Mapleson, 1962; Mushin et al., 1969). If, however, the pressure of the pressure generator is high, a large gradient exists between ventilator and alveoli, and characteristics of a constant-flow generator result. In both pressure and volume cycling, it is the pressure at the ventilator or the volume leaving the ventilator and not conditions in the lung which determine the cycling. When one is using time- or volume-

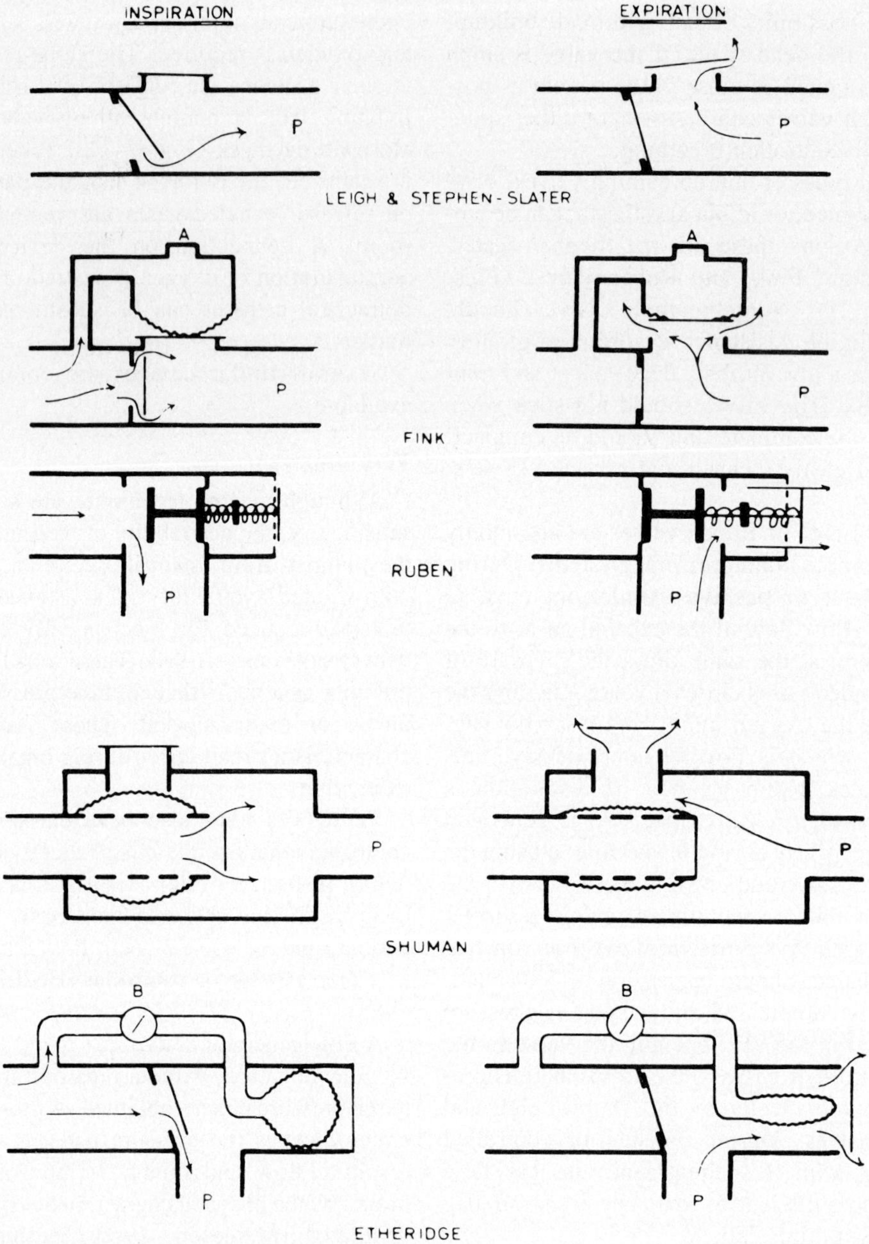

Figure 7–20. Diagrams illustrate the working principles of some common nonrebreathing valves. *P* refers to the patient end of the valve. *A* (Fink) marks the vent that is opened during spontaneous respiration to ensure that the pressure within the chamber remains at atmospheric. *B* (Etheridge) is a three-way tap that occludes the bypass tube and vents the balloon to atmosphere during spontaneous respiration. (From Sykes, M.K.: Nonrebreathing Valves. Br. J. Anaesth., 31:450, 1959.)

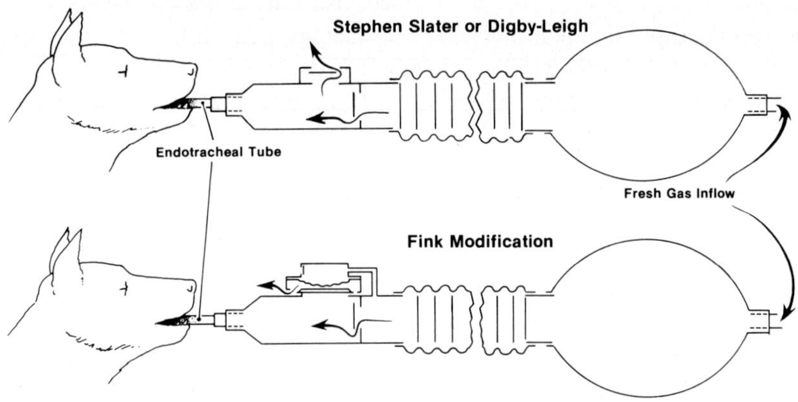

Figure 7–21. Two types of nonrebreathing apparatus, showing relationship of reservoir bag, corrugated tubing, valve, and endotracheal tube.

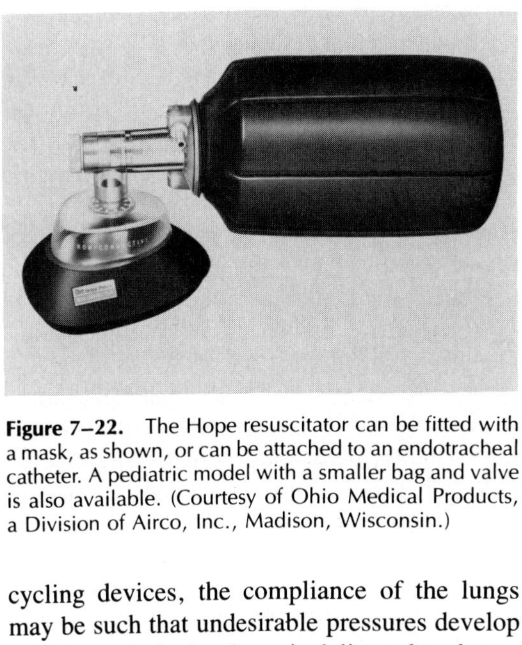

Figure 7–22. The Hope resuscitator can be fitted with a mask, as shown, or can be attached to an endotracheal catheter. A pediatric model with a smaller bag and valve is also available. (Courtesy of Ohio Medical Products, a Division of Airco, Inc., Madison, Wisconsin.)

cycling devices, the compliance of the lungs may be such that undesirable pressures develop before the desired volume is delivered or the set time elapses. Such units should therefore be fitted with a pressure-limiting device. Ventilators (assistors) may also be patient-cycled and are triggered by any slight spontaneous respiratory effort. During exhalation many ventilators are pressure generators. In all ventilators, the inhalation phase should be brief and exhalation should be of sufficient duration to allow the alveolar pressure to return to that of the atmosphere. Expiratory resistance will delay this return to atmospheric pressure and should therefore be minimal, unless an elevated end-expiratory pressure is required.

Although various patterns of flow and pressure have been used throughout the respiratory cycle, these are considered of secondary importance (Hunter, 1962). When a constant-flow generator is used, the alveolar pressures depend on the compliance, reduced compliance resulting in increased alveolar pressure. If the ventilator is time- or volume-cycled, there is no change in the total ventilation. If it is pressure-cycled, an increase in airway resistance or reduction in compliance hastens the onset of the triggering pressure, shortens the inspiratory phase, and reduces tidal volume. When expiration is also pressure-cycled, it is similarly affected, and minute volume remains unchanged (Mapleson, 1962). Reduced compliance under such circumstances reduces both the tidal volume and the time required to inflate the lungs. Increased airway resistance, on the other hand, slows inflation but may not reduce tidal volume. With the advent of closed chest cardiac massage (compression), a serious disadvantage has arisen with the pressure-cycled ventilator. Forceful compression of the chest during cardiac resuscitation triggers the ventilator, which consequently cycles at a rate too rapid to achieve effective pulmonary ventilation. The use of high-frequency ventilation may, in the future, offset this problem.

With the increasing emphasis upon intensive care and upon the use of intermittent positive-pressure breathing in human medicine, often for prolonged periods, criteria for desirable ventilators have been designated (Hedley-Whyte, 1968). Desirable features include reliability, permitting prolonged use with minimal maintenance, and ability to produce pulmonary ventilation with a low mean intrathoracic pressure. Loss of positive pressure should be immediate once the inspiratory phase is complete, and intermittent mandatory ventilation, humidification, and the use of air-oxygen mixtures should be available. Patient triggering to permit assisted ventilation may also be used but often requires too great an effort to trigger during use in small animals. In the event of failure of the ventilator, it should be possible to ventilate manually. Criteria for animal ventilators together with the necessary pressure and flow requirements have yet to be fully established. However, many human models are satisfactory for small animals and even for immature larger animals. For large animals, ventilators should be capable of supplying 250 L per minute or more so that tidal volumes of 15 to 22 ml/kg can be delivered in 2 to 3 seconds with an inspiratory:expiratory ratio of 1:2 and a respiratory rate of 6 to 8 per minute (Riebold et al., 1979, 1982). Satisfactory pulmonary ventilation implies maintenance of a normal arterial carbon dioxide tension. Elevated $Paco_2$ values indicate hypoventilation, whereas low $Paco_2$ values result from hyperventilation. Adequate ventilation should therefore maintain a normal arterial pH. Oxygen provided during ventilation should be sufficient to maintain normal Pao_2 values. Should oxygen tension be inadequate, the inspired oxygen concentration may be increased or end expiratory pressure elevated to increase FRC.

In animals, ventilators are used predominantly for short periods. The need to use varying mixtures of air and oxygen or to humidify the inspired gas is thus less essential than in humans. It is, however, important to appreciate that bypass of normal humidifying mechanisms of the upper respiratory tract by an endotracheal tube or tracheostomy induces increased mucus viscosity, damages ciliated cells of the tracheobronchial tree, inhibits mucociliary motility, and reduces static compliance (Chalon, 1974).

Cytologic studies of endotracheal aspirates indicate that no patient should receive gases with a relative humidity of less than 60% if a procedure is expected to last over one hour. Humidity of gases delivered by various types of nonrebreathing circuits is especially low. Such circuits therefore require the introduction of vaporizers, nebulizers, and heat and moisture exchangers, such as the Garther heat and moisture exchanger, the Bird cold water nebulizer, or the Bennett electrically heated cascade humidifier. Humidity should not be so great that wetting of the ventilator occurs during the expiration phase with consequent bacterial growth, nor should the water temperature in the vaporizer exceed 1° C above ambient (Chalon, 1974). Since prolonged use of high concentrations of oxygen may be hazardous, consideration should be given to the use of air or air-oxygen mixtures under such circumstances. Although simplicity of control may be less essential in human medicine, this is most desirable in animal use since trained personnel may not be available to operate the equipment.

A mechanical ventilator was used during animal anesthesia as early as 1923. A sudden insufflation technique was used, and exhalation occurred around the tracheal tube (Jones, 1964). Subsequently, numerous ventilators have been used with animals, especially dogs. Pressure-cycled ventilators include the PR-3, incorporating the Burns valve (Dameron and Greene, 1950), and various Bird models. Other ventilators include the Air-Shields Ventimeter (time-cycled), Knight-Wood (constant-flow, time-cycled) (Knight and Wood, 1951), Harvard pump (constant-flow, volume-cycled), North American Drager large and small animal ventilators (volume-cycled), Metomatic small animal fluidic ventilator (volume- or pressure-cycled), and Monaghan 300 s/m ventilator (volume-cycled).

Indications for subatmospheric pressure during exhalation encouraged the development of such ventilators as the Seeler and Stanton (Seeler and Good, 1953; Jones, 1964). Anesthetic may be administered while these and other ventilators are in use, either by the bag-in-bottle principle (see Chap. 11) or by including a vaporizer in the system (Clarke et al., 1957; Jones, 1964; Steffey and Berry, 1977).

In addition to these units, numerous other resuscitators have been used in animal anesthesia. They include the E & J, Bennett, and those constructed in the laboratory as reported by Sewell (1962) and by Clarke et al. (1957).

In the case of the Bird ventilators, several models are available offering various accessories, including a spirometer for determination of tidal volume, nebulizer, and anesthetic vaporizer (Fig. 7–23). Commonly used Bird ventilators are, during inhalation, flow generators that are time- and pressure-cycled, although other cycling options are available. The constant flow of inspiratory gases can be varied, the range depending upon the model, and the inspiratory phase may be terminated at selected pressures. The expiratory phase is constant (atmospheric) pressure generated and time- or patient-cycled. In the Bird Mark 9, a flow of up to 272 L per minute is possible. The units may, if required, be triggered by the inspiratory effort of the patient, with the end of the expiratory phase triggered by selecting varying degrees of negative pressure, or by the duration of this phase. Entrainment valves are incorporated for mixing room air with oxygen. The resulting air-oxygen mixture varies markedly, however, owing to fluctuating downstream resistance. Pressure cycling can be replaced by volume limiting in some models. For specific instructions on operation of the Bird Mark 7 and Mark 9, the reader is referred to the text by Sechzer (1965).

The Bird Mark 9 is the most suitable ventilator for use in a wide variety of animal species, especially large animals. Other units used in large animals include 1) the Vetaspirator (see Fig. 3–13),* 2) a method using a vacuum cleaner motor and rheostat, and 3) the Hudson demand valve. The Vetaspirator provides intermittent positive pressure ventilation (IPPV). Since it is capable only of gas flows of 150 L/min, it is inefficient for large horses. The modified vacuum cleaner requires a one-way valve

*See Appendix A

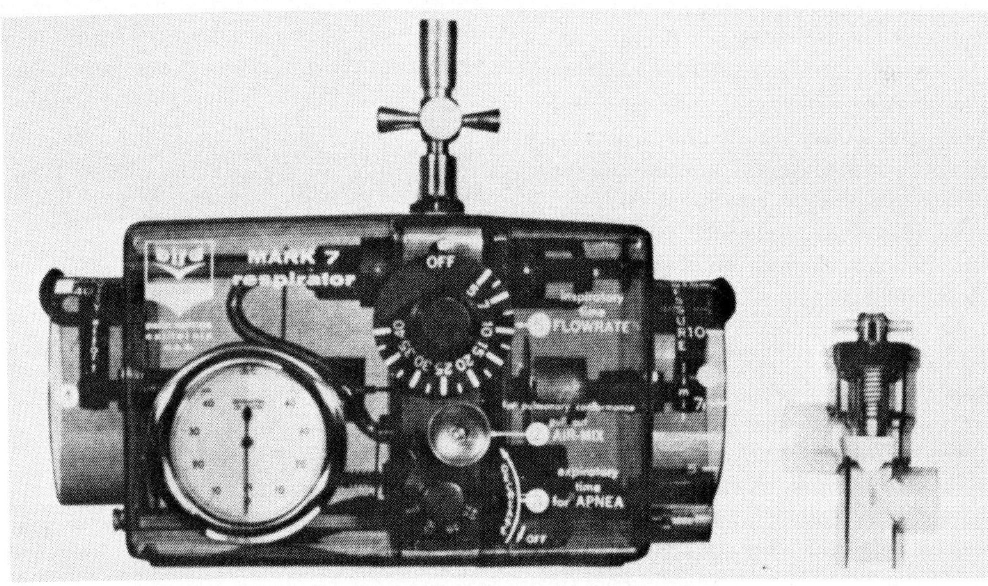

Figure 7–23. The Bird Mark 7 ventilator and expiratory-valve assembly. This device, which delivers up to 80 L per minute, is suitable for small animals, swine, sheep, and goats. (From Mushin, W.W., Rendell-Baker, L., Thompson, P.W., and Mapleson, W.W.: *Automatic Ventilation of the Lungs,* 2nd ed. F.A. Davis Co., Philadelphia, 1969.)

to regulate air flow and an electrical source (Levy and Gillespie, 1972). It can generate high gas flows and produce effective ventilation with air. Riebold et al. (1979) have described use of a Hudson demand valve in the horse. When operated with a gas supply pressure of 50 psi, this valve delivers 200 L/min and, at a supply pressure of 80 psi, it provides flow rates exceeding 275 L/min. The demand valve is triggered by spontaneous respiration, thereby providing assisted ventilation. Alternatively, IPPV may be administered by manual compression of a control button. If the airway pressure reaches 54 cm H_2O, oxygen flow will cease.

In pressure-cycled ventilators, cycling may be delayed, may fail, or may be more rapid than normal. Gas leaks delay or stop the development of triggering pressures; cycling therefore fails during either inhalation or exhalation. Cycling failure also results from obstruction of the pressure-sensitive diaphragm with aspirated mucus. A mucus trap between the animal and the resuscitator mechanism obviates this. Rapid cycling indicates a reduced tidal volume owing to elevation of airway resistance or reduced compliance. Very rapid cycling indicates a complete airway obstruction.

High airway resistance results from too small endotracheal tubes or adapters, bending of the tube, too long a tube, overinflation of the cuff, accumulation of secretions in the airway, and gas flow rates exceeding the critical flow rate. When one is using a mask, soft tissue obstruction of the nasopharynx may cause cycling failures. Rapid cycling due to reduced compliance also results from compression of the thorax, intrathoracic retractors, packs, fluids, and atelectasis, or occlusion of a bronchus by an endotracheal tube.

Atelectasis can result from surgical manipulation, from excessive negative pressure, from bronchial occlusion, and from inadequate inflation pressures. During mechanical ventilation, progressive adherence of lung surfaces may predispose to atelectasis, and maximal inflation of the lungs should be carried out at regular intervals to reestablish a normal tidal volume (''sigh'' at least every 15 minutes). Use of relatively high tidal volumes or continuous positive pressure ventilation obviates this problem. Should reduced tidal volume be indicated by an increased cycling rate in pressure-cycled ventilators, this should be corrected by establishing a free airway which is as wide, straight, smooth, and short as possible; by curtailing excessive gas flow; by increasing cycling pressures; and by minimizing factors decreasing compliance. In larger species, it may be advantageous to increase thoracic compliance by using muscle relaxants.

Criticism of the constant-flow generator, which is pressure-cycled, is based primarily on its susceptibility to variations in airway resistance and compliance. The resulting variations in cycling rate, however, serve to monitor changes in both these factors. Just as degrees of obstruction are illustrated by increased cycling rates, so leaks are indicated by reduced or absent cycling. Leaks and changes in resistance and compliance may not be so readily detectable in equipment utilizing time- or volume-cycled mechanisms. Likewise, if ventilation is pressure-cycled, overdistension with pulmonary damage is unlikely.

When the anesthesiologist is assisting spontaneous respiration with patient-triggered ventilators (assistors), the animal determines the respiratory rhythm. During controlled respiration, spontaneous respiratory efforts may hinder ventilator rhythm. Control of respiration is most easily accomplished after administration of muscle relaxants or intravenous barbiturates. With the former, spontaneous respiration is suppressed or absent; with the latter, the threshold to stimulation of the respiratory centers is elevated, and apnea due to hyperventilation or to maximal stimulation of Hering-Breuer reflexes may be induced. When spontaneous respiration is again desired, ventilation is reduced, and IMV, nonrebreathing, or diffusion techniques are initiated. Varying periods may be required before spontaneous breathing is initiated. These can be minimized by progressively reducing pulmonary ventilation for a few minutes prior to terminating mechanical ventilation and by maintaining a minimal anesthetic level.

REFERENCES

Acheson, F., Bull, A.B., and Glees, P.: Electroencephalogram of the Cat after Intravenous Injection of Lidocaine and Succinylcholine. Anesthesiology, 17:802, 1956.

Atkinson, R.S., Rushman, G.B., and Lee, J.A.: *A Synopsis of Anaesthesia,* 8th ed. Year Book Medical Publishers Inc., Chicago, 1977.

Baratz, R.A., Philbin, D.M.,and Patterson, R.W.: Plasma Antidiuretic Hormone and Urinary Output during Continuous Positive-Pressure Breathing in Dogs. Anesthesiology, 34:510, 1971.

Bernhard, W.F., Tank, E.S., Frittelli, G., and Gross, R.E.: Feasibility of Hypothermic Perfusion under Hyperbaric Conditions in Surgical Management of Infants with Cyanotic Congenital Heart Disease. J. Thorac. Cardiovasc. Surg., 46:651, 1963.

Boerema, I., Meyne, N.G., Brummelkamp, W.H., Bouma, S., Mensch, M.H., Kamermans, F., Hanf, M.S., and Van Aalderen, W.: Life Without Blood. Arch. Chir. Neerl., 11:70, 1959.

Chalon, J.: Humidity Control in Anesthetic Circuitry and Ventilators. Refresher Courses in Anesthesiology, 2:27, 1974.

Clarke, N.P., Zuidema, G.D., and Smith, G.D.: A Method of Producing Controlled Automatic Inhalation Anesthesia. J.A.V.M.A., 130:347, 1957.

Dameron, J.T., and Greene, D.G.: Use of the Burns Valve as Simple Respirator for Intrathoracic Surgery in the Dog. J. Thorac. Cardiovasc. Surg., 20:706, 1950.

Dejours, P.: *Respiration.* Oxford University Press, New York, 1966.

Downs, J.G., and Modell, J.H.: Patterns of Respiratory Support Aimed at Pathophysiologic Conditions. Refresher Courses in Anesthesiology, 5:71, 1977.

Draper, W.B., and Whitehead, R.W.: Diffusion Respiration in the Dog Anesthetized by Pentothal Sodium. Anesthesiology, 5:262, 1944.

Dripps, R.D., Eckenhoff, J.E., and Vandam, L.D.: *Introduction to Anesthesia: Principles of Safe Practice,* 3rd ed. W.B. Saunders Co., Philadelphia, 1967.

Fairley, H.B.: Respiratory "Fine Tuning" PEEP, CPAP, IMV, etc. *Annual Refresher Course Lectures,* Lecture #103. Am. Soc. Anesthes., 1978.

Gallagher, J.J.: Alternatives to Conventional Ventilation. *Annual Refresher Course Lectures,* Lecture #230. Am. Soc. Anesthes., 1981.

Gerst, P.H.: The Effects of Positive Pressure Lung Inflation Upon Pulmonary Vascular Dynamics. J. Thorac. Cardiovasc. Surg., 42:607, 1961.

Gillespie, J.R.: Long Term Oxygen Therapy in Veterinary Medicine. Am. Anim. Hosp. Assoc. Proc. 39th, 284, 1972.

Gillespie, J.R., and Martin, D.B.: Long-term Oxygen Cage Therapy for Hypoxemic Dogs. J.A.V.M.A., 156:717, 1970.

Grenvik, A., Snyder, J.V., and Powner, D.J.: Circulatory Effects of Mechanical Ventilation. Refresher Courses in Anesthesiology, 5:99, 1977.

Hall, K.D.: Principles of Hyperbaric Medicine. *Annual Refresher Course Lectures,* Lecture #140. Am. Soc. Anesthes., 1968.

Hall, L.W.: *Wright's Veterinary Anaesthesia and Analgesia,* 7th ed. Williams & Wilkins, Baltimore, 1971.

Hall, S.V., Johnson, E.E., and Hedley-Whyte, J.: Renal Hemodynamics and Function with Continuous Positive-Pressure Ventilation in Dogs. Anesthesiology, 41:452, 1974.

Hartsfield, S.M., Gendreau, C.L., Smith, C.W., Rouse, G.P., and Thurman, J.C.: Endotracheal Intubation by Pharyngotomy. J. Am. Anim. Hosp. Assoc., 13:71, 1977.

Hedley-Whyte, J.: Use of Mechanical Ventilators. *Annual Refresher Course Lectures,* Lecture #133. Am. Soc. Anesthes., 1968.

Hunter, A.R.: The Duration of Inspiration during Artificial Ventilation of the Lungs. Anaesthesia, 17:3, 1962.

Irwin, R.L., Draper, W.B., and Whitehead, R.W.: Urine Secretion during Diffusion Respiration after Apnea from Neuromuscular Block. Anesthesiology, 18:594, 1957.

Johnson, E.E., and Hedley-White, J.: Continuous Positive-Pressure Ventilation and Choledochoduodenal Flow Resistance. J. Appl. Physiol., 39:937, 1975.

Jones, E.W.: Mechanical Ventilation During Intravenous and Inhalation Anaesthesia of the Dog. In *Small Animal Anesthesia.* Edited by O. Graham-Jones. Pergamon Press, London, 1964, p. 205.

Knight, G.C., and Wood, C.R.: An Apparatus for Providing Positive Pressure Ventilation of the Lungs. J. Physiol., 133:3P, 1951.

Kopecky, F.A., Rayburn, C.J., Whitehead, R.W., and Draper, W.B.: A Study of Anuria Occurring during Apnea under Diffusion Respiration. Am. J. Physiol., 168:131, 1952.

Levy, W., and Gillespie, J.R.: Emergency Ventilator for Resuscitating Horses. J.A.V.M.A., 161:57, 1972.

Manley, S.V., and McDonell, W.N.: A New Circuit for Small Animal Anesthesia; the Bain Coaxial Circuit. J. Am. Anim. Hosp. Assoc., 15:61, 1979.

Mapleson, W.W.: The Effects of Changes of Lung Characteristics on the Functioning of Automatic Ventilators. Anaesthesia, 17:300, 1962.

Modell, J.H.: Inhalation Therapy. *Annual Refresher Course Lectures,* Lecture #137. Am. Soc. Anesthes., 1968.

Morgan, B.C., Martin, W.E., Hornbein, T.F., Crawford, E.W., and Guntheroth, W.G.: Hemodynamic Effects of Intermittent Positive Pressure Respiration. Anesthesiology, 27:584, 1966.

Mushin, W.W., Rendell-Baker, L., Thompson, P.W., and Mapleson, W.W.: *Automatic Ventilation of the Lungs,* 2nd ed. F.A. Davis Co., Philadelphia, 1969.

Pedersoli, W.M., and Krista, L.M.: Alterations in Tracheal Epithelium in Dogs Due to Endotracheal Intubation. Vet. Anesth., 6:34, 1979.

Riebold, T.W., Evans, A.T., and Robinson, N.E.: Emergency Ventilation in the Horse. Proc. 25th Ann. Convention Am. Assoc. Eq. Practitioners, Miami Beach, Florida, December, 1979.

Riebold, T.W., Goble, D.O., and Geiser, D.R.: *Large Animal Anesthesia.* Iowa State University Press, Ames, Iowa, 1982.

Rochford, J.D.: In *General Anesthesia,* Vol. II. Edited by F.T. Evans, and T.C. Gray. Butterworth and Co., Ltd., London, 1959.

Sechzer, P.H.: *The Bird Respirator.* D.H. White & Co., Houston, 1965.

Seeler, H.W., and Good, D.R.: Automatic Resuscitator. J. Aviation Med., 24:63, 1953.

Sewell, W.H.: A Respirator for Experimental Intrathoracic Surgery. Surg. Gynecol. Obstet., 114:760, 1962.

Shapiro, B.A., Harrison, R.A., and Trout, C.A.: *Clinical*

Applications of Respiratory Care, 2nd ed. Year Book Medical Publishers, Chicago, Illinois, 1979.

Steffey, E.P., and Berry, J.D.: Flow Rates from an Intermittent Positive Pressure Breathing/Anesthetic Delivery Apparatus for Horses. Am. J. Vet. Res., 38:685, 1977.

Sugioka, K., Davis, D.A., Hinternhoff, M., McKnight, R.L., and Grosskreutz, D.C.: Oxygen and Carbon Dioxide Tensions as Factors in Respiration after Apnea from Hyperventilation. Anesthesiology, 23:776, 1962.

Sullivan, S.F., Patterson, R.W., and Papper, E.M.: Posthyperventilation Hypoxia. J. Appl. Physiol., 22:431, 1967.

Sykes, M.K.: Nonrebreathing Valves. Br. J. Anaesth., 31:450, 1959.

Waltz, R.C., Hubay, C.A., Ankeney, J.L., and Merrill, J.: Experimental Study of Pulmonary Histo-pathology following Positive and Negative Pressure Respirations. Surg. Gynecol. Obstet., 99:580, 1954.

Webb, A.I., and Warren, R.G.: Hazards and Precautions Associated with the Use of Compressed Gases. J.A.V.M.A., 181:1491, 1982.

Wycoff, C.C.: Manufacture of an Endotracheal Catheter Cuff. Anesthesiology, 8:643, 1947.

CHAPTER 8

Preanesthetic Agents

Preanesthetic agents are so named because they are usually given to prepare the patient for administration of an anesthetic agent. In this regard they are used to:

1. reduce the amount of general anesthetic needed and increase the margin of safety (Fig. 8–1);
2. calm the patient so that anesthesia can be administered without fright or struggling;
3. reduce secretions of the salivary glands and mucous glands of the respiratory tract, thus maintaining a free airway;
4. reduce gastric and intestinal motility and prevent vomiting while the patient is under anesthesia;
5. block the vagovagal reflex, thus preventing cardiac slowing or arrest; and
6. reduce pain, struggling, and crying during the recovery period.

Many preanesthetic agents are capable of producing analgesia, sedation, or narcosis of the patient to a degree that will enable minor procedures to be carried out without general anesthesia. Their use in combination with local anesthesia helps to restrain the patient and to allay apprehension during surgical procedures. Employing such a combination sometimes helps avoid the dangers of general anesthesia.

Whether preanesthetics are used depends to a degree upon personal preference, and the type of practice in which one is engaged. When one is accustomed to using these agents routinely, the procedure is seldom discontinued. In brachycephalic dogs, it is foolhardy to attempt general anesthesia without administration of a drug to reduce secretions. It is equally unwise to induce general anesthesia in the horse without preanesthetic tranquilization to insure a calm induction and to minimize struggling during recovery.

A variety of drugs are used as preanesthetic agents. Pharmacologically they fall into the following groups: anticholinergics, tranquilizers,

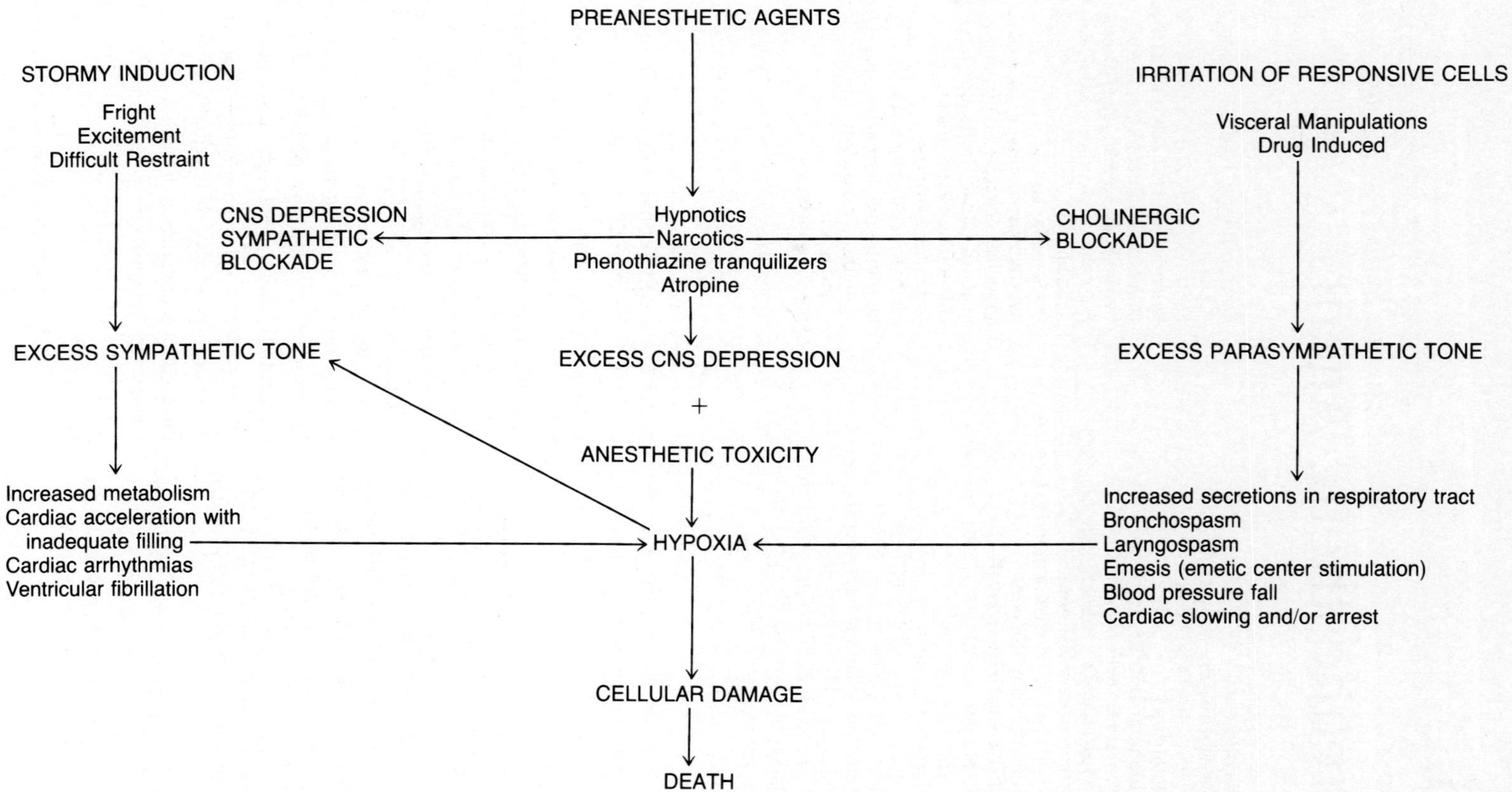

Figure 8–1. Actions of preanesthetic agents. Adverse effects of stormy induction and/or irritation of responsive cells can be blocked by proper use of preanesthetic agents. Conversely, preanesthetic agents can produce excessive central nervous system depression which, combined with anesthetic depression, may prove fatal.

opiate and nonopiate analgesics, and tranquilizer-narcotic combinations.

ANTICHOLINERGICS

Atropine Sulfate, U.S.P.

Atropine is obtained by extraction from leaves of the plant *Atropa belladonna*. It is also produced synthetically.

Atropine blocks acetylcholine at the postganglionic terminations of cholinergic fibers in the autonomic nervous system. This diminishes secretion of mucus in the mouth, throat, and respiratory tract, and dilates the bronchi. Atropine increases the dead space, both anatomic and physiologic, and may accentuate postoperative hypoxemia from ventilation-perfusion impairment (Atkinson et al., 1977). Motor and secretory activity in the gastrointestinal tract are reduced, and vagus inhibition of the heart is prevented. In therapeutic doses, atropine does not produce significant blood pressure changes. It blocks the cholinergic fibers of the short ciliary nerves, relaxing the sphincter muscle of the iris, and allowing dilation of the pupil. It does not dilate the pupils of birds because their irides are composed of striated muscle (Goodman and Gilman, 1958). Atropine sulfate (0.02 mg/kg subcutaneously) reduces tear formation in both awake and anesthetized dogs (Gelatt et al., 1975; Ludders and Heavner, 1979). It also suppresses the muscarinic action of anticholinesterases used to reverse nondepolarizing muscle relaxants.

Atropine may be given subcutaneously, intramuscularly, or intravenously, the latter method being used when a quick effect is desired. Since its action is rapid, it can be given shortly before induction of anesthesia. When given intravenously, atropine has 1) an initial central vagal stimulating action, 2) an intermediate vagotonic action on the conducting mechanism of the heart, and 3) the classic parasympatholytic action (Adriani, 1964). Its use should be avoided in cases in which tachycardia already exists.

The dose of atropine sulfate is rather arbitrary. As a preanesthetic in large animals, 0.2 mg/100 lb is recommended intravenously, intramuscularly, or subcutaneously. Doses as high as 32.0 mg have been used for this purpose in horses.

The dose of atropine for swine is 0.03 to 0.04 mg/lb. Sheep and goats require much higher doses, 15 mg/50 lb prior to anesthesia and 3 to 6 mg every 15 minutes thereafter. Even with these doses excessive salivation may occur and secretions may become more viscid.

Jones (1957) recommends 0.02 mg/lb for dogs. At the rate of 0.5 mg/kg administered intravenously, atropine causes excitement in dogs (Hatch, 1967). In contrast, doses as high as 1.0 mg/kg may be used in cats (Stoliker, 1969). The minimum lethal dose in this species is 30.0 mg/kg (Cloetta, 1908). Harrison and Vanik (1963) found that atropine possessed little effect on laryngospasm produced by ether inhalation in cats (see Chap. 21).

Hatch (1967) determined that preanesthesia with massive doses of atropine (0.5 mg/kg IV) reduced the required amount of thiopental by about 25% and doubled the period of anesthesia. If given intravenously as dogs were arousing from thiopental anesthesia, atropine caused reanesthetization and the duration of sleep increased 163%. Using a smaller dose (0.044 mg/kg SQ), Klide et al. (1974) produced the same results.

Muir (1978) studied changes in cardiac rate and rhythm in dogs treated with atropine prior to, during, and after anesthetic induction with thiamylal sodium and maintenance with 1% halothane in 50% nitrous oxide and 50% oxygen. The incidence of cardiac dysrhythmias and sinus tachycardia was significantly higher prior to and after anesthetic induction in dogs given atropine, compared with dogs receiving none. Second-degree atrioventricular block was the most frequent dysrhythmia prior to anesthesia in dogs treated with atropine. Most dysrhythmias were observed during anesthetic induction and early maintenance. The most common dysrhythmias during these periods were unifocal ventricular premature depolarizations and ventricular bigeminy. Muir concluded that while atropine may be lifesaving in cases of profound sinus bradycardia with hypotension, indiscriminate use of atropine prior to every anesthesia is not warranted.

De Moor (1968) injected 22 horses intramuscularly with 6 mg/100 kg of atropine. He found a highly significant decrease in arterial oxygen tension and a significant fall in packed cell volume. No change was seen in arterial oxygen saturation or acid-base status or in the blood levels of glucose, lactate, or pyruvate. The lactate/pyruvate ratio was not affected, and there was no excess lactate production.

In ponies, Ducharme and Fubini (1983) found intravenous doses of 0.044 mg/kg and 0.176 mg/kg of atropine sulfate stopped intestinal motility and produced colic in 30% of ponies injected. Similar clinical results in horses have been reported by this group and others.

Atropine degradation and elimination vary among animal species. The cat, rat, and rabbit can destroy large quantities of atropine because they have atropine esterase in the liver (Godeaux and Tonnesen, 1949; Stormont and Suzuki, 1970). In the dog, atropine disappears quickly from the blood, part being excreted in the urine unchanged or as tropine and part being unaccounted for.

Routine administration of atropine as a preanesthetic agent has declined in recent years owing to its detrimental effects. Selective use with specific agents is still recommended.

Glycopyrrolate (Robinul-V)

Glycopyrrolate is a synthetic quaternary ammonium anticholinergic agent. It is prepared as an injectable solution containing 0.2 mg/ml, and may be given intravenously, intramuscularly, or subcutaneously. The dosage for dogs is 0.005 mg/lb (1 ml/40 lbs).

Glycopyrrolate inhibits the action of acetylcholine on structures innervated by postganglionic cholinergic nerves, and on smooth muscles that respond to acetylcholine and lack cholinergic innervation. It reduces the volume and free acidity of gastric secretions, intestinal motility, and pharyngeal, tracheal, and bronchial secretions. It has a longer lasting effect than atropine.

In anesthetized dogs, intravenous doses of 0.0023 to 0.0045 mg/lb markedly reduce intestinal tone and inhibit moderately the amplitude of intestinal contraction. At this dose level there is essentially no effect on respiration, arterial blood pressure, or cardiac rate. Bradycardia, hypertension, and intestinal hyperactivity from peripheral vagal stimulation are reduced. The polar ammonium moiety of glycopyrrolate limits its passage across lipid membranes such as the blood-brain barrier in contrast to the belladonna alkaloids, which are nonpolar.

After subcutaneous or intramuscular administration, the peak effect occurs in 30 to 45 minutes. Vagal blocking lasts for 2 to 3 hours and the antisialagogue effect persists for up to 7 hours. When the drug is injected intravenously, the action is evident within one minute.

Glycopyrrolate is indicated as a preoperative agent to reduce salivary, tracheobronchial, and pharyngeal secretions, and to reduce the volume and free acidity of gastric secretion. It also blocks cardiac vagal inhibitory reflexes during induction of anesthesia and intubation.

Short et al. (1974) have recommended use of glycopyrrolate to prevent acid regurgitation and aspiration, which result in sudden tachycardia, tachypnea, cyanosis, marked hemodynamic changes (Mendelson's syndrome), and occasionally death during anesthesia. They found that glycopyrrolate produced a higher pH of gastric secretions and reduced intestinal smooth muscle activity, thus reducing the likelihood of regurgitation. Glycopyrrolate should not be administered to pregnant bitches. Excretion may be prolonged in animals with impaired renal or gastrointestinal function. The LD_{50} in dogs is 25.0 mg/kg intravenously.

TRANQUILIZERS

Major subgroups of tranquilizers used in veterinary medicine include the phenothiazines, butyrophenones, and benzodiazepines. These have proved useful in a wide variety of conditions in animals, namely:

1) as preanesthetic sedatives;
2) to relieve anxiety in hospitalized animals;
3) to restrain refractory animals during examination or large animals during shipment;

4) to prevent animals from licking wounds or chewing bandages and splints; and
5) as an antiemetic for carsickness or prior to administration of anthelmintics.

When used as preanesthetic agents, the tranquilizers are usually administered intravenously, although the intramuscular and oral routes may be used. The latter two are not as fast or reliable. Intravenous injection should be made at least 15 minutes prior to administration of a general anesthetic agent. This allows time for the animal to receive the full effect prior to induction of anesthesia. Doses of phenothiazine tranquilizers above the optimal dose rate provide little additional tranquilization.

Injection should be made slowly. As tranquilization develops, the animal relaxes and hangs its head; the ears may droop. In cattle and horses, the penis is relaxed and partially extruded. The dog may lie down; the eyes are usually glazed, and the membrana nictitans protrudes. Occasionally, acute toxic symptoms are seen, particularly in horses, in which intracarotid injection occasionally occurs accidentally. Among these are extreme depression, hypotension, tremors, dyspnea, muscle spasticity, hyperirritability, convulsions, ataxia, and death. Epinephrine is contraindicated in treatment of the hypotension, norepinephrine or phenylephrine being the drugs of choice. Although there are few reports of animals dying from intravenous administration of tranquilizers, deaths have occurred. Because of the occasional complications of intravenous administration in the horse, many choose only the intramuscular route of administration. An occasional animal may become aggressive or may show other evidence of central nervous stimulation. Generally, these agents are not as effective in cats as in other animals.

Phenothiazine tranquilizers may potentiate the toxicity of organophosphates and the activity of procaine hydrochloride. Their use is contraindicated in cardiovascular and hepatic disease. In male large animals, persistent or permanent paraphimosis may occur. Narcotic- or anesthetic-induced respiratory and cardiac depression is potentiated.

Advantages of preanesthetic tranquilizers are:

1. The animal is easier to handle during induction of anesthesia.
2. The required amount of general anesthetic is reduced.
3. The antiemetic action inhibits vomiting.
4. Alpha blockade (phenothiazines only) helps prevent shock.
5. The animal is protected by phenothiazines from ventricular arrhythmias and cardiac fibrillation, especially those that are epinephrine-induced.
6. Recovery from anesthesia is smooth and free from struggling and vocalization.
7. Little delay is necessary between administration of preanesthetic and anesthetic agent.
8. No narcotic license is needed.

Disadvantages of tranquilizer administration are:

1. Tranquilizers do not produce true analgesia.
2. Occasional severe or even fatal reactions may occur.
3. The cost is many times greater than that for combined morphine and atropine.
4. Persons handling tranquilizers may become sensitized resulting in urticaria and pruritus.
5. When administered to animals in shock or to those with cardiovascular disease, alpha blockade may produce fatal hypotension.
6. Permanent-penile protrusion may occur in male large animals following administration of phenothiazine-type agents.

Chlorpromazine Hydrochloride Injection, U.S.P.

Chlorpromazine can be considered the prototype of the phenothiazine derivatives. It is a whitish-gray, water-soluble powder marketed for oral use in 10-, 25-, and 50-mg tablets, and for intramuscular and intravenous injection in sterile solution containing 25 mg/ml. A syrup containing 10 mg/5 ml is also available.

Chlorpromazine possesses four main pharmacologic properties: 1) central depressant action,

2) antiemetic action, 3) alpha-adrenergic blocking effect, and 4) enhancing effect on the activity of analgesics, anesthetics, and sedatives. The central depressant activity probably is on the ascending reticular formation of the midbrain which controls the centers for vomiting and temperature. The drug also has ganglionic blocking, antihistaminic, anticholinergic, anti-5HT, anticonvulsive, and quinidine-like actions. Owing to its effect on temperature control and to peripheral vasodilation, the body temperature may fall significantly, especially in small laboratory animals. Its antiemetic action is believed to be due to depression of the emetic chemoreceptor trigger zone and the vomiting reflex centrally. In addition, the volume of gastric secretion is lowered, and the small intestine, bladder, and uterus are relaxed.

Intravenous injection of 2 to 5 mg/kg of chlorpromazine in anesthetized dogs causes a decrease in the respiratory rate, increased tidal volume, and an overall decreased oxygen consumption (Bourgeois-Gavardin et al., 1955). No consistent changes in renal function occur in dogs when they are given 50 mg of chlorpromazine intravenously, except for a moderate increase in urine volume and sodium excretion. In cats chlorpromazine (4.4 mg/kg) produces tranquilization for over 8 hours (Davis and Donnelly, 1968), but does not lower the pain threshold.

Chlorpromazine produces effects similar to those of a stressing agent, in that blood eosinophils and lymphocytes decrease and adrenal ascorbic acid content decreases simultaneously.

The hypotensive effect of chlorpromazine may produce shock. It antagonizes and sometimes reverses the alpha (vasoconstrictor) action of epinephrine and other sympathomimetic amines. Epinephrine should not be used under these circumstances because its beta effect may result in further lowering of blood pressure. Norepinephrine or phenylephrine are the most suitable vasopressor agents for use in this situation.

Paradoxically, it has been reported that dogs were completely protected against the lethal effect of hemorrhagic shock by intravenous administration of chlorpromazine at a rate of 2 mg/kg, before or immediately after hemorrhage. This is presumably due to the alpha blocking effect on the peripheral vasculature, which improves blood flow and tissue oxygenation. Treated dogs exhibited none of the usual signs of shock. In addition, shock resulting from injection of irritants into the cerebral peduncles of dogs was modified and mortality reduced by intravenous chlorpromazine, either before or after the procedure.

The fate of chlorpromazine in the body is not completely clear, but the main metabolite appears to be chlorpromazine sulfoxide, which can be found in the urine of dogs. The sulfoxide undergoes further metabolism to an unidentified product. The biological half-life is estimated to be 6 hours (Salzman and Brodie, 1956).

Chlorpromazine, when used in surgery, is expected to 1) facilitate restraint during induction of anesthesia, 2) reduce the volume of general anesthetic required, 3) prevent vomiting, 4) improve muscle relaxation, and 5) eliminate struggling and crying during recovery. A dosage schedule for various species is listed in Table 8–1.

No deaths occurred in dogs given 50 mg/kg (22.6 mg/lb) of body weight subcutaneously or 100 mg/kg (45.4 mg/lb) orally (Courvoisier et al., 1953). It has no ill effect on fetuses in utero (Macko et al., 1958). In another study, when 200 mg were given orally to pregnant bitches for 7 days prior to whelping, normal full-term pups were delivered.

Estrada (1956) reported a reaction in a 25-lb terrier given 6 mg/lb at a rapid rate. Opisthotonus, urination, and collapse occurred. The animal regained its ability to stand about 30 minutes after injection but remained depressed for several hours. According to Burch (1957), perivascular infiltration of chlorpromazine solution in dogs causes swelling and pain.

Promazine Hydrochloride (Sparine)

Promazine has the same basic structure as chlorpromazine but lacks a chlorine atom on the phenothiazine nucleus. It is a white crystalline salt, readily soluble in water and alcohol. Solutions are stable indefinitely. It is supplied in solution for intravenous and intramuscular in-

TABLE 8–1. Chlorpromazine: Route of Administration and Dose Range (mg/lb)

				Average Dose		
	IV Range	*IM Range*	*Oral Range*	*IV*	*IM*	*Oral*
Dog	0.25 to 2.0	0.5 to 3.0	0.25 to 4.0	0.5	1.0	1.5
Cat	0.25 to 2.0	1.0 to 3.0	1.0 to 4.0	0.5	1.0	1.5
Chinchilla			1–3 drops syrup			1–3 drops
Birds						
Parakeets			1 drop syrup			1 drop
Large birds			0.25			0.25
Horse	0.1	0.5 to 1.8		0.1	0.75	
Cattle	0.1 to 0.5	0.5 to 1.0		0.15	0.3	
Sheep and Goat	0.25 to 2.0	1.0 to 3.0		0.5	1.0	1.0

Dosing varies from 1 to 4 times daily depending on the type of case and the desired results. (Data obtained from Pitman-Moore Company, Washington Crossing, New Jersey.)

jection and in tablets of 25, 50, and 100 mg for oral therapy.

In general, the effects of promazine are similar to those of chlorpromazine, though less hypnosis and fewer side effects have been reported.

The intravenous dose of preanesthetic promazine in the dog is 1 to 3 mg/lb. The amount of barbiturate necessary for anesthesia is thereby reduced one-third to one-half. Gupta et al. (1970) have used promazine (3 mg/lb intravenously) plus lidocaine hydrochloride injected along the abdominal midline for cesarotomy in the bitch. No depression of fetuses was reported, and 98% of puppies delivered in 94 cesarotomies were alive.

Promazine has proved to be a safe and efficient preanesthetic agent for dogs (Weberlein et al., 1959; Knowles, 1957; Krawitz, 1957) and primates (Green, 1979). It has been used extensively as a tranquilizer for horses and other large animals. The intravenous dose for horses and cattle is approximately 0.5 mg/lb. It should not be used in animals intended for human consumption.

TABLE 8–2. Dosage of Triflupromazine Hydrochloride

Animal	*Total Daily Parenteral Dosage*
Dogs	0.5–1 mg/lb intravenously 1–2 mg/lb intramuscularly
Cats	2–4 mg/lb intramuscularly
Cattle	5 mg/100 lb intravenously up to maximum dose of 40 mg
Horses	10–15 mg/100 lb intravenously or intramuscularly up to maximum dose of 100 mg
Hogs	40 mg/100 lb intravenously 60 mg/100 lb intramuscularly
Sheep	1 mg/2 lb intravenously up to a maximum dose of 40 mg
	Total Daily Oral Dosage
Dogs	1–2 mg/lb
Cats	1–2 mg/lb

(Courtesy of E. R. Squibb & Sons, New York.)

Triflupromazine Hydrochloride (Vetame)

Triflupromazine is a phenothiazine-type tranquilizer containing fluorine. The pH of a 2% solution is 4.1; it precipitates from aqueous solutions at a pH of 6.4. The parenteral form is marketed in brown bottles to protect it from decomposition by light. It is also available in 10- and 25-mg tablets for oral administration.

Triflupromazine has about 10 times the antiemetic effect of chlorpromazine and 3 to 5 times the tranquilizing potency. Its side effects are essentially equivalent to those of chlorpromazine. On rare occasions, it may stimulate dogs to chew on any object close at hand. This effect, though alarming, is transitory.

The recommended intravenous dosage for the dog is 0.5 to 1 mg/lb (Table 8–2). When triflupromazine is used as a preanesthetic, the dosage of barbiturate is generally one-half to two-thirds of that usually required. The intravenous LD_{50} for the dog is 16.7 ± 4.2 mg/kg.

Jha et al. (1961) reported erratic results following administration to goats. In doses of 0.5 mg/lb, respiration and blood pressure were usually depressed, while heart rate was increased.

In clinical practice, triflupromazine has proved to be comparable to promazine in its effects.

Acepromazine Maleate

Acepromazine, a phenothiazine derivative, is a potent neuroleptic agent with low toxicity. It is the most widely used tranquilizer and is the one of choice in the horse and most other species. It is available in solution containing 10 mg/ml of acepromazine maleate plus 0.36% sodium citrate, 0.075% citric acid, 1.0% benzyl alcohol, and water for injection. Tablets containing 10 and 25 mg of acepromazine maleate are also available.

This drug has been found particularly valuable in dogs, horses, and cats and has been given to a wide variety of wild animal species. Federal law prohibits its use in animals intended for human consumption. When the drug is given intramuscularly, intravenously, or subcutaneously, the following doses are generally effective:

Dogs: 0.25–0.5 mg/lb
Cats: 0.5–1.0 mg/lb
Horses: 2.0–4.0 mg/100 lb

If tablets are given orally, the following dosages are recommended:

Dogs: 0.25–1.0 mg/lb
Dosage may be repeated as required
Cats: 0.5–1.0 mg/lb
Dosage may be repeated as required.

The LD_{50} in mice intravenously is 61.37 mg/kg, subcutaneously 130.5 mg/kg, and orally 256.8 mg/kg. In dogs, 40 mg/kg daily produced no deleterious effects.

Acepromazine produces a central nervous depression with sedation, muscular relaxation, and a reduction in spontaneous activity. When used as a preanesthetic agent, it lowers the amount of general anesthetic ordinarily required. It possesses antiemetic, anticonvulsant, antispasmodic, hypotensive, and hypothermic properties (Pugh, 1964). It will reduce or prevent the hyperthermic response in susceptible swine exposed to halothane (McGrath et al., 1980).

Ballard et al. (1982) studied acepromazine pharmacokinetics in horses and found a high degree of protein binding, an elimination half-life of 184.8 minutes, and a detectable plasma level at 8 hours. Penile prolapse occurred at intravenous doses of 0.01 mg/kg to 0.4 mg/kg and was dose-related. Hematocrit levels were significantly lowered, and respiration was de-

TABLE 8–3. Dosage of Propiopromazine Hydrochloride

Small Animals
DOGS:
Tranquilization: 0.2 to 1.0 mg/lb intravenously or intramuscularly
Preanesthetic: 0.5 to 1.5 mg/lb intravenously. A small-bore syringe, such as a tuberculin syringe, should be used in smaller breeds.
CATS:
Tranquilization: 0.5 to 2.0 mg/lb intravenously or intramuscularly.
Preanesthetic: 0.5 to 2.5 mg/lb intravenously. A small-bore syringe, such as a tuberculin syringe, should be used in smaller animals.
Large Animals
EQUINES:
Tranquilization or Preanesthetic: 0.05 to 0.1 mg/lb intravenously.
Standards and Thoroughbreds ONLY:
0.05 mg/lb intravenously.
Stallions over 2 years of age should not be injected.
CATTLE:
Tranquilization or Preanesthetic: 0.1 to 0.5 mg/lb intravenously or intramuscularly.
Injections in very young calves (less than two weeks) should be avoided, since their degree of response is variable and cannot be predicted well.
Milk taken from dairy animals within 12 hours, or one milking (whichever is longer), after the last injection must not be used for human consumption. Do not administer to cattle being shipped to slaughter. Cattle must not be treated within 72 hours of slaughter for human consumption.
SWINE:
Tranquilization or Preanesthetic: 0.25 to 0.5 mg/lb intravenously or intramuscularly.
SHEEP:
Tranquilization or Preanesthetic: 0.5 mg/lb intravenously.

pressed. Locomotor and behavioral responses were also reduced.

Acepromazine is effective in preventing cardiac arrhythmias and ventricular fibrillation. When used as a preanesthetic in dogs in doses of 0.4 to 1.0 mg/kg IV, it protects against arrhythmias produced by thiamylal, methohexital, and thiopental. Furthermore, if halothane or methoxyflurane is given following these agents, acepromazine will protect against epinephrine and norepinephrine-induced arrhythmias (Wiersig et al., 1974; Muir et al., 1975; Szabuniewicz et al., 1975).

Garland and White (1968) have reported apnea and syncope in four brachycephalic dogs following intravenous administration of 0.25 mg/lb of acepromazine. All of these dogs recovered, two after intravenous injection of methylamphetamine hydrochloride and a soluble steroid. Bartels et al. (1977) noted that seizures occurred in all animals that received acepromazine prior to subarachnoid metrizamide injection for myelography.

Persistent paraphimosis may follow use of acepromazine in horses.

Propiopromazine Hydrochloride (Tranvet)

Propiopromazine, a phenothiazine derivative, is a yellow odorless powder that is readily soluble in water and alcohol. Its effects are similar to those of other phenothiazine derivatives in that it has an antiemetic effect, causes epinephrine reversal, and lowers blood pressure in animals under pentobarbital anesthesia. It is somewhat more sedative, and it produces greater potentiation of barbiturates and a greater degree of motor deficit than chlorpromazine.

An intravenous dose of 1 mg/lb in dogs causes ataxia, pupillary constriction, decreased activity, and slight prolapse of the nictitating membrane. The same effects are produced in cats and monkeys. If it is administered prior to thiopental or pentobarbital anesthesia, the amount of anesthetic required is reduced and the sleeping time prolonged (Table 8–3).

Propiopromazine has proved clinically to be a safe and efficient tranquilizer with effects lasting in some instances as long as 2 to 3 days. Persistent paraphimosis may occur after its use in the horse.

Piperacetazine (Psymod)

Piperacetazine is a phenothiazine derivative that has tranquilizing and sedative action in dogs and cats. It is supplied in sterile solution for injection and as tablets for oral administration. When used as a preanesthetic agent, it should be given intravenously. Each milliliter of solution contains piperacetazine hydrochloride, 2 mg; ascorbic acid, 2 mg; sodium chloride, 4 mg; and sodium bisulfite, 2 mg.

Piperacetazine produces a tranquilizing effect with minimal drowsiness and ataxia. Sedation develops in 10 to 15 minutes when the drug is given intravenously and in approximately 45 minutes on intramuscular or subcutaneous administration. Recovery usually occurs within 4 to 6 hours.

Piperacetazine has tranquilizing and antiemetic effects 35 and 50 times greater than those of chlorpromazine, respectively, in dogs. For tranquilization and as a preanesthetic, the recommended dosage in dogs and cats is 1 mg/20 lb (Bowman, 1976). For marked sedation, the dosage can be increased to 1 mg/5 lb administered intravenously, intramuscularly, or subcutaneously. In veterinary use, the greatest value of piperacetazine is probably its antipsychotic and behavior-modifying properties (Mandelker, 1979).

At least 25 mg/kg IV is required to produce acute toxicity in dogs, and no lethal effects have been observed with up to 100 mg/kg orally.

Ethyl Isobutrazine (Diquel)

Ethyl isobutrazine is a phenothiazine derivative with properties similar to those of other members of this group. It potentiates anesthesia and analgesia, reducing the dose of pentobarbital approximately 30% in recommended dosage.

Ethyl isobutrazine is available in solution containing 25 mg/ml and in tablets of 10 and 50 mg. For small animals, the oral and intramuscular dosages are 2 to 5 mg/lb; the intravenous dosage is 1 to 2 mg/lb.

Droperidol

Droperidol, a butyrophenone derivative, is a short-acting neuroleptic. In the dog, it produces sedation with decreased motor activity and tranquilization similar to that produced by phenothiazine derivatives. It has a wide margin of safety (Table 8–4). Tremors, muscle spasticity, and hyperirritability occur with high doses administered intravenously (5 to 10 mg/lb). When the drug was given to hyperthermia-susceptible pigs, 20 mg/kg prolonged the reaction time to halothane (McGrath et al., 1980).

Droperidol inhibits learned responses and antagonizes the CNS stimulatory effects of amphetamine and vomiting produced by apomorphine. It has adrenergic-blocking properties, preventing arrhythmias produced by epinephrine and also its hypertensive effects. In the anesthetized dog, the blood pressure falls with little or no change in cardiac output after intravenous administration. The respiratory depressant effects of morphine-like compounds are antagonized. Droperidol potentiates the actions of barbiturates, reducing the anesthetic dose. The principal use of droperidol has been as a component of Innovar Vet, a mixture with fentanyl (discussed subsequently). It is especially advantageous in this mixture, since its sedative and antiemetic effects are complemented by antagonism of the respiratory depressant action of the narcotic.

Azaperone (Stresnil)

Azaperone is a neuroleptic of the butyrophenone series. It is probably the most potent and specific sedative available for swine. It also has been used in capture and control of a wide variety of exotic species of animals (see Chap. 18).

Given intramuscularly to swine, it produces psychomotor sedation without narcosis. The animal becomes quiet and indifferent to its surroundings but remains conscious. Within a few minutes after injection, the animal lies down in sternal or lateral recumbency. Peak effect is reached in about 15 minutes in young animals and in 30 minutes with adults. At dose rates of 1 to 2 mg/kg, young animals are recumbent for 1 to 2 hours, whereas older animals are affected for 3 to 4 hours.

Azaperone has been used in aggressive sows to allow piglets to be accepted, and is used to prevent "porcine stress syndrome" due to handling or transport. It may be used as premedication for cesarean section with local anesthesia (2 to 4 mg/kg), or for general anesthesia (2 mg/kg).

TABLE 8–4. Comparison of Chlorpromazine and Droperidol

	Chlorpromazine	*Droperidol*
Neuroleptic activity in rats		
Lowest active dose level	0.16 mg/kg	0.01 mg/kg
Potency	1	16
Duration of action	intermediate	short
Relative potency as:		
Antagonist of amphetamine	1	30
Antagonist of apomorphine	1	90
Antishock agent	1	16
Hypothermic agent	1	⅓
Hypotensive agent	+ + +	+
Ataxia-inducing agent	+ + +	+
Therapeutic ratio	850	68,000
Neuroleptic activity in dogs		
Inhibition of learned reflexes s.c.	1	400
Antiemetic activity s.c.	1	1000

(After Marsboom, R., and Mortelmans, J.: *Small Animal Anaesthesia.* Proceedings of Symposium by the British Small Animals Veterinary Association and the Universities Federation for Animal Welfare. Edited by G. Jones. The Macmillan Co., New York, 1964.)

TABLE 8–5. Tranquilizing Dose of Diazepam in Several Species

Species	*Route*	*Dose (mg/lb)*
Cattle	IM	0.25–0.5
Sheep	IM	0.25–0.5
Swine	IM	0.25–0.5
Chickens	IM	2.5–5.0
Turkeys	IM	2.5–5.0
Deer	Oral	2.5
Beaver	Oral	2.5
Porcupine	Oral	2.5

Azaperone (0.4 mg/kg) plus metomidate (2.5 mg/kg) intravenously produces complete anesthesia in pigs for as long as 2 hours and can be prolonged by further injections of metomidate (see Chaps. 13, 18).

Azaperone has antishock and adrenolytic activity. It is metabolized in the liver; approximately 13% is excreted in the feces (Heykants et al., 1971).

Azaperone is sold in a concentration of 40 mg/ml. It is not available in the United States.

Diazepam (Valium)

Diazepam, a benzodiazepine compound, has calming, muscle-relaxant, and anticonvulsant activities in animals (Table 8–5). It is useful as a preanesthetic agent, for relief of skeletal muscle spasm, and for convulsive seizures (Wauquier et al., 1979). It is an excellent preanesthetic agent for animals with a history of CNS disorders. Diazepam has been used with a wide variety of other agents such as inhalation anesthetics, muscle relaxants, pentazocine, morphine, xylazine, and ketamine (see Chap. 13). Each ml contains 5 mg diazepam with 40% propylene glycol, 10% ethyl alcohol, 5% sodium benzoate and benzoate acid as buffers, and 1.5% benzyl alcohol as preservative. The pH of the injectable form is 6.4 to 6.9.

In animals, diazepam appears to act on parts of the limbic system, the thalamus, and the hypothalamus to produce calming effects. It was found to reduce neural firing in the hippocampus, suggesting this location as a site of action (Olds and Olds, 1969). Mohler and Okada (1977) discovered high-affinity benzodiazepine receptors in the CNS, which were associated mainly with synaptic membranes.

Pentobarbital has been shown to increase the affinity of diazepam for the benzodiazepine receptor (Skolnick et al., 1981). The major muscle relaxant actions of the benzodiazepines occur in the CNS. This may be at the spinal level, resulting in enhancement of presynaptic activity, and at supraspinal sites, probably in the brain stem reticular formation (Schallek et al., 1972). Diazepam also produces an effect at the neuromuscular synapse which may involve direct muscle depression (Dretchen et al., 1971). The effects of diazepam occur at neuronal pathways in which γ-aminobutyric acid (GABA) is the transmitter, and GABA is essential for the effects (Costa and Giudotti, 1979).

Uptake of diazepam in the brain is reached within one minute after injection. The drug readily passes the placental barrier and is found in the fetal circulation. Protein binding has been calculated at 96% (van der Kleijn et al., 1971). Diazepam is metabolized by demethylation and hydroxylation in man, dogs, and rats to N-desmethyldiazepam, 3-hydroxydiazepam, and oxazepam. These metabolites are all pharmacologically active (Schallek et al., 1972). Essentially all of the urinary products are conjugated metabolites. Approximately 70% of an administered dose is excreted in urine and 10% in feces.

Diazepam solution should be injected slowly to prevent the possibility of venous thrombosis, and extreme care should be taken to avoid intra-arterial administration or extravasation. Care should be used in administering diazepam to ill patients and to those with limited cardiac and pulmonary reserve. There is an increased risk of congenital malformations associated with diazepam during early pregnancy. It may increase cough reflex and laryngospasm and is not recommended for obstetric use. It is contraindicated in glaucoma.

In clinical doses there are minimal respiratory and cardiac effects. Very high intravenous doses cause a slight decrease in respiration, blood pressure, and left ventricular stroke work. An increase in heart rate and decrease in cardiac output can also occur. Muir et al. (1982) determined the cardiopulmonary, behavioral, and pharmacokinetic properties of diazepam in horses. Cardiopulmonary dynamics were unchanged with doses of 0.05 to 0.4 mg/kg IV. Doses exceeding 0.2 mg/kg frequently produced recumbency. Smaller doses resulted in muscular fasciculations, weakness, and ataxia. Diazepam half-life values ranged from 6.94 to 21.6 hours.

The toxicity of diazepam is relatively low, no acute hepatotoxic or nephrotoxic effects being apparent. In rabbits the LD_{50} for intravenous diazepam is 60 mg/kg. Overdosage should be treated with supportive measures including intravenous fluids and an adequate airway. Hypotension may be alleviated by the use of levarterenol or metaraminol. Physostigmine (0.25 to 1.50 mg/kg IV or IP) has been reported to be a highly potent antidote in rats, rabbits, and cats (Nagy and Decsi, 1978). Atropine may be given concurrently to reduce parasympathetic stimulation, without altering the antidotal effect. Lukas and Griffiths (1982) were able to precipitate withdrawal symptoms in baboons after as few as 7 days of diazepam treatment.

TABLE 8–6. Summary of the Actions of Prototypical Agonists, Antagonists, and Agonist-Antagonists at Hypothetical Subtypes of Opioid Receptor

Compound	*Receptor Types**		
	μ	κ	σ
Morphine	Ag†	Ag	—
Naloxone‡	Ant	Ant	Ant
Pentazocine	Ant	Ag	Ag
Nalorphine	Ant	pAg	Ag
Buprenorphine	pAg		—
Propiram	pAg		—
N-allyl-normetazocine	Ant		Ag

*The μ receptor is thought to mediate supraspinal analgesia, respiratory depression, euphoria, and physical dependence; the κ receptor, spinal analgesia, miosis, and sedation; the σ receptor, dysphoria, hallucinations, and respiratory and vasomotor stimulation.

†Ag = agonist; Ant = competitive antagonist; pAg = partial agonist, the absence of an entry means that the compound has not yet been fully studied; — = no significant action.

‡ Naloxone is more potent in antagonizing the effects of μ agonists than κ or σ agonists and is thus thought to have the highest affinity for the μ receptor.

(From Jaffee, J.H. and Martin, W.R.: Opioid Analgesics and Antagonists. In *The Pharmacological Basis of Therapeutics,* 6th ed. Macmillan Publishing Co., Inc., New York, 1980.)

OPIATES AND NONOPIATE ANALGESICS

Opiates produce their analgesic effect by interacting with opiate receptors designed for the naturally-occurring endorphins (see Chap. 4). Three mechanisms appear to be involved: 1) inhibition of pain transmission in the dorsal horn, 2) inhibition of somatosensory afferents at supraspinal levels, and 3) activation of descending inhibitory pathways (Pert, 1981).

Studies of narcotic substances have led to recognition of multiple types of opiate receptors with differing characteristics (Chang et al., 1979; Pasternak et al., 1980). Some of these have been designated σ, κ, and μ (Martin et al., 1976; Gilbert and Martin, 1976). The effects of several agonists, antagonists, and agonist-antagonists on these receptors are shown in Table 8–6. Narcotic antagonists are discussed in Chapter 20.

Morphine Sulfate, U.S.P.

Morphine is the prototype narcotic agonist. Its chief pharmacologic effect is analgesia. Morphine produces a fast and marked increase in serotonin (5-HT) synthesis, which correlates with its analgesic effect (Godefroy et al., 1980). The site of action is probably the nucleus raphe magnus-spinal system. Subarachnoid injection of morphine produces prolonged increases in the pain thresholds of rats, rabbits, cats, and primates without affecting motor function (Yaksh et al., 1979). Morphine also affects the medullary centers, the respiratory, cough, and vasomotor centers being depressed, while the vomiting center is stimulated. With therapeutic doses, there is a reduction in the basal metabolic rate resulting in a temperature drop of 1 to 3° F.

Depression of the respiratory centers results in decreased respiratory minute volume and increased alveolar carbon dioxide tension. Both hypercarbia and hypocarbia appear to increase morphine concentrations and prolong its half-life in the brain over those values found during normocarbia (Finck et al., 1977; Nishitateno et al., 1979). In most species, morphine does not significantly depress the myocardium, rate and rhythm are usually unaltered, and there is no significant effect on cardiac output. Histamine release causes peripheral vasodilation. According to Krantz and Carr (1951), when morphine is given intravenously to the dog and cat, leg volume increases indicating capillary bed dilatation and accounting for blood pressure fall. In the dog, there is also a marked bradycardia.

Morphine has significant antidiuretic effects in the dog (Bidwai et al., 1975), probably due to release of antidiuretic hormone.

A useful action of morphine is its direct stimulatory effect on the vomiting center. The sphincters of the gastrointestinal tract are stimulated causing an overall action that is constipating; increased intestinal peristalsis tends to combat this effect. Dogs given parenteral morphine usually defecate soon after administration.

The reflex centers of the spinal cord are stimulated. This should be remembered when the use of cord stimulants is contemplated, since spinal convulsions will result. Morphine is contraindicated in strychnine poisoning for the same reason (Jones, 1957). Morphine produces an irregular effect on the brain depending upon the species in which it is administered. Because of this, the use of morphine as a preanesthetic agent is confined almost entirely to the dog. Individual variations also occur among members of the same species. In the cat, morphine in high doses (20.0 mg/kg) produces mania with tonic convulsions that may last for hours and terminate fatally. This is due to dopamine release in the CNS (Dasmana et al., 1972). Stimulation is also seen in the horse and mouse.

Davis and Donnelly (1968) have re-examined the effects of morphine in the cat. They found that at a dose of 0.1 mg/kg subcutaneously no excitement occurred and that analgesia lasting over 4 hours was produced. At 1.0 mg/kg, mydriasis, salivation, and some anxiety were evident.

Use of morphine in horses has not been accepted because it produces excitement, which could be dangerous to the animal and its handlers. Kalpravidh et al. (1984*a*) determined the analgesic and behavioral effects of morphine (.66 mg/kg IM) in ponies. Morphine produced good analgesia for superficial pain (2 hours), but only slight effect on visceral pain. Morphine caused highly significant increases in heart rate and systolic, diastolic, and mean blood pressures for 4 hours. Central venous pressure was increased slightly. Cardiac arrhythmias were not detected. Significant increases in respiratory rate were also observed. Shivering or tremors and restlessness were produced, which these authors believed might be due to dopamine release.

Klein and Baetjer (1974) gave combined morphine (.75 mg/kg) and xylazine (1.2 mg/kg) intravenously in horses. The restraint produced was considered to be superior to that produced by xylazine alone. Sweating, tremors, and cutaneous wheals were observed and attributed to the morphine.

In most species, morphine is inactivated by the liver to morphine 3-0-glucuronide, which is eliminated in the urine. Morphine stimulates secretion of antidiuretic hormone from the posterior lobe of the pituitary and is contraindicated in uremia, since it has been shown that urine production may be reduced as much as 90%.

The toxicity of morphine for the dog varies widely depending upon the age and condition of the animal. According to Jones (1957), the fatal subcutaneous or intravenous dose of morphine sulfate varies from 50 to 100 mg/lb of body weight. Booth (1961) states that doses of 400 to 500 mg/kg of body weight have been given to the dog without fatality, provided pentobarbital sodium was given intravenously to counteract the spinal convulsions that resulted. Fatal doses of morphine sulfate in the dog cause death from respiratory depression. Morphine is contraindicated in dogs suffering from traumatic or hemorrhagic shock and often proves fatal if this rule is ignored. Death is due to severe depression of blood pressure, cardiac output, and lowered oxygen consumption (Powers et al., 1947). The action of morphine can be reversed by the narcotic antagonists (see Chap. 20).

Morphine sulfate solution containing 15 mg (.25 gr)/ml is available for injection. Hypodermic tablets containing .25 gr of morphine sulfate are less commonly used. These are dissolved in sterile distilled water. Morphine is usually injected subcutaneously or intramuscularly, but may be given by slow intravenous infusion. The dosage for dogs varies widely; Booth (1961) has recommended the use of 2.5 mg/lb of body weight as a preanesthetic. Four and one-half mg/lb of body weight reduces the dose of pentobarbital sodium to one-third that usually given. Since morphine administered subcutaneously or intramuscularly does not produce its effect immediately, it should be given at least 30 minutes prior to induction of anesthesia. Following administration, dogs should be put on a run so they can eliminate.

Morphine is less widely used as a preanesthetic agent for dogs than in the past. It is usually given in combination with atropine. The dose remains the same whether given with atropine, scopolamine, or alone. From the standpoint of cost, morphine is cheaper to use as a preanesthetic agent than are other morphine substitutes or tranquilizers. The dosage and effects of morphine for several species are listed in Table 8–7.

Morphine has been used as the sole analgesic and narcotic agent for cesarean section in the bitch. When used for this purpose, morphine sulfate is given at a rate of 4 mg/lb of body weight. In old or debilitated animals, which are poor risks, this dose should be reduced. Morphine narcosis produces hypersensitivity to noise, and spinal reflexes are easily stimulated causing rigidity of the limbs. For this reason loud noises should be avoided. The bitch can be placed in sternal recumbency immediately following the operation.

Since morphine crosses the placenta, fetal respiration is depressed, but the puppies are quickly able to nurse. The bitch, however, is ataxic for as long as 18 hours postoperatively and will not care for the puppies. Care must be exercised to see that she does not lie on them and crush them. When this procedure is used, therefore, a narcotic antagonist (see Chap. 20) should be given to speed recovery of the mother and puppies.

Morphine-Apomorphine Narcosis

A combination of morphine sulfate and apomorphine hydrochloride, a dopamine agonist, can be given for deep narcosis in the dog, thus allowing painful surgical procedures to be undertaken without general anesthesia. One of the chief uses for this mixture has been in cesarean section, though it is quite effective in many other situations.

A conventional dose of morphine is administered and followed in 30 minutes with .025 to .10 gr of apomorphine, depending upon the size of the dog. The two drugs may be given simultaneously if desired, though more strenuous vomiting is produced. The pharmacologic action of the mixture has not been well explained;

TABLE 8–7. Effect of Morphine in Various Species

Species	*Dose and Route of Administration*	*Effect*
Mouse	0.1 mg/g S.Q.	Excitatory
Rat	5 mg/kg S.Q.	Soporific
Rabbit	5 mg/kg S.Q.	Soporific
	20 mg/kg S.Q.	Narcotic
Cat	0.5 mg/kg I.V., IM., S.Q., Oral	Excitatory
Monkey *(Macacus rhesus)*	2 mg/kg	Soporific
	10 mg/kg	Narcotic
	20 mg/kg	May be lethal
Chimpanzee	4 mg/kg	Soporific
Dog	10 mg/kg S.Q.	Narcotic
	50 mg/kg S.Q.	Deep narcotic (24 hours)

(From data of Krueger, H., Eddy, N.B., and Sumwalt, M.: *The Pharmacology of the Opium Alkaloids.* Part I. U.S. Public Health Service, 1941.)

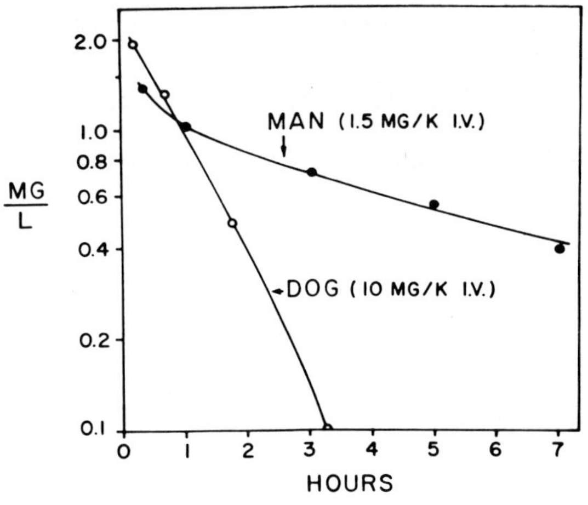

Figure 8–2. Plasma levels of meperidine in man and dog. (From Burns, J.J.: Role of Biotransformation. In *Uptake and Distribution of Anesthetic Agents*. Edited by E.M. Papper and R.J. Kitz. McGraw-Hill Book Co., Inc., New York, 1963.)

however, it appears to be a synergism. Little has been written regarding this technique and its safety, though no fatalities have been reported (Anonymous, 1952).

Apomorphine in the aforementioned dose can also be given to potentiate and prolong anesthesia in dogs beginning to recover from morphine-pentobarbital.

Meperidine Hydrochloride, U.S.P. (Demerol, Isonipecaine, Pethidine)

Meperidine hydrochloride was synthesized by Eisleb and Schaumann in 1939. It is a white crystalline powder, the free base exhibiting a strong alkaline reaction, the hydrochloride being neutral. It is commonly marketed as a solution containing 50 mg/ml or as 50-mg tablets.

The analgesic effect of meperidine is not as great as that of morphine, and plasma levels in the dog drop rapidly (Fig. 8–2). It has a spasmolytic effect similar to atropine and reduces salivary and respiratory secretions. Meperidine is used as a preanesthetic narcotic agent to quiet the animal and make it more tractable on induction. It decreases the amount of general anesthetic needed and reduces postoperative pain. It does not cause nausea, vomiting, or defecation in most animals. However, Scott et al. (1947) report it stimulates the small bowel. It is destroyed for the most part in the liver, a small amount being excreted in the urine.

When meperidine is given intravenously to dogs, there is a fall in blood pressure due to peripheral vasodilation (Gruber et al., 1941) and decreased left ventricular pressure (Frye, 1974). Rapid intravenous administration must be avoided, since the drug stimulates the central nervous system and causes convulsions.

The subcutaneous dose of meperidine as a preanesthetic agent for dogs is 10 mg/kg to 10 mg/lb. One hundred mg is equal to the analgesic effect of 10 mg of morphine sulfate. Meperidine administered as a preanesthetic agent should be given 30 minutes prior to anesthesia in order for its full effect to develop prior to induction.

Another use for meperidine is in dogs that prematurely begin to arouse from anesthesia. When it is administered intramuscularly to these animals (5 mg/kg), anesthesia is prolonged, and recovery is free of struggling and crying. Meperidine can also be used as the sole agent for cesarean section in dogs. The dosage for this purpose is 15 mg/lb.

The action of meperidine is reversed by narcotic antagonists (see Chap. 20).

Booth and Rankin (1954), in a study of the effects of meperidine in the cat, indicate that the dosage is 5 to 10 mg/kg of body weight administered subcutaneously. Animals so treated were tractable and easier to handle though the depression produced was not marked. Using the technique of Ercoli and Lewis to measure the pain threshold, researchers could not prove that analgesia was produced in the cat. Davis and Donnelly (1968) found that meperidine was rapidly metabolized in the cat. When 11 mg/kg were given intramuscularly, analgesia was apparent at 2 hours but not at 30 minutes or 4 hours.

The dosage of meperidine for preanesthesia in the horse is 0.5 to 2.0 mg/lb. It may be combined at the lower dosage with 18 mg/lb of promazine. This reduces the amount of barbiturate needed by one-third. Although it does not have a marked sedative action, its analgesic and spasmolytic effects make it a suitable preanesthetic for horses having colic.

Some have recommended its preanesthetic use in swine, although others have found it to have no sedative effect. It may also be used for postoperative analgesia.

Methadone Hydrochloride, U.S.P. (Methadone, Amidone, Dolophine)

Methadone hydrochloride is a synthetic analgesic and narcotic agent unrelated to morphine. It is a white odorless crystalline compound that is water-soluble. A 1% aqueous solution has a pH of 5.8, and under ordinary conditions its solutions are stable. It is active orally and parenterally. Toxicity by the oral, subcutaneous, and intravenous routes is approximately in the ratio of 3:2:1 respectively (Table 8–8). Narcotic antagonists reverse the toxic action (see Chap. 20).

Vomiting, salivation, incoordination, and muscular weakness are observed in dogs receiving high doses for extended periods. There is no disturbance in hematopoiesis, nonprotein nitrogen, or bromsulphalein liver function values, and the urine is free of albumin and sugar (Reutner and Gruhzit, 1948). Metabolism of the drug is obscure, about one-fourth being excreted in the urine.

Both clinical and experimental studies indicate that methadone stimulates the respiratory rate. Burroughs (1953) states that on intravenous administration in dogs relaxation follows with partial to complete loss of postural control, generalized depression, copious salivation, and frequently defecation within a few minutes. Generalized depression accompanied by an increase in the pain threshold is seen for 2 to 6 hours. During this period high-pitched noises stimulate the animal to attempt to retain postural control.

The dose of methadone for dogs is 1 mg/kg administered intravenously or subcutaneously. When the latter route is used, at least one-half hour should elapse before induction of anesthesia. The barbiturate dose is reduced approximately one-half. When given at this rate, methadone alone can be used for analgesia and narcosis for many minor surgical procedures and for restraint.

Burroughs (1953) recommends its use for cesarean section, supplementing methadone analgesia with epidural procaine and local infiltration at the incision site. Depression of the fetuses is minimal, and the bitch remains conscious throughout the procedure. This method can also be used for hysterectomies on adult dogs affected with pyometra.

Methadone combined with a phenothiazine tranquilizer has been used in horses (see Methadone-Promazine and Methadone-Acepromazine).

Oxymorphone Hydrochloride (Numorphan)

Oxymorphone hydrochloride is a semisynthetic narcotic analgesic with a potency approximately 10 times that of morphine (Eddy and Lee, 1959). It is supplied in two strengths, 1.0 and 1.5 mg/ml in sodium chloride solution (0.8%), sodium hydrosulfite (not more than 0.1%), methylparaben (0.18%), and propylparaben (0.02%) as preservatives.

Oxymorphone can be safely administered to dogs, cats, monkeys, ocelots, rodents, and lions by any parenteral route of administration (Table 8–9). In dogs, oxymorphone (0.09 mg/lb) ap-

TABLE 8–8. Summary of Acute Toxicity Studies of Methadone in Dogs

Route of Administration	*Animals (No.)*	*SAD* (mg/kg)*	*MTD† (mg/kg)*	*LD_{50}‡ (mg/kg)*
Oral	21	35.0	50.0	75.0
Subcutaneous	22	15.0	25.0	50.0
Intravenous	27	10.0	17.5	27.0

*Surgical anesthetic dose.
†Maximum tolerated dose, survival of 100% of the animals.
‡Lethal dose, 50, death of 50% of the animals.
From Reutner, T.F., and Gruhzit, O.M.: Methadon, A New Analgesic. J.A.V.M.A., 113:448, 1948.)

TABLE 8–9. Dosage of Oxymorphone Hydrochloride

Animal	*Body Weight (lbs)*	*Oxymorphone Dose IM, SC, or IV (mg)*
Dogs	2 to 5	0.75
	5 to 15	0.75 to 1.5
	15 to 30	1.5 to 2.5
	30 to 60	2.5 to 4.0
	60	4.0
Cats	small	0.4 to 0.75
	large	0.75 to 1.5

(From Palminteri, A.: Oxymorphone, an Effective Analgesic in Dogs and Cats. J.A.V.M.A., 143:160, 1963.)

TABLE 8–10. Comparison of Meperidine and Fentanyl

	Meperidine	*Fentanyl*
Analgesic activity		
Mice SC	1	500
Rats SC	1	300
Man SC	—	500–1000
Peak effects		
Mice, rats, dogs, man		
Duration	+ + + +	+
Intensity	+	+ + +
Acute toxicity		
Mice SC	1	25
Rats SC	1	30
Therapeutic ratio		
Mice SC	1	200
Rats SC	1	10

(After Marsboom, R., and Mortelmans, J.: *Small Animal Anaesthesia*. Proceedings of Symposium by the British Small Animals Veterinary Association and the Universities Federation for Animal Welfare. Edited by G. Jones. The Macmillan Co., New York, 1964.)

pears to produce more tranquilization and less hypnosis than morphine (Nytch, 1964). Respiratory depression is not marked, and there is little depression of the cough reflex. The anesthetic dose of barbiturates is reduced one-third to two-thirds. When combined with a tranquilizer, it produces neuroleptanalgesia, the effect depending upon the tranquilizer used and the dosage of the two drugs. When combined with triflupromazine, moderately profound neuroleptanalgesia results. Chlorprothixen plus oxymorphone produces an even more profound effect. When combined with propiopromazine, a prolonged effect results. If 1.5 mg (1 ml) of oxymorphone is given intravenously combined with either 20 mg (1 ml) of triflupromazine, 12.5 mg (1 ml) of chlorprothixen, or 12.5 mg (0.25 ml) of propiopromazine, a profound effect can be obtained in a 20- to 40-lb dog or large cat (Palminteri, 1966). If more analgesia is needed, the oxymorphone dose can be increased. For routine use, equal volumes of oxymorphone and triflupromazine or chlorprothixen are given intravenously. Onset of analgesia usually occurs within 1 minute. Animals so treated are responsive to loud noise.

If arousal from the mixture is desired, the narcotic can be antagonized by levallorphan, nalorphine, or naloxone. One mg (1 ml) of levallorphan or 5 mg (1 ml) of nalorphine are used either intravenously or intramuscularly. The dosage of naloxone is 0.4 mg/1.5 mg of oxymorphone and is given by any parenteral route.

Fentanyl Citrate and Carfentanil

Fentanyl is approximately 500 times more potent than meperidine on a weight basis (Table 8–10). It has a rapid onset of action following intravenous or intramuscular injection. Analgesia, sedation, and respiratory depression develop in 3 to 8 minutes depending on the species. Fentanyl produces behavioral effects similar to those of other narcotics, such as analgesia, sedation with decreased motor activity, ataxia, and exaggerated response to loud auditory stimuli. It has a short duration of action, the peak effect lasting less than 30 minutes. The actions of fentanyl can be reversed by the narcotic antagonists (see Chap. 20).

The respiratory effects are not consistent, ranging from depression with occasional apnea to hyperventilation. Peak respiratory depression is usually noted 5 to 15 minutes after injection. In dogs anesthetized with pentobarbital, the rate and tidal volume decrease sharply following intravenous injection. As with morphine, panting may occur.

Although fentanyl is a short-acting narcotic analgesic, respiratory depression has been seen in the postanesthetic period several hours after the last dose. Hug and Murphy (1979) found that fentanyl, which is a highly lipophilic drug, equilibrated rapidly between plasma and CSF. There was close correlation between the concentrations of fentanyl in plasma and CSF and the intensity of respiratory depression. Repeated injections of fentanyl led to accumulation with increased ventilatory depression.

Fentanyl is a basic drug, and an increase in pH shifts the equilibrium to favor the unionized moiety. This makes fentanyl more lipid-soluble and increases penetration through the blood-brain barrier. Furthermore, it increases nonspecific brain tissue binding. The reverse is true with respiratory acidosis. Ainslie et al. (1979) found that the brain-blood ratios of fentanyl were highest with hypocarbia and lowest with hypercarbia. At 35 minutes postadministration, when clinical analgesia may be considered terminated, hypocarbic brain levels of fentanyl were double those of normocarbia. This may be due, to a large extent, to higher serum fentanyl concentrations and reduced washout because of decreased blood flow. Higher brain fentanyl levels, to a small but unknown extent, may result from increased blood-brain penetration due to increased lipid solubility and increased brain tissue binding during alkalosis.

Intravenous or intramuscular injection of fentanyl produces bradycardia in either awake or anesthetized dogs and rabbits due to an increase in vagal tone. This seems to have little effect on cardiac output or blood pressure at normal dose levels (Green, 1979). Administration of atropine at the rate of 0.02 mg/lb prevents bradycardia. In dogs anesthetized with barbiturates, intravenous fentanyl (0.04 mg/kg) produces a fall in blood pressure with a gradual return to near-normal levels. This occurs in both vagotomized and nonvagotomized dogs, indicating that hypotension is not a function of changing heart rate. Histamine release rarely occurs. Extreme care should be exercised if fentanyl is administered to animals that have already received barbiturates. Bradycardia, hypotension, and respiratory depression may occur and may be difficult to reverse.

Liu et al. (1976) administered large doses of fentanyl (0.05 to 2 mg/kg) and fentanyl plus N_2O to dogs to determine the cardiovascular effects. Fentanyl caused a dose-related increase in heart rate which was significant at 0.05 mg/kg. Cardiac output, PVR, and systolic, diastolic, and mean arterial blood pressures also decreased, while stroke volume increased. These changes became significant at 0.1 mg/kg for diastolic blood pressure, 0.15 mg/kg for cardiac output and mean blood pressure, 0.25 mg/kg for stroke volume and systolic blood pressure, and at 1.25 mg/kg for peripheral vascular resistance. N_2O after fentanyl did not significantly change any parameter, although stroke volume, cardiac output, and heart rate usually increased and PVR decreased. The changes appeared to be less profound than those produced by equianalgesic doses of morphine. They suggested that this combination might be an attractive alternative to morphine-oxygen anesthesia in critically ill human patients.

Fentanyl, unlike morphine, usually does not produce vomiting in dogs; however, the anal sphincter is relaxed, and frequently there is defecation. This is considered undesirable by many practitioners who do not use the drug for this reason.

Fentanyl has been used in ponies and horses, but has not proved to be particularly effective as an analgesic unless combined with xylazine. Pippi and Lumb (1979) found that fentanyl (0.055 mg/kg) and xylazine (1.1 mg/kg) in combination were significantly better than xylazine alone in obtunding visceral pain for up to 4 hours.

When fentanyl is used alone, a dosage of 0.2 mg/kg produces recumbency in ponies but not surgical anesthesia. A dose of 0.1 mg/kg was not found to be particularly effective in controlling superficial, deep, or visceral pain.

Fentanyl combined with droperidol is marketed as Innovar-Vet (see p. 190). It has been combined with fluanisone in rabbits, rats, swine, primates, dogs, mice, hamsters, and guinea pigs. It may also be used to supplement xylazine, metomidate, or short-acting barbiturates (Green, 1979). For wild animals especially, it has been combined with azaperone (10 mg/dl fentanyl with 80 mg/ml azaperone).

Carfentanil (R33799), a congener of fentanyl, is 12,000 to 18,000 times more potent than meperidine and has been termed "superfentanyl." Because of its potency, it can be administered by swabbing or spraying the buccal or nasal mucosa (Port et al., 1982, 1983). It is available in 1-ml ampules containing 10 mg of drug. It has been used almost exclusively for capture of exotic species of animals (see Chap. 18). Its action is reversed by the usual morphine antagonists, cyprenorphine (M285) or deprenorphine (M5050) probably being the drugs of choice. According to De Vos (1978), in free-ranging wild animals its potency compared to etorphine and fentanyl is approximately 20:15:1, respectively.

Thiambutene Hydrochloride (Themalon)

Thiambutene hydrochloride is a white powder, highly soluble in water. Aqueous solutions may be boiled, but they do not withstand autoclaving and turn brown if kept for a few days. Solutions injected subcutaneously cause little reaction, and a local anesthetic action is produced. When the drug is given orally, the stomach is irritated, and vomiting usually occurs.

The drug closely resembles morphine in its pharmacologic effects, which are chiefly analgesic and hypnotic. It produces a greater insensitivity to pain than can be obtained with morphine. It does not cause vomiting when injected parenterally. Salivation is produced in some dogs due, in part, to depression of the swallowing reflex. This can be prevented by administration of atropine. Evacuation of the bowel often occurs.

High intravenous doses depress the vasomotor center with immediate hypotension. The respiration may be increased or decreased by therapeutic doses, higher doses causing slowing. It crosses the placenta and depresses fetal respiration. This, however, can be rapidly reversed with narcotic antagonists. Occasional idiosyncrasy occurs in dogs characterized by hysteria, vocalization, and convulsions. This is not a problem if the drug is used in conjunction with diazepam (Green, 1979).

When given subcutaneously, it is about one-fifth as active as morphine sulfate and 3 to 4 times more active than meperidine on a weight basis. Doses of 5 to 20 mg/kg give a wide range of effect from mild analgesia and sedation to deep narcosis. The action starts within 5 to 10 minutes, reaches a peak within 30 minutes, and lasts for 1 to 10 hours. Hysterical animals require much greater doses, 50 mg/kg subcutaneously sometimes being necessary to produce deep narcosis.

When injected intravenously, 1 to 5 mg/kg produce narcosis within a few minutes. Recovery occurs more rapidly than with subcutaneous administration, being complete within 15 minutes to 3 hours depending upon the dose.

When thiambutene is injected intravenously in dogs anesthetized with pentobarbital, blood pressure falls immediately, and there is brief apnea and spasm of the small intestine.

A series of 120 dogs were given thiambutene for restraint required during examination or surgery under local anesthesia, or for premedication prior to general anesthesia (Owen, 1955*a*). Thiambutene was injected either intravenously at a rate of 2 mg/lb over a period of approximately 1 minute or subcutaneously at the rate of 10 mg/lb. Table 8–11 summarizes the narcotic effects seen in 79 dogs. The depth of narcosis varied, but usually lasted for periods of up to 2½ hours. The onset occurred after 5 to 10 minutes and reached its peak about 30 minutes later. Changes in the pulse rate varied and were not considered significant. The respiratory rate decreased in some dogs and increased in others. The body temperature was lowered. Thiambutene narcosis was effectively ended by the injection of 1 mg/lb of nalorphine intravenously.

In pyometra, regardless of the condition of the bitch, thiambutene (2 mg/lb) was given intravenously over a period of 1 minute (Owen, 1955*b*). Ten to 15 minutes later, thiopental was given intravenously. The narcosis produced by thiambutene was satisfactory in 21 of 22 cases of pyometra. Temporary spasticity and apnea developed in one instance. The chief advantage was reduction in the amount of barbiturate required and shortening of the period of narcosis, along with elimination of postanesthetic excitement. The duration of anesthesia was so short that ether or additional thiopental had to be given in 60% of the animals anesthetized. With one injection of thiopental, anesthesia averaged 29 minutes.

This drug has been used extensively in dogs and in capture of feral animals; it is contrain-

TABLE 8–11. Summary of the Narcotic Effects of Thiambutene in the Dog

Route of Administration and Dose	Narcotic Effect			
	Light	Medium	Deep	Total
Intravenous (2 mg/lb)	10	23	19	52
Subcutaneous (10 mg/lb)	9	9	9	27

(From Owen, L.N.: The Narcotic Effects of Thiambutene in the Dog and Its Antagonism by Nalorphine. Vet. Rec., 67:561, 1955.)

dicated in cats. It is not available in the United States.

Etorphine Hydrochloride (M-99)

Etorphine hydrochloride, an oripavine derivative, has been used extensively for restraint of wild animals. It is chemically related to morphine, and its use requires a narcotic license. When given subcutaneously, etorphine is 80 to 1,000 times more potent than morphine depending upon the test situation. Etorphine is supplied in vials containing 10 or 20 mg.

Etorphine is administered intramuscularly in the shoulder or hip area with either a hand-held syringe or a syringe dart (see Chap. 3). There is a species variation in susceptibility to etorphine. Among the more sensitive species are the elephant, hippopotamus, rhinoceros, tapir, bear, and primates. With medium doses, most animals remain on their feet but can be approached safely (Harthoorn, 1966). Deaths occasionally occur after injection. Other drugs that have been used in combination with etorphine are acepromazine, scopolamine, promazine, methotrimeprazine, and phencyclidine. There is no evidence that incompatibility with these drugs occurs.

In ungulates, etorphine produces tachycardia, elevated blood pressure, depression of respiration and the cough center, suppression of rumen movements, total analgesia, loss of reflexes without loss of consciousness, depression of body temperature, and loss of visual accommodation.

The actions of etorphine resemble those of morphine in rodents, cats, dogs, and monkeys, producing analgesia, catatonia, respiratory depression, antidiuresis, reduced gastrointestinal motility, and blockade of conditioned reflexes. In mice and rats, it causes excitement; in rats, dogs, cats, and monkeys, bradycardia and hypotension occur. It does not cause excitement or vomiting in the dog (Blane et al., 1967). Etorphine (7.5 μg/kg) combined with methotrimeprazine (6.0 mg/kg) has been used successfully for neuroleptanalgesia in dogs, pigs, calves, rats, guinea pigs, rabbits, and mice. In all these species cardiac arrhythmias and respiratory depression were greater than with equianalgesic doses of fentanyl-fluanisone (Green, 1979).

The effects of etorphine can be antagonized with nalorphine or diprenorphine. The dose of the former is in a ratio (etorphine/nalorphine) of 1:10 to 1:20, or 1:1 to 1:2 for diprenorphine (Burkhart, 1967). Higher doses of antagonists are not advantageous and may produce protracted recovery times. The dose of antagonist should be given intravenously for quick response. Reversal should occur within 10 minutes after administration, although Gray (1968) has reported as long as 6 to 8 hours may be required. Relapse after reversal has been reported (VanLaun, 1977). The extreme potency of the drug makes it dangerous to handle, and accidental self-administration has occurred.

Levorphanol Tartrate (Levo-Dromoran)

Levorphanol tartrate is a highly potent, long lasting synthetic analgesic with properties and actions similar to those of morphine (Casey, 1971). It produces a degree of analgesia equal to that of morphine and greater than that of meperidine at far smaller doses than either. From 6 to 8 hours of pain relief can be expected with levorphanol whether given orally or by injection, depending upon species. Its safety margin is about equal to that of morphine, but it is less likely to produce nausea, vomiting, and constipation.

In humans, it is used in alleviating pain due to biliary and renal colic, myocardial infarction, and severe trauma, intractable pain due to cancer and other tumors, as a preanesthetic, and for postoperative pain relief. It has not been used to any extent in animals.

To prevent or to counteract narcotic-induced respiratory depression (particularly in parturients and neonates, or during nitrous oxide-oxygen anesthesia with narcotic supplementation), levorphanol can be combined with levallorphan tartrate, a narcotic antagonist. Levorphanol/levallorphan (SQ or IV) is given in the ratio of 10:1. This combination prevents respiratory depression without significantly reducing the pain relief provided by levorphanol. When given to an equine induced-colic model at 0.03 mg/kg IM, levorphanol produced a slight degree of analgesia for 4 hours (Kalpravidh et al., 1984*a*). No analgesia for superficial pain was observed at this dose level. Systolic, diastolic, and mean blood pressures, heart and respiratory rates, central venous pressure, body temperature, and blood gas parameters remained within normal limits. Motor activity was stimulated.

In the mouse, the LD_{50} is 40.9 ± 5.0 mg/kg IV. In the rat it is 27.1 ± 9.4 mg/kg IV, 120.3 ± 99.8 mg/kg SQ, and 163.5 ± 48.0 mg/kg PO. The LD_{50} IV in the rabbit is 20.0 ± 3.8 mg/kg. Levorphanol is approximately 50% bound to plasma proteins. In the rat biotransformation is almost complete, only 1 to 2% of the total dose being excreted intact. Levorphanol probably passes freely into milk and through the placental barriers. The half-life in rat brain and plasma is 2.1 and 1.2 hours respectively.

Butorphanol Tartrate (Stadol, Dorphanol, Torbutrol)

Butorphanol is a synthetic analgesic with both narcotic agonist and antagonist properties. It is 3 to 5 times more potent than morphine. Its narcotic antagonist activity is about equipotent with nalorphine or about 50 times less potent than naloxone (Pircio et al., 1976). The dose of naloxone required to reverse butorphanol effects in animal studies was higher than that required to antagonize complete narcotic agonists.

The effects of butorphanol on respiratory parameters resemble those seen with morphine but, unlike the latter, respiratory depressant activity appears to reach a "ceiling" beyond which higher doses do not produce an appreciably greater effect. In rats, butorphanol subcutaneously produced a small increase in arterial blood CO_2 and a decrease in the pH. When doses from 2.5 to 10 mg/kg were given, the latter produced no appreciable change in these parameters over the 2.5 mg/kg dose. In anesthetized dogs, approximately equianalgesic intravenous doses of butorphanol (0.75 mg/kg) and morphine (3 mg/kg) rapidly decreased mean arterial blood pressure, but morphine produced a more marked decrease (77% vs. 21% at 1 to 2 minutes after injection) (Schurig et al., 1978). In contrast, Sederberg et al. (1981) found butorphanol infusions (0.1 and 0.2 mg/kg/min) produced significant decreases in heart rate, blood pressure, and cardiac output. Addition of nitrous oxide further depressed cardiac function. They indicated that butorphanol is not a good alternative to morphine or fentanyl as a narcotic anesthetic in dogs.

In anesthetized dogs, equianalgesic intravenous doses of butorphanol (0.025 mg/kg) and morphine (0.1 mg/kg) had spasmogenic effects, increasing duodenal activity. The maximum effect obtained with butorphanol, however, was only about 13% of that with morphine (Roebel et al., 1977). Butorphanol did not produce any significant changes in bile flow, whereas morphine produced a dose-related significant reduction in flow.

When given intravenously (0.5 mg/kg), butorphanol produced only mild sedation in dogs and no changes in blood histamine concentrations (Pircio et al., 1976). In guinea pigs and dogs, butorphanol is 115 times more effective than codeine or dextromethorphan in suppressing electrically stimulated or pathologic cough (Cavanaugh et al., 1976). High doses of butorphanol (5 to 30 mg/kg subcutaneously) produce a dose-related diuretic response associated with decreased urinary excretion of antidiuretic hormone (Miller, 1975).

Robertson et al. (1981) have studied the cardiopulmonary and behavioral effects of butorphanol in horses. Butorphanol was administered intravenously at 0.1, 0.2, and 0.4 mg/kg. No significant changes were seen in heart rate, mean and diastolic arterial blood pressure, mean and diastolic pulmonary arterial blood pressure, or cardiac output. Systolic arterial blood pressure was significantly elevated in horses receiving 0.2 mg/kg. No changes were observed in electrocardiographic intervals, respiratory rate, arterial blood gas values, or pH. The behavioral changes with large doses of intravenous butorphanol were predominantly excitatory.

Kalpravidh et al. (1984*a,b*) investigated the effects of intravenous and intramuscular butorphanol on induced equine colic and superficial pain models. Good analgesia for visceral pain was afforded by 0.22 mg/kg IM for 4 hours, and by 0.10 mg/kg IV for 30 minutes. The optimal dose IV was believed to be between 0.10 and 0.20 mg/kg. Motor activity in the horses was increased.

A combination of butorphanol (0.1 mg/kg IV) plus xylazine (1.1 mg/kg IV) will allow standing surgical procedures in horses for approximately 30 minutes (Robertson and Muir, 1983).

In dogs, doses of 0.1 to 0.3 mg/kg reduced enflurane minimum alveolar concentration (MAC) in a dose-dependent fashion. Additional doses did not result in further reduction of MAC, indicating a "ceiling effect" (Murphy and Hug, 1981).

Distribution of the drug in animals is mainly to excretory organs and fatty or highly perfused tissues. In women, butorphanol readily passes into the fetus. Butorphanol is extensively metabolized in humans, approximately 90% to hydroxybutorphanol and 10% to norbutorphanol, neither of which appears to have analgesic activity. Excretion occurs primarily in the urine (70%) with some biliary elimination (11 to 14%).

The LD_{50} of butorphanol in mice intravenously, subcutaneously, and orally was 40 to 57 mg/kg, 299 to 432 mg/kg, and 395 to 527 mg/kg, respectively. Corresponding figures for rats were 17 to 20 mg/kg, 622 to 852 mg/kg, and 570 to 756 mg/kg. In dogs, the LD_{50} following intravenous, intramuscular, or oral administration was 10 to 50 mg/kg, 17 to 29 mg/kg, and greater than 50 mg/kg respectively. The oral LD_{50} in monkeys was more than 50 mg/kg.

Pentazocine Lactate (Talwin, Fortral)

Pentazocine, a member of the benzomorphan series,* is a white crystalline substance, soluble in acidic solutions. It is packaged in 1-ml ampules and 10-ml multiple-dose vials. Sodium chloride and acetone sodium bisulfate have been added, along with methylparaben as a preservative. The pH is adjusted to between 4 and 5 with lactic acid and sodium hydroxide.

Pentazocine is an analgesic having agonist-antagonist properties (see Table 8–6). In man, the analgesic potency of 30 mg of pentazocine is equal to 10 mg of morphine. It has the potential for abuse in humans, and its use is regulated by the Drug Enforcement Administration in the United States.

Pentazocine has minimal effect on the cardiovascular system and is a mild respiratory depressant. It has been found to be an effective analgesic in horses, dogs, pigs, primates, rabbits, and rats. The doses for horses are 0.5 to 3.0 mg/kg IV and 0.5 to 6.0 mg/kg IM, for pigs 2.0 mg/kg IM, and for dogs 2.0 mg/kg. Effects are observed within 15 minutes and last for as long as 2 hours (Green, 1979).

Roughly 80% of a dose of 1 mg/kg is excreted in 24 hours in rats and monkeys. About 70% is found in urine and 10% in feces. Intramuscular doses of up to 4 mg/kg four times a day are tolerated by dogs with some sedation and loss of postural reflexes. Higher doses produce moderate salivation, tremors, and mydriasis, whereas high doses (20 mg/kg) cause tremors and convulsions. Monkeys and cats exhibit similar symptoms.

When used to treat an induced colic model, the intravenous injection of 0.25 to 2 mg/lb of pentazocine in the horse produced analgesia for

*Also known as benzazocine series.

15 to 30 minutes. Intramuscular injections of 0.25 to 3 mg/lb produced analgesia for 5 to 160 minutes depending upon the dose. Doses above 2 mg/lb produced ataxia and muscle tremors (Lowe, 1969).

The usual narcotic antagonists are not effective against pentazocine-induced respiratory depression; however, naloxone hydrochloride has been found to be a specific antagonist for pentazocine (Kallos and Smith, 1968).

Xylazine Hydrochloride (Rompun)

Xylazine, 2(2,6-dimethylphenylamino)-4H-5,6-dihydro-1,3-thiazine-hydrochloride), is a potent non-narcotic sedative and analgesic as well as a muscle relaxant. Sedative and analgesic activity are related to central nervous system depression mediated by stimulation of α_2-receptors (Hsu, 1981); muscle relaxant effect is based on inhibition of intraneural transmission of impulses in the central nervous system. Xylazine hydrochloride is available for small animals in 2% solution and for large nonruminant animals in 10% solution. The pH is adjusted to 5.5 ± 0.3.

Xylazine was first used in Germany (Sagner et al., 1968) and has since been found satisfactory for use in a wide variety of domestic and exotic species. It is currently approved for use in dogs, cats, horses, deer, and elk in the United States. Dosages for several species are listed in Table 8–12. When xylazine is used as a preanesthetic agent, the amount of barbiturate or thiobarbiturate subsequently employed should be reduced by one-third to one-half of the estimated dose. The halothane requirement for anesthesia (MAC) is reduced nearly 40% (Tranquilli et al., 1983).

Principal effects develop within 10 to 15 minutes after intramuscular injection, and within 3 to 5 minutes following intravenous administration. After intramuscular injection, peak plasma concentrations are reached in horses, cattle, sheep, and dogs within 12 to 14 minutes. After intravenous administration, the systemic half-life is 23 minutes for sheep, 30 minutes for dogs, 36 minutes for cattle, and 50 minutes for horses (Garcia-Villar et al., 1981). A sleep-like state, the depth of which is dose-dependent, is usually maintained for 1 to 2 hours, while analgesia lasts from 15 to 30 minutes (Mozier, 1972).

TABLE 8–12. Xylazine Dosages

	mg/kg of body weight	
	Intravenous	*Intramuscular*
Horse	0.5 –1.1	1–2
Cattle*	0.03–0.1	0.1–0.2
Sheep*	0.05–0.1	0.1–0.3
Goats*	0.01–0.5	0.05–0.5
Pig	—	2–3
Dog	0.5 –1	1–2
Cat	0.5 –1	1–2
Birds	—	5–10

*Lower dosage should be used if sedation without recumbency is desired.
(From Knight, A.P.: Xylazine. J.A.V.M.A., 176:454, 1980.)

A combination of atropine (0.05 mg/kg IM) followed in ten minutes by acepromazine (0.5 mg/kg IM) and xylazine (2.2 mg/kg IM) has been recommended for use in dogs by Cronin et al. (1983). This combination gives excellent muscle relaxation with consistent loss of the righting reflex, deep sedation, and moderate analgesia.

Klide et al. (1975) studied the cardiopulmonary effects in dogs (Fig. 8–3). They found that heart rate decreased significantly along with aortic flow. There was an initial increase in blood pressure and peripheral vascular resistance. Muir and Piper (1977) found an initial positive inotropic response after administration of 1.1 mg/kg intravenously to dogs. This effect was followed by a return to or significant decrease from baseline recordings at faster heart rates, or later times following xylazine administration (30 and 60 minutes). Cardiac contractility was reduced by xylazine at heart rates greater than 150/min.

Klide et al. (1975) did not find any changes in pH, Pa_{O_2}, or Pa_{CO_2} in dogs following xylazine administration intravenously (1.1 mg/kg) or intramuscularly (2.2 mg/kg). They believed that this indicated no changes in alveolar ventilation or acid-base status.

Ponder and Clark (1980) reported dose-dependent depression of thermoregulation with decreases in body temperature in cats receiving xylazine (1 to 4 mg/kg SC or 0.5 to 2 mg/kg

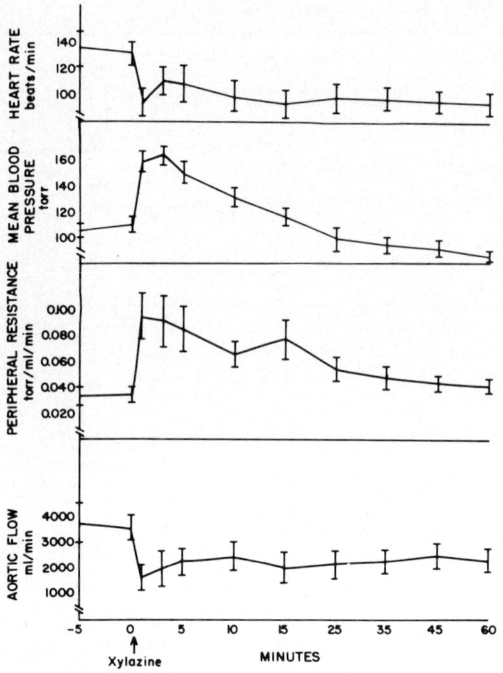

Figure 8–3. Heart rate, blood pressure, peripheral resistance, and aortic flow in 6 dogs given xylazine (1.1 mg/kg) intravenously. (From Klide, A.M., Calderwood, H.W., and Soma, L.R.: Cardiopulmonary Effects of Xylazine in Dogs. J.A.V.M.A., 36:931, 1975.)

IV). Changes were maximal 3 to 4 hours after injection and persisted for at least 12 hours. A hyperthermic response was observed in xylazine-treated cats in a 32° C environment. Hypothermia has also been reported in rats, and in nonhuman primates when xylazine is used in combination with ketamine. Xylazine induces hyperglycemia in cats and dogs, resulting from inhibition of insulin secretion and an increase in the glucagon/insulin ratio (Feldberg and Symonds, 1980; Benson et al., 1983). Hsu et al. (1981) produced a dose-dependent (0.01 to 1.0 mg/kg IV) mydriasis in cats with xylazine, which could be antagonized by yohimbine (0.5 mg/kg IV). Mydriasis was believed to be due to CNS inhibition of parasympathetic tone to the iris by postsynaptic α_2-adrenergic receptors.

Hoffman (1974) has administered xylazine intravenously to horses requiring restraint, sedation, or analgesia prior to a variety of clinical procedures. Sedation and analgesia were good to excellent in 88 and 81%, respectively, without adverse effects from single or repeated doses. Maximal sedation occurred in approximately 3 minutes and lasted 30 to 40 minutes. Optimal dosage was found to be 1.1 mg/kg. He concluded that xylazine is a useful restraining agent for horses because of its speed of onset, brief duration of action, and consistency of action, regardless of breed, age, sex, or temperament variations. Ketamine-xylazine anesthesia in horses is described in Chapter 13.

When xylazine was compared with several narcotics, Pippi and Lumb (1979) and Kalpravidh et al. (1984*a*) found it to be significantly more effective in obtunding deep pain in ponies. Xylazine (1.1 mg/kg) combined with fentanyl (0.055 mg/kg) was significantly better for control of visceral pain than xylazine alone (2.2 mg/kg) or xylazine combined with meperidine or oxymorphone (Pippi and Lumb, 1979).

Baker (1974) has made the following recommendations for use of xylazine in ruminants:

1. The dosage should be only one-tenth to one-fifth of the dose recommended for horses.
2. Five to 15 mg/100 lb seems to be the most effective and safest dosage to use.
3. The small animal product (20 mg/ml) should be used on ruminants under 50 lb for more accurate dosage.
4. The solution recommended for horses (100 mg/ml) may be diluted to 25 mg/ml with distilled water if the small animal product is not available.
5. An insulin or tuberculin syringe should always be used for smaller ruminants (calves, sheep, and goats) for more accurate dosage.
6. If given intravenously, the lower dosage levels should always be used initially.
7. Debilitated animals or animals with quiet temperament do not require the dosage that a high-strung animal requires.
8. There is no currently available antidote for xylazine, which makes it extremely important that overdosage not occur.

The intravenous dose of xylazine for beef cows and calves is 0.05 mg/lb. This dose should be diluted in saline and given over a 2- to 3-

minute period. The intramuscular dose is 0.10 mg/lb. For bulls the dose is less (0.05 mg/lb IM). When supplemented with local anesthesia, 8 mg/lb intravenously provides light sedation for standing surgeries.

In calves, the hemodynamic effects of sedative doses of xylazine (0.22 mg/100 kg IM) include immediate and prolonged reductions in heart rate, cardiac output, arterial blood pressure, and left ventricular dp/dt max (Campbell et al., 1979). Stroke volume initially decreases and then returns within 15 minutes to baseline values. Total peripheral resistance, end-diastolic left ventricular pressure, end-diastolic left ventricular volume, and left ventricular residual fraction increase after drug administration. These changes indicate that xylazine depresses the myocardium. The hypertensive response, seen in other species, has not been observed in calves. Only small doses of xylazine are required for sedation of calves compared to those required for other species.

When xylazine (0.2 mg/kg) was given intravenously to beef cattle, it resulted in the rapid onset (15 minutes) of hyperglycemia (Eichner et al., 1979). Plasma glucose values increased to 195 mg/dl at 15 minutes and 3 hours, respectively. Concomitantly, plasma insulin concentrations fell from 23 μU/ml before xylazine to 5.8 μU/ml and 2.4 μU/ml at 15 minutes and 3 hours, respectively. According to Hsu and Hummel (1981), the hyperglycemia and hypoinsulinemia are mediated by α_2-adrenergic receptors in pancreatic β-cells which inhibit insulin release. Twenty percent decreases in percentage of hemoglobin, RBC count, and packed cell volume were also observed by Eichner et al. (1979). Plasma urea nitrogen was significantly increased within 3 hours postadministration (11.5 mg/dl vs. 6.7 mg/dl). Because of these changes, alternative methods of anesthesia should be used in instances where biopsy material is to be obtained for studies of carbohydrate metabolism.

Ketamine-xylazine anesthesia in cattle is described in Chapter 13.

Swine are resistant to xylazine, requiring 20 to 30 times the ruminant dose. It is not widely used in this species because of the poor results obtained.

Xylazine has a wide margin of safety. Increasing dosages do not in general increase the degree of sedation but rather the duration of effect. Ten times the recommended dose is tolerated by dogs, cats, and horses; however, this amount results in muscle tremors, bradycardia with partial atrioventricular block, and reduced respiratory rate. Movement in response to sharp auditory stimuli may also be observed (Mozier, 1972). Unlike morphine, it does not cause excitement in cats. Bradycardia is produced by activation of presynaptic α_2-adrenergic receptors (Hsu et al., 1981). Kerr et al. (1972*a,b*) have indicated that xylaine-induced second-degree A-V block can be abolished by prior intravenous administration of 0.011 mg/kg or more of atropine sulfate. They recommended use of the minimal effective dose of atropine, larger doses tending to produce a marked tachycardia and hypertension, which appeared to be dose-related.

Emesis occurs occasionally in dogs and frequently in cats soon after xylazine is administered. Acute abdominal distension occasionally occurs in large dogs given xylazine intravenously or intramuscularly. Affected dogs usually weigh more than 50 lb (Haskins, 1979). Abdominal distension may be due to aerophagia, or may be related to the parasympatholytic activity of the drug, which results in gastrointestinal atony with accumulation of gas. Some of these dogs require emergency treatment several hours following injection. For this reason it should not be used in Great Danes, Irish setters, basset hounds, and other dogs prone to bloat (Folkers, 1980). This feature also makes xylazine sedation undesirable when one is taking upper GI radiographs, since it may cause the stomach to fill with gas and make roentgenogram interpretation less certain.

Xylazine-induced bradycardia may occasionally lead to heart block and death in dogs (Folkers, 1980). If xylazine is used in dogs as a preanesthetic prior to halothane, it causes an increased probability of cardiac arrhythmias and lowers the threshold to ventricular fibrillation. This reaction may be due to its ability to potentiate cardiac sensitization to epinephrine (Muir et al., 1975). Sudden deaths in horses following xylazine administration have been reported by Clarke and Hall (1969) and Fuentes (1978). Violent seizures followed by collapse may occur on inadvertent injection into the carotid artery. Fatalities in healthy mature goats have followed a dose of 10 mg (Baker, 1974). Ruminants regurgitate and become tympanitic under its effect. Appropriate precautions to prevent aspiration are essential when doses inducing recumbency are used. Xylazine is also contraindicated in the last trimester of pregnancy in cattle, since abortion may occur.

A combination of 4-aminopyridine (0.3 mg/kg) and yohimbine (0.125 mg/kg) intravenously will antagonize a dose of 2.2 mg/kg of xylazine in dogs (Hatch et al., 1982). These dogs can walk in less than 2 minutes, and the total recovery time is reduced to 30 minutes. The same dosage of these drugs intravenously will antagonize xylazine sedation in cattle (Kitzman et al., 1982).

Doxapram (2 mg/kg IM) reverses xylazine-atropine sedation in dogs. However, relapses, muscular and postural abnormalities, and dangerous and unpredictable aggressive behavior have been reported following its use (Hatch, 1983).

Care should be taken by persons using xylazine, because it can be absorbed through wounds or mucous membranes and causes serious effects.

TRANQUILIZER-NARCOTIC COMBINATIONS

Fentanyl Citrate-Droperidol (Innovar-Vet)

A combination of fentanyl citrate and droperidol is sold as Innovar-Vet. It is used to produce neuroleptanalgesia. This is a state of central nervous system depression and analgesia produced without the use of barbiturates or volatile agents. In dogs, the combination produces sufficient analgesia and sedation to allow surgery, but still permits an auditory response.

The commercial mixture is supplied in 20-ml multiple-dose vials. Each ml contains 0.4 mg of fentanyl and 20 mg of droperidol, with 1.8 mg of methylparaben and 0.2 mg of propylparaben as preservatives. Lactic acid is added for pH adjustment to approximately 3.1. Because it contains fentanyl, a narcotic license is necessary for its purchase and use.

The combination of the two agents produces an intense action of relatively short duration with each agent exerting its own effects. In general, tranquilizers have no analgesic properties, some being considered antianalgesic (Moore and Dundee, 1961). In mice, the analgesic actions of fentanyl are enhanced by droperidol without an increase in toxicity.

In dogs, the mixture produces sedation, analgesia, immobilization, respiratory depression or panting, adrenergic blockade, a fall in blood pressure, and bradycardia. Vomiting is not produced, although defecation frequently occurs.

Fentanyl-droperidol has wide application for use in painful procedures to be performed on dogs. Advantages are ease of administration, wide margin of safety, quiet recovery, partial reversibility with narcotic antagonists, and tolerance by animals in a poor physical state. Although it is possible to perform radical surgery using neuroleptanalgesia produced by this combination, most surgeons prefer general anesthesia. Because the mixture potentiates general anesthetics, the dosage of barbiturates should be reduced from one-third to one-half the regular dosage. When it is used as a preanesthetic agent, the recommended dosage is 1 ml/15 to 20 lbs intramuscularly or 1 ml/25 to 60 lb intravenously, followed in 10 minutes by intravenous injection of barbiturate. With this method, induction of general anesthesia is smooth, and recovery occurs without excitement. The combination has been used with a wide variety of barbiturates, and local and general anesthetics.

Franklin and Reid (1965) reported that fentanyl-droperidol reduced the amount of thiamylal needed to produce and to maintain general anesthesia up to 90%. In a series of 355 cases in which the combination was used alone, 4 dogs died within 24 hours postoperatively. These deaths were not attributed to the drug combination since the dogs had shown routine recovery and had become ambulatory prior to death. Soma and Shields (1964) reported use of fentanyl-droperidol in 100 dogs for a variety of procedures. One death occurred postoperatively in a dog operated upon for pyometra.

Hamlin et al. (1968) used intravenous fentanyl-droperidol (1 ml/25 lbs) followed within 15 seconds by intravenous pentobarbital sodium (3 mg/lb). Surgical anesthesia was produced and lasted 30 to 45 minutes. Dogs could walk with a staggering gait in 77 ($\pm$ 12) minutes; complete recovery occurred in 176 ($\pm$ 34) minutes. Heart rate and cardiac output were reduced, which these authors interpreted as indicating that more cardiac reserve was left available to the animal. They stated that the dog maintained its "normal physiologic reflexes" at least to the same degree as with morphine-chloralose anesthesia, while at the same time fentanyl-droperidol-pentobarbital was easier to administer. The most undesirable complication was diarrhea in 25% of the dogs anesthetized.

Fentanyl-droperidol was administered intravenously, alone or with atropine sulfate (0.02 or 0.04 mg/kg), to determine if stable neuroleptanalgesia could be produced in the dog (Buckhold et al., 1977). Given alone, the combination caused significant increases in peripheral vascular resistance and mean arterial pressure at 5 minutes followed by a decrease in these values over the next 30 minutes. Left ventricular dp/dt increased significantly 15 and 30 minutes after injection. In dogs given atropine mixed with fentanyl-droperidol intravenously, heart rate increased significantly and stroke volume decreased. Significant initial increases occurred in diastolic and mean arterial blood pressures, ventricular contractility, and coronary blood flow. The dose of 0.02 mg/kg of atropine was believed optimal; when 0.04 mg/kg was given, large inotropic and chronotropic effects were produced.

Fentanyl-droperidol/N_2O anesthesia has been shown to limit experimental cerebral edema in dogs (Smith and Marque, 1976).

Occasionally, the desired degree of depression is not produced by a standard dose of fentanyl-droperidol. This is particularly true in the larger breeds. Aggressiveness during the recovery period and other changes in disposition have been noted in a few instances following its use. Prolonged effects lasting for several days have been observed, particularly where overdose occurred. Other undesirable effects produced include defecation, salivation, and bradycardia, which may be prevented by pretreatment with atropine, respiratory depression or panting, and spontaneous movements or movements in response to auditory stimuli. Overdosage produces a high incidence of spontaneous movements or even clonic convulsions with extensor rigidity.

Use of narcotic antagonists results in immediate reversal of the effects of fentanyl, including analgesia (see Chap. 20). This technique is often used on completion of the desired period of neuroleptanalgesia to lighten the depression.

Booth et al. (1982) found that a mixture of 4-aminopyridine (0.5 mg/kg) and naloxone hydrochloride (0.04 mg/kg), administered intravenously, markedly antagonized the CNS effects of 1 ml/9 kg of droperidol-fentanyl. All dogs could stand immediately and walk without evidence of tranquilization or ataxia.

Currently, fentanyl-droperidol is sold for use in dogs only and is not to be used in food-producing animals. It causes an undesirable central nervous stimulation in cattle, sheep, cats, and horses. Its action in swine is similar to that in dogs (DeYoung et al., 1970) (see Chap. 18).

Meperidine-Acepromazine

Warner (1968) has described the use of meperidine and acepromazine in combination for neuroleptanalgesia. Equal volumes of the two drugs are mixed in the same syringe for intramuscular administration to cats and subcutaneous or intravenous administration to dogs. Eight- to 10-lb cats are given one-quarter to one-half of the combination, which requires 10 to 15 minutes for full effect. Large dogs (45 lb and over) are given 1 ml of the mixture, whereas 15- to 35-lb dogs receive one-half ml. For rapid onset, the combination can be given intravenously and may be given "to effect."

Schauffler (1968) has used a combination of meperidine hydrochloride and acepromazine hydrochloride for sedation and mild analgesia of horses. The intravenous dose for a 1000-lb horse is 100 mg of acepromazine and 500 mg of meperidine.

Methadone-Promazine

Both Roberts (1968) and Schauffler (1969) have described use of methadone hydrochloride combined with a phenothiazine tranquilizer intravenously in horses. Roberts' "lytic cocktail" consists of 40 mg (1.25 ml of 32 mg/ml of solution) of atropine sulfate combined with 20 ml (10 mg/ml) of methadone hydrochloride. One ml of this solution/50 kg is combined with 5 ml (250 mg) of promazine hydrochloride in a syringe.

Methadone-Acepromazine

Schauffler (1969) has used methadone (50 mg) and acepromazine (50 mg) combined in the same syringe for a 1000-lb horse. Either this or the aforementioned combination furnishes a more effective and reliable chemical restraint for horses than a phenothiazine tranquilizer alone.

A dose of 0.5 mg of methadone and 0.5 mg of acepromazine per pound of body weight has been used in both dogs and cats (Schauffler, 1970). The two drugs are mixed in the same syringe and administered intravenously or intramuscularly. When they are given intravenously, the effect is noted in approximately 30 seconds, is most pronounced in 15 minutes, and subsides in 3 to 12 hours. Occasionally animals may be sedated as long as 3 days. Defecation does not occur as with fentanyl-droperidol. Narcotic antagonists reverse the effect of methadone.

Etorphine-Acepromazine and Etorphine-Methotrimeprazine (Immobilon, L.A. and S.A.)

Etorphine has been combined with acepromazine for use in large animals, and with methotrimeprazine for small animals. The large animal preparation contains 2.45 mg of etorphine and 10.0 mg of acepromazine/ml. The small animal form contains 0.074 mg of etorphine and 18.0 mg of methotrimeprazine/ml. Unfortunately, both preparations have been termed Immobilon,* thus creating confusion in the literature. The large animal mixture has been found most useful in horses, and in chemical restraint of wild and zoo animals (see Chap. 18). In addition, it is diluted and used in small animals. Neither combination is available in the United States. Table 8–13 sets forth the dosage and effects of these combinations.

TABLE 8–13. Dosage and Effects of Immobilon

Species	*Dosage (ml/50 kg)*	*Route*	*Time to Effect (min)*	*Time to Walk* (min)*
Horses†	0.5	I.M., I.V.	3–4 (I.M.)	1–4
Pigs†	0.5	I.M., I.V.	3–5 (I.M.)	1–10
Dogs‡	0.12 mg/kg	I.M.	2–10	1–30
	0.06 ml/kg	I.V.		

*After I.V. injection of diprenorphine
†'Immobilon LA'.
‡'Immobilon SA'.
(From Green, C.J.: *Animal Anaesthesia*. Laboratory Animals, Ltd., London, 1979.)

In horses, etorphine-acepromazine has been used as the sole agent for immobilization during short operations, such as castration. When it is given intravenously, recumbency quickly occurs. Care should be exercised to prevent injury as the animal goes down. When the combination is given intramuscularly, horses may exhibit excitement prior to recumbency. Muscular tremors, rigidity, sweating, mydriasis, reduction in intestinal peristalsis, and respiratory depression may also occur. Initially the cardiac rate and blood pressure rise; the latter subsequently falls, probably due to the α-blocking action of acepromazine (Bogan et al., 1978). Priapism in horses after use of this combination has been reported by Pearson and Weaver (1978).

Boyd and Ducker (1975) have given etorphine-acepromazine (0.10 to 0.15 ml of L.A.) to sheep, and reported that if the animal's head is lowered, passive regurgitation occurs. This is attributed to cessation of esophageal and stomach movements produced by the combination. They recommend maintaining the cranial end of the animal close to horizontal.

Hermansen and Larsen (1974) found that

*See Appendix A for manufacturer.

etorphine-acepromazine produced no effect on systolic blood pressure, and a slight fall in diastolic pressure in dogs. A significant bradycardia was noted during neuroleptanalgesia, and tachycardia occurred during arousal when etorphine was antagonized by diprenorphine. Bradycardia could be prevented by administration of atropine and tachycardia by propranolol.

Diprenorphine reversal of the effects of etorphine allows quicker recovery and is recommended (see Chap. 20). The dosage for all species is 0.272 mg/kg IV by slow injection. Horses may sometimes become restless and excited 6 to 8 hours following immobilization/reversal; in donkeys this may occur within 2 to 3 hours (Dobbs and Ling, 1972).

The etorphine-methotrimeprazine combination for small animals has not been widely accepted. It must not be used in cats. In dogs, it produces neuroleptanalgesia and hyperglycemia. Naloxone (0.6 to 0.8 mg/kg) produces reversal of the respiratory and cardiovascular depression of the etorphine, but the action of naloxone is short, and relapse tends to occur within 10 to 15 minutes (Dodman and Waterman, 1978). Diprenorphine reversal is therefore recommended.

OTHER PREANESTHETICS

A number of other agents may be used as preanesthetics. Included among these are several drugs listed in Chaper 13.

REFERENCES

Adriani, J.: *Appraisal of Current Concepts in Anesthesiology,* Vol. 2. The C.V. Mosby Company, St. Louis, 1964.

Ainslie, S.G., Eisele, J.H.,Jr., and Corkill, G.: Fentanyl Concentrations in Brain and Serum during Respiratory Acid-Base Changes in the Dog. Anesthesiology, 51:293, 1979.

Anonymous: Morphine-Apomorphine Analgesia. A Clinical Review. J. Small Anim. Med., 1:220, 1952.

Atkinson, R.S., Rusman, G.B., and Lee, J.A.: *A Synopsis of Anaesthesia,* 8th ed. Year Book Medical Publishers, Chicago, 1977.

Baker, J.S.: Use of Rompun (Xylazine) in Ruminants. Purdue Veterinary Notes No. 83. Purdue University, Lafayette, Indiana, 1974.

Ballard, S., Shults, T., Kownacki, A.A., Blake, J.W., and Tobin, T.: The Pharmacokinetics, Pharmacological Responses and Behavioral Effects of Acepromazine in the Horse. J. Vet. Pharmacol. Therap., 5:21, 1982.

Bartels, J.E., Braund, K.G., and Redding, R.W.: An Experimental Evaluation of a Non-ionic Agent Amipaque (Metrizamide) As a Neuroradiologic Medium in the Dog. J. Am. Vet. Rad. Soc., 18:117, 1977.

Benson, G.J., Thurmon, J.C., and Tranquilli, W.J.: Effect of Xylazine Hydrochloride upon Plasma Glucose and Serum Insulin in Adult Pointer Dogs. Proc. Scientific Mtg., American College of Veterinary Anesthesiologists, Atlanta, Georgia, 1983.

Bidwai, A.V., Stanley, T.H., Bloomer, H.A., and Blatnik, R.A.: Effects of Anesthetic Doses of Morphine on Renal Function in the Dog. Anesth. Analg., 54:357, 1975.

Blane, G.F., Boura, A.L.A., Fitzgerald, A.E., and Lister, R.E.: Actions of Etorphine Hydrochloride (M-99). A Potent Morphine-like Agent. Br. J. Pharmacol. Chemother., 30:11, 1967.

Bogan, J.A., MacKenzie, G., and Snow, D.H.: An Evaluation of Tranquilizers for Use with Etorphine as Neuroleptanalgesic Agents in the Horse. Vet. Rec., 103:471, 1978.

Booth, N.H.: Personal Communication. Colorado State University, Fort Collins, Colorado, 1961.

Booth, N.H., Hatch, R.C., and Crawford, L.M.: Reversal of the Neuroleptanalgesic Effect of Droperidol-Fentanyl in the Dog by 4-Aminopyridine and Naloxone. Am. J. Vet. Res., 43:1227, 1982.

Booth, N.H., and Rankin, A.D.: Evaluation of Meperidine Hydrochloride in the Cat. Vet. Med., 49:249, 1954.

Bourgeois-Gavardin, M., Nowill, W.K., Margolis, G., and Stephen, C.R.: Chlorpromazine: A Laboratory and Clinical Investigation. Anesthesiology, 16:829, 1955.

Bowman, B.M.: Piperacetazine: A Clinical Survey. Pract. Vet., 48:30, 1976.

Boyd, J.S., and Ducker, M.J.: Passive Regurgitation in the Use of Immobilon. Vet. Rec., 96:250, 1975.

Buckhold, D.K., Erickson, H.H., and Lumb, W.V.: Cardiovascular Response to Fentanyl-Droperidol and Atropine in the Dog. Am. J. Vet. Res., 38:479, 1977.

Burch, G.R.: Quoted in Laboratory and Clinical Reports on Thorazine. Pitman-Moore Co., Indianapolis, 1957.

Burkhart, R.L.: Evaluation of M-99 (Etorphine) and Antagonists, Nalorphine, and M-285 (Cyprenorphine) in Wild Animals. Research and Development Agricultural Division, American Cyanamid Co., Princeton, N.J., 1967.

Burroughs, H.E.: Methadone Narcosis in Dogs. J. Small. Anim. Med., 1:301, 1953.

Campbell, K.B., Klavano, P.A., Richardson, P., and Alexander, J.E.: Hemodynamic Effects of Xylazine in the Calf. Am. J. Vet. Res., 40:1777, 1979.

Casey, A.F.: The Structure of Narcotic Analgesic Drugs. In *Narcotic Drugs: Biochemical Pharmacology.* Edited by D.H. Clouet, Plenum Press, New York, 1971.

Cavanaugh, R.L., Gylys, J.A., and Bierwagen, M.E.: Antitussive Properties of Butorphanol. Arch. Int. Pharmacodyn. Ther., 220:258, 1976.

Chang, K-J., Cooper, B.R., Hazum, E., and Cuatrecasas, P.: Multiple Opiate Receptors: Different Regional Distribution in the Brain and Differential Binding of Opiates and Opioid Peptides. Mol. Pharmacol., 16:91, 1979.

Clarke,K.W., and Hall, L.W.: "Xylazine"—A New Sedative for Horses and Cattle. Vet. Rec., 85:512, 1969.

Cloetta, M.: On the Behavior of Atropine in Animal Species with Different Sensitivities. Arch. f. Exp. Path. U. Pharmak., 23:119, 1908.

Costa, E., and Giudotti, A.: Molecular Mechanisms in the Receptor Action of Benzodiazepines. Ann. Rev. Pharmacol. Toxicol., 19:531, 1979.

Courvoisier, S., Fournel, J., Ducrot, R., Kolsky, M., and Koetschet, P.: Pharmacodynamic Properties of 10-(2-Dimethylaminopropyl)-2-Chlorophenothiazine Hydrochloride. Arch. Int. Pharmacodyn., 92:305, 1953.

Cronin, M.F., Booth, N.H., Hatch, R.C., and Brown, J.: Acepromazine-Xylazine Combination in Dogs: Antagonism with 4-Aminopyridine and Yohimbine. Am. J. Vet. Res., 44:2037, 1983.

Dasmana, K.M., Dixit, K.S., Jaju, B.P., and Gupta, M.L.: Role of Central Dopaminergic Receptors in Manic Response of Cats to Morphine. Psychopharmacologia, 24:380, 1972.

Davis, L.E., and Donnelly, E.J.: Analgesic Drugs in the Cat. J.A.V.M.A., 153:1161, 1968.

DeMoor, A.: Influence of Atropine on Arterial Oxygen Tension, Acid-base Status and Tissue Hypoxia in the Conscious Horse. Zbl. Vet. Med., A, 15:494, 1968.

De Vos, V.: Immobilisation of Free-Ranging Wild Animals Using a New Drug. Vet. Rec., 103:64, 1978.

DeYoung, D.W., Lumb, W.V., and Sawyer, D.C.: An Inhalation Anesthesia Technique for Miniature Swine. Vet. Med./Small Anim. Clin., 65:339, 1970.

Dobbs, H.E., and Ling, C.M.: The use of Etorphine/Acepromazine in the Horse and Donkey. Vet. Rec., 91:40, 1972.

Dodman, N.H., and Waterman, A.E.: Clinical Observations on the Antagonism of Immobilon by Nalaxone in Dogs. Vet. Rec., 103:334, 1978.

Dretchen, K., Ghoneim, M.M., and Long, J.P.: The Interaction of Diazepam with Myoneural Blocking Agents. Anesthesiology, 34:463, 1971.

Ducharme, N.G., and Fubini, S.L.: Gastrointestinal Complications Associated with the Use of Atropine in Horses. J.A.V.M.A., 182:229, 1983.

Eddy, N.B., and Lee, L.E., Jr.: The Analgesic Equivalence to Morphine and Relative Side Action Liability of Oxymorphine (14-hydroxydihydromorphinone). J. Pharm. Exp. Ther., 125:116, 1959.

Eichner, R.D., Prior, R.L., and Kvasnicka, W.B.: Xylazine-Induced Hyperglycemia in Beef Cattle. Am. J. Vet. Res., 40:127, 1979.

Estrada, E.: Clinical Uses of Chlorpromazine in Veterinary Medicine. J.A.V.M.A., 128:292, 1956.

Feldberg, W., and Symonds, H.W.: Hyperglycaemic Effect of Xylazine. J. Vet. Pharmacol. Ther., 3:197, 1980.

Finck, A.D., Berkowitz, B.A., Hempstead, B.S., and Ngai, S.H.: Pharmacokinetics of Morphine: Effects of Hypercarbia on Serum and Brain Morphine Concentrations in the Dog. Anesthesiology, 47:407, 1977.

Folkers, E.R.: Xylazine Precaution. J.A.V.M.A., 176:956, 1980.

Franklin, I., and Reid, J.S.: Clinical Use of a Combination of Fentanyl and Droperidol in Dogs. Vet. Med./Small Anim. Clin., 60:922, 1965.

Frye, E.: Cardiovascular Effects of High Dosages of Fentanyl, Meperidine, and Naloxone in Dogs. Anesth. Analg., 53:40, 1974.

Fuentes, V.O.: Sudden Death in a Stallion after Xylazine Medication. Vet. Rec., 102:106, 1978.

Garcia-Villar, R., Toutain, P.L., Alvinerie, M., and Ruckebusch, Y.: The Pharmacokinetics of Xylazine Hydrochloride: An Interspecific Study. J. Vet. Pharmacol. Ther., 4:87, 1981.

Garland, J.E., and White, K.B.: Unusual Reactions to Acetyl Promazine. Vet. Rec., 83:641, 1968.

Gelatt, K.N., Peiffer, R.L., Jr., Erickson, J.L., and Gum, G.G.: Evaluation of Tear Formation in the Dog, Using a Modification of the Schirmer Tear Test. J.A.V.M.A., 166:368, 1975.

Gilbert, P.E., and Martin, W.R.: The Effects of Morphine and Nalorphine-like Drugs in the Nondependent, Morphine-dependent and Cyclazocine-dependent Chronic Spinal Dog. J. Pharmacol. Exp. Ther., 198:66, 1976.

Godeaux, J., and Tonnesen, M.: Investigations into Atropine Metabolism in the Animal Organism. Acta Pharmacol. Toxicol., 5:95, 1949.

Godefroy, F., Weil-Fugazza, J., Coudert, D., and Besson, J.M.: Effect of Acute Administration of Morphine on Newly Synthesized 5-Hydroxytryptamine in Spinal Cord of the Rat. Brain Res., 199:415, 1980.

Goodman, L.S., and Gilman, A.: *The Pharmacological Basis of Therapeutics,* 2nd ed. The Macmillan Co., New York, 1958.

Gray, C.: Comments on M-99. Am. Assoc. Zoo Vet., Washington, D.C., March 25, 1968.

Green, C.J.: *Animal Anaesthesia.* Laboratory Animals Ltd., London, 1979.

Gruber, C.M., Hart, E.R., and Gruber, C.M., Jr.: The Pharmacology and Toxicology of the Ethyl Ester of 1-Methyl-4-Phenyl-Piperidine-4-Carboxylic Acid (Demerol). J. Pharmacol. Exp. Ther., 73:319, 1941.

Gupta, B.N., Moore, J.A., and Conner, G.H.: The Use of Promazine Hydrochloride in Cesarean Section in the Dog. Lab. Anim. Care, 20:474, 1970.

Hamlin, R.L., Ginaven, S.M.,and Smith, C.R.: Fentanyl Citrate-Droperidol and Pentobarbital for Intravenous Anesthesia in Dogs. J.A.V.M.A., 152:360, 1968.

Harrison, G.A., and Vanik, P.E.: The Effect of Atropine on Laryngeal Spasm before and during Cyclopropane Inhalation in Cats Anesthetized with Urethane. Br. J. Anaesth., 35:760, 1963.

Harthoorn, A.M.: Restraint of Undomesticated Animals. J.A.V.M.A., 149:875, 1966.

Haskins, S.C.: Abdominal Distention Associated with Xylazine Use. Mod. Vet. Pract., 60:433, 1979.

Hatch, R.C.: Effects of Doxapram in Dogs Given Atropine and Xylazine. J.A.V.M.A., 183:948, 1983.

Hatch, R.C.: Restraint, Preanesthetic Medication, and Postanesthetic Medication of Dogs with Chlorpromazine and Atropine. J.A.V.M.A., 150:27, 1967.

Hatch, R.C., Booth, N.H., Clark, J.D., Crawford, L.M., Kitzman, J.V., and Wallner, B.: Antagonism of Xylazine Sedation in Dogs by 4-Aminopyridine and Yohimbine. Am. J. Vet. Res., 48:1009, 1982.

Heard, W.T.: Personal Communication. Denver, Colorado, 1962.

Hermansen, K., and Larsen, J.-J.: Some Pharmacological Properties of the Combination of Etorphine and Acepromazine (Immobilon) and the Morphine Antagonist, Diprenorphine, in the Dog. Acta Pharmacol. Toxicol., 34:189, 1974.

Heykants, J., Symoens, J., and Marsboom, R.: On the

Distribution and Metabolism of Azaperone (R 1929) in the Rat and Pig. Part III: Distribution of Azaperone and Its Metabolites in the Pig. Arzneimittelforsch (Drug Res.)., 21:1357, 1971.

Hoffman, P.E.: Clinical Evaluation of Xylazine as a Chemical Restraining Agent, Sedative, and Analgesic in Horses. J.A.V.M.A., 164:42, 1974.

Hsu, W.H.: Xylazine-Induced Depression and Its Antagonism by Alpha Adrenergic Blocking Agents. J. Pharmacol. Exp. Ther., 218:188, 1981.

Hsu, W.H., Betts, D.M., and Lee, P.: Xylazine-induced Mydriasis: Possible Involvement of a Central Postsynaptic Regulation of Parasympathetic Tone. J. Vet. Pharmacol. Ther., 4:209, 1981.

Hsu, W.H., and Hummel, S.K.: Xylazine-Induced Hyperglycemia in Cattle: A Possible Involvement of α_2-Adrenergic Receptors Regulating Insulin Release. Endocrinology, 109:825, 1981.

Hug, C.C., and Murphy, M.R.: Fentanyl Disposition in Cerebrospinal Fluid and Plasma and Its Relationship to Ventilatory Depression in the Dog. Anesthesiology, 50:342, 1979.

Jha, S.K., Lumb, W.V., and Johnston, R.F.: Some Effects of Triflupromazine Hydrochloride on Goats. Am. J. Vet. Res., 22:915, 1961.

Jones, L.M.: *Veterinary Pharmacology and Therapeutics,* 2nd ed. The Iowa State College Press, Ames, Iowa, 1957.

Kallos, T., and Smith, T.C.: Naloxone Reversal of Pentazocine-Induced Respiratory Depression. J.A.M.A., 204:932, 1968.

Kalpravidh, M., Lumb, W.V., Wright, M., and Heath, R.B.: Effects of Butorphanol, Flunixin, Levorphanol, Morphine, and Xylazine in Ponies. Am. J. Vet. Res., 45:217, 1984*a*.

Kalpravidh, M., Lumb, W.V., Wright, M., and Heath, R.B.: Analgesic Effects of Butorphanol in Horses: Dose Response Studies. Am. J. Vet. Res., 45:211, 1984*b*.

Kerr, D.D., Jones, E.W., Holbert, D., and Huggins, K.: Comparison of the Effects of Xylazine and Acetylpromazine Maleate in the Horse. Am. J. Vet. Res., 33:777, 1972*a*.

Kerr, D.D., Jones, E.W., Huggins, K., and Edwards, W.C.: Sedative and Other Effects of Xylazine Given Intravenously to Horses. Am. J. Vet. Res., 33:525, 1972*b*.

Kitzman, J.V., Booth, N.H., Hatch, R.C., and Wallner, B.: Antagonism of Xylazine Sedation by 4-Aminopyridine and Yohimbine in Cattle. Am. J. Vet. Res., 43:2165, 1982.

Klein, L.V., and Baetjer, C.: Preliminary Report: Xylazine and Morphine Sedation in Horses. Vet. Anesth., 3:2, 1974.

Klide, A.M., Calderwood, H.W., and Soma, L.R.: Cardiopulmonary Effects of Xylazine in Dogs. Am. J. Vet. Res., 36:931, 1975.

Klide, A.M., Rives, C., and Peters, J.: Effect of Atropine Sulfate on Thiopental-Induced Sleeping Time in the Dog. J.A.V.M.A., 35:1029, 1974.

Knowles, J.O.: Clinical Experience with Tranquilizing Agents. J.A.V.M.A., 130:10, 1957.

Krantz, J.C., Jr., and Carr, C.J.: *The Pharmacologic Principles of Medical Practice,* 2nd ed. Williams & Wilkins, Baltimore, 1951.

Krawitz, L.: A Safer Technique for the Induction of General Anesthesia in Small Animals. Vet. Med., 52:442, 1957.

Liu, W.S., Bidwai, A.V., Stanley, T.H., and Isern-Amaral, J.: Cardiovascular Dynamics After Large Doses of Fentanyl and Fentanyl Plus N_2O in the Dog. Anesth. Analg., 55:168, 1976.

Lowe, J.E.: Pentazocine for the Relief of Abdominal Pain in Ponies. Proc. 15th Ann. Convention, Am. Assoc. Equine Pract., Houston, Texas, 1969.

Ludders, J.W., and Heavner, J.E.: Effect of Atropine on Tear Formation in Anesthetized Dogs. J.A.V.M.A., 175:585, 1979.

Lukas, S.E., and Griffiths, R.R.: Precipitated Withdrawal by a Benzodiazepine Receptor Antagonist (Ro 15-1788) after 7 Days of Diazepam. Science, 217:1161, 1982.

Macko, E., Scheidy, S.F., and Tucker, R.G.: Chlorpromazine in the Dog. Vet. Med., 53:378, 1958.

Mandelker, L.: Clinical Use of Piperacetazine to Modify Behavior in Dogs and Cats: A Practitioner's Viewpoint. Vet. Med./Small Anim. Clin., 74:505, 1979.

Martin, W.R., Eades, C.G., Thompson, J.A., Huppler, R.E., and Gilbert P.E.: The Effects of Morphine and Nalorphine-like Drugs in the Nondependent and Morphine-dependent Chronic Spinal Dog. J. Pharmacol. Exp. Ther., 197:517, 1976.

McGrath, C.J., Rempel, W.E., Addis, P.B., and Crimi, A.J.: Prophylactic Use of Major Tranquilizers in Prevention of Malignant Hyperthermia in Swine. Vet. Anesth., 8:28, 1980.

Miller, M.: Inhibition of ADH Release in the Rat by Narcotic Antagonists. Neuroendocrinology, 19:241, 1975.

Mohler, H., and Okada, T.: Benzodiazepine Receptor: Demonstration in the Central Nervous System. Science, 198: 849, 1977.

Moore, J., and Dundee, J.W.: Alterations in Response to Somatic Pain Associated with Anesthesia: VII. The Effects of Nine Phenothiazine Derivatives. Br. J. Anaesth., 33:422, 1961.

Mozier, J.: Personal Communication. Animal Health Division, Chemagro Corporation, Stilwell, Kansas, 1972.

Muir, W.W.: Effects of Atropine on Cardiac Rates and Rhythm in Dogs. J.A.V.M.A., 172:917, 1978.

Muir, W.W., and Piper, F.S.: The Effect of Xylazine on Indices of Myocardial Contractility in the Dog. Am. J. Vet. Res., 38:931, 1977.

Muir, W.W., Sams, R.A., Huffman, R.H., and Noonan, J.S.: Pharmacodynamic and Pharmacokinetic Properties of Diazepam in Horses. Am. J. Vet. Res., 43:1756, 1982.

Muir, W.W., Werner, L.L., and Hamlin, R.L.: Effects of Xylazine and Acetylpromazine upon Induced Ventricular Fibrillation in Dogs Anesthetized with Thiamylal and Halothane. Am. J. Vet. Res., 36:1299, 1975.

Murphy, M.R., and Hug, C.C., Jr.: "Ceiling Effect" of Butorphanol (Stadol) as an Anesthetic Supplement. Anesthesiology, *55,* Abstract 260, 1981.

Nagy, J., and Decsi, L.: Further Studies on the Site of Action of Diazepam: Anticonvulsant Effect in the Rabbit. Neuropharmacology, 18:39, 1979.

Nishitateno, K., Ngai, S.H., Finck, A.D., and Berkowitz, B.A.: Pharmacokinetics of Morphine: Concentrations in the Serum and Brain of the Dog during Hyperventilation. Anesthesiology, 50:520, 1979.

Nytch, T.F.: Clinical Observations on the Preanesthetic Use

of Oxymorphone and Its Antagonist, N-allyl-noroxymorphone, in Dogs. J.A.V.M.A., 145:127, 1964.

Olds, M.E., and Olds, J.: Effects of Anxiety-Relieving Drugs on Unit Discharges in Hippocampus, Reticular Midbrain, and Preoptic Area in the Freely Moving Rat. Int. J. Neuropharmacol., 8:87, 1969.

Owen, L.N.: The Narcotic Effects of Thiambutene in the Dog and Its Antagonism by Nalorphine. Vet. Rec., 67:561, 1955*a*.

Owen, L.N.: Thiambutene-Thiopentone Anaesthesia for Hysterectomy in Pyometra of the Bitch. Vet. Rec., 67:580, 1955*b*.

Palminteri, A.: Oxymorphone—An Aid to Outpatient Practice. Mod. Vet. Pract., 47:68, 1966.

Pasternak, G.W., Childes, S.R., and Snyder, S.H.: Opiate Analgesia: Evidence for Mediation by a Subpopulation of Opiate Receptors. Science, 208:314, 1980.

Pearson, H., and Weaver, B.M.Q.: Priapism After Sedation, Neuroleptanalgesia and Anesthesia in the Horse. Equine Vet. J., 10:85, 1978.

Pert, A.: Neuropharmacology of Analgesics. Surg. Pract. News, 10:10, 1981.

Pippi, N.L., and Lumb, W.V.: Objective Tests of Analgesic Drugs in Ponies. Am. J. Vet. Res., 40:1082, 1979.

Pircio, A.W., Gylys, J.A., Cavanagh, R.L.,Buyniski, J.P., and Bierwagen, M.E.: The Pharmacology of Butorphanol, a 3, 14-Dihydroxymorphinan Narcotic Antagonist Analgesic. Arch. Int. Pharmacodyn. Ther., 220:231, 1976.

Ponder, S.W., and Clark, W.G.: Prolonged Depression of Thermoregulation after Xylazine Administration to Cats. J. Vet. Pharmacol. Ther., 3:203, 1980.

Port, J.D., Stanley, T.H., and Steffey, E.M.: Narcotic Inhalation Anesthesia. Anesthesiology, 57:A344, 1982.

Port, J.D., Stanley, T.H., Steffey, E.P., and Henrickson, R.: Carfentanil: The Primate Experience. Proc. Scientific Mtg., American College of Veterinary Anesthesiologists, Atlanta, Georgia, 1983.

Powers, S., Reed, C., and Gregersen, M.I.: The Effects of Morphine on Dogs in Hemorrhagic and Traumatic Shock. Am. J. Physiol., 148:269, 1947.

Pugh, D.M.: Acepromazine in Veterinary Use. Vet. Rec., 76:439, 1964.

Reutner, T.F., and Gruhzit, O.M.: Methadon, A New Analgesic. J.A.V.M.A., 113:448, 1948.

Roberts, D.: The Role of Glyceryl Guaiacolate in a Balanced Equine Anesthetic. Vet. Med. Small Anim. Clin., 63:157, 1968.

Robertson, J.T., and Muir, W.W.: A New Analgesic Drug Combination in the Horse. Am. J. Vet. Res., 44:1667, 1983.

Robertson, J.T., Muir, W.W., and Sams, R.: Cardiopulmonary Effects of Butorphanol Tartrate in Horses. Am. J. Vet. Res., 42:41, 1981.

Roebel, L.E., Baryla, U.M., and Buyniski, J.P.: The Effects of Butorphanol and Morphine on Terminal Bile Duct and Duodenal Activity in Anesthetized Dogs. Pharmacologist, 19:241, 1977.

Sagner, F., Hoffmeister, F., and Kroneberg, G.: Pharmakolog, Grundlagen eines neuartigen Praparates fur Analgesie, Sedation und Relaxation in der Veterinarmedizin (BAY VA 1470) (Fundamentals of a New Type of Preparation for Analgesia, Sedation and Relaxation in Veterinary Medicine [Bay VA 1470].) Dtsch. tierarztl. Wochenschr., 75:565, 1968.

Salzman, N.P., and Brodie, B.B.: Physiological Disposition and Fate of Chlorpromazine and a Method for Its Estimation in Biological Material. J. Pharm. Exp. Ther., 118:46, 1956.

Schallek, W., Schlosser, W., and Randall, L.O.: Recent Developments in the Pharmacology of the Benzodiazepines. Adv. Pharmacol. Chemother., 10:119, 1972.

Schauffler, A.F.: Acepromazine and Meperidine: New Drug Combination Aids in Equine Restraint. Mod. Vet. Pract., 49:43, 1968.

Schauffler, A.F.: Better Equine Restraint. Mod. Vet. Pract., 50:46, 1969.

Schauffler, A.F.: Use of Acetylpromazine-Methadone in Dogs. Mod. Vet. Pract., 51:72, 1970.

Schurig, J.E., Cavanaugh, R.L., and Buyniski, J.P.: Effect of Butorphanol and Morphine on Pulmonary Mechanics, Arterial Blood Pressure and Venous Plasma Histamine in the Anesthetized Dog. Arch. Int. Pharmacodyn. Ther., 233:296, 1978.

Scott, C.C., Chen, K.K., Kohlsteadt, K.G., Robbins, E.B., and Israel, F.W.: Further Observations on the Pharmacology of Dolophine (Methadon, Lilly). J. Pharm. Exp. Ther., 91:147, 1947.

Sederberg, J., Stanley, T.H., Reddy, P., Liu, W., Port, D., and Gillmor, S.: Hemodynamic Effects of Butorphanol-Oxygen Anesthesia in Dogs. Anesth. Analg., 60:715, 1981.

Short, C.E., Paddleford, R.R., and Cloyd, G.D.: Glycopyorrolate for Prevention of Pulmonary Complications During Anesthesia. Mod. Vet. Pract., 55:194, 1974.

Skolnick, P., Moncada, V., Barker, J.L., and Paul, S.M.: Pentobarbital: Dual Actions to Increase Brain Benzodiazepine Receptor Affinity. Science, 211:1448, 1981.

Smith, A.L., and Marque, J.J.: Anesthetics and Cerebral Edema. Anesthesiology, 45:64, 1976.

Soma, L.R., and Shields, D.R.: Neuroleptanalgesia Produced by Fentanyl and Droperidol. J.A.V.M.A., 145:897, 1964.

Stoliker, H.E.: Personal Communication. Parke-Davis and Co., Detroit, Michigan, 1969.

Stormont, C., and Suzuki, Y.: Atropinesterase and Cocainesterase of Rabbit Serum: Localization of the Enzyme Activity in Isozymes. Science, 167:200, 1970.

Szabuniewicz, M., Davis, R.H., Jr., and Wiersig, D.O.: Prevention of Methoxyflurane and Thiobarbiturate Cardiac Sensitization of Catecholamines in Dogs. Pract. Vet., 47:12, 1975.

Tranquilli, W.J., Thurmon, J.D., Benson, G.J., Corbin, J.E., and Davis, L.E.: Halothane Sparing Effect of Xylazine in Dogs and Subsequent Reversal with Tolazoline. Proc. Scientific Mtg., American College of Veterinary Anesthesiologists, Atlanta, Georgia, 1983.

van der Kleijn, E., van Rossum, J.M., Muskens, E.T.J.M., and Rijntjes, N.V.M.: Pharmacokinetics of Diazepam in Dogs, Mice and Humans. Acta Pharmacol. Toxicol., 29:109, 1971.

Van Laun, T.: Anaesthetizing Donkeys. Vet. Rec., 100:391, 1977.

Warner, H.E.: New Drug Combination for Small Animal Restraint. Mod. Vet. Pract., 49:20, 1968.

Wauquier, A., Ashton, D., and Melis, W.: Behavioral Analysis of Amygdaloid Kindling in Beagle Dogs and the Effects of Clonazepam, Diazepam, Phenobarbital, Diphenylhydantoin, and Flunarizine on Seizure Manifestation. Exp. Neurol., 64:579, 1979.

Weberlein, M.K., McClumpha, C.A., Brengle, L.A., Lickfeldt, W.E., and Dawson, H.A.: Promazine in Canine Medicine. J.A.V.M.A., 134:518, 1959.

Wiersig, D.O., Davis, R.H., Jr., and Szabuniewicz, M.: Prevention of Induced Ventricular Fibrillation in Dogs Anesthetized with Ultrashort Acting Barbiturates and Halothane. J.A.V.M.A., 165:341, 1974.

Yaksh, T.L., Wilson, P.R., Kaiko, R.F., and Inturrisi, C.E.: Analgesia Produced by a Spinal Action of Morphine and Effects Upon Parturition in the Rat. Anesthesiology, 51:386, 1979.

CHAPTER 9

General Anesthesia

General anesthesia may be defined as complete unconsciousness. When inducing this state, however, the anesthesiologist requires the following components: unconsciousness, insensitivity to pain, loss of motor power, relaxation, and absence of reflex response. The degree to which these are required for specific procedures varies. The anesthesiologist must therefore select the most suitable drugs and be able to assess the degree to which the varying effects are induced. The progressive changes resulting from administration of anesthetic drugs are classified in four stages. Recognition of signs characteristic of these stages allows the anesthesiologist to determine whether the required degree of suppression has been achieved, or whether it is insufficient or too much, and to compare observations with those of others.

STAGES OF GENERAL ANESTHESIA

For descriptive purposes, general anesthesia has been divided into four stages depending upon neuromuscular signs exhibited by the patient (Table 9–1). It should be emphasized that no clear division exists between stages, one blending into the next. In addition, variation in response among patients is to be expected. Preanesthetic medication, adequacy of oxygenation, carbon dioxide retention, and physical status of the patient all modify the signs. Patient response is also governed by the anesthetic that is being administered, considerable variation existing between agents.

Stage I. This is termed the stage of analgesia or voluntary movement, and is defined as lasting from initial administration to loss of consciousness. Although it is sometimes termed the stage of analgesia, pain sensation still exists. Some analgesia may occur, however, in the deeper phases of this stage. In any case, this stage is the most variable. Deviations result from the anesthetic used, from variations in the temperament and condition of the patient, from the manner in which the animal is restrained, and from the rate of induction. A nervous animal is bound to resist restraint. Should the anesthetic necessitate the use of a mask or be irritating to the upper airway, fear with consequent resistance by the patient will be accentuated. Excited, apprehensive animals may struggle violently and voluntarily hold their breath for short periods. Epinephrine release causes a strong rapid heartbeat and pupillary dilation. Salivation is frequent in some species, as are urination and defecation. With the approach of stage II, the animal becomes progressively ataxic, loses its ability to stand, and assumes lateral recumbency. Initially it is able to turn or lift its head without support. This righting reflex is, however, lost in stage II.

Stage II. This is called the stage of delirium or involuntary movement. As the central nervous system (CNS) becomes depressed, the patient loses consciousness and all voluntary control is lost. This feature marks the change from stage I. By definition, this stage lasts from loss of consciousness to the onset of a regular pattern of breathing. As a result of anesthetic depression of the CNS, reflexes initiated become more

TABLE 9–1. Characteristics of the Stages of General Anesthesia

System Affected	Characteristic Observed	Stage of Anesthesia: *I*	*II*	*III* Plane *1* *Light*	*III* Plane *2* *Medium*	*III* Plane *3* *Medium*	*III* Plane *4* *Deep*	*IV*
Cardiovascular	Pulse*	tachycardia		progressive bradycardia†				weak or imperceptible
	Blood pressure*	hypertension		normal	increasing hypotension			shock level
	Capillary refill	1 sec or less			progressive delay			3 sec or more
	Dysrhythmia probability	+ + +	+ + +	+ +	+		+ +	+ + + +
Respiratory	Respiratory rate*	irregular or increased		progressive decrease‡			slow irregular	ceased, may gasp terminally
	Respiratory depth*	irregular or increased		progressive decrease			irregular	ceased
	Mucous membrane, skin color	normal					cyanosis#, pale to white	
	Respiratory action	may be breath holding		thoracoabdominal, abdominal			diaphragmatic	ceased
	Cough reflex	+ + + +	+ + +	+	lost			
	Laryngeal reflex	+ + + + may vocalize		lost				
	Intubation possible	no		yes				

Gastrointestinal	Salivation	+ + + +	+ + +	+	diminished, absent, except in ruminants	absent
	Oropharyngeal reflex	+ + + +	+ + +	+	lost	
	Vomition probability	+ + +	+ + +	+	very slight	
	Reflux (regurgitation) potential	none		increases with relaxation		+ + + +
	Tympany (rumen, cecum)	none		potential increases with duration of anesthesia		
Ocular	Pupils	dilated		normal or constricted, progressive dilation		acutely dilated
	Corneal reflex	normal	+ + +	diminishes, lost (horse may persist)		absent
	Lacrimation	normal	+ + +	+	diminishes, absent	absent
	Photomotor reflex	normal	+ + +	+	diminishes, absent	absent
	Palpebral reflex	normal	+ + +	+	diminishes, absent	absent
	Eyeball position	normal	variable	fixed (ventromedial dog and cat) fixed (central)		
	Nystagmus	+ + + + especially horse, cow			+	none
Musculoskeletal	Jaw tone	+ + + +	+ + + +	decreased, minimal		lost
	Limb muscle tone	+ + + +	+ + + +	decreased, minimal		lost
	Abdominal muscle tone	+ + + +	+ + + +	+ +	decreased, minimal	lost
	Sphincters (anus, bladder)	may void,		progressive relaxation		control lost
Nervous	Sensorium	+ + +	+	lost		
	Pedal reflex§	+ + + +	+ + + +	decreased	absent	
	Reaction to surgical manipulation	+ + + +	+ + + +	+	none	

*Surgical stimulation causes increased heart rate, blood pressure, respiratory rate, and depth via autonomic responses that persist in plane 2. Vagal reflexes due to visceral traction persist in plane 3.

†Especially with halothane and methoxyflurane; does not occur with ether.

‡Tachypnea may occur with halothane; rate may be maintained with ether.

§Varies with efficiency of analgesia; lost during plane 1 to 2 with methoxyflurane, during plane 3 in barbiturate anesthesia.

#Cyanosis is not apparent until cardiac arrest if O_2 is used.

+ to + + + + = degree present.

primitive and exaggerated. The patient reacts to external stimuli by violent reflex struggling, breath holding, tachypnea, and hyperventilation. Continued epinephrine release causes a fast strong heartbeat, cardiac arrhythmias may occur, and the pupils may be widely dilated. During this stage, the animal may whine, cry, bellow, or neigh, depending upon the species concerned. In some species, especially ruminants and felines, salivation may be excessive; in the dog, cat, and goat, vomiting may be evoked. In view of the exaggerated reflex responses during this stage, stimulation of any kind should be avoided.

Stage III. This is the stage of surgical anesthesia and is characterized by unconsciousness with progressive depression of the reflexes. Muscular relaxation develops, and respirations become slow and regular. Vomiting and swallowing reflexes are lost.

In human anesthesiology, this stage has been further divided into planes 1 to 4 to give finer differentiation. Others have suggested the simpler classification of light, medium, and deep. Light anesthesia persists until eyeball movement ceases, medium is characterized by progressive intercostal paralysis, and deep by diaphragmatic respiration (Lee and Atkinson, 1968).

Stage IV. In this stage, the nervous system is extremely depressed, and respirations cease. The heart continues to beat only for a short time. Blood pressure is at the shock level, capillary refill of visible mucous membranes is markedly delayed, and the pupils are widely dilated. The anal and bladder sphincters relax. Death quickly intervenes unless immediate resuscitative steps are taken.

If the anesthetic is withdrawn and artificial respiration is initiated before heart action stops, these effects may be overcome and the patient will go through the various stages in reverse.

The stages just described are best seen when ether or other inhalant anesthetics are administered, probably because considerable time is required for an anesthetic concentration to accrue in the central nervous system. This allows the various signs to become apparent. With intravenous anesthetics or the concurrent use of preanesthetic sedatives, the time between stages is shorter, and many signs are often inapparent.

SIGNS OF ANESTHESIA

Respiration. Respiratory minute volume increases during stage I. Breath holding may occur in stage I, especially if preanesthetic sedation is not used. As anesthetic depression increases to stage II, the respirations become irregular, and breath holding commonly occurs. With the onset of stage III, breathing once again becomes regular. The depth of respiration at this time depends on the respiratory threshold to stimulation; surgical manipulation, for instance, stimulates, whereas premedication depresses respirations. If barbiturates are used for either preanesthetic sedation or induction, early respiratory depression occurs. This is especially apparent in the horse, in which irregular respirations occur early in stage II of barbiturate anesthesia. As stage III increases, there is progressive weakening of the intercostal muscles and the diaphragm. Consequently, the intercostals, because they operate at a mechanical disadvantage, ultimately appear to be paralyzed (Gray, 1960). The depth of respiration thus declines progressively, thoracic movement decreases, respiration becomes largely or entirely abdominal, and the rate may increase. At the same time, the interval between inspiration and expiration is prolonged at the expense of the former. With an overdosage, respiration becomes entirely abdominal and diaphragmatic contraction causes the abdomen to bulge during inspiration and the thorax to collapse. During expiration, the reverse occurs, the anterior excursion of the diaphragm causing the thorax to expand. With progressive overdosage, diaphragmatic movements become smaller, respiratory exchange diminishes further, there is lack of oxygen, and respirations are gasping and ultimately cease. In the dog, oral and cervical movements may be observed during this stage.

Circulation. Safe anesthesia not only requires regular effective ventilation, but also a steady heart rate and adequate blood pressure in the face of surgical stimulation. Cardiovascular signs are therefore as important as those of the respiratory system in assessing anesthetic depth and safety. Although blood pressure may be monitored by indirect methods (see Chap. 19), or by direct arterial puncture, the animal anesthesiologist is often not able to measure pressure. He must depend on the pulse rate, or bleeding at the surgical site, and on induction of momentary blanching by compressing an exposed mucous membrane (such as the conjunctiva, oral mucosa, or tongue) to give some indication of the circulatory status of the patient. The mucous membranes may show pallor as a result of hemorrhage or shock and cyanosis due to hypoxia. In rodents, feet, ears, and muzzles are observed for such signs; in poultry it is necessary to examine the comb and/or wattles; in rats and rabbits the color of light reflected from the eye is helpful.

During stages I and II, the pulse is strong and accelerated. Arrhythmias sometimes occur during stage II. In stage III, the pulse rate is regular and usually slightly accelerated. In halothane anesthesia, progressive bradycardia occurs. Pain stimulation in light stage III may induce tachycardia or even arrhythmias. As the depth of anesthesia increases, blood pressure declines, and the pulse is weak. With the onset of overdosage, arrhythmias occur.

Ocular Signs. These signs include eyeball position and movement, photomotor reflexes and pupillary size, lacrimation, and corneal and conjunctival reflexes. Although ocular signs are often helpful, they are variable and should never replace observation of respiratory and circulatory signs. Eyeball position and movement are especially valuable in horses and cattle in which nystagmus occurs with the onset of stage II and continues through light surgical anesthesia. In light and medium surgical anesthesia in the dog, cat, and pig, the eyeballs are turned downward. The eyelids during this time are usually closed. The pupillary size is modified by the degree of light and by premedication with such drugs as morphine and atropine. The pupils are dilated during stage II, but thereafter constricted. Constriction is especially marked during barbiturate anesthesia. In deep anesthesia or stage IV, pupillary dilatation indicates overdosage. Reflex constriction of the pupil on exposure to light stimuli (photomotor reflex) is lost on transition from light to medium surgical anesthesia. It has been suggested that the pupillary light reflex may indicate the degree of anesthetic depression when other reflexes are obtunded by muscle-relaxant drugs (Croft, 1961).

Lacrimation is no longer observed in the deeper stages of surgical anesthesia. Because the eyes may also be open in deep anesthesia, the cornea appears dull and is subject to the adverse effects of drying. To protect against this hazard, ointment should be applied to the eyes or they should be taped closed after anesthesia has been induced. The palpebral reflex, which is a blink induced by touching the eyelids, is lost as medium surgical anesthesia develops. Blinking induced by gently touching the conjunctiva or cornea (corneal reflex) is variable, but is usually lost shortly after the palpebral reflex. In the horse, however, the corneal reflex may persist throughout stage III.

Pharyngeal and Upper Airway Reflexes. Suppression of these reflexes is of particular importance for endotracheal intubation and for induction of anesthesia in animals with full stomachs, such as ruminants. Coughing and laryngospasm in response to intubation are lost in light surgical anesthesia, but persist into medium anesthesia in the cat. The intensity of these responses varies with the animal species concerned: especially intense in the cat, and relatively mild in cattle and horses. The swallowing and vomiting reflexes disappear with the onset of stage III; like the laryngeal reflexes, the swallowing reflex persists into medium anesthesia in the cat.

Other Signs. After an initial increase during stage II, muscle tone progressively declines as indicated by relaxation of the abdominal muscles, decreasing efficiency of the intercostal muscles, and reduced resistance to passive flexion of the limbs. In lean animals with short-hair coats, abdominal muscle relaxation may be such that the profile of viscera is readily apparent. The contour of the rumen may become visible in some ruminants. In cats, detectable extensor tone, in response to passive flexion of the limb by pushing on the digits, persists into medium surgical anesthesia. Generally, limb muscles are relaxed in light anesthesia whereas abdominal muscles are not well relaxed until anesthesia is deep. The tone of the anal sphincter of the horse is a good indicator of relaxation in this species. During stage II the sphincter is tight, but as anesthetic depth increases, the sphincter relaxes so that in deep surgical anesthesia it may gape to such an extent that feces can be observed in the anal canal. Concomitant with progressive dilatation, the anal sphincter gradually loses ability to contract in response to mechanical stimulation in medium to deep surgical anesthesia. The anal reflexes are not commonly used as anesthetic signs in other species. Deliberate anal dilatation induces an increase in respiratory rate; this respiratory reflex is lost during light stage III.

In the canine, response to opening the jaw is considered to be a useful sign by many anesthesiologists. During transition from stage II to stage III, passive opening of the mouth may elicit yawning, a response especially likely in barbiturate anesthesia. Resistance to opening the mouth fully is lost in medium anesthesia. The digital (pedal) reflex in which the limb is flexed in response to painful stimulation of the digits or interdigital region is also a useful guide to the depth of anesthesia in the dog, cat, and rat. This reflex is lost as transition from light to medium surgical anesthesia occurs. Head shaking in response to ear pinching is a helpful sign in cats, rabbits, and guinea pigs and is lost with the onset of surgical anesthesia. Twitching of the whiskers in response to this same stimulus is lost as light anesthesia progresses to medium. Painful stimulation by pinching the tail of rodents and snakes, and the wattles or combs of birds, is a useful indicator of the onset of surgical anesthesia.

Encephalographic changes are discussed in Chapter 19.

ALVEOLAR CONCENTRATION OF ANESTHETIC AND ANESTHETIC DEPTH

In the 1930s, Guedel and several other workers compared anesthetic response and potency. Robbins (1946) related anesthetic concentration required to induce apnea (LD_{50}) to that which induced loss of righting reflexes, and Courtin et al. (1950) compared responses with electroencephalographic changes. It was not until Merkel and Eger (1963) related stimulus, response, and dose to alveolar partial pressure, and thereby anesthetic partial pressure in the brain, that a consistent indicator of potency became available. As an index of comparison, Merkel and Eger (1963) utilized the minimal alveolar concentration (MAC) of an anesthetic required to keep a dog from gross movement in response to a painful stimulus. Anesthetic dose was thus expressed as multiples of MAC, an expression that was found to be consistent in both man and animals.

Subsequently, the use of this measure of anesthetic potency has become widely accepted (Tables 9–2, 9–3, 9–4). The subject has been reviewed by Quasha et al. (1980). The following information concerning MAC has been, unless otherwise indicated, abstracted from this review.

In animals, MAC is determined by maintenance of a consistent end-tidal anesthetic concentration for 15 minutes in an attempt to achieve equilibrium between alveolar gas, arterial blood, and the brain. The animal is then stimulated by means of a tail clamp or by a subcutaneous electrical current (50 volts at 50 cycles/sec for 10 msec). If there is no response, the anesthetic concentration is reduced and the procedure repeated. The end-tidal anesthetic concentration midway between that allowing movement and that preventing it is MAC 1.0. In man, the stimulus used is a surgical incision. Multiple patients are tested over a range of alveolar anesthetic concentrations, and the concentration at which 50% of patients respond to the stimulus is called MAC 1.0.

With this consistent measure of potency, it became possible to determine the degree to which various factors affect anesthetic potency. Duration of up to 500 minutes of halothane anesthesia in dogs did not affect MAC, but acute and chronic tolerance to nitrous oxide with cross-tolerance to cyclopropane and isoflurane has been observed in mice. MAC varies slightly ($\pm$ 10%) during the circadian cycle in rats and mice, being greatest during the greatest period

TABLE 9–2. Anesthetic Potencies (MAC) of Various Anesthetics in Different Species (and Classes) of Animals*

	Man	Monkey		Dog	Horse	Cat	Rabbit	Rat	Mouse	Toad	Newt	Goldfish
		Java	*Stump-tail*									
Halothane	0.73 0.74 0.77	1.15	0.89	0.86 0.87	0.88	0.82 1.14	0.82	1.11† 1.13† 1.17†		0.67		0.76
Enflurane	1.68	1.84		2.2 2.06	2.12	1.2						
Isoflurane	1.15	1.28		1.28	1.31	1.63		1.38†				
Methoxyflurane	0.16			0.23 0.24		0.23		0.27†		0.22		0.13
Cyclopropane	9.2			15.9 17.5 20.6		19.7		20.5†		9.0		
Fluroxene	3.4			6.0 6.57				4.22				
Ethylene	67							132				
Diethyl ether	1.92			3.04 3.29		2.1			3.2	1.64		2.20
Nitrous oxide	105‡		200	188 222		255		136	146 150	82.2		
Chloroform				0.77					0.78			0.63

*All values are expressed as percentages of one atmosphere. The observed variance in MACs among species is in part due to variations in the techniques used in measuring MAC, as well as some variability in the ages, temperatures, and circadian cycles of the subjects tested. The stimulus used to obtain MAC in man was either a surgical incision or an electrical pulse. In the dog and horse, either a tail clamp or an electrical pulse was used. Monkeys, cats, rabbits, and rats were tested with a tail clamp. The stimulus in mice and newts was a rotating chamber, and the end point was loss of righting reflex. Toads were stimulated with a clamp to the lower extremity. Goldfish were electrically stimulated. End-tidal anesthetic concentrations were measured in man, monkey, dog, horse, cat, rabbit, and rat where indicated, † whereas for all other subjects inspired anesthetic concentration was used.

‡Winter, P.M., Hornbein, T.F., and Smith, G.: Hyperbaric Nitrous Oxide Anesthesia in Man: Determination of Anesthetic Potency (MAC) and Cardiorespiratory Effects. Abstracts of Scientific Papers. Annual Meeting, American Society of Anesthesiologists, 1972, pp. 103–104.

(Adapted from Quasha, A.L., Eger, E.I., II, and Tinker, J.H.: Determination and Application of MAC. Anesthesiology, 53:315, 1980.)

TABLE 9–3. The Means and Standard Deviations of Various Physiologic Parameters at Different Alveolar Concentrations of Halothane during Spontaneous Respiration in Dogs

	MAC 1.0	*MAC 1.5*	*MAC 2.0*	*MAC 2.5*	*MAC 3.0*	*MAC 3.5*	*MAC 4.0*	*R-1.0*
Number of dogs represented by data	6	6	6	6	5	4	1	6
Mean arterial pressure (mm Hg)	119 ± 10	96 ± 14	76 ± 10	64 ± 12	67 ± 8	75 ± 16	64	121 ± 3
Mean venous pressure (cm H_2O)	−0.6 ± 2.3	−0.5 ± 2.1	+1.8 ± 3.2	+4.8 ± 4.0	+54 ± 2.5	+11.8 ± 4.5	+9.5	+0.7 + 3.2
Cardiac output (l/min)	1.99 ± 0.52	1.75 ± 0.41	1.66 ± 0.40	1.49 ± 0.48	1.67 ± 0.24	1.06 ± 0.33	1.63	2.20 ± 0.47
Total peripheral resistance (dynes sec/cm^5)	5,100 ± 1,320	4,680 ± 1,140	3,780 ±730	3,540 ± 1,100	3,100 ± 520	3,750 ± 1,000	2,800	4,580 + 960
Cardiac rate	127 ± 27	124 ± 23	117 ± 22	114 ± 18	124±11	132 ± 20	110	122 ±13
Respiratory rate	23.3 ± 8.0	22.0 ± 5.7	21.2 ± 4.2	18.7 ± 9.7	19.5 ±18	3.0 ± 5.2	6.0	32.3 ± 7.5
Tidal volume (ml)	161 ± 39	148 ± 43	120 ± 37	97 ± 50	105 ± 21	15 ± 26	90	143 ±28
Minute volume (l/min)	3.43 ± 0.66	3.03 ± 0.40	2.86 ± 0.46	2.08 ± 1.02	1.96 ± 1.05	0.18 ± 0.31	0.54	4.50 ± 0.86
Arterial P_{CO_2} (mm Hg)	41.3 ± 3.2	46.7 ± 2.9	54.5 ± 4.8	69.3 ± 9.5	82.4 ± 12.7	115 ± 31	88	44.5 ± 5.6
Arterial buffer base excess (mEq/l)	−2.25 ± 3.5	−3.1 ± 1.9	−3.7 ±1.4	−5.5 ± 1.6	−6.0 ± 1.8	−7.4 ± 1.6	−6.0	−4.4 ± 1.7
Arterial pH	7.349 ± 0.103	7.289 ± 0.066	7.228 ± 0.082	7.127 ± 0.071	7.070 ± 0.075	6.950 ± 0.117	7.050	7.281 ± 0.037
Arterial P_{O_2} (mm Hg)	519 ± 49	503 ± 32	470 ± 41	456 ± 39	460 ± 35	433 ± 45	453	432 ± 63

R-1.0 indicates recovery values at MAC 1.
(From Merkel, G., and Eger, E.I.: A Comparative Study of Halothane and Halopropane Anesthesia. Anesthesiology, 24:345, 1963.)

TABLE 9–4. The Means and Standard Deviations of Various Physiologic Parameters at Different Alveolar Concentrations of Halothane during Controlled Ventilation in Dogs

	MAC 1.0	*MAC 1.5*	*MAC 2.0*	*MAC 2.5*	*MAC 3.0*	*MAC 3.5*	*MAC 4.0*	*R-1.0*
Number of dogs represented by data	6	6	6	6	5	3	2	6
Mean arterial pressure (mm Hg)	111 ± 22	108 ± 22	91 ± 21	65 ± 26	59 ± 24	65	56	118 ± 10
Mean venous pressure (cm H_2O)	+1.1 ± 0.6	+2.3 ± 2.4	+4.3 ± 1.6	+6.0 ± 0.9	+7.1 ± 0.6	+7.7	+10.5	+3.7 ± 1.1
Cardiac output (l/min)	1.82 ± 0.49	1.45 ± 0.37	1.11 ± 0.32	0.87 ± 0.32	0.75 ± 0.24	0.69	0.53	1.65 ± 0.56
Total peripheral resistance (dynes sec/cm^5)	5,490 ± 2,440	6,230 ± 2,100	6,870 ± 1,600	5,800 ± 2,210	5,050 ± 2,300	7,070	7,330	6,003 ± 2,000
Cardiac rate	118 ± 27	106 ± 15	109 ± 15	106 ± 9	106 ± 9	120	114	105 ± 14
Respiratory rate	14.2 ± 2.2	13.9 ± 2.8	13.8 ± 2.6	13.4 ± 2.2	12.7 ± 1.7	13.3	12.0	13.3 ± 1.7
Tidal volume (ml)	392 ± 51	372 ± 25	350 ± 28	355 ± 32	361 ± 31	333	345	342 ± 34
Minute volume (l/min)	5.48 ± 0.79	5.12 ± 0.56	4.81 ± 0.57	4.68 ± 0.42	4.54 ± 0.17	4.33	4.14	4.50 ± 0.57
Arterial P_{CO_2} (mm Hg)	33.2 ± 3.4	32.2 ± 3.6	33.5 ± 4.2	33.4 ± 1.6	33.9 ± 3.3	36.3	32.5	35.8 ± 7.3
Arterial buffer base excess (mEq/l)	−1.4 ± 2.1	−0.25 ± 2.1	+0.7 ± 3.1	+0.3 ± 4.1	−0.3 ± 4.5	+0.3	−2.5	−0.4 ± 2.6
Arterial pH	7.426 ± 0.035	7.451 ± 0.037	7.446 ± 0.070	7.446 ± 0.046	7.430 ± 0.041	7.413	7.413	7.415 ± 0.059
Arterial P_{O_2} (mm Hg)	434 ± 57	468 ± 31	482 ± 26	469 ± 47	485 ± 22	461	470	482 ± 26

R-1.0 indicates recovery values at MAC 1.0.
(From Merkel, G., and Eger, E.I.: A Comparative Study of Halothane and Halopropane Anesthesia. Anesthesiology, 24:346, 1963.)

of metabolic activity. Similar variations have been observed between other species. Pregnancy reduces halothane (rats, sheep) and isoflurane (sheep) MAC, an effect that is apparently not entirely due to elevated plasma progesterone levels.

Levels of $Paco_2$ from 15 to 95 torr had no effect on halothane MAC in dogs; higher values were increasingly narcotic. Neither metabolic acidosis nor alkalosis had any marked effect. Oxygen had no effect upon halothane MAC in dogs between Pao_2 values of 38 to 500 mm Hg. Below 38 mm Hg MAC was decreased. In hyperventilated, hypothermic toads breathing 100% oxygen, halothane and methoxyflurane requirements were reported to be increased.

Progressive reduction of halothane MAC occurred in dogs as mean arterial blood pressure was reduced to 50 to 20 mm Hg. Increased mean arterial pressure (50 to 100%) significantly increased canine halothane MAC during ephedrine infusion, but not during phenylephrine, metaraminol, methoxamine, norepinephrine, or epinephrine administration. This is believed to support the hypothesis that anesthetic requirement is related to the release of CNS catecholamines. Drugs such as alpha-methyldopa and reserpine, which suppress central and peripheral catecholamines, have been shown to produce dose-related reductions in canine halothane MAC values. Conversely, drug-induced increases of CNS catecholamines have been found to increase halothane MAC requirements.

Halothane MAC values have been shown to decline with patient age (Fig. 9–1). This decline parallels reduced cerebral blood flow, cerebral oxygen consumption, and neuronal density. Cerebral oxygen consumption is also influenced by body temperature. Hypothermia ($\lessapprox$ 28° C) in dogs reduces cyclopropane, diethyl ether, fluroxene, halothane, and methoxyflurane MACs rectilinearly. Similar effects have been observed during cyclopropane and halothane anesthesia in rats (Fig. 9–2). As for hyperthermia, halothane MAC increases 8% per degree from 37.3° to 40.7°C; above 42°C MAC decreases. Although MAC values are also influenced by variations in oxygen consumption due to deviations in thyroid function, changes are less than those associated with body temperature, because cer-

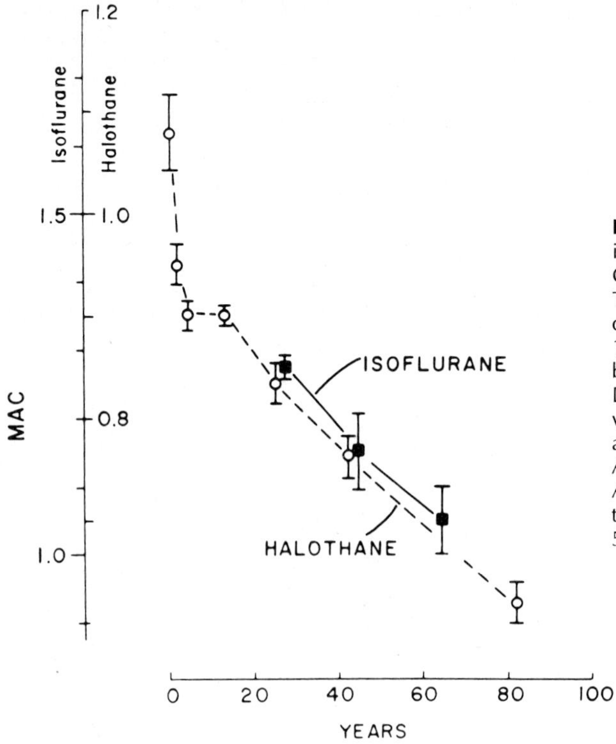

Figure 9–1. MACs for halothane and isoflurane in humans decrease with increasing age. (From Gregory, G.A., Eger, E.I., II, and Munson, E.S.: The Relationship between Age and Halothane Requirement in Man. Anesthesiology, 30:488, 1969, and Stevens, W.C., Dolan, W.M., Gibbons, R.T., White, A., Eger, E.I., II, Miller, R.D., DeJong, R.H. and Elashoff, R.M.: Minimum Alveolar Concentrations (MAC) of Isoflurane with and without Nitrous Oxide in Patients of Various Ages. Anesthesiology, 42:197, 1975. In Quasha, A.L., Eger, E.I., II, and Tinker, J.H.: Determination and Application of MAC. Anesthesiology, 53:315, 1980.)

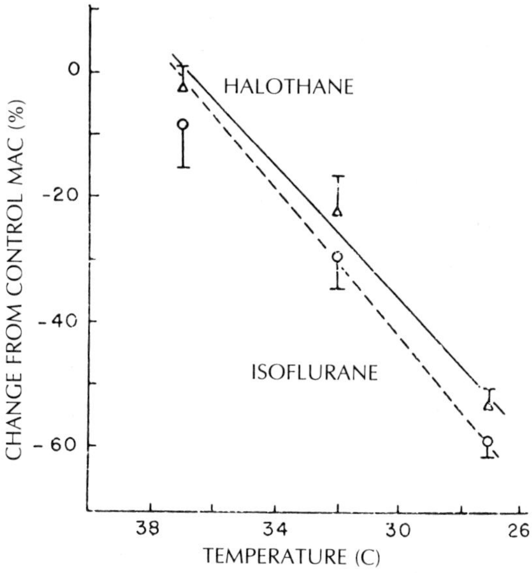

Figure 9–2. Effects of temperature on halothane (Δ) and isoflurane (O) MACs in tracheotomized rats breathing spontaneously. Mean values ± SE are shown. (From Vitez, T.S., White, P.F., and Eger, E.I., II: Effects of Hypothermia on Halothane MAC and Isoflurane MAC in the Rat. Anesthesiology, 41:80, 1974.)

ebral oxygen consumption is unaffected by thyroid function.

Magnesium sulfate has been used extensively with chloral hydrate for large animal anesthesia (see Chap. 13). Although magnesium salts depress skeletal muscle function, any anesthetic effect is believed to be due to cerebral hypoxia. Halothane and cyclopropane potencies vary directly with CSF calcium ion concentrations, and lithium administration has been reported to decrease MAC and to enhance morphine analgesia. Although potassium levels do not appear to influence halothane MAC in dogs, changes in serum electrolytes or osmolality do appear to alter anesthetic requirements when accompanied by changes in brain sodium (Fig. 9–3).

Narcotics in rats (meperidine, morphine) produce a reduction in MAC. This effect increases in a log-dose fashion to the maximal doses used (60 mg/kg and 8 mg/kg respectively). Pentazocine, however, has little additional benefit above a dose of 20 mg/kg. Halothane MAC

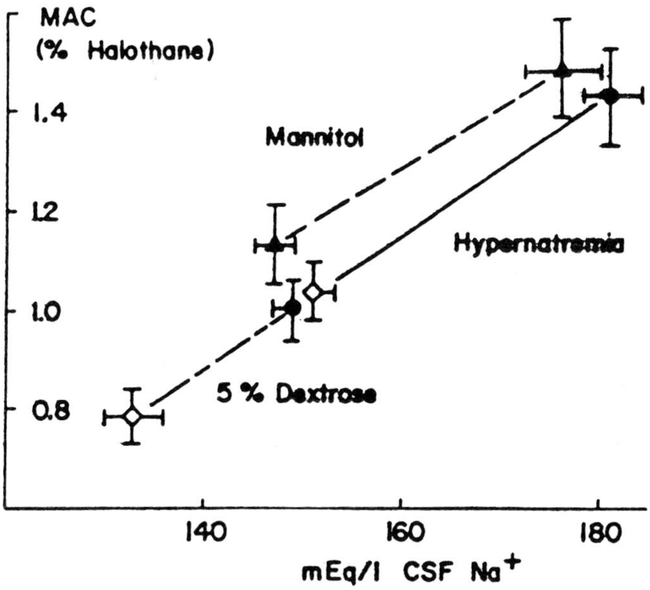

Figure 9–3. The CSF sodium concentration was altered by intravenous administration of mannitol, hypertonic saline solution, or 5% dextrose. Halothane requirement (MAC) in dogs increased with increasing CSF sodium and decreased with decreasing sodium. (From Tanifuji, Y., and Eger, E.I., II: Brain Sodium, Potassium, and Osmolality: Effects on Anesthetic Requirement. Anesth. Analg., 57: 404, 1978.)

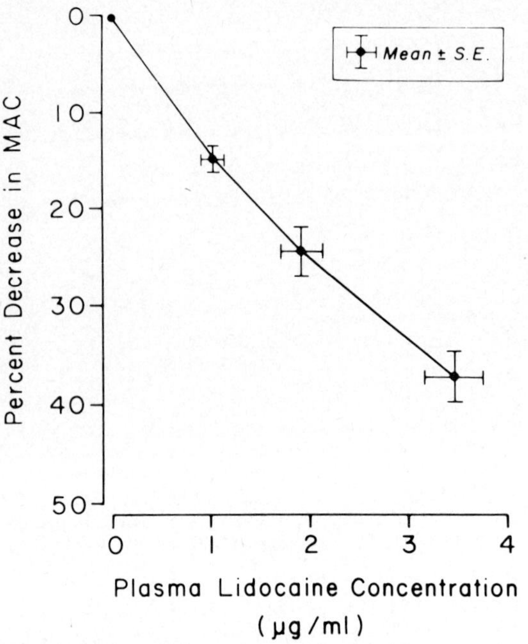

Figure 9–4. Enflurane MAC in dogs decreases as a function of plasma lidocaine concentration. (From Himes, R.S., Jr., Munson, E.S., and Embro, J.W.: Enflurane Requirement and Ventilatory Response to Carbon Dioxide during Lidocaine Infusion in Dogs. Anesthesiology, 51:131, 1979.)

values in dogs have been shown to decrease progressively with morphine tolerance.

Non-narcotic premedicants (amobarbital, barbital, pentobarbital, chlorpromazine, diazepam, hydroxyzine, ketamine) likewise have an anesthetic sparing effect in various species. On the other hand, small doses of promethazine (0.1 to 0.15 mg/kg) do not affect halothane MAC in dogs. Halothane MAC is decreased by pancuronium (man) and by lidocaine (arterial concentrations of 1 to 4 mg/ml in dogs) (Fig. 9–4). Results have been conflicting concerning the effect of naloxone, and large doses of physostigmine and neostigmine were found to decrease halothane MAC in dogs. Combinations of inhalation anesthetics are generally additive.

The curves for anesthetic dose versus CNS response are parallel, so that the ratios of anesthetic concentrations producing more or less CNS depression than that occurring at MAC 1.0 are relatively constant. In view of the preceding information and the availability of monitors of end-tidal anesthetic concentration, the use of MAC as a guideline for the selection and maintenance of anesthetic concentrations is beneficial. MAC may be used to gauge the margin of safety of an anesthetic relative to the MAC values at which specific effects occur. In addition, MAC permits quantitation of anesthetic effect of specific drugs in varying clinical situations.

TABLE 9–5. Return of Reflexes in Dogs Following Large Intravenous Doses of Barbiturates*

	Sodium Pentobarbital 35 mg/kg	*Sodium Thiopental 30 mg/kg*
Wink reflex	2.0 (1–3)	2.3 (1–3)
Corneal reflex	4.1 (2–7)	4.6 (2–8)
Swallowing reflex	7.7 (6–9)	7.2 (6–8)
Endotracheal reflex	4.6 (3–6)	3.7 (2–4)
Patellar reflex	1.3 (1–3)	1.3 (1–3)
Respiratory reflex	3.2 (2–4)	3.6 (2–5)
Movement reflex	6.5 (5–8)	6.2 (5–7)
Spontaneous movement	6.7 (5–8)	7.6 (6–9)
Head-righting reflex	8.9 (8–9)	8.5 (8–9)
Walking	10.0	10.0
Freedom from ataxia	11.0	11.0

*The first reflex to reappear was ranked 1, and as others returned they were ranked consecutively. Mean rank is indicated in the first column and range in the second.

Wink reflex—contraction of orbicularis oculi induced by a tap on the inner canthus of the eye.

Corneal reflex—contraction of the orbicularis oculi when the cornea is touched with cotton.

Swallowing reflex—swallowing movement produced by separating the jaws and pulling the tongue.

Endotracheal reflex—coughing produced by vigorous movement of an endotracheal tube within the trachea.

Patellar reflex—extension of the leg when the quadriceps tendon is tapped.

Respiratory reflex—a change in the respiratory pattern produced by forceful and rapid dilation of the anal sphincter.

Movement reflex—movement of an extremity produced by forceful and rapid dilation of the anal sphincter.

Spontaneous movement—movement of an extremity without a provoking stimulus.

Head-righting reflex—ability of the animal to maintain its head in an upright position without support.

(From Maynert, E.W.: The Usefulness of Clinical Signs for the Comparison of Intravenous Anesthetics in Dogs. J. Pharmacol. Exp. Ther., 128:182, 1960.)

RECOVERY FROM ANESTHESIA

As anesthetic drugs are eliminated from the brain, the degree of anesthesia lightens, and reverse progress through the stages of anesthesia occurs. Induction techniques are usually selected and carried out to minimize the duration of stage II, in which excitement and motor activity may occur. During recovery, however, stage II is prolonged, so that every effort should be made to avoid stimulation of the animal at this time. This stage of recovery is of particular concern when large animals are anesthetized. Horses are especially subject to excitement and struggling during this stage, although the use of preanesthetic sedation can do much to minimize this.

Maynert (1960) conducted an extensive study of the reflexes in dogs as they arouse from pentobarbital and thiopental (Table 9–5). No individual reflex was always found to reappear in the same order when all were tested. From this investigation, Maynert concluded that the intensity of neurologic derangement could best be estimated using a scale containing six levels of depression:

Level 0—Freedom from ataxia
Level 1—Ability to walk though ataxic
Level 2—Presence of the head-righting reflex
Level 3—Presence of spontaneous movement, the movement reflex, or the swallowing reflex
Level 4—Presence of one or more of the following reflexes: wink, corneal, endotracheal, or respiratory
Level 5—Only the patellar reflex present

CONCLUSION

The question arises of how best to judge the various stages of anesthesia, particularly when so many modifying factors must be taken into account. *The experienced anesthesiologist finds himself relying less on classical signs of anesthesia and more on the patient's response to stimuli.* These stimuli may be produced by the surgeon or the anesthesiologist himself and may cause responses in respiration, circulation, or muscle tone. Needless to say, effective anesthesia is that which just obliterates the patient's response to painful stimuli without depressing vital functions.

REFERENCES

Courtin, R.F., Bickford, R.G., and Faulconer, A., Jr.: Classification and Significance of Electroencephalographic Patterns Produced by Nitrous Oxide-Ether Anesthesia During Surgical Operations. Proc. Staff Meet., Mayo Clin., 25:197, 1950.

Croft, P.G.: The Photomotor Reflex as an Indicator of Consciousness in the Immobilized Dog. J. Small Anim. Pract., 2:206, 1961.

Gray, T.C.: A Reassessment of the Signs and Levels of Anaesthesia. Irish J. Med. Sci., 419:499, 1960.

Lee, J.A., and Atkinson, R.S.: *A Synopsis of Anaesthesia,* 6th ed. Williams & Wilkins, Baltimore, 1968.

Maynert, E.W.: The Usefulness of Clinical Signs for the Comparison of Intravenous Anesthetics in Dogs. J. Pharmacol. Exp. Ther., 128:182, 1960.

Merkel, G., and Eger, E.I.: A Comparative Study of Halothane and Halopropane Anesthesia. Anesthesiology, 24:346, 1963.

Quasha, A.L., Eger, E.I., II, and Tinker, J.H.: Determination and Application of MAC. Anesthesiology, 53:315, 1980.

Robbins, B.H.: Preliminary Studies of the Anesthetic Activity of Fluorinated Hydrocarbons. J. Pharmacol. Exp. Ther., 86:197, 1946.

CHAPTER 10

The Inhalation Anesthetics

ADVANTAGES AND DISADVANTAGES OF INHALATION ANESTHESIA

Inhalation anesthesia has two distinct advantages: 1) The agents used are primarily exhaled through the lungs; therefore, recovery from anesthesia is not dependent solely upon redistribution within the body and detoxification mechanisms. In poor-risk patients, this is particularly helpful. 2) Because these agents are rapidly exhaled, the anesthesiologist has good control of the level of anesthesia and can quickly alter the depth at any time.

Certain disadvantages also are inherent with these agents: 1) They require constant surveillance by an anesthesiologist during administration, 2) some are explosive and inflammable, 3) some irritate body tissues, and 4) chronic exposure to some inhalant anesthetic mixtures is hazardous to operating room personnel.

METABOLISM OF VOLATILE ANESTHETIC AGENTS

For many years, it was believed that volatile anesthetics were not metabolized in the body, but were eliminated by exhalation and in urine, feces, and sweat (see Chap. 2).

Studies with radioactive-labeled anesthetics have revealed that a small percentage of most agents is metabolized and that the metabolites are eliminated in exhaled air and in urine (Table 10–1).

TABLE 10–1. Results of In Vivo Metabolism of Volatile Anesthetics in Rats

Anesthetic	*% Recovery as CO_2*	*% Recovery of Isotope in Urine*
C^{14}-Chloroform	4–5	0–2
Diethyl-l-C^{14}-ether	4.0	2.0
C^{14}-Halothane $C^{14}F_3CClBrH$	0.48	1.0–2.5
C^{14}-Methoxyflurane $C^{14}H_3OCF_2CCl_2H$	1.0–4.0	3.5–6.0

Values indicate 24-hour recoveries from a single dose of anesthetic given I.P.

(From Chenoweth, M.B.: Physiologic and Biochemical Responses to Methoxyflurane Anesthesia. In *Experimental Animal Anesthesiology.* Edited by D.C. Sawyer. U.S.A.F. School of Aerospace Medicine, Brooks Air Force Base, Texas, 1965.)

Subanesthetic doses of halothane, methoxyflurane, cyclopropane, enflurane, and isoflurane have been administered to swine, and the amount of hepatic metabolism has been measured by comparing concentrations of blood in the portal vein with those in the hepatic veins (Sawyer et al., 1971; Halsey et al., 1971). A high percentage of halothane (35%) and methoxyflurane (52%) passing through the liver was metabolized, whereas little enflurane (12%) and no cyclopropane or isoflurane was metab-

TABLE 10–2. Historical and Clinical Data on the Inhalation Anesthetic Agents

Agent	*Nitrous Oxide*	*Diethyl Ether*	*Methoxyflurane*	*Enflurane*	*Halothane*	*Isoflurane*	*Chloroform*
Chemical formula	N_2O	$(C_2H_5)_2O$	$CHCl_2CF_2$-O-CH_3	CFHCl-CF_2-O-CF_2H	$CF_3CHBrCl$	CF_3CHCl-O-CF_2H	$CHCl_3$
Discovery	1772 by Priestley	1540 by Cordus	1958 by Larsen	1963 by Terrell	1956 by Suckling	1965 by Terrell	1831 by Guthrie, Liebig, and Souberian independently
First observation of narcotic properties	1799 by Davy	1796 by Beddoes	1958 by Larsen, Chenoweth, and Shea	1963 by Krantz	1956 by Raventos	1965 by Krantz and Rudd	1847 by Flourens
First used clinically in man	1844 by Wells	1842 by Long 1846 by Morton	1960 by Van Poznak and Artusio	1966 by Virtue	1956 by Johnson	1971 by Dobkin et al.	1847 by Simpson
Type of compound	Oxide of nitrogen	Saturated ether	Halogenated ether	Halogenated ether	Halogenated hydrocarbon	Halogenated ether	Chlorinated hydrocarbon
Molecular weight	44.02	74.12	145.979	184.5	197.30	184.5	119.39
Boiling point °C	−89.5	34.6	104.65	56.5	50.2	48.5	61.3
Vapor density (Air = 1) at 25°C	1.53	2.56	5.7	6.4	6.9	6.4	4.12
Vapor pressure (torr) 18°C	Completely gaseous state at 20°C	—	20.3	156.3	224.1	218.7	—
20°C		444	22.8	171.8	244.1	239.5	166
22°C		—	25.5	188.6	265.5	261.8	—
24°C		—	28.4	206.6	288.3	285.8	—
26°C		—	31.7	226.1	312.7	311.5	—
Commercial preparation	Decomposition of ammonium nitrate by heat	Dehydration of ethanol with sulfuric acid	Base catalyzed, addition of $CF_2=CCl_2$ to methanol	Base catalyzed, addition of methanol to CF_2CFCl, chlorination and fluorination	Stepwise halogenation of trichlorethylene	Reaction of CF_2HCl and trifluoroethanol and chlorination	Chlorination of acetone or alcohol
Impurities that may be present in crude product	Higher oxides of nitrogen; nitrogen; ammonia	Peroxides; aldehydes	Methyl chloroacetate, dimethyl carbonate, 1, 1, 1, 2-tetrachloro-2,2-difluoroethane	Various halogenated ethers	HCl, HBr, other halogenated hydrocarbons	Various halogenated ethers	Phosgene Hydrogen chloride Acetone
Stabilizing agent added	None	None; trace C_2H_3OH present from manufacture	0.01% butylated hydroxytoluene	None	0.01% thymol	None	0.01% phenyl alpha naphthalamine
Reaction with soda lime	Stable	Traces of aldehydes may be formed	Decomposes	Stable	Decomposes	Stable	Converted to salt of formic acid when warmed

Partition coefficients at 37°C							
Blood/gas	0.47	15.2	12.0	1.9	2.3	1.4	10.3
Brain/gas	0.50	12.1	22.1	2.6	4.1	2.6	8.4
Fat/gas	1.22	—	890.0	105	185.0	60.0	—
Liver/gas	0.38	—	24.8	3.8	7.2	—	—
Muscle/gas	0.54	—	20.0	3.0	6.0	5.2	—
Oil/gas	1.4	65.0	930.	98.5	224.0	91.0	265.0
Water/gas	0.47	15.6	4.5	0.8	0.7	0.61	3.8
Rubber/gas at 23°C	1.2	—	630	74	120	62.0	—
Potency (ethyl ether = 1)	0.15:1	1:1	8:1	—	4:1	—	3:1
% Conc. of Inhaled Mixture for:							
Analgesia	35–40	—	0.2–0.4	0.5	—	0.4	—
Anesthesia	85–90	3.5–4.5	0.4–1.0	1.5–2.5	0.8–1.2	0.8–1.5	1.35–1.65
Respiratory Arrest	—	6.7–8.0	3.0–4.0	—	3.6–4.0	—	2
Minimum alveolar concentration (MAC) %	105 (man) 200 (monkey 188 (dog) 255 (cat) 136 (rat) 146 (mouse) 82.2 (toad)	1.92 (man) 3.04 (dog) 2.1 (cat) 3.2 (mouse) 1.64 (toad) 2.20 (goldfish)	0.16 (man) 0.23 (dog) 0.23 (cat) 0.27 (rat) 0.22 (toad) 0.13 (goldfish)	1.68 (man) 1.84 (monkey) 2.2 (dog) 2.12 (horse) 1.2 (cat)	0.74 (man) 0.89 (monkey) 0.87 (dog) 0.88 (horse) 0.82 (cat) 0.82 (rabbit) 1.13 (rat) 0.67 (toad) 0.67 (goldfish)	1.15 (man) 1.28 (monkey) 1.28 (dog) 1.31 (horse) 1.63 (cat) 1.38 (rat)	0.77 (dog) 0.78 (mouse) 0.63 (goldfish)
Flammable range in vol-%							
Air	Will support combustion only	1.85–36.5	7.0	Nonflammable in usual anesthetic concentrations at room temperature	Nonflammable in usual anesthetic concentrations at room temperature	Nonflammable in usual anesthetic concentrations at room temperature	Oxidized by flame $2CHCl_3 + O_2\Delta \rightarrow 2COCl_2 + 2HCl$
O_2		2.10–82.0	5.4	Nonflammable as above	Nonflammable as above	Nonflammable as above	Nonflammable in all concentrations with oxygen at room temperature
70% N_2O/30% O_2			4.0	5.8	4–5	7.0	
Ignition temperature in °C							
Air	Will support combustion only	304°	453°	None		None	
O_2		180°		None	1000° with 20–22.5 vol-%	None	

(Courtesy of Dr. William H.L. Dornette and Ohio Medical Products with additions from Eger, E.I., II: Isoflurane (Forane), A Compendium and Reference. Ohio Medical Products, Madison, Wisconsin, 1981; Anonymous: Ethrane (Enflurane), A Compendium and Reference. Ohio Medical Products, Madison, Wisconsin, 1979; Quasha, A.L., Eger, E.I., II, and Tinker, J.H.: Determination and Applications of MAC. Anesthesiology, 53:315, 1980; and Larsen, E.R.: Personal communication, Dow Chemical U.S.A., Midland, Michigan, 1982) olized. As the concentration of halothane was increased, a smaller fraction of the total was metabolized, indicating that high concentrations may depress the metabolic mechanism. Sawyer and associates and Halsey and co-workers suggested that, since toxic effects of anesthetics may be due to their metabolites, cyclopropane and isoflurane are less toxic than halothane or methoxyflurane.

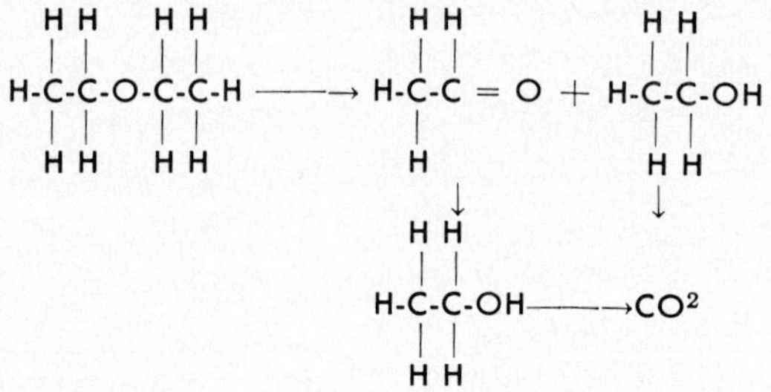

Figure 10–1. Metabolic pathway of diethyl ether. (From Chenoweth, M.B.: Physiologic and Biochemical Responses to Methoxyflurane Anesthesia. In *Experimental Animal Anesthesiology.* Edited by D.C. Sawyer. U.S.A.F. School of Aerospace Medicine, Brooks Air Force Base, Texas, 1965.)

METHODS OF ADMINISTRATION

Inhalation anesthetics are divided into *volatile liquids* and *gases* according to their physical state. The common liquids are ethyl ether, halothane, methoxyflurane, enflurane, and isoflurane (Table 10–2). The common gas is nitrous oxide. All gaseous agents are administered by means of a closed, semiclosed, or semiopen system (see Chap. 11). Volatile liquid agents are administered by various methods that include insufflation, open nonrebreathing, and semiopen, semiclosed, and closed systems.

VOLATILE LIQUID ANESTHETICS

Ether, U.S.P. (Ethyl Ether; Diethyl Ether; $(C_2H_5)_2O$)

Ethyl ether was synthesized by Valerius Cordus in Germany in 1540. Ether, as it is commonly called, is a colorless highly volatile liquid with a pungent odor and irritating vapor. The vapor is 2.6 times heavier than air; inflammable and explosive mixtures are therefore more likely to accumulate close to the floor. For practical purposes, ether is *always* explosive. Because of the explosion hazard, ether should *never* be stored in a conventional refrigerator; it must be explosion-proof.

Ether oxidizes in the presence of air or oxygen to form peroxides and aldehydes, which are toxic. In addition, peroxides may rarely cause explosions. Because light causes oxidation, ether is stored in sealed metal containers coated inside with copper or another metal that combines with oxygen. This preferential absorption by the metal prevents oxidation.

Ether may be given by all commonly used methods for administration of inhalant anesthetics. Use in a closed system minimizes dispersal of an explosive mixture into the operating room. With the exception of methoxyflurane, it has the longest induction time of the inhalation anesthetics, varying from 3 to 10 minutes depending upon the concentration administered, the method of administration, premedication, physical status of the patient, and other variable factors. The concentration necessary for anesthesia is 3.5 to 4.5% by volume in the inhaled mixture; 6.7 to 8.0% causes respiratory failure. For rapid induction, higher concentrations are necessary to saturate the blood. Since vaporization of ether causes rapid cooling with marked reduction of attainable vapor concentrations (see Fig. 11–22), the high gas flow rates necessary for large animal anesthesia make adequate ether vapor concentrations difficult to maintain. It is therefore usually impossible to anesthetize horses and cattle by administering ether via open or semiopen systems. Under such circumstances, use of a closed or semiclosed system with an in-circuit vaporizer or a copper kettle is desirable.

Over 80% of ether is exhaled, the remainder being metabolized (see Table 10–1, Fig. 10–1) or eliminated in feces, urine, and other body fluids. Complete desaturation of the body is slow, requiring over 24 hours (Fig. 10–2).

Ether irritates all tissues, and this accounts for many of the effects seen during and after anesthesia. Because it irritates the mucous membranes of the respiratory tract, breath-holding

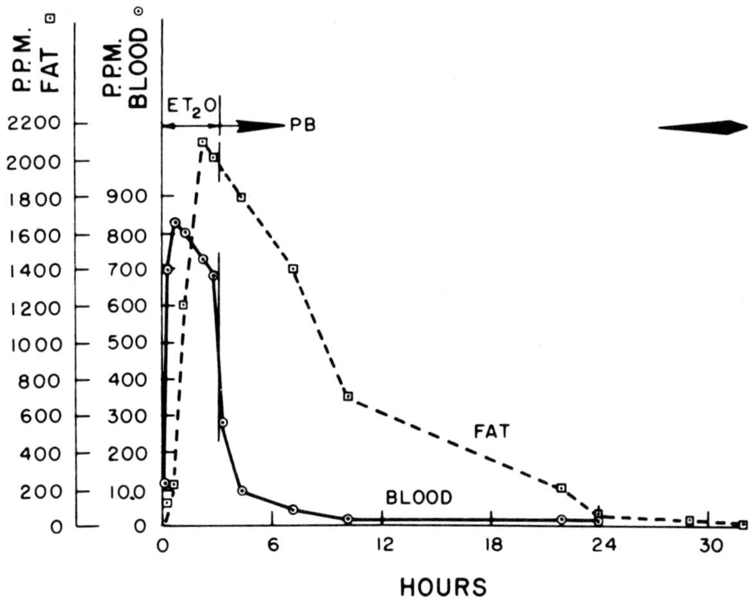

Figure 10–2. Blood and fat levels of diethyl ether in dogs. *ET_2O*, diethyl ether; *PB*, pentobarbital sodium. (From Chenoweth, M.B.: Physiologic and Biochemical Responses to Methoxyflurane Anesthesia. In *Experimental Animal Anesthesiology*. Edited by D.C. Sawyer. U.S.A.F. School of Aerospace Medicine, Brooks Air Force Base, Texas, 1965.)

by the patient is common during induction. Ether administered by the semiopen drop method leads to inhalation of high concentrations of vapor with paralysis of the respiratory centers. Removal of the mask and artificial respiration will resuscitate most of these patients; however, most deaths from ether anesthesia occur during induction. The flow of saliva and mucus increases, which may interfere with respiration. This also lowers resistance of the lung tissue to infection and increases susceptibility to postoperative pneumonia.

Ether irritates kidney tissues and reduces urine output during anesthesia. MacNider (1920, 1921, 1922) has shown that the effect varies with age. Dogs 4 to 11 years old have marked reduction in urine output or even complete anuria after 1 hour of anesthesia. Ten percent dextrose solution injected intravenously before ether administration has a protecting effect. Albuminuria and tubular casts are common in the postanesthetic period.

The effect on the liver is minimal. Histologically, centrilobular glycogen depletion and slight fatty changes have been noted in dogs anesthetized for 3-hour periods on 5 consecutive days (Stephen et al., 1958). Bromsulphalein tests in these animals were unaltered.

There is no demonstrable effect on cardiac muscle histologically. However, disturbances of rhythm and extrasystoles frequently occur, particularly on induction. Cardiac output is increased during induction because of epinephrine release. During light surgical anesthesia, output is increased about 20% above normal, and blood pressure is normal or slightly elevated (Blalock, 1928). Deep surgical anesthesia is accompanied by a progressive fall in blood pressure due to beginning paralysis of the vasomotor centers and decreased cardiac output. In the stage of medullary paralysis, the centers are affected in the following order: respiratory, vasomotor, and cardiac.

Anemia and icterus are occasionally seen after anesthesia. It is not certain whether this is due to the effect upon the blood or liver. The most obvious change in the blood is a hyperglycemia, which may be sufficiently high to produce glycosuria. There is hemoconcentration with an increase in the red cell count and hemoglobin, accompanied by a decrease in plasma volume. Leukocytosis also occurs, the polymorphonuclear leukocytes increasing relatively and absolutely. Progressive acidosis develops through loss of bicarbonate (due to excretion of sodium with acetone bodies) and retention of carbon dioxide through decreased respiration.

Contraindications for ether anesthesia are acute or chronic respiratory infections, acidosis, kidney or liver disease, shock, and lack of equipment and facilities for an explosive anesthetic.

The advantages of ether are that it gives good muscular relaxation, has a wide margin of safety, is initially a respiratory stimulant, and does not depress the circulation at the usual level of anesthesia. It is stable, easily preserved, relatively inexpensive, and can be administered with minimal equipment.

In horses, cattle, sheep, and swine, anesthesia can be economically maintained, providing ether is administered via a semiclosed or closed system. Recovery is usually complete within 1 hour after administration ceases.

The disadvantages include a long induction period accompanied by excitement, slow recovery, irritation to all tissues, flame and explosion hazards, and extreme difficulty of induction in large animals. Recovery is slow compared with halogenated hydrocarbons, and in horses the use of tranquilizers to control emergence struggling is indicated. Ether is an irritant to all tissues and during induction causes profuse salivation and secretion of mucus, especially in ruminants, swine, and cats. Ether is inflammable and explosive, factors that are important to consider in closed environments when large volumes of vapor are being dissipated during large animal anesthesia. Furthermore, most facilities and equipment available for large animals are not designed for explosive anesthetic agents.

Ether is a safe agent in the hands of the inexperienced anesthesiologist.

Methoxyflurane (Metofane; Penthrane; $CHCl_2CF_2OCH_3$)

Methoxyflurane is a clear colorless liquid that will not explode in any concentration at room temperature. It will explode at higher temperatures and at concentrations above those used clinically. It can be employed safely with the electric cautery. If it is used with high concentrations of nitrous oxide, the flammability limit is lowered (Table 10–3).

TABLE 10–3. Flammability Limits of Methoxyflurane

Atmosphere	*Lower Flammability Limit (%)*
Air	7.0
O_2	5.4
50% N_2O–50% O_2	4.6
70% N_2O–30% O_2	4.0
80% N_2O–20% O_2	3.6
100% N_2O	2.7

(From Chenoweth, M.B.: Physiologic and Biochemical Responses to Methoxyflurane Anesthesia. In *Experimental Animal Anesthesiology.* Edited by D.C. Sawyer. U.S.A.F. School of Aerospace Medicine, Brooks Air Force Base, Texas, 1965.)

Methoxyflurane vaporizes 10 times more easily than water; 1 g requires 58.5 cal of heat, whereas 584.9 cal of heat at 20°C are required to evaporate 1 g of water. Methoxyflurane thus vaporizes without absorbing much heat from the vaporizer. The temperature of the vaporizer does not fall as rapidly as it would with agents such as ether that have a higher latent heat of vaporization. In normal room temperatures, therefore, reduced vapor concentrations due to evaporative cooling are less of a problem than with ether. Vaporization is, however, inefficient in out-of-circuit vaporizers when environmental temperatures are below 70°F. At its saturated vapor pressure, a limited number of anesthetic molecules are presented to the patient, and induction is relatively slow. To increase the number of molecules carried to the patient, a higher volume of gas must be delivered; therefore, induction flows should be high. The concentration of methoxyflurane is limited by its saturated vapor pressure (25 mm Hg at 21°C) to a maximum of 3.5% at 23°C (73°F). Under normal temperature and pressure, no vaporizer can deliver a greater concentration. It is significant that this concentration is the same as that for induction; hence, initial overdose is difficult. Maintenance of anesthesia can be accomplished with concentrations of 0.4 to 1.0%. Because methoxyflurane boils at 104°C at 760 mm Hg, it can be used in hot climates without excessive loss of agent through rapid evaporation.

The specific gravity is 1.4006 at 37°C, which is important when the agent is used with in-circle vaporizers. Water vapor from the patient and from the chemical reaction of carbon dioxide with soda lime tends to condense on all colder surfaces within the system. This causes water condensation on the vaporizing wick, the surface of the methoxyflurane, and other metal and glass components of the vaporizer. Since methoxyflurane is heavier than water, the latter accumulates above methoxyflurane in the vaporizer and saturates the wick. This impedes further vaporization, and maintenance of anesthesia becomes difficult. For this reason, each patient should be started with a dry wick, and any condensed water on the methoxyflurane should be absorbed onto a paper towel from the surface of the liquid. Out-of-circle vaporizers do not pose this problem.

Methoxyflurane is highly rubber-soluble (Eger and Brandstater, 1963). Both induction and recovery may be prolonged due to uptake and release of methoxyflurane from rubber in the anesthetic circuit. It will also extract rubber, thus accelerating its aging.

Methoxyflurane does not react to light, but the antioxidant may slowly break down, producing a brown color. This will not affect its qualities or safety, but may stain the wick in vaporizers.

The use of methoxyflurane in veterinary medicine has been extensively reviewed by Hezel (1976). Methoxyflurane produces good analgesia and muscle relaxation. The action of curariform drugs is potentiated to about the same degree as with diethyl ether.

The classic eye signs are of no value in determining the stages of anesthesia. The pupils change little, and the eyeballs become fixed early. Respiratory rate, pulse, and degree of reflex activity are the best criteria.

Methoxyflurane may be administered by any of the commonly used systems for administration of inhalant anesthetics. Like halothane, its expense is such that it requires administration with minimal waste. Partial or complete rebreathing techniques are therefore preferred for larger dogs and large animals. When one is using such techniques, an in-circuit wick vaporizer is commonly employed, although out-of-circuit calibrated vaporizers such as the Pentec,* Copper Kettle, and Vernitrol* are advantageous (see Chap. 11). In view of the limits of vaporization of methoxyflurane, simple bubble vaporizers may be used out-of-circuit or in nonrebreathing systems. Induction with methoxyflurane alone is slow, especially when rebreathing techniques are used, and requires approximately 10 minutes. Induction by nonrebreathing techniques is possible in less than 5 minutes in dogs and even in small calves.

Salivation is not stimulated. Respirations are at first slightly increased followed by a progressive decrease in rate and minute volume with deepening anesthesia. This leads to acidosis if anesthesia is maintained over long periods.

The heart is sensitized to epinephrine, but to a much smaller degree than with halothane. Use of atropine, nitrous oxide, ouabain, or thiopental with methoxyflurane does not result in synergistic cardiac sensitization to catecholamines (Pedersoli et al., 1978). Blood pressure falls progressively and is directly related to the depth of anesthesia. Heart rate is reduced slightly or not at all. Decrease in cardiac output is probably due to depression of myocardium, depressed tension of atrial and papillary muscles, and reduced peripheral resistance (Hezel, 1976). During long periods of anesthesia, shock levels will be reached.

The tone and motility of the gastrointestinal tract are decreased; increased salivation is not generally seen, with the possible exception of cats and some brachycephalic breeds of dogs. Vomiting is not observed in dogs fed before receiving anesthesia, but has been observed in one species of monkey (Hezel, 1976).

No change in blood cells or coagulation time has been reported. The blood sugar is slightly reduced when breathing is augmented.

Methoxyflurane concentrations in the blood rise and fall fairly rapidly in direct relationship to the amount administered. The fat concentra-

*See Appendix A for manufacturer.

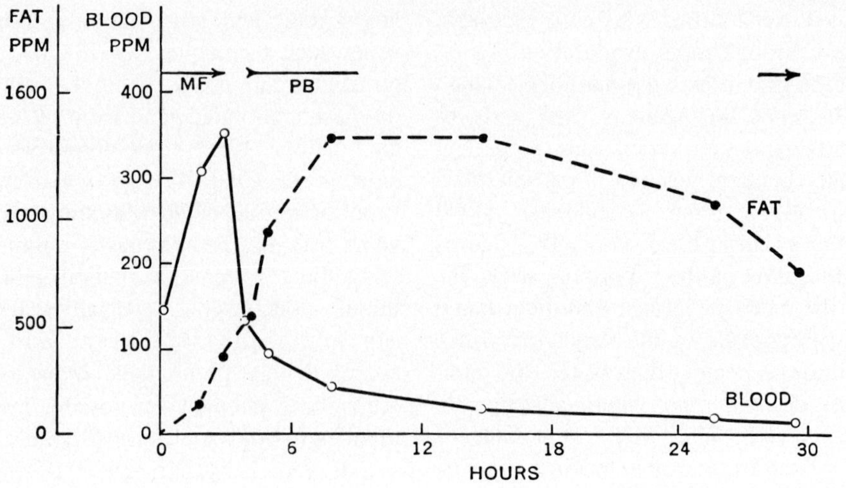

Figure 10–3. Methoxyflurane concentrations in blood and fat of a dog during and following 3 hours of anesthesia. *MF,* methoxyflurane (Penthrane); *PB,* pentobarbital sodium. (From Chenoweth, M.B., Robertson, D.N., Erley, D.F., and Golhke, R.: Blood and Tissue Levels of Ether, Chloroform, Halothane and Methoxyflurane in Dogs. Anesthesiology, 23:101, 1962.)

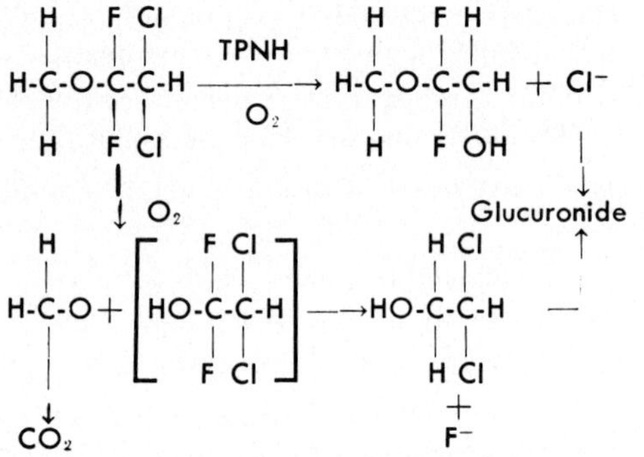

Figure 10–4. Metabolic pathway of methoxyflurane. (From Chenoweth, M.B.: Physiologic and Biochemical Responses to Methoxyflurane Anesthesia. In *Experimental Animal Anesthesiology.* Edited by D.C. Sawyer. U.S.A.F. School of Aerospace Medicine, Brooks Air Force Base, Texas, 1965.)

tion rises for about 2 hours after administration even though the blood level falls. Thirty hours later there is still a measurable amount of methoxyflurane in the blood; and the fat concentration is still high (Fig. 10–3). The odor of the drug can be detected in the breath for many hours since most is eliminated through the lungs. Some methoxyflurane is metabolized (see Table 10–1, Fig. 10–4). Defluorination of methoxyflurane is enhanced by enzyme induction (Mazze et al., 1974).

Advantages claimed for methoxyflurane are lack of explosive capability, good muscle relaxation with freedom from side effects and toxicity, a high margin of safety in both large and small animals, and analgesia extending into the postanesthetic period.

Because emergence is generally quiet, the slower recovery period in relation to halothane is generally not a problem; unless heavily sedated, most small animals are able to stand within 1 hour. With horses, in which rapid smooth recovery is highly desirable, an average recovery period of 1 to 1½ hours (Heinze, 1965) is a disadvantage when compared with halothane. Like other general anesthetics, methoxyflurane crosses the placental barrier and depresses the newborn. Other disadvantages are slow induction, depression of blood pressure, and respiratory acidosis during long periods of anesthesia. Studies in the pregnant ewe revealed that at 1.0 and 1.5 MAC there were slight to moderate falls in maternal blood pressure, cardiac output, and uterine blood flow, but no serious fetal deterioration. At 2.0 MAC there were marked decreases in these parameters, with fetal hypoxemia and mixed respiratory and metabolic acidosis (Smith et al., 1975).

Both renal and hepatic toxicity have been reported in man following methoxyflurane administration. Pezzi et al. (1966), Crandell et al. (1966), Austin and Villandry (1967), Elkington et al. (1968), and Crandell and MacDonald (1968) have all reported a syndrome characterized by high urine output, hypernatremia, elevated blood urea nitrogen, and dehydration. In most cases, recovery occurred in 10 to 20 days, but in a few the blood urea nitrogen remained elevated for months. This syndrome in man has been attributed to metabolic degradation of methoxyflurane, with production of inorganic fluoride and oxalic acid, which are nephrotoxic. It may be induced by tetracycline administration either immediately before or after methoxyflurane administration (Kuzucu, 1970). Liver damage in man following methoxyflurane has been reported by Lindenbaum and Leifer (1963), Kataoka (1965), Durkin et al. (1966), and Klein and Jeffries (1966).

Bergeron et al. (1966) could find no deleterious effects on renal hemodynamics or tubular handling of water in dogs after moderately deep methoxyflurane anesthesia. While urine fluoride is increased in dogs during and after anesthesia, nephrotoxicity does not occur (Pedersoli, 1977*a,b*; Brunson et al., 1979).

Cale et al. (1962), studying the hepatic effects of methoxyflurane in dogs, consistently found a watery vacuolation of liver cord cells that was reversible. Jaundice in a dog following 4 hours of methoxyflurane anesthesia has been reported by Soma (1965). Douglas et al. (1964) have reported jaundice and elevated serum SGOT and bilirubin values in 3 horses 24 hours after the animals received methoxyflurane in a closed system.

Because of its safety for the patient and ease of administration, methoxyflurane has become the most popular inhalation anesthetic for small animals in the United States.

Enflurane (Ethrane; $CFHCl\text{-}CF_2\text{-}O\text{-}CF_2H$)

Enflurane is 2-chloro-1,1,2-trifluoroethyl difluoromethyl ether, a nonflammable anesthetic agent. It is a clear, colorless, stable liquid with a mild sweet odor. It does not decompose in contact with soda lime and does not attack aluminum, tin, brass, iron, or copper.

Induction and recovery from anesthesia with enflurane are rapid. It does not stimulate excess salivation or tracheal-bronchial secretions, or affect bronchomotor tone. The level of anesthesia can be changed rapidly. Ventilation is reduced as the depth of anesthesia increases. Blood pressure decreases with induction, but returns to near normal with surgical stimulation. In dogs, progressive increases in depth of anesthesia produce increasing hypotension (Klide, 1976). Cardiac rhythm generally remains stable, and there is no significant bradycardia.

The compatibility of enflurane and epinephrine has been studied in dogs by Krivosic et al. (1979). They anesthetized dogs with 1%, 2%, 3%, 4%, and 5% enflurane and then gave epinephrine by intravenous infusion for 5 minutes (1.4 μg/kg/min). No relationship was observed between the inspired enflurane concentrations and the onset of cardiac arrhythmias. Arrhythmias occurred in 23 of 50 dogs tested at all concentrations. These included premature ventricular contractions, bigeminy, trigeminy, and atrioventricular block. Significant differences between quantities of epinephrine necessary to provoke arrhythmias at the varying depths of anesthesia were not found, indicating that depth of anesthesia did not influence development of arrhythmias.

The potency of enflurane, halothane, and isoflurane was compared in horses (Table 10–4) by Steffey et al. (1977). Cardiovascular and respiratory parameters with enflurane anesthesia in horses are shown in Table 10–5. In studies on 6 ponies, Orsini and Taylor (1980) concluded that enflurane had no great advantage over halothane with respect to cardiopulmonary effects or margin of safety. Advantages included smooth, unusually rapid induction and emergence, and a lower level of biotransformation.

The concentration of enflurane delivered during anesthesia should be known. This may be determined by using either specifically calibrated enflurane vaporizers or vaporizers from which flows can be easily calculated. Generally, maintenance concentration should not exceed 3%. If a vaporizer not specifically calibrated for enflurane is used, delivered concentration may be estimated using the nomograph in Figure 10–5.

TABLE 10–4. Anesthetic Potency in Horses

Item	*Enflurane*	*Halothane*	*Isoflurane*
Age (years)	3.4 ± 0.5	2.6 ± 0.2	2.8 ± 0.3
Rectal temp (C)	38.0 ±0.1	37.9 ± 0.1	38.0 ± 0.2
MAC (volumes %)	2.12 ± 0.06	0.88 ± 0.03	1.31 ± 0.07
[(Insp-ET/ET)] × 100	10 ± 1	21 ± 3	17 ± 2
Apneic concentration (volumes %)	4.91 ± 0.32 (6)	2.37 ± 0.10 (6)	3.23 ± 0.15 (6)
Anesthetic index	2.26 ± 0.16 (6)	2.60 ± 0.13 (6)	2.33 ± 0.12 (6)

Mean ± standard error is given; n = 10 horses unless indicated differently in parentheses; Insp = inspired concentration; ET = end-tidal concentration; MAC = minimal alveolar concentration; anesthetic index = apneic concentration/MAC.

(From Steffey, E.P., Howland, D., Giri, S., and Eger, E.I., II: Enflurane, Halothane, and Isoflurane Potency in Horses. Am. J. Vet. Res., 38:1037, 1977.)

Muscle relaxation is generally good, and if greater relaxation is required, muscle relaxants may be used. All commonly employed relaxants are compatible with enflurane. The nondepolarizing relaxants are markedly potentiated. Deepening anesthesia may produce twitching in various muscle groups. This can be terminated by reducing the anesthetic concentration.

Increasing depth of anesthesia with enflurane produces a change in the electroencephalogram characterized by high voltage and fast frequency. This progresses through spike-dome complexes alternating with periods of electrical silence to frank seizure activity (Michenfelder and Cucchiara, 1974). The latter may or may not be associated with motor movement. Temporary behavioral changes have been reported in cats following enflurane anesthesia (Julien and Kavan, 1972).

Clark et al. (1979) exposed dogs and monkeys to anesthetic (1.5 MAC) and subanesthetic (1/100 MAC) levels of enflurane for 3 hours on alternate days for 4 weeks. They found that arterial blood pressure was lower (60 to 85 mm Hg) with enflurane than with halothane (70 to 105 mm Hg). Exposure to enflurane had no effect on ophthalmologic, bone marrow, hematologic, urinalysis, or clinical chemistry parameters. No serum enzyme abnormalities or increased BSP retention were observed in dogs treated with enflurane. Enflurane did not produce renal or hepatotoxicity in dogs or monkeys.

Reproduction studies in rats and rabbits indicate that enflurane is safe in pregnant animals.

TABLE 10–5. Enflurane Anesthesia in Horses

Variables	MAC *1.0*	MAC *1.5*	MAC *2.0*
Heart rate (beats/minute)	38 ± 2	39 ± 2	35 ± 4 (4)
Systolic arterial pressure (mm of Hg)	111 ± 12	91 ± 4	55 (2)
Respiratory frequency (breaths/minute)	6 ± 1	6 ± 1	8 ± 2 (4)
Pa_{O_2} (mm of Hg)	341 ± 50	164 ± 35	135 ± 38 (4)
Pa_{CO_2} (mm of Hg)	67 ± 2	73 ± 6	77 ± 13 (4)
Arterial pH	7.270 ± 0.020	7.240 ± 0.030	7.214 ± 0.076 (4)
Base excess (mEq/L)	0.5 ± 1.3	−0.5 ± 1.4	−1.4 ± 1.9 (4)
Inspired O_2 (%)	95.8 ± 0.2	96 ± 0	96 ± 0 (4)
Rectal temperature (C)	38.0 ± 0.3	37.6 ± 0	37.5 ± 0.3 (4)
Hematocrit (%)*	32.3 (3)	37.0 (3)	39.3 ± 6.6 (3)
Plasma proteins (g/dl)*	7.6 (3)	7.7 (3)	7.8 ± 0.3 (3)

Mean ± standard error is given; n = 5 horses unless indicated differently in parentheses.

MAC = Minimal alveolar concentration.

*Hematocrit and plasma protein concentration in awake horses was 37.3 ± 5.7% and 8.3 ± 0.0 g/dl, respectively.

(From Steffey, E.P., Howland, D., Giri, S. and Eger, E.I., II: Enflurane, Halothane, and Isoflurane Potency in Horses. Am. J. Vet. Res., 38:1037, 1977.)

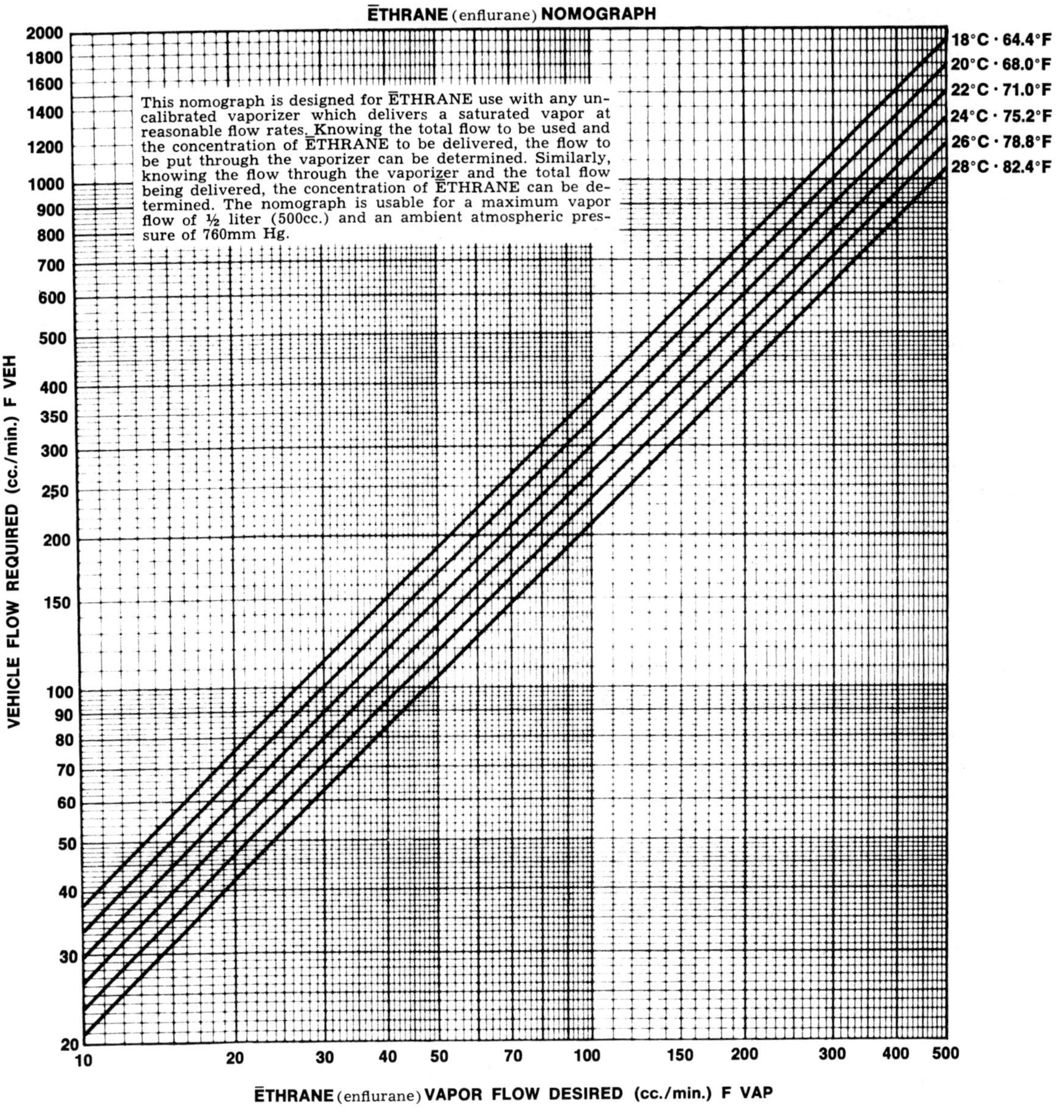

Figure 10–5. Knowing the total flow to be used (F_{TOT}), multiply this by the percent concentration V/V of Ethrane to be delivered to obtain Ethrane vapor flow (F_{VAP}). Locate this value on the horizontal scale and project a vertical line to intersect the sloped line representing vaporizer temperature. From this intersection, project a horizontal line to the vertical scale and read the corresponding value of the required vehicle flow (F_{VEH}) (flow through vaporizer). Set this rate on the vaporizer flowmeter. The diluent flow $F_{DIL} = F_{TOT} - F_{VAP} - F_{VEH}$. Calculate the diluent flow and distribute it as desired among flowmeters that do not supply the vaporizer. (Courtesy of Ohio Medical Anesthetics, a Division of Airco, Inc., Madison, Wisconsin.)

In man, at least 2.42% of administered enflurane undergoes biotransformation. Organic and inorganic fluorides are excreted in the urine for several days (Chase et al., 1971).

Halothane (Fluothane; $CF_3CHClBr$)

Halothane is a clear, colorless, volatile liquid with a nonirritating odor. Some decomposition occurs when it is exposed to light, so the liquid is stabilized by addition of 0.01% (w/w) thymol and stored in amber glass bottles. It is unaffected by warm soda lime and can be used in closed systems. Halothane is *nonexplosive* and *nonflammable* when mixed in high concentrations with oxygen.

Halothane vapor in concentrations of 2 to 4% produces stage III, plane 2 to 3 anesthesia in dogs and monkeys in 2 to 5 minutes. When the anesthesiologist is inducing halothane anesthesia in large animals, production of a minimal alveolar anesthetic concentration may be delayed due to the need for saturation of large circuit and patient volumes. Surgical anesthesia is maintained by inhalation of 0.8 to 1.2% mixtures, depending on whether preanesthetic agents are administered. On this basis, it is estimated that halothane is about twice as potent as chloroform and 4 times as potent as diethyl ether. Recovery occurs rapidly and, with prolonged anesthesia, is frequently complete in 10 to 20 minutes (Fig. 10–6). Even in horses and cattle premedicated with tranquilizers and induced with intravenous thiobarbiturate, recovery is rapid when anesthesia is maintained with halothane. Emergence struggling during recovery from halothane anesthesia is rarely a problem.

The action of halothane on the cardiovascular system is somewhat controversial. All investigators agree that a definite hypotension is produced (a decline of 20 to 40 mm Hg in the dog), but the mechanism is in question. It has been explained as 1) a ganglionic blocking action, 2) a central vasomotor depression, and 3) a direct depression of the myocardium. Following reduction in concentration of the drug, the blood pressure rapidly returns to normal levels, indicating lack of permanent damage to the cardiovascular system. In prolonged anesthesia, cardiovascular depression tends to lessen. Dogs under anesthesia have hyperemic mucous membranes, but bleeding in the operative field is not excessive. Many authors have commented on the absence of shock in both man and most animals anesthetized with this agent. In rhesus and stump-tailed macaques, halothane has a greater cardiovascular depressant effect than in dogs or man (Lees et al.,1971; Steffey et al., 1974).

Bradycardia due to vagal stimulation follows administration of halothane. Bradycardia increases with the depth of anesthesia, and is usually not a problem when lighter planes of surgical anesthesia are maintained (Table 10–6, Fig. 10–7). In deeper planes severe bradycardia occurs. Heart rates ranging from 12 to 20 per minute have been reported in 12 horses with concomitant respiratory rates of 4 to 6 per minute and systolic arterial pressures from 66 to 74 mm Hg (Vasko, 1962). Nodal rhythms, ven-

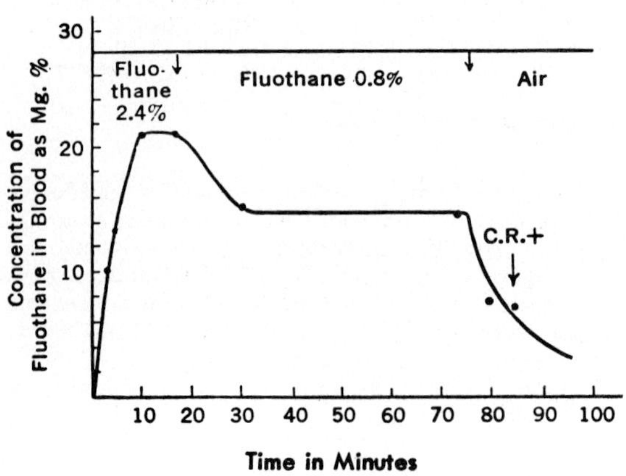

Figure 10–6. Concentration of halothane (Fluothane) in the blood of a dog during anesthesia. *C.R.*, Corneal reflex. (From Raventos, J.: The Action of Fluothane—A New Anesthetic. Br. J. Pharmacol., 11:394, 1956.)

TABLE 10–6. Heart Rates of Conscious and Anesthetized Horses

Heart rate (beats/min)	*Conscious (18)†*	*Anesthetized**	
		Halothane (19)†	*Ether (8)†*
Mean	44.4	48.2	62.8
S.E.	2.28	2.6	2.84
Range	24–60	32–70	44–76
P‡	—	>0.20	<0.001
P§	—	—	<0.01

*After one hour's anesthesia.

†Figures in parentheses indicate the number of animals.

‡The significance of differences between mean values for halothane and ether anesthesia compared with conscious animals as determined by *t* tests.

§The significance of differences between mean values of halothane compared to ether anesthesia as determined by *t* tests.

(From Tavernor, W.D., and Lees, P.: The Influence of Propranolol on Cardiovascular Function in Conscious and Anesthetized Horses. Arch. Int. Pharmacodyn., 180:89, 1969.)

tricular tachycardia, and varying degrees of arrhythmia were observed in 7 of the horses. Variations of cardiac rhythm are usually associated with carbon dioxide accumulation, hypoxia, catecholamine release, and overdosage. Halothane causes a decrease in myocardial blood flow, especially during hypotension, and an increase in vascular resistance within the myocardium (Vance et al., 1979). Although overdosage should be avoided, the bradycardia can be prevented by atropine, and many therefore prefer to premedicate with this drug. If, however, a cardiac or pulse monitor is used, progressive slowing of the heart rate does provide a useful warning that the degree of anesthesia is deep.

Hillidge and Lees (1977) determined the effects of thiopental-halothane and thiopental-ether anesthesia on left ventricular function in ponies. With both combinations, peak ventricular systolic pressure was reduced through a 120-minute period of anesthesia. The maximal effect occurred within the first 30 minutes. Reduction of peak systolic pressure was greatest in halothane-anesthetized animals. Left ventricular end-diastolic pressure was increased similarly with both ether and halothane. The durations of left ventricular systole and the periods of isometric tension development and isotonic contraction were reduced slightly during ether anesthesia, but the changes were usually insignificant. In ponies anesthetized with halothane, these variables increased significantly. The cardiovascular effects in horses of adding N_2O to halothane are shown in Figure 10–13 under the section on Nitrous Oxide.

Halothane sensitizes the myocardial conduction system to the action of epinephrine and norepinephrine, and arrhythmias may result (Hall and Norris, 1958). These can largely be prevented by premedication with acetylpromazine (Wiersig et al., 1974). Methoxamine and phenylephrine have traditionally been vasopressors of choice with halothane, because they have been shown to produce a blood pressure rise without alteration in cardiac rhythm. In thiamylal-halothane anesthetized dogs, Bednarski and Muir (1983) found the order of arrhythmogenicity of three catecholamines to be: epinephrine > dobutamine > dopamine (see Chap. 20). Should catecholamine-induced arrhythmias occur during halothane anesthesia, these may be effectively treated with propranolol (Tavernor and Lees, 1969).

In anemic dogs receiving halothane anesthesia, no differences were observed in cardiac output, blood pressure, heart rate, left ventricular end-diastolic pressure, or arterial base excess. It was concluded that halothane is a safe anesthetic during severe anemia (Loarie et al., 1979).

In animals, both the amplitude and frequency of respiratory movements are decreased with halothane. This results in progressive respiratory acidosis (Fig. 10–8). Inhalation of high concentrations produces apnea, which is easily reversible, but deaths in dogs, monkeys, cattle, sheep, horses, and swine have been reported. During experimental asphyxia of the sheep fetus, compensatory cerebrovascular dilation is impaired by maternal halothane anesthesia (Palahniuk et al., 1980). Respiratory failure precedes cardiac failure by a considerable margin. Because of its potency, the depth of halothane anesthesia can be altered with several respirations.

Salivary, mucous, and bronchial secretions

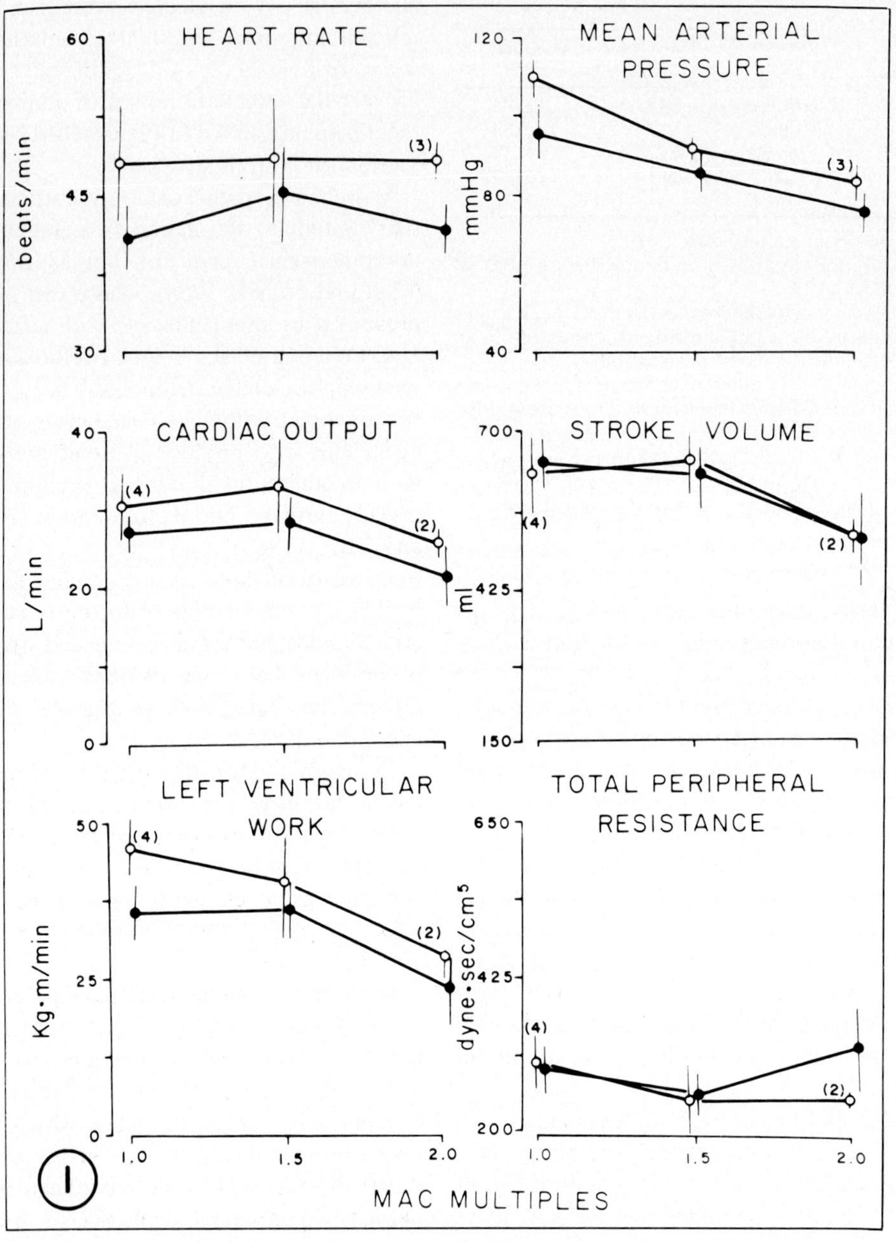

Figure 10–7. Cardiovascular effects of halothane (●) and isoflurane (○) in five horses during spontaneous ventilation. The $\overline{X} \pm 1$ SEM are indicated and the number of observations, if not five, are indicated in parentheses. MAC = minimal alveolar concentration. Significant differences ($P > 0.05$) are not present between isoflurane and halothane at equipotent doses (i.e. equal MAC multiple). (From Steffey, E.P. and Howland, D.: Comparison of Circulatory and Respiratory Effects of Isoflurane and Halothane Anesthesia in Horses. Am. J. Vet. Res., 41:821, 1980.)

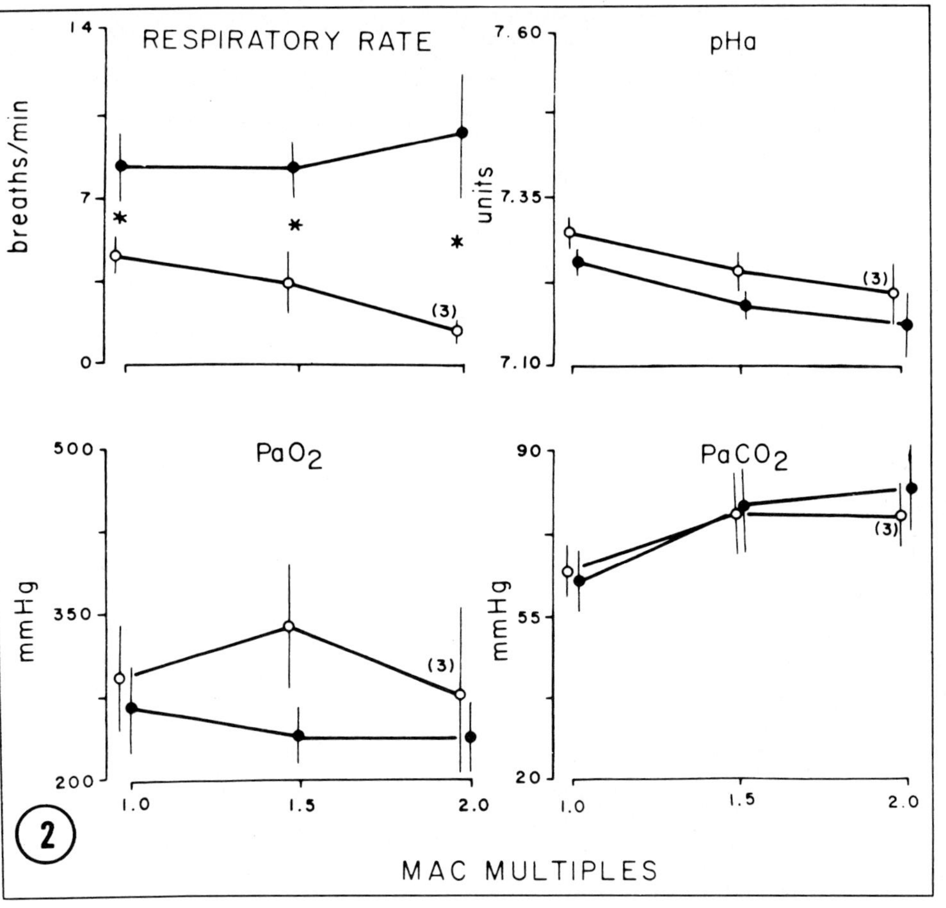

Figure 10–8. Effects of halothane (●) and isoflurane (○) in five horses during spontaneous ventilation. The $\bar{X} \pm 1$ SEM are indicated and the number of observations, if not five, are indicated in parentheses. Stars (*) indicate a significant difference ($P < 0.05$) between isoflurane and halothane anesthesia. (From Steffey, E.P. and Howland, D.: Comparison of Circulatory and Respiratory Effects of Isoflurane and Halothane Anesthesia in Horses. Am. J. Vet. Res., 41:821, 1980).

are absent during halothane anesthesia. Laryngospasm is not produced. Halothane significantly reduces bronchospasm (increased pulmonary resistance) resulting from administration of Ascar's antigen, and depresses mucociliary clearance (Hirshman and Bergman, 1978; Forbes and Gamsu, 1979). Vomiting is rarely a complication.

Minimal pathologic changes have been found in the livers of dogs, monkeys, horses, and sheep anesthetized for long periods, but nothing comparable to those seen following chloroform. Results of liver and kidney function tests following 3 hours of halothane anesthesia for 5 consecutive days were within normal limits (Stephen et al., 1958). Following 2 hours of surgical plane anesthesia in horses, Wolff et al. (1967) found slight centrilobular necrosis and glycogen depletion 2 days after anesthetic administration (Fig. 10–9).

Fatalities due to liver necrosis have been reported in man. Despite many such reports, a retrospective study failed to incriminate halothane specifically (Bunker, 1966). There is evidence, however, that repeated exposure to halothane may cause recurrent episodes of hepatitis. A recent report indicates that severe hepatic necrosis in man probably has a frequency of 1:20,000 to 35,000 anesthesias (Nimmo, 1980). Rapidly repeated exposures are

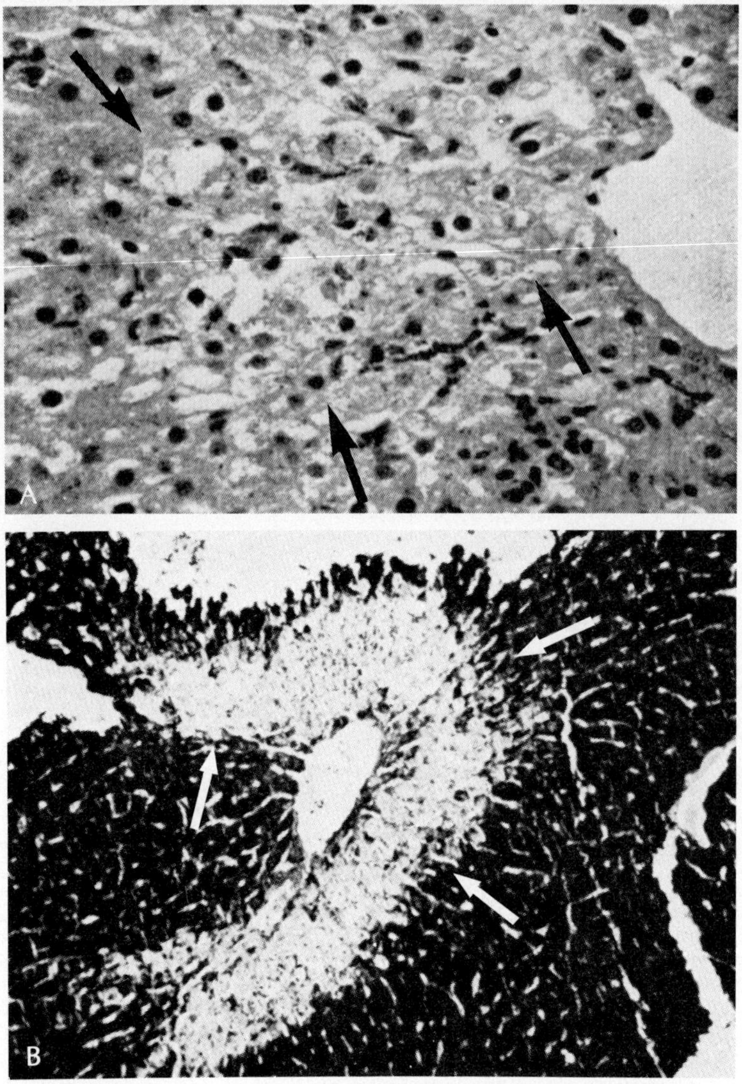

Figure 10–9. *A,* Centrilobular hepatic necrosis (arrows) in biopsy section from horse 2 days after halothane anesthesia. H&E stain; ×435. *B,* Centrilobular glycogen depletion in same horse. Periodic acid-Schiff reaction; ×100. (From Wolff, W.A., Lumb, W.V., and Ramsay, K.: Effects of Halothane and Chloroform Anesthesia on the Equine Liver. Am. J. Vet. Res., 28:1367, 1967.)

most frequently incriminated (Walton et al., 1976). Recurrent hepatitis due to halothane sensitization has been reported in an anesthetist (Klatskin and Kimberg, 1969). Sensitivity of certain strains of swine and occasional horses and dogs to halothane-triggered malignant hyperthermia has been observed (Jones et al., 1970) (see Chap. 21).

Halothane can be administered by mask, but it is difficult to control the level of anesthesia since small changes in concentration markedly change the depth. Both open and semiopen systems are wasteful of the agent and therefore almost prohibitive in cost, in all but very small dogs, cats, and small laboratory animals. Halothane is best used in a closed or semiclosed system with temperature-compensated vaporizers to give accurate control of the anesthetic concentration. When such techniques are used in the horse, it has been found that 2.2 to 8.7

ml of halothane per 100 lb of body weight are required to maintain anesthesia for 1 hour (Jones et al., 1962). Induction is accomplished by direct administration of vapor with a mask or anesthetic chamber, or by intravenous injection of a thiobarbiturate, followed by maintenance with halothane through an endotracheal catheter. The latter method of induction is usually preferred. When one is using thiobarbiturate induction techniques, however, it may be difficult to achieve smooth transition from intravenous to inhalation anesthesia owing to respiratory depression and ineffective alveolar ventilation. In such cases, assisted respiration or use of nitrous oxide in oxygen is advantageous. Nitrous oxide-oxygen mixtures are frequently given concurrently with halothane to potentiate analgesia. The anesthetizing effect of nitrous oxide at concentrations permitting adequate oxygenation (75% N_2O or less) in healthy dogs, cats, monkeys, and horses is relatively small (Table 10–7). In calves, use of 50% N_2O in inspired gases reduces halothane MAC from 0.76 vol. % with 100% O_2 to 0.59 vol % (Steffey and Howland, 1979). Whatever the induction technique, preanesthetic tranquilizers markedly cut the cost of halothane anesthesia, facilitate maintenance of an even plane of anesthesia, and assure a quiet recovery.

Halothane has been used in animals in combination with a wide variety of preanesthetic and anesthetic agents (Lumb, 1959; Jones et al., 1962). Succinylcholine, tubocurarine, gallamine, or pancuronium have been administered with halothane, but succinylcholine may be contraindicated, at least in horses (see Chap. 14).

Because halothane produces rapid induction and recovery, it is currently the most popular inhalation agent for use in large animals by partial or complete rebreathing techniques. In large animals, complications have included postanesthetic myopathy due to recumbency, faulty limb position, and impaired circulation (see Chap. 21).

Halothane is rapidly eliminated from the body, most being exhaled while a small portion is metabolized (Table 10–1, Fig. 10–10). See also Chapter. 2.

Halothane anesthesia causes increases of serum bromide in man (Tinker et al., 1976), horses (DeMoor et al., 1978), and dogs (Pedersoli, 1980). In man and horse, the highest concentrations occurred 48 to 72 hours after anesthesia, whereas in the dog, the highest concentration was at 24 hours. Bromide is a psychoactive ion that enters the chloride pool and is slowly excreted. Sedative or psychoactive levels of serum bromide thus become possible with repeated use of halothane anesthesia on a daily basis, or when other factors increase bromide intake or decrease excretion.

Isoflurane (Forane; $CF_3CHCl\text{-}O\text{-}CF_2H$)

Isoflurane is a new volatile liquid halogenated inhalation agent. It is nonflammable and nonexplosive, stable without a preservative, and nonreactive with soda lime. It has a mildly pungent ethereal odor. Its vapor pressure is almost

TABLE 10–7. Alveolar Halothane Concentration at 1.0 MAC with Increasing Concentrations of N_2O

Percent N_2O	0	25	50	75
		Percent Halothane at 1.0 MAC		
Dog	0.87 ± 0.02	0.74 ± 0.0	0.65 ± 0.01	0.57 ± 0.02
Cat	1.14 ± 0.03	0.98 ± 0.03	0.92 ± 0.03	0.79 ± 0.03
Monkey (*M. actoides*)	0.89 ± 0.02	0.76 ± 0.02	0.67 ± 0.02	0.56 ± 0.03
Horse	0.93 ± 0.04	0.82 ± 0.05	0.70 ± 0.05	—

± = Standard error

(From Steffey, E.P., and Howland, D.: Potency of Halothane-N_2O in the Horse. Am. J. Vet. Res., 39:1141, 1978 and Steffey, E.P., Gillespie, J.R., Eger, E.I., II, Berry, J., and Munson, E.S.: The Anesthetic Potency (MAC) of Nitrous Oxide in the Dog, Cat, and Monkey *(M. actoides)*. J. Appl. Physiol., 36:530, 1974.)

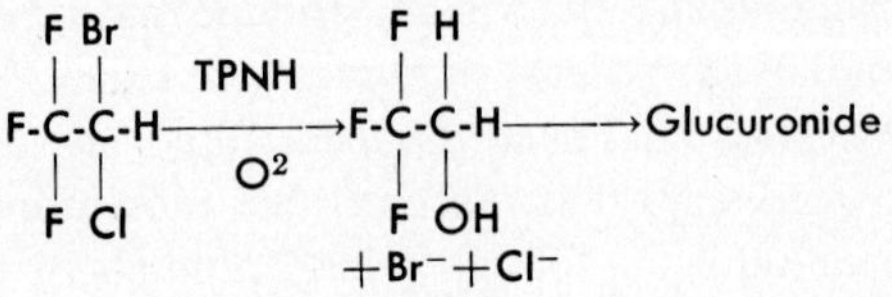

Figure 10–10. Metabolic pathway of halothane. (From Chenoweth, M.B.: Physiologic and Biochemical Responses to Methoxyflurane Anesthesia. In *Experimental Animal Anesthesiology.* Edited by D.C. Sawyer. U.S.A.F. School of Aerospace Medicine, Brooks Air Force Base, Texas, 1965.)

identical to that of halothane, enabling the use of isoflurane in halothane vaporizers.

The MAC for isoflurane does not change with duration of anesthesia. In addition, MAC varies only a small amount between species, being lowest in primates (1.28%) and highest in cats (1.635%). The anesthetic index* is 2.5 for dogs, 2.4 for cats, and 2.33 for horses (Steffey and Howland, 1977; Steffey et al., 1977).

Steffey and his associates have extensively studied the effects of isoflurane in horses (Steffey, 1978; Steffey et al., 1979; Steffey and Howland, 1980). They found that long-term and/or profound anesthesia with isoflurane produced minimal changes in blood counts and biochemical values. When compared with enflurane, isoflurane causes less reduction in cardiovascular function, and cardiac rhythm remains stable (see Fig. 10–7). A dose-dependent reduction in respiratory rate occurs with isoflurane, and changes in respiratory rate in horses are indicative of anesthetic depth (see Fig. 10–8).

In the dog, isoflurane depresses cardiopulmonary function less than enflurane (Klide, 1976). It has less tendency to sensitize the heart to sympathomimetic amines than does halothane (Tucker et al., 1974) (Fig. 10–11). Isoflurane is a profound respiratory depressant in both dogs and cats, and produces a dose-dependent increase in $Paco_2$ (Table 10–8).

Isoflurane increases cerebral blood flow and intracranial pressure. The latter can be reduced by decreasing $Paco_2$. Isoflurane enhances the action of muscle relaxants. This effect is greater than that occurring with halothane.

*The alveolar concentration required to produce at least 60 seconds of apnea divided by MAC.

Studies by Murphy et al. (1973) indicate that isoflurane can initiate fatal hyperthermia in susceptible swine. The propensity for this phenomenon is equal to that of enflurane and less than that of halothane.

Studies in rats, guinea pigs, dogs, monkeys, and horses indicate that isoflurane is not a significant hepatotoxin. Renal blood flow, glomerular filtration rate, and urinary flow are reduced.

Three pathways for metabolism of isoflurane have been proposed. All three produce organic and inorganic fluoride as end products, although the amount of the latter is minute. The metabolism of isoflurane is far less than with any other modern halogenated agent.

Isoflurane has not been released for veterinary use in the United States, but is used in human patients. Because of its desirable features, it probably will be employed soon in animal anesthesia.

Chloroform, U.S.P. ($CHCl_3$)

Because of cardiovascular, hepatic, and renal toxicity, chloroform is no longer used in clinical anesthesia. For information concerning it, the reader is referred to the first edition of this text.

Ethyl Chloride, U.S.P. (C_2H_5Cl) and Trichloroethylene, U.S.P. (Trichlorethylene; Trilene; Trimar; Chlorylene; Westrosol; $CCl_2 = CHCl$)

Both ethyl chloride and trichlorethylene have been used as inhalation anesthetics. Their disadvantages include cardiotoxicity, poor muscle relaxation, and sensitization to epinephrine. For these reasons, they have been supplanted by newer, safer agents. For information concerning them, the reader is referred to the first edition of this text.

For information concerning ethyl chloride as a local anesthetic, see Chapter 15.

ANESTHETIC GASES

Nitrous Oxide, U.S.P. (N_2O)

Nitrous oxide is a colorless, sweet-tasting, nonirritating gas that is 1.53 times heavier than air. It is nonflammable, though it will support

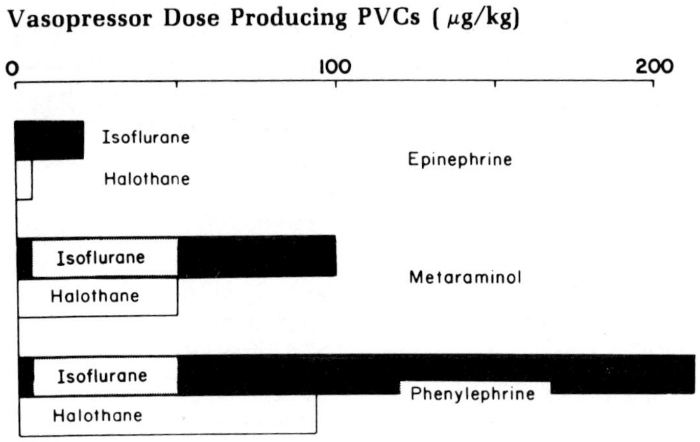

Figure 10–11. Dogs given 1.2 MAC isoflurane develop premature ventricular contractions (PVCs) at higher doses of epinephrine, metaraminol or phenylephrine than dogs given 1.2 MAC halothane. (From Tucker, W.K., Rakstein, A.D., and Munson, E.S.: Comparison of Arrhythmic Doses of Adrenaline, Metaraminol, Ephedrine and Phenylephrine During Isoflurane Anaesthesia in Dogs. Br. J. Anaesth., 46:392, 1974.)

TABLE 10–8. Isoflurane Anesthesia in 8 Spontaneously Breathing Cats (Mean ± SE)

	MAC *Multiples*			
	1.0	*1.5*	*2.0*	*2.4**
Mean aortic pressure (mm Hg)	85 ± 9[a,b,c]	61 ± 3[b]	53 ± 3	64 ± 7 (7)
Heart rate (beats/min)	148 ± 7[a]	134 ± 6[c]	137 ± 5[c]	161 ± 10 (7)
Respiratory frequency (breaths/min)	36 ± 5[a,c]	27 ± 2[c]	28 ±2[c]	0 (7)
Pa_{O_2} (mm Hg)	483 ± 19[c]	459 ± 19[c]	439 ± 23	349 ± 39 (6)
Pa_{CO_2} (mm Hg)	35 ±2[a,b,c]	40 ± 2[b,c]	61 ± 3[c]	117 ± 10 (6)
pHa	7.37 ± 0.02[a,b,c]	7.32 ± 0.02[b,c]	7.16 ± 0.03[c]	6.94 ± 0.03 (6)
Base excess (mEq/L)	−4.5 ± 1.4[b,c]	−5.3 ± 1.0[b,c]	−7.4 ± 1.3[c]	−10 ± 1.9 (6)
Packed cell volume (%)	34 ± 2	35 ± 1	36 ± 1	37.5 ± 2 (6)
Plasma proteins (g/dl)	5.7 ± 0.3[c]	5.6 ± 0.4	5.4 ± 0.3	5.2 ± 0.4 (6)
Esophageal temperatures (C)	37.9 ± 0.2	37.9 ± 0.2	37.8 ± 0.2	37.9 ± 0.2 (7)

Parentheses indicate n if less than 8.
*Measurements taken after 60 seconds of apnea.
[a]Significantly different from 1.5 MAC.
[b]Significantly different from 2.0 MAC.
[c]Significantly different from 2.4 MAC.
(From Steffey, E.P., and Howland, D., Jr.: Isoflurane Potency in the Dog and Cat. Am. J. Vet. Res., 38:1833, 1977.)

combustion. The gas is produced by heating ammonium nitrate to about 250°C. It is com-

$$NH_4NO_3 \xrightarrow[\Delta]{} N_2O + 2H_2O$$

pressed into liquid at a pressure of about 30 atmospheres and marketed in cylinders at 650 to 800 psi. Nitrous oxide is administered with a semiclosed or closed system with oxygen.

Nitrous oxide is exhaled unaltered from the lungs. It is an innocuous agent when used with adequate oxygen, dogs having been anesthetized as long as 72 hours without harm. It is considered the safest of the inhalant anesthetics, but has been shown to cause teratogenic effects in rats (Lane et al., 1980). There is a mild leukocytosis that persists less than 24 hours after administration has ceased.

Nitrous oxide must be given in at least 80% concentration to produce anesthesia. *A common cause for death when using N_2O is failure to add sufficient O_2 to the anesthetic mixture* (see Chap. 23). It should be pointed out that the body must have at least 15% oxygen or progressive hypoxia develops. Symptoms and lesions that have developed following anesthesia have been attributed to hypoxia and asphyxia.

Because it is nonexplosive, nonirritating, quickly absorbed, and eliminated, nitrous oxide is one of the best available gaseous agents if used with sufficient oxygen. Its chief disadvantage is lack of potency.

To obtain the maximum effects from nitrous oxide, it should not be unnecessarily diluted with either oxygen or nitrogen, and the animal must be saturated with the nitrous oxide. Initial administration of a high concentration with minimal rebreathing is therefore necessary to eliminate the nitrogen from the system (Fig. 10–12). Once this has been accomplished, the degree of

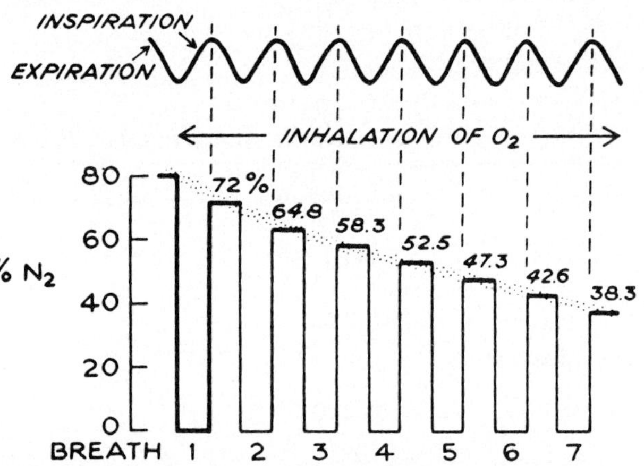

F.R.C. INCLUDING D.S. ml.	3150	3150	3150	3150	3150	3150	3150
ALVEOLAR T.V. ml	350	350	350	350	350	350	350
% DILUTION OF F.R.C.	10%	10%	10%	10%	10%	10%	10%
% N_2 IN ALVEOLI BEGINNING INSPIRATION	80	72	64.8	58.3	52.5	47.3	42.6
DECREASE IN % N_2	8	7.2	6.48	5.83	5.25	4.73	4.26
% N_2 IN ALVEOLI END INSPIRATION	72	64.8	58.3	52.5	47.3	42.6	38.3

Figure 10–12. Pulmonary N_2 washout curve. A man with uniform distribution of inspired gas breathes O_2 at constant alveolar tidal volume of 350 ml; the N_2 concentration of inspired and expired gas is recorded continuously by a N_2 meter. The plateaus represent expired *alveolar* gas (after washout of anatomic dead space). This N_2 washout curve is a single exponential curve. The alveolar N_2 concentrations at the beginning and end of each inspiration show a 10% dilution with each breath. (From Comroe, J.H.: *Physiology of Respiration*. Year Book Medical Publishers, Chicago, 1974.)

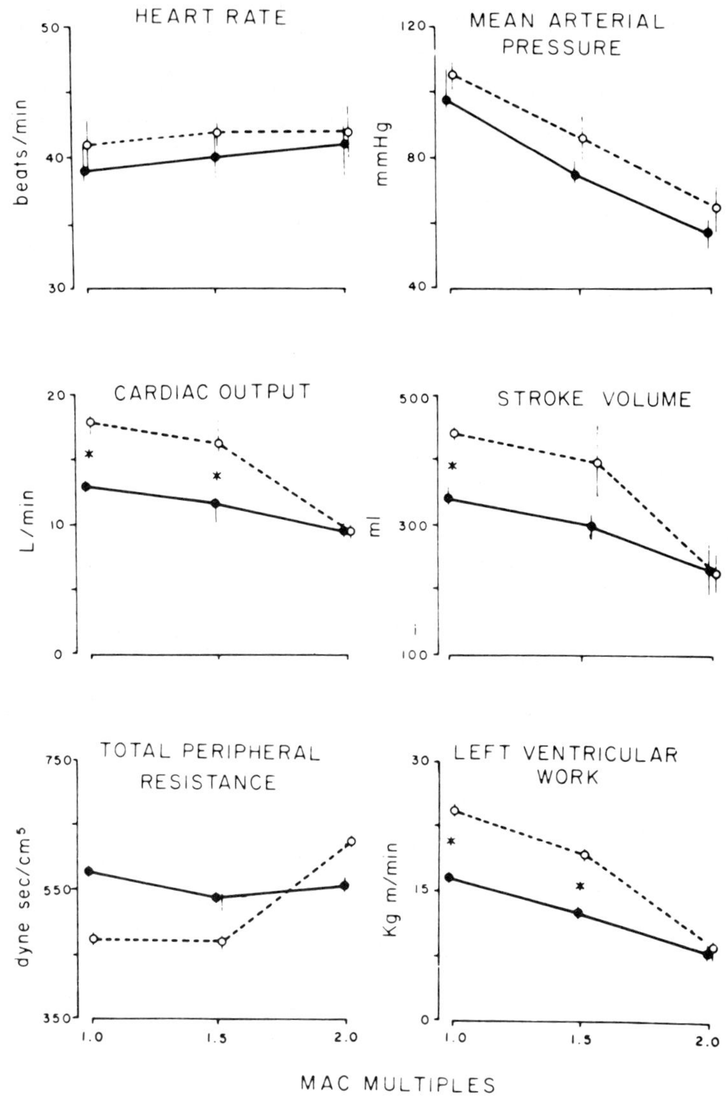

Figure 10–13. The cardiovascular effects of halothane-O_2 (closed circles, solid line) and halothane-50% N_2O-O_2 (open circles, dotted line) in horses during controlled ventilation. The mean ± SEM are shown and * = $P < 0.05$. (From Steffey, E.P., and Howland, D.: Potency of Halothane-N_2O in the Horse. Am. J. Vet. Res., 39:1141, 1978.)

rebreathing can be increased, although it is important to realize that at low gas inflow rates, oxygen consumption may reduce the oxygen content of respired gases to subminimal levels (see Respiratory and Anesthetic Gases, Chap. 19). Diffusion of nitrous oxide into the alveoli during recovery from prolonged nitrous oxide administration may likewise induce hypoxia by dilution of the alveolar oxygen concentration. This phenomenon has been termed ''diffusion anoxia.''

Nitrous oxide alone provides inadequate anesthesia except for the most minor operation; therefore, it is not commonly used as the sole anesthetic agent. However, nitrous oxide-oxygen mixtures (4:1 to 1:1) are useful for vaporization and supplementation of volatile liquid anesthetics during administration by partial rebreathing. Addition of N_2O reduces the amount of volatile agent required. The reduction in concentration of halothane produced by addition of N_2O is shown in Table 10–7. The degree of reduction varies with species. High flow rates have been advocated with mixtures of N_2O-O_2 plus volatile agents. Virtue et al. (1979), on the other hand, have shown that concentrations of anesthetic agents in operating rooms can be materially reduced by using low flow rates, and the cost for anesthesia can be drastically reduced.

Because of its good analgesic properties and innocuous character, N_2O is frequently used with a small amount of volatile liquid anesthetic in poor-risk patients. Addition of N_2O to anesthesia produced by a volatile liquid agent reduces the required concentration of the latter. This, in turn, has a sparing effect on cardiopulmonary function (Fig. 10–13).

Another advantage of N_2O combined with a volatile agent is that induction is accelerated by the "second gas" effect (Epstein et al., 1964; Stoelting and Eger, 1969). In this situation, N_2O is rapidly diffused to and absorbed from the lung, and as this occurs the rate of delivery of the second agent to the alveoli is increased. The net effect is that the arterial tension of the second gas rises more quickly in the presence of N_2O.

With preanesthetic narcotics, such as meperidine, fentanyl, or oxymorphone, N_2O-O_2 (1:1, 2:1 or 3:1) is often adequate to maintain light planes of anesthesia following intravenous barbiturate induction. Other agents such as ketamine and xylazine or mixtures containing these agents (see Chaps. 8 and 13) also are satisfactory with N_2O. Muscle relaxants may be added to the preceding combinations to achieve immobilization; however, care must be taken that adequate analgesia is provided.

Administration of 60% nitrous oxide to dogs has been shown to increase cerebral metabolism and cerebral blood flow, with EEG slowing (Sakabe et al., 1978). Nitrous oxide has little effect on somatosensory evoked potentials, and for this reason is often used in combination with narcotics when potentials are being recorded (Fialho and Lumb, 1980).

Nitrous oxide is 32 times more soluble in blood than is nitrogen and, therefore, can replace N_2 in blood and other biologic solvents. Because of this greater solubility, organs containing gas increase in volume during N_2O administration. Steffey et al. (1979) demonstrated this phenomenon in the bowels of dogs and horses, and found that the distention could not be reversed in a few minutes. The same phenomenon occurs in patients with pneumothorax.

The need to use high concentrations (50% or more) of nitrous oxide necessitates special consideration of potential environmental hazards (see Chap. 21). Epidemiologic studies of anesthetists, anesthesiologists, and dentists have suggested higher risks of spontaneous miscarriage, liver disease, and other serious health problems, although these individuals were also exposed to other anesthetic gases. Animal studies have revealed slow recovery of testicular function after chronic exposure in mice, bone marrow changes in rats, changes in lysosomal cells in lungs of mice, and damage to cortical cells in the occipital region of rats (Anonymous, 1980).

Cyclopropane, U.S.P. (Trimethylene; C_3H_6) and Ethylene, U.S.P. ($CH_2{=}CH_2$)

Cyclopropane and ethylene have never been widely used in veterinary anesthesia in the United States because 1) both are flammable and explosive, and 2) veterinarians have not had suitable facilities in which to use these agents. The advent of newer halogenated hydrocarbons has virtually obviated their use. For a description of these agents, the reader is referred to the first edition of this text.

Carbon Dioxide (CO_2)

Carbon dioxide is used as an anesthetic gas for laboratory animals (see Chaps. 6 and 18).

PHYSICAL PROPERTIES OF MEDICAL GASES

Gases that are liquefied when compressed in cylinders are nitrous oxide, cyclopropane, and carbon dioxide. Gases that are nonliquefied include oxygen, helium, carbon dioxide-oxygen mixtures, helium-oxygen mixtures, and ethylene.

Pressure in cylinders containing liquefied compressed gas and vapor in equilibrium is de-

FIGURE 10–15. Net contents of cylinders for all gases.*†

Cylinder Color Code

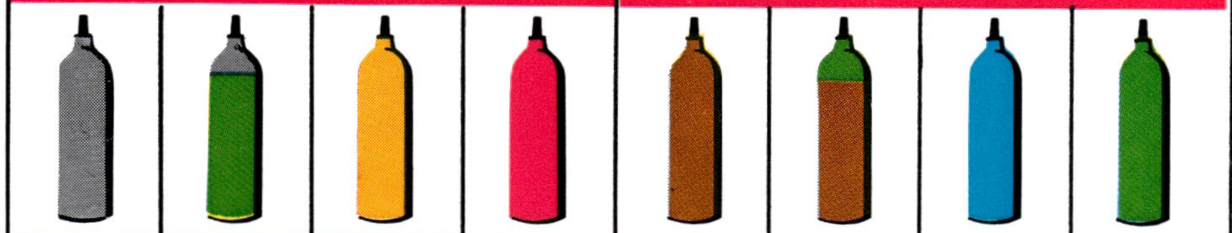

Size	CO_2	CO_2-O_2	$(CH_2)_3$	C_2H_4	He	He-O_2	N_2O	O_2	Cylinder Dimensions	Weight of Empty Cylinder (lbs.)
G	3200 gals.	1400 gals.		2800 gals.	1100 gals.	1126 gals.	3655 gals.	1400 gals.	$8\frac{1}{2} \times 55''$	100
M		800 gals.		1600 gals.			2000 gals.	800 gals.	$7 \times 47''$	66
E		165 gals.		330 gals.			420 gals.	165 gals.	$4\frac{1}{4} \times 29\frac{3}{4}''$	15
D	250 gals.	95 gals.	230 gals.	200 gals.	80 gals.	82 gals.	250 gals.	95 gals.	$4\frac{1}{4} \times 20\frac{1}{4}''$	$10\frac{1}{4}$
B		40 gals.		100 gals.			100 gals.	40 gals.	$3\frac{1}{4} \times 16\frac{1}{2}''$	$5\frac{3}{4}$
A	50 gals.	20 gals.		40 gals.	15 gals.	15 gals.	50 gals.	20 gals.	$3 \times 10\frac{3}{4}''$	$2\frac{1}{2}$
†DD			230 gals.						$3\frac{3}{4} \times 23\frac{1}{4}''$	$8\frac{3}{4}$
†BB			100 gals.						$2\frac{3}{4} \times 19\frac{3}{4}''$	4
†AA			40 gals.						$2\frac{3}{4} \times 11''$	3

* Courtesy of Ohio Chemical & Surgical Equipment Co.

† Cyclopropane cylinders may be chrome plated and bear orange labels.

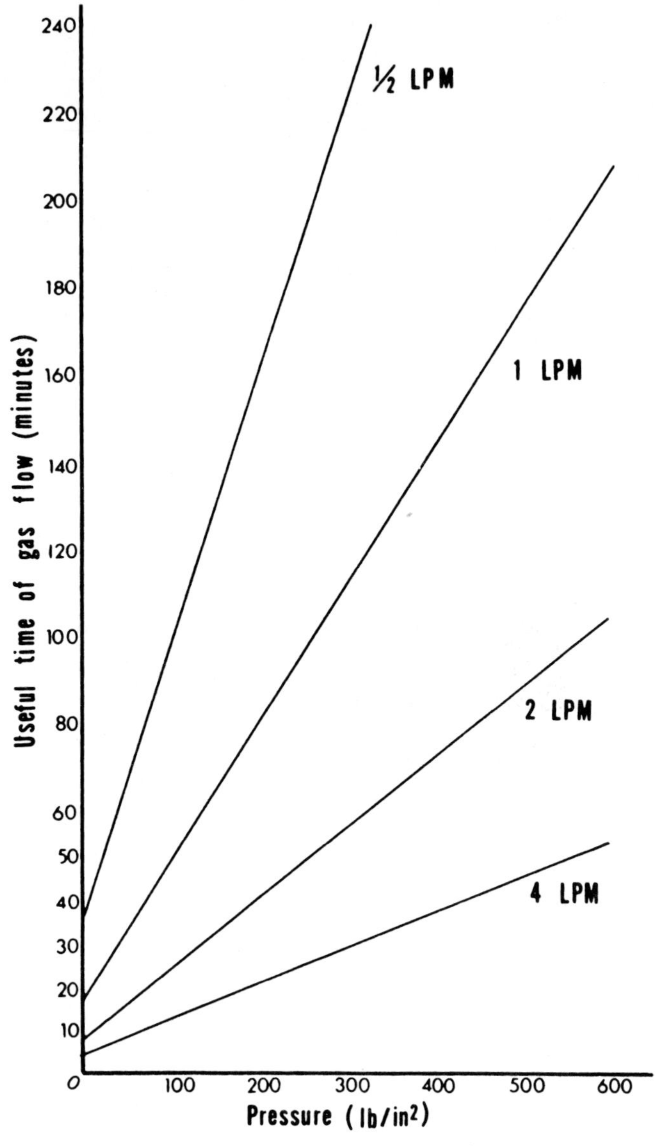

Figure 10–14. Estimated useful time remaining for an E cylinder of nitrous oxide when the pressure is less than 700 psi and the cylinder is equilibrated at a room temperature of 22 degrees C (71.6 F) at the beginning of use. (From Haskins, S.C., and Sansome, A.L.: A Timetable for Exhaustion of Nitrous Oxide Cylinders Using Cylinder Pressure. Vet. Anesth., 6:6, 1979.)

termined by the vapor pressure of the liquid at the existing temperature, and has no relation to the amount of liquid remaining in the cylinder. At a constant temperature, pressure in a cylinder filled with liquefied compressed gas remains approximately constant until all the liquid has been exhausted, at which time the pressure drops as the remaining gas is withdrawn. Pressure in a cylinder containing liquefied compressed gas, therefore, is not an indication of the amount of remaining gas. This can be determined only by weighing the cylinder.

Haskins and Sansome (1979) have studied the emptying time of nitrous oxide cylinders that register less than 700 psi at room temperature. Figure 10–14 indicates the remaining useful time of E cylinders.*

The pressure in cylinders charged with non-

*See the section on Physical Properties of Medical Gases for further discussion.

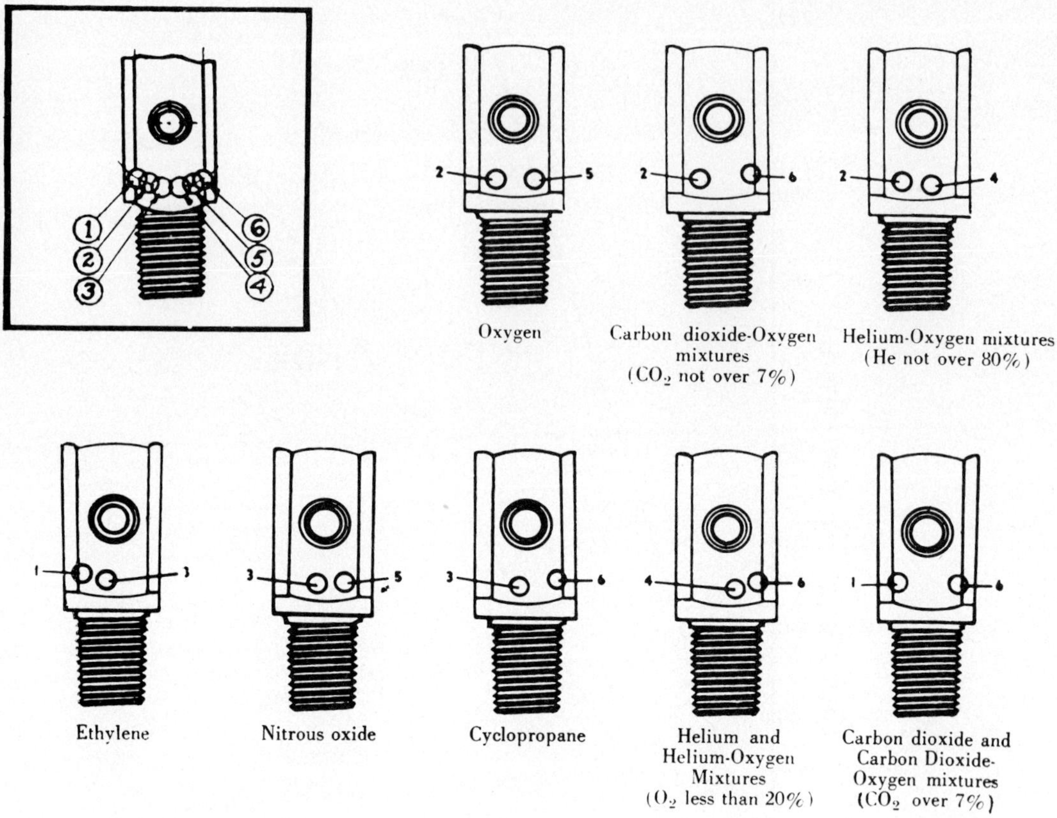

Figure 10–16. Pin index safety system. (Courtesy of Ohio Chemical and Surgical Equipment Company.)

liquefied compressed gas is related to the temperature and the amount of gas remaining in the cylinder. With the temperature constant, if the pressure is reduced by one-half, the cylinder will be approximately one-half full.

Cylinder sizes and approximate contents for the various gases are shown in Figure 10–15.

REGULATIONS CONCERNING MEDICAL GASES

Interstate shipment of compressed gases is regulated by the United States Government under the provisions of an Act of Congress dated March 4, 1921. This Act states that cylinders containing medical gases that are shipped in commerce are subject to the jurisdiction of the Interstate Commerce Commission and must comply with ICC specifications.* In addition, medical gases are also regulated by the Federal Food, Drug and Cosmetic Act. This Act states that medical gases must conform to the standards of the *Pharmacopeia of the United States* and must be appropriately labeled.

A cylinder color code entitled *Simplified Practice Recommendation R176-41 of the Bureau of Standards* has been published by the U.S. Department of Commerce. The code stipulates a cylinder color for each gas to enable quick recognition of cylinder content.

*The ICC cylinder specifications and regulations have been reprinted by the Bureau of Explosives of the Association of American Railroads as "Interstate Commerce Commission Regulations for Transportation of Explosives and Other Dangerous Articles by Land and Water in Rail Freight Service and by Motor Vehicle (Highway) and Water Including Specifications for Shipping Containers." This pamphlet is available from the Bureau of Explosives, 30 Vesey Street, New York, New York 10007.

Kind of Gas	*Cylinder Color*
Oxygen	Green
Carbon Dioxide	Gray
Nitrous Oxide	Light Blue
Cyclopropane	Orange
Helium	Brown
Ethylene	Red
Carbon Dioxide and Oxygen	Gray and Green
Helium and Oxygen	Brown and Green

It should be remembered, however, that the preceding color code is to be used only as a guide. The primary identification of the cylinder content is *always* the label.

PIN INDEX SYSTEM

To prevent inadvertent connection of the wrong gas to an anesthetic machine, the American Standard Connection No. 860 pin index safety system has been developed (Fig. 10–16). The system consists of two pins protruding from the yoke of the anesthesia machine. These pins must fit into matching holes in the gas cylinder. Each gas is assigned a specific code for the two-pin holes, thus preventing attachment of the wrong kind of gas cylinder to the yoke.

Disposal of waste anesthetic gases from operating rooms is discussed in Chapter 11.

REFERENCES

Anonymous: Nitrous Oxide Hazards. FDA Drug Bulletin 10:15, 1980.

Austin, W.H., and Villandry, P.J.: Methoxyflurane and Renal Function. Anesthesiology, 28:637, 1967.

Bednarski, R.M., and Muir, W.W.: Arrhythmogenicity of Dopamine, Dobutamine, and Epinephrine in Thiamylal-Halothane Anesthetized Dogs. Am. J. Vet. Res., 44:2341, 1983.

Bergeron, J.L., Shinaberger J.H., Frederickson, E.L., Martinez, F.J., and Buckalew, V.M.: The Effect of Methoxyflurane (M) Anesthesia on Renal Tubular Handling of Water. Paper presented at the Southern Anesthesia Society Meeting, 1966.

Blalock, A.: The Effects of Ether, Chloroform, and Ethyl Chloride Anaesthetics on the Minute Cardiac Output and Blood Pressure. Surg. Gynecol. Obstet., 46:72, 1928.

Brunson, D.B., Stowe, C.M., and McGrath, C.J.: Serum and Urine Inorganic Fluoride Concentrations and Urine Oxalate Concentrations Following Methoxyflurane Anesthesia in the Dog. Am. J. Vet. Res., 40:197, 1979.

Bunker, J.P.: Summary of the National Halothane Study: Possible Association between Halothane Anesthesia and Postoperative Hepatic Necrosis. J.A.M.A., 197:775, 1966.

Cale, J.O., Colby, R.P., and Jenkins, M.T.: Hepatic and Renal Effects of Methoxyflurane in Dogs. Anesthesiology, 23:248, 1962.

Chase, R.E., Holaday, D.A., Fiserova-Bergerova, V., Saidman, L.J., and Mack, F.E.: The Biotransformation of Ethrane in Man. Anesthesiology, 35:262, 1971.

Clark, G.C., Kesterson, J.W., Coombs, D.W., Cherry, C.P., Prentice, D.E., and Kohn, F.E.: Comparative Effects of Repeated and Prolonged Inhalation Exposure of Beagle Dogs and Cynomolgus Monkeys to Anaesthetic and Subanaesthetic Concentrations of Enflurane and Halothane. Anaesth. Scand. (Suppl.), 71:1, 1979.

Crandell, W.B., and MacDonald, A.: Nephropathy Associated with Methoxyflurane Anesthesia. J.A.M.A., 205:174, 1968.

Crandell, W.B., Pappas, S.G., and MacDonald, A.: Nephrotoxicity Associated with Methoxyflurane Anesthesia. Anesthesiology, 27:591, 1966.

DeMoor, A., Van Den Hende, C., Moens, Y., and Desmet, P.: Increased Plasma Bromide Concentration in the Horse after Halothane Anesthesia. Am. J. Vet. Res., 39:1624, 1978.

Douglas, T.A., Jennings, S., Longstreeth, J., and Weaver, A.D.: Methoxyflurane Anesthesia in Horses and Cattle. Vet. Rec., 76:615, 1964.

Durkin, M.G., Brick, I.E., and Schreiner, G.E.: Fatal Hepatic Necrosis Following Penthrane Anesthesia. Gastroenterology, 50:420, 1966.

Eger, E.I., and Brandstater, B.: Solubility of Methoxyflurane in Rubber. Anesthesiology, 24:679, 1963.

Elkington, S.G., Goffinet, J.A., and Conn, H.O.: Renal and Hepatic Injury Associated with Methoxyflurane Anesthesia. Ann. Intern. Med., 69:1229, 1968.

Epstein, R.M., Rackow, H., Salanitre, E., and Wolf, G.L.: Influence of the Concentration Effect on the Uptake of Anesthetic Mixtures: The Second Gas Effect. Anesthesiology, 25:364, 1964.

Fialho, S.A.G., and Lumb, W.V.: Anesthesia for Spinal Trauma and Recording Somatosensory Evoked Potentials. Vet. Anesth., 8:18, 1980.

Forbes, A.R., and Gamsu, G.: Depression of Lung Mucociliary Clearance by Thiopental and Halothane. Anesth. Analg., 58:387, 1979.

Gilman, A.G., Goodman, L.S., and Gilman, A.: *The Pharmacological Basis of Therapeutics,* 6th ed. Macmillan Publishing Company, Inc., New York, 1980.

Hall, K.D., and Norris, F.H., Jr.: Fluothane Sensitization of Dog Heart to Action of Epinephrine. Anesthesiology, 19:631, 1958.

Halsey, M.J., Sawyer, D.C., Eger, E.I., II, Bahlman, S.H., and Impelman, D.M.K.: Hepatic Metabolism of Halothane, Methoxyflurane, Cyclopropane, Ethane and Forane in Miniature Swine. Anesthesiology, 35:43, 1971.

Haskins, S.C., and Sansome, A.L.: A Timetable of Exhaustion of Nitrous Oxide Cylinders Using Cylinder Pressure. Vet. Anesth., 6:6, 1979.

Heinze, C.D.: Methoxyflurane Anesthesia in Large Animals. J.A.V.M.A., 147:1411, 1965.

Hezel, W.M.: Use of Methoxyflurane in Veterinary Medicine. Pract. Vet., 48:(1, 2, 3) 4, 1976.

Hillidge, C.J., and Lees, P.: Left Ventricular Systole in Conscious and Anesthetized Horses. Am. J. Vet. Res., 38:675, 1977.

Hirshman, C.A., and Bergman, N.A.: Halothane and Enflurane Protect Against Bronchospasm in an Asthma Dog Model. Anesth. Analg., 57:629, 1978.

Jones, E.W., Burnap, T.K., Nelson, T.E., Anderson, I.L., and Kerr, D.D.: Preliminary Studies on Fulminant Hyperpyrexia in a Family of Swine. Proceedings, Annual Meeting, Am. Soc. Anesthes., 1970.

Jones, E.W., Vasko, K.A., Hamm, D., and Griffith, R.W.: Equine General Anesthesia: Use of Halothane for Maintenance. J.A.V.M.A., 140:148, 1962.

Julien, R.M., and Kavan, E.M.: Electrographic Studies of a New Volatile Anesthetic Agent: Enflurane (Ethrane). J. Pharmacol. Exp. Ther., 183:393, 1972.

Kataoka, Y.: Liver Necrosis after Methoxyflurane Anesthesia. Jpn. J. Anesth., 14:1158, 1965.

Klatskin, G., and Kimberg, D.V.: Recurrent Hepatitis Attributable to Halothane Sensitization in an Anesthetist. N. Engl. J. Med., 280:515, 1969.

Klein, N.C., and Jeffries, G.H.: Hepatotoxicity after Methoxyflurane Administration. J.A.M.A., 197:207, 1966.

Klide, A.M.: Cardiopulmonary Effects of Enflurane and Isoflurane in the Dog. Am. J. Vet. Res., 37:127, 1976.

Krivosic, R., Besse, M.D., Bosznai, Z., and Moreau, D.: Compatibility of Enflurane and Adrenalin—Experiments in the Dog. Anaesth. Scand. (Suppl.), 71:52, 1979.

Kuzucu, E.Y.: Methoxyflurane, Tetracycline, and Renal Failure. J.A.M.A., 211:1162, 1970.

Lane, G.A., Nahrwold, M.L., Tait, A.R., Taylor-Busch, M., and Cohen, P.J.: Anesthetics as Teratogens: Nitrous Oxide is Fetotoxic, Xenon is not. Science, 210:899, 1980.

Lees, M.H., Hill, J., Ochsner, A.J., III, and Thomas, C.: Regional Blood Flows of the Rhesus Monkey During Halothane Anesthesia. Anesth. Analg., 50:270, 1971.

Lindenbaum, J., and Leifer, E.: Hepatic Necrosis Associated with Halothane Anesthesia. N. Engl. J. Med., 268:525, 1963.

Loarie, D.J., Wilkinson, P., Tyberg, J., and White, A.: The Hemodynamic Effects of Halothane in Anemic Dogs. Anesth. Analg., 58:195, 1979.

Lumb, W.V.: Closed-Circuit Halothane Anesthesia in the Dog. J.A.V.M.A., 134:218, 1959.

MacNider, W. deB: Naturally Nephropathic Animals: The Ability of an Alkaline Solution to Influence the Amount of Stainable Lipoid Material that Appears in the Kidney Following the Use of a General Anesthetic. J. Pharmacol. Exp. Ther., 20:365, 1922.

MacNider, W. deB.: A Preliminary Paper on the Relation Between the Amount of Stainable Lipoid Material in the Renal Epithelium and the Susceptibility of the Kidney to the Toxic Effect of the General Anesthetics. J. Pharmacol. Exp. Ther., 17:289, 1921.

MacNider, W. deB.: A Study of the Anurias Occurring in Normal Animals During the Use of the General Anesthetics. J. Pharmacol. Exp. Ther., 15:249, 1920.

Mazze, R.I., Hitt, B.A., and Cousins, M.J.: Effect of Enzyme Induction with Phenobarbital on the In Vivo and In Vitro Defluorination of Isoflurane and Methoxyflurane. J. Pharmacol. Exp. Ther., 190:523, 1974.

Michenfelder, J.D., and Cucchiara, R.F.: Canine Cerebral Oxygen Consumption during Enflurane Anesthesia and its Modification during Induced Seizures. Anesthesiology, 40:575, 1974.

Murphy, F.L., Nelson, T.E., Strobel, G.E., and Jones, E.W.: A Comparison of Halothane, Isoflurane, Enflurane, and Fluroxene in Triggering Malignant Hyperthermia in Susceptible Swine. Abstr. of Scientific Papers, Annual Meeting, Am. Soc. Anesthesiologists, 1973, p. 181.

Nimmo, W.S.: Editorial. Drug Reactions and the Liver. Br. J. Anaesth., 52:1059, 1980.

Orsini, J.A., and Taylor, J.I.: Enflurane Anesthesia in the Pony: A Comparative Study Between Enflurane and Halothane. Cornell Vet., 70:50, 1980.

Palahniuk, R.J., Doig, G.A., Johnson, G.N., and Pash, M.P.: Maternal Halothane Anesthesia Reduces Cerebral Blood Flow in the Acidotic Sheep Fetus. Anesth. Analg., 59:35, 1980.

Pedersoli, W.M.: Blood Serum Inorganic, Ionic Fluoride, Tetracycline, and Methoxyflurane in Dogs. J. Am. Anim. Hosp. Assoc., 13:242, 1977*a*.

Pedersoli, W.M.: Serum Bromide Concentrations During and After Halothane Anesthesia in Dogs. Am. J. Vet. Res., 41:77, 1980.

Pedersoli, W.M.: Serum Fluoride Concentration, Renal, and Hepatic Function Test Results in Dogs with Methoxyflurane Anesthesia. Am. J. Vet. Res., 38:949, 1977*b*.

Pedersoli, W.M., Rezakhani, A., and Edjtehadi, M.: Possibility of Catecholamine-Induced Ventricular Fibrillation in Dogs Anesthetized with Methoxyflurane. J. Am. Anim. Hosp. Assoc., 14:126, 1978.

Pezzi, P.J., Frobese, A.S., and Greenberg, S.R.: Methoxyflurane and Renal Toxicity. Lancet, 1:823, 1966.

Sakabe, T., Kuramoto, T., Inoue, S., and Takeshita, H.: Cerebral Effects of Nitrous Oxide in the Dog. Anesthesiology, 48:195, 1978.

Sawyer, D.C., Eger, E.I., II, Bahlman, S.H., Cullen, B.F., and Impelman, D.: Concentration Dependence of Hepatic Halothane Metabolism. Anesthesiology, 34:230, 1971.

Smith, J.B., Manning, F.A., and Polahniuk, R.J.: Maternal and Foetal Effects of Methoxyflurane Anaesthesia in the Pregnant Ewe. Can. Anaesth. Soc. J., 22:449, 1975.

Soma, L.R.: Personal communication. University of Pennsylvania, Philadelphia, 1965.

Steffey, E.P.: Enflurane and Isoflurane Anesthesia: A Summary of Laboratory and Clinical Investigations in Horses. J.A.V.M.A., 172:367, 1978.

Steffey, E.P., Gillespie, J.R., Berry, J.D., Eger, E.I., II, and Rhode, E.A.: Cardiovascular Effects of Halothane in the Stump-Tailed Macaque During Spontaneous and Controlled Ventilation. Am. J. Vet. Res., 35:1315, 1974.

Steffey, E.P., and Howland D., Jr.: Comparison of Circulatory and Respiratory Effects of Isoflurane and Halothane Anesthesia in Horses. Am. J. Vet. Res., 41:821, 1980.

Steffey, E.P., and Howland, D., Jr.: Halothane Anesthesia in Calves. Am. J. Vet. Res., 40:372, 1979.

Steffey, E.P., and Howland, D., Jr.: Isoflurane Potency in the Dog and Cat. Am. J. Vet. Res., 38:983, 1977.

Steffey, E.P., Howland, D., Giri, S., and Eger, E.I., II: Enflurane, Halothane, and Isoflurane Potency in Horses. Am. J. Vet. Res., 38:1037, 1977.

Steffey, E.P., Johnson, B.H., Eger, E.I., II, and Howland, D., Jr.: Nitrous Oxide: Effect on Accumulation Rate and Uptake of Bowel Gases. Anesth. Analg., 58:405, 1979.

Steffey, E.P., Zinkl, J., and Howland, D., Jr.: Minimal Changes in Blood Cell Counts and Biochemical Values Associated with Prolonged Isoflurane Anesthesia of Horses. Am. J. Vet. Res., 40:1646, 1979.

Stephen, C.R., Margolis, G., Fabian, L.W., and Bourgeois-Gavardin, M.: Laboratory Observations with Fluothane. Anesthesiology, 19:770, 1958.

Stoelting, R.K., and Eger, E.I., II: An Additional Explanation for the Second Gas Effect: A Concentration Effect. Anesthesiology, 30:273, 1969.

Tavernor, W.D., and Lees, P.: The Influence of Propranolol on Cardiovascular Function in Conscious and Anesthetized Horses. Arch. Int. Pharmacodyn., 180:89, 1969.

Tinker, J.H., Gandolfi, A.J., and Van Dyke, R.A.: Elevation of Plasma Bromide Levels in Patients Following Halothane Anesthesia: Time Correlation with Total Halothane Dosage. Anesthesiology, 44:194, 1976.

Tucker, W.K., Rackstein, A.D., and Munson, E.S.: Comparison of Arrhythmic Doses of Adrenaline, Metaraminol, Ephedrine and Phenylephrine During Isoflurane and Halothane Anesthesia in Dogs. Br. J. Anaesth., 46:392, 1974.

Vance, J.P., Brown, D.M., Smith, G., and Thornburn, J.: Canine Coronary Blood Flow Responses to Hypoxaemia: The Influence of Halothane. Br. J. Anaesth., 51:193, 1979.

Vasko, K.A.: Preliminary Report on the Effects of Halothane on Cardiac Action and Blood Pressure in the Horse. Am. J. Vet. Res., 23:248, 1962.

Virtue, R.W., Escobar, A., and Model, J.: Nitrous Oxide Levels in Operating Room Air with Various Gas Flows. Can. Anaesth. Soc. J., 26:313, 1979.

Walton, B., Simpson, B.R., Strunin, L., Doniach, D., Perrin, J., and Appleyard, A.J.: Unexplained Hepatitis Following Halothane. Br. Med. J., 1:1171, 1976.

Wiersig, D.O., Davis, R.H., Jr., and Szabiniewicz, M.: Prevention of Induced Ventricular Fibrillation in Dogs Anesthetized with Ultrashort Acting Barbiturates and Halothane. J.A.V.M.A., 165:341, 1974.

Wolff, W.A., Lumb, W.V., and Ramsay, K.: Effects of Halothane and Chloroform Anesthesia on the Equine Liver. Am. J. Vet. Res., 28:1366, 1967.

CHAPTER 11

Methods and Equipment for Administration of Inhalation Anesthetics

INTRODUCTION

The route by which inhaled anesthetics are transported to and from the cells of the central nervous system is similar to that utilized for the transport of oxygen and carbon dioxide. It is not surprising, therefore, that the methods for administration of inhalation anesthetics are similar to those by which oxygen is administered (see Chap. 7). Since inhalation anesthetics are often expensive and their accumulation within the operating room environment is undesirable, exhaled anesthetics are often reutilized. Systems by which anesthetics are inhaled are commonly classified according to both the degree of rebreathing of expired gases and the use of reservoir bags, carbon dioxide absorbent, and unidirectional valves within the system.

METHODS

The methods by which inhalation anesthetics are administered conform to the following fundamental systems: open-insufflation, semiopen without nonrebreathing valves, semiopen with nonrebreathing valves, semiclosed, and closed.

Open-Insufflation

The insufflation technique is similar to that used for administration of oxygen via catheter or mask (see Chap. 7). With this system, anesthetic gas or vapor, together with air and/or oxygen, is delivered to the mouth or trachea by a mask or catheter (Fig. 11–1). The technique was used first by Elsberg in 1910 (Hewer, 1923–1924). If the gas flow is approximately twice the minute volume* and is delivered into the trachea, there will be little or no rebreathing. Inhaled gases include room air as well as those from the delivery tube. Exhalation occurs

*Tidal Volume—Dog, 14 ml/kg; cat, 5 ml/kg; white rabbit, 2.3 ml/kg; white rat, 8 ml/kg; mouse 7.5 ml/kg (Kleinman and Radford, 1964). Minute volume = tidal volume × respirations per minute.

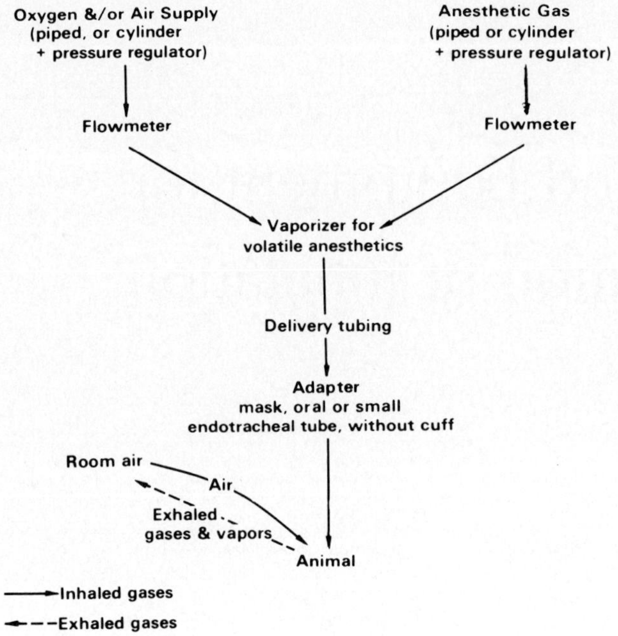

Figure 11–1. Insufflation system. Suitable anesthetics for use in this system include halothane, methoxyflurane, and nitrous oxide.

around the catheter or mask. The catheter should, therefore, be small and should not restrict the airway. This technique is simple, safe, and has minimal dead space and restriction to breathing (providing a small catheter is used). It does not require valves, a carbon dioxide absorber, or a reservoir bag. Disadvantages include waste of gas and anesthetic, drying of the airway, loss of body heat, variable anesthetic concentration due to dilution with room air, pollution of the environment with anesthetic gases, and inability to control or assist breathing. The technique is suitable for small laboratory animals in which airway resistance and dead space may assume major significance and in which the amount of gas and anesthetic lost to the environment is insignificant.

Administration by insufflation is usually by means of an endotracheal catheter and is therefore used for maintenance of anesthesia after induction by other methods. Induction can, however, be achieved by attaching a loose-fitting mask to the system and permitting exhalation around the periphery of the mask. In such a case, preanesthetic sedation and premedication with atropine are often indicated to prevent excessive salivation and possible cardiac arrhythmias. Instillation of ophthalmic ointment into the conjunctival sac to protect the eyes from high concentrations of anesthetic vapor is also advantageous.

While the open drop system and cones are often included in this category, in animals there is usually significant rebreathing, and inclusion in semiopen systems without valves seems more appropriate.

Semiopen Systems without Nonrebreathing Valves

In semiopen systems, exhaled gases pass to the surrounding atmosphere, and some may be rebreathed; the degree to which this occurs is determined by the gas flow rate (Dripps et al., 1967). There is no chemical absorption of carbon dioxide. This category includes the following techniques: semiopen drop, anesthetic boxes or chambers, Ayre's T-tube and related modifications, and Mapleson systems. These systems are generally termed semiclosed—without carbon dioxide absorption in British texts (Atkinson et al., 1977).

Semiopen Drop. A volatile anesthetic is dripped onto a towel or absorbent material, such as gauze or cotton, placed within a cone or mask. Several masks are available, particularly for dogs and cats. Anesthetic is dispensed by a

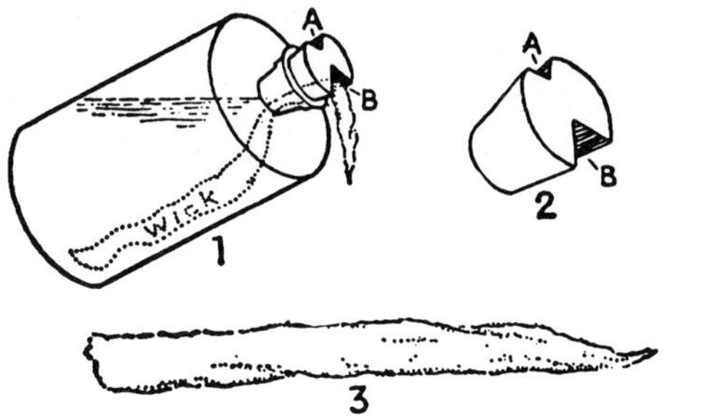

Figure 11–2. Equipment for semiopen drop administration. *1*, Container of anesthetic liquid. *2*, Cork with small notch (A) and large notch (B). *3*, Wick, strip of gauze, cotton, or piece of pipe cleaner long enough to reach to bottom of container. (From American Medical Association: *Fundamentals of Anesthesia*, 3rd ed. W.B. Saunders Co., Philadelphia, 1954.)

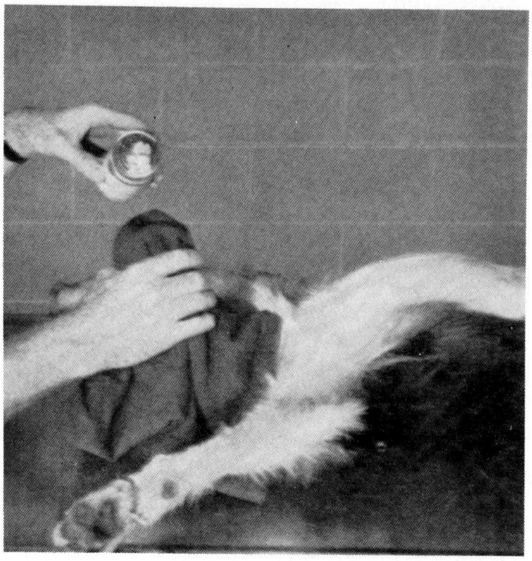

Figure 11–3. A simple mask for semiopen drop administration can be made from a towel folded over patient's face.

dropper bottle or syringe (Fig. 11–2), and a towel or mask is applied to the face of the animal (Fig. 11–3). Anesthetics administered by the semiopen drop technique include chloroform, ether, halothane, and methoxyflurane. In the case of the latter two, cost restricts their use to small dogs, cats, and small laboratory animals. Environmental pollution is a hazard. This technique is suitable for induction of small laboratory animals where restraint is not a problem. In any event, preanesthetic sedation is indicated to minimize struggling and to facilitate a smooth induction. It is also advisable to premedicate with atropine and to instill ophthalmic ointment into the conjunctival sac to protect the eyes.

The tendency is to attempt rapid induction in order to pass quickly through the stage of reflex activity, with its concomitant excitement. This practice often results in the inhalation of dangerously high concentrations of anesthetic. In addition, hypoxia and high carbon dioxide levels are produced in the patient, thereby creating an additional hazard. Since induction by the semiopen drop method is thus usually a combination of anesthesia and asphyxia, the introduction of oxygen under the mask is desirable.

Once the patient passes through stage II, the drip is slowed. Anesthesia is maintained by administration at a slow rate, the mask remaining on the patient during the maintenance period. If anesthesia becomes too deep, the mask should be completely removed.

This technique was at one time commonly used for administration of chloroform to large animals. A towel was wrapped about the nostrils or a large animal mask applied. The anesthetic was dripped onto the towel, or 10 to 40 ml were placed on cotton or on a sponge in the mask.

Anesthetic Boxes or Chambers. A wide variety of boxes and chambers for administration of volatile liquid anesthetic agents have been used. They vary from the simple bell jar, under which a cotton pledget soaked with anesthetic is inserted along with the patient, to elaborate chambers that provide constant circulation of gases and carbon dioxide absorption. The advantages of a chamber are: 1) It requires no restraint; therefore, anesthesia can be induced without an assistant. 2) It presents a professional appearance to the owner. 3) Anesthetic emergencies are minimized. 4) If explosive agents are used, the danger of explosion is reduced.

Most boxes or chambers are made of glass or transparent plastic, thereby allowing visualization of the patient during induction of anesthesia. The anesthetic may be insufflated into the chamber or poured on cotton, gauze, or a sponge and placed in the chamber. The equipment is usually simple. If the anesthetic is insufflated into the chamber, a gas source, flowmeter, and vaporizer are required. In animals such as primates, a cage or catching box may be used. These chambers should be no larger than needed to contain the animal. Stiles (1959) has described an ether box made from an aquarium (Fig. 11–4). An elaborate chamber for anesthetizing animals from the size of mice to that of cats has been described by Zauder and Orkin (1959) (Fig. 11–5). This chamber, which was designed principally for experimental testing of anesthetic agents, provides for constant circulation of gases and carbon dioxide absorption. In addition, it is airtight, has ports for sample removal, and is vented to the outside by means of rubber tubing.

Boxes and chambers have their greatest application in anesthesia of cats, laboratory animals, and various species of wild animals, such as skunks. An airtight anesthesia cage has been used for induction of halothane anesthesia in small bears (Day, 1964).

The chief disadvantage of anesthetic chambers is that maintenance of anesthesia must be achieved by some other means. In most, there is almost complete rebreathing with no carbon dioxide absorption, and it is difficult to perform manipulative procedures within the box while anesthetic is being administered. With larger species, the size of chamber required necessitates the use of large quantities of anesthetic, and there is an appreciable delay before adequate concentrations are achieved.

Ayre's T-Tube. This device consists of a piece of tubing with a small side inlet for the anesthetic gas mixture (Fig. 11–6). One end of the tubing is attached to an endotracheal tube or mask, while the other is open to the atmosphere and is virtually an extension of the endotracheal tube. The open end of the tube serves as a reservoir for the anesthetic mixture, tending to prevent its dissemination into the room air during the expiratory pause. If the capacity of the reservoir tube equals one-third of the tidal volume, the total gas flow into the system necessary to prevent dilution of the inspired anesthetic mixture with room air is about twice the respiratory minute volume (Ayre, 1956). Such a flow also minimizes rebreathing. A nomogram (see Fig. 6–2) is used to estimate the tidal volume, and the length of the reservoir portion of the tube is adjusted by addition of a length of rubber tubing.

This technique is useful for maintenance of anesthesia in small dogs and laboratory animals. Rebreathing is minimal, provided gas flow is adequate, there is no increase in airway resistance, and the equipment required is simple and inexpensive. Anesthetic cost is not a factor when this technique is used on small animals with low minute volumes. Operating room ventilation should be adequate to avoid hazardous environmental pollution, or an exhaust system should be used. With a cuffed endotracheal tube, the system can be used for controlled ventilation by intermittent brief occlusion of the open end of the reservoir limb of the T-tube. Further modifications of the Ayre's T-tube system include the Norman mask elbow, the Bain circuit (a modification of the Norman mask elbow), and the Kuhn system (see Fig. 7–19). All of these modifications incorporate a reservoir bag while the Bain circuit and the Norman mask elbow are especially designed to minimize dead space.

Magill System. This system utilizes a constant flow of anesthetic mixture, a reservoir bag, having a capacity approximately 8 times that of the tidal volume, corrugated tubing (internal diameter > airway diameter) between the bag and mask or endotracheal tube adapter, and an exhalation valve located as close to the animal as possible. It is essentially identical to a nonrebreathing system described in the next section with exclusion of the nonrebreathing valve. Rebreathing is minimal when the flow of oxygen-anesthetic mixture exceeds the respiratory minute volume (Atkinson et al., 1977).

In this system the gas flow is reduced, so that there is economy in the use of anesthetic. Carbon dioxide absorption is not required, and rebreathing is limited. Dependence on valves is minimal, with little resistance, and assisted ventilation is possible by manual compression of the reservoir bag. To prevent accumulation of carbon dioxide, gas flows should be increased considerably during assisted ventilation. The system is suitable for dogs and cats; loss of

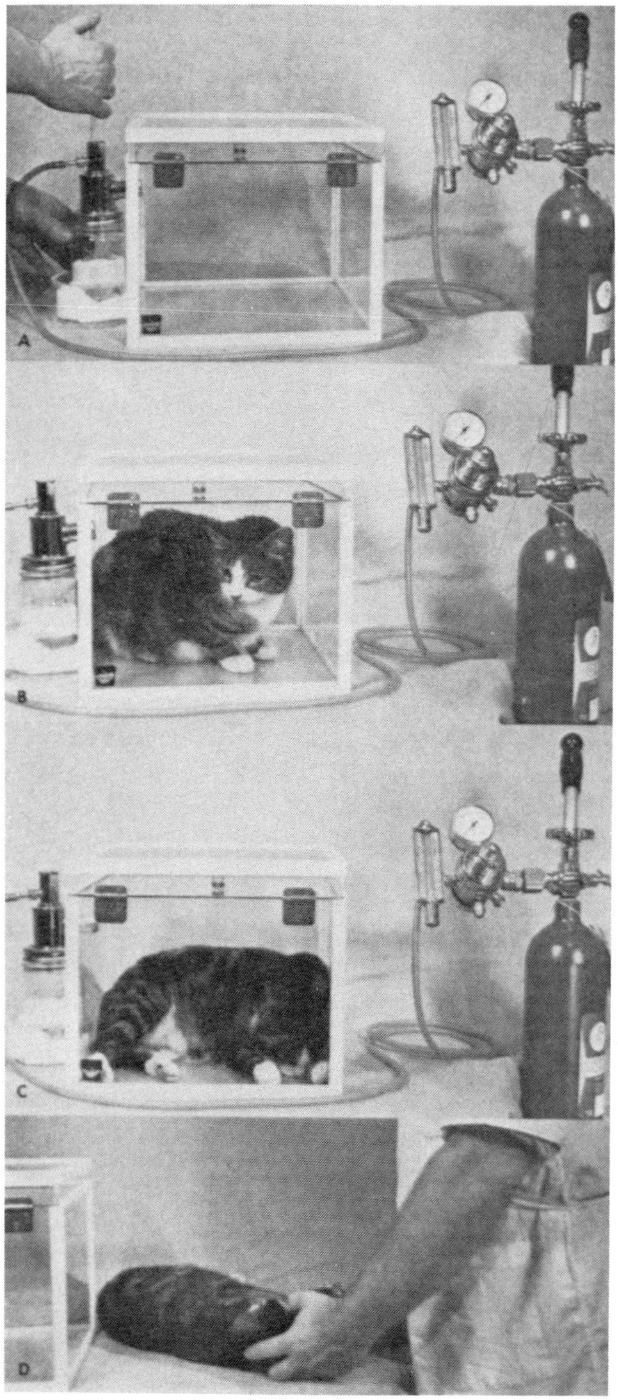

Figure 11–4. Induction of anesthesia with an ether box. *A*, The equipment consists of a plastic box, nebulizer, and oxygen cylinder with reduction valve and flowmeter. Inside the pint jar below the nebulizer is a 3-oz. bottle containing 20 ml of ether, with a plastic suction tube extending from the bottom of the nebulizer into the bottle containing the ether. *B*, Cat is placed in the box and the lid closed. They seldom offer resistance, usually remaining quiet in a crouching position. Oxygen is allowed to flow for approximately 2 minutes at a rate of 3 to 4 liters per minute, or until the ether is gone from the bottle. Salivation may occur but is seldom excessive. *C*, Induction of anesthesia is complete approximately 9 minutes after the start of oxygen flow. *D*, The cat is removed from the box, and anesthesia is continued with an ether cone. (From Stiles, S.W.: Induction of Ether Anesthesia in Cats. J.A.V.M.A., 134:275, 1959.)

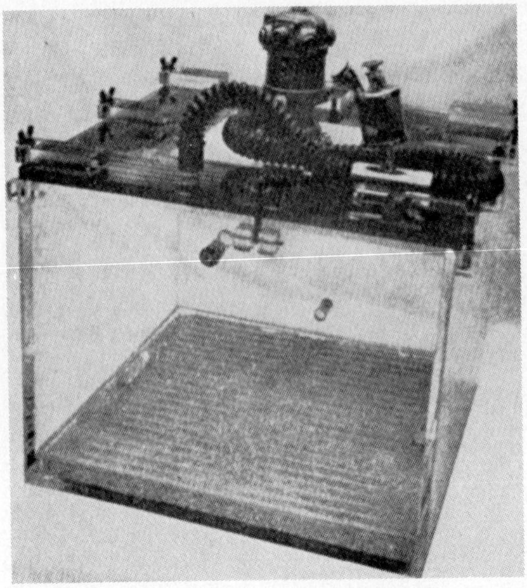

Figure 11–5. An elaborate anesthetic chamber that provides for constant circulation of gases and carbon dioxide absorption. (From Zauder, H.L., and Orkin, L.R.: Chamber for Anesthetization of Small Animals. Anesthesiology, 20:708, 1959.)

anesthetic and gas is excessive in larger animals. Precautions should be taken to overcome environmental pollution.

Mapleson Systems. With the proliferation of various systems, Mapleson, in 1954, classified the various circuits into five basic types (Fig. 11–7). These were summarized with associated techniques by Rayburn (1981).

In this classification, the Mapleson A circuit was the same as the Magill system. Circuits B and C were similar, except for the length of the corrugated tubing. Circuit D functioned in a manner similar to the Jackson-Rees circuit, which was an Ayre's T-piece, modified by addition of a double-ended bag. Circuit E was essentially the Ayre's T-piece. The Jackson-Rees circuit was later classified as the Mapleson F system. In these systems, it appeared that fresh gas flow should be three times the respiratory minute volume to prevent rebreathing in a T-piece containing an expiratory limb volume greater than the patient's tidal volume. This was thought to be true, irrespective of whether controlled or spontaneous ventilation was used. Based on blood gas determinations, these flow rates have subsequently been shown to be excessive. With a change from emphasis on prevention of rebreathing to maintenance of normal blood gases, new techniques have been derived. The alveolar carbon dioxide can be predicted for semiopen circuits by:

$$F_{A}CO_2 = \frac{V_{CO_2}}{V_F}$$

(where $F_{A}CO_2$ = the fraction of alveolar CO_2, V_{CO_2} = minute CO_2 production, and VF = fresh gas flow per minute). Providing minute alveolar ventilation is met and mixing of fresh gas flow and exhaled alveolar gas is complete, then whichever is less, fresh gas flow or ventilation, will be the major controlling factor for CO_2 elimination.

In 1972 Bain and Spoerel developed a streamlined Mapleson D-type semiopen (co-axial) circuit in which the fresh gas flow tube was positioned inside the corrugated expiratory tube (see Chap. 7). Using this system, they noted that if minute ventilation was three times the minute fresh gas flow, 95% mixing of the gases occurred. Subsequently, they found that the required fresh gas to maintain Pa_{CO_2} at 40 mm Hg was 2.5 L per square meter of body surface area per minute. By using this value for the fresh

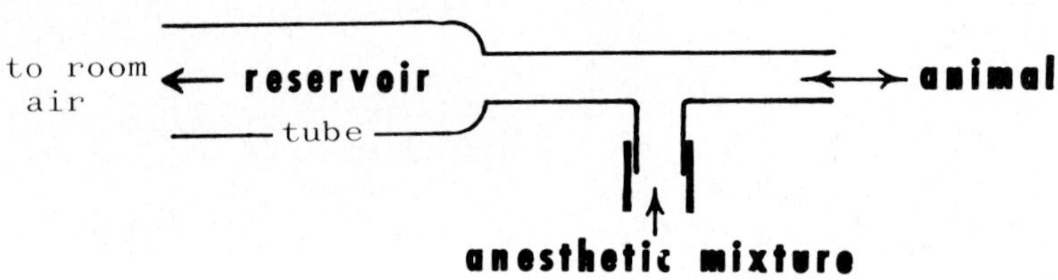

Figure 11–6. Ayre's T-tube. (From Jones, E.W.: *Anesthesia in Laboratory Animals: Equipment.* Fed. Proc., 28:1570, 1969.)

A.
B.
C.
D.
E.
F.

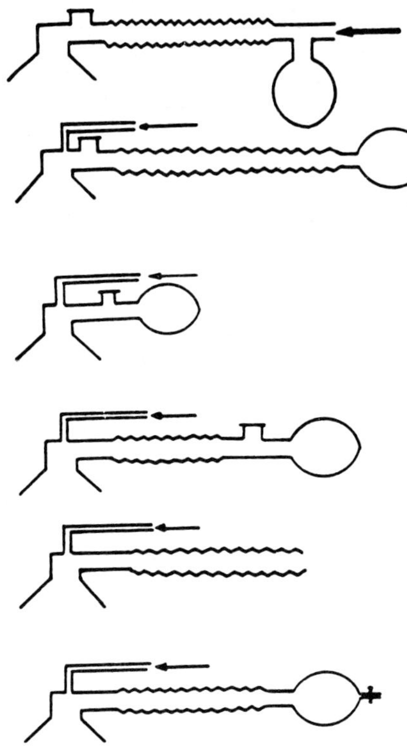

Figure 11–7. Mapleson classification of circuits. See text for descriptions. (From Rayburn, R.L.: Pediatric Anesthesia Circuits. Annual Refresher Course Lectures, Lecture No. 117. Am. Soc. Anesth., 1981.)

gas flow and a minute ventilation of three times the fresh gas flow (usually tidal volume was 12 to 15 ml/kg), one could make the Mapleson D semiopen co-axial circuit achieve normocapnia in both pediatric and adult human patients. This technique has been called Controlled Partial Rebreathing Anesthesia Method (CPRAM) (Rayburn and Watson, 1980). It has several advantages. It allows use of the semiopen Mapleson-type co-axial circuit, which is easily cleaned, has no valves, and is easily scavenged. Soda lime, with its attendant disadvantages, is eliminated. The method works equally well in patients of all sizes. Since fresh gas flow controls the carbon dioxide, rather than ventilation, minute ventilation may be generous to prevent atelectasis. The heat and humidity of the inspired gases are excellent, and have been found superior to the semiclosed and closed circle methods. Humidity in most patients is adequate (relative humidity 60%) without the need for humidifiers. During spontaneous respiration, the partial rebreathing techniques have less advantage, and flows are less clearly defined. Some recommend that, using co-axial circuits, fresh gas flows should be 2.5 to 3 times the minute ventilation, i.e., the circuit is used as a nonrebreathing technique. Others have recommended a flow of 100 ml/kg per minute in the adult human. Others have found a fresh gas flow of 4 L per square meter per minute to be satisfactory in larger children and adult humans. Parameters for animals have yet to be established.

Lamplugh et al. (1979) have reported upon the Mapleson E circuit (Ayre's T-piece) for controlled ventilation in laboratory dogs under anesthesia. In dogs weighing 13 to 20 kg, normocapnia was produced by a fresh gas flow of 100 to 150 ml/kg with a respiratory frequency of 20 and a tidal volume of 500 to 650 ml. A fresh gas flow of 1300 to 1950 ml/minute for a 13-kg dog with a minute ventilation volume of 10 to 13 L produced normocapnia during mechanical ventilation, providing the minute volume of ventilation was at least three times the fresh gas flow. Hypoxemia was not a problem even at a high Pa_{CO_2}, as long as oxygen in the fresh gas flow was 30% or more. Another advantage of the high minute volume to fresh gas flow ratio was the increased humidity of the inhaled gases. A relative humidity of 96% at a temperature of 27° C was measured during steady-state anesthesia with normocapnia. During oxygen/halothane anesthesia of cats utilizing an Ayre's T-piece system, Rawlings and Moreland (1978) recommended a flow rate of one L per minute in cats weighing an average of 2.4 kg. Respiratory minute volume was not reported.

Semiopen Systems with Nonrebreathing Valves

In this method, inspired and expired gases are separated by a valve as close to the animal as possible, rebreathing is minimal, and the animal breathes only the anesthetic mixture delivered. Use of a reservoir bag between the valve and gas source is desirable. In this way, anesthetic and oxygen flow into the reservoir bag during expiration and are conserved until they are required during the next inspiration. The gas and anesthetic flow rate has only to equal the minute volume rather than peak inspiratory flow rates. This system has been described previously for administration of oxygen (see Chap. 7), and is illustrated schematically in Figure 11–8. Basic equipment required includes an oxygen and anesthetic supply with pressure regulators, flowmeters, a vaporizer for volatile anesthetics, a reservoir bag, nonrebreathing valve, adapter, and a mask or endotracheal tube with inflatable cuff.

A nonrebreathing valve and reservoir bag may also be used in conjunction with a mechanical ventilator and vaporizer, thereby providing a system suitable for nonrebreathing techniques with or without mechanical ventilation (Jones, 1964).

A functional classification for nonrebreathing valves has been proposed, according to whether the valve is used mainly for spontaneous respiration, controlled ventilation, or both. Valves used for spontaneous breathing include the Stephen-Slater and the Digby-Leigh. Valves solely for controlled ventilation are usually intended for use with respirators or with resuscitation apparatus, and are not generally used for anesthesia. Valves intended for spontaneous or controlled ventilation include the Fink, Lewis-Leigh, Ruben, Frumin, Steen, Sierra, Ambu-Hesse, Ambu, and Laerdal. During spontaneous respiration, the reservoir bag in such systems is maintained at approximately three-fourths full at the beginning of inspiration, and the fresh gas flow is set to the patient's minute volume. During controlled ventilation, the flow of gases is set at the desired minute volume with ventilation controlled by compression of the reservoir bag. To obviate the development of high pressures in the circuit as a result of high fresh gas flows, a pressure release valve may be incorporated. The Fink and Lewis-Leigh valves allow the anesthesiologist to make an adjustment to convert from spontaneous to controlled ventilation and vice versa. Problems associated with such semiopen nonrebreathing systems include 1) loss of heat and humidity, 2) sticky valves, 3) variation in minute volume during spontaneous respiration requiring frequent adjustment of gas flow to prevent collapse or overdistension of the

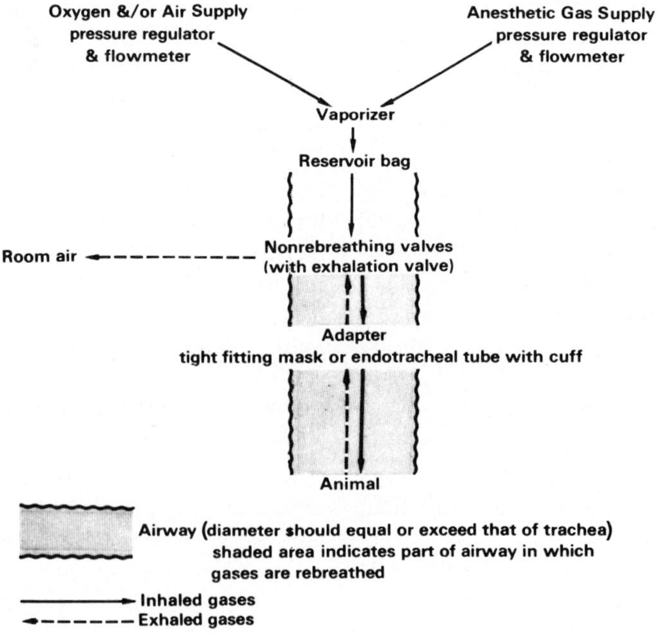

Figure 11–8. Semiopen nonrebreathing system. Suitable anesthetics include chloroform, ether, halothane, methoxyflurane, and nitrous oxide.

reservoir bag, 4) the need to have the valve close to the patient's mouth with the possibility of occlusion by surgical drapes, 5) pollution of the operating room environment with exhaled gases, and 6) the relatively large dead space in the system when used on small animals. Thus, these valves are less frequently used in favor of the more popular Mapleson-type systems (see previous discussion).

Inhalers fitted with nonrebreathing valves are modifications of a nonrebreathing system. In this case, air is inhaled from the atmosphere through a low-efficiency drawover-type vaporizer. Bubble vaporizers increase the resistance to inhalation and should not be used. Since the inspired air vaporizes the anesthetic, a reduction in ventilation reduces the amount of anesthetic vaporized. Exhaled gases pass to the outside. The addition of a self-inflating bag to such a system permits manually controlled ventilation.

A similar system (EMO) has been described by Hall (1978). It was originally developed in 1959 for human ether/air anesthesia, but was found safe, effective, and inexpensive for anesthesia in dogs. The inspiratory flow rate of cats and small dogs was, however, too low to provide satisfactory vaporization of ether, requiring addition of a temperature-compensated vaporizer. Anesthesia with spontaneous breathing gave normal oxygen tensions in the arterial blood. When it was used with relaxant drugs and intermittent positive pressure ventilation with air, hyperventilation was required to maintain normal oxygen tensions.

Administration through a nonrebreathing system is simple; the composition of the inspired mixture is constant once the concentration is set. If the reservoir bag does not collapse on inspiration, the gas inflow equals or exceeds the minute volume, and rebreathing is minimal. Use of this system obviates the need for carbon dioxide absorption, thereby eliminating the complications that may result from ineffective absorption with carbon dioxide accumulation. Induction by this technique is more rapid than by closed and semiclosed rebreathing techniques in which inhaled anesthetic mixtures are diluted by exhaled gases, washout of normal gases from the lungs is slowed, and production of anesthetic concentrations within the alveoli is delayed.

Although a nonrebreathing system wastes more anesthetic than one in which rebreathing occurs, this is minimized by using a reservoir bag and by adjusting the gas inflow to approximate the minute volume. Gas flows are such that waste is not usually a problem in anesthesia of laboratory animals, although in long operations loss of moisture may be.

Loss of gas and anesthetic to the room air does preclude the use of such a system in instances where explosive mixtures are used in larger animals, and where scavenging systems cannot be used, for anesthetic is hazardous in room air. A nonrebreathing system has nevertheless been found useful for anesthetizing sows up to 300 lb body weight and for anesthetizing calves up to 1 month old.

Should anesthesia be induced by a nonrebreathing system, preanesthetic sedation, premedication with atropine sulfate, and application of ophthalmic ointment to the eyes are indicated. The animal is restrained, a mask is applied snugly to the face, the head is extended to minimize possible soft tissue obstruction of the upper airway, and the delivery of anesthetic mixture is commenced. To minimize mechanical dead space, the mask should be as small as possible. A gas flow sufficient to prevent collapse of the reservoir bag during inspiration is adequate. The vaporizer is adjusted to deliver an induction dose of anesthetic vapor. Use of methoxyflurane generally means that the vaporizer is fully open, whereas for halothane a 3% setting may be used in dogs and cats and a setting as high as 10% in large animals. Once laryngeal reflexes are obtunded, it is preferable to maintain anesthesia by endotracheal administration. In the event that assisted or controlled breathing is required, this can be performed by intermittent compression of the reservoir bag.

Semiclosed and Closed Systems

All conventional anesthesia machines* can be used for both semiclosed and closed techniques. These techniques differ only by the extent to

*See Equipment section for components.

which exhaled gases are rebreathed, by the degree of carbon dioxide absorption necessary, and by the flow of new gases required. In the semiclosed (partial rebreathing) technique, gases are partly exhaled to the atmosphere and partly rebreathed. A relatively high fresh gas flow is thus required. Carbon dioxide is removed chemically from the portion that is rebreathed. In closed administration, on the other hand, rebreathing of exhaled gases is complete, carbon dioxide is absorbed, and only sufficient oxygen is added to the system to satisfy metabolic needs and inadvertent leaks. In comparison to the semiclosed system, this is thus a low-flow system. Equipment for closed and semiclosed administration is assembled as *to-and-fro* (single-phase) or *circle* (two-phase) systems.

Closed-circuit anesthetic equipment with carbon dioxide absorption was first described by Snow in 1850 and reintroduced for use in animals by Jackson in 1915. The clinical use of this to-and-fro (single-phase) system in man was reported by Waters in 1924 (Waters, 1926). The system consists of a mask or endotracheal tube with adapter, an exhalation valve, a canister of carbon dioxide absorbent, a rebreathing bag, and a supply of oxygen and anesthetic vapor or gas (Fig. 11–9). Exhaled gases pass through the carbon dioxide absorber into the reservoir bag, from which they return via the same route to be inhaled once again. Fresh gases are usually added to the system by a connector close to the mask or endotracheal tube adapter, where an adjustable exhalation valve is also located. This valve permits the system to be flushed and allows partial exhalation to the room environment when desired. It also serves to prevent overdistension of the reservoir bag.

The circle (two-phase) system was developed by B. Sword in 1926 (Sword, 1930). In this system, gases flow in a circular route that may be considered to have an exhalation and inhalation phase. One-way flow of gases is assured by unidirectional valves. The system (Fig. 11–10) includes the following: a mask or an endotracheal tube and adapter, a Y-connector with exhalation valve, inhalation and exhalation hoses, unidirectional valves, a reservoir bag, a carbon dioxide absorber, a supply of oxygen and anesthetic gases, and a vaporizer. The latter may be incorporated in the line supplying gases (out-of-circuit) or may be within the anesthetic circuit (in-circuit), in which case exhaled gases pass through the vaporizer.

Since the completely closed system requires only the addition of sufficient oxygen to satisfy metabolic needs and permits reuse of exhaled anesthetic gases, it is especially economical of gases and anesthetic. The risk of explosion, when flammable anesthetics are used, is reduced, and exposure of operating room personnel to anesthetic gases is limited. Reuse of exhaled gases also conserves body moisture and heat. Nevertheless, adequate humidification of anesthetic gases in circle systems is frequently lacking, and efforts to correct this have not gained wide acceptance. Most methods require humidifiers that may become contaminated and are cumbersome. Other modifications to increase humidity include passing the fresh gas flow through the soda lime before it goes to the patient.

The closed system is not without its disadvantages. The efficiency of carbon dioxide absorption diminishes with time (Lund et al., 1956). Absorbent must be periodically replaced, and even at maximum efficiency absorption is far from perfect. Carbon dioxide absorption generates heat, which may be excessive, especially in the to-and-fro system. In this system the absorber must be as close to the animal as possible in order to minimize equipment dead space, whereas, in the circle system dead space is only that space from the Y-connector to the patient. In both to-and-fro and circle systems, however, dead space is an undesirable factor that must be considered when anesthetizing dogs or other small animals that weigh less than 30 lbs.

Use of these systems also increases resistance to breathing, which becomes increasingly hazardous in smaller and poor-risk patients. During inspiration, increased resistance accentuates intrapulmonary negative pressure and the potential for pulmonary edema, while expiratory resistance may impair venous return, thereby reducing cardiac output. Other disadvantages of the closed system include: possible cross-infec-

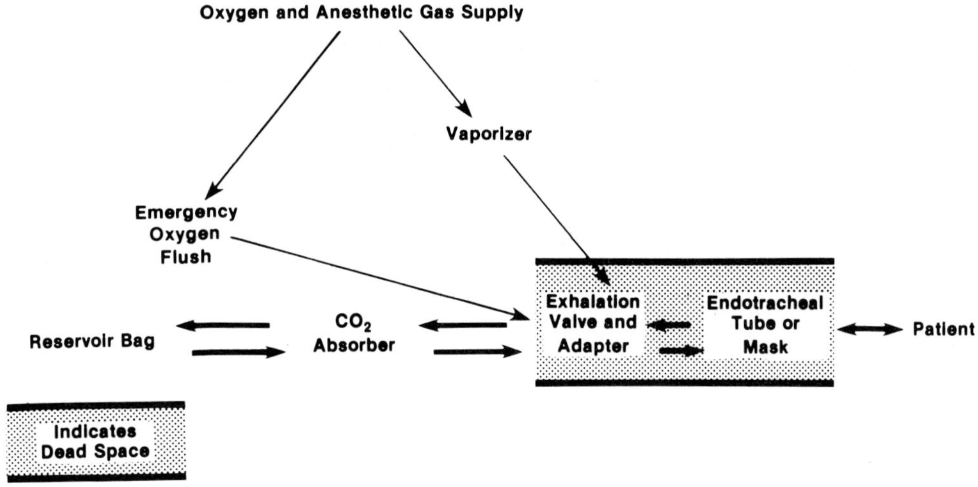

Figure 11–9. To-and-fro (single-phase) system derives its name from the flow of inhaled and exhaled gases back and forth through the CO_2 (soda lime) absorber.

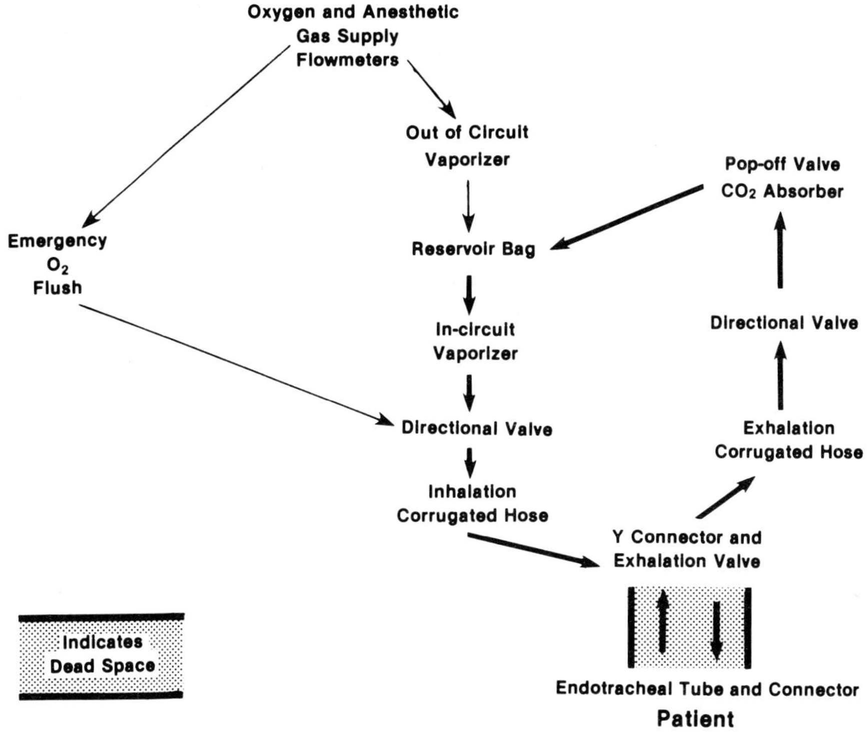

Figure 11–10. Circle (two-phase) system for closed and semiclosed administration techniques. Shaded area indicates the part of the airway in which gases are rebreathed. This system derives its name from the flow of gases around the circle (arrows).

tion from animal to animal; dilution of anesthetic mixture with exhaled gases, thereby delaying attainment of minimal anesthetic concentrations in the alveoli; and the need to use low gas flow rates. In the latter instance, some vaporizers and flowmeters are inefficient or even ineffective when low rates are used.

In a 32-liter large animal circle anesthesia circuit, fresh gas inflow rates of 3, 6, and 12 liters per minute required 10.7, 5.3, and 2.7 minutes, respectively, to achieve a 63% change in inspired halothane concentration (Steffey and Howland, 1977). Much of this delay can be offset by a high flow technique. However, this imposes significant waste, and additional requirements for waste gas scavenging. In some instances halothane vaporizers become inefficient not only at low gas flows, but also at high flow rates, e.g., 12 L per minute and greater. To obtain adequate anesthetic concentrations during induction, some anesthesiologists have injected liquid anesthetic directly into the system (1 ml liquid equals approximately 200 ml vapor).

Because mechanical support of respiration during use of circle systems in large animals also presents physical difficulties, it has become necessary to utilize large specially designed mechanical ventilators. These ventilators generally follow the bag-in-bottle or drum principle (Fig. 11–11). Schatzmann (1978) reported that in the horse a respiratory minute volume of 92 ml/kg maintains a normal carbon dioxide partial pressure, in contrast to previous reports of 185 ml/kg by Weaver and Walley (1975).

Although additional devices are continually

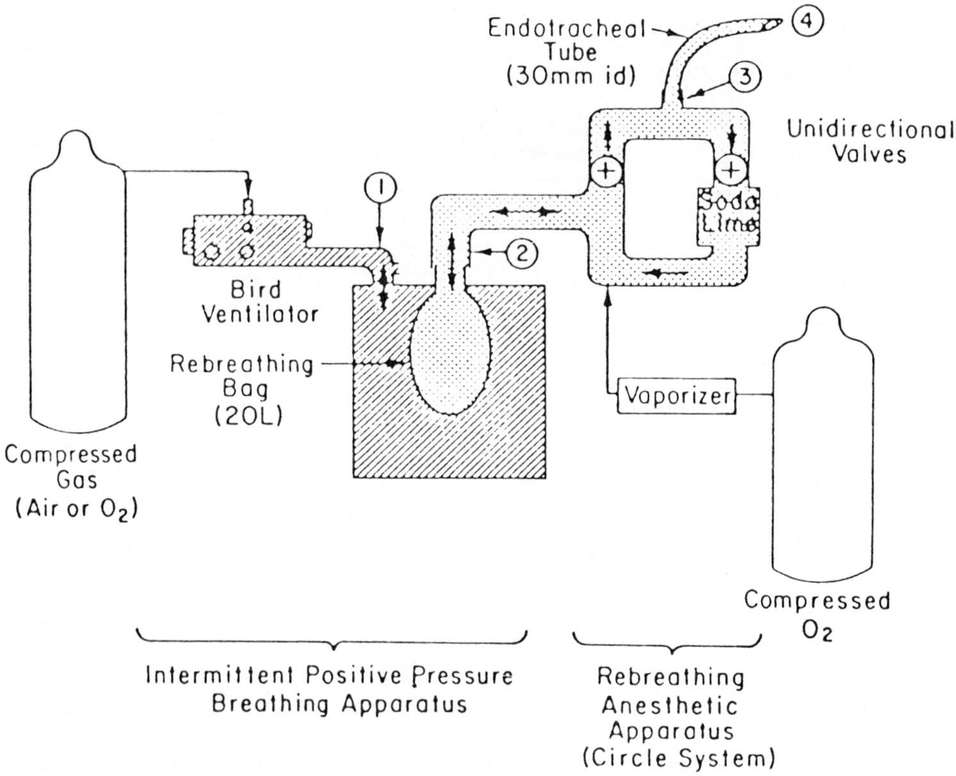

Figure 11–11. Schematic of an equine intermittent positive pressure breathing and anesthetic delivery apparatus. The rebreathing bag of the anesthetic apparatus is contained within an air-tight drum ("bag-in-bottle" principle) and is rhythmically compressed by the ventilator. Gas from the ventilator does not mix with those in the anesthetic apparatus. For determination of flow rate measurements, internal diameters of the apparatus are 21 mm at location 1, 53 mm at location 2, and 30 mm at locations 3 and 4. (From Steffey, E.P., and Berry, J.D.: Flow Rates from an Intermittent Positive Pressure Breathing/Anesthetic Delivery Apparatus for Horses. Am. J. Vet. Res., 38:685, 1977.)

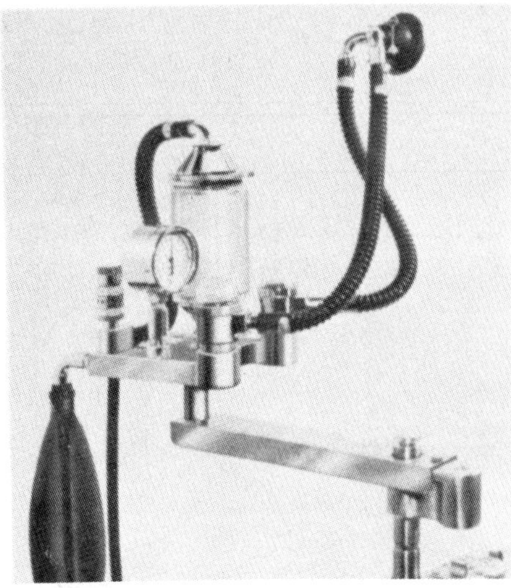

Figure 11–12. A modification of the Bloomquist infant circle absorber. (Courtesy of Foregger Company, Roslyn Heights, New York.)

added to the anesthetic machine, its basic design has not changed significantly since the first closed-circuit system was developed. A significant advance has been the utilization of calibrated vaporizers, which have not been completely satisfactory. Because the Kettle system requires significant calculation to deliver known concentrations, it is less frequently used. The more sophisticated calibrated vaporizers are prone to failure and require periodic calibration. Additions to the anesthetic machine have been made to prevent back-flow into the vaporizer, to prevent failure of the oxygen system, to control vaporizer temperature, to provide mechanical ventilation, and to monitor such information as minute ventilation, inspiratory pressure, and concentration of various gases and vapors.

Despite these additions, the needs of the anesthesiologist relative to anesthetic machine design have only recently been reexamined (Cooper et al., 1978). The objectives of these authors were to eliminate the human factors problems associated with present anesthesia apparatus, and to provide a foundation for developing new techniques in anesthesia management. Their prototype machine does all that a conventional machine does, and in addition performs numerous monitoring activities. The system is electronic, incorporating controlled proportioning of oxygen and nitrous oxide, liquid anesthetic injection systems for atomizing inhalant anesthetics directly into the gas stream, and bar-graph and digital display screens indicating not only the specific delivery components of the system, but also airway pressure and expired oxygen concentrations. It was also designed with a display screen to indicate numerous other patient variables. The machine and control console are operated under software control by a microcomputer based on an INTEL 80/80 microprocessor. Program routines examine machine status and control settings and warn the operator of changing conditions, such as loss of oxygen or nitrous oxide supply, hypoxic mixture selection, or failing battery voltage.

EQUIPMENT

To understand the mechanics of operating anesthesia machines, a knowledge of the parts and their functions is essential. Despite their diversity in appearance, all machines contain the same essential components. Thus, knowing how to run one machine allows one to operate other brands with little difficulty.

The wide range of animal sizes obviously necessitates different equipment for varying sizes. Functional requirements for various components of the to-and-fro and circle circuits are discussed below. Certain generalities about appropriate equipment can be made. Human pediatric units or modifications thereof (Fig. 11–12) are suitable for small animals (5 to 30 lbs). Conventional human anesthetic systems or their equivalent (Fig. 11–13) are suitable for animals from 30 to approximately 300 lbs body weight. For larger animals, specially designed equipment is necessary (Figs. 11–14, 11–15).

Masks

The simplest mask consists of an ordinary hand towel folded to fit the patient's face. Another inexpensive method for making a mask is to remove both ends from a tin can. It is then wrapped with gauze by repeatedly running the gauze through the center hole and around the

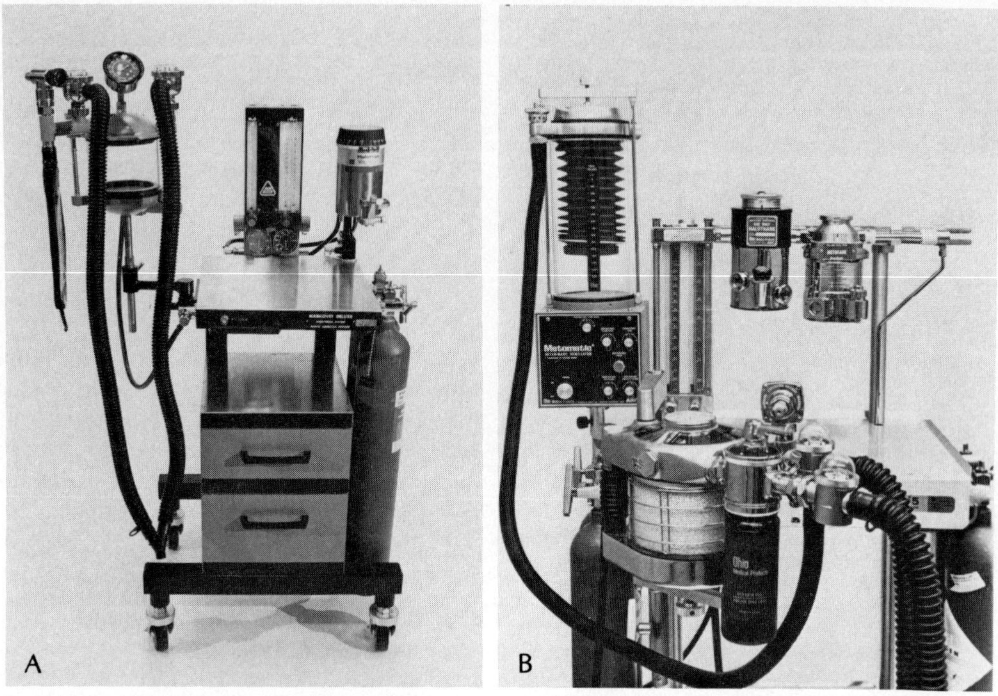

Figure 11–13. *A*, Small animal circle system with Vapor out-of-circuit vaporizer (Narkovet Deluxe, North American Dräger, Telford, Pennsylvania). In use, the "pop-off" valve adjacent to the left dome valve at the top of the illustration attaches to a scavenging system. The unit is equipped for use of nitrous oxide. (Courtesy of North American Dräger Company, Telford, Pennsylvania.) *B*, Small animal circle system with halothane and methoxyflurane out-of-circuit vaporizers and in-circuit wick vaporizer. The rebreathing bag is replaced by a bag-in-bottle ventilator, and the unit is equipped for use of nitrous oxide. (Courtesy of Pitman-Moore, Inc., Washington Crossing, New Jersey.)

outside, until the can is covered. A piece of cotton is placed in one end, and anesthetic is dripped on it.

A variety of masks are available commercially. Most are made of metal or plastic, clear plastic having the advantage that the patient's face is visible to the anesthetist (Fig. 11–16). Few masks are available for large animals, but the need for these is less since induction by inhalation is not commonly used. Masks of this size, however, may be made from plastic waste containers or bottles. Masks are likewise generally not available for laboratory animals, but can be constructed from plastic syringe containers or plastic beakers. Tube connectors are glued to the mask, and a diaphragm to prevent gas escape around the face is constructed from a finger cot. The balloon ends of Simplex IV administration sets may also be used.

In any case, masks should provide a snug seal about the animal's face and should contain minimal space. Air space between the mask and the animal's face constitutes mechanical dead space and is likely to impair effective ventilation. This is especially so in small dogs, cats, and laboratory animals.

Airways

Inspiration and exhalation should be accomplished with minimal resistance. Use of an airway that is too small has the same consequences as a partial respiratory obstruction. Respiratory effort is increased; negative intrapulmonary pressure is increased during inhalation; gaseous exchange is impaired, and pulmonary edema may develop.

Resistance to gas flow through a tube is increased especially by reduction in tube diameter, by increased gas flow rates, by the onset of turbulent flow, and to a lesser degree by tube length. It is essential, therefore, that airways

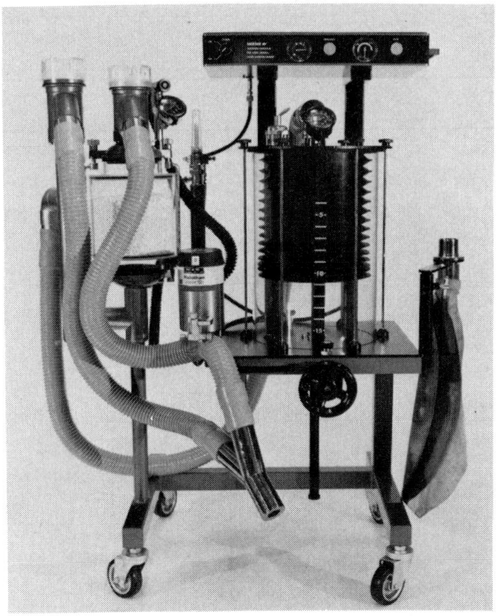

Figure 11–14. Large animal circle system with Vapor out-of-circuit vaporizer. The unit includes a bag-in-bottle type ventilator for controlled ventilation. (Courtesy of North American Dräger Company, Telford, Pennsylvania.)

should have a wide bore and be as short as possible. They should also have smooth walls, with gradual bends and no constrictions, since these predispose to turbulent flow and increased resistance (Figs. 11–17, 11–18).

Animal anesthesiologists must anesthetize animals of greatly differing sizes. They must therefore take great care to ensure that the equipment they use has an adequate airway. A good rule of thumb is that the airway should exceed the tracheal diameter. The only exception is, of course, the endotracheal tube, which should be as large as practical (see Chap. 7). In addition to the connecting hoses (corrugated to avoid kinking), the lumen of connectors, adapters, and valves should also equal or exceed that of the trachea. It is thus apparent that while human gas machines are suitable for small animals, large animals such as horses and cattle require much larger airways. A 2-inch internal diameter airway is considered necessary for such animals (Hansson and Johannisson, 1958; Jones et al., 1962).

Should any doubt exist regarding adequacy of the airway, the nature of the respirations and thoracic excursions should be carefully observed. In the event the airway is inadequate, inspiratory effort will compare with that observed due to obstruction from any other cause.

Valves

A variety of valves are incorporated in anesthesia machines. Their placement varies, depending upon the manufacturer. Generally, they can be divided into two types: 1) unidirectional valves, which control the direction of flow in the circuit (inhalation and exhalation valves), and 2) expiratory (overflow, pressure relief, "pop off") valves, which allow controlled escape of gases from the system.

All valves should be freely movable and

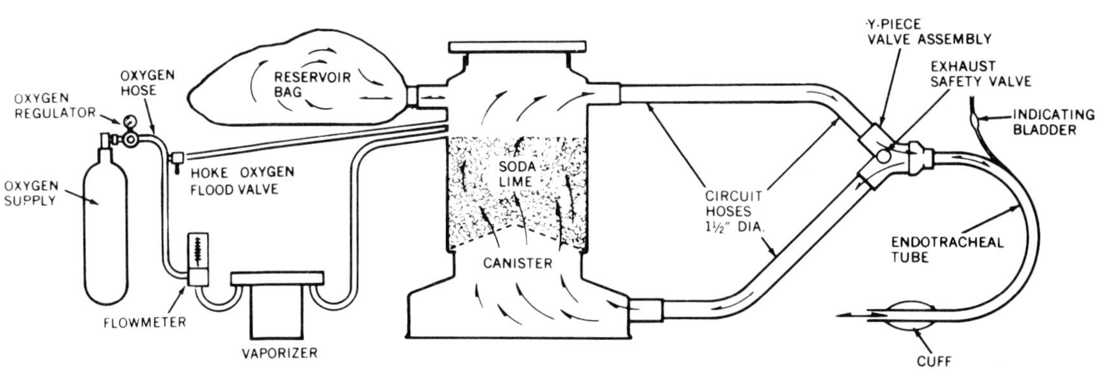

Figure 11–15. Circuit diagram of the Snyder circle system large animal anesthesia machine. This equipment is compact and portable for field use. Arrows indicate direction of gas flow around the circle. (Courtesy of Summit Hill Laboratories, Avalon, New Jersey.)

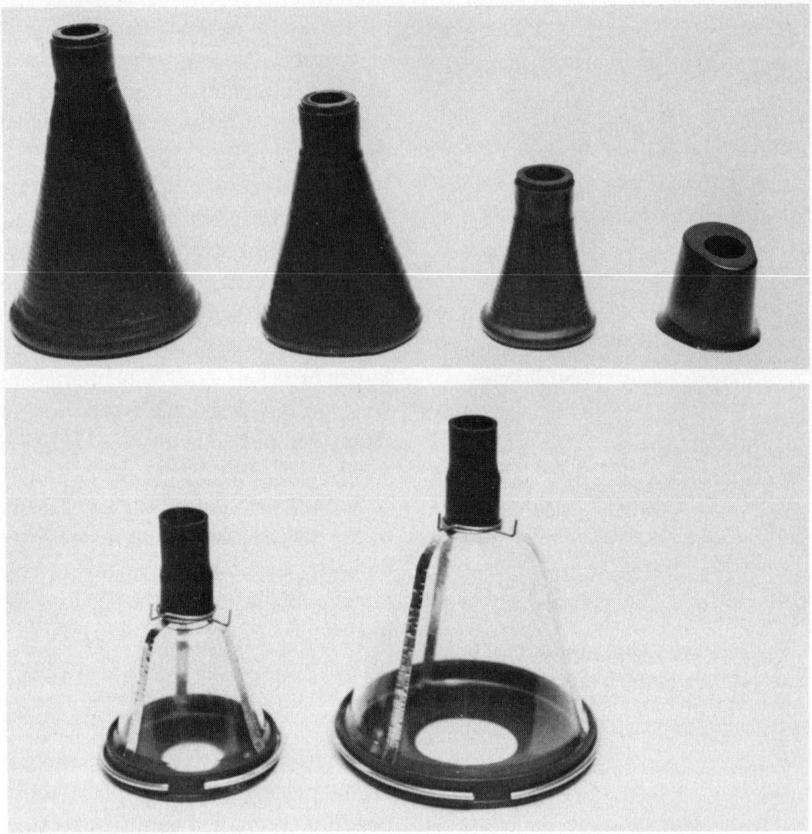

Figure 11–16. Small animal masks of varying sizes. The nontransparent masks are designed to minimize dead space within. (Courtesy of North American Dräger Company, Telford, Pennsylvania.)

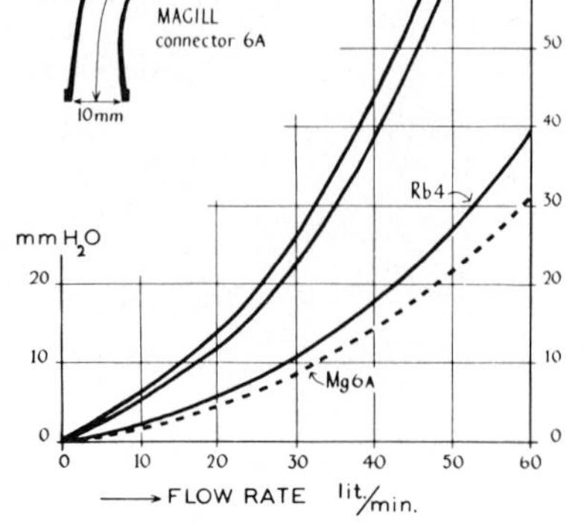

Figure 11–17. Resistance of several endotracheal connectors as a function of the flow rate. The three curves marked "Rb" refer to the Rowbotham connectors; their sizes are entered on the inset table. The curved Magill ("Mg") connector offers less resistance to flow than all three angular Rowbotham connectors. (From Macintosh, R., Mushin, W.W., and Epstein, H.G.: *Physics for the Anaesthetist,* 3rd ed. Blackwell Scientific Publications, Oxford, England, 1963.)

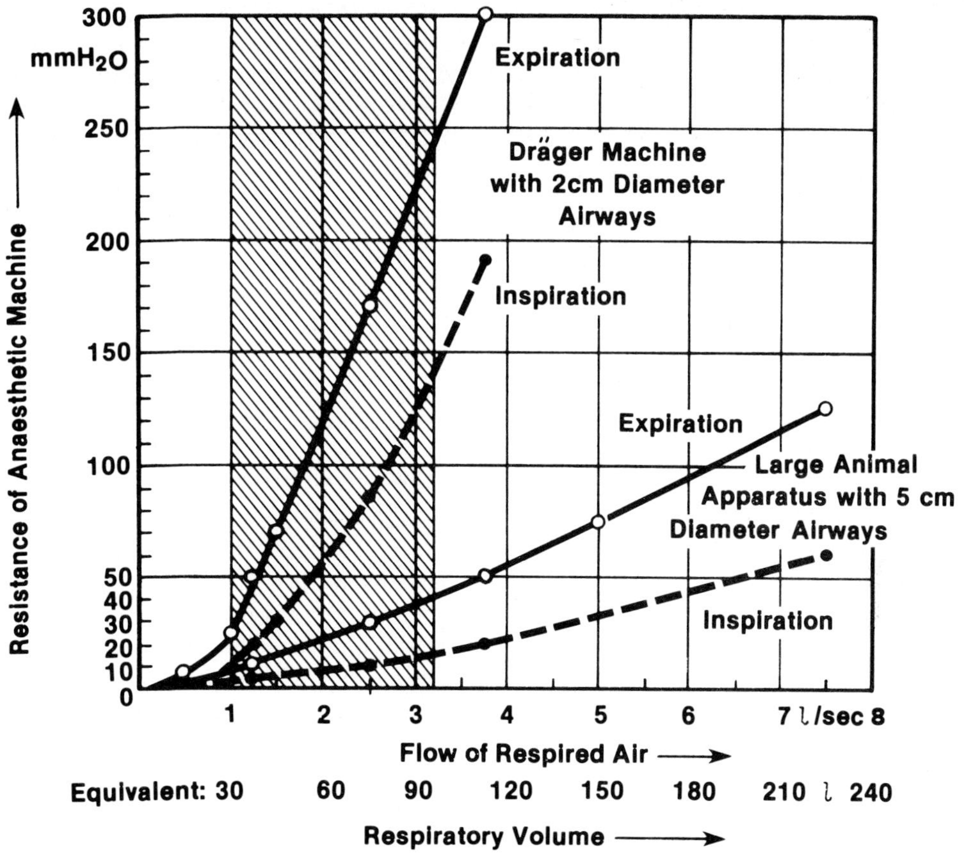

Figure 11–18. Respiratory resistance in circle absorber with different diameters of airways. The shaded area respresents the range of normal respiration in the horse: 8 to 16 respirations/min with tidal volume of 4000 to 6000 ml (equals 32 to 96 liters minute volume). (From Westhues, M., and Fritsch, R.: *Animal Anaesthesia, General Anaesthesia*. Oliver and Boyd, Edinburgh, 1965.)

should have an airway diameter in excess of the diameter of connecting tubes. Placement of unidirectional valves in the Y-connector of circle systems minimizes the mechanical dead space. The Foregger small animal unit, a modification of the standard Bloomquist infant circle absorber, is so arranged. The Columbia pediatric circle valve* (Rackow and Salanitre, 1968) is a Y-connector incorporating unidirectional valves (Fig. 11–19). The valve has a dead space of only 0.5 ml. Resistance at 2 to 3 L/min of air is minimal and less than 1 cm H_2O at 15 L/min of air. An expiratory (overflow) valve is placed just distal to the unidirectional valve of the expiratory limb. When studying the effects of inflow and overflow on valve placement in the economy of the circle system, Eger and Ethans (1968) found the arrangement of unidirectional and overflow valves previously described (Rackow and Salanitre, 1968) preferable. Preferred inflow of new gases is between the absorber and the inspiratory unidirectional valve (Brown et al., 1964). If unidirectional valves are not situated in the Y-connector, dome valves are used. These are transparent domes containing disc valves that are visible when in operation (see Fig. 11–13). Malfunction is readily detected, and resistance is minimal.

Expiratory valves are one-way, usually spring-loaded, and should have minimal resistance to breathing when fully open. The valve should be located as close to the patient as possible. If complete rebreathing is desired, the

*See Appendix A.

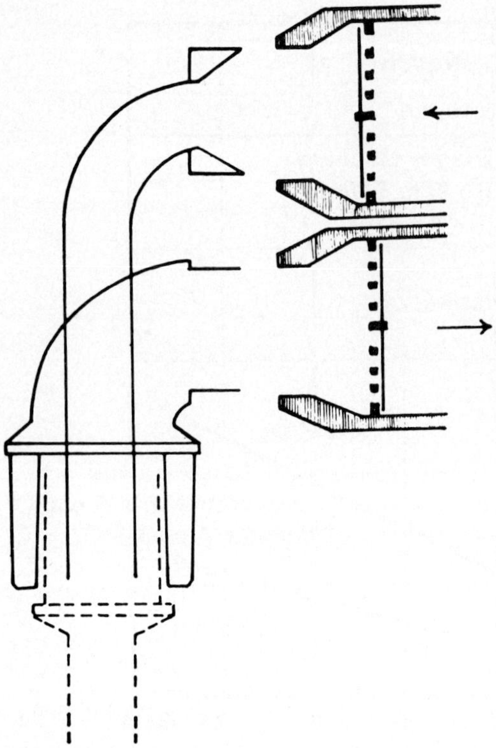

Figure 11–19. Columbia pediatric circle valve. A two-way respiratory valve (Zechman et al., 1965) is used (shaded portion of figure). To this is added a valve body made from an endotracheal tube adapter modified by adding a concentric 8.5-mm tube to divide inspiratory and expiratory pathways. When an endotracheal tube adapter is attached to the valve, inspiratory and expiratory pathways are divided into approximately equal cross-sectional areas. (From Rackow, H., and Salanitre, E.: A New Pediatric Circle Valve. Anesthesiology, 29:833, 1968.)

valve is closed, and the fresh gas flow is adjusted to just meet the patient's metabolic needs. In partial rebreathing, the valve is opened to allow some exhaled gas to escape to the atmosphere. The degree of rebreathing is determined by the extent to which the valve is opened. If nonrebreathing is desired, the valve is opened fully. With partial and nonrebreathing techniques, the fresh gas flow must be increased proportionally in order to maintain expansion of the rebreathing bag.

To enable assisted or controlled respiration to occur, the expiratory valve must be partially or completely closed; otherwise, adequate volume cannot be maintained in the rebreathing bag, despite increased fresh gas flow. If positive end-expiratory pressure (PEEP) is required, the expiratory valve may be replaced by a PEEP valve, although in semiclosed systems most of the resistance to expiration already resides in the expiratory valve.

The need for scavenging systems has necessitated the development of a new type of expiratory valve that can be connected to an exhaust system. These valves replace the conventional valve on older machines or attach to the tail of the rebreathing bag. These scavenging valves have generally been found to have a lower resistance (Nott and Norman, 1978).

Carbon Dioxide Absorbers

In the to-and-fro system, absorption is most efficient when the tidal volume of the patient equals air space in the canister filled with absorbent. Efficiency decreases when the air space is more or less than the tidal volume; thus, small canisters should be used with small patients and large canisters with large patients (Fig. 11–20). For sustained absorption in circle filters, it is most important to have the air space greater than the tidal volume. In a canister properly packed with 4- and 8-mesh absorbent granules, approximately half the volume consists of intergranular space. Selection of 4- to 8-mesh granules provides a compromise between minimal resistance to the passage of gases through the absorber and adequate surface area of absorbent for removal of carbon dioxide.

Neither circle nor to-and-fro units will remove all the carbon dioxide for any length of time. For years the ill effects of hypercapnia were not appreciated, but now it is known that high carbon dioxide blood levels predispose to ventricular fibrillation. Since certain patients tolerate incomplete removal of carbon dioxide better than others, the objective is total removal of carbon dioxide from the system.

Soda lime, the agent that absorbs carbon dioxide, is not a specific chemical compound. It varies in fragility, porosity, moisture content, and carbon dioxide absorptive capacity, according to the manufacturer.

Soda lime is essentially a mixture of sodium and calcium hydroxide, that furnishes free OH^-

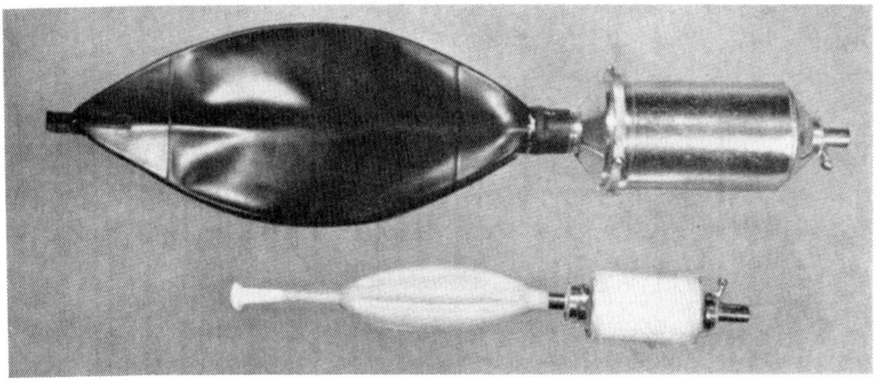

Figure 11–20. A conventional size to-and-fro canister and rebreathing bag is shown (top) in comparison to one used for small dogs and cats (bottom).

ions. The chemical reaction occurring in the canister is caused by carbon dioxide combining with water to form carbonic acid, which is then neutralized by the base.

$$2CO_2 + 2H_2O \longrightarrow 2H_2CO_3 \longrightarrow 4H + 2CO_3$$
$$2NaOH \longrightarrow 2OH + 2Na$$
$$Ca(OH)_2 \longrightarrow 2OH + Ca$$
$$\downarrow$$
$$4H_2O + Na_2CO_3 + CaCO_3$$

Absorption of carbonic acid does not easily occur because it is a weak, poorly ionized substance. Because the distance between granules of soda lime is relatively great, carbon dioxide molecules can pass between the granules. In addition, some that do contact the soda lime are not converted to carbonic acid. Therefore, some carbon dioxide passes through soda lime and returns to the patient. The concentration of carbon dioxide in the system thus gradually increases as alkali on the surface of the granules is converted to carbonates. Adriani and Rovenstine (1941) have arbitrarily selected 0.5% carbon dioxide as the average point where patients will show signs of hypercapnia.

Soda lime must contain 15 to 20% moisture in order to be efficient. Additional moisture caused by humidification of gases in the system does not increase the efficiency.

Today, considerable attention is paid to the production of soda lime. Moisture content is controlled. Potassium hydroxide, which is more active chemically than sodium hydroxide, is added in small quantities to improve absorption. Silicates, which confer hardness but decrease efficiency, have been eliminated. The reaction of sodium carbonate and calcium hydroxide to regenerate sodium hydroxide keeps pace with carbon dioxide absorption in the soda limes commercially available.

There is no difference in efficiency when canisters are placed in the horizontal or vertical position. Horizontal canisters should, however, be tightly packed to avoid a space through which absorbent is bypassed (channeling). A center tube in the canister, to diffuse gases through the soda lime, likewise makes no appreciable difference. The to-and-fro filter is dependent upon tidal volume, which varies considerably. The circle filter offers more efficient absorption if a large-capacity canister is used. Some canisters are divided into two equal-sized compartments that are interchangeable. As one half becomes exhausted, the other half is shifted into position and the exhausted half replenished.

In the most efficient systems, 1 g of soda lime absorbs 175 ml of carbon dioxide. The ordinary single canister absorbs 100 to 125 ml of carbon dioxide/g of soda lime. The total hours of effective use of soda lime are roughly proportional to the amount used. Once exhausted, soda lime does not regenerate upon being aerated and, therefore, should be discarded.

Baralyme (80% calcium hydroxide with 20% barium hydroxide) may be used as an alternative to soda lime. It is said to be less caustic and to produce less heat than soda lime.

Most absorbents (soda lime and Baralyme) contain an indicator, such as ethyl violet, which changes color as exhaustion occurs (usually this is from white or pink to violet). This color change may, however, revert on standing and therefore is not reliable. The color change is due to a shift in pH to the acidic side. Used soda lime also becomes hard and flintlike when crumbled between the fingers, and this test can be used to help determine when it is exhausted. Under ordinary conditions, the average canister is effective for 3 to 6 hours of continuous anesthesia.

If the absorbent inadvertently becomes exhausted during an operation, the patient will develop hypercapnia *with no evidence of cyanosis*. The pulse rate increases, the blood pressure rises and ultimately falls, the depth of respirations increases, and there is increased oozing in the surgical wound. As a result of increased pulmonary ventilation, the reservoir bag tends to collapse. If the condition is allowed to progress, hypercapnia increases the depth of anesthesia, and acidosis induces cardiac arrhythmias and arrest. It is imperative, therefore, that the condition of the absorbent be checked before each anesthetic period and occasionally during prolonged anesthesia. It is unwise to await the onset of signs of depletion of the absorbent. Should any doubt exist, fresh absorbent should always be used.

Owing to the water incorporated in the absorbent granules and the heat of carbon dioxide neutralization by soda lime, the humidity of the gases leaving the absorber is increased. Inhaled gases are also humidified by exhaled water, which rains out in the mechanical dead space of the system and is revaporized. Despite warm gases exhaled by the patient in a circle system, most heat in the system (approximately 75%) is due to neutralization of carbon dioxide by soda lime (Chalon, 1974). Humidity in a circle system is obviously modified by the amount of fresh gas flow, ventilation rate, tidal volume, volume of carbon dioxide exhaled, and previous use of the system. Nomograms are available that enable calculation of humidity in the system. Reducing the fresh gas flow raises the humidity, an advantage of the low flow technique. The smaller the patient, the drier the inhaled gases. With average patients, values of 30 to 60% relative humidity have been reported; it may take as much as an hour and a half for such maximal humidification to occur.

In to-and-fro systems in which the absorber is near the patient's airway, fully saturated vapor may be inhaled after approximately 30 minutes. The temperature may be as high as 42° C (Fig. 11–21), which is sufficient to eliminate the loss of body heat by the lungs. It is a hazard in warm environments (Chalon, 1974). Furthermore, with the close proximity of the absorber, there is the potential for soda lime to be inhaled by the patient.

Rebreathing or Reservoir Bag

The rebreathing bag acts as a reservoir for gases during the pause between respiratory excursions and accommodates the fluctuating volume and pressure of the closed and semiclosed systems. The bag size should allow for these volume fluctuations without collapsing or overdistending; at the same time, respirations should cause obvious movement of the bag and permit evaluation of respiratory activity. A bag size 8 to 10 times the tidal volume is therefore indicated (Adriani, 1962). An excessively large bag, especially in large animal equipment, will prolong the equilibration time between gas flowing into the circuit and the inspired gas. Compliance of the bag should be such that resistance to breathing is not excessive. This is of special concern in small dogs, cats, and laboratory animals. Since gases are moved in and out of the bag by the patient's own respiratory efforts, the internal diameter of the neck of the bag should equal or exceed that of the airway. Some bags are also provided with an additional outlet from

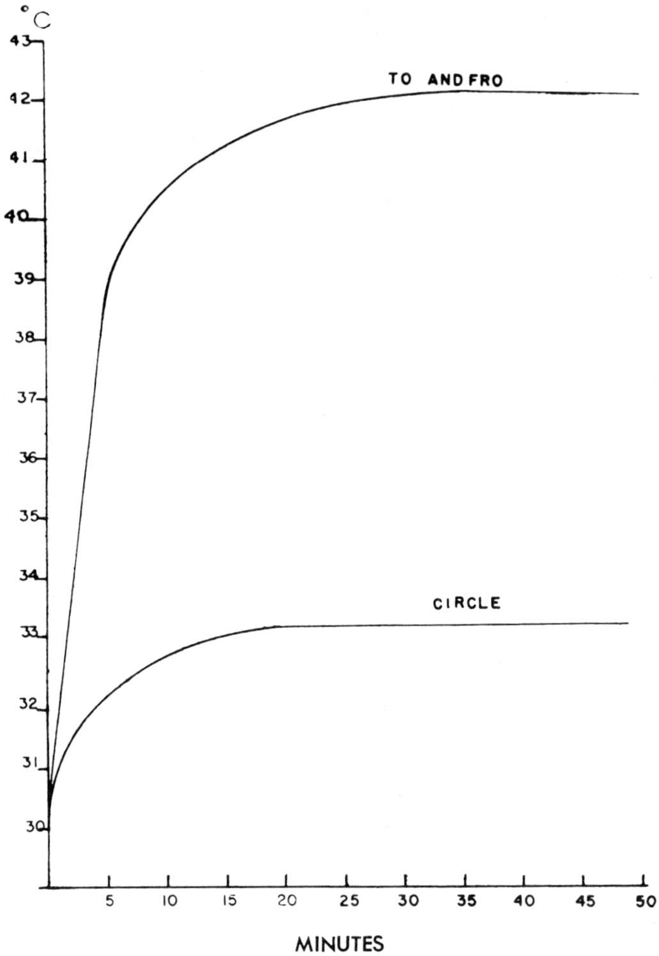

Figure 11–21. Comparison under identical ventilating conditions of temperatures in mask using circle filter (Foregger with 30″ × 1¼″ corrugated tubing) and to-and-fro (13 × 8 cm brass canister). The time in minutes required to reach a steady state is also shown. (From Adriani, J.: *The Chemistry and Physics of Anesthesia,* 2nd ed. Charles C Thomas, Springfield, Illinois, 1962.)

which water can be drained or through which gases can be added.

Vaporizers

If volatile liquid anesthetic agents are used in a gas machine, it is necessary to have some form of vaporizer to volatilize them.

Oxygen flowing through the vaporizer becomes partially or completely saturated with anesthetic vapor, which is then carried to the patient. Oxygen thus acts as a transport mechanism for these agents, in addition to satisfying the patient's oxygen requirements.

The output of a vaporizer is basically dependent upon the vapor pressure of the anesthetic at a given temperature. Figure 11–22 shows the vapor pressures of commonly used anesthetics at various temperatures. As the temperature rises, the vapor pressure rises and, other factors remaining constant, output of the vaporizer rises also.

Four types of simple vaporizers are commonly employed for anesthetic liquids. Listed in order of increasing efficiency, they are surface, wick, bubble, and drip (Fig. 11–23).

In surface (drawover) vaporizers, oxygen passes over the liquid anesthetic and in the process displaces vapor rising from the liquid. This

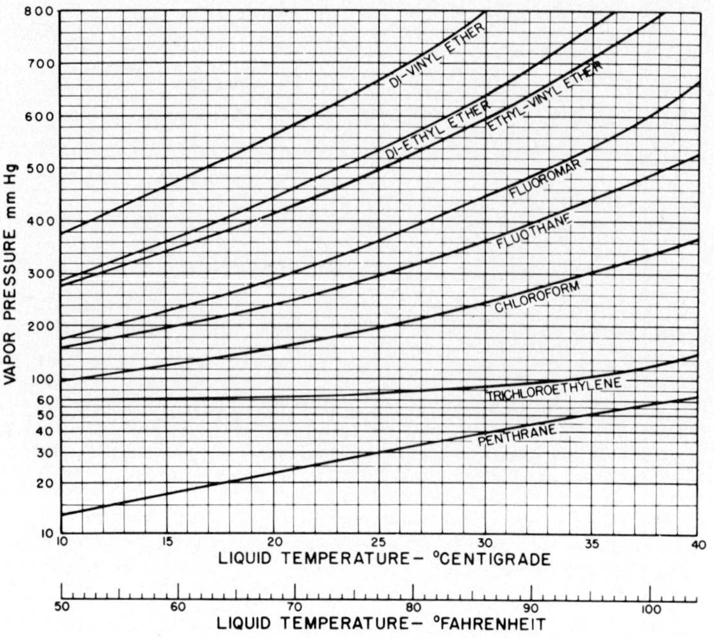

Figure 11–22. Vapor pressure graph. As the temperature of the liquid anesthetic rises, the vapor pressure increases. High temperatures tend to produce dangerously high concentrations of anesthetic in vaporizers that are not temperature-compensated. Penthrane = methoxyflurane; fluothane = halothane; fluoromar = fluroxene.

reduces the partial pressure of the vapor, and liquid begins to evaporate to restore the vapor pressure. Heat required for vaporization (latent heat of vaporization) is extracted from unevaporated liquid and the vaporizer jar itself, thus lowering their temperature and reducing the vapor pressure of the remaining liquid. For this reason, simple vaporizers are reduced in efficiency as time elapses and the liquid anesthetic cools.

Wick vaporizers contain cotton fibers partially immersed in the anesthetic to increase the area of contact between gas and liquid. The cotton fibers have greater affinity for water than for anesthetic and absorb exhaled water vapor, if present, to the exclusion of anesthetic liquid.

Bubble vaporizers direct the gas flow through the anesthetic and thus increase the amount of vapor entrained. These also tend to develop a falling output due to cooling of the anesthetic liquid. They are used out-of-circuit.

The drip method employs a reservoir containing the anesthetic agent. A valve controls the release of liquid and the rate of flow can be seen in a drip chamber. The agent is allowed to drop at a metered rate onto a copper screen from

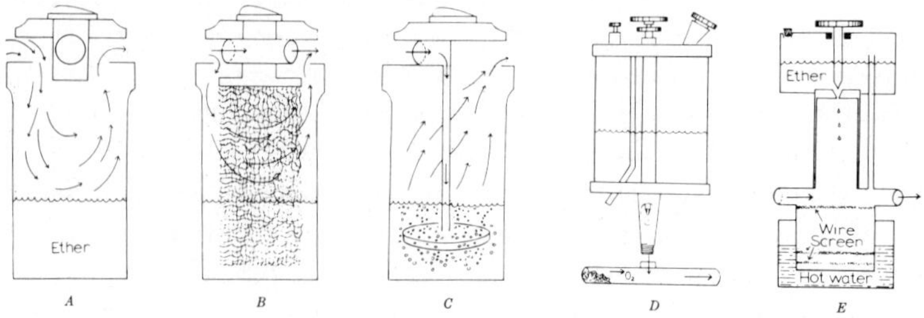

Figure 11–23. Vaporizers in order of increasing efficiency: *(A)* surface, *(B)* wick, *(C)* bubble, and *(D, E)* drip. Arrows indicate direction of gas flow.

which it evaporates. The screen is often incorporated in a soda lime canister, and absorption of carbon dioxide produces heat, which in turn vaporizes the anesthetic.

Some refinements have been developed to overcome the loss of efficiency that occurs in vaporizers during prolonged periods of anesthesia. These include immersion of the vaporizer in a second container of warm water (e.g., EMO) or use of a heavy thermoconductive sheath for the vaporization chamber (Foregger Copper Kettle, Dräger Vapor).

Saturation vaporizers, such as the Copper Kettle and Vernitrol, produce the maximum vapor output that can be achieved at any given temperature (see Fig. 11–22). To determine anesthetic flows from a saturation vaporizer, the following formula is used:

$$\frac{\text{Vapor pressure}}{\text{Atmospheric pressure}} \times 100\% = \%\text{ of total volume}$$

For example, at 21 ° C (70° F), the vapor pressure of halothane is 253.9 mm Hg.

$$\frac{253.9\text{ mm Hg}}{760\text{ mm Hg}} \times 100\% = 33\%\text{ of total volume}$$

Because the output of a saturation vaporizer usually exceeds the required concentration, it is diluted with bypass oxygen to produce a working concentration. If a saturation vaporizer containing halothane at 21° C has an oxygen flow of 100 ml per minute passing through it and 33% of the total output is halothane vapor, then the total output is 150 ml per minute.

$$\begin{aligned} 100\text{ ml/min of } O_2\ (66\%) &= 100\text{ ml/min } O_2 \\ \text{Halothane vapor } (33\%) &= \underline{\ 50\text{ ml/min}} \\ \text{Total output}\quad & \ \ 150\text{ ml/min} \end{aligned}$$

Since 33% halothane vapor far exceeds the quantity that is safe for induction, it must be diluted to a usable concentration. If 3% halothane is desired, the necessary calculation can be accomplished using the following formula:

$$\begin{aligned} 3\%\ x &= 50\text{ ml/min halothane} \\ 100\%\ x &= 1665\text{ ml/min total flow} \end{aligned}$$

$$(50\text{ ml/min halothane} + 1615\text{ ml/min } O_2)$$

This type of calculation is most easily done with a slide rule furnished with the vaporizer.

Use of a saturation vaporizer at high ambient temperatures is potentially dangerous unless the anesthetist is aware of the vaporizer's capabilities. For example, at 68° F a saturation vaporizer cannot produce more than 3.0% methoxyflurane vapor, which is the concentration used for induction (see Fig. 11–22). At 95° F the output is 6.6%, a more dangerous concentration. When one is using halothane in a saturation vaporizer, the temperature effect is even more pronounced.

Because of their extreme potency and/or the need for economy, special precision vaporizers have been developed for metering halothane, methoxyflurane, and similar anesthetics (Fig. 11–24). Vaporizers of this type are calibrated in percentage of a specific anesthetic by volume in the mixture delivered. They include Fluotec,* Pentec,* Fluomatic,* and Drager Vapor.* The Copper Kettle* and Vernitrol* also permit precision vaporization of various anesthetics. The Vapor and Fluotec Mark III are especially desirable when small animals are anesthetized and gas flow rates are less than 1 L per minute, for these vaporizers provide known halothane concentrations at low gas flow rates.

Among factors affecting precision direct-reading vaporizers are viscosity, density, and flow rate of the carrier gases. Some are also affected by back pressure and retrograde flow, temperature of the anesthetic liquid, deterioration due to corrosion, and accumulation of preservatives or other foreign materials within the vaporizer. Vaporizers are calibrated with oxygen. Different carrier gases with different viscosities and densities alter the distribution of gas flow within the vaporizer. Haskins and Knapp (1980) found that halothane output for the Fluotec Mark III, using air, nitrous oxide/oxygen, (50%/50%), and nitrous oxide (100%), decreased an average of 87.9%, 85.4%, and 70.9% respectively, when compared with halothane/oxygen output. They reported that similar findings for the Vapor and the Fluomatic vaporizers have been encountered. A total gas flow of 2 L per minute was used. The qualitative

*See Appendix A

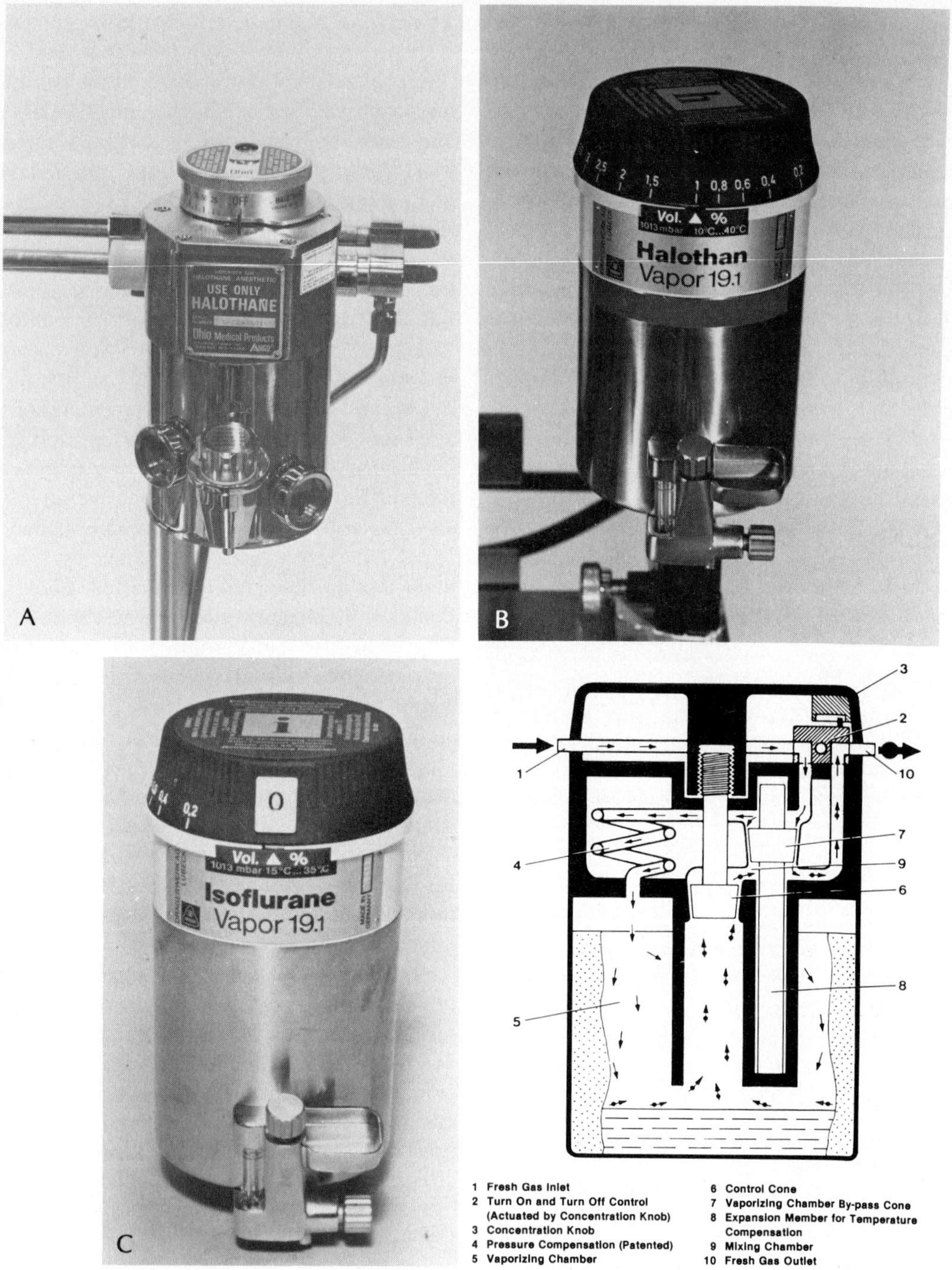

D

Figure 11–24. Three types of calibrated temperature-compensated out-of-circuit vaporizers. *A*, Ohio, and *B*, Vapor for halothane. *C*, Vapor for isoflurane. *D*, A cross-sectional diagram of the Vapor. *1*, Fresh gas inlet; *2*, Turn on and turn off control (actuated by concentration knob); *3*, concentration knob; *4*, Pressure compensation (patented); *5*, Vaporizing chamber; *6*, Control cone; *7*, Vaporizing chamber by-pass cone; *8*, Expansion member for temperature compensation; *9*, Mixing chamber; *10*, Fresh gas outlet. (*A* is from Ohio Medical Products, Madison, Wisconsin, and *B*, *C*, and *D* are from North American Dräger, Telford, Pennsylvania).

effect of the carrier gas on the output is the same with flow rates up to 5 L per minute.

When vaporizers are connected in series (for example, a halothane vaporizer downstream from a methoxyflurane vaporizer), cross-contamination of the vaporizers can occur, especially if an agent of high volatility is placed upstream from an agent of low volatility. They should, therefore, be connected in parallel.

In-circuit vaporizers are generally unsuitable for administration of halothane because known concentrations cannot be administered and dangerously high concentrations are likely. Vaporizers of relatively low efficiency, such as the Goldman,* may, however, be used in-circuit. The advantages and disadvantages of in-circuit and out-of-circuit vaporizers are outlined in Table 11–1.

Precision vaporizers, similar to those used for halothane, are available for administration of methoxyflurane. These are the Pentec* and Pentomatic.* They should *never* be used for halothane because the percentage of halothane delivered is far greater than the dial setting for percentage of methoxyflurane (Fig. 11–25). Similar vaporizers are available for enflurane and isoflurane. Since the vapor pressure of the latter is similar to that of halothane, isoflurane can, with precautions, be used in halothane vaporizers. The Copper Kettle and Vernitrol may also be used; in fact, these latter two vaporizers can be used to deliver known concentrations of any volatile anesthetic.

Methoxyflurane may also be administered with a bubble-type vaporizer; these, however, are not calibrated. If an in-circuit vaporizer is to be used, it must be of the drawover or wick type in order to avoid high resistance to breathing. These vaporizers are especially suitable for administration of ether or methoxyflurane.

*See Appendix A.

Flowmeters

Flowmeters indicate the rate at which anesthetic gases and oxygen flow to the patient.

TABLE 11–1. Comparison of Vaporizer Outside (VOC) and Inside (VIC) the Breathing Circuit

VOC	VIC
VENTILATION	
1. Changes in ventilation do not affect the output of the vaporizer.	1. An increase in ventilation due to light anesthesia automatically increases the inspired concentration.
2. An increase in ventilation reduces inspired concentration because of an increased uptake of anesthetic agent by the animal and a constant output of the vaporizer.	2. Sudden changes in ventilation can produce dangerously high inspired concentrations.
3. Assisted or controlled ventilation can be used with a greater degree of safety.	3. Assisted or controlled ventilation at any given setting greatly increases inspired concentrations.
FRESH GAS FLOW	
1. For any setting, the lower the fresh gas flow the lower is the amount of anesthetic inspired.	1. For any setting, the lower the fresh gas flow the higher the inspired concentration.
2. The lower the fresh gas flow, the greater the economy.	2. The lower the fresh gas flow, the greater the economy.
3. Economy does not introduce the risk of high concentrations.	3. Economy is at the expense of potentially high inspired concentrations.
VAPORIZER	
1. High-efficiency vaporizers are essential.	1. Low-efficiency vaporizers can be used.
2. Known concentrations can be delivered to the breathing circuit, and the inspired concentration can be estimated with no difficulty.	2. Calibrated vaporizers are meaningless because ventilation affects the inspired concentration to a marked degree.

(Adapted from Soma, L.R., and Klide, A.M.: Techniques and Equipment for Inhalation Anesthesia in Small Animals. J.A.V.M.A., 152:957, 1968.)

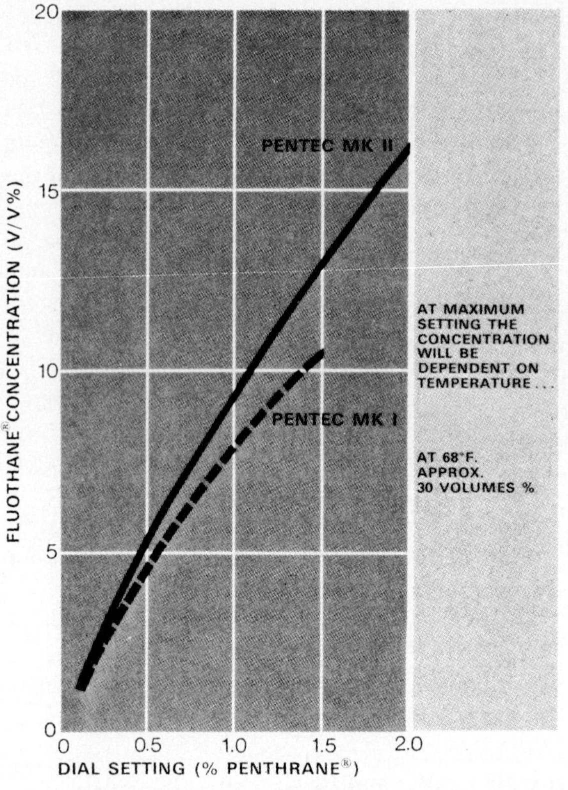

Figure 11–25. Typical performance of Pentec vaporizers, designed for use with methoxyflurane (Penthrane), when filled with halothane (Fluothane). Lethal concentrations of halothane are easily achieved at dial settings that are safe for methoxyflurane. Oxygen flow is 5 liters/minute at normal room temperature.

Those commonly used are either 1) the fixed orifice flowmeter, or 2) the variable orifice flowmeter.

With the first type, gas under pressure is forced through a standard orifice. This causes a pressure differential on either side of the orifice. If a manometer is placed so that one limb is upstream to the orifice and the other limb downstream, the pressure drop across the orifice can be measured on the manometer. The ''wet flowmeter,'' which in years past was standard equipment on the Foregger apparatus, is an example of this type (Fig. 11–26,*F*). Depression of water in the upstream limb of the manometer is calibrated as flow rate on the manometer tube. This type of flowmeter is highly efficient, provided the orifice is kept clean and the water level remains constant.

Variable orifice flowmeters are of several types, but the basic principle in their operation is the same. The differential between upstream and downstream pressures remains constant, whereas the diameter of the orifice varies. The rate of flow is directly proportional to the size of the orifice; the larger the size, the greater the flow and *vice versa*.

The variable orifice flowmeter, sometimes called the Thorpe tube, consists of a tapered glass tube containing a ball, bobbin, rotor, or other type of float. The inside diameter of the tube enlarges from the bottom upward, so that when gas enters at the bottom the rotor is elevated to the point where gas escapes around the rotor. The rotor then floats free in the tube suspended by the flow of gas. If gas flow is increased, the float rises within the tube. The tube is calibrated, and the float height indicates flow rate.

As gas flows through the tube and passes the float, a pressure drop occurs. The difference in the upstream and downstream pressure is equal to the weight of the float, and an equilibrium is reached. If the flow rate is increased, the float again rises until the pressure differential equals the weight of the float, at which point a new equilibrium is established.

Some flowmeters are calibrated to function with the tube placed at an angle, compensation

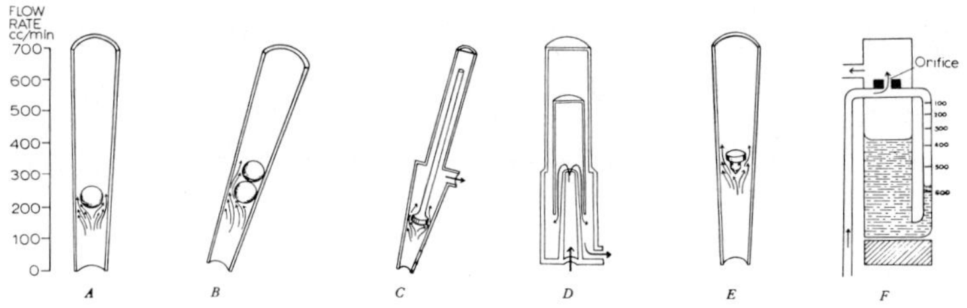

Figure 11–26. Several types of flowmeters. Arrows indicate direction of gas flow. In "dry" flowmeters (*A* through *E*), a float is suspended on the stream of gas. As flow increases, the float rises. Calibration of the tube enables measurement of flow rate. *F* is a "wet" flowmeter containing distilled water. As gas flows through the orifice, a pressure differential is created on the two columns of water. This differential is measured as gas flow on the small calibrated tube.

being made for the effect of friction between float and tube wall. Others are accurate only when the tube is vertical and the float rotates freely in the tube. Anesthetic machines equipped with the latter usually have a built-in leveling device that must be adjusted each time the equipment is moved.

Manometers

If open chest surgery is to be performed, a manometer is desirable. Connected to the rebreathing system, it serves to prevent harmful overexpansion of the lungs. Both spring-operated and water types are available. Spring types are usually used in conjunction with an expiratory valve, the valve being set to release whenever pressure in the system exceeds that desired. With water manometers, gas is automatically vented through the manometer when pressure exceeds the setting. With spontaneous breathing, the setting is usually 15 to 18 cm of water.

Regulators

Regulators are attached between the source of compressed gas and the flowmeter. They permit the flowmeter to provide a constant gas flow despite variations of pressure and temperature within the cylinder of compressed gas. They also serve to supply a constant pressure of oxygen for the operation of ventilators (see Chap. 7).

Operation of Semiclosed and Closed Systems

When administration of anesthetic by one of these techniques is planned, the following steps are performed:

1. The machine and system are checked to determine that everything is working properly. A routine suggested by Dorsch and Dorsch (1977) includes the following:
   a. Close the flow control valves. If one is open when a cylinder valve is opened, the indicator may shoot to the top, stick in this position, and remain unnoticed. Even in piped systems, it is essential to verify that emergency oxygen and nitrous oxide are available in case the pipe system fails. Turn the oxygen cylinder valve only sufficiently to verify that pressure is 500 PSIG or greater; then close the valve. Repeat this procedure for the nitrous oxide cylinder, the pressure of which should be 700 PSIG or greater. Where piped gas is not available, check both oxygen and nitrous oxide tanks to verify that one cylinder is full (oxygen 2100 PSIG, nitrous oxide 780 PSIG), and that the other tank has an adequate pressure as described previously. Close the full reserve cylinder valve and leave the new cylinder valve wide open. Connect pipeline hoses and turn on the oxygen alarm (if available).

   Check each flowmeter to see that the indicator moves smoothly, does not stick, and returns to zero when the flow control valve is closed. Check vaporizers for liquid level and a tight filler cap; add more liquid agent if necessary. Check the machine for leaks. The authors recommend attaching a pressure gauge from a standard blood pressure apparatus to the machine outlet (immediately distal to the vaporizers), and opening the flow control valve until pressure of 22 mm Hg (30 cm water) is maintained on the gauge. Do this with the vaporizers turned on. The leak rate should be less than 50 ml per minute. If it is greater, turn the vaporizers off and repeat the test, since leaks commonly occur in the vaporizer. If the leak persists, the machine should not be used until repaired. After checking for leaks, turn off the flowmeter and vaporizer.

Check the absorber to see that it is not turned off or partially bypassed and that the absorbent is not exhausted. Absorbent showing signs of exhaustion when rested may revert to pre-exhaustion color; this change is not accompanied by any significant recovery of absorptive function, and color will return soon after it is put into use. It is therefore better to check absorbent at the end of use. A label on the absorber to indicate duration of use is advisable.

b. Check for proper gas flow by having the anesthesiologist or technician breath through the system twice, first to check unidirectional valves for proper movement, next to see that the reservoir bag inflates and deflates. Turn on and calibrate the oxygen analyzer, if one is to be used.

c. Test the remainder of the system for leaks and function of the expiratory valve by closing the valve, occluding the Y-piece, and filling the reservoir bag via the oxygen flush valve until a pressure of 30 cm of water is present on the manometer. The pressure should be maintained and not fall quickly. Open the valve, and the pressure should fall rapidly. Obviously, if a leak is found, the system should be checked carefully.

d. Check the scavenging system. Make sure that the scavenging device is connected to the expiratory valve and that the disposal system is connected. An emergency resuscitation bag should be available, so that when a problem occurs that cannot be corrected quickly, it is possible to ventilate the patient with at least 21% oxygen (room air) while the system is repaired.

2. Endotracheal catheters of appropriate sizes are checked to insure that the lumen is patent and that the cuff does not leak.

3. The patient is premedicated (if indicated), and anesthesia is induced by intravenous thiobarbiturate, by administration of ketamine, or by neuroleptanalgesia or similar combination. Anesthesia may also be induced by inhalation from a mask.

4. An endotracheal catheter is inserted and the cuff inflated and clamped.

5. The adapter of the catheter is connected to the gas machine.

6. Oxygen is run into the system in sufficient quantity to inflate the reservoir bag to approximately one-half to two-thirds capacity. If immediate administration of anesthetic is desired, the system may be briefly flushed and charged with anesthetic mixture. Once the unit is in use, the gas flow is adjusted to maintain partial inflation of the bag and to produce the anesthetic concentration (MAC) for induction or maintenance as indicated. The degree to which a high or low flow technique will be used depends upon the depth of anesthesia already induced, patient size, status of anesthetic waste disposal, need for controlled or assisted ventilation, use of nitrous oxide, and personal preferences of the anesthesiologist. When a closed technique is used, the oxygen flow is adjusted to a rate estimated to meet the metabolic requirements of the animal (50 to 250 ml per minute in most dogs, for instance). Should only partial rebreathing be required, the gas flow must be considerably increased, owing to loss through the opened expiratory valve. Initially, adjustment of gas flow to provide a stable degree of distension of the bag may be difficult, especially when a complete rebreathing technique is used. Too much overdistends the bag; too little results in collapse. In either instance, respiratory resistance is increased. After stabilization of the gas flow, variation of bag distension is indicative of a change in respiratory minute volume and, therefore, the degree of anesthesia, the efficiency of carbon dioxide absorption, or the level of pain stimulation.

7. When one is using complete rebreathing, it may be necessary to add additional anesthetic intermittently, since many vaporizers are ineffective or inaccurate when the gas flow through them is small, no system is entirely air-tight, and the rubber goods absorb anesthetics. Anesthetic is administered continuously in partial rebreathing techniques.

8. If assisted or controlled breathing is required, the bag is compressed until the chest expands adequately; it is then released and the procedure repeated. The duration of the expiratory pause should be at least twice that of inspiration. When a partial rebreathing technique is used, it may be necessary either to increase the degree of rebreathing by partially closing the expiratory valve or to increase the gas flow rate. Increased fresh gas flow decreases rebreathing and predisposes to hypocapnia during controlled ventilation; humidity in the circuit will also be low. When an in-circuit vaporizer is used, its output should be reduced during controlled ventilation to prevent increased delivery of anesthetic.

9. Should anesthesia become too deep and rapid elimination of anesthetic from the circuit be required, the vaporizer or anesthetic gas is turned off, the expiratory valve opened, the bag compressed and emptied, and the system refilled with oxygen by means of the emergency flush control. This procedure is repeated several times, thereby flushing anesthetic from the system. Respiration is assisted during this time to facilitate elimination of the anesthetic.

When one is using rebreathing techniques, it is important to realize that the oxygen as well as the anesthetic mixture is diluted by exhaled gases. The degree of dilution increases as the fresh gas flow decreases relative to the respiratory minute volume (Fig. 11–27).

10. When anesthesia is to be terminated, the anesthetic is turned off, the expiratory valve is opened, and the anesthetic mixture is flushed from the system with oxygen. As the patient recovers from anesthesia, the adapter of the endotracheal catheter can be disconnected from the gas machine. The catheter should be allowed to remain in position until the swallowing reflex returns. This is especially important in the ruminant, which may otherwise aspirate rumen con-

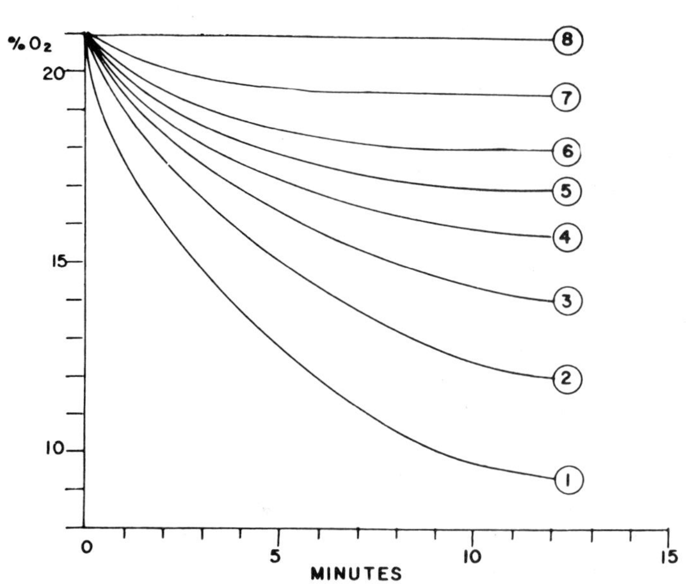

Figure 11–27. Curves indicate the rapidity of decline in inspired oxygen tension of a subject having a minute volume of 8 liters per minute breathing from a semiclosed inhaler. Gas mixture contained 21% oxygen at flow rates in liters per minute indicated by the figure in a circle. Mixtures used at low flow rates must contain more than 1 part oxygen to 4 of other gas or vapors. (From Adriani, J.: *The Chemistry and Physics of Anesthesia,* 2nd ed. Charles C Thomas, Springfield, Illinois, 1962.)

tents or saliva, and in animals (brachycephalic breeds of dogs, Equidae) in which soft tissue obstruction of the upper airway is common.

11. An alternate method of induction is by means of a mask connected to the anesthetic circuit. Preanesthetic sedation should be administered first. The animal is restrained, and the mask is held snugly over the animal's face while anesthetic mixture is inhaled from the system. The lesser the degree of rebreathing, the more rapid is induction, since the induction mixture is not diluted by exhaled gases. A high-flow technique (fresh gas flow greater than minute volume) is used. Once the residual air in the lungs is replaced with anesthetic mixture, the amount of rebreathing can be increased as required.

With the relatively large apparatus volume of the circle system, gases are not rapidly circulated by the small tidal volume of small patients. This theoretically delays changes in the depth of anesthesia. Modifications of the circle system have been designed, therefore, to overcome this problem for human pediatric patients. Ultimately a miniaturized circle system was developed, such as the Bloomquist. In this system, the fresh gas flow was introduced in the expiratory side of the circuit. Humidity was improved, but there were increases both in resistance to expiration and in the chances of soda lime inhalation. Several different sizes of soda lime canisters were required, depending upon the size of the patient. A more recent modification utilized the exothermic reaction of the carbon dioxide and soda lime to heat a vaporizer and thereby to improve humidity in the circuit.

Just as problems associated with small patients have influenced modifications of the basic circle system, the needs of large animals have imposed the necessity for design modification. When one is inducing inhalation anesthesia in large animals, economy dictates maximal rebreathing. In this case, filling the anesthetic circuit with a high concentration of anesthetic vapor is advantageous. If, for instance, a 10% Fluotec vaporizer is available, the system may be filled with 10% halothane vapor prior to application of the mask. The concentration of anesthetic vapor in the system may also be increased by dropping a measured amount of liquid anesthetic into the reservoir bag (1 ml volatile anesthetic = approximately 200 ml vapor). Since irregular respirations and even voluntary breath holding are common during induction, it is essential that this be differentiated from possible respiratory obstruction or arrest. Observation of both the reservoir bag and thorax for adequate excursion is therefore imperative. When reflex apnea presents a problem, assisted ventilation may be helpful. In fact, provided oxygen is being administered, restraint and relaxation may be achieved by injection of succinylcholine followed by anesthesia induced by controlled ventilation. Whatever the method of induction by inhalation, once this is achieved, maintenance by endotracheal administration is desirable.

Selection of Semiclosed or Closed Techniques

During the late 1950s low flow rate (closed) systems for inhalation anesthesia without reliance upon specific concentrations of anesthetic agents were commonplace (Hamilton, 1980). With the advent of halothane anesthesia, high-flow, essentially nonrebreathing, techniques became common. With halothane, out-of-circuit vaporizers were needed, especially when controlled ventilation was used. The function of these out-of-circuit precision vaporizers was enhanced by high flow rates. Their use was further encouraged by the concept of MAC and by the consistency of its dose-effect relationship. Concern that low fresh gas flows of nitrous oxide and oxygen in a circle system may contribute to a dangerous FIO_2 also supported high flow rates. Consequently, the increasing precision of anesthetic delivery and of the dosage required to induce and maintain anesthesia promoted increasing reliance on the machine and vaporizer setting. More recently, there has been a resurgence of interest in low flow anesthesia owing to the need to decrease operating room contamination, to maintain normocapnia in the face of ventilation, and to maintain relative humidity at 60% or greater (Hamilton, 1980). In large animal anesthesia, low flow techniques have been essential due to the need for economy in a system that would otherwise require gas flow rates equal to or greater than the minute volume. The influence of flow rate upon economy is well illustrated in Figure 11–28.

When low flow techniques are employed in large animal anesthesia, nitrogen accumulation in the circuit has been a concern. Tevik et al. (1969) found in the horse that oxygen flow rates of 1.5 to 2.5 L per minute were sufficient to meet oxygen requirements of the normal anesthetized horse, which was breathing spontaneously. The closed system was not flushed with oxygen during the anesthetic period, and nitrogen accumulated from 23 to 57% after two hours. The authors recommend, in the average horse, using an oxygen flow rate of 2.5 L per minute, periodically flushing the rebreathing bag with oxygen two to four times during the first 15 minutes of anesthesia (every half hour thereafter), and assisting respiration to remove excess CO_2.

The inspired breath from an anesthetic circuit is comprised of previously expired gas, fresh gas, or usually a mixture of the two. The higher the flow rate (i.e., the more fresh gas added), the more each inspiration comprises new gas. On the other hand, the lower the flow rate, the more the inhaled gas is previously breathed gas. Since uptake of the anesthetic agent is high during induction, the exhaled gas contains relatively little anesthetic agent. Dilution of anesthetic in the fresh gas flow is thus significant if a large fraction of rebreathing occurs. When the uptake of oxygen and the anesthetic agent become equal, then inspired/expired equilibrium is achieved. Beyond this point in time, for instance with nitrous oxide, oxygen uptake is greater than anesthetic uptake, the expired gas is rich in nitrous oxide, and the inspired concentration of nitrous oxide is higher than that metered (Hamilton, 1980). With high flow rates, this effect makes little difference. It is

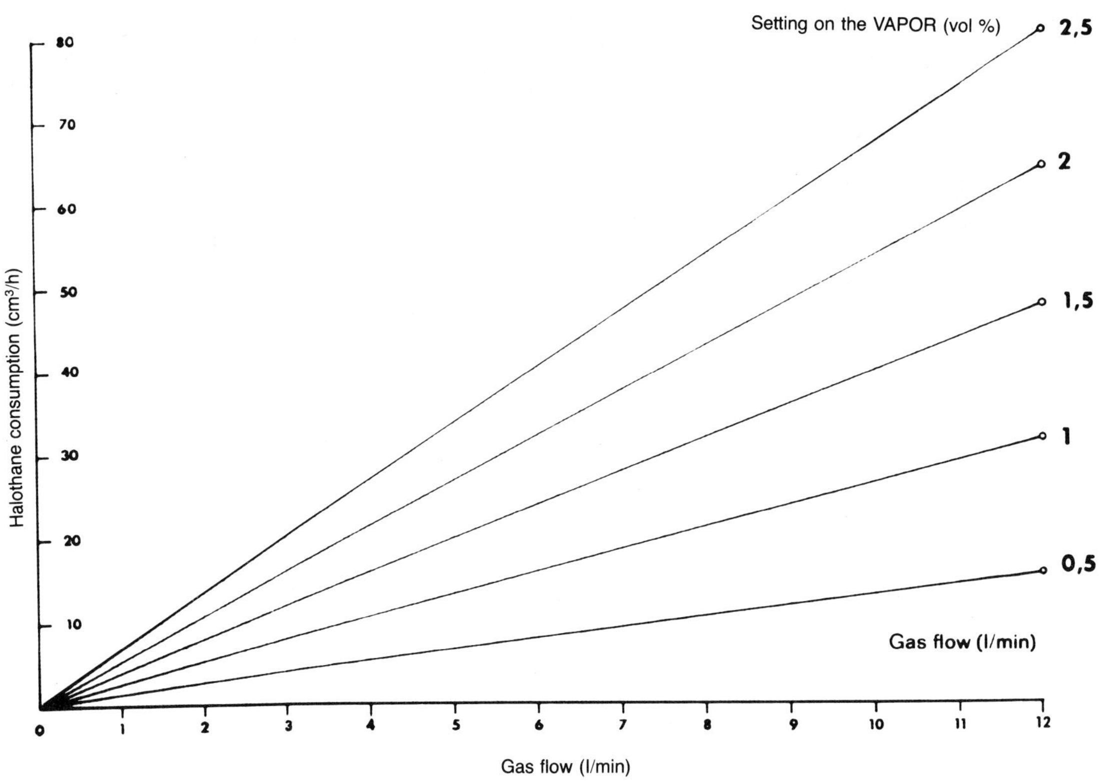

Figure 11–28. Halothane consumption as a function of the concentration and the gas flow (at 20° C and 760 mm Hg). (Courtesy of North American Dräger Company, Telford, Pennsylvania.)

also obvious that the lower the flow rate, the longer it takes for a change in metered concentration to result in a comparable change in inspired concentration, the greater the difference between inspired concentration and metered concentration, and the less one can rely on flowmeter and vaporizer settings. In practice, one should thus use high gas flow rates to achieve MAC values in a reasonable time.

Once induction has been achieved, a low flow system is utilized. Oxygen flow is reduced to that necessary to satisfy metabolic needs (4 ml/kg), and nitrous oxide is added in a quantity sufficient to maintain the desired concentration (Hamilton, 1980). One must monitor the following: 1) the concentration of oxygen in the inspired gas, 2) the fullness of the reservoir bag, which indicates the presence or absence of a leak or indicates if the supply of gas is equal, less, or greater than the uptake of either oxygen or anesthetic agent, and 3) the adequacy of the level of anesthesia. If nitrous oxide is used in combination with halothane or other volatile anesthetics, similar principles are utilized, but it is essential to appreciate that metered concentration of anesthetics may need to be much higher. For instance, at low flow settings it may be necessary to deliver as much as 10% of halothane. Ten percent of a total flow of 500 ml of gas is only 50 ml of vapor added to the anesthetic system per minute. Changes in concentration within the total system would therefore be slow. With such a low flow system, potent inhalation agents may be added continuously in small amounts or intermittently in small bursts. When a continuous technique is used, the amount of anesthetic needed should decrease with time. When the metered technique is used, the intervals between bursts of agent become progressively longer with time. Conversion to a high flow system is appropriate for rapid reduction in the level of anesthesia.

Other workers have attempted more precise determination of flow rates in a closed system by use of mathematical formulas based upon kinetics of uptake and distribution of anesthetic agents (Lowe, 1981). In a totally closed system, precise monitoring of metabolic oxygen consumption (fresh oxygen flow required to maintain a steady concentration) has benefits. Any decrease in metabolic oxygen consumption from that predicted on the basis of body weight and temperature constitutes an oxygen deficit, and the underlying cause should be corrected to avoid metabolic acidosis. Decreased oxygen consumption has been observed clinically during periods of diminished cardiac output or vasoconstriction, and with tourniquets and aortic cross-clamping. Lowe (1981) indicated that metabolic oxygen consumption oscillates plus or minus 10% following bolus injections of opiates, but does not vary significantly with the concentrations of volatile agents required for clinical anesthesia, i.e., 1.3 MAC or less.

After considering the advantages and disadvantages of the fully closed circuit, it is readily apparent that many of the disadvantages can be overcome by dissipating some exhaled gases to the outside. Use of a partial rebreathing technique reduces the accumulation of carbon dioxide and heat and also limits the dilution of inhaled anesthetic mixtures with exhaled air. In small animals in which equipment dead space may constitute a significant proportion of the tidal volume, the increased gas flow tends to flush exhaled gases from this dead space. Therefore, the degree of compromise between virtual nonrebreathing and complete rebreathing is contingent upon the relative significance of economy, contamination of room air with anesthetic, and the disadvantages of a fully closed system. In small animals, gas flows approaching or even in excess of the respiratory minute volume do not create an economic burden (Fig. 11–28), whereas equipment dead space may well be excessive. In large domestic animals, however, in which respiratory minute volumes often exceed 100 L per minute, a considerable degree of rebreathing is obviously essential, and oxygen flow rates are often adequate for metabolic needs only.

CARE OF THE ANESTHETIC MACHINE

Although most anesthetic machines require little maintenance, the various detachable components of the circuit do require thorough washing and sterilization. Anesthetic apparatus may harbor pathogenic microorganisms that are a potential threat to the anesthetized patient. During a nosocomial outbreak of *Klebsiella* spp. in a veterinary hospital, the organism was cultured from endotracheal catheters (Heath, 1983). Certainly conditions favor transfer when the same apparatus is used consecutively for several patients, although recognizable morbidity from cross-infection by contaminated anesthetic equipment is rare.

Several reports suggest anesthesia machines as sources of infection, but these are mostly inconclusive. Studies of six anesthetic machines in routine use on patients colonized with gram-negative bacilli and patients not colonized failed to reveal significant contamination of the machines. Bacterial species most commonly recovered were environmental in origin. Machines were subjected to routine hygienic management. The surface of the machine was wiped with a damp cloth and then wiped with alcohol. Soda lime was changed prior to each use. Disposable corrugated tubing, bag, plastic "Y" piece and elbow connectors, and sterile mask or endotracheal tube were used (du Moulin and Saubermann, 1977). These authors believe routine sterilization and cleaning procedures currently in use are adequate. Others, however, have expressed significant concern (Beck, 1978; Craig et al., 1975). The latter authors report that if ethylene oxide sterilization is not available, detachable components of anesthetic breathing circuits can be "pasteurized" by washing in a standard automatic clothes-washing machine supplied with hot water at 170° F (76.5° C). If ethylene oxide is used for sterilization, thorough elimination of the gas by at least six poststerilization vacuums is recommended (Atkinson et al., 1977).

Endotracheal tubes, catheters, face masks, and reservoir bags should be thoroughly washed in soap and water and rinsed after each use. Sterilization is desirable by boiling, chemical sterilization (ethylene oxide, 0.1% chlorhexidine), or pasteurization (75° C for 10 minutes). Circle absorbers, if not sterilized by ethylene oxide or gamma radiation, should be frequently dismantled, cleaned, and wiped with alcohol (Atkinson et al., 1977). The anesthetic machine itself should also be wiped with alcohol. Precision vaporizers should be cleaned and adjusted periodically according to the manufacturers' recommendations.

SAFETY PRECAUTIONS

Explosions and fires in the operating room are an occupational hazard with the anesthetist who uses volatile liquid or gaseous anesthetic agents.* An explosion occasionally causes death of the patient. In man, the ratio of explosions to anesthetic periods for the following three agents is listed by Collins (1976) as:

Ether	1:58,000
Ethylene	1:41,000
Cyclopropane	1:25,000

Veterinarians are particularly haphazard in their handling of explosive anesthetic agents. The fact that explosions do occur in veterinary hospitals is attested by the following newspaper article published in 1956.

Injured in Hospital Explosion Dr. ______ Reported in Fair Condition

Three men were injured, two seriously, when an ether bottle exploded in the operating room of a northside animal hospital yesterday morning.

Two of the men suffered multiple lacerations when particles of the exploded glass bottle scattered through the operating room of the ______ Small Animal Hospital.

The third man was treated at the hospital and released.

Another veterinarian said he was outside the operating room when he heard the explosion and the men started rushing by him.

Officers are uncertain what caused the blast. Dr. ______was filling a pint glass jar with ether when the explosion occurred. ______told deputies that they were operating on an animal and that Dr. ______was forcing ether mixed with oxygen to the animal. The dog was not hurt.

*A color film entitled "Fire and Explosion Hazards from Flammable Anesthetics" is available from Graphic Services, United States Department of Interior, Bureau of Mines Central Experiment Station, 4800 Forbes Avenue, Pittsburgh, Pennsylvania 15213.

The lights in the operating room were smashed and blood from the injured men was smeared on the walls. The ether bottle was made of heavy plated glass.

Commonly used inhalation anesthetic agents that are nonflammable and nonexplosive at normal temperatures are nitrous oxide, chloroform, halothane, enflurane, isoflurane, and methoxyflurane. When anesthetic mixtures of any of the others are made, the mixture passes into the explosive range. All except ethylene are more dense than air so that they tend to pool along the floor. Ethylene, on the other hand, rises rather than falls.

Explosion may occur when the following four conditions are present:

1. a flammable substance;
2. oxygen, either in air, in nitrous oxide, or in the pure form;
3. an explosive mixture of 1 and 2; and
4. an ignition source, such as
   a. open flame (cigarettes, cigars, pipes, or gas burners),
   b. electric sparks (cauteries, electric switches, clippers, endoscopic equipment, fans, surgical lamps, suction pumps, defective wiring), or
   c. static electricity (wool blankets, rubber goods, clothing, hair, plastics, tearing adhesive).

Static electricity is the most important ignition source. Electrical charges are developed on various surfaces by friction. This results in potential differences between surfaces and, when the proper distance separates the two, a spark jumps the gap.

Clothing of silk, wool, or plastic develops static electricity. Cotton clothing does not. Leather shoes should be worn; rubber-soled shoes insulate the wearer, allowing a charge to develop on the body. Rubber mats have the same effect and should never be used. Gases flowing through dry tubing develop a charge on the tubing; therefore, anesthetic gases should not be blasted through tubes of anesthetic machines.

Other precautions that should be taken include the following:

1. Leaks in anesthetic equipment should be prevented.
2. Electrical switches and outlets should be at least 5 feet above the floor.
3. Anesthetic gases should be vented outside the building.
4. Circulation of air through the operating room should be adequate to dissipate agents that escape.
5. Intercoupling of patient, operating table, gas machine, and anesthesiologist should be performed. This dissipates charges of static electricity that may develop.
6. Humidity above 65% discharges nearly all static charges; therefore, operating areas should not be dehumidified.
7. When one is purchasing operating room equipment, it should be made certain that motors meet underwriter approval for use under explosive conditions and that conductive casters are used on all types of apparatus.
8. In construction of new hospitals, installation of sparkproof electrical connections and conductive floors should be considered if explosive anesthetics are to be used.

WASTE GAS DISPOSAL

Without proper control measures, high concentrations of waste anesthetic gases may develop in the operating room. These have been shown to be toxic for personnel. Based upon three large retrospective surveys in the United States and United Kingdom, consistent findings include: 1) an increase in spontaneous abortion among female physicians who work in the operating room, 2) an increase in birth defects in live-born children of women physicians exposed to the operating room, compared to nonanesthetist physicians, and 3) a significantly increased incidence of liver disease in male anesthetists (Whitcher, 1977). These observations are supported by experimental evidence in rats and other animals in which there was decreased survival upon chronic exposure to trace concentrations of various anesthetics. Trace concentrations of halothane during gestation cause decreased performance in solving maze problems. Ultrastructural changes have been described in the rat brain, liver, and kidney as a result of a single maternal exposure to halothane during fetal life. Exposure to 20% nitrous oxide causes testicular damage in rats, and skeletal abnormalities are regularly caused by chronic exposure to anesthetic concentrations of various inhalation anesthetics. Performance of humans in completing complex tasks has been reported to be compromised upon acute exposure to trace concentrations of nitrous oxide and mixtures of this gas with other potent agents. Other investigators have cited stress as a possible alternative cause for these occupational problems (Whitcher, 1977).

Other problems identified in operating room personnel that may be related to occupational exposure to inhalation agents include a higher incidence of involuntary infertility, of lymphoid and reticuloendothelial malignancies, and of renal disease; decreased mental activity, fatigue, and irritability also occur. It should be appreciated that the anesthesiologist, located near the source of the greatest leak (the popoff valve), breathes up to 10 times more anesthetic than persons elsewhere in the operating room. Personnel exposed to these agents continue to exhale them for considerable periods, for instance, nitrous oxide 3 to 7 hours, halothane 7 to 64 hours, and methoxyflurane 30 hours. Fluoride ions are detectable in the urine of operating room personnel up to 6 hours after exposure (Anderson, 1980).

A survey of veterinary practices in eastern Colorado indicated that exposure to waste halogenated anesthetic gases was less than in human hospitals (2 vs. 10 ppm) (Wingfield et al., 1981). Semiclosed anesthesia systems were most commonly used, with scavenging systems being used in only 3 of 28 practices. The mean estimated weekly exposure for small animal practitioners was 5.3 hours; animal technicians had slightly higher weekly exposure times. Other workers have indicated that staff and students have higher exposure times (Dreesen et al., 1981). One-third of 156 samples taken within various operating rooms exceeded the recommended maximum of 2 ppm of halothane. Methoxyflurane levels in 33 samples were not detectable or were below 2 ppm. During a period when a scavenging system was inoperable, an average of 36 ppm of halothane occurred.

In 1982, Ward and Byland monitored the operating rooms of 14 veterinary hospitals for waste methoxyflurane (MOF)and N_2O. Four of the rooms exceeded the recommended maximum MOF concentration of 2 ppm after 1 hour or more of anesthetic administration. The average MOF concentration for the 14 rooms was 2.3 ppm (range 0.7 to 7.4 ppm). Three of four rooms in which N_2O was administered exceeded the recommended level of 25 ppm (average 138 ppm). Scavenging, where used, reduced the levels of both MOF and N_2O to acceptable levels. Charcoal filters in use on some anesthesia machines were not effective in reducing MOF levels. Venting waste MOF vapors onto the floor did not reduce exposure of personnel.

Milligan et al. (1982) also found excessively high concentrations of halothane, MOF, and N_2O in a veterinary recovery room after use of these agents in dogs. They caution that personnel holding or working closely with recovering animals are exposed to high concentrations of anesthetic gas exhaled by the patient.

The evidence for toxicity is such that control measures to hold occupational exposure to the lowest feasible levels are indicated. Waste scavenging is only one of several facets for a clean air program for operating rooms. Others include the ventilation and air conditioning system of the operating rooms. If the air conditioning system is of a nonrecirculating type with an air exchange rate in the order of 12 to 15 changes per hour, waste gases can be dumped into the system anywhere in the exhaust side with assurance that they will pass to the outside atmosphere. In the recirculating type, only a small amount of fresh air is added, and typically there are about five air changes per hour, the remainder being recycled air with a total air exchange of approximately 20 changes per hour. With the increased efficiency of bacterial filters, recirculated systems in human operating rooms have become more popular. In the exhaust side of the system, the degree of negative pressure increases as the exhaust fan is approached; if waste gases are introduced at the grill, negative pressure is minimal and usually does not interfere with anesthetic breathing systems. If the waste is dumped where negative pressure is significant, the anesthetic breathing bag may collapse, and pressure equalization necessary to prevent this is required (Whitcher, 1977).

At the anesthetic machine, the waste gas must be trapped before significant atmospheric pollution occurs. This necessitates an airtight enclosure around the expiratory valve with tubing connected to the disposal system. If a ventilator is used, it is necessary to connect the scavenging outlet from the ventilator to the effluent from the scavenging expiratory valve. Scavenging adapters are also available for nonrebreathing valves. The simplest disposal system leads the waste gas from the scavenging trap directly to the outside, through a wall or window or into a nonrecirculating air conditioning system. The waste may also be scavenged via a central vacuum system. Ideally, this should be separate from that provided for surgical suction, and it cannot be used for flammable agents. The exhaust from the compressor must be vented to a disposal site away from fresh air intakes or personnel. Venting waste gases from the expiratory valve to the floor is ineffective because air conditioning and ventilating systems keep the atmosphere agitated. Where waste disposal is provided by a negative pressure or exhaust system, interfacing or pressure balancing between the anesthetic system and the disposal system is required. Appropriate pressure balancing can be provided by the design of the expiratory valve or by special separate pressure-balancing impedance valves. If negative pressure in the waste system is high, frequent adjustment of the expiratory valve to prevent evacuation of the breathing system is required (Whitcher, 1977).

In addition to an adequate scavenging system, equipment maintenance is also necessary. Leaks especially should be held to a minimum; they commonly occur from vaporizers, expiratory valves, around endotracheal tubes and masks, and from swivel Y-connectors. Despite the aforementioned measures, only by determining the degree of pollution can one be assured that a control program is adequate. Air samples obtained in the operating room may be sent to commercial laboratories or, alternatively, an infrared analyzer may be used to measure nitrous oxide and the various potent inhalation agents. Room samples should be aspirated into a closed container and taken, both from the general room environment and from the breathing zone, within 6 to 10 inches of the nose of operating room personnel. Where no analyzer is available, air may be monitored by servicing organizations responsible for preventive maintenance of anesthetic equipment.

REFERENCES

Adriani, J.: *The Chemistry and Physics of Anesthesia,* 2nd ed. Charles C Thomas, Springfield, Illinois, 1962.

Adriani, J., and Rovenstine, E.A.: Experimental Studies on Carbon Dioxide Absorption for Anesthesia. Anesthesiology, 2:1, 1941.

Anderson, I.L.: *Anesthesiology Lecture Notes,* Mississippi State University, 1980.

Atkinson, R.S., Rushman, G.B., and Lee, J.A.: *A Synopsis of Anaesthesia,* 8th ed. Year Book Medical Publishers, Chicago, 1977.

Ayre, P.: The T-piece Technique. Br. J. Anaesth., 28:521, 1956.

Bain, J.A., and Spoerel, W.E.: A Streamlined Anesthetic System. Can. Anaesth. Soc. J., 19:26, 1972.

Beck, W.C.: Sterilization of Anesthetic Apparatus. (Letter to the Editor) Anesthesiology, 48:387, 1978.

Brown, E.S., Seniff, A.M., and Elam, J.O.: Carbon Dioxide Elimination in Semiclosed Systems. Anesthesiology, 25:31, 1964.

Chalon, J.: Humidity Control in Anesthetic Circuitry and Ventilators. Refresher Courses in Anesthesiology, 2:27, 1974.

Collins, V.J.: *Principles of Anesthesiology,* 2nd ed. Lea & Febiger, Philadelphia, 1976.

Cooper, J.B., Newbower, R.S., Moore, J.W., and Trautman, E.D.: A New Anesthesia Delivery System. Anesthesiology, 49:310, 1978.

Craig, D.B., Cowan, S.A., Forsyth, W., and Parker, S.E.: Disinfection of Anaesthesia Equipment by a Mechanized Pasteurization Method. Can. Anaesth. Soc. J., 22:219, 1975.

Day, P.W.: Techniques of Bear Anesthesia Applicable to Research. Experimental Animal Anesthesiology Symposium, U.S.A.F. School of Aerospace Medicine, Brooks Air Force Base, Texas, 1964.

Dorsch, J.A., and Dorsch, S.E.: Your Anesthesia Apparatus: Friend or Foe? Annual Refresher Course Lectures, Am. Soc. Anesthesiol., Lecture #203, 1977.

Dreesen, D.W., Jones, G.L., Brown, J., and Rawlings, G.A.: Monitoring for Trace Anesthetic Gases in a Veterinary Teaching Hospital. J.A.V.M.A., 179:797, 1981.

Dripps, R.D., Eckenhoff, J.E., and Vandam, L.D.: *Introduction to Anesthesia: Principles of Safe Practice,* 3rd ed. W.B. Saunders Co., Philadelphia, 1967.

Eger, E.I., II, and Ethans, C.T.: The Effects of Inflow, Overflow and Valve Placement on Economy of the Circle System. Anesthesiology, 29:93, 1968.

Hall, L.W.: The E.M.O. System in Small Animal Anaesthesia. J. Small Anim. Pract., 19:385, 1978.

Hamilton, W.K.: Low Flow Systems Without Calculus (or even Algebra). Refresher Courses in Anesthesiology, 8:79, 1980.

Hansson, C.H., and Johannisson, D.: Inhalation Anesthesia with Automatic Artificial Respiration during Succinylcholine Relaxation in Large Animals. Nord. Vet. Med., 10:469, 1958.

Haskins, S.C., and Knapp, R.G.: Effect of Various Carrier Gases on the Halothane Output of the Fluotec Mark III Vaporizer. Am. J. Vet. Res., 41:153, 1980.

Heath, R.B.: Personal Communication. Colorado State University, Fort Collins, 1983.

Hewer, C.L.: The Endo-Tracheal Administration of Nitrous Oxide-Oxygen-Ethanesal as the Routine Anaesthetic of Choice for Major Surgery. Br. J. Anaesth., 1:113, 1923–1924.

Jackson, D.E.: A New Method for the Production of General Analgesia and Anaesthesia with a Description of the Apparatus Used. J. Lab. Clin. Med., 1:1, 1915. (Reproduced in "Classical File" Survey of Anesthesiology, 9:98, 1965.)

Jones, E.W.: Mechanical Ventilation During Intravenous and Inhalation Anaesthesia of the Dog. Proceedings of a Symposium held in London, July, 1963. Pergamon Press, Long Island City, New York, 1964.

Jones, E.W., Vasko, K.A., Hamm, D., and Griffith, R.W.: Equine General Anesthesia: Use of Halothane for Maintenance. J.A.V.M.A., 140:148, 1962.

Lamplugh, G., Jones, R.S., and Snowdon, S.L.: The Mapleson E Circuit and Controlled Ventilation Using An Air System in Dogs. J. Small Anim. Pract., 20:557, 1979.

Lee, J.A., and Atkinson, R.S.: *A Synopsis of Anaesthesia,* 6th ed. Williams & Wilkins, Baltimore, 1968.

Lowe, H.J.: Closed System Anesthesia, How to Do It. Annual Refresher Course Lectures. Am. Soc. Anesthesiol, Lecture #242, 1981.

Lund, I., Andersen, K.L., and Erikson, H.: Efficiency of Carbon Dioxide Absorption by Soda Lime in a Closed System. Br. J. Anaesth., 28:13, 1956.

Milligan, J.D., Sablan, J.L., and Short, C.E.: Waste Anesthetic Gas Concentrations in a Veterinary Recovery Room. J.A.V.M.A., 181:1540, 1982.

du Moulin, G. C., and Saubermann, A.J.: The Anesthesia Machine and Circle System are not Likely to be Sources of Bacterial Contamination. Anesthesiology, 47:353, 1977.

Nott, M.R., and Norman, J.: Resistance of Heidbrink-Type Expiratory Valves. Br. J. Anaesth., 50:477, 1978.

Rackow, H., and Salanitre, E.: A New Pediatric Circle Valve. Anesthesiology, 29:833, 1968.

Rawlings, C.A., and Moreland, S.: Oxygen Flow Rates Through a Non-Rebreathing System for Feline Anesthesia. J. Small Anim. Pract., 19:583, 1978.

Rayburn, R.L.: Pediatric Anesthesia Circuits, Annual Refresher Course Lectures. Soc. Anesthesiol., Lecture #117, 1981.

Rayburn, R.L., and Watson, R.L.: Humidity in Children and Adults Using the Controlled Partial Rebreathing Anesthesia Method. Anesthesiology, 52:291, 1980.

Schatzmann, U.: Investigations of the Applicability of Controlled Ventilation during Routine Anesthesia in the Horse. J. Eq. Med. Surg., 2:453, 1978.

Steffey, E.R., and Howland, D.: Rate of Change of Halothane Concentration of Large Animal Circle Anesthetic System. Am. J. Vet. Res., 38:1993, 1977.

Stiles, S.W.: Induction of Ether Anesthesia in Cats. J.A.V.M.A., 134:275, 1959.

Sword, B.C.: Closed-Circle Method of Administration of Gas Anesthesia. Curr. Res. Anesth., 9:198, 1930.

Tevik, A., Sharpe, J., Nelson, A.W., Berkley, W.E., and Lumb, W.V.: Effect of Nitrogen in a Closed Circle System With Low Oxygen Flows for Equine Anesthesia. J.A.V.M.A., 154:166, 1969.

Ward, G.S., and Byland, R.R.: Concentrations of Methoxyflurane and Nitrous Oxide in Veterinary Operating Rooms. Am. J. Vet. Res., 43:360, 1982.

Waters, R.M.: Advantages and Technique of Carbon Dioxide Filtration with Inhalation Anesthesia. Anesth. Analg., 5:160, 1926.

Weaver, B.M.Q., and Walley, R.V.: Ventilation and Cardiovascular Studies During Mechanical Control of Ventilation of Horses. Eq. Vet. J., 7:9, 1975.

Whitcher, C.E.: Control of Occupational Exposure to Inhalation Anesthetics—Current Status. Annual Refresher Course Lectures. Am. Soc. Anesthesiol., Lecture #206, 1977.

Wingfield, W.E., Raby, D.L., Bucham, R.M., and Gunther, B.J.: Waste Anesthetic Gas Exposures to Veterinarians and Animal Technicians. J.A.V.M.A., 178:399, 1981.

Zauder, H.L., and Orkin, L.R.: Chamber for Anesthetization of Small Animals. Anesthesiology, 20:707, 1959.

CHAPTER 12

The Barbiturates

Barbituric acid was first prepared by Conrad and Gutzeit in 1882. In 1903, Fischer and von Mering introduced a derivative, diethyl barbituric acid (veronal, barbital), for use as a hypnotic agent. Fischer is believed to have named the drug veronal from the Latin *vera* since he thought it to be the "true" hypnotic.

CHEMICAL STRUCTURE

The barbiturates all contain a pyrimidine nucleus resulting from the condensation of malonic acid and urea (Fig. 12–1). Barbituric acid itself has no hypnotic activity. Substituting alkyl or aryl groups on the R_1 or R_2 positions (Fig. 12–2) produces various compounds with hypnotic activity. Replacement of the oxygen atom in position X by a sulfur atom produces the ultrashortacting thiobarbiturates.

Substituted R_1–R_2 derivatives of barbituric acid behave as weak acids and unite with fixed alkalies to form soluble salts. These salts hydrolyze in water to varying degrees and form alkaline solutions. Those commonly employed in veterinary medicine have a pH of 10 or above, and for this reason may cause severe tissue damage and slough if injected perivascularly in any appreciable quantity.

CLASSIFICATION

The barbiturates have been classified into four groups according to duration of action (Fig. 12–3, Tables 12–1, 12–2): long, intermediate, short, and ultrashort. All of those used for clin-

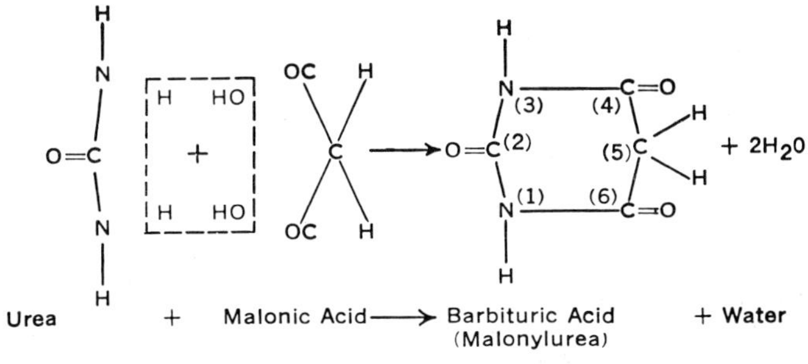

Figure 12–1. Formation of barbituric acid from urea and malonic acid.

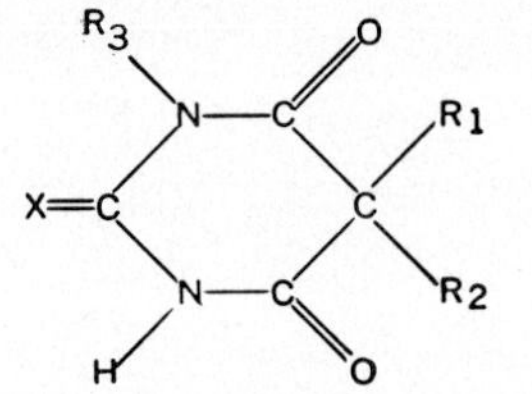

Figure 12–2. General formula of the barbiturates.

ical anesthesia fall in the short or ultrashort classification, whereas those used for sedation or control of convulsions are of long or intermediate action.

GENERAL PHARMACOLOGY

Racemic mixtures of the barbiturates are used as both hypnotics and general anesthetics. The principal effect of a barbiturate is depression of the central nervous system by interference with passage of impulses to the cerebral cortex.

Barbiturates act directly on CNS neurons in a manner similar to that of the inhibitory transmitter γ-aminobutyric acid (GABA). Barbiturate anesthesia is thought to be produced by the combined effect of enhanced inhibition and diminished excitation. Using mouse spinal cord

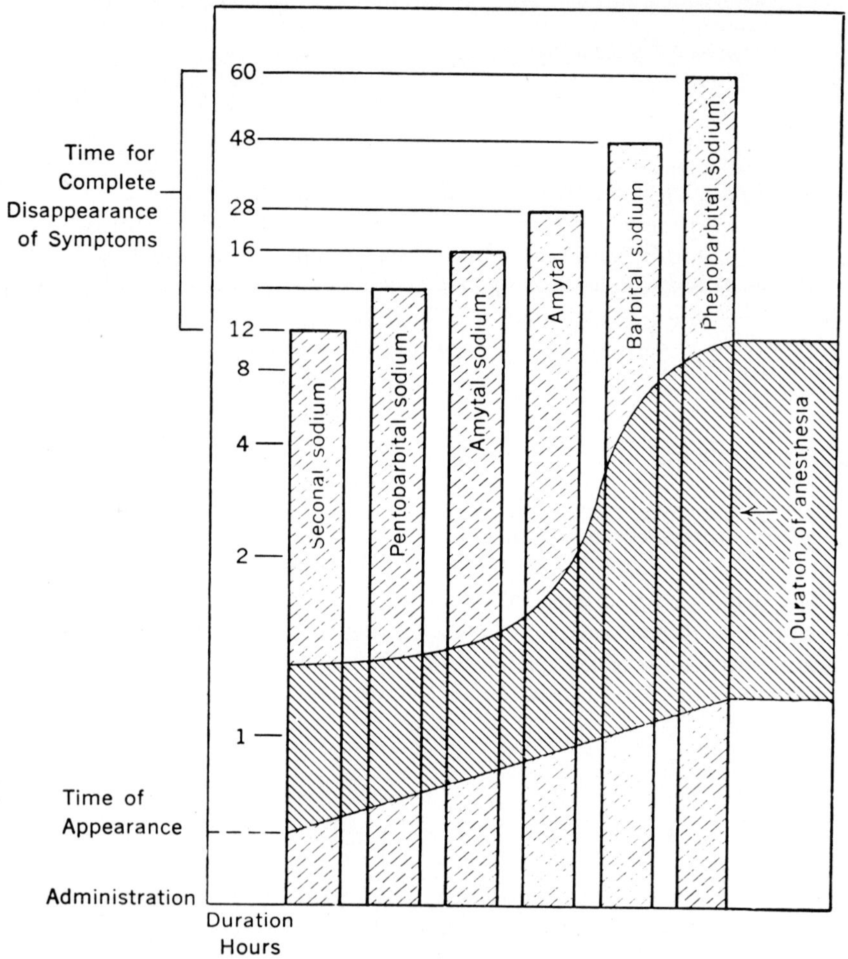

Figure 12–3. Time of appearance, duration of anesthesia, and time needed for complete disappearance of symptoms after oral administration of equivalent single anesthetic doses in animals. (From Jones, L.M.: *Veterinary Pharmacology and Therapeutics*, 4th ed. Iowa State University Press. Ames, Iowa, 1977.)

TABLE 12–1. Names, Status, Chemical Structures, Duration of Action, and Excretion of the Barbiturates

Barbiturate	*Status*	*Commercial Names or Synonyms*	R_1	R_2	R_3	X	*Duration of Action*	*Organ of Degradation and/or Excretion*
Allylbarbituric Acid	N.F.	Sandoptal	allyl	isobutyl	H	O	Intermediate	III
Amobarbital	U.S.P	Amytal	ethyl	isoamyl	H	O	Intermediate	III
Aprobarbital	N.F.	Alurate	allyl	isopropyl	H	O	Intermediate	II
Barbital	N.F.	Veronal, Barbitone	ethyl	ethyl	H	O	Long	I
Butabarbital*	N.N.R.	Butisol	ethyl	*sec*-butyl	H	O	Intermediate	—
Butallylonal*	N.F.	Pernoston	2-bromallyl	*sec*-butyl	H	O	Intermediate	II
Butethal	N.F.	Neonal	ethyl	*n*-butyl	H	O	Intermediate	II
Cyclobarbital	N.F.	Phanodorn	ethyl	cyclohexenyl	H	O	Short	II
Cyclopal	—	—	allyl	cyclopentenyl	H	O	Short	II
Diallylbarbituric Acid	N.F.	Dial	allyl	allyl	H	O	Long	II
Hexethal*	N.N.R.	Ortal	ethyl	*n*-hexyl	H	O	Intermediate	III
Hexobarbital†	N.F.	Evipal, Hexobarbitone	methyl	cyclohexenyl	CH_3	O	Ultrashort	IV
Kemithal†	—	—	allyl	cyclohexenyl	H	S	Ultrashort	IV
Mephobarbital	N.F.	Mebaral	ethyl	phenyl	CH_3	O	Long	II
Pentobarbital	U.S.P.	Nembutal	ethyl	1-methylbutyl	H	O	Short	III
Phenobarbital	U.S.P.	Luminal, Phenobarbitone	ethyl	phenyl	H	O	Long	I
Probarbital*	N.F.	Ipral	ethyl	isopropyl	H	O	Intermediate	III
Propallylonal	—	Nostal	isopropyl	2-bromallyl	H	O	Intermediate	III
Secobarbital*	U.S.P.	Seconal	allyl	1-methylbutyl	H	O	Short	III
Thiamylal†	N.N.R.	Surital	allyl	1-methylbutyl	H	S	Ultrashort	IV
Thiopental†	U.S.P.	Pentothal	ethyl	1-methylbutyl	H	S	Ultrashort	IV
Vinbarbital*	N.F.	Delvinal	ethyl	1-methyl-1-butenyl	H	O	Intermediate	II

*Employed principally as the sodium salt.
†Used for intravenous anesthesia, as sodium salt.
I Mainly excreted by kidney.
II Degraded by liver and excreted by kidney.
III Degraded by liver.
IV Absorbed by body fat, degraded by liver, and excreted by kidney.
(Adapted from Goodman, L.S., and Gilman, A.: *The Pharmacological Basis of Therapeutics,* 2nd ed. Macmillan Publishing Co., New York, 1958.)

TABLE 12–2. Historical and Clinical Data of the Oxybarbiturates and Thiobarbiturates

Agent	*OXYBARBITURATES*				*THIOBARBITURATES*		
(Generic Name)	*Pentobarbital*	*Secobarbital*	*Hexobarbital*	*Methohexital*	*Thiamylal*	*Thiopental*	*Thialbarbitone*
Trade Name	Nembutal Sodium Registered by Abbott Laboratories	Seconal Sodium Registered by Eli Lilly & Co.	Evipal Sodium Registered by Parke, Davis & Co.	Brevital Registered by Eli Lilly & Co.	Surital Sodium Registered by Parke, Davis & Co.	Pentothal Sodium Registered by Abbott Laboratories	Kemithal Sodium Registered by Fort Dodge Laboratories
Chemical Name	Sodium 5-ethyl-5(1-methylbutyl)-barbiturate	Sodium 5-allyl-5-(1-methylbutyl)-barbiturate	Sodium 1,5-dimethyl-5-(1-cyclohexenyl)-barbiturate	Sodium a-dl-1-methyl-5-allyl-5-(1-methyl-2-pentynyl)-barbiturate	Sodium 5-allyl-5-(1-methylbutyl)-2-thiobarbiturate	Sodium 5-ethyl-5-(1-methylbutyl)-2-thiobarbiturate	Sodium 5-allyl-5-(2-cyclohexenyl)-2-thiobarbiturate
Formula	$C_{11}H_{17}N_2O_3Na$	$C_{12}H_{17}N_2O_3Na$	$C_{12}H_{15}N_2O_5Na$	$C_{14}H_{17}N_2O_3Na$	$C_{12}H_{17}N_2O_2SNa$	$C_{11}H_{17}N_2O_2SNa$	$C_{13}H_{15}O_2N_2SNa$
Discovery of Compound	1930 by Volwiler	1930 by Shonle	1932 by Krepp and Taub	1955 by Doran	1929 by Dox	1929 by Taburn and Volwiler	1938 by Carrington
Discovery of Anesthetic or Relaxant Properties	1930 by Volwiler and Tabern	1931 by Swanson	1932 by Weese and Scharpff	1955 by Gibson	1933 by Gruhzit	1933 by Tatum	1946 by Carrington and Raventos
Type of Compound	5-substituted barbiturate	5-substituted barbiturate	N-substituted barbiturate	N-5-substituted barbiturate	5-substituted thiobarbiturate	5-substituted thiobarbiturate	5-substituted thiobarbiturate
Molecular Weight	248.26	260.27	258.25	284.0	276.33	264.23	286.3
Buffer Employed	None	None	None	Sodium carbonate	6% Sodium carbonate	6% Sodium carbonate	None

Preservative or Stabilizing Agent Used	None	Phenol, 0.25% and polyethylene glycol 200, 50%	None	None	None	None	None
Thermostability	Precipitates on heating	Precipitates on heating	Free acid melts at 146° C	Deteriorates when boiled	Precipitates when boiled	Precipitates when boiled	Thermolabile
Chemostability	Solution stable indefinitely	Solution stable up to 18 mo in sealed container; decomposes on exposure to air	Solution stable for 48 hrs if tightly stoppered	Solution stable at room temperature for 6 mo	Solution stable for 48–72 hrs if tightly stoppered	Solution stable for 48–72 hrs if tightly stoppered	Solution stable 7 days; indefinitely if frozen
Onset of Action Duration of Action	30–60 sec 1–2 hrs	30–60 sec 1–2 hrs	30–60 sec 15–30 min	10–30 sec 5–15 min	20–30 sec 10–15 min	20–30 sec 10–15 min	20–30 sec 15–45 min
Route and/or Organ of Detoxification or Elimination	Detoxified by the liver	Detoxified by the liver	Detoxified by the liver	Detoxified by the liver	Absorbed by fat and detoxified by the liver	Absorbed by fat and detoxified by the liver	Absorbed by fat and detoxified by the liver
Usual Mode of Administration	Intravenous, intrathoracic, intraperitoneal	Intravenous	Intravenous	Intravenous	Intravenous	Intravenous	Intravenous, intrathoracic, intraperitoneal
Specific Pharmacologic Antagonist	Yohimbine plus 4-aminopyridine will partially antagonize pentobarbital and probably other barbiturates. Oxygen administration and artificial respiration recommended in respiratory arrest.						
pH of Solution	6%-pH 10.0–10.3	5%-pH 9.8–10.1	2.5%-pH 8.5–10.5	5%-pH 10.4–11.4	2.5%-pH 10.5–11	2.5%-pH 10.5–11	10%-pH 10.6

(Adapted from data compiled by Dr. W.H.L. Dornette and published by the Ohio Chemical and Surgical Equipment Company.)

tissue cultures, MacDonald and Barker (1978) were able to demonstrate that barbiturate anesthetics and barbiturate anticonvulsants possess qualitative and quantitative differences that explain their different clinical effects. They suggested that the distinction between an anesthetic and an anticonvulsant barbiturate depends on the concentration at which amino acid modulation and GABA-mimetic activities occur. If both effects are present at similar concentrations, the agent will have anesthetic properties, whereas, if the threshold for modulatory activity is lower, the agent will be an effective anticonvulsant, with sedation only at toxic doses.

Nicoll and Iwamoto (1978) demonstrated that ganglionic transmission was approximately 20 times more sensitive to pentobarbital than was axonal conduction. The fast excitatory postsynaptic potential (EPSP) was approximately 10 times more sensitive to pentobarbital than were the slow potentials (slow EPSP and slow IPSP). Phenobarbital also exerted some degree of selectivity toward the fast EPSP. The authors stated that anesthetic concentrations of pentobarbital selectively block the fast EPSP, and that blockade of ganglionic transmission is solely mediated by a postsynaptic action.

They believed that a selective postsynaptic block of the nicotinic action of acetylcholine fully accounted for the depressant effects of anesthetic concentrations of pentobarbital on ganglionic transmission. This selective depression on the nicotinic action of acetylcholine could occur by various molecular mechanisms. They theorized that barbiturates depress receptor function by altering the binding of acetylcholine or by increasing desensitization, and that barbiturates might be acting at some step after receptor activation by decreasing ion-channel conduction.

In hypnotic doses, the barbiturates have little effect upon respiration, whereas in anesthetic doses, respiration is depressed. Overdoses produce respiratory paralysis and death. With anesthetic doses, there is cardiovascular depression, both centrally and peripherally, with a fall in blood pressure.

In hypnotic doses, barbiturates have little effect on the basal metabolic rate. With anesthetic doses, basal metabolism is depressed, resulting in lowered body temperature.

Leukocyte counts, packed-cell volumes, and differential counts were determined in 12 normal and 6 splenectomized dogs following pentobarbital, thiopental, thiamylal, and methohexital anesthesia (Usenik and Cronkite, 1965). Decrease in leukocytes was significant in both normal and splenectomized dogs. The packed-cell volume decreased only in the normal animals, presumably owing to splenic sequestration of red blood cells. There was no significant change in the differential counts (Tables 12–3 and 12–4).

The oxidation of pentobarbital, hexobarbital, and amobarbital is noncompetitively inhibited by halothane, methoxyflurane, and diethyl ether in anesthetic concentrations (Brown and Vandam, 1971). Saturation of the enzyme system by the anesthetic appears responsible. Chloramphenicol, a microsomal inhibitor, can markedly prolong recovery from barbiturate anesthesia.

Barbiturates administered during the prenatal period can produce permanent alterations in sexual maturity of hamsters and rats (Clemens et al., 1979; Gupta et al., 1980), and perhaps an increased incidence of congenital malformations in humans (Aase, 1974; Barr et al., 1974).

DISTRIBUTION OF BARBITURATES

Barbiturates diffuse throughout the body, penetrating cell walls and crossing the placenta. The extent of ionization, the extent of lipid solubility (partition coefficient), and the extent of protein binding are the three most important factors in distribution and elimination of barbiturates.

Barbiturates are sodium salts of barbituric acid derivatives. When dissolved in water, they ionize. The degree of ionization is determined by the pH of the solution and the dissociation constant (pK_a) of the agent. This dissociation constant is the pH at which the compound exists in equal quantities in the dissociated (ionized or polar) and undissociated (unionized or nonpolar) forms (Fig. 12–4). For a barbiturate to penetrate the lipoid of cell membranes, it must be

TABLE 12–3. Leukocyte Counts and Packed-Cell Volumes in 12 Normal Dogs Following Barbiturate Anesthesia

	Pentobarbital		*Thiopental*		*Thiamylal*		*Methohexital*	
Time in minutes	*Leukocytes × 10³*	*PCV, %*	*Leukocytes × 10³*	*PCV, %*	*Leukocytes × 10³*	*PCV, %*	*Leukocytes × 10³*	*PCV, %*
−30	13.7 ± 1.5*	50 ± 1.2	12.4 ± 1.0	49 ± 1.2	12.5 ± 1.1	48.5 ± 1.5	13.4 ± 1.4	50 ± 1.4
Anesthesia 0	13.6 ± 1.5	48 ± 1.5	12.2 ± 0.9	47 ± 1.0	12.7 ± 1.0	48 ± 1.2	13.5 ± 1.4	49 ± 1.1
+30	10.8 ± 1.3	40 ± 1.2	10.8 ± 1.0	40 ± 1.4	10.8 ± 1.0	41 ± 1.2	10.9 ± 1.2	42 ± 0.7
+60	10.9 ± 1.3	40 ± 1.5	10.7 ± 0.9	40 ± 1.6	10.1 ± 1.0	41 ± 1.4	11.0 ± 1.4	42 ± 1.0
+120	10.7 ± 1.4	40 ± 1.4	10.9 ± 1.1	42 ± 1.6	10.3 ± 1.1	43 ± 1.2	11.1 ± 1.2	44 ± 1.0
+180	10.8 ± 1.3	41 ± 1.0	11.3 ± 1.2	42 ± 1.3	10.7 ± 1.1	43 ± 1.2	10.9 ± 1.4	44 ± 1.1

*Mean ± standard deviation.

(From Usenik, E.A., and Cronkite, E.P.: Effects of Barbiturate Anesthetics on Leukocytes in Normal and Splenectomized Dogs. Anesth. Analg., 44:167, 1965.)

TABLE 12–4. Leukocyte Counts and Packed-Cell Volumes in 6 Splenectomized Dogs (2 Trials/Dog) Following Pentobarbital Anesthesia

Time in Minutes	*Leukocytes × 10³*	*PCV, %*
−30	14.2 ± 1.0*	46.5 ± 1.6
Anesthesia 0	13.9 ± 1.0	46 ± 1.9
+30	11.6 ± 1.1	45 ± 1.8
+60	11.2 ± 1.0	45 ± 1.8
+120	11.0 ± 1.1	45 ± 1.8
+180	11.0 ± 1.0	45 ± 1.9

*Mean ± standard deviation.

(From Usenik, E.A., and Cronkite, E.P.: Effects of Barbiturate Anesthetics on Leukocytes in Normal and Splenectomized Dogs. Anesth. Analg., 44:167, 1965.)

pK_a = dissociation constant

or

pH at which equal amount of drug is in ionized and unionized forms.

$$HA \rightleftharpoons H^+ + A^-$$

Barbiturate	pK_a
Thiopental	7.4
Secobarbital	7.9
Pentobarbital	8.0

Figure 12–4. Dissociation of barbiturates.

in the undissociated or nonpolar form (Fig. 12–5). The more acidic the solution containing the drug, the more undissociated form that exists and the greater the amount that can penetrate cell membranes to produce deeper anesthesia. The reverse is also true; the more alkaline the solution, the greater the dissociation and the less cell penetration that occurs.

At a blood pH of 7.4, a barbiturate assumes a "normal" distribution within the cells of the central nervous system and produces the desired degree of anesthesia. A change in blood pH, however, may lead to a change in the depth of anesthesia. An increase in acidity, such as commonly occurs with respiratory or metabolic acidosis, increases the depth. An increase in alkalinity, caused by hyperventilation or administration of alkalinizing agents, increases dissociation. As a result, barbiturate migrates outward from the cells to the plasma, and anesthesia will lighten (Waddell and Butler, 1957). Alkalinization of the urine also decreases tubular reabsorption.

The undissociated form has a high affinity for nonpolar solvents. This varies between compounds as shown in Table 12–5. The highly

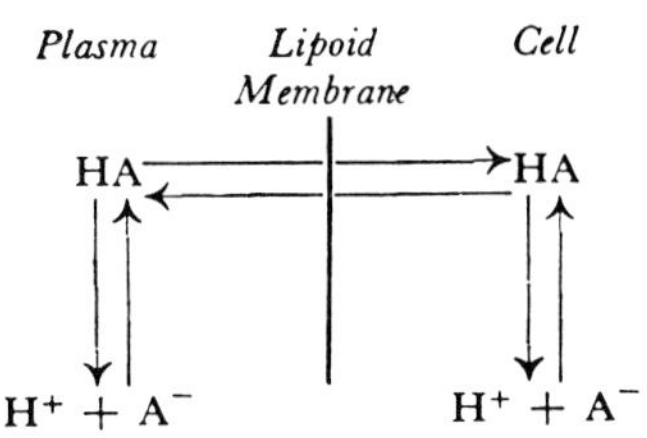

Figure 12–5. Barbiturate dissociation. Cell membrane is permeable only to undissociated (un-ionized) barbiturate.

lipid-soluble agents have a rapid onset and are short-acting. They are rapidly metabolized and also easily reabsorbed by the kidney tubules.

A reversible bond develops to plasma proteins, chiefly albumin, the degree of which agrees roughly with the partition coefficient. Because cerebrospinal fluid is practically protein-free, it contains less barbiturate than plasma (Table 12–6). Organ tissues contain a slightly higher level of barbiturate, while fat contains very high concentrations. Highly lipid-soluble compounds penetrate brain tissue quite rapidly, reaching equilibrium with 2 or 3 circulations of blood. Gray matter of the brain is penetrated rapidly, with white matter being slower to reach equilibrium (Table 12–7).

Termination of barbiturate anesthesia is produced by physical redistribution (see Chap. 2), metabolic degradation, and renal excretion. Again, the solubility coefficient dictates the chief route of elimination. Short-acting agents with a high solubility coefficient are largely reabsorbed from the kidney tubules. Their action ceases when they are metabolically transformed into inactive substances, principally in the liver. Long-acting agents with low lipid-solubility are chiefly excreted through the kidneys.

Maynert and Van Dyke (1950) studied barbiturate distribution using barbital labeled with N^{15}. They found that barbital is not destroyed or metabolized in the body. As much as 85% of both barbital and phenobarbital may be recovered from the urine over several days following administration. The short-acting barbiturates (pentobarbital, amobarbital, and secobarbital) are destroyed principally by the liver. Their rapid destruction in the body accounts for their short action.

The ultrashort-acting barbiturates are quickly redistributed, which accounts for their short duration of action. They, too, are then metabolized over a longer period.

THE "GLUCOSE EFFECT"

A unique reanesthetizing action, termed the "glucose effect," has been observed in animals recovering from barbiturate anesthesia that were subsequently given glucose. A species variation in susceptibility to this effect has been demonstrated; guinea pigs, chickens, pigeons, rabbits, and hamsters are susceptible; dogs are intermediate, and mice, rats, goldfish, and tadpoles are refractory or negative. Intermediates in the glycolysis of glucose and in the Krebs cycle have been shown to have the same effect. The "glucose effect" presumably occurs with most barbiturates and thiobarbiturates, but not with inhalation or other anesthetics. Glucose causes a decrease in activity of the components

TABLE 12–5. Barbiturates: Relation Between Physicochemical Factors, Distribution, and Fate

Barbiturate	*Partition Coefficient**	*Plasma Protein Binding†*	*Brain Protein Binding‡*	*Delay in Onset of Activity§*	*Excreted by Kidney¶*	*Degradation by Liver Slices#*	*pKa‖*
Barbital	1	0.05	0.06	22	65–90	—	7.8
Phenobarbital	3	0.20	0.19	12	30	—	7.3
Pentobarbital	39	0.35	0.29	0.1	—	0.21	8.0
Secobarbital	52	0.44	0.39	0.1	—	0.28	7.9
Thiopental	580	0.65	0.50	—	—	0.38	7.4

*(Concentration in methylene chloride):(concentration in aqueous phase) of the nonionized form at approximately 25° C.

†Binding of 0.001 M barbituric acids by 1% bovine serum albumin in M/15 phosphate buffer at pH 7.4; fraction bound.

‡Fraction of barbiturate bound by rabbit brain homogenates.

§Minutes until anesthesia after intravenous injection in mice.

¶Approximate percentage of total dose excreted unchanged in urine of man.

#Fraction degraded in vitro by liver slices in 3 hours.

‖Ionization exponent at 25° C.

(From Goodman, L.S., and Gilman, A. (Eds.): *The Pharmacological Basis of Therapeutics,* 4th ed. Macmillan Publishing Co., New York, 1970.)

TABLE 12–6. Rates of Passage of Drugs from Bloodstream into CSF of Dogs and Degrees of Ionization of Drugs at pH 7.4

Drug	*Percent Un-ionized at pH 7.4*	*Permeability Coefficient**	*Heptane-Water Partition Coefficient of Un-ionized Form of Drug*
Barbital	55.7	0.026	0.002
Thiopental	61.3	0.50	3.3
Pentobarbital	83.4	0.17	0.05

*The higher the permeability coefficient, the more rapid the rate of entry into the CSF.

(From Shanker, L.S.: Penetration of Drugs into the Central Nervous System. In *Uptake and Distribution of Anesthetic Agents*. Edited by E.M. Papper, and R.J. Kitz. McGraw-Hill Book Co., Inc., New York, 1963.)

TABLE 12–7. Influence of Carbon Dioxide on Penetration of Brain by Drugs

	CONCENTRATION IN BRAIN		
Area	*Hyper-capnic Acidosis*	*Hypo-capnic Alkalosis*	*Relative Pene-tration*
	Urea (1 hr)		
Gray	0.40	0.16	2.50
White	0.12	0.05	2.40
	Phenobarbital (½ hr)		
Gray	1.20	0.72	1.67
White	1.08	0.40	2.70
	Salicylic acid (1 hr)		
Gray	0.44	0.11	4.00
White	0.38	0.04	9.50

Concentration in brain is expressed as a fraction of levels in plasma (relative penetration: brain fractions under conditions of hypercapnia to brain fraction under conditions of hypocapnia). Note the disproportionate increase in penetration of white matter by salicylic acid under conditions of hypercapnia. Gray: cerebral cortex; white: cerebral white matter.

(From Roth, L.J., and Barlow, C.F.: Drugs in the Brain. Science, 134:22, 1961. Copyright 1961 by the American Association for Advancement of Science.)

TABLE 12–8. Relative Ability of Glucose, Sodium Lactate, and Epinephrine to Cause Anesthetic Rebound* in Dogs Recovering from Thiopental Anesthesia.

Drug and Dosage	*Dogs Given Injections (No.)*	*Dogs Rebounded (No.)*	*Dogs Rebounded (%)*	*Average Increase in Sleep Time (%)*
Glucose, 600.0 mg/kg	18	2	11.1	47.9
Sodium lactate, 60.0 mg/kg	18	7	38.9	48.9
Epinephrine, 0.1 mg/kg	13	11	84.6	38.8
Saline solution, 1.0 ml/kg	12	0	0	0

*Apparent reanesthetization as indicated by loss of voluntary and involuntary movements and possible loss of pedal reflexes.

(From Hatch, R.C.: The Effect of Glucose, Sodium Lactate and Epinephrine on Thiopental Anesthesia in Dogs. J.A.V.M.A., 148:135, 1966.)

of the microsomal electron chain resulting in decreased microsomal metabolism (Peters and Strother, 1972).

Hamlin et al. (1965) studied the "glucose effect" on respiration and EEG in dogs following pentobarbital administration. They could find no evidence of significant deepening of anesthesia as judged by cortical depression, decreasing rate or depth of respiration, or decrease in minute volume.

Epinephrine given intravenously to dogs or mice also causes a return of sleep on awakening from hexobarbital or chloral hydrate anesthesia. Norepinephrine is less effective in producing this effect (Lamson et al., 1952). This phenomenon presumably is due to increased glucose levels in the blood and should be remembered when the use of epinephrine is considered in barbiturate-anesthetized dogs.

Hatch (1966) studied the effect of glucose, sodium lactate, and epinephrine on thiopental anesthesia in dogs (Table 12–8). It was his observation that the "glucose effect" was not of practical concern as long as these drugs were used at the proper time and in a therapeutic dose.

Heavner and Bowen (1968) found that an injection of epinephrine or isoproterenol caused reanesthetization of thiopental-anesthetized dogs. This was not observed with methohexital-anesthetized dogs. They theorized that this effect could be due to a peripheral analgesic action of epinephrine since this drug depressed the sensory electroneurogram of the superficial radial nerve.

THERAPEUTIC USES OF BARBITURATES

Barbiturates are used for three purposes:

1. *Sedation and hypnosis*. In this respect, they have been supplanted, in most instances, by tranquilizers.
2. *Anticonvulsant*. The ability of barbiturates to depress the motor cortex has been utilized to treat convulsions associated with poisoning, particularly strychnine, "running fits," distemper encephalitis, and overdosage of local anesthetics.
3. *Anesthesia*. Barbiturates are most frequently used for this purpose in veterinary medicine.

ADDICTION TO BARBITURATES

Although barbiturate addiction can be produced in animals, it is by its very nature self-limiting; however, in man repeated oral use of barbiturates as soporifics or sedatives may become habit-forming. For this reason, legislation in many countries prohibits use of these drugs without a prescription. Veterinarians should be acquainted with applicable laws regarding their use and sale to avoid infraction and to prevent liability.

OXYBARBITURATES

Phenobarbital Sodium, U.S.P. (Phenobarbitone, Luminal)

Phenobarbital was synthesized in 1912 in Germany and marketed under the trade name Luminal. It is a long-acting barbiturate, and advantage has been taken of its prolonged action in treating various convulsive disorders (see Fig. 12–3). In control of convulsions due to distemper encephalitis, it appears to be as effective as any of the newer drugs and considerably cheaper. Because it is excreted slowly in the urine, it tends to be cumulative. An oral "loading dose" should be administered first, followed by a daily maintenance dose. In the average dog (10 kg), this would be 1 gr initially followed by .25 gr three times a day. Loss of motor coordination results from overdose; when this occurs, the dose should be reduced.

Serial assays on serum, saliva, and cerebrospinal fluid (CSF) have shown considerable daily fluctuation of phenobarbital levels, even after several weeks of therapy. A gradually increasing phenobarbital concentration occurs in the three fluids up to dosages of 9.0 mg/kg. Serum or saliva assays can accurately indicate the phenobarbital concentration in CSF (Skinner et al., 1980).

In convulsions due to strychnine poisoning, if anesthesia needs to be maintained for a long time, phenobarbital solution may be given intravenously "to effect" in the same manner as one would administer pentobarbital sodium.

Phenobarbital is a hepatic microsomal enzyme inducer. Concomitant administration of phenobarbital and digoxin can shorten the biological half-life of the latter by approximately 30% (Breznock, 1975).

Pentobarbital Sodium, U.S.P. (Nembutal)

Pentobarbital sodium came into general use as an anesthetic agent for dogs and cats in the early 1930s. It slowly supplanted ether and ACE mixture, administered by open mask methods, as the anesthetic of choice. By 1940 its use was widespread. Today, it has largely been supplanted by the inhalation anesthetics.

Commercial preparations of pentobarbital are racemic mixtures. Administration of subanesthetic doses is often associated with stimulation of the central nervous system and preanesthetic excitation. The (+) isomer of pentobarbital causes a transient period of hyperexcitability before depressing the CNS, whereas the (−) isomer produces relatively smooth and progressively deeper hypnosis (Huang and Barker, 1980).

Studies of the cellular mechanisms underlying this phenomenon have revealed that the drug depresses neuronal excitability in various ways (Mathers and Barker, 1980). Two depressant effects appear to be caused primarily by the (−)

isomer of the drug. One of these involves an increase in Cl^- conductance. It is possible that the effects of (−) pentobarbital are mediated through activation of γ-aminobutyric acid (GABA) receptors. The drug opens ion channels whose conductance is similar to that of GABA-activated channels, but these channels remain open five times as long.

Pentobarbital sodium occurs as a white powder or cystalline granules. It is freely soluble in water or alcohol. It forms a clear, colorless solution that is marketed under several trade names.

Aqueous solutions have an alkaline pH and may precipitate on standing, but the drug can be redissolved by addition of alkali such as sodium hydroxide. Commercial solutions for anesthesia contain 64 mg (1 gr) of pentobarbital sodium per milliliter of solution. The calculated dosage for dogs and cats is 13 mg (.20 gr) per pound of body weight or 1.0 ml/5 lb of body weight; however, it should be emphasized that pentobarbital is given "to effect."

Following a single intravenous dose of pentobarbital, there is early depression of blood pressure. The heart rate increases for 10 to 20 minutes and then stabilizes or decreases. Cardiac output is variable, while peripheral vascular resistance increases (Fig. 12–6).

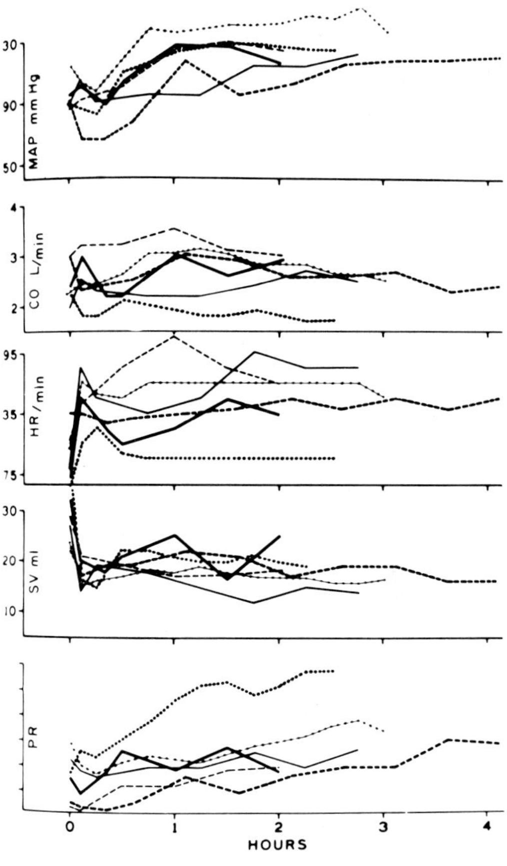

Figure 12–6. Long-term changes from pentobarbital in 6 dogs. MAP = mean arterial pressure; CO = cardiac output; HR = heart rate; SV = stroke volume; and PR = peripheral resistance. Note large and abrupt increase in heart rate and decrease in stroke volume at the onset of the experiments. (From Olmsted, F., and Page, I.H.: Hemodynamic Changes in Dogs Caused by Sodium Pentobarbital Anesthesia. Am. J. Physiol., 210:817, 1966.)

Priano et al. (1969) examined the cardiovascular responses to pentobarbital anesthesia in 12 dogs. Unanesthetized control values were compared with anesthetized values taken at 30-minute intervals for 2½ hours. The following variables were measured: systolic, diastolic, and mean aortic blood pressures; central venous pressure, heart rate, initial ventricular impulse, and cardiac output; and arterial Po_2, Pco_2, and pH. From these, stroke volume, pulse pressure, and peripheral resistance were calculated (Table 12–9).

Systolic blood pressure, initial ventricular impulse, stroke volume, pulse pressure, central venous pressure, Pao_2, pH, and body temperature were all depressed. Heart rate and $Paco_2$ were elevated as was peripheral resistance from 1½ hours on. Cardiac output was decreased after 1 hour. Mean arterial pressure was significantly decreased during induction, but had returned to control values by the 30-minute observations. Priano et al. concluded that "barbiturates render a preparation pathologic rather than physiologic."

MacConnell (1969) studied the effect of barbiturates on regional blood flows. Electromagnetic flow probes were placed on the ascending aorta, superior mesenteric artery, left renal artery, and femoral and celiac arteries. He found the hemodynamic responses to intravenous pentobarbital in pentobarbital-anesthetized dogs to be decreases in contractile force (17.4%) (as measured by strain gauges attached to the heart), arterial blood pressure (4.8%), and renal blood

TABLE 12–9. Cardiovascular Responses to Pentobarbital Anesthesia in 12 Dogs

		TIME AFTER PENTOBARBITAL					
Parameters	*Control*	*0 hr*[a]	*½ hr*	*1 hr*	*1½ hr*	*2 hr*	*2½ hr*
Systolic blood pressure	142 ± 3	116 ± 5[c]	123 ± 4[c]	121 ± 3[c]	122 ± 3[c]	124 ± 3[c]	130 ± 3[c]
(mm Hg)	100%[b]	82 ± 3	87 ± 3	86 ± 3	86 ± 2	88 ± 2	92 ± 2
Mean blood pressure	108 ± 4	95 ± 4[c]	104 ± 4	106 ± 3	108 ± 2	111 ± 3	117 ± 3
(mm Hg)	100%	89 ± 4	97 ± 4	99 ± 4	101 ±3	104 ± 4	109 ± 4
Diastolic blood pressure	83 ± 3	80 ± 4	89 ± 4	93 ± 3[c]	95 ± 2[c]	90 ± 3[c]	105 ±3[c]
(mm Hg)	100%	98 ± 5	109 ± 5	115 ± 6	117 ± 5	122 ± 6	127 ± 6
Pulse pressure (mm Hg)	59 ± 2.6	36 ± 2.4[c]	34 ± 1.9[c]	28 ± 2.2[c]	27 ± 1.9[c]	26 ± 1.3[c]	25 ± 1.4[c]
Central venous pressure (mm Hg)	+1.44 ± 0.7	+0.14 ± 0.4[c]	−0.4 ± 0.4[c]	−1.00 ± 0.5[c]	−1.25 ± 0.5[c]	−1.08 ± 0.5[c]	−1.55 ± 0.6[c]
Heart rate (beats/min)	96 ± 5	157 ± 5[c]	153 ± 7[c]	157 ± 8[c]	141 ± 7[c]	135 ± 7[c]	146 ±10[c]
	100%	167 ± 9	165 ± 11	168 ± 9	155 ± 10	146 ± 11	157 ± 12
Initial ventricular impulse	7 ± 0.4	9 ± 0.4[c]	9.8 ± 0.5[c]	10.1 ±1[c]	12.5 ± 0.9[c]	13.8 ± 1[c]	14.7 ± 0.9[c]
(angle in °)	100%	130 ± 6	142 ± 8	147 ± 15	180 ± 11	193 ± 11	212 ± 11
Cardiac output (L/min)	1.734 ± 0.15	1.834 ± 0.14	1.811 ± 0.09	1.502 ± 0.11[c]	1.324 ± 0.12[c]	1.195 ± 0.10[c]	1.172 ± 0.09[c]
	100%	111 ± 8	111 ± 8	90 ± 5	79 ± 6	71 ± 5	70 ± 5
Stroke volume (ml/beat)	18.6 ± 2	11.8 ± 1[c]	12.3 ± 1[c]	10.1 ± 1[c]	9.5 ± 1[c]	9.4 ± 1[c]	8.9 ± 1[c]
	100%	66 ± 4	68 ± 3	54 ± 2	51 ± 1	50 ± 3	47 ± 4
Total peripheral resistance	5287 ± 558	4574 ± 385	4819 ± 419	6200 ± 551	7370 ± 696[c]	8535 ± 942[c]	8864 ± 928[c]
(dynes-sec/cm⁵)	100%	91 ± 7	95 ± 6	124 ± 11	142 ± 8	163 ± 10	168 ± 8
pO_2 (mm Hg)	93.5 ± 3	60 ± 5[c]	70 ± 3[c]	73.5 ± 6[c]	70 ± 6[c]	77 ± 4[c]	75 ± 5[c]
	100%	61 ± 5	72 ± 4	75 ± 7	80 ± 6	79 ± 5	76 ± 6
pCO_2 (mm Hg)	30.9 ± 0.8	40.9 ±3[c]	44 ± 2[c]	41 ± 3[c]	38 ± 3[c]	38 ± 3[c]	38 ± 3[c]
	100%	132 ± 9	141 ± 5	133 ± 8	121 ± 7	123 ± 9	123 ± 7
pH arterial	7.38 ± 0.01	7.27 ± 0.03[c]	7.27 ± 0.03[c]	7.29 ± 0.03[c]	7.30 ± 0.02[c]	7.30 ± 0.03[c]	7.32 ± 0.03[c]
Temperature (°C)	38.8 ± 0.2	38.7 ± 0.2[c]	38.5 ± 0.2[c]	38.1 ± 0.2[c]	37.9 ± 0.2[c]	37.6 ± 0.2[c]	37.4 ± 0.2[c]

[a]0, time values taken 3 to 5 min after pentobarbital IV.
[b]Each value indicates mean ± S.E. with % of control ± S.E. below.
[c]Denotes statistically significant changes with $P < .05$.

(From Priano, L.L., Traber, D.L., and Wilson, R.D.: Barbiturate Anesthesia: An Abnormal Physiologic Situation. J. Pharmacol. Exp. Ther., 165:126, 1969.)

flow (8.4%), and increases in cardiac output (4.8%) and superior mesenteric artery flow (14.1%). The decreased arterial blood pressure was believed to be due to vasodilation of major vascular beds, and the increased cardiac output due to increased venous return.

Respiration is initially depressed and gradually increases during recovery. The respiratory parameters have been analyzed by Hamlin and Smith (1967) (Table 12–10).

Light pentobarbital anesthesia has little influence on renal hemodynamics. Deep anesthesia depresses renal function, both blood and urine flow, by circulatory depression and also by reflex vasoconstriction. Pentobarbital also sharply inhibits water diuresis by stimulating release of antidiuretic hormone (Blake, 1957).

A striking and constant leukopenia that reaches its height in approximately 90 minutes is found in dogs (Graca and Garst, 1957). Leukocyte counts drop to 20% of control values (Fig. 12–7). After 90 minutes, cell numbers rise gradually so that at 190 minutes the mean value is 39% of the control. Although the absolute differential white count decreases, there is a relative lymphocytosis that reaches its peak at 90 minutes and then returns to normal.

The red cells decrease also, the lowest count being reached 30 minutes following injection, with a reading of 84.6% of control values. The count returns to normal in 130 minutes. Hemoglobin and hematocrit values show corresponding changes. Hausner et al. (1938) have shown radiographically that pentobarbital, amobarbital, and thiopental produce dilatation of the spleen, which presumably accounts for the decrease in erythrocytes. Maximum dilatation usually occurs 20 to 30 minutes after injection of the anesthetic. Sedimentation rate and coagulation time are both increased, while prothrombin time is decreased. Oddly, oral administration of pentobarbital sodium in sedative doses does not affect the blood constituents in the same fashion.

In some animals, the effect produced by pentobarbital anesthesia is difficult to differentiate from shock produced in other ways and may actually terminate with death of the animal. Size of the dose and method of its administration are the major factors in variation of response to

TABLE 12–10. Respiratory Measurements in 77 Pentobarbital-Anesthetized Dogs

Value No.	*All Dogs*	*Males*	*Females*
1) Weight (kg)	19.06(8.49)	20.99(8.38)	16.75(8.16)
2) Age (yr)	5.80(4.74)	6.38(4.87)	5.09(4.55)*
3) DV (cm)	20.84(3.95)	21.30(3.82)	20.29(4.08)
4) L (cm)	13.41(2.47)	13.67(2.36)	13.10(2.59)
5) Temperature (C)	38.29(0.8)	38.29(0.6)	38.29(0.9)
6) Respiratory rate (breaths/min)	13.56(10.77)	15.50(12.38)	11.23(8.02)
7) Oxygen consumption ($\Delta\ O_2$ = ml/min)	120.46(44.08)	127.31(42.47)	112.23(45.17)
8) Tidal volume (V_T = ml)	202.47(100.84)	198.88(81.64)	206.77(121.06)
9) Neg (mm of Hg)	−3.06(1.87)	−3.23(2.09)	−2.87(1.58)
10) Inspiration duration (sec)	1.13(0.48)	1.12(0.50)	1.13(0.46)
11) Expiration duration (sec)	0.54(0.36)	0.55(0.33)	0.53(0.39)
12) DV/L	1.57(0.22)	1.57(0.20)	1.57(0.25)
13) V_M (ml/min)	2,415.6(2,144.4)	2,923.2(2,585.7)	1.806.4(1,231.4)*
14) Oxygen consumption/kg of body weight	6.82(2.33)	6.44(1.60)	7.29(2.94)
15) V_T/kg	11.05(4.46)	9.96(3.17)	12.35(5.40)*
16) Value 15/value 9	−4.77(2.95)	−4.38(2.87)	−5.24(3.02)
17) Value 10/value 11	2.51(1.21)	2.40(1.11)	2.65(1.33)
18) Value 10/value 15	0.11(0.05)	0.12(0.05)	0.10(0.03)
19) Value 11/value 15	0.05(0.03)	0.06(0.04)	0.05(0.03)

DV = Transthoracic distance in dorsoventral dimension at sixth intercostal space; L = transthoracic distance in lateral dimension at sixth intercostal space; V_M = minute volume; and V_T = tidal volume.

*Means and standard deviations of all values of respiration for all dogs, for males, and for females are recorded. All values analyzed were shown by the *chi*-square statistic to be distributed normally. Those values marked by an asterisk are ones that differ significantly ($p < 0.05$) between males and females.

(From Hamlin, R.L., and Smith, C.R.: Characteristics of Respiration in Healthy Dogs Anesthetized with Sodium Pentobarbital. Am. J. Vet. Res., 28:173, 1967.)

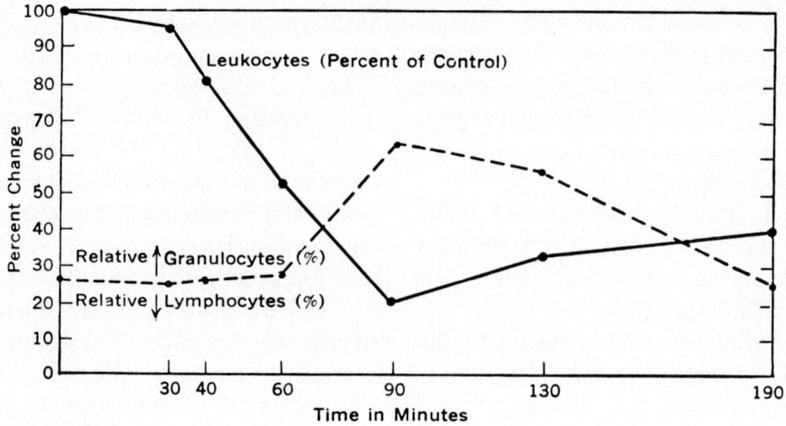

Figure 12–7. The relative percent change in white cell counts with intravenous pentobarbital sodium anesthesia in 12 dogs as compared to control levels in unanesthetized dogs. The relative percent distribution cf lymphocytes and granulocytes is shown on the same scale.(From Graca, J.G., and Garst, E.L.: Early Blood Changes in Dogs Following Intravenous Pentobarbital Anesthesia. Anesthesiology, 18:461, 1957.)

pentobarbital. In addition, individual variations undoubtedly exist. Roughly one of four animals given a dose of 30 mg/kg develops side effects that may mimic some phases of experimental shock (Mylon et al., 1943).

On intraperitoneal administration, the peak concentration in the blood is reached more slowly than with intravenous injection, and the portion of drug absorbed into the portal system is subjected to early destruction in the liver. When a 2.5% aqueous solution is given intraperitoneally in a dose of 30 mg/kg of body weight, the anesthesia produced usually is not accompanied by impaired renal function, and effective renal plasma flow occurs. Arterial blood pressure is elevated in dogs so anesthetized, with a mean of 146.7 mm Hg (Corcoran and Page, 1943).

Pentobarbital freely crosses the placental barrier and enters the fetus. For this reason, its use for cesarean section results in high mortality in the newborn. These animals are viable at birth, but usually do not recover from anesthesia, are unable to nurse, and die within the first 24 to 48 hours postoperatively.

Given pentobarbital containing N^{15} orally, dogs excrete about 60% of the total dose of N^{15} in the urine during the first 24 hours (Van Dyke et al., 1947). Over 92% of the N^{15} is excreted as metabolic products derived from the drug, and only 3% is in the form of pentobarbital.

Davis et al. (1973) studied the disappearance of pentobarbital from the blood of intact and bilaterally nephrectomized dogs. They found that the rate of elimination is totally dependent upon biotransformation of pentobarbital by the liver. The absence of renal function per se does not seem to alter the pharmacokinetics of pentobarbital; however, the sensitivity of a patient to the action of barbiturates may be increased by uremia. This phenomenon is probably due to the decreased capacity of plasma protein to bind acidic drugs. In dogs anesthetized with methoxyflurane and then nephrectomized, elimination was reduced for the first 24 hours, presumably by inhibition induced by the methoxyflurane.

Glucose treatment causes a twofold increase in the elimination constant for pentobarbital in mice, which is associated with a twofold increase in sleeping time. There is no significant difference in blood pentobarbital levels at waking between glucose-treated and control animals, indicating that the prolongation is due to decreased pentobarbital metabolism (Peters and Strother, 1972).

Injection of glucose in dogs awakening from pentobarbital anesthesia causes return of the anesthetic state in 25% of the animals, no response in 25%, and in the remaining 50% a doubtful response (Lamson et al., 1951). This phenomenon probably has killed some dogs unwittingly treated for postoperative shock with intravenous glucose.

The duration of surgical anesthesia with pentobarbital varies widely with individual animals, averaging about 30 minutes. Complete recovery usually occurs in 6 to 18 hours. Occasional animals, particularly cats, may not rouse for as long as 24 to 72 hours.

Pentobarbital is seldom used alone to produce anesthesia in cattle and horses, owing to the prolonged recovery period and the production of marked respiratory depression. It has been administered by slow intravenous injection (15 to 30 mg/kg) in foals and young cattle. Because of excessively prolonged recovery, pentobarbital should not be administered to animals under 1 month of age. In adult cattle, anesthesia has been induced with 14 mg/kg intravenously; half of the dose is injected rapidly, the animal is positioned on its sternum, and the remainder is injected slowly to effect (Toosey, 1959). Pentobarbital may be administered with chloral hydrate (see Chap. 13) or thiopental sodium to the adult horse (Jones et al., 1960).

Pentobarbital can be used to induce anesthesia in goats before administration of inhalant anesthetics (Linzell, 1964). The full intravenous anesthetic dose is 30 mg/kg, which in adult goats maintains anesthesia for approximately 20 minutes. Anesthesia could be further maintained by doses of 6 to 36 mg/kg/hr of pentobarbital. Linzell preferred, however, to maintain anesthesia with cyclopropane or halothane. He injected one-half to two-thirds of the computed anesthetic dose intravenously into the standing goat. After the goat fell to the ground, induction was continued until the jaws were fully relaxed, at which time the animal was intubated and inhalant anesthetic was administered. The induction and intubation dose ranged from 10 to 42 mg/kg (mean 21 ± 5 mg/kg). Because commercial preparations contain 20% propylene glycol, which causes hemolysis and hematuria in goats, Linzell used 60 mg of pentobarbital sodium per ml in 10% ethanol in saline. A similar technique for intravenous pentobarbital in sheep has been described by Harrison (1964). Like goats, sheep rapidly metabolize pentobarbital, and additional doses are required to maintain anesthesia for periods longer than 20 to 30 minutes. Harrison recommends that the sheep be restrained sitting on its buttocks for induction. One injects 4 to 5 ml of pentobarbital (60 mg/ml) rapidly, intravenously, in the average sheep. Additional anesthetic is administered slowly until the jaw is relaxed, the pupil is constricted, and the corneal reflex is weak. The average dose of pentobarbital sodium is 24.2 mg/kg (116 cases, range 10.7 to 53.9 mg/kg) with the average body weight 40.9 kg (range 14.0 to 82.4 kg). In all ruminants, immediate intubation to prevent aspiration of regurgitated rumen contents is essential.

In swine, 10 to 30 mg/kg intravenously provides anesthesia for 15 to 45 minutes. If anesthesia is induced until reflex response to surgical stimulation is abolished, respiratory depression is often severe, and apnea may occur. Pentobarbital is sometimes administered to small swine by intraperitoneal injection (Hall, 1971). Swine up to 20 kg receive 30 mg/kg, and those between 20 and 30 kg receive 24 mg/kg. The technique is not recommended.

Animals awakening from pentobarbital anesthesia tend to exhibit the same signs as when they are anesthetized, except in reverse order. These include crying, shivering, involuntary running movements, thrashing, increased respiratory movements followed by recovery of the righting reflex, and later, ability to stand with a staggering gait (see Table 9–5). Because recovery is slow, without preanesthetic agents these actions may become so exaggerated that the animal injures itself through contact with the cage or stall or causes wound disruption. Greyhounds are notable for this effect. Show animals have been known to break canine teeth, much to the embarrassment of the veterinarian. Administration of a narcotic or a tranquilizer is *always* indicated in cases of emergence excitement.

Recently it has been shown that yohimbine plus 4-aminopyridine will antagonize pentobarbital anesthesia in dogs preanesthetized with atropine-xylazine or atropine-acepromazine (Hatch et al., 1983) (see Chap. 20).

Pentobarbital in excessive dosage is often given intravenously for euthanasia. Appendix C contains directions for preparing such a solution.

Methohexital Sodium (Brevital)

Methohexital sodium is an ultrashort-acting barbiturate, which is unique in that it contains no sulfur atom and hence is not a thiobarbiturate. Its short duration is probably due to redistribution rather than to rapid metabolism in the tissues. Blood concentrations necessary to produce anesthesia are approximately one-half those required with thiopental or thiamylal.

According to the manufacturer, a double dose rapidly administered intravenously causes temporary apnea. The lethal dose is said to be approximately 2.5 times greater than the median anesthetic dose. Animals that die show respiratory failure followed by cardiac failure.

Methohexital sodium is supplied as 500 mg of dry powder in rubber-stoppered vials. It is diluted with water or normal saline to form a 2.5% solution for injection. Solutions are said to be stable for as long as 6 months at room temperature.

The dosage for the dog or cat is 1 ml/5 lb of body weight of 2.5% solution. Half of the estimated dose is injected intravenously at a rapid rate, following which administration is continued to effect. Surgical anesthesia for 5 to 15 minutes is obtained by an initial injection. More prolonged anesthesia can be maintained by intermittent administration or continuous drip. Recovery is quick and may be accompanied by muscular tremors and violent excitement, which detract from the usefulness of the drug. Dogs are usually ambulatory 30 minutes after administration ceases.

Methohexital has been used alone and with several preanesthetics in horses (Table 12–11). Even with preanesthetic sedation, the recovery period is characterized by muscle tremors and struggling (Grono, 1966). For this reason, the anesthesia produced is undesirable except when followed by administration of an inhalant anesthetic. Under these circumstances, it proves to be an ideal agent for induction since its effects are shortlasting. One injection provides just sufficient time for intubation and administration of the inhalant before its effect ceases, leaving the horse anesthetized with only the inhalant. The dose for induction in the horse is approximately 1 g/350 lb of a 10% solution. It must be given rapidly or anesthesia will not be achieved.

Methohexital has been used for induction of anesthesia in calves at the rate of 2.8 to 4.5 mg/kg. A smooth, rapid induction allowing endotracheal intubation was produced (Robertshaw, 1964). In adult cattle, the dose for induction is 0.6 g/100 kg (Monahan, 1964).

A high percentage of the metabolites of methohexital is excreted in the bile of both dogs and rats (Welles et al., 1963). When C^{14}-labeled methohexital is administered to dogs, 30.1% of the radioactivity can be found in the feces; in rats 82.7% is found. In the dog, 21.7% is excreted in bile and urine in the first hour and 52.4% in 8 hours.

THIOBARBITURATES

Thiopental Sodium, U.S.P. (Pentothal)

Thiopental was the first thiobarbiturate to gain popularity as an anesthetic agent for animals. It is the thio analogue of pentobarbital sodium, and only differs in that the number two carbon has a sulfur atom attached to it instead of an oxygen atom. Thiopental sodium is a yellow crystalline powder that is unstable in aqueous solution or when it is exposed to atmospheric air. For this reason, it is dispensed in sealed containers as a powder buffered with sodium carbonate. It is usually mixed with sterile water or saline to form 2.5%, 5.0%, 6.4% (1 gr/ml), or 10% solutions. Thiopental solutions should be stored in a refrigerator at 5 to 6° C (41 to 42° F) to retard deterioration. As solutions age, they become turbid and crystals precipitate. This results in progressive loss of activity, but does not increase toxicity of the drug. Since the potency is decreased, larger quantities of solution must be used to produce the desired effect (Robinson, 1947).

Taylor et al. (1952) studied the metabolism of thiopental and found it to be exceedingly complex. Following injection with thiopental containing radioactive sulfur (S^{35}), monkeys produce at least 12 different metabolic products

TABLE 12–11. Effect of Methohexital Sodium on the Horse Following Premedication with Morphine, Meperidine, or Promazine (Using 4 Horses per Treatment)

Premedication	Induction Time (sec)		Duration (min)		Time to Stand (min)		Number of Horses and Type of Recovery*
	Mean	Range	Mean	Range	Mean	Range	
Nil	26	23–32	4	3–5.5	21	15–29	4+ + +
Meperidine†	18	10–25	6	3–16	18	11–30	2+ + + 2+ +
Morphine†	16	10–20	5	2–9	19	10–27	2+ + + 1+ + 1+
Meperidine Morphine	20	20–21	5	2–7	17	10–34	2+ + + 1+ + 1+
Promazine†	32	25–35	9	7–10	12	9–16	4+ + +
Promazine Meperidine	21	13–30	10	7–13	18	9–26	1+ + 3+
Promazine Morphine	24	20–30	7	4–9	27	22–30	1+ + 3+
Promazine Meperidine Morphine	27	21–35	8	6–11	17	5–30	1+ + 3+

*+ Hyperesthesia; + + mild paddling; + + + severe paddling.

†The dose rates used in this trial were: meperidine 1 mg/lb body weight subcutaneously; morphine sulphate one-third gr/100 lb body weight; promazine 0.25 mg/lb body weight; methohexital sodium 1 g/300 to 400 lb body weight.

(From Grono, L.R.: Methohexital Sodium Anaesthesia in the Horse. Aust. Vet. J., 42:398, 1966.)

that are excreted in the urine. About 86% is found in the urine within 4 days after intravenous injection; small amounts are also found in the tissues and feces.

The initial toxic effect produced by thiopental is a marked depression of the respiratory centers. Both rate and amplitude are affected. Rawlings and Kolata (1983) found that five minutes after administration of thiopental there were increases in heart rate, aortic pressure, peripheral vascular resistance, and left ventricular systolic and end-diastolic pressures. Bigeminy was common. Others have found high rates of cardiac arrhythmias associated with thiobarbiturate anesthesia (Muir, 1977), which were accentuated by xylazine, halothane, methoxyflurane, and epinephrine (Wiersig et al., 1974; Szabuniewicz et al., 1975; Muir et al., 1975). These arrhythmias, which occurred in up to 80% of dogs, included sinus tachycardia, bigeminy, extrasystoles, ventricular tachycardia, multifocal ventricular tachycardia, and ventricular fibrillation. Administration of lidocaine boluses (8.8 mg/kg) concurrently with thiopental (11 mg/kg) reduced the cardiopulmonary depressive effects of the latter, and has been suggested for anesthetic induction of patients with cardiopulmonary disease (Rawlings and Kolata, 1983).

Booker et al. (1952) determined that there is a prominent hyperglycemia, increase in lactic acid and amino acids of the blood, and decrease in liver glycogen during prolonged thiopental anesthesia. Insulin was shown to prevent the decrease of liver glycogen or to favor increased storage of liver glycogen. Furthermore, increased glycogen storage in the liver seemed to favor destruction of thiopental, as evidenced by the fact that increased amounts of thiopental were necessary to maintain surgical anesthesia when insulin was administered. Animals on a high-protein diet or high-carbohydrate diet were also found to require more thiopental for surgical anesthesia than animals maintained on a "normal diet."

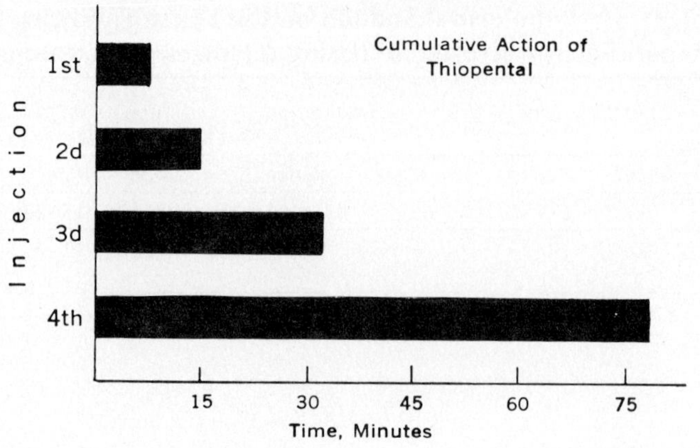

Figure 12–8. The average duration of anesthesia after successive hourly intravenous injections of equal doses of thiopental to dogs. (From data of Wyngaarden, J.N., Woods, L.A., Ridley, R., and Seevers, M.H.: Anesthetic Properties of Sodium-5-allyl-5-(1-methylbutyl)-2-thiobarbiturate (Surital) and Certain Other Thiobarbiturates in Dogs. J. Pharmacol. Exp. Ther., 95:322, 1949.)

Repeated doses of thiopental have a cumulative effect, as shown in Figure 12–8. Prolonged periods of anesthesia may result from this effect if numerous doses are administered.

Brodie et al. (1952) believed that thiopental has an ultrashort action not because it is rapidly metabolized, but because it is rapidly redistributed and becomes localized in body fat. As concentrations in the plasma, muscle, and viscera fall, the thiopental level in fat continues to rise (see Fig. 2–7). Saidman and Eger (1966), on the other hand, found an appreciable amount was metabolized in the dog's liver, and this fraction played an important role in the early rapid reduction of arterial thiopental levels.

Anderson and Magee (1956) have shown the same effect occurs after a fatty meal. A high chylomicron level in the blood produces a significant reduction in sleeping time. They believed that because thiopental is in more intimate contact with chylomicrons and a smaller diffusion distance is present, blood fat is more potent than depot fat in reducing thiopental sleeping time.

The effect of thiopental on several physiologic parameters in horses has been investigated by Tyagi et al. (1964). The leukopenia, hyperglycemia, elevated arterial P_{CO_2}, and decreased arterial P_{O_2} (Table 12–12), are comparable to changes observed in other species.

For small animals, 1.25%, 2.5%, 5.0%, and 6.4% (1 gr/ml) solutions of thiopental are used depending upon the animal's size. Whenever convenient, the more dilute solutions should be used since overdosage is less likely, and irritation is less in the event of accidental perivascular injection. As in other species, thiopental may be used in the dog and cat as the sole anesthetic or for induction prior to inhalation anesthesia. For rapid induction of anesthesia of short duration, the dose is 6 to 8 mg/kg. Should 10 to 20 minutes of surgical anesthesia be required, the dose range is 20 to 30 mg/kg. One-third of the estimated dose is injected rapidly within 15 seconds, and the remainder is administered slowly to effect. Recovery (to standing) usually requires 1 to 1½ hours. Additional doses may be administered to prolong anesthesia when required. Excessive use will, however, saturate the tissues and cause a prolonged emergence. When induction is preceded by preanesthetic sedation, a dose range of 10 to 20 mg/kg is used. As in other species, too large a dose prior to inhalation anesthesia depresses respirations and impairs the uptake of inhaled gases. The use of thiopental is contraindicated in the neonate and in feline porphyria (Hall, 1971).

Thiopental is commonly used for rapid induction of anesthesia in the horse. After preanesthetic sedation with a suitable tranquilizer (e.g., promazine, acepromazine—see Chap. 8),

TABLE 12–12. Mean Values of the Parameters Listed Below Following a Single Intravenous Anesthetic Dosage of Thiopental Sodium in 8 Horses*

	Preanesthetic Value	*Minutes after Administering Anesthesia*			*Statistical Differences*
		5	*15*	*25*	
Leukocyte count cell/mm³	9,700	7,800	7,500	6,100	§
Packed-cell volume (vol %)	32	31	30.5	31	
Blood glucose (mg %)	82.1	85.0	91.2	103.1	§
Heart rate† (per min)	61	85	95	81	§
Blood pressure‡ (mm Hg) Systolic/diastolic	158/117	188/153	173/141	176/140	§
Respiratory rate‡ (per min)	29	8	14	21	§
O_2 content of arterial blood (vol %)	19.2	19.0	18.2	18.4	‖
O_2 content of venous blood (vol %)	14.3	13.5	13.0	12.8	‖
CO_2 content of arterial blood (vol %)	43.3	44.2	49.9	49.2	§
Arterial blood (pH)	7.39	7.31	7.21	7.22	§
Plasma level of thiopental Na (mg/L)	—	49.3	37.1	35.8	§

*To produce surgical anesthesia, 9 to 17 mg/kg were required.
†Mean values in 6 horses because of equipment failure.
‡Mean values in 5 horses because of equipment failure.
§Statistically significant difference at the 1% level before and after administration of thiopental sodium.
‖Statistically significant difference at the 5% level before and after administration of thiopental sodium.
(From Tyagi, R.P.S., Arnold, J.P., Usenik, E.A., and Fletchers, T.F.: Effects of Thiopental Sodium (Pentothal Sodium) Anesthesia on the Horse. Cornell Vet., 54:584, 1964.)

6 to 15 mg/kg of thiopental are injected intravenously. If injected as rapidly as possible via a 20-gauge 1½-inch needle, 6.0 to 9.0 mg/kg are adequate. The smaller dose is used prior to the use of inhalant anesthetics, while the larger dose is used when a short period of surgical anesthesia is required. After sedation with 0.25 mg/lb of promazine, the rapid intravenous injection of 3.74 mg/lb of thiopental in a 10% aqueous solution was found to produce a mean duration of surgical anesthesia of 6.5 minutes and a recovery period (to standing) of 45.8 minutes (Jones et al., 1960).

Approximately 20 to 30 seconds after completion of the injection, the horse inspires deeply. At this time, the head rope should be grasped securely and the head extended and pulled down slightly. This usually prevents the horse from falling backward. By pulling on both the head and tail at the time of induction, one can usually dictate the side on which the horse falls. Since the horse may occasionally fall heavily, animals with full stomachs should not be induced in this manner, for gastric rupture may result. In the event that a longer duration of anesthesia is required, larger doses are used, half being injected rapidly and the remainder slowly after the horse is recumbent. Anesthesia may also be prolonged by combination of the thiopental with glyceryl guaiacolate (see Chap. 14). Occasionally an induction dose of thiopental is injected in the horse without apparent effect. This usually results from perivascular injection, inadequate dosage, or too slow an injection. Since the margin of safety is large, the procedure may be repeated without ill effect, although recovery may be prolonged. If preanesthetic sedation is inadequate, emergence struggling and floundering may occur. The recovery period (to standing) is prolonged if limb movement is restricted by bandages, splints, or casts.

To facilitate subsequent intubation, an induction dose of thiopental may be immediately followed, before the animal falls, by intravenous injection of 0.15 mg/kg of succinylcholine chloride. This has the same disadvantage as the use of succinylcholine alone, namely tachycardia, cardiac arrhythmia, and apnea. Rapid induction with thiopental alone, on the other hand, induces a moderate tachycardia, a slight reduction in mean arterial blood pressure, and a short period of respiratory depression (Tavernor and Lees, 1970). Rapid intravenous injection of thiopental is usually followed by slow irregular respirations and sometimes brief periods of apnea (up to 1 or 2 minutes). Should apnea occur, a sharp slap on the thoracic wall usually initiates spontaneous respiration. Since recovery may be unduly prolonged, the use of thiopental is contraindicated in the newborn foal. This rapid injection technique is also contraindicated in animals in shock or in those with uncompensated cardiovascular disease.

Similar doses of thiopental may be given in the same manner to induce anesthesia in the bovine. Once anesthesia is induced, endotracheal intubation to prevent possible aspiration of rumen contents is essential. The possibility of this is reduced by positioning the animal so that the anterior thoracic region is higher than any other part of the body. As in the newborn foal, use of thiopental is contraindicated in the neonatal calf.

Thiopental is also used in doses of 8 to 30 mg/kg in small ruminants. Rapid intravenous induction can be achieved with 8 to 12 mg/kg,

TABLE 12–13. Suggested Minimal Surgical Dose (m.s.d.) of 5% Pentothal Sodium Solution as a Basis for Judging Initial Rapid Injection Dosage in Swine

	Amt. of 5% Pentothal Sodium, Intravenous	
Size of Animal (lb)*	*Calculated m.s.d. (ml/lb)*	*Actual Amt. to Give Rapidly (ml/lb)*
10–50	0.1	0.05
50–100	0.09	0.045
100–200	0.08	0.04
200–300	0.07	0.035
300–400	0.06	0.03
400–600	0.05	0.025

*Thrifty animals; unthrifty animals require less anesthetic per unit of body weight.

(From Muhrer, M.E.: Restraint of Swine with Penthothal Sodium. J.A.V.M.A., 117:293, 1950.)

whereas larger doses are given by slow intravenous injection to effect. The latter technique provides 10 to 20 minutes of surgical anesthesia.

The dose of thiopental required to induce anesthesia in swine is even more variable. Muhrer (1950) has indicated that the minimal dose required to induce surgical anesthesia varies from 2.5 mg to 5.0 mg/kg in a 5% solution (Table 12–13). He injected only half this amount rapidly, and the remainder more slowly over the next several minutes. Even during light anesthesia, respiratory depression, irregular breathing, and apnea commonly occur in swine.

Thiamylal Sodium, N.N.R. (Surital)

Thiamylal sodium is the thio analogue of the barbiturate, secobarbital sodium. It differs from thiopental sodium in that the ethyl radical of the latter (on R_1) is replaced by an allyl radical. According to Swanson (1951), it was first synthesized by Shonle and his associates. Thiamylal sodium is marketed as a mixture with sodium carbonate, the mixture being prepared by adding thiamylal sodium and sodium carbonate to just enough sodium hydroxide solution to dissolve the salts. The pH is adjusted to between 10.7 and 10.9. The solution is made to volume with water, filtered, sterilized, and lyophilized. The finished product consists of pale yellow, hygroscopic, agglutinated masses of crystals with no pronounced odor. On addition of distilled water, it readily dissolves forming a clear yellow solution with a pH of 10.3 (in 2.5% solution). Solutions have a pungent odor that has been described as that of sulfur or garlic. Reduction in pH of the solution results in precipitation of the drug; a few drops of alkali redissolve precipitated material. According to Helrich et al. (1950), normal saline is the preferred diluent. They state that solutions of thiamylal and saline have been kept for as long as 14 days without loss of potency or change in appearance.

Wyngaarden et al. (1947) compared the action of thiamylal and some other thiobarbiturates in dogs and found that the anesthetic potency of thiamylal was 1.5 compared to 1 for thiopental. Thiamylal was found to be less cumulative than thiopental as shown in Figure 12–9.

Swanson (1951) found that no tolerance developed to thiamylal from repeated administration every other day for 4 weeks. The pulse rate slowed and the blood pressure was reduced. No inhibition of the vagus in dogs was observed following anesthetic doses as occurs with some other barbiturates. Thiamylal was considered less cardiotoxic than thiopental by Woods et al. (1947) who studied their actions in both heart-lung preparations and intact dogs. Significant increases in heart rate, arterial blood pressure, left ventricular peak pressure, and myocardial oxygen consumption are produced by 8.0 mg/kg administered intravenously (Nagel et al., 1979). A common cardiac dysrhythmia occurring on intravenous administration of thiamylal sodium is ventricular bigeminy (ventricular premature depolarization coupled to the preceding sinus beat). This appears to originate in the ventricle distal to the bundle of His (Muir, 1977). Most investigators have found thiamylal to be more arrhythmogenic than thiopental. Because of its arrhythmogenic effect, Musselman (1976) stated that thiamylal is contraindicated in any dog with impaired cardiac function. For additional information on thiobarbiturate arrhythmias, see the section on Thiopental Sodium.

With a dose of 8.0 mg/kg, respiratory rate is not significantly changed although the tidal volume and minute volume are decreased. This results in significant increases in arterial P_{CO_2} with decreases in pH and P_{O_2} (Nagel et al., 1979). Depression of respiration is pronounced on rapid intravenous injection. When dogs are given excessive doses of thiamylal or thiopental by continuous injection, the respiratory rate and amplitude progressively decrease, but blood pressure does not drop significantly until respiratory arrest occurs. Then it drops precipitously (Woods et al., 1949). Dogs artificially respired will tolerate 1½ to 3½ times the dose

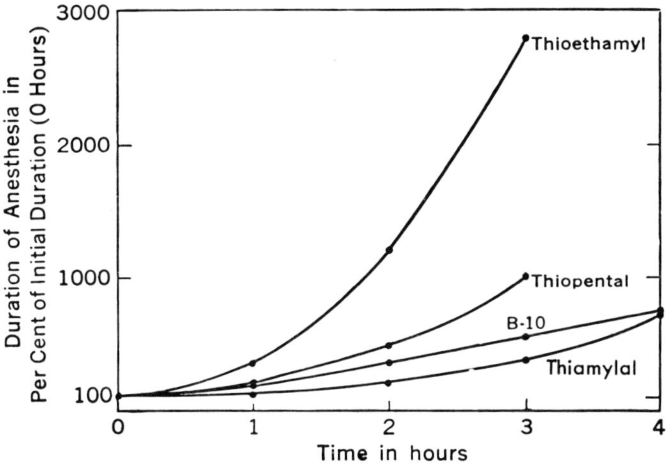

Figure 12–9. Cumulative action of hourly injections of four thiobarbiturates. Time values on the abscissa represent the hour on which injections were administered. (From Wyngaarden, J.B., Woods, L.A., Ridley, R., and Seevers, M.H.: Anesthetic Properties of Sodium-5-allyl-5-(1-methylbutyl)-2-thiobarbiturate (Surital) and Certain Other Thiobarbiturates in Dogs. J. Pharmacol. Exp. Ther., 95:326, 1949.)

of thiamylal tolerated with spontaneous respiration. Artificially ventilated animals show a gradual decline in blood pressure to low levels. With overdose, hypoxia secondary to respiratory failure is the cause of death.

Shideman et al. (1947) studied the role of the liver in degradation of the thiobarbiturates. By producing liver damage with carbon tetrachloride, they demonstrated that it plays an important role in detoxification of thiopental and thiamylal. This fact was confirmed in a second experiment that reduced liver blood flow by production of an Eck's fistula.

The effect of dog collars containing dichlorovos on thiamylal anesthesia in dogs has been investigated by Ritter et al. (1970). After wearing collars for 7 days, the animal had significant reduction in plasma cholinesterase but not in red blood cell cholinesterase. When the dog was anesthetized, Po_2 was slightly but not significantly reduced and Pco_2 was increased by an amount that had borderline significance. It was concluded that no significant synergism occurred between the two agents.

Reutner and Gruhzit (1948) repeatedly injected groups of dogs with 15, 17.5, 20, 22.5, and 25 mg/kg of thiamylal, some dogs receiving as many as 18 injections over 49 days. Red, white, and differential blood cell counts and hemoglobin values remained unchanged. Urine specimens were free of sugar and albumin throughout the test period. Likewise, the total blood nonprotein nitrogen, blood sugar, and bromsulfalein liver function tests remained normal.

Since thiamylal sodium is similar in its action to thiopental, it is used in a like manner. Thiamylal for use in small animals is usually prepared as a 4% or weaker solution by adding sterile water or saline to 1 g of powder. A dose of 17.5 mg/kg (0.125 gr/lb) intravenously produces surgical anesthesia in dogs for approximately 15 minutes, with complete recovery in about 3 hours. If anesthesia of longer duration is desired, repeated increments can be administered. It has been used with a wide variety of preanesthetic agents and muscle relaxants with excellent results. After tranquilization, thiamylal is commonly used as an induction agent prior to inhalation anesthesia in horses and cattle. The dose for rapid induction is 3.0 to 3.5 mg/lb. Intravenous injection of a 5 or 10% solution is made with an 18- or 20-gauge needle. The animal usually relaxes within 15 to 20 seconds and remains recumbent for 20 to 40 minutes. Provision should be made for artificial respiration when thiamylal is used in this manner, since apnea may be produced. Depending upon dose rate and size, doses of 10 to 20 mg/kg are usually satisfactory in ruminants and swine.

Thiamylal was found to be best for analyses of spontaneous electrical activity in the monkey brain when compared with phencyclidine, etorphine, etorphine plus methotrimeprazine and tiletamine (Hinko et al., 1970).

Because of its low toxicity, thiamylal is used in young, aged, and poor-risk patients. It has won universal acclaim for its safety and is probably the most widely used thiobarbiturate in small animal and equine practice.

ADMINISTRATION OF BARBITURATES

Intravenous Injection

Barbiturates are administered by several routes depending upon the anesthesiologist, the patient, and the effect desired. For anesthesia, the intravenous route is preferable since the anesthetic can be given "to effect." Because of wide variation in patient response, this type of dose control is desirable. With intrathoracic, intraperitoneal, and intramuscular administration, control is difficult since a precalculated dose must be given. The oral route is slow and unpredictable, and therefore is used chiefly when sedation is sought.

Care should be taken in selection of needles and syringes for administration. In large species of animals, 12- to 20-gauge 1½- to 2-inch needles are used, depending upon the quantity of anesthetic that must be injected rapidly to carry the patient through the excitement stage. When large quantities are to be injected, a vascular catheter* is preferred. In smaller animals, 20- to 24-gauge needles aid in venipuncture and

*See Appendix A for manufacturers.

help slow the rate of injection. There is a careless tendency to use large syringes on very small animals. This is dangerous because the dose cannot be accurately controlled. A syringe of size commensurate with the dose should always be employed; use of large syringes with small doses is an invitation to disaster.

In many practices, an indwelling venous catheter is inserted prior to anesthetic administration. This is used for anesthetic injection and subsequent fluid administration during operation. It also helps ensure that inadvertent perivascular injection does not occur when animals are transported.

In small animals (less than 10 pounds), it is advisable to dilute the anesthetic with sterile water. By making a 100% dilution, or larger, more accurate dose control is achieved.

When intravenous injection is to be made, hair over the vein may be removed with clippers or scissors and the skin prepared by swabbing with a suitable antiseptic. The latter procedure, in addition to cleaning the area, tends to distend the vein.

For intravenous anesthesia, the cephalic vein on the anterior aspect of the forelimb is most commonly used in small animals. In dogs, second choice is generally the saphenous vein on the lateral surface of the hind limb just proximal to the hock. In cats, the femoral vein on the inner surface of the thigh is second choice. Other veins less frequently used are the jugular and the marginal vein of the ear. In dogs already anesthetized, the lingual veins on the ventral surface of the tongue are easily accessible. These veins tend to bleed rather profusely, however, following venipuncture. In horses, cattle, and sheep, the jugular vein is used almost exclusively. In swine, the marginal vein of the ear or the anterior vena cava is most commonly employed.

In the dog, if injection is to be made into the cephalic vein of the right foreleg, the assistant stands by the animal's left side with his left arm circling the neck and his right arm extended over the dog's back. The right hand grasps the right foreleg just below the elbow (Fig. 12–10A). The right index finger is extended over the dorsal surface of the limb, the thumb is held around the ventral surface of the leg and, by compressing thumb and forefinger, the vein is occluded causing it to distend with blood. The wrist is turned slightly so that the skin covering the dorsal aspect of the foreleg and the cephalic vein is rotated outward. The anesthesiologist grasps the paw of the right foot with his left hand and, if the vein is not easily seen, by rapidly squeezing the paw several times, he pumps blood from the paw to distend the vein. If the carpus is flexed acutely, the vein is stretched tightly over the underlying muscles and rolling is prevented. Good technique demands that the needle used for injection be threaded into the vein so that the hub is at the site of venipuncture. The leg and syringe are both held in the left hand during injection so they will move as a unit if the animal moves. This prevents accidental retraction of the needle from the vein.

Persons experienced with administration of barbiturates to dogs and cats usually estimate the weight of the animal and draw an excess of solution into a syringe. The first one-third to one-half of the dose is rapidly injected while the anesthesiologist watches the animal's facial expression closely. As injection is made, the animal often licks its lips as though tasting the drug. Frequently, dogs move the head from side to side as the anesthetic effect begins. These movements are seen early in the course of administration and indicate more drug must be given. The eyes begin to lose their alert expression, and the animal then relaxes. At this point, it is usually best to lay the patient on its side without restraint so that the rate and depth of respiration can be observed.

As injection is continued, the anesthesiologist can, with his thumb and forefinger placed behind the canine teeth, open the animal's jaw. If in a light state of anesthesia, the patient will further open the jaw, curl the tongue, and simulate a yawn. At this point, the corneal and pedal reflexes are still present and the animal is not in a state of surgical anesthesia. Administration of anesthetic should be continued cautiously and in small amounts, with careful attention paid to the respiration and reflexes. Surgical anesthesia is reached when the pedal reflex is abolished.

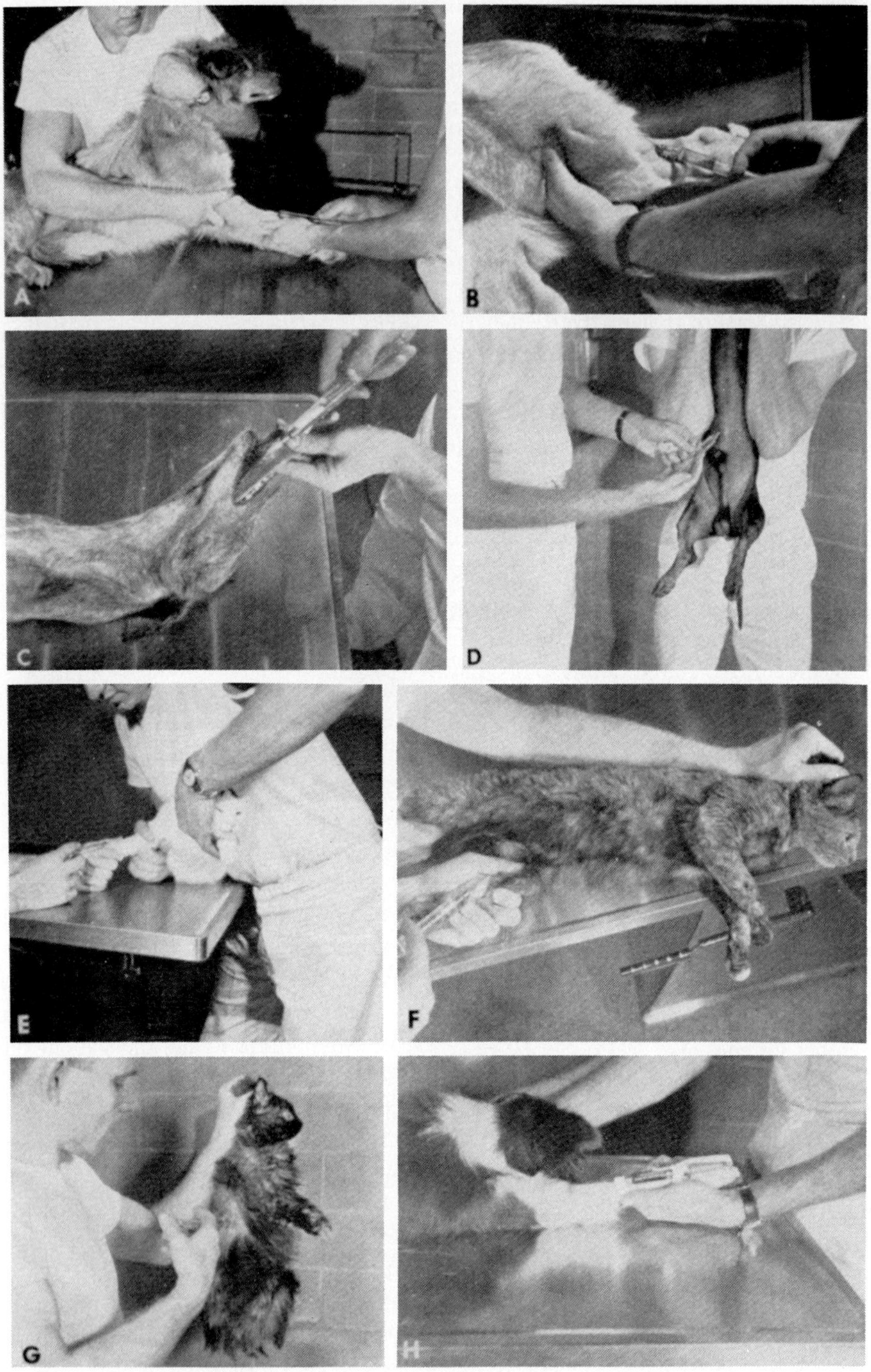

Figure 12–10. Methods of parenteral administration of barbiturates. *A*, Cephalic vein, dog. *B*, Saphenous vein, dog. *C*, Sublingual vein, dog. *D*, Intraperitoneal injection, dog. *E*, Cephalic vein, cat. *F*, Femoral vein, cat. *G*, Intrathoracic injection, cat. *H*, Method of taping syringe to limb for intermittent injections.

At this point, further administration of drug is dangerous.

One should constantly bear in mind that anesthesia is most safely accomplished when the final portion is administered quite slowly. In many small animal practices, it is routine procedure to anesthetize the animal lightly, and then to tape the syringe containing the agent to the limb (Fig. 12–10H). A short piece of tape is applied parallel to the barrel and plunger of the syringe to prevent venous backpressure from pushing the plunger out of the barrel. At this point the animal is clipped, scrubbed, and prepared for surgery. Then the final dose of anesthetic is administered. The syringe is left in position throughout the operation so that small increments can easily be given as needed.

When barbiturates are given intravenously to horses, cattle, and other large animals, care should be taken to prevent injury to the animal when it collapses. Horses should be haltered and held by attendants, since if care is not exercised they may fall over backward. The attendants should pull forward on the halter, and the head should be caught as the animal falls to prevent its hitting the ground with damaging force.

Intraperitoneal Injection

Intraperitoneal injection has been employed extensively in the past, but has the disadvantage that the dose cannot be as accurately controlled as it can by intravenous administration. Usually with this method, the animal is restrained by an assistant, who holds it in a vertical position against his body with the abdomen facing the anesthesiologist. An area just lateral to the umbilicus is clipped and a suitable antiseptic applied. The needle is then thrust through the abdominal wall and the injection made (Fig. 12–10D). The dose for intraperitoneal administration is calculated in the same manner as the intravenous dose. The peak concentration in the blood is reached more slowly, and drug absorbed into the portal system is subject to early destruction in the liver (Corcoran and Page, 1943).

Intramuscular Injection

Under unusual circumstances, such as when wild animals are anesthetized, intramuscular or subcutaneous injection of barbiturates may be indicated. Because of their high alkalinity, there is a tendency for tissue necrosis to develop following this procedure.

Bleicher (1958) has advocated intramuscular pentobarbital sodium for basal and general anesthesia in laboratory dogs. The solution is injected in the rectus femoris muscle, care being taken to avoid the sciatic nerve. Up to 8 ml of standard pentobarbital solution has been injected in one site. For basal anesthesia prior to ether, 20 mg/kg of body weight are used; for moderate anesthesia, 30 mg/kg, and for surgical anesthesia of 1 to 2 hours, 40 mg/kg are administered. Induction requires about 15 minutes, and anesthesia reaches its height about 30 minutes following injection. While this procedure is not generally acceptable in small animal practice, in certain situations it may prove expedient.

Intrathoracic Injection

Because of difficulty in restraining cats and other small species for intravenous injection, some individuals prefer to anesthetize them by injecting a barbiturate intrathoracically. The technique in cats has been described by Sternfels (1955) who used 4% thiamylal and injected 1 ml/5 lb of body weight. He stated that the injection should be made posterior and dorsal to the heart at the level of the eighth rib using a 25-gauge one-half-inch needle (Fig. 12–10G). With thiamylal, anesthesia develops in 4 to 6 minutes and lasts 15 to 45 minutes. No excitement occurs on induction or recovery.

Niemeyer (1958) advocated the use of pentobarbital intrathoracically and indicated that the site of injection is not too important. He preferred a low thoracic approach, 1 cm below and 1 cm behind the flexed elbow joint, and used the same dose as for intravenous anesthesia. On the other hand, Holzworth (1958) strongly opposed intrathoracic administration of anesthetic to cats, stating that there is bound to be some risk to the heart, pericardium, and lung and that barbiturate is irritating to the serosal surfaces. The latter fact can be confirmed on necropsy of animals destroyed with intrathoracic barbiturates. Enold (1962) found pleural thickening, bronchitis, and coagulative necrosis of the lung on examination of experimentally injected cats.

ADMINISTRATION OF THIOBARBITURATES

In general, thiobarbiturates are administered intravenously in the same manner as oxybarbiturates. Thiobarbiturates produce more respiratory depression on induction than oxybarbiturates; often one-third of the calculated dose causes the patient to collapse and respiration to stop. This transient apnea is alarming to those not aware of this reaction. When it occurs, injection of anesthetic should be suspended until spontaneous rhythmic respirations resume. This usually occurs as soon as the blood carbon dioxide level rises and stimulates the respiratory center. Injection is then continued using the same signs to determine the depth of anesthesia as are used with oxybarbiturates.

Intrathoracic injection of thiamylal in cats has been advocated by Sternfels (1955), whereas intraperitoneal and intramuscular injections of the same strength do not produce sufficient anesthesia for surgical procedures. This is probably due to slower absorption.

BARBITURATE SLOUGH

Occasionally, an animal may struggle during induction of barbiturate anesthesia and some of the drug may be administered perivascularly. This should be avoided because a tissue slough may develop. Experienced anesthetists prevent barbiturate slough by threading the needle into the vein. This procedure makes it unlikely that the needle will come out of the vein if the syringe is jarred or the animal moves. Sloughs due to anesthesia require 2 to 4 weeks to heal and leave an unsightly scar. Nothing can infuriate an owner more than development of a slough in his animal.

If it is suspected that barbiturate solution has been injected perivascularly, the area should be infiltrated with 1 or 2 ml of 2% procaine solution. According to Elder and Harrison (1944), procaine is effective in this condition for two reasons. First, procaine is a vasodilator and prevents vasospasm in the area; it thus aids in dilution and absorption of the barbiturate. Second, procaine is broken down by an alkaline medium and in this reaction the alkali (barbiturate) is neutralized. Some may also inject a corticosteroid or nonsteroidal anti-inflammatory drug, and/or use hot packs or hydrotherapy.

REFERENCES

Aase, J.M.: Anticonvulsant Drugs and Congenital Abnormalities. Am. J. Dis. Child., 127:758, 1974.

Anderson, E.G., and Magee, D.F.: A Study of the Mechanism of the Effect of Dietary Fat in Decreasing Thiopental Sleeping Time. J. Pharmacol. Exp. Ther., 117:281, 1956.

Barr, M., Jr., Poznanski, A.K., and Schmikel, R.D.: Digital Hypoplasia and Anticonvulsants During Gestation: A Teratogenic Syndrome? J. Pediatr., 84:254, 1974.

Blake, W.D.: Some Effects of Pentobarbital and Anesthesia on Renal Hemodynamics, Water and Electrolyte Excretion in the Dog. Am. J. Physiol., 191:393, 1957.

Bleicher, N.: Intramuscular Nembutal in Canine Anesthesia. Vet. Med., 53:372, 1958.

Booker, W.M., Maloney, A.H., Tureman, J.R., and Ratliff, C.: Some Metabolic Factors Influencing the Course of Thiopental Anesthesia in Dogs. Am. J. Physiol., 170:168, 1952.

Breznock, E.M.: Effects of Phenobarbital on Digitoxin and Digoxin Elimination in the Dog. Am. J. Vet. Res., 364:371, 1975.

Brodie, B.B., Bernstein, E., and Mark, L.C.: The Role of Body Fat in Limiting the Duration of Action of Thiopental. J. Pharmacol. Exp. Ther., 105:424, 1952.

Brown, B.R., and Vandam, L.D.: A Review of Current Advances in Metabolism of Inhalation Anesthetics. Ann. N.Y. Acad. Sci., 179:235, 1971.

Clemens, L.G., Popham, R.V., and Ruppert, P.H.: Neonatal Treatment of Hamsters with Barbiturate Alters Adult Sexual Behavior. Dev. Psychobiol., 12:49, 1979.

Corcoran, A.C., and Page, I.H.: Effects of Anesthetic Dosage of Pentobarbital Sodium on Renal Function and Blood Pressure in Dogs. Am. J. Physiol., 140:234, 1943.

Davis, L.E., Baggot, J.D., Davis, C.A.N., and Powers, T.E.: Elimination Kinetics of Pentobarbital in Nephrectomized Dogs. Am. J. Vet. Res., 34:231, 1973.

Elder, C.K., and Harrison, E.M.: Pentothal Sodium Slough: Prevention by Procaine Hydrochloride. J.A.M.A., 125:116, 1944.

Enold, G.L.: Pathologic Effects of Intrathoracic Barbiturate Anesthesia in Cats. J.A.V.M.A., 140:795, 1962.

Graca, J.G., and Garst, E.L.: Early Blood Changes in Dogs Following Intravenous Pentobarbital Anesthesia. Anesthesiology, 18:461, 1957.

Grono, L.R.: Methohexital Sodium Anaesthesia in the Horse. Aust. Vet. J., 42:398, 1966.

Gupta, C., Sonawane, B.R., and Yaffe, S.J.: Phenobarbital Exposure in Utero: Alterations in Female Reproductive Function in Rats. Science, 208:508, 1980.

Hall, L.W.: *Wright's Veterinary Anesthesia and Analgesia,* 7th ed. Bailliere Tindall, London, 1971.

Hamlin, R.L., Redding, R.W., Rieger, J.E., Smith, R.C., and Prynn, B.: Insignificance of the "Glucose Effect" in Dogs Anesthetized with Pentobarbital. J.A.V.M.A., 146:238, 1965.

Hamlin, R.L., and Smith, C.R.: Characteristics of Respiration in Healthy Dogs Anesthetized with Sodium Pentobarbital. Am. J. Vet. Res., 28:173, 1967.

Harris, J.R., and Hyder, N.: The Use of Secobarbital Sodium and Mephenesin as an Anesthetic for Dogs. J.A.V.M.A., 123:297, 1953.

Harrison, F.A.: The Anaesthesia of Sheep Using Pentobarbitone Sodium and Cyclopropane. In *Small Animal Anaesthesia*. Pergamon Press, London, 1964.

Hatch, R.C.: The Effect of Glucose, Sodium Lactate, and Epinephrine on Thiopental Anesthesia in Dogs. J.A.V.M.A., 148:135, 1966.

Hatch, R.C., Clark, J.D., Booth, N.H., and Kitzman, J.V.: Comparison of Five Preanesthetic Medicaments in Pentobarbital-Anesthetized Dogs: Antagonism by 4-Aminopyridine, Yohimbine, and Naloxone. Am. J. Vet. Res., 44:2312, 1983.

Hausner, E., Essex, H.E., and Mann, F.C.: Roentgenologic Observations of the Spleen of the Dog under Ether, Sodium Amytal, Pentobarbital Sodium and Pentothal Sodium Anesthesia. Am. J. Physiol., 121:387, 1938.

Heavner, J.E., and Bowen, J.M.: Influence of Adrenergic Agents on Recovery of Dogs from Anesthesia. J.A.V.M.A., 29:2133, 1968.

Helrich, M., Papper, E.M., and Rovenstine, E.A.: Surital Sodium: A New Anesthetic Agent for Intravenous Use. Preliminary Clinical Evaluation. Anesthesiology, 11:33, 1950.

Hinko, P.J., Wendt, W., Wollin, L.R., and Massopust, L.C.: Neurophysiologic and Behavioral Effects of Certain Anesthetics Administered Intramuscular in the Rhesus Monkey (Macaca mulatta). Am. J. Vet. Res., 31:1661, 1970.

Holzworth, J.: Intrathoracic Administration of General Anesthesia. Mod. Vet. Pract., 39:48, 1958.

Huang, L.Y.M., and Barker, J.L.: Pentobarbital: Stereospecific Actions of (+) and (−) Isomers Revealed on Cultured Mammalian Neurons. Science, 207:195, 1980.

Jones, E.W., Johnson, L., and Heinze, C.D.: Thiopental Sodium Anesthesia in the Horse: A Rapid Induction Technique. J.A.V.M.A., 137:119, 1960.

Lamson, P.D., Greig, M.E., and Hobdy, C.J.: Modification of Barbiturate Anesthesia by Glucose, Intermediary Metabolites, and Certain Other Substances. J. Pharmacol. Exp. Ther., 103:460, 1951.

Lamson, P.D., Greig, M.E., and Williams, L.: Potentiation by Epinephrine of the Anesthetic Effect in Chloral and Barbiturate Anesthesia. J. Pharmacol. Exp. Ther., 106:219, 1952.

Linzell, J.L.: Some Observations on General and Regional Anesthesia in Goats. In *Small Animal Anaesthesia*. Pergamon Press, London, 1964.

MacConnell, H.L.: The Effect of Barbiturates on Regional Blood Flows. Can. Anaesth. Soc. J., 16:1, 1969.

MacDonald, R.L., and Barker, J.L.: Different Actions of Anticonvulsant and Anesthetic Barbiturates Revealed by Use of Cultured Mammalian Neurons. Science, 200:775, 1978.

Mathers, D.A., and Barker, J.L.: (−) Pentobarbital Opens Ion Channels of Long Duration in Cultured Mouse Spinal Neurons. Science, 209:507, 1980.

Maynert, E.W., and Van Dyke, H.B.: The Absence of Localization of Barbital in Divisions of the Central Nervous System. J. Pharmacol. Exp. Ther., 98:184, 1950.

Monahan, C.M.: The Use of Methohexitone for Induction of Anaesthesia in Large Animals. Vet. Rec., 76:1333, 1964.

Muhrer, M.E.: Restraint of Swine with Pentothal Sodium. J.A.V.M.A., 117:293, 1950.

Muir, W.W.: Electrocardiographic Interpretation of Thiobarbiturate-Induced Dysrhythmias in Dogs. J.A.V.M.A., 170:1419, 1977.

Muir, W.W., Werner, L.L., and Hamlin, R.L.: Effects of Xylazine and Acetylpromazine upon Induced Ventricular Fibrillation in Dogs Anesthetized with Thiamylal and Halothane. Am. J. Vet. Res., 36:1299, 1975.

Musselman, E.E.: Arrhythmogenic Properties of Thiamylal Sodium in the Dog. J.A.V.M.A., 168:145, 1976.

Mylon, E., Winternitz, M.C., and De Suto-Nagy, G.J.: Studies on Therapy in Traumatic Shock. Am. J. Physiol., 139:313, 1943.

Nagel, M.L., Muir, W.W., and Nguyen, K.: Comparison of the Cardiopulmonary Effects of Etomidate and Thiamylal in Dogs. Am. J. Vet. Res., 40:193, 1979.

Nicoll, R.A., and Iwamoto, E.T.: Action of Pentobarbital on Sympathetic Ganglion Cells. J. Neurophysiol., 41:977, 1978.

Niemeyer, K.H.: Intrathoracic Anesthesia. Mod. Vet. Pract., 39:12, 1958.

Peters, M., and Strother, A.: A Study of Some Possible Mechanisms by Which Glucose Inhibits Drug Metabolism in Vivo and in Vitro. J. Pharmacol. Exp. Ther., 180:151, 1972.

Priano, L.L., Traber, D.L., and Wilson, R.D.: Barbiturate Anesthesia: An Abnormal Physiologic Situation. J. Pharmacol. Exp. Ther., 165:126, 1969.

Rawlings, C.A., and Kolata, R.J.: Cardiopulmonary Effects of Thiopental/Lidocaine Combination during Anesthetic Induction in the Dog. Am. J. Vet. Res., 44:144, 1983.

Reutner, T.F., and Gruhzit, O.M.: Surital Sodium, a New Anesthetic and Hypnotic: Studies in Dogs. J.A.V.M.A., 113:357, 1948.

Ritter, C., Hughes, R., Snyder, G., and Weaver, L.: Dichlorovos-Containing Dog Collars and Thiamylal Anesthesia. Am. J. Vet. Res., 31:2025, 1970.

Robertshaw, D.: Methohexital Sodium Anaesthesia in Calves. Vet. Rec., 76:357, 1964.

Robinson, M.H.: Deterioration of Solutions of Pentothal Sodium. Anesthesiology, 8:166, 1947.

Saidman, L.J., and Eger, E.I.: The Effect of Thiopental Metabolism on Duration of Anesthesia. Anesthesiology, 27:118, 1966.

Shideman, F.E., Kelly, A.R., and Adams, B.J.: The Role of the Liver in the Detoxication of Thiopental (Pentothal) and Two Other Barbiturates. J. Pharmacol. Ther., 91:331, 1947.

Skinner, S.F., Robertson, L.T., Artero, M., and Gerding, R.K.: Longitudinal Study of Phenobarbital in Serum, Cerebrospinal Fluid, and Saliva in the Dog. Am. J. Vet. Res., 41:600, 1980.

Sternfels, M.: Intrathoracic Anesthesia in Cats. Vet. Med., 50:365, 1955.

Swanson, E.E.: Sodium 5-Allyl-5-(1-Methylbutyl)-2-Thiobarbiturate, A Short Acting Anaesthetic. J. Pharm. Pharmacol., 3:112, 1951.

Szabuniewicz, M., Davis, R.H., and Wiersig, D.O.: Prevention of Methoxyflurane and Thiobarbiturate Cardiac Sensitization to Catecholamines in Dogs. Practicing Vet., 47:12, 1975.

Tavernor, W.D., and Lees, P.: The Influence of Thiopentone and Suxamethonium on Cardiovascular and Respiratory Function in the Horse. Res. Vet. Sci., 11:45, 1970.

Taylor, J.D., Richards, R.K., and Tabern, D.L.: Metabolism of S^{35} Thiopental (Pentothal). J. Pharmacol. Exp. Ther., 104:93, 1952.

Toosey, M.B.:The Uses of Concentrated Pentobarbitone Sodium Solution in Bovine Practice. Vet. Rec., 71:24, 1959.

Tyagi, R.P.S., Arnold, J.P., Usenik, E.A., and Fletcher, T.F.: Effects of Thiopental Sodium (Pentothal Sodium) Anesthesia on the Horse. Cornell Vet., 54:584, 1964.

Usenik, E.A., and Cronkite, E.P.: Effects of Barbiturate Anesthetics on Leukocytes in Normal and Splenectomized Dogs. Anesth. Analg., 44:167, 1965.

Van Dyke, H.B., Scudi, J.V., and Tabern, D.L.: The Excretion of N^{15} in the Urine of Dogs after the Administration of Labeled Pentobarbital. J. Pharmacol. Exp. Ther., 90:364, 1947.

Waddell, W.J., and Butler, T.C.: The Distribution and Excretion of Phenobarbital. J. Clin. Invest., 36:1217, 1957.

Welles, J.S., McMahon, R.E., and Doran, W.J.: The Metabolism and Excretion of Methohexital in the Rat and Dog. J. Pharmacol. Exp. Ther., 139:166, 1963.

Wiersig, D.O., Davis, R.H., and Szabuniewicz, M.: Prevention of Induced Ventricular Fibrillation in Dogs Anesthetized with Ultrashort Acting Barbiturates and Halothane. J.A.V.M.A., 165:341, 1974.

Woods, L.A., Wyngaarden, J.B., Rennick, B., and Seevers, M.H.: The Cardiovascular Effects of Sodium Pentothal and Sodium 5-Allyl-5-(1-Methylbutyl)-2-Thiobarbiturate in the Dog. Fed. Proc., 6:387, 1947.

Woods, L.A., Wyngaarden, J.B., Rennick, B., and Seevers, M.H.: Cardiovascular Toxicity of Thiobarbiturates: Comparison of Thiopental and 5-Allyl-5-(1-Methylbutyl)-2-Thiobarbiturate (Surital) in Dogs. J. Pharmacol. Exp. Ther., 95:328, 1949.

Wyngaarden, J.B., Woods, L.A., and Seevers, M.H.: The Cumulative Action of Certain Thiobarbiturates in Dogs. Fed. Proc., 6:388, 1947.

CHAPTER 13

Other Methods for Producing General Anesthesia

Although the anesthetic agents previously described are those most commonly employed, several miscellaneous agents and techniques may be used for general anesthesia, particularly under special circumstances. Ketamine, especially, has widespread use in both domestic and feral species. Chloral hydrate and mixtures of chloral hydrate, magnesium sulfate, and pentobarbital sodium, while less desirable than thiobarbiturate induction and inhalation maintenance, are still commonly used in large domestic animals, especially the horse. Several drugs used for anesthesia of laboratory animals do not find application in routine clinical use. Among them are chloral hydrate, chlorobutanol, chloralose, urethan, paraldehyde, and magnesium sulfate. Tribromoethanol has been used in several wild species.

Electronarcosis has not proved to be a useful clinical modality. Acupuncture has gained some adherents, chiefly for chronic pain relief rather than for surgical anesthesia. Hypothermia has had limited use in veterinary teaching institutions, principally for cardiac surgery.

The techniques most generally used are combinations of drugs. Because there are a myriad of these combinations, only a few are described.

KETAMINE HYDROCHLORIDE (VETALAR, KETASET)

Dissociative anesthetics are those that induce anesthesia by interrupting flow of information from the unconscious to the conscious parts of the brain, instead of depressing all brain centers. Phencyclidine was the first of these agents used clinically for veterinary anesthesia. Because of its abuse potential, it is no longer available. The reader is referred to the previous edition of this text for information concerning its use. Ketamine is an analogue of phencyclidine, with a shorter duration of action (Table 13–1).

The ketamine molecule exists as two optical isomers or enantiomers. This racemic mixture is currently used clinically; however, in animals the (+) isomer produces hypnosis lasting nearly twice as long as the (−) isomer (Marietta et al., 1977; Ryder et al., 1978). The racemic mixture is intermediate in effect. Analgesia with the (+) isomer is more profound, and there is less locomotor activity after anesthesia (White et al.,

TABLE 13–1. The Overt Effects of Phencyclidine (P) and Ketamine (K)

Species	*Compound*	*Excitation*	*Dysergia*	*Catalepsy*	*Anesthesia*	*Convulsion*	*Duration*
Pigeon	P	−	+	+	−	+	Long
	K	−	+	+	+	−	Short
Mouse	P	+	+	+	−	+	Long
Rat	K	+	+	+	+	−	Short
Guinea pig	P	−	+	+	−	+	Long
	K	−	+	+	−	−	Short
Rabbit	P	−	+	+	−	−	Long
	K	−	+	+	−	−	Short
Cat	P	−	+	+	+	Rare	Long
	K	−	+	+	+	Rare	Short
Dog	P	−(+?)	+	+	Poor	+	Long
	K	−(+?)	+	+	Poor	+	Short
Monkey	P	−	+	+	+	+	Long
	K	−	+	+	+	Very rare	Short
Man	P	−	+	+	+	?	Long
	K	−	+	+	+	?	Short

(From Chen, G.: The Pharmacology of Ketamine. Anaesthesiologie und Wiederbelebung, Bd. 40, Ketamine. hrsgb. Kreuscher. Springer, Berlin, Heidelberg, New York, 1969.)

1980). Ketamine enters the brain rapidly, and the brain/plasma concentration ratio becomes constant in less than one minute after rapid IV administration (Cohen et al., 1973). Rapid redistribution of the drug from brain to other tissues may account for its short action. In the cat, approximately 87% is excreted unchanged in the urine (Eads, 1974). It is rapidly metabolized in the liver of most other animal species, with as many as four metabolites excreted in the urine. The metabolites may contribute a small additive effect to the anesthetic action of the drug. Chloramphenicol will prolong recovery (Bree et al., 1975). Ketamine rapidly crosses the placental barrier.

When used alone, ketamine fails to produce good skeletal muscle relaxation, can lead to a stormy recovery, and frequently causes convulsions in dogs and occasionally in cats. To eliminate these side effects, many veterinarians use diazepam, acepromazine, xylazine, thiobarbiturates, or inhalation anesthetics concurrently with ketamine.

Ketamine, as the sole anesthetic agent, has been administered principally to cats and man, although its use in mice, rats, dogs, pigeons, primates, and exotic species has been reported (Chen et al., 1966; Bree and Gross, 1969; Kaump et al., 1969; Wright, 1982). In cats it produces profound anesthesia, allowing a wide variety of painful procedures depending upon the dose administered.

Mild cardiac stimulation and respiratory depression occur. Folts et al. (1975) found that ketamine produced an increase in heart rate and cardiac work in dogs. A significant increase in coronary blood flow also occurred, but appeared to be insufficient to meet the metabolic demands of the myocardium, as the coronary sinus oxygen content decreased,

Because ketamine increases blood pressure and intracranial pressure, it should not be used in head injuries or intraocular surgery. The eyes usually remain open with the pupils dilated so that a good view of the fundus can be obtained with an ophthalmoscope. Because they remain open, the eyes should be protected with an ophthalmic ointment. The pharyngeal and laryngeal reflexes remain active as does somatic muscle tone. Salivation commonly occurs; atropine should be administered to control secretions. Nausea, vomiting, and anorexia have not been observed. During anesthesia and the recovery phase, tonic-clonic spasms of varying severity frequently occur. For this reason, external stimuli should be avoided, and the animals should not be sent home until fully recovered. Use of acepromazine (0.025 mg/lb) mixed with ketamine tends to prevent this problem.

Ketamine is available in sterile aqueous solution for injection, each milliliter containing 100 mg of base with 1:10,000 benzethonium chloride added as preservative. The intramuscular dose of ketamine for cats varies from 5 to 20 mg/lb depending upon the condition and age of the patient and the procedure to be performed. Following injection, the cat becomes recumbent in 1 to 8 minutes. The duration of anesthesia is approximately 30 to 45 minutes. If necessary, additional ketamine may be administered to prolong anesthesia. A total dose of over 50 mg/lb is not recommended because prolonged anesthesia results. Immature animals may exhibit shorter anesthetic periods. Intravenous administration of 2 to 4 mg per pound of body weight has also been found satisfactory in dogs and cats. Premedication with 0.5 mg of promazine or 0.1 mg of acepromazine per pound of body weight is necessary in dogs to avoid coincident confusional states (Jones, 1972).

A constant intravenous infusion of 0.1% ketamine in 5% dextrose solution has been used effectively in dogs (Brasmer, 1980). The animals are first given 0.011 mg/kg of atropine and 0.5 to 1.0 mg/kg of acepromazine. Induction of anesthesia is accomplished at 120 to 150 drops/minute, and maintenance is at 15 to 30 drops/minute.

Intramuscular injection of 100 mg/lb has been suggested as a safe dosage for several species of birds (Kittle, 1971).

There are no known contraindications to use of ketamine in combination with other anesthetic agents, but the dose of the latter must be reduced accordingly. Physostigmine salicylate has been used as a ketamine antidote. At least in man, however, when administered in the early stages of spontaneous recovery from ketamine, physostigmine is in some ways synergistic and will prolong recovery of orientation and consciousness (Drummond et al., 1979). Hatch et al. (1983) found that a mixture of 0.6 mg/kg of 4-aminopyridine and 0.25 mg/kg of yohimbine would partially antagonize a dose of 20 mg/kg of ketamine in cats, terminating the anesthesia but not the cataleptic effect.

Ketamine has been used extensively as an anesthetic in humans and has a high potential for drug abuse. Inadvertent injection of 30 mg into a technician, caused by a struggling cat, has been reported by Sawyer (1980). Hallucinations, blurred vision, and weakness persisted for approximately 45 minutes.

Because of its ease of administration, ketamine is widely used as an anesthetic for many procedures in a variety of species.

KETAMINE-DIAZEPAM

Taylor (1983) has used diazepam and ketamine for short-term anesthesia in dogs. The combination is preceded by administration of 0.02 mg/lb of atropine sulfate subcutaneously. The dosage is 0.25 to 0.5 mg/lb of diazepam and 0.5 to 1.0 mg/lb of ketamine, administered intravenously mixed in one syringe. For longer anesthesia, acepromazine plus ketamine may be used. In this combination, 0.1 ml/lb of acepromazine is mixed with the preceding dosage of ketamine.

Diazepam-ketamine anesthesia has been used in man for open heart surgery (Hatano et al., 1976; Kumar et al., 1978; Jackson et al., 1978). Pretreatment with diazepam has been shown to prevent the increase in plasma catecholamines associated with ketamine administration.

For approximately one hour of profound anesthesia in dogs, Heath (1982) has recommended a mixture of diazepam, ketamine, and meperidine. These are given separately as follows: diazepam, 0.125 mg/lb, IV; ketamine, 3 to 4 mg/lb, IV; and meperidine hydrochloride, 2 to 3 mg/lb, IV. This mixture is particularly effective for deep oral surgery where the cough reflex must be obtunded. Because ventilation is reduced, the animal, when possible, should be intubated and ventilated.

A different technique is to administer 0.02 mg/lb of atropine subcutaneously followed by 0.2 mg/lb of diazepam and 1.0 mg/lb of ketamine intravenously. Ketamine can be repeated at one-half the dosage as needed. For better muscle relaxation, 0.07 mg/lb of succinylcholine can be added (Brasmer, 1980).

KETAMINE-XYLAZINE

Administration of xylazine and ketamine together tends to produce anesthesia that blends the best features of both agents. Many animal species have been anesthetized satisfactorily with this combination.

When one combines xylazine with ketamine in cats, the ketamine dose is reduced to about one-third of that required if ketamine is used alone or in combination with acepromazine. Recovery following xylazine-ketamine anesthesia in cats is considerably shorter than if ketamine is used alone, and the combination produces good muscle relaxation without convulsions. Recovery is smooth, although personality changes are occasionally observed. Postrecovery emesis is frequent, but can be controlled with atropine. An ophthalmic ointment should be applied to the patient's eyes to prevent exposure keratitis when the mixture is being used.

Xylazine (20 mg/ml) is injected intramuscularly at a rate of 1 mg/lb. Emesis usually follows in 4 to 8 minutes. Ketamine is injected at a dosage of 5 mg/lb approximately 10 minutes after xylazine. Surgical anesthesia follows the latter injection within 3 to 5 minutes. Faulk (1978) reported that the mean sleeping time in 16 cats was 125 ± 35 minutes. Faulk (1978) has also given cats a 1-ml mixture containing 10 mg of xylazine and 50 mg of ketamine. When the mixture is given intramuscularly at a rate of 0.1 ml/lb, a high percentage of cats will vomit within six minutes after injection. Unless the patient has been fasted prior to anesthesia, the xylazine-ketamine mixture may be undesirable, and Faulk recommends that xylazine precede ketamine because of its emetic properties. Surgical anesthesia occurs within 10 minutes after injection, making induction with the combination slower than if ketamine alone is used.

Kirkpatrick (1978) has administered xylazine-ketamine to over 200 dogs. Xylazine (1 mg/lb IM) was followed in 10 minutes by ketamine (5 mg/lb IM). This combination produces muscle relaxation and analgesia for a period of 25 to 50 minutes. If shorter anesthesia is required, the ketamine dosage can be reduced to 2 to 4 mg/lb.

Complications include insufficient anesthesia, which occurs particularly in high-strung smaller breeds. These dogs may suffer repeated seizures during induction or may fail to reach an adequate anesthetic plane. In these animals, mask induction with methoxyflurane is used. Small ketamine doses seem to produce a greater tendency toward seizure; therefore, dogs receiving reduced doses are left to rest quietly in their cage until anesthesia is complete, which usually requires 5 minutes.

In large breeds (60 lbs and over), complications have included reduced body temperature and hypoxia. For this reason, the dose of xylazine is usually reduced by one-third, and ketamine dosage is also reduced to 3 to 5 mg/lb. Because of seizures, this anesthetic technique should not be used in front of clients. Excessive salivation sometimes occurs and can be controlled with atropine.

Two dogs are known to have died within 24 hours of receiving this mixture. No cause was ascertained for these deaths.

In a two-year dental study in dogs, Stephenson et al. (1978) anesthetized dogs biweekly utilizing xylazine-ketamine anesthesia. Blood calcium, phosphorus, glucose, urea nitrogen, uric acid, cholesterol, total protein, albumin, total bilirubin, alkaline phosphatase, serum glutamic-oxaloacetic transaminase (SGOT), and creatinine were studied. Fifteen minutes before administration of xylazine-ketamine, 0.25 mg of atropine sulfate was given intramuscularly. Xylazine (2 mg/kg) and ketamine (5.5 mg/kg), mixed in a common syringe, were administered intramuscularly. Anesthesia was induced in approximately 10 minutes and averaged approximately 30 minutes. Recovery occurred after 1 to 2 hours.

Serum chemistry values generally remained within normal ranges. Alkaline phosphatase and glucose values for individual dogs exceeded these ranges at times. Periodically 4 of the 17 subjects exhibited transitory CNS stimulation resembling a mild epileptiform seizure. The authors believed that these could have been avoided had the xylazine preceded the ketamine injection.

Muir et al. (1977) have used xylazine (1.1

mg/kg) administered intravenously prior to or simultaneously with ketamine hydrochloride (2.2 mg/kg) in horses. They found that this combination produced excellent short-term analgesia and light anesthesia. Cardiac output, arterial blood pressure, pulmonary arterial pressure, central venous pressure, and pulmonary arterial wedge pressure remained within normal limits. Respiratory acidosis tended to develop with time. Induction and recovery were smooth and excitement-free.

When xylazine was administered (1.1 mg/kg), there were obvious signs of sedation within 30 to 60 seconds. The horse's head lowered, the lower lip drooped, and the animal became incoordinate. All horses remained standing with this dose. Three to five minutes later, ketamine (2.2 mg/kg) was administered, and the animals collapsed without struggling to a laterally recumbent position within 30 to 60 seconds. At this stage, the horses could easily be intubated. The period of analgesia appeared to last approximately 16 minutes and was somewhat dependent upon the breed of horse, hot-blooded horses having a shorter duration of analgesia. As the horse recovered, it rolled to its sternum before standing. Excitement was not evident, and all horses were able to return to their stalls within 5 minutes of recovery.

In a second group of horses, xylazine was mixed with ketamine in the same syringe, and the anesthetic period and recovery were similar to that described for the first group. The mean time to standing recovery was 23 minutes. In a third group of horses given the same dose of xylazine but a higher dose (6.6 mg/kg) of ketamine, the analgesia was not as long as in the lower-dose groups, averaging 12 minutes. However, the time to standing recovery was prolonged (93 minutes) and marked by extreme incoordination, muscular tremor, rigidity, sweating, hypertension, tachycardia, oculogyric movements, and excitement. Some of these horses had to be resedated with intravenous xylazine.

Purohit et al. (1981) studied the effects of ketamine-xylazine on the ECG, respiratory rate, and electroencephalogram (EEG) of horses. Six of six horses injected with 1.1 mg/kg of xylazine IV developed second-degree atrioventricular block in approximately 23 seconds. Ketamine was injected 3 minutes later (2.2 mg/kg IV), and the AV block disappeared approximately 90 seconds thereafter in four horses. The remaining two had second-degree AV block through a 15- to 18-minute recording period. Xylazine depressed heart rates an average of 29.3%. After ketamine administration, they increased or remained unchanged. The horses sedated with xylazine exhibited hypersynchronous EEG patterns; ketamine administration caused an increase in high-voltage slow activity.

All horses went into sternal and then lateral recumbency within 90 seconds after ketamine administration.

The hemodynamic and respiratory effects of this combination appear to be a synthesis of the pharmacologic activities of both drugs. Xylazine alone is known to produce a decrease in arterial blood pressure after initially producing a transient rise. These actions may be due to α_2-receptor stimulation followed by profound and prolonged bradycardia. Ketamine causes an outflow of electrical activity in the limbic-hypothalamic centers to the autonomic nervous system through the medullary center. Thus, ketamine tends to produce increases in cardiac output, blood pressure, and heart rate.

Kaka et al. (1979) studied the pharmacokinetics of ketamine in horses. They found that if it is given to xylazine-treated horses at the rate of 2.2 mg/kg by rapid IV injection, the minimum anesthetic plasma concentration of 1.15 μg/ml is reached in approximately 12 minutes.

Since xylazine is considered to be the sedative of choice in cattle, it has been combined in this species with ketamine for its immobilizing, profound analgesic effect, as well as its sedative qualities. Xylazine (0.2 mg/kg IM) was administered 10 minutes prior to ketamine (5 mg/kg IV or 10 mg/kg IM) or simultaneously with it. Intramuscularly, the initial bradycardia associated with xylazine administration was not observed. Anesthesia was characterized by good muscular relaxation and a smooth uncomplicated recovery lasting 20 to 25 minutes. Duration was longer (35 minutes) in calves receiving concurrent xylazine and ketamine, and was

85 minutes after the last injection of maintenance doses of ketamine (5 mg/kg IM) (Waterman, 1981).

Xylazine-ketamine has also been used in several laboratory and exotic species (see Chap. 18).

KETAMINE-XYLAZINE-GUAIFENESIN

Muir et al. (1978) used a combination of intramuscular xylazine (2.2 mg/kg) plus intravenous guaifenesin (55 mg/kg in 5% dextrose) and ketamine (17 mg/kg) for short-term anesthesia (23 ± 8 minutes) in horses. This combination was also satisfactory for induction of general anesthesia with halothane or enflurane.

ALTHESIN (SAFFAN)

Althesin is a combination of two steroids: alphaxalone and alphadolone acetate. The solubility of alphaxalone (9 mg/ml) is increased by alphadolone acetate (3 mg/ml) and by 20% w/v polyoxyethylated castor oil (Cremophor EL). The combination of the two steroids has an exceptionally high therapeutic index (30.6). It has little cumulative effect (Fig. 13–1); the duration of anesthesia varies with species (Fig. 13–2). Administration of the combination before or after barbiturates is not advised. Adverse effects when used with other anesthetic drugs have not been reported.

In the cat, a dose of 9 mg/kg is recommended for intravenous administration and 12 to 18 mg/kg for intramuscular administration. Intravenous injection produces relaxation in approximately 9 seconds and surgical anesthesia in about 25 seconds. Intramuscular administration produces variable results but may be useful in fractious animals. The onset after intramuscular injection occurs in 6 to 12 minutes and lasts for approximately 15 minutes. A quiet area for induction is desirable. In the fractious cat, where drugs can be administered intramuscularly, ketamine is the drug of choice, since althesin is less reliable by this route (Jones, 1979).

Althesin has a neutral pH and does not produce pain or inflammation when injected perivascularly or intramuscularly. Additional doses can be given to prolong anesthesia without cumulative effects, and recovery is rapid. In contrast to ketamine, althesin produces good muscular relaxation. Dodds and Twissell (1972) found that althesin has a slightly protective effect against epinephrine-induced arrhythmias in the cat's heart. Urination, defecation, muscle tremors, paddling, salivation, and hyperesthesia have been reported as side effects. Edema of the feet, ears, and muzzle occur in approximately 25% of cats injected, but is usually transient and disappears within 2 hours. This condition apparently occurs in females more often than in males. Antihistamine administration reduces this possibility.

Child et al. (1971) stated that in the dog and some other canidae, polyoxyethylene derivatives of hexitol anhydride partial fatty acid esters produce an allergic response. This response is manifest by a prolonged fall in blood pressure and a positive skin wheal if the drug is injected intradermally. Urticaria and erythema are believed to be the result of release of histamine or histamine-like substances. Cremophor EL, a nonionic polyoxyethylated emulsifying agent used as the vehicle in althesin, elicits the same response. Watkins and Clark (1978) have discussed adverse reactions in man and state that an allergic reaction can occur due to either the vehicle (polyoxyethylated castor oil) or either of the two steroids. The reaction can be of the true hypersensitivity type, which requires previous exposure to the drug, or of the complement activation type, which requires no previous sensitization.

Hall (1972) reviewed the use of althesin in horses, sheep, and swine. Horses developed unacceptable violent paddling and galloping movements during recovery. These could be suppressed by prior administration of xylazine (1 mg/kg). The minimum dose of althesin for induction of anesthesia was approximately 1.2 to 1.34 mg/kg in the unpremedicated horse. Xylazine increased the recovery time from 20 to 34 minutes.

The dose of althesin for sheep is approximately 2.2 mg/kg intravenously. This produces light surgical anesthesia for 8 to 15 minutes. The average maintenance dose to produce sur-

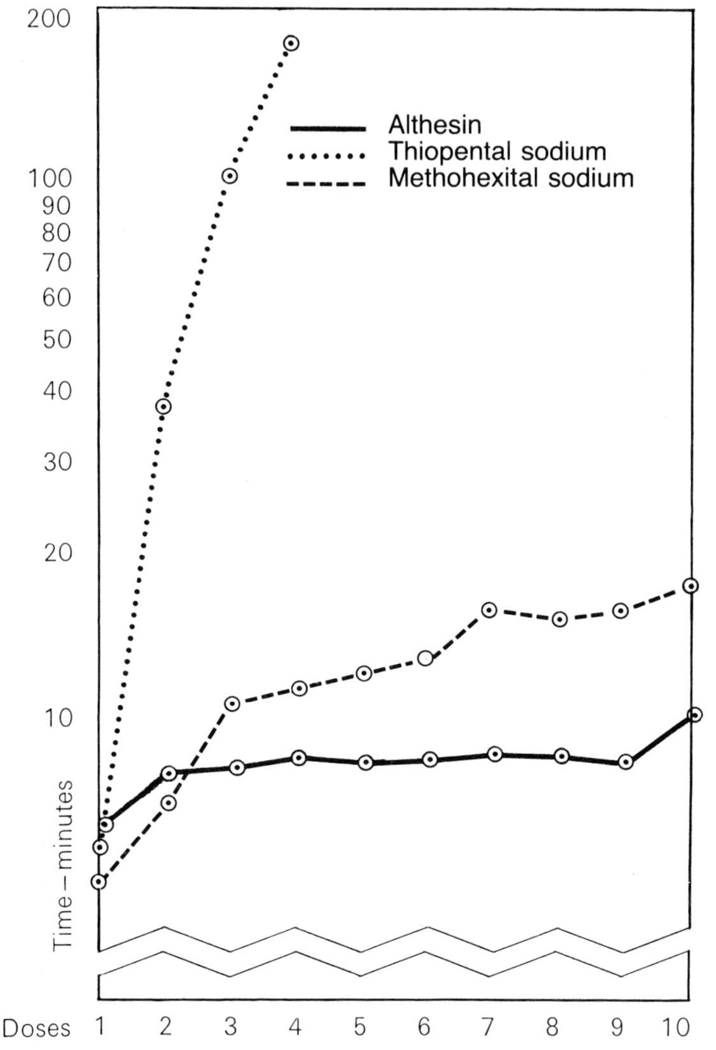

Figure 13–1. Duration of loss of righting reflex in mice given repeated intravenous doses of althesin and other anesthetics. Second and subsequent doses given 30 seconds after return of the righting reflex. Five mice per group. (After Child, K.J., Currie, J.P., Davis, B., Dodds, M.G., Pearce, D.R., and Twissell, D.J.: The Pharmacological Properties in Animals of CT 1341—A New Steroid Anaesthetic. Br. J. Anaesth., 43:2, 1971.)

gical anesthesia for a 3-hour period is 0.23 mg/kg/minute. Sheep given althesin had bradycardia with a decrease in systolic and diastolic pressures of 20 to 35% of preinjection levels. Left ventricular end-diastolic pressure was elevated and cardiac ouput was decreased. These parameters returned to normal within 6 to 8 minutes after injection. A depression of dp/dt max was observed also. Camburn (1982) has successfully used althesin followed by halothane-N_2O for a variety of operations in ruminants (goats, sheep, young calves).

The dose of althesin for pigs is approximately 6 mg/kg to produce 10 to 15 minutes of anesthesia. In pigs known to develop malignant hyperthermia under anesthesia, althesin did not cause this phenomenon, and Hall (1972) suggested that it can be used safely in animals known to be susceptible to this condition.

Pickerodt et al. (1972) found that althesin produced a fall in cerebral blood flow accompanied by a fall in intracranial pressure in baboons.

Child et al. (1972) studied the metabolism

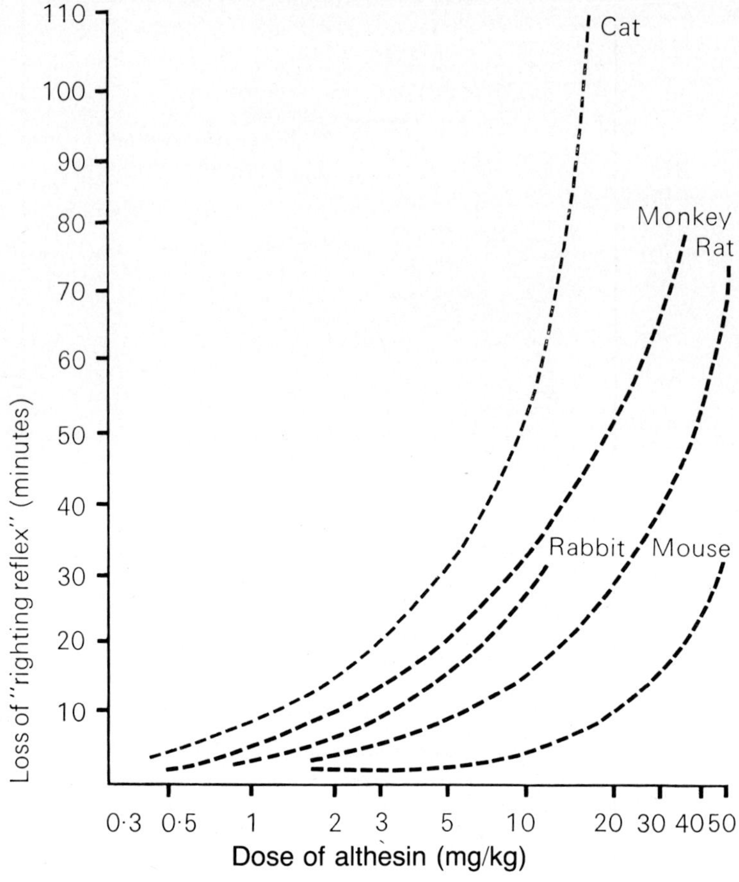

Figure 13–2. Anesthetic activity of althesin in different species. (After Child, K.J., Currie, J.P., Davis, B., Dodds, M.G., Pearce, D.R., and Twissell, D.J.: The Pharmacological Properties in Animals of CT 1341—A New Steroid Anaesthetic. Br. J. Anaesth., 43:2, 1971.)

and excretion of althesin in the rat. They stated that neither of the two steroids is extensively protein-bound by the serum of rat, cat, horse, or man. Approximately 60 to 70% of a radioactive dose of alphaxalone or alphadolone acetate is excreted as metabolic products in the feces during the five days following intravenous injection; the other 20 to 30% appears in the urine during the same period.

ALTHESIN-FENTANYL-PANCURONIUM

Michalot et al. (1980) have administered althesin-fentanyl-pancuronium anesthesia to dogs for 24 hours and produced only minimal hemodynamic changes. Ten dogs weighing 10 to 20 kg were anesthetized with althesin (5 ml IV) and were maintained by continuous infusion of althesin 0.2 ml/kg/hr, fentanyl 8 μg/kg/hr, and pancuronium bromide 64 μg/kg/hr in lactated Ringer's and 10% dextrose solutions. The infusion rate was 4 ml/kg/hr. The dogs were intubated and the lungs ventilated with room air using a preset volume ventilator at 12 bpm. Body temperature was maintained by a thermoregulated heating blanket.

Cardiac parameters in which there were no significant changes included cardiac index, heart rate, right ventricular end-diastolic pressure, systolic arterial pressure, total systemic vascular resistance, pulmonary arteriolar resistance, and arterial blood gases. The only significant changes found throughout the 24-hour period were in mean pulmonary arterial pressure and pulmonary capillary wedge pressure.

The technique was remarkably stable hemodynamically. Values under althesin-fentanyl-pancuronium anesthesia were similar to those observed with a single injection of althesin. The choice of the dog as an animal model might be questioned since Cremophor EL, the solvent for althesin, may cause anaphylactic reaction in dogs. In this study, none of the dogs showed signs of hypersensitivity.

CHLORAL HYDRATE, U.S.P.

Liebrich, who introduced chloral hydrate as a hypnotic in 1869, thought that because it released chloroform in vitro it would do the same in vivo. This has subsequently been proved a misconception.

Chloral hydrate occurs as colorless translucent crystals that volatilize on exposure to air with an aromatic, penetrating odor. It has a bitter, caustic taste. One gram of the crystals dissolves in 0.25 ml of water. It may be administered orally, or solutions may be injected intravenously or intraperitoneally. It irritates the gastric mucosa and may cause vomiting if not diluted in water, but is readily absorbed from the gastrointestinal tract. A small amount of chloral hydrate is excreted unchanged in the urine. The greater portion is reduced to trichlorethyl alcohol, a less potent hypnotic, and this in turn is conjugated with glycuronic acid to form urochloralic (trichlorethylglycuronic) acid, which has no hypnotic property. The latter is excreted in the urine. In animals with liver damage, chloral hydrate may be found in larger quantities and urochloralic acid in smaller quantities in the urine.

Chloral hydrate depresses the cerebrum with loss of reflex excitability. In subanesthetic doses, motor and sensory nerves are not affected. Chloral hydrate is a good hypnotic, but a poor anesthetic; the amount needed to produce anesthesia approaches the minimal lethal dose, and it produces deep sleep that lasts for several hours. It has weak analgesic action. In hypnotic doses, the medullary centers are not affected. Anesthetic doses of chloral hydrate depress the vasomotor center severely, resulting in a fall in blood pressure. Hypnotic doses depress respiration, and anesthetic doses markedly depress the respiratory center. Death from chloral hydrate administration is caused by progressive depression of the respiratory center. The margin of safety is such that it is not a satisfactory surgical anesthetic.

Chloral hydrate is not used for small animal anesthesia and has lost most of its popularity as a general anesthetic in large animals. Its continued use in large animals depends on the simplicity of administration and on the duration of effect of the induction dose—an interval adequate for many routine procedures. It is relatively inexpensive, and may be combined with barbiturates. Despite these advantages, it is a poor anesthetic, as large doses are necessary to induce general anesthesia, and it is irritant when inadvertently injected outside the vein. Although dangerous sequelae may result from accidental injection of chloral hydrate solution into perivenous tissues, care during injection usually avoids this. Use of a vascular catheter obviates this hazard. The concentration of the chloral hydrate solution should not be too high; 7 to 12% w/v aqueous solutions are generally used.

Doses reported for intravenous chloral hydrate vary extensively, probably due both to the rate of administration and to varying interpretations of the depth of resulting anesthesia. The recommended intravenous dose for chloral hydrate in the horse varies from 2 to 3 g/100 lb as a sedative and up to 10 g/100 lb for general anesthesia.

The solution is commonly administered at 15 to 30 g/minute and is given until the horse is about to fall, at which time the intravenous tubing is disconnected and the animal is restrained in recumbency. If necessary, additional anesthetic is administered slowly until the desired degree of sedation or anesthesia is achieved. Because of conversion to trichloroethanol and slow passage across the blood-brain barrier, anesthetic depression increases for several minutes after initial induction. Therefore, additional doses should not be administered immediately. The chief disadvantage with chloral hydrate is that the dose required to induce general anesthesia is such that recovery is prolonged. For this reason, the drug is usually used to induce a degree of narcosis, and analgesia is produced by means of local or regional anesthetics. Studies by Stopiglia (1962) indicate that premedication with tranquilizers reduces the amount of chloral hydrate required, facilitates induction, and minimizes struggling during recovery.

The time required for horses to stand after cessation of administration varies from 1 to 4 hours and is similar in duration to that observed during use of a combination of chloral hydrate and magnesium sulfate. If anesthesia is maintained for longer than is usual and maintenance doses are necessary, the recovery period may be greatly prolonged. The nature of the recovery period varies; if left undisturbed, the horse often passes quietly into a hypnotic state, remaining thus until it is ready to stand. Excitement and struggling during recovery are not uncommon and can be minimized by use of tranquilizers.

Chloral hydrate is also occasionally used to induce narcosis or anesthesia in cattle and swine. In the former, it has been replaced with xylazine. The dose required is similar to that for horses. In cattle, premedication with atropine sulfate and early intubation are indicated.

Chloral hydrate may also be administered to horses and cattle by stomach tube to induce varying degrees of sedation or narcosis (3 to 6 g/100 lb body weight).

CHLORAL HYDRATE AND MAGNESIUM SULFATE

A combination of chloral hydrate and magnesium sulfate is commonly used by those who use chloral hydrate. Mixtures of 1 (Vladutin, 1939), 2 (Danks, 1943), and 3 parts (Coffee, 1949) of chloral hydrate to 1 part of magnesium sulfate have been recommended. The following advantages for the mixture are claimed (Danks, 1947): 1) It results in more rapid and quieter induction. 2) It increases the anesthetic depth. 3) It reduces the toxicity of the chloral hydrate and is less irritant.

A comparison of the use of chloral hydrate alone and 2:1 and 1:1 mixtures with magnesium sulfate in the horse failed to reveal obvious differences (Jones, 1949). The dose of chloral hydrate when used with magnesium sulfate and the resulting degree of anesthesia in the horse are illustrated in Figure 13–3.

CHLORAL HYDRATE, MAGNESIUM SULFATE, AND PENTOBARBITAL SODIUM

Millenbruck and Wallinga (1946) described the use of a mixture of chloral hydrate, magnesium sulfate, and pentobarbital sodium for induction and maintenance of anesthesia in horses. After trying several combinations of these drugs, they found the following mixture to be preferable: chloral hydrate 1 oz, magnesium sulfate 0.5 oz, pentobarbital sodium 100 gr., distilled water to make 1000 ml. They claimed this mixture had the following advantages: 1) no excitement during induction, 2) no emergence struggling and floundering, 3) complete immobility during the short period (15 to 30 minutes) of anesthesia followed by 1½ hours for recovery, 4) a wide margin of safety, and 5) economy. The mixture is administered in the same manner as combinations of chloral hydrate and magnesium sulfate. It has also been used for anesthesia of birds.

There seems to be little merit in the use of chloral hydrate alone or in combination, in view of the tranquilizers, analgesics, and anesthetics now available.

CHLOROBUTANOL, U.S.P. (CHLORETONE)

Chlorobutanol occurs as colorless crystals that are sparingly soluble in water and readily soluble in alcohol. It has been administered orally or intravenously for anesthesia in laboratory animals. The LD_{50} for dogs is 238 mg/kg orally. It formerly was used as a sedative and hypnotic, but currently is used chiefly as a preservative for various solutions, particularly those for parenteral administration.

CHLORALOSE

Chloralose is prepared by heating anhydrous glucose and trichloroacetaldehyde (anhydrous chloral) in a water bath. Both alpha and beta chloralose are formed, the alpha form being the active fraction. It has been used in studies of the baroreceptor reflexes since it produces a

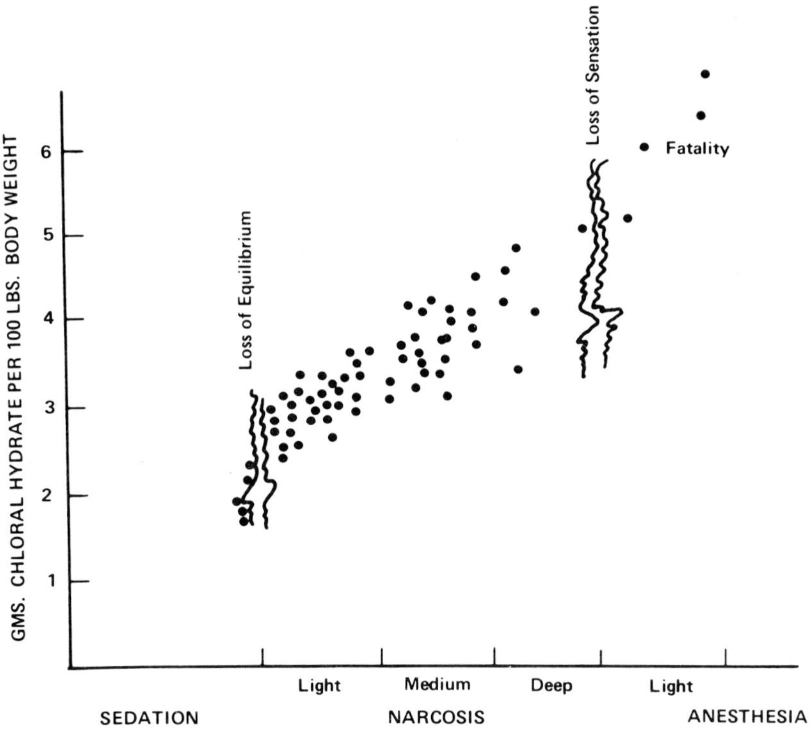

Figure 13–3. Chloral hydrate and magnesium sulfate anesthesia (2:1) in the horse. Dose of chloral hydrate used and degree of anesthesia obtained in clinical cases.

higher blood pressure and more active reflexes than other agents (Brown and Hilton, 1956).

Chloralose is usually prepared as a 1.0% aqueous solution. Heat is necessary to dissolve the drug, but solutions should not be boiled. The intravenous anesthetic dose for dogs of α-chloralose is approximately 0.11 g/kg. For adult cats, it is 36 mg/lb (King and Unna, 1954).

Harding et al. (1979) determined the effects of pentobarbital and α-chloralose anesthesia on recordings made from sensorimotor cerebral cortical neurons in the cat. They found that α-chloralose offered a broader view of the neuronal contents of the cortex, and of potential routes of afferent influence, than pentobarbital, and that neither yields the same view as in the awake unanesthetized cat. Chloralose is still considered valuable for maintenance of basal narcosis for long periods in nonsurvival experiments.

URETHAN, N.F. (URETHANE, ETHYL CARBAMATE)

Urethan is prepared by heating urea with alcohol under pressure or by warming urea nitrate with alcohol and sodium nitrite. The drug is marketed in the crystalline state. One gram dissolves in 0.5 ml of water, the aqueous solution being neutral. It is most often used as an anesthetic in laboratory animals and fish. The lethal intravenous dose for rabbits is 2.0 g/kg. The dose for dogs and cats is 0.6 to 2.0 g. Up to 500 mg/kg may be used as a hypnotic dose.

Urethan is mutagenic, carcinostatic, and carcinogenic (Auerbach, 1967). Mice given urethan develop an exceptionally high incidence of lung tumors, regardless of the route of administration. Tumors also develop in treated rats and rabbits. There are no known instances where lung tumors have developed in humans from urethan. However, until further work is done, concern over the health of individuals in prolonged contact with urethan or its solutions is justified (Wood, 1956).

PARALDEHYDE, U.S.P.

Paraldehyde is a polymer of acetaldehyde. In hypnotic doses, it has a wide margin of safety because it depresses only the cerebrum and not the medullary centers. When it is given to dogs at a rate of 2 ml/kg/minute intravenously, a 9% aqueous solution may cause hemoglobinuria. The LD_{50} for dogs is 3.5 g/kg. It has also been used as an hypnotic for rabbits, baboons, porpoises, and amphibians. However, better drugs are now available (Green, 1979).

MAGNESIUM SULFATE

Dilute aqueous solutions of magnesium sulfate can be used to produce surgical anesthesia in small animals; however, all parts of the central nervous system are depressed, and the result is often fatal respiratory arrest. For this reason, and since it is relatively inexpensive, the drug is used principally for euthanasia, a saturated solution being administered intravenously. Its effect, however, is not as desirable as that achieved with the barbiturates, animals sometimes showing a period of excitement prior to collapse.

Magnesium sulfate is also used in combination with chloral hydrate and pentobarbital for anesthesia of horses, cattle, swine, and birds (see Chap. 18).

Magnesium anesthesia can be counteracted by intravenous injection of a soluble calcium salt such as calcium gluconate or calcium chloride. Animals so treated show an immediate and almost total recovery. Combined neostigmine (0.35 to 0.63 mg/kg) and pentylenetetrazol (10 mg/kg) intravenously produce the same result in rabbits (Borglin and Lindsten, 1949).

About 70% of injected magnesium sulfate is excreted by the kidneys in 48 hours.

METOMIDATE (HYPNODIL)

Metomidate hydrochloride (R7315) is a hypnotic agent with muscle relaxant properties. Its hypnotic effect is exerted on mammals, birds, reptiles, and fish (see Chap. 18). Given alone, it induces sleep without analgesia. General anesthesia can be produced by combining it with neuroleptics or analgesics.

It is available in powdered form, which dissolves readily in water to make 1% or 5% solutions. These solutions have a pH of 2.9 and 2.4, respectively. Combined with azaperone (see Chap 8), metomidate produces anesthesia in swine for approximately 2 hours (Dimigen and Reetz, 1970). Respiration slows and deepens. With rapid intravenous injection, apnea may occur. The cardiovascular system remains stable. When metomidate is used for cesarean section in sows, the piglets are usually alert at delivery.

ETOMIDATE (AMIDATE)

Etomidate, a congener of metomidate (above), contains 2 mg/ml of the drug in 35% ethylene glycol. It should be refrigerated at 2 to 8° C until used, and should not be frozen or exposed to extreme heat. The brain stem reticular formation appears to be the site of hypnotic activity. No analgesia is produced.

Etomidate in powder and injectable forms has been used as an anesthetic for exotic species of animals. It has recently been introduced in the United States as an induction agent for poor-risk human patients because it does not depress the cardiovascular and respiratory systems or release histamine.

Single injections produce relatively brief hypnosis. In dogs, dosages of 1.5 and 3.0 mg/kg lasted 8 ± 5 and 21 ± 9 minutes, respectively (Nagel et al., 1979). The duration of hypnosis is directly dose-related. The anesthetic indices in rats and dogs when given intramuscularly are 26.4 and 15.9, respectively. Etomidate is rapidly hydrolyzed in the liver and also excreted in the urine.

Etomidate is compatible with other common preanesthetic agents. Venous pain is common on injection in humans, and myoclonia may occur without administration of premedication.

TRICAINE METHANESULFONATE (MS-222)

Tricaine methanesulfonate, a crystalline water-soluble powder, is marketed under the commercial name, MS-222. It is used as an anesthetic to immobilize amphibia, fish, and other cold-blooded animals by complete bathing of small subjects, by gill spraying in large fish, or by injecting larger species (see Chap. 18). It exerts a prompt, intense action and has a low degree of toxicity, being approximately three times less toxic than procaine and about 10 times less toxic than cocaine. A 1:1000 solution may be autoclaved without loss of narcotic properties or increase in toxicity.

HYPOTHERMIA

As the body temperature of a warm-blooded animal falls, metabolism is reduced and, therefore, the need for oxygen is diminished. Bigelow et al. (1950) found that oxygen uptake in dogs is reduced by approximately 50% at 30° C and 65% at 25° C. Fuhrman et al., in 1950, showed that the metabolic rate of isolated slices of rat heart was reduced 90% by lowering the temperature to 10° C. Gott et al. (1962) determined that the potassium-arrested heart at 37° C utilized four times as much glycogen and produced three times as much lactic acid as the heart at 17° C. In addition, the ATP level was reduced twice as far in normothermic hearts. Thus the heart, brain, liver, or other vital organs can survive at a low temperature for a considerably increased period when deprived of all or a portion of their blood supply. Hypothermia may be artificially produced in the entire body, or in only a portion such as the heart or head. While it has been tried in many situations, it has found its greatest usefulness in surgery of the heart and central nervous system (Swan et al., 1953).

It would seem that the colder an animal was made to become, the less oxygen would be required by a given organ. It has been shown, however, that the reduction of oxygen consumption varies for different organs. For example, the work done by the heart at 26 to 27° C is little less than that at normal temperature, and while the general oxygen uptake by the body at this temperature is reduced to 40% of normal, that of the heart is still 50%. Bering et al. (1956), working with monkeys, found little change in cerebral oxygen uptake until a temperature of 31° C is reached. At this point it falls sharply, and through the next 4° there is a drop of about 25%. Below 27° C oxygen consumption continues to fall but at a much slower rate. The relationship of cerebral oxygen consumption to temperature is sigmoid rather than linear (Fig. 13–4).

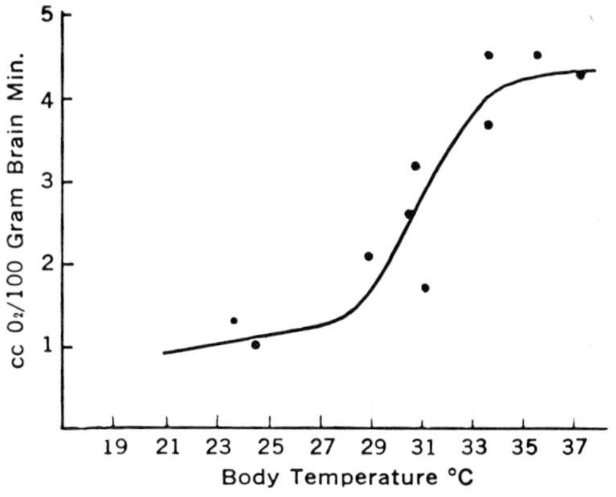

Figure 13–4. Relation of oxygen uptake by the brain to temperature. (From Bering, E.A., Jr., Taren, J.A., McMurray, J.D., and Bernhard, W.F.: Surg. Gynecol. Obstet., 102:134, 1956.)

Several species of warm-blooded animals have been subjected to drastic hypothermia. It is possible to cool small laboratory animals to 0° C, and even lower, followed by recovery. Andjus and Lovelock (1955) reported 80 to 100% recovery in rats after cooling to temperatures just above the freezing point with cardiac and respiratory arrest for 1 hour. Smith (1956) kept golden hamsters "on ice" with circulatory arrest for up to 7 hours. These animals even survived supercooling to −5 or −6° C. When the circulation has been maintained with a pump-oxygenator, dogs have survived cooling to 1.5° C (Gollan et al., 1955). Niazi and Lewis (1957) anesthetized 6 adult monkeys with thiopental and reduced the body temperature to between 4 and 9° C. Cardiac standstill occurred

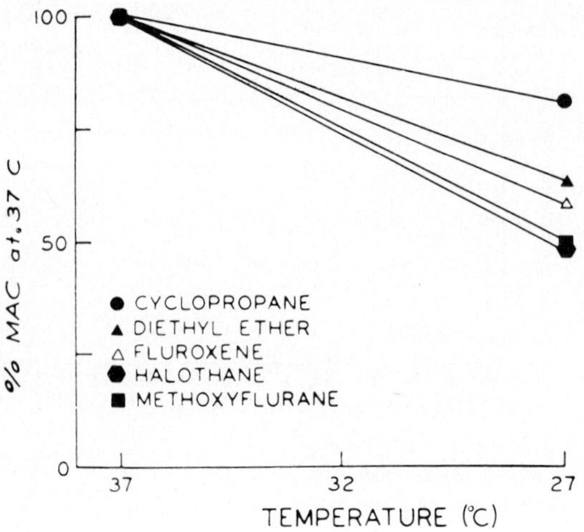

Figure 13–5. The percentage decline between 37 and 27° C of the minimum alveolar concentration (MAC) required for anesthesia. Cyclopropane, the least oil-soluble agent, declines least, and halothane and methoxyflurane, the most soluble, decline most. (From Regan, M.J., and Eger, E.I.: Effect of Hypothermia in Dogs on Anesthetizing Apneic Doses of Inhalation Agents. Anesthesiology, 23:689, 1967.)

when the body temperature reached 14 to 11° C and lasted for periods of 42 minutes to 2 hours. Five of the monkeys survived and appeared normal.

In order to induce the hypothermic state as quickly as possible, it is necessary to control shivering since it is an important mechanism in protection against cold. Shivering is induced by an increased temperature gradient between cold receptors in the skin and centers in the hypothalamus (Davis and Mayer, 1955). Even without visible shivering, there is general hypertonicity of the skeletal muscles, which results in increased metabolic, heart, and respiratory rates. Shivering can be prevented by deep anesthesia, or light anesthesia with curarization or tranquilization with a phenothiazine. The latter drugs are thought to exert their effect through a peripheral action on muscle fibers and on the hypothalamic temperature control center.

The effect of hypothermia on anesthetizing and apneic doses of inhalation agents in dogs was studied by Regan and Eger (1967). They found that moderate hypothermia produced a rectilinear decrease in anesthetic requirements (MAC) for cyclopropane, diethyl ether, fluroxene, halothane, and methoxyflurane (Fig. 13–5). Moderate hypothermia also reduced the concentration of anesthetic required to produce apnea. Munson (1970) found the same phenomenon occurred in rats given cyclopropane or halothane. However, the magnitude of changes was much greater indicating, perhaps, a species variation. There is little difference between halothane, pentobarbital, and chloralose in their effects on whole-body oxygen consumption during surface cooling in dogs (Westenskow et al., 1979) (Fig. 13–6).

Three methods of whole-body cooling have been utilized: 1) surface, 2) body cavity, and 3) extracorporeal. Surface cooling is usually accomplished by directly immersing the unprotected body in ice water or by placing the body on a mattress* through which ice water is circulated. Hyperventilation is maintained throughout the procedure to keep the blood pH on the alkaline side of normal. This has been shown to reduce cardiac arrhythmias and fibrillation. Below 28° C (82.4° F) no anesthetic is needed, and the patient is maintained on artificial ventilation alone. Active cooling is stopped when approximately two-thirds of the desired temperature fall has been accomplished. Otherwise, the temperature continues to drop once the desired degree of hypothermia has been reached.

Body cavity cooling is accomplished by pouring cold saline solution into the open thoracic cavity (Blades and Pierpont, 1954). This method has the disadvantage of being slow and requiring large volumes of saline solution.

Extracorporeal cooling can be accomplished by running blood from a cannulated artery through a heat exchanger using cold tap water as the cooling medium. A pump is required to force the blood through the system. Thrombosis is prevented by administration of heparin.

Extracorporeal cooling has been used to lower the brain temperature below that of the general body temperature. Kimoto et al. (1956) developed this method in dogs, cannulating the carotid artery so that the blood could pass through a cooling coil and return to the distal artery.

*See Appendix A for manufacturer.

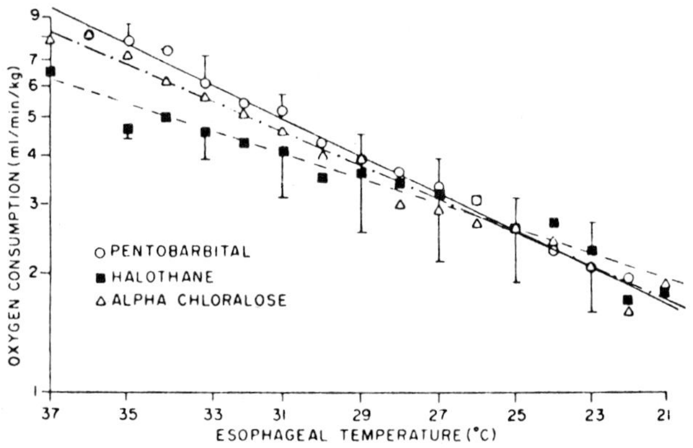

Figure 13–6. Whole-body oxygen consumption vs esophageal temperature during surface cooling in dogs. The least-squares best-fit lines are shown for three anesthetics: pentobarbital, halothane, and alpha-chloralose. Each point represents the mean, each bar 1 SD. (From Westenskow, D.R., Wong, K.C., Johnson, C.C. and Wilde, C.S.: Physiologic Effects of Deep Hypothermia and Microwave Rewarming: Possible Application for Neonatal Cardiac Surgery. Anesth. Analg., 58:397, 1979.)

With this technique, the brain temperature is lowered to 14° C while body temperature remains at 31 to 32° C.

Extracorporeal cooling carries with it the dangers of hemolysis and interference with the blood coagulation mechanism. It also presents the hazard of thrombosis. The most obvious advantage is that it provides the best control over body temperature, and rewarming can be carried out quickly and efficiently by running warm water through the heat exchanger.

Warming also may be accomplished by covering the patient with electric blankets or by using warm water baths. Microwave rewarming has been used experimentally (Westenskow et al., 1979).

Since hypothermic anesthesia is a form of general anesthesia, it has all the risks involved in this procedure. In addition, it has its own hazards which may be grouped under 1) the circulatory system, 2) the skin and internal organs, and 3) the metabolism.

Blood pressure falls during hypothermia, due to decreased cardiac output, whereas peripheral vascular resistance increases. Occasionally, severe drops in blood pressure may occur. The fall in heart rate seen with hypothermia is due to depression of the SA node and bundle of His. These conduction changes are manifested by a prolonging of the PR interval, spreading of the QRS complex, and lengthening of the ST interval. In dogs a cardiac crisis occurs between 23 and 15° C. This is characterized by cessation of sinus rhythm, intense bradycardia, ventricular extrasystoles, and ventricular fibrillation or standstill. Atropine does not relieve the bradycardia. Ventricular fibrillation has been shown to occur most often when the temperature of the heart muscle is below 28° C and when the heart is manipulated. Because fibrillation rapidly depletes cardiac muscle energy stores without circulating the blood, it is detrimental and should be prevented, if possible. It occurs less frequently in young animals than in adults. Hypercapnia with acidemia, hyperkalemia, and myocardial hypoxia appear to cause fibrillation also.

The incidence of spontaneous ventricular fibrillation has been shown to vary with the anesthetic used to initiate hypothermia. Pentobarbital results in a higher incidence than does thiopental or ether (Covino et al., 1954). Cyclopropane produces a high rate of arrhythmias (Steinhaus et al., 1959). Sands et al. (1980) reported that for surface-induced (ice-water immersion) hypothermia (18 to 20° C rectal temperature) in dogs and children, ether administered in 100% O_2 was superior to halothane, isoflurane, and fluroxene. In dogs, they found that halothane-ether azeotrope in 95% O_2 and 5% CO_2 was as effective as ether and eliminated the danger of ether explosion.

Several cardioplegic solutions have been used to stop the heartbeat and to prevent fibrillation (Table 13–2). Hypothermia plus cardioplegia is more protective of cardiac tissue than hypothermia alone (Hess et al., 1980; Rosenfeld et al., 1980). Combined with deep hypothermia, cardioplegia allows 30 minutes of cardiac arrest without heart-lung bypass.

An important blood change during hypothermia is prolongation of clotting time. In ad-

TABLE 13–2. Composition of Preservation Solutions

Modified Extracellular Solution		*Modified Collins Solution*		*Blood Cardioplegia*	
*Component**	*Concentration*	*Component**	*Concentration*	*Component**	*Quantity*
0.9% Sodium chloride	80 mEq/L	Dibasic potassium phosphate	57.5 mEq/L	Beef lung heparin	3,000 U
Potassium chloride	40 mEq/L	Hydrochloric acid	10 mEq/L	Blood	300 ml
Sodium bicarbonate	25 mEq/L	Magnesium sulfate	8.1 mEq/L	Lactated Ringer's	180 ml
Monobasic potassium phosphate	1.2 mEq/L	Sodium bicarbonate	10 mEq/L	Potassium chloride	18 mEq
Mannitol	100 mEq/L	Glucose	139 mEq/L	CPD additive solution	10 ml
		Mannitol	100 mEq/L	THAM (tromethamine)	4 mEq base

*Components listed in the order in which they are added.
CPD = citrate-phosphate-dextrose.
(From Swanson, D.K., Drifek, J.H., and Kahn, D.R.: Improved Myocardial Preservation at 4°C. Ann. Thorac. Surg., 30:519, 1980.)

dition, there is a decrease in platelets, hemoconcentration with sludging, reduction in eosinophil and leukocyte counts, with a fall in the mean corpuscular hemoglobin concentration.

Prolonged hypothermia has been shown to have a detrimental effect on primates, cats, and dogs (Michenfelder and Milde, 1977; Steen et al., 1979; Steen et al., 1980). In dogs held at 29° C for 24 hours, cardiac output and whole-body oxygen consumption decreased progressively to 7% and 28% of control, respectively. Cerebral blood flow and cerebral oxygen consumption responded similarly. On rewarming, cardiovascular collapse with severe tissue hypoxia and metabolic acidosis occurred. Cerebral blood flow became grossly inadequate with depletion of brain energy stores.

Knocker (1955) has shown that hypothermia causes severe damage to the liver, kidneys, and adrenal glands in dogs when temperatures of around 25° C are maintained for hours. Short periods of cooling, however, do not appear to cause demonstrable damage.

Hypothermia has been used for surgery of the heart and great vessels, brain, and spinal cord, and in some other surgical procedures. It also has been advocated in treatment of shock, stroke, cerebral and spinal contusion, and in prevention of brain damage following a severe hypoxic episode. The chief factor limiting its use alone in heart surgery is the danger of hypoxic brain damage. For this reason older patients and those with cardiac defects requiring extensive repair should be managed with heart-lung bypass. In neurosurgery, hypothermia may be combined with induced hypotension. Although hypothermia has been used in dogs for removal of heartworms and repair of cardiac anomalies, its use is not widespread. This is probably because many veterinarians are not aware of the simplicity of the technique and do not appreciate its potential.

Induction of Hypothermia in the Dog

To produce hypothermia in the dog, a phenothiazine tranquilizer may be given intravenously as a preanesthetic agent. A thiobarbiturate is injected for general anesthesia, following which an endotracheal catheter is inserted and an inhalant anesthetic is used for maintenance. A slow intravenous drip of Ringer's lactate or 5% dextrose is started, and a muscle relaxant is given in the drip tubing to abolish respirations. Controlled respiration is then started.

Unless a cooling mattress is available, the animal is positioned in a sink, bathtub, or other container, with its head above water (Fig. 13–7). Electronic thermometer probes are placed in the esophagus at heart level and in the

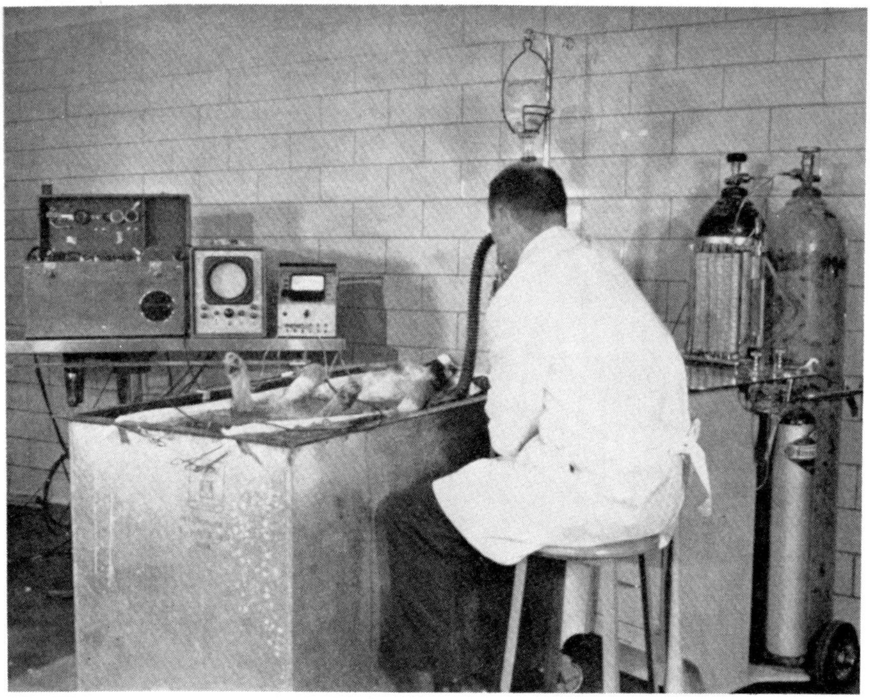

Figure 13–7. Induction of hypothermia in a dog. An electrocardiograph with coupled oscilloscope (left) monitors the heart. A multichannel thermometer, with probes in the patient's esophagus and rectum, determines temperature of the patient's body and the water bath. Oxygen and halothane are administered by means of the gas machine at right.

rectum, and electrodes of an ECG machine are attached to the feet. From this point, constant monitoring of the ECG on an oscilloscope is desirable, since cardiac fibrillation may occur at any time during the cooling period and requires immediate corrective measures.

Ice water is used for rapid cooling. It should be constantly agitated by hand or with a pump. The dog should be removed from the bath before the desired body temperature is reached, since it will continue to decline after removal from the water.

After removal, the dog should be dried with towels and placed on an inactive heating pad during the operative period. Rewarming can then be started as soon as closure of the surgical wound is begun. As anesthesia is discontinued and shivering commences, the body temperature quickly begins to rise. If the operation is short, rewarming in a water bath may be necessary along with administration of atropine and neostigmine to reverse the muscle relaxant.

CARDIOPULMONARY BYPASS TECHNIQUES

As previously mentioned, in order to do lengthy intracardiac surgery, various bypass techniques have been developed. The advantage is that the surgeon is able to directly visualize the operative field within the bloodless heart. Moderate hypothermia alone does not allow this procedure for more than 10 minutes. Cardiopulmonary bypass may be performed in conjunction with hypothermia or without the latter; however, the use of extracorporeal circulation with hypothermia and cardioplegia reduces the work load of the heart and enables periods of surgery for as long as two hours.

Heart-lung machines consist essentially of

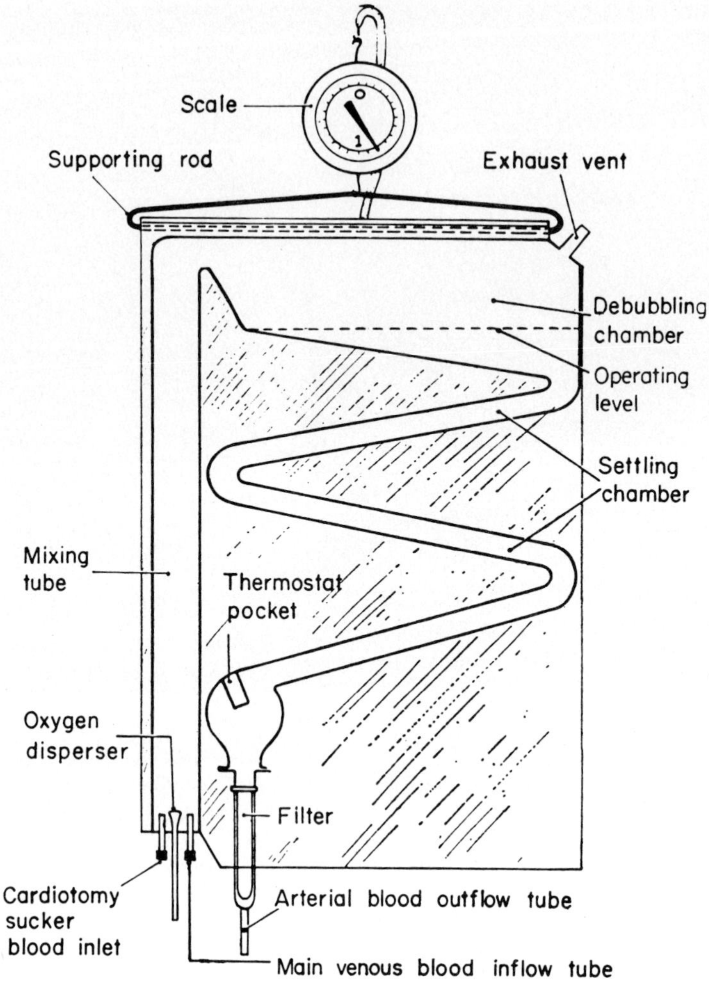

Figure 13–8. Schematic drawing of a plastic sheet oxygenator suspended from a spring scale. Venous blood from the patient enters the bottom of the mixing tube where it is oxygenated. It then flows through the debubbling chamber and into the settling chamber, from which it is pumped to the patient. The scale makes it possible to maintain a constant blood volume in the unit. Heat loss is controlled by directing infrared heat lamps on the settling chamber. (From Gott, V.L., Sellers, R.D., DeWall, R.A., Varco, R.L., and Lillehei, C.W.: A Disposable Unitized Plastic Sheet Oxygenator for Open Heart Surgery. Dis. Chest, 32:615, 1957.)

three pieces of equipment: an oxygenator that is a substitute for the patient's lungs, a pump (or pumps) that substitutes for the heart, and a heat exchanger for cooling and warming the blood. The simplest oxygenators are those in which oxygen is bubbled directly through the blood; these are available as disposable units (Fig. 13–8). Other more complicated oxygenators may incorporate a heat exchanger (Fig. 13–9).

To initiate cardiopulmonary bypass, a thoracotomy is performed and the patient is heparinized by intravenous administration of 1.5 mg/kg/ of heparin. The oxygenator and tubing are primed with Ringer's lactate solution. Catheters are inserted in the anterior and posterior venae cavae, and blood is run through the oxygenator, cooled in the heat exchanger, and pumped into the aorta directly or via the femoral artery (Fig. 13–10). In dogs, flow rates during pumping seldom exceed 75 ml/kg/minute. The aorta is clamped distal to the sinus of Valsalva to prevent retrograde flow. A cardioplegic solution is infused into the left ventricle to produce

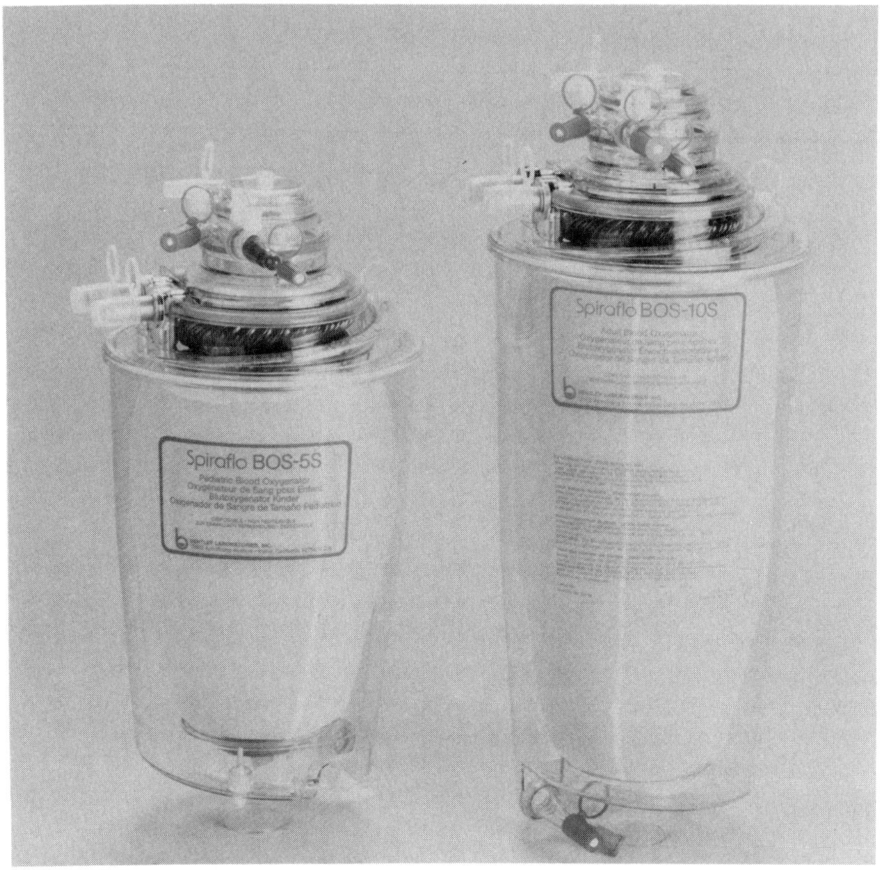

Figure 13–9. Pediatric (left) and adult (right) oxygenators. These have the advantages of small size, low priming volume, and increased gas exchange capability. A heat exchanger is incorporated in the device. (Courtesy of Bentley Laboratories, Inc., Irvine, California.)

cardiac standstill (see Table 13–2). Reperfusion of the solution should be performed every 20 to 30 minutes (Lucas et al., 1980). As the heart is opened, blood is removed from it by suction and returned to the system through a separate inlet.

When cardiac surgery is completed, the aortic clamp is removed, blood in the oxygenator is pumped into the patient, the cannulas are removed, and the chest incision is closed.

With this technique the heart may withstand ischemia for two hours or more. When the operation is complete, the clamp is removed from the aorta and blood from the heart-lung machine flushes out the cardioplegic solution. Use of potassium cardioplegia at normothermia does not produce myocardial preservation.

Deep hypothermia alone (7° C) has been used to cause cardioplegia. On rewarming, many hearts spontaneously resume a normal beat, and those that fibrillate can be successfully managed with massage and electrical defibrillation. Since effective heart action stops at temperatures below 25° C, no attempt at electrical defibrillation should be made until the heart temperature rises to 28° C.

Protamine sulfate is given intravenously to neutralize the anticoagulant effect of heparin. It is available in 1% solution. The dose is one to two times the amount of heparin previously administered. Occasionally, protamine may cause a dangerous hypotension.

ELECTRONARCOSIS

Electrical stimulation of the brain can activate either opiate or nonopiate pain control path-

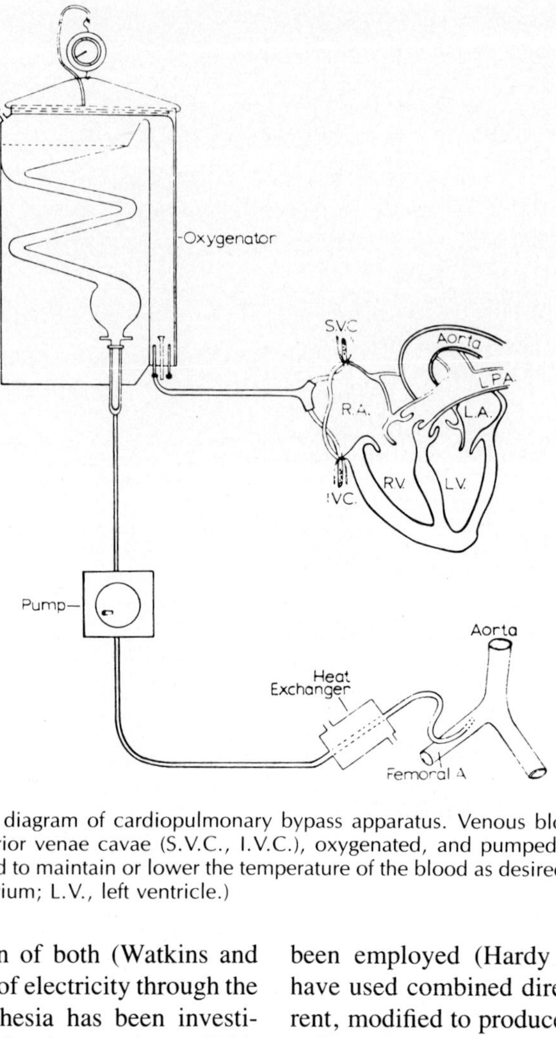

Figure 13–10. Schematic diagram of cardiopulmonary bypass apparatus. Venous blood is collected by gravity from the superior and inferior venae cavae (S.V.C., I.V.C.), oxygenated, and pumped into the femoral artery. A heat exchanger may be used to maintain or lower the temperature of the blood as desired. (R.A., right atrium; R.V., right ventricle; L.A., left atrium; L.V., left ventricle.)

ways, or a combination of both (Watkins and Mayer, 1982). Passage of electricity through the brain to produce anesthesia has been investigated for many years. In the veterinary field, clinical trials were conducted by Sir Frederic Hobday in England as early as 1932. Despite extensive research, much remains to be learned about this technique before it can be applied generally for animal anesthesia. Early workers were bothered by respiratory depression, hyperthermia, convulsions, and fatalities. Electronarcosis may be of greatest use in situations where prolonged anesthesia is required for experimental purposes.

Most instruments deliver the current through needle electrodes applied to the head (Fig. 13–11). Direct, pulsating direct, and alternating current have been used to produce electronarcosis. Alternating current of 700 cycles, 35 to 50 milliamperes, and approximately 40 volts has been employed (Hardy et al., 1961). Others have used combined direct and alternating current, modified to produce a rectangular wave of 1.0 to 1.4 milliseconds duration, with a frequency of 100 waves per second (Smith et al., 1961*a*). Continuous electrode contact is important to maintain anesthesia. *Individual variation among animals requires that the current be adjusted for each according to the response observed.*

Electrical anesthesia is characterized by convulsions on induction unless a muscle relaxant is first administered. An exception to this is the method of Smith et al. (1961*a*), which employs direct current for induction and then both direct and alternating current. Profuse salivation develops on induction and continues throughout. This can be counteracted by use of atropine. Endotracheal intubation should always be performed. Hyperthermia, probably due to disturb-

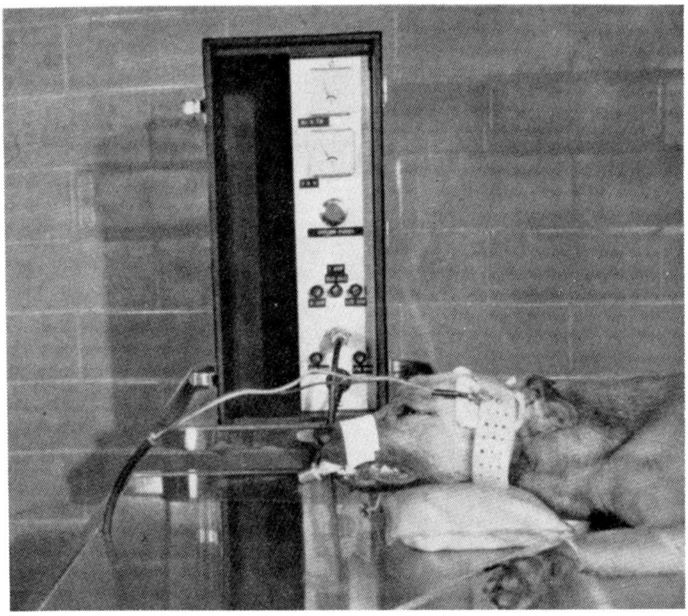

Figure 13–11. Electronarcosis. An electrode is placed on either side of the head and held with a latex strap. Contact is enhanced by use of plastic foam pads soaked with ECG electrode solution. An alternative method is the use of subcutaneously placed needle electrodes. An endotracheal catheter is inserted to maintain a patent airway. (Courtesy of Dr. R.A. Herin, Colorado State University, Fort Collins, Colorado.)

ance of the thermoregulatory center in the hypothalamus, is commonly seen. The EEG immediately following anesthesia is decreased in amplitude and increased in frequency, but returns to normal within 30 minutes. Brain lesions have been found following electronarcosis (Herin, 1968), and skin burns from the electrodes have been reported (Smith et al., 1961*b*).

Electrical anesthesia appears to produce severe stress as evidenced by an increased plasma level of hydroxycorticoids, epinephrine, and norepinephrine (Fig. 13–12). The blood pressure rises sharply and then gradually falls to near normal levels (Fig. 13–13). The clotting time, sedimentation rate, hemoglobin, hematocrit, and total and differential white blood cell counts do not differ from preinduction values (Herin, 1963). There is little effect on blood oxygen; blood carbon dioxide content and pH are lowered, while blood glucose rises. It has been suggested that electrical anesthesia, which produces an uninhibited response of the adrenal medullary and cortical systems, may be more desirable than an anesthetic, such as pentobarbital, which depresses this response (McNeil and Hardy, 1959).

It is difficult to assess the depth of electrical anesthesia in dogs or other species. Muscle relaxation varies from adequate to poor. Pain induced by surgery may cause body movements in animals that appear unconscious. The photomotor reflex is probably the best means of determining the depth of anesthesia if a large dose of atropine has not been used (see Chap. 14).

Analgesia persists for several minutes following removal of the current, and the animal often appears hypnotized. A slight stimulus may then cause arousal, following which the animal resumes all normal activities. Because arousal occurs rapidly once the current is cut off, a stand-by power source should be available in case the regular supply fails.

Advantages of electronarcosis are economy and immediate recovery of the patient when the current is turned off. Currently, suitable equipment and standardized techniques for its clinical application are not available. It is used occa-

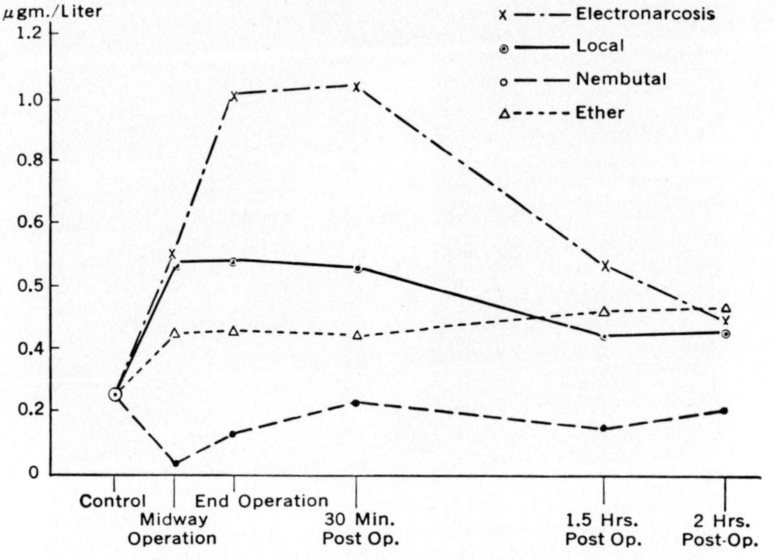

Figure 13–12. Epinephrine secretion in response to a standard laparotomy; a comparison of different agents for anesthesia. The points on each curve represent the average values from 7 dogs. Electronarcosis and laparotomy produced the greatest rise in epinephrine secretion, with response to procaine and to ether next in order, respectively. Nembutal (pentobarbital) depressed the epinephrine level of plasma despite the associated surgery. (From Hardy, J.D., Carter, T., and Turner, M.D.: Catechol Amine Metabolism. Ann. Surg., 150:669, 1959.)

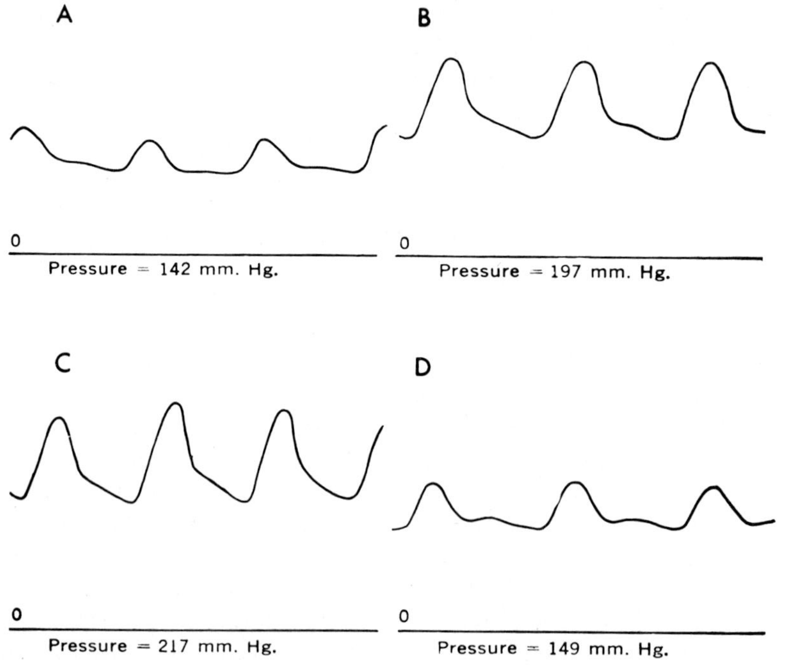

Figure 13–13. Mean femoral artery blood pressure in a dog under electronarcosis: *A*, preinduction; *B*, induction; *C*, beginning surgical anesthesia; and *D*, 15 minutes after onset of surgical anesthesia. (Courtesy of Dr. R.A. Herin, Colorado State University, Fort Collins, Colorado.)

sionally in research laboratories when an experimental protocol requires anesthesia without the use of drugs.

HYPNOSIS

Certain species of animals are highly susceptible to hypnosis (immobility reflex). These include arthropods, amphibians, reptiles, birds, guinea pigs, and rabbits (Klemm, 1976). This modality is seldom used in animal anesthesia. For induction in rabbits, see Chapter 18.

REFERENCES

Andjus, R.K., and Lovelock, J.E.: Reanimation of Rats from Body Temperatures Between 0 and 1° C by Microwave Diathermy. J. Physiol., 128:541, 1955.

Auerbach, C.: The Chemical Production of Mutations. Science, 158:1141, 1967.

Bering, E.A., Jr., Taren, J.A., McMurray, J.D., and Bernhard, W.F.: Studies on Hypothermia in Monkeys. II. The Effect of Hypothermia on the General Physiology and Cerebral Metabolism of Monkeys in the Hypothermic State. Surg. Gynecol. Obstet., 102:134, 1956.

Bigelow, W.G., Lindsay, W.K., Harrison, R.C., Gordon, R.A., and Greenwood, W.F.: Oxygen Transport and Utilization in Dogs at Low Body Temperatures. Am. J. Physiol., 160:125, 1950.

Blades, B., and Pierpont, H.C.: A Simple Method for Inducing Hypothermia. Ann. Surg., 140:557, 1954.

Borglin, N.E., and Lindsten, T.: On the Combined Effect of Neostigmine and Pentamethylenetetrazol or Beta-Phenylisopropylamine on Magnesium Anaesthesia. Acta Pharmacol., 5:309, 1949.

Brasmer, T.H.: Personal communication. Kaneohe, Hawaii, 1980.

Bree, M.M., and Gross, N.B.: Anesthesia of Pigeons with CI-581 (Ketamine) and Pentobarbital. Lab. Anim. Care, 19, 500, 1969.

Bree, M.M., Park, J.S., and Short, C.E.: Responses of Cats to Ketamine-Antibiotic Combinations. Vet. Med. Small Anim. Clin., 70:1309, 1975.

Brown, R.V., and Hilton, J.G.: The Effectiveness of the Baroreceptor Reflexes under Different Anesthetics. J. Pharmacol. Exp. Ther., 118:198, 1956.

Camburn, M.A.: Use of Alphaxalone-Alphadolone in Ruminants. Vet. Rec., 111:166, 1982.

Chen, G., Ensor, C.R., and Bohner, B.: The Neuropharmacology of 2-(0-Chlorophenyl)-2-Methyl-aminocyclohexanone Hydrochloride. J. Pharmacol. Exp. Ther., 152:332, 1966.

Child, K.J., Currie, J.P., Davis, B., Dodds, M.G., Pearce, D.R., and Twissell, D.J.: The Pharmacological Properties in Animals of CT 1341—A New Steroid Anaesthetic Agent. Br. J. Anaesth., 43:2, 1971.

Child, K.J., Harnby, G., Gibson, W., and Hart, J.W.: Metabolism and Excretion of Althesin (CT 1341) in the Rat. Postgrad. Med. J., 48:(Suppl. 2) 37, 1972.

Coffee, W.M.: Anesthesia and Restraint of Large Animals. J.A.V.M.A., 114:290, 1949.

Cohen, M.L., Chan, S.-L., Way, W.L., and Trevor, A.J.: Distribution in the Brain and Metabolism of Ketamine in the Rat after Intravenous Administration. Anesthesiology, 39:370, 1973.

Covino, B.G., Charleson, D.A., and D'Amato, H.E.: Ventricular Fibrillation in the Hypothermic Dog. Am. J. Physiol., 178:148, 1954.

Danks, A.G.: Anesthesia in Horses and Swine. Cornell Vet., 33:344, 1943.

Danks, A.G.: Personal communication. Cornell University, 1947.

Davis, T.R.A., and Mayer, J.: Nature of the Physiological Stimulus for Shivering. Am. J. Physiol., 181:669, 1955.

Dimigen, J., and Reetz, I.: Versuche zur Schmerzausschaltung beim Schwein mit Neurolaptikum Azaperon und dem Hypnotikum Metomidat. Dtsch. Tierarztl. Wochenschr., 77:470, 1970.

Dodds, M.G., and Twissell, D.J.: Effect of Althesin (CT 1341) on Circulatory Responses to Adrenaline and on Halothane-Adrenaline Cardiac Dysrhythmias in the Cat. Postgrad. Med. J., 48:(Suppl. 2) 17, 1972.

Drummond, J.D., Brebner, J., Galloon, S., and Young, P.S.: A Randomized Evaluation of the Reversal of Ketamine by Physostigmine. Can. Anaesth. Soc. J., 26:1979.

Eads, F.E.: Personal communication. Parke, Davis & Company, Detroit, 1974.

Faulk, R.H.: Xylazine and Ketamine Synergism for Ultrashort Anesthesia in Cats. Feline Pract., 8:15, 1978.

Folts, J.D., Afonso, S., and Rowe, G.G.: Systemic and Coronary Haemodynamic Effects of Ketamine in Intact Anaesthetized and Unanaesthetized Dogs. Br. J. Anaesth., 47:686, 1975.

Fuhrman, G.J., Fuhrman, F.A., and Field, J.: Metabolism of Rat Heart Slices, With Special Reference to Effects of Temperature and Anoxia. Am. J. Physiol., 163:642, 1950.

Gollan, F., Tysinger, D.S., Jr., Grace, J.T., Kory, R.C., and Meneely, G.R.: Hypothermia of 1.5° C in Dogs Followed by Survival. Am. J. Physiol., 181:297, 1955.

Gott, V.L., Bartlett, M., Long, D.M., Lillehei, C.W., and Johnson, J.A.: Myocardial Energy Substances in the Dog Heart During Potassium and Hypothermic Arrest. J. Appl. Physiol., 17:815, 1962.

Green, C.J.: *Animal Anaesthesia*. Laboratory Animals Ltd., London, 1979.

Hall, L.W.: Althesin in the Larger Animal. Postgrad. Med. J., 48:(Suppl. 2) 55, 1972.

Harding, G.W., Stogsdill, R.M., and Towe, A.L.: Relative Effects of Pentobarbital and Chloralose on the Responsiveness of Neurons in Sensorimotor Cerebral Cortex of the Domestic Cat. Neuroscience, 4:369, 1979.

Hardy, J.D., Turner, M.D., and McNeil, C.D.: Electrical Anesthesia. III. Development of a Method and Laboratory Observations. J. Surg. Res., 1:152, 1961.

Hatano, S., Dadove, M.S., Keane, D.M., Boggs, R.E., and El-Naggar, M.A.: Diazepam-Ketamine Anaesthesia for Open Heart Surgery "Micro-Mini" Drip Administration Technique. Anaesthetist, 25:457, 1976.

Hatch, R.C., Booth, N.H., Kitzman, J.V., Wallner, B.M., and Clark, J.D.: Antagonism of Ketamine Anesthesia in Cats by 4-Aminopyridine and Yohimbine. Am. J. Vet. Res., 44:417, 1983.

Heath, R.B.: Personal communication. Colorado State University, Fort Collins, 1982.

Herin, R.A.: Electroanesthesia: A Review of the Literature (1819–1965). Act. Nerv. Super, 10:439, 1968.

Herin, R.A.: Electrical Anesthesia in the Dog. J.A.V.M.A., 142:865, 1963.

Hess, M.L., Krause, S.M., and Greenfield, L.J.: Assessment of Hypothermic, Cardioplegic Protection of the Global Ischemic Canine Myocardium. J. Thorac. Cardiovasc. Surg., 80:293, 1980.

Jackson, A.P., Dhadphale, P.R., Callaghan, M.L., and Alseri, S.: Haemodynamic Studies During Induction of Anaesthesia for Open Heart Surgery Using Diazepam and Ketamine. Br. J. Anaesth., 50:375, 1978.

Jones, E.M.: Unpublished data. Oklahoma State University, 1972.

Jones, E.M.: Unpublished data. Oklahoma State University, 1949.

Jones, R.S.: Injectable Anaesthetic Agents in the Cat: A Review. J. Small Anim. Pract., 20:345, 1979.

Kaka, J.S., Klavano, P.A., and Hayton, W.L.: Pharmacokinetics of Ketamine in the Horse. Am. J. Vet. Res., 40:978, 1979.

Kaump, D.H., Kurtz, S.M., Fisken, R.A., Schardein, J.L., Roll, D.E., and Reutner, T.F.: Toxicology of Ketamine. Proc. Internat. Symposium on Ketamine. (University of Mainz, February, 1968.) Springer-Verlag, Berlin, 1969.

Kimoto, S., Sugie, S., and Asano, K.: Open Heart Surgery under Direct Vision with the Aid of Brain-Cooling by Irrigation. Surgery, 39:592, 1956.

King, E.E., and Unna, K.R.: The Action of Mephenesin and Other Interneuron Depressants on the Brain Stem. J. Pharmacol. Exp. Ther., 111:293, 1954.

Kirkpatrick, R.M.: Use of Xylazine and Ketamine as a Combination Anesthetic. Canine Pract., 5:53, 1978.

Kittle, E.L.: Ketamine HCl as an Anesthetic for Birds. Mod. Vet. Pract., 52:40, 1971.

Klemm, W.R.: Use of the Immobility Reflex ("Animal Hypnosis") in Neuropharmacological Studies. Pharmacol. Biochem. Behav., 4:85, 1976.

Knocker, P.: Effects of Experimental Hypothermia on Vital Organs. Lancet, 2:837, 1955.

Kumar, S.M., Kothary, S.P., and Zsigmond, E.K.: Plasma Free Norepinephrine and Epinephrine Concentrations Following Diazepam-Ketamine Induction in Patients Undergoing Cardiac Surgery. Acta Anaesth. Scand., 22:593, 1978.

Lucas, S.K., Elmer, E.B., Flaherty, J.T., Prodromos, C.C., Bulkley, B.H., Gott, V.L., and Gardner, T.J.: Effect of Multiple-Dose Potassium Cardioplegia on Myocardial Ischemia, Return of Ventricular Function, and Ultrastructural Preservation. J. Thorac. Cardiovasc. Surg., 80:102, 1980.

Marietta, M.P., Way, W.L., Castognoli, N., Jr., and Trevor, A.J.: On the Pharmacology of the Ketamine Enantiomorphs in the Rat. J. Pharmacol. Exp. Ther., 202:157, 1977.

McNeil, C.D., and Hardy, J.D.: Electrical Anesthesia: Some Metabolic Observations and Comparisons. Surg. Forum, 9:394, 1959.

Michalot, G., Girardet, P., Grimbert, F., Plasentin, D., and Stieglitz, P.: 24-Hour Althesin-Fentanyl Anesthesia in Dogs. Time Course of Haemodynamic Changes. Br. J. Anaesth., 52:19, 1980.

Michenfelder, J.D., and Milde, J.H.: Failure of Prolonged Hypocapnia, Hypothermia or Hypertension to Favorably Alter Stroke in Primates. Stroke, 8:87, 1977.

Millenbruck, E.W., and Wallinga, M.H.: A Newly Developed Anesthetic for Horses. J.A.V.M.A., 108:148, 1946.

Muir, W.W., Skarda, R.T., and Milne, D.W.: Evaluation of Xylazine and Ketamine Hydrochloride for Anesthesia in Horses. Am. J. Vet. Res., 38:195, 1977.

Muir, W.W., Skarda, R.T., and Sheehan, W.: Evaluation of Xylazine, Guaifenesin, and Ketamine Hydrochloride for Restraint in Horses. Am. J. Vet. Res., 39:1274, 1978.

Munson, E.S.: Effect of Hypothermia on Anesthetic Requirement in Rats. Lab. Anim. Care, 20:1109, 1970.

Nagel, M.L., Muir, W.W., and Nguyen, K.: Comparison of the Cardiopulmonary Effects of Etomidate and Thiamylal in Dogs. Am. J. Vet. Res., 40:193, 1979.

Niazi, S.A., and Lewis, F.J.: Profound Hypothermia in the Monkey with Recovery After Long Periods of Cardiac Standstill. J. Appl. Physiol., 10:137, 1957.

Pickerodt, V., McDowall, D.G., Coroneos, N.J., and Keaney, N.P.: Effect of Althesin on Carotid Blood Flow and Intracranial Pressure in the Anaesthetized Baboon: Preliminary Communication. Postgrad. Med. J., 48:(Suppl. 2) 58, 1972.

Purohit, R.C., Mysinger, P.W., and Redding, R.W.: Effects of Xylazine and Ketamine Hydrochloride on the Electroencephalogram and the Electrocardiogram in the Horse. Am. J. Vet. Res., 42:615, 1981.

Regan, M.J., and Eger, E.I.: Effect of Hypothermia in Dogs on Anesthetizing and Apneic Doses of Inhalation Agents. Anesthesiology, 23:689, 1967.

Rosenfeldt, F.L., Hearse, D.J., Cankovic-Darracott, S., and Braimbridge, M.V.: The Additive Protective Effects of Hypothermia and Chemical Cardioplegia During Ischemic Cardiac Arrest in the Dog. J. Thorac. Cardiovasc. Surg., 79:29, 1980.

Ryder, S., Way, W.L., and Trevor, A.J.: Comparative Pharmacology of the Optical Isomers of Ketamine in Mice. Eur. J. Pharmacol., 49:15, 1978.

Sands, M.P., Dillard, D.H., Hessel, E.A., II, and Miller, D.W., Jr.: Improved Anesthesia for Deep Surface-Induced Hypothermia: The Halothane-Diethyl Ether Azeotrope. Ann. Thorac. Surg., 29:123, 1980.

Sawyer, D.C.: A Ketamine Experience: Unintentional Injection of Ketamine HCL into a Human. J. Am. Small Anim. Assoc., 16:123, 1980.

Smith, A.U.: Resuscitation of Hypothermic, Supercooled and Frozen Mammals. Proc. R. Soc. Med., 49:357, 1956.

Smith, R.H., Goodwin, C., Fowler, E., Smith, G.W., and Volpitto, P.P.: Electronarcosis Produced by a Combination of Direct and Alternating Current. A Preliminary Study. Anesthesiology, 22:163, 1961*a*.

Smith, R.H., Gramling, Z.W., Smith, G.W., and Volpitto, P.P.: Electronarcosis by Combination of Direct and Alternating Current. 2. Effects on Dog Brain as Shown by EEG and Microscopic Study. Anesthesiology, 22:970, 1961*b*.

Steen, P.A., Milde, J.H., and Michenfelder, J.D.: The Detrimental Effects of Prolonged Hypothermia and Rewarming in the Dog. Anesthesiology, 52:224, 1980.

Steen, P.A., Soule, E.H., and Michenfelder, J.D.: The Detrimental Effect of Prolonged Hypothermia in Cats and Monkeys With and Without Regional Cerebral Ischemia. Stroke, 10:522, 1979.

Steinhaus, J.E., Siebecker, K.L., and Kimmey, J.R.: Comparative Effects of Anesthetic Agents on Cardiac Irritability During Hypothermia. J.A.M.A., 169:76, 1959.

Stephenson, J.C., Blevins, D.I., and Christie, G.J.: Safety of Rompun/Ketaset Combination in Dogs: A Two-Year Study. Vet. Med. Small Anim. Clin., 73:303, 1978.

Stopiglia, A.V.: Contribuicão para o Estudo da Anestesia Genal de Equideos. Fac. de Med. Vet., Universidad de São Paulo, Brasil, 1962.

Swan, H., Zeavin, I., Holmes, J.H., and Montgomery, V.: Cessation of Circulation in General Hypothermia. Ann. Surg., 138:360, 1953.

Taylor, R.A., Rucker, N.C., and Lumb, W.V.: Ketamine, Diazepam, and Acetylpromazine for General Anesthesia in the Dog. Submitted to J. Am. Anim. Hosp. Assoc., 1983.

Vladutin, O: Hydrate de Chloral Associe au Sulfate de Magnesium dans l'Anesthesia Generale du Cheval. Abst. Rec. Med. Vet., 115:236, 1939.

Waterman, A.E.: Preliminary Observations on the Use of a Combination of Xylazine and Ketamine Hydrochloride in Calves. Vet. Rec., 109:464, 1981.

Watkins, J., and Clark, R.S.J.: Report of a Symposium: Adverse Responses to Intravenous Agents. Br. J. Anaesth., 50:1159, 1978.

Watkins, L.R., and Mayer, D.J.: Organization of Endogenous Opiate and Nonopiate Pain Control Systems. Science, 216:1185, 1982.

Westenskow, D.R., Wong, K.C., Johnson, C.C., and Wilde, C.S.: Physiologic Effects of Deep Hypothermia and Microwave Rewarming: Possible Application for Neonatal Cardiac Surgery. Anesth. Analg., 58:397, 1979.

White, P.F., Ham, J., Way, W.L., and Trevor, A.J.: Pharmacology of Ketamine Isomer in Surgical Patients. Anesthesiology, 52:231, 1980.

Wood, E.M.: Urethane as a Carcinogen. Progressive Fish Culturist, 18:135, 1956.

Wright, M.: Pharmacologic Effects of Ketamine and Its Use in Veterinary Medicine. J.A.V.M.A., 180:1462, 1982.

CHAPTER 14

The Muscle Relaxants and Other Adjuvants to Anesthesia

THE MUSCLE RELAXANTS

A number of drugs can be used in conjunction with anesthetic agents to produce more complete muscle relaxation. On occasion, their use alone may be indicated; for example, they may be used to relax the patient for endotracheal intubation.

Muscle relaxation can be effected in three ways:

1) Administration of drugs acting centrally, such as the intravenous or inhalant anesthetics, produces muscle relaxation. These drugs depress the central nervous system; this is reflected as a decreased activity of the ventral horn cells of the spinal cord, causing lowered muscle tone. However, certain disadvantages are found when profound muscular relaxation is produced in this manner. Depression of the vasomotor and respiratory centers may result in severe hypotension and hypoxia.

2) Local anesthetics produce muscle relaxation if injected directly into a muscle or around the nerve that supplies it. Transmission of impulses that maintain muscular tone is thus abolished. Certain disadvantages pertain here also; namely, restraint may be a problem with this type of anesthesia, and with epidural or spinal anesthesia, hypotension may result due to paralysis of sympathetic nerves.

3) A third means of producing muscle relaxation is with drugs known as *muscle relaxants*. All muscle relaxants produce their effect on the neuromuscular junction, except mephenesin and guaifenesin, which act upon synapses in the spinal cord.

Since curare was first used to produce muscle relaxation, the term *curariform* has been applied to the action of this group of drugs. Actually, from the pharmacologic standpoint they are divided into three categories:

1. Depolarizing Agents
    a. Decamethonium (Syncurine, C-10)
    b. Succinylcholine (Anectine, Suxamethonium)
2. Nondepolarizing Agents
    a. Tubocurarine chloride, U.S.P.
    b. Metocurine iodide, U.S.P. (Metubine)
    c. Gallamine (Flaxedil)
    d. Benzoquinonium (Mytolon)
    e. Hexafluorenium (Mylaxen)
    f. Pancuronium (Pavulon)
3. Miscellaneous

a. Mephenesin (Myanesin, Tolserol)
b. Guaifenesin (Gecolate, Glycodex)

When a motor nerve impulse arrives at the terminal nerve fibers, acetylcholine is liberated. The acetylcholine reacts with a protein receptor substance on the specialized end-plate region of the muscle fiber. It thus produces a change in permeability of the membrane in the end-plate region to all ions, causing a variation in the resting potential of the end-plate known as the end-plate potential. As the end-plate potential reaches a critical level, it fires, producing an electrical wave propagated along the sarcolemma known as the muscle action potential (see Figs. 4–10, 4–11, 4–12, 4–13). Once the action is produced, acetylcholine is then hydrolyzed to acetic acid and choline by an enzyme, cholinesterase, which is found in the end-plate region.

Transmission of the nerve impulse may be interfered with in several ways:

1. Anything that interferes with release of acetylcholine interferes with transmission of the nerve impulse. Procaine, magnesium ions, or deficiency of calcium ions will slow or stop production of acetylcholine at the nerve terminal.
2. Delay in breakdown of acetylcholine at the end-plate region causes persistent depolarization of the membrane, and transmission of subsequent impulses is impossible. Delay of breakdown can be caused by anticholinesterase drugs such as neostigmine and edrophonium.
3. Agents that produce depolarization and continue to persist at the end-plate will stop transmission of impulses at the neuromuscular junction. Among drugs that act in this manner are decamethonium (C-10) and succinylcholine; these are not hydrolyzed by cholinesterase. The persistent nature of the block by these drugs has been explained on the basis that it is a total depolarization and also that a decreased sensitivity to acetylcholine exists at the end-plate. Regardless of cause, these drugs produce an initial depolarization of the end-plate region *(phase I block)* and are termed *depolarizing agents*. A peculiar effect seen after the prolonged administration of depolarizing drugs is termed *dual or phase II block*. Depolarization of the muscle fibers occurs first, followed gradually by repolarization, so that the type of block changes until it exhibits the characteristics of a nondepolarizing block.
4. A fourth type of block is produced by drugs, such as tubocurarine, which have affinity for the protein molecules of the motor end-plate receptors. These drugs combine loosely with the end-plate receptors and prevent excitation of the muscles by acetylcholine. This block is referred to as ''competitive inhibition'' since these drugs compete with acetylcholine for the end-plate receptor sites. In addition to tubocurarine, many other drugs competitively inhibit the action of acetylcholine and the term *nondepolarization block* is used to describe the action of these agents.

Autoradiographs have identified the receptors at the neuromuscular junction. In the postjunctional membrane, they are concentrated on the crests of the junctional folds in exact alignment with the release sites for vesicles in the nerve endings. The receptors are made of proteins in dynamic association with the channels through which ions flow, the lipids of the membrane, cholinesterase, and other proteins. The end-plate receptor is a biologic amplifier responding to two ions of acetylcholine by opening a channel through which thousands of sodium, calcium, and potassium ions flow across the end-plate membrane.

It is not known whether the channel is part of the receptor or is formed by a separate protein and ionophore. Functionally, it appears that there is a paired complex, the receptor recognizing acetylcholine and the ionophore passing ions. The receptor-ionophore complex is in the lipid matrix of the postjunctional membrane, with a molecule of acetylcholinesterase adjacent to it (Fig. 14–1). The receptor penetrates the cell membrane, protruding into both extracellular and intracellular spaces.

Subunits of the receptor bind agonists and

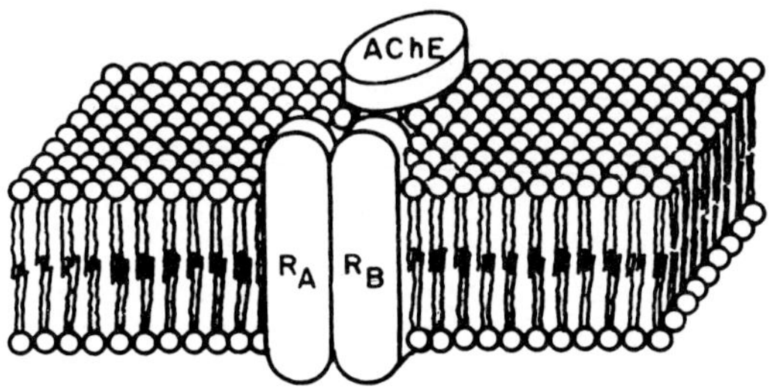

Figure 14–1. Sketch of membrane with receptor-ionophore and cholinesterase in lipid bilayer. (From Standaert, F.G.: Neuromuscular Transmission—What is a Cholinergic Receptor? Annual Refresher Course Lectures. Am. Soc. Anesthesiologists Ann. Mtg., 1980.)

antagonists and form the "recognition" part of the complex. The recognition units exist in two forms, one able to be activated, the other desensitized. The receptor that can be activated binds acetylcholine, undergoing a change in conformation that contributes to channel opening. The desensitized form does not respond by opening an ion channel, although it has a high affinity for acetylcholine. A continuous, spontaneous interchange occurs between activatable and desensitized conformation. Anything tending to shift the equilibrium toward the desensitized state or to speed production of desensitized units reduces the ability of acetylcholine to open ion channels and to depolarize the end-plate. This then reduces neuromuscular transmission. The cholinergic agonists, including acetylcholine, succinylcholine, and decamethonium, tend to promote the desensitized state.

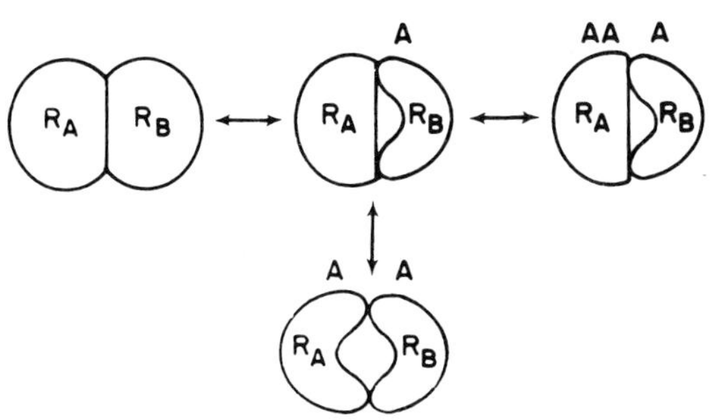

Figure 14–2. Sketch of receptor units (R_A + R_B). A, agonist; AA, antagonist. Channel opens when A units are bound to both receptor units. (From Standaert, F.G.: Neuromuscular Transmission—What is a Cholinergic Receptor? Annual Refresher Course Lectures. Am. Soc. Anesthesiologists Ann. Mtg., 1980.)

The nondepolarizing compounds (tubocurarine and gallamine, many local and inhaled anesthetics, lidocaine, diethyl ether, and halothane) also tend to promote the desensitized state. The phase II blockade produced by depolarizing relaxants is probably due in part at least to desensitized receptors. Desensitization cannot be overcome by anticholinesterases; rather, they encourage desensitization. It appears that receptor units are paired and that an ion channel opens only when both units are in the activated form and are bound to acetylcholine (Fig. 14–2). When either unit is unoccupied, desensitized, or bound to an agonist, the channel will not open. To block acetylcholine, therefore, an antagonist must occupy only one of the two activatable units.

Under normal conditions, an ion channel activated by an agonist opens cleanly, remains open for about a millisecond, and closes quickly. The ionophore of the end-plate does not discriminate among cations, and they move through the channel simultaneously. Sodium and calcium flow into the cell while potassium flows out. Because more ions move in than out, there is a net influx causing depolarization of the end-plate membrane. Acetylcholine released by a single nerve impulse opens simultaneously about 500,000 channels, and the sum of the currents flowing through these develops the end-plate potential.

Many drugs easily affect the ionophore. All agonists open the channel, but for different durations. Tubocurarine competes with acetylcholine for receptors and thus reduces the number of channel openings and depolarization of the end-plate. Anticholinesterases prolong the lifetime of acetylcholine, enhancing its capacity to compete for receptors. When the ionophore channels open, they also admit drugs. Decamethonium may pass completely through and enter the cell, but most bind near the entrance and block it. Local anesthetics bind and unbind so quickly that a channel may be plugged and unplugged several times during a single open period. Tubocurarine, gallamine, or other depolarizing relaxants may enter and plug the channel. Atropine and phencyclidine appear to hinder opening and closing of channels, whereas

TABLE 14–1. Drugs Affecting the Neuromuscular Junction

Drug	*Animal*[1]	*Neuromuscular Blocking Potency mg (cation)/kg*	*LD_{50} mg (cation)/kg*	*Antagonist or Antidote*	*Other Effects*
Gallamine triethiodide (Flaxedil)	Man	0.45–0.6		Neostigmine, edrophonium	Histamine release; parasympathetic stimulation
	Cat	0.3–1.1			
	Dog	0.25	0.5	Edrophonium	
	Mouse	1.2	1.9–2.7		
	Rabbit	0.2–0.3	0.4	Neostigmine	
	Rat		3.3		Histamine release
	Frog[2]	6 and 36			
Succinylcholine chloride U.S.P. (Sucostrin; Quelicin; Anectine)	Man	0.1–0.3		Plasma cholinesterase	Anticholinesterase, nicotinic; initial stimulation of muscular contraction
	Cat	0.05–0.1			Nicotinic; initial stimulation of muscular contraction
	Dog	0.1	0.15	Plasma cholinesterase	Anticholinesterase
	Mouse	0.05–0.1	0.25		
	Rabbit	0.1	0.5		
	Sparrow	5.0	10.0		Contracture
	Frog[2]	2.5			Nicotinic; contracture
	Man	0.08–0.19		Neostigmine, edrophonium	Cardiovascular; histamine release
	Cat	0.12–0.23			Histamine release; ganglion blocking

Tubocurarine chloride, U.S.P. (d-Tubocurarine chloride: Tubarine)	Dog	0.08–0.15	0.38	Edrophonium	Ganglion blocking
	Monkey	0.06			
	Mouse	0.06–0.09	0.11–0.15		
	Rabbit	0.09–0.15	0.165	Neostigmine	Ganglion blocking
	Rat	0.04–0.06	0.08		Histamine release
	Chick	0.13			
	Frog[2]	1.4, 4.1 and 7.5	>20.0	Acetylcholine	
Metocurine iodide, U.S.P. (Metubine iodide)	Man	0.027		Edrophonium, neostigmine	
	Cat	0.02			Ganglion blocking; histamine release
	Mouse	0.08–0.1	0.16		
	Rabbit	0.01–0.015	0.02	Neostigmine	
	Rat	0.009	0.025–0.03	Neostigmine	Histamine release
	Frog[2]	0.94	14.4		
Pancuronium bromide (Pavulon)	Dog	0.015			
	Cat	0.013		Neostigmine	
	Pig	0.01		Pyridostigmine	
	Goat	0.01		Edrophonium	
	Sheep	0.005			
	Horse	0.1			
	Man	0.024			
	Mouse	0.03	0.047 0.167 SQ		
	Rat		0.153		
	Rabbit	0.008	0.016		

[1]Unless otherwise indicated, drug administered by intravenous injection. [2]Ventral lymph sac injection. (Adapted from *Handbook of Biological Data*. Edited by W.S. Spector. W.B. Saunders Co., Philadelphia, 1956.)

lipid-soluble materials, including inhaled anesthetics, barbiturates, diazepam, and ketamine, speed closing. Since anything that reduces ion flow reduces depolarization, drugs that enter the channels or hasten closing impair neuromuscular transmission. Channel blockage is not alleviated by anticholinesterases.

The receptor-ionophore complex is located in the lipid matrix of the end-plate membrane. The lipid membrane is fluid and can accommodate changes in conformation of the proteins. Fluidity of the lipids is required for the proteins to function and many drugs, including the inhaled anesthetics and barbiturates, dissolve in the membrane, changing its fluidity. These compounds thus interfere with the recognition function of the receptor, the transition from desensitized to activatable conformation, and opening and closing of the ion channel.

From the foregoing, one can see that many drugs are capable of influencing neuromuscular transmission or of interacting with traditional relaxants. It explains why gallamine is not exactly like tubocurarine, and decamethonium is different from acetylcholine. It also explains why local, inhaled, and injected anesthetics can influence neuromuscular transmission (Standaert, 1980).

In all species of animals, relaxant drugs produce approximately the same sequence of muscle relaxation. The facial muscles, the jaw, and the tail are affected first, usually within 30 to 60 seconds after intravenous injection. This is followed by paralysis of the neck and limb muscles, and then the swallowing and phonatory muscles. The abdominal musculature is affected next, followed by the intercostal muscles. The diaphragm is last to become paralyzed; when this occurs, unless artificial respiration is performed, the animal will die of respiratory failure. The recovery pattern is in the reverse order. Table 14–1 summarizes the activity and actions of these drugs in various species.

Early workers attempted to give a dose that would just paralyze the abdominal musculature without paralyzing the diaphragm. It was found, however, that this procedure reduced the respiratory minute volume to the point that artificial respiration was necessary. Therefore, at the present time the dose of relaxant is not determined on this basis; rather, enough is given to paralyze all respiratory muscles and controlled respiration is routinely administered.

Because muscle relaxants produce a paralysis of the respiratory muscles, their use without a means for controlled respiration is dangerous and foolhardy. *Oxygen should always be available when these drugs are used.*

With the possible exception of guaifenesin, *none of the muscle relaxants produces analgesia;* thus, though an animal may be completely immobilized it feels all painful stimuli. For this reason, analgesics or anesthetics should always be administered concurrently. When a relaxant is used with light general anesthesia, it is difficult to distinguish, by the usual voluntary muscle reflexes, between true unconsciousness and consciousness masked by immobilization (Croft, 1961). The photomotor reflex (contraction of the pupil of the eye on stimulation with a bright light) can be used as a differential test provided not more than 0.032 mg/kg of atropine has been given as premedication. For best results, the eyes should be covered for a short period prior to stimulation.

Administration of the "mycin" drugs will potentiate the effects of neuromuscular blocking agents (Table 14–2). As an action potential arrives at the nerve terminal, it produces an influx of Ca^{++} that in turn triggers the discharge of acetylcholine from storage vesicles into the junctional cleft. The aminoglycoside antibiotics have been found to decrease the availability of Ca^{++} at the axonal terminal and thus interfere with the excitation-secretion coupling process. This group also acts on the postjunctional membrane, reducing its sensitivity to acetylcholine by competitively blocking the nicotinic cholinergic receptors.

General anesthetics, such as ether, pentobarbital, halothane, and methoxyflurane, also have direct depressant effects on the somatic myoneural junction. Skeletal muscle relaxants, including succinylcholine, tubocurarine, gallamine, and pancuronium, block the cholinergic receptors of skeletal muscle. These interrelationships explain why aminoglycoside antibiot-

TABLE 14–2. Interaction of Antibiotics, Muscle Relaxants, Neostigmine, and Calcium

	Neuromuscular Block from Antibiotic Alone Antagonized by		*Increase in Neuromuscular Block of*		*Neuromuscular Block from Antibiotic and Tubocurarine Antagonized by*	
	Neostigmine	*Calcium*	*Tubocurarine*	*Succinylcholine*	*Neostigmine*	*Calcium*
Neomycin	sometimes	sometimes	yes	yes	usually	usually
Streptomycin	sometimes	sometimes	yes	yes	usually	usually
Gentamicin	sometimes	yes‡	yes	*	sometimes	yes‡
Kanamycin	sometimes	sometimes	yes	yes	sometimes	sometimes
Paromomycin	yes‡	yes‡	yes	*	yes‡	yes‡
Viomycin	yes‡	yes‡	yes	*	yes‡	yes‡
Polymyxin A	no	no	yes	*	no	no
Polymyxin B	no†	no	yes	yes	no†	no
Colistin	no	sometimes	yes	yes	no	sometimes
Tetracycline	no	*	yes	no	partially	partially
Lincomycin	partially	partially	yes	*	partially	partially
Clindamycin	partially	partially	yes	*	partially	partially

*Not studied
†Block augmented by neostigmine
‡In spite of this, difficulty with antagonizing the block from these antibiotics is still likely to occur
(From Smith, N.T., Miller, R.D., and Corbascio, A.N.: *Drug Interactions in Anesthesia*. Lea & Febiger, Philadelphia, 1981.)

ics act synergistically with other drugs and chemicals that inhibit release of acetylcholine from the nerve terminal, or prevent the coupling of acetylcholine with postjunctional receptors (Adams et al., 1976).

When a neuromuscular blocking agent is given, it is estimated that as much as 90% of the muscle receptors must be blocked before muscle twitch is abolished. Recovery of diaphragmatic movement from the effects of injection of a curariform agent requires only 5% of the diaphragmatic muscle receptors to be free in dogs and 18% in cats (Waud and Waud, 1972). Thus, more than 80% of the receptors can still be blocked by the neuromuscular agent. This becomes clinically important, particularly in the postoperative period, since a patient may gain control of spontaneous respiration and voluntary muscles despite the fact that only a small percentage of muscle receptors are free for interaction with acetylcholine. If the patient is then given another drug that depresses neuromuscular function, such as an aminoglycoside, serious respiratory complications can occur. Anesthetic deaths in humans, cats, and at least one dog have been reported from this phenomenon.

Pittinger and Morris (1953, 1955) demonstrated that tubocurarine, gallamine, and succinylcholine are transmitted across the placenta in pregnant bitches to the puppies, whereas decamethonium is not. At delivery, depression of puppies was noted following administration of succinylcholine and gallamine.

Winnie and Collins (1965) have described the *doxapram test* for differential diagnosis of apnea in man following the use of general anesthesia and muscle relaxants. This test is used to differentiate between apnea due to *central depression* and that caused by *peripheral neuromuscular blockade*. In apneic patients, injection of 2 mg/kg of doxapram (see Chap. 20) evokes a marked respiratory response if the cause of the apnea is central depression. If there is no response, the cause is persistent neuromuscular block. If the patient breathes spontaneously but with inadequate tidal volume, the doxapram test serves as an intermediate step in distinguishing residual central depression from partial curarization. If persistent partial curarization is the cause, doxapram produces an increased respiratory rate but a decreased tidal volume. This is because the partially paralyzed respiratory muscles cannot respond further, while the respiratory center responds with an increased rate.

The effects of muscle relaxants can also be gauged by use of a nerve stimulator (Katz,

1965). For purposes of comparison, the stimulation site, duration, and frequency should all be constant (see Chap. 19).

AGENTS PRODUCING DEPOLARIZATION BLOCK

Depolarization block differs from nondepolarization block as follows:

1. Paralysis is preceded by transient stimulation of the muscle fibers thought to be caused by initial depolarization. This muscle twitching may be visible in animals.
2. Antagonists to the nondepolarizing agents tend to potentiate the depolarizing drugs; hence, they may prolong their initial (phase I) action.
3. In nerve-muscle preparations, it can be shown that after partial paralysis due to a nondepolarizing drug, loss of induced tetanus is rapid, whereas after paralysis caused by depolarizing agents, induced tetanus is maintained.
4. The depolarizing agents probably never produce a pure neuromuscular block. In dogs, they cause both depolarization and nondepolarization. In contrast, the nondepolarizing relaxants always have a pure nondepolarizing action.
5. The depolarizing relaxants have been shown to affect the red muscle fibers more than the white in the cat, rat, and mouse; the nondepolarizing agents have an opposite effect.

Succinylcholine Chloride Injection, U.S.P. (Anectine; Suxamethonium; Sucostrin; Quelicin)

Succinylcholine is a white odorless solid, marketed as an aqueous solution with a pH of 3.2 to 3.5. Warm solutions at a pH of 7.4 hydrolyze appreciably. Opened vials of solution gradually lose potency.

Succinylcholine is prepared as a chloride or an iodide anhydrous salt; the chloride is 1½ times as potent as the iodide. Because it is similar chemically to two molecules of acetylcholine, it is sometimes referred to as diacetylcholine.

With its structural resemblance to acetylcholine, succinylcholine can stimulate cholinoceptive loci nicotinic receptors, sympathetic and parasympathetic ganglia, and muscarinic receptors in SA and AV nodes. The net autonomic effects may vary, but they usually result in accentuation of autonomic tone in the nondominant side of the autonomic nervous system (Lebowitz and Savarese, 1980). Thus, sinus bradycardia or tachycardia may occur; the latter is more frequent. Vagal stimulation with bradycardia is especially likely if repeated IV doses are given. Successive administration can also result in junctional rhythms, ventricular escape beats, asystole, and arrest. Stimulation of cardiac muscarinic receptors, ganglionic stimulation, and direct myocardial effects have been incriminated. Prevention thus includes intravenous atropine, ganglion-blocking drugs, and pretreatment with nondepolarizers. Succinylcholine has been shown to lower the threshold to catecholamine-induced arrhythmias in the dog and monkey (Lebowitz and Savarese, 1980). Ventricular arrhythmias may also be initiated by the release of potassium associated with succinylcholine-induced depolarization. Succinylcholine-induced ventricular arrhythmias may be facilitated by conditions in which the threshold of cardiac muscle to depolarization is lowered (e.g., patients treated with digitalis, catecholamines, or tranquilizers). Under such circumstances, administration of a small dose of a nondepolarizing agent first may make cardiac arrhythmias less likely (Savarese and Kitz, 1975). Other consequences of succinylcholine administration are stimulation of other cholinoceptive sites, such as autonomic ganglia and muscarinic receptors, with increased intraocular and intragastric pressure (Savarese and Kitz, 1975).

Succinylcholine is free from the usual complications of muscle relaxants such as hypotension, tachycardia, histamine release, bronchospasm, and urticaria. Lack of cumulative effect permits almost instantaneous change in the degree of muscle relaxation. It is rapidly hydrolyzed and usually produces no residual respiratory paralysis. The chief disadvantage is that the effective dose and duration of effect are inconsistent between individuals.

Succinylcholine produces depolarization of the motor end-plate. The muscles of the eyes are affected first, followed by the muscles of the throat, peripheral muscles, intercostal muscles, and lastly the diaphragmatic musculature. A general uncoordinated muscular twitching accompanies the depolarizing action. In man this produces pain, not during the main action of the drug but in the recovery period, the pain outlasting the period during which the drug is known to be present in the body.

Of the muscle relaxants, only succinylcholine has a rapid rate of destruction, due to hydrolysis in the serum where no membranes have to be passed in order to reach the hydrolyzing enzyme. Less than 2% of an injected dose of succinylcholine appears in the urine. Plasma cholinesterase (pseudocholinesterase) hydrolyzes succinylcholine quickly to form succinylmonocholine and choline. Succinylmonocholine then is broken down into choline and succinic acid. Acetylcholinesterase (true cholinesterase of erythrocytes) cannot hydrolyze succinylcholine. Because it relies on metabolism for elimination, a large dose of succinylcholine must be given if a sufficient concentration is to reach the end-plate and produce neuromuscular block. In turn, if its metabolism is delayed due to decreased activity of plasma cholinesterase, prolonged recovery may result (Waud, 1981).

The liver is probably the site of synthesis of true (red cell, brain, muscle) and pseudo (plasma) cholinesterase production. The physiologic function of plasma cholinesterase remains uncertain, but it may be to hydrolyze butyrylcholine and prevent its nicotinic action when it is produced during fatty acid degeneration (Clitherow et al., 1963). This is supported by the observation of a seasonal variation in plasma cholinesterase in horses paralleling the seasonal variation in fat metabolism, both being maximal in late summer (Strelitz, 1944). It has been shown that it will hydrolyze succinylcholine, succinylmonocholine, neostigmine, procaine, and amethocaine.

The duration of action of succinylcholine varies widely, depending upon the species and the inherent plasma cholinesterase level (Stowe, 1955). Horse plasma contains 8 to 10 times as much cholinesterase as cow plasma (Stowe et al., 1958). Using whole blood, Palmer et al. (1965) found the mean Δ pH units/hr for horses was 0.39 (range 0.18 to 0.60) and for Angora goats 0.14 (range 0.04 to 0.24). Radeleff and Woodard (1956) found little or no plasma cholinesterase in cattle and sheep. Erythrocytic cholinesterase activity in cattle was 0.46 Δ pH units/hr and in sheep 0.16. These values are 54% and 19% respectively of those reported for man. According to Hall et al. (1953), plasma cholinesterase activity in the dog shows a wide range of variation depending on the breed. Hazelwood and Heath (1976) found that dogs had the highest plasma cholinesterase level, followed in descending order by rabbits, pigs, calves, and sheep.

Robertson (1966) has discussed factors altering plasma cholinesterase. In malnutrition, liver disease, chronic anemia, cancer, cardiac failure, and severe acute infection, plasma cholinesterase activity is reduced. In liver disease, administration of succinylcholine may produce prolonged apnea.

Therapeutic radiation diminishes plasma cholinesterase, whereas it is increased in hypertension and diabetes. Low cholinesterase values are found in severely burned patients. Robertson (1966) has shown that pregnant women have a reduction in plasma cholinesterase activity beginning at 10 weeks of gestation. In humans, atypical cholinesterase and even total lack of the enzyme have been reported.

Exposure to organophosphorus compounds reduces cholinesterase activity by combination between organic phosphates and the esteratic site of plasma cholinesterase. Organophosphate anthelmintics, by depressing plasma cholinesterase activity, markedly increase the susceptibility of animals, especially horses, to succinylcholine (Himes et al., 1967; Ward and Glicksberg, 1971; Short et al., 1971). This decreased tolerance develops within minutes following organophosphate treatment and persists for five days to one month. Organophosphate-impregnated flea collars worn by dogs and cats may produce the same result.

Theoretically, pralidoxime chloride,* by reactivating phosphorylated cholinesterase, is of value in treatment (Woodward, 1957; Himes et al., 1967). The dose, which must be administered within 36 hours of exposure, is approximately 11 mg/kg. Irwin et al. (1956) have shown in dogs that calcium may also be of benefit for succinylcholine-induced apnea.

Plasma cholinesterase is inhibited by other drugs including hexafluorenium, neostigmine, pyridostigmine, pancuronium, echothiophate, nitrogen mustards, trimethophan, promethazine, diphenhydramine, and chlorpromazine (Waud, 1981). Phenothiazines cause exacerbation of the symptoms seen in poisoning by anticholinesterase insecticides, and anticholinesterases potentiate behavioral changes induced by chlorpromazine. Procaine has been shown to intensify the myoneural action of succinylcholine if injected after the relaxant. The action is antagonized if procaine is injected before administration of succinylcholine.

In rabbit hearts, succinylcholine increases the effect of digitalis on the conduction system and makes the ventricle more irritable. This effect may range from occasional ectopic ventricular foci to fibrillation. Tubocurarine will reverse ventricular arrhythmias occurring after digitalis toxicity or those produced by succinylcholine in the digitalized heart. Dowdy et al. (1965) believe that succinylcholine is contraindicated in digitalized patients or those having high serum calcium or low serum potassium levels. A nerve impulse releases more acetylcholine if the concentration of calcium is increased, yet calcium decreases the degree of depolarization produced by acetylcholine (Waud, 1981).

*See Appendix A.

Using nerve-muscle preparations, Hansson (1958) demonstrated the relative susceptibility to succinylcholine of horses, cattle, pigs, and dogs (Fig. 14–3) and compared this with other dosage information for these species (Table 14–3).

In adult rabbits, a dose of 0.5 mg/kg is necessary for complete paralysis. Intravenous doses of up to 340 mg/kg are required to produce fetal depression, while 570 mg/kg are required to produce flaccid paralysis of fetuses 3 to 6 minutes after injection (Kivisselgaard and Moya, 1961).

In the dog and cat, depolarization of skeletal muscle by succinylcholine is accompanied by an increased plasma concentration and urinary excretion of potassium (Stevenson, 1960). This effect becomes less marked in the dog when repeated doses are administered (Fig. 14–4). It is accentuated by massive tissue trauma, burns, denervated muscle, and intra-abdominal infection (Lebowitz and Savarese, 1980).

Minimal doses may produce muscular tremors in dogs, particularly in the head and front limbs. On intravenous injection approach-

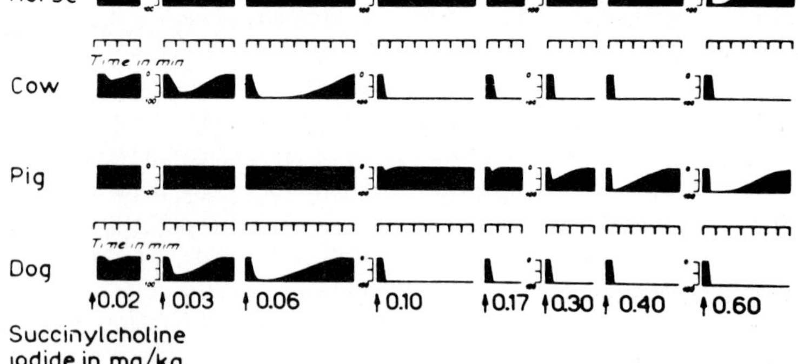

Figure 14–3. Schematic representation of the results obtained with the neuromuscular preparations in the horse, cow, pig, and dog, showing the duration and degree of paralysis of the muscle twitch caused by different doses of succinylcholine during barbiturate anesthesia. (From Hansson, C.H.: Studies on the Effect of Succinylcholine in Domestic Animals. Nord. Vet. Med., 10:201, 1958.)

TABLE 14–3. Comparisons between Dose, Duration and Tolerance of Succinylcholine Iodide

Species	*Min. Block Dose in Mg per Kg Body Weight*	*Time for Complete Restitution of the Twitch in Minutes at Min. Blocking Dose*	*Tolerance for SCh per Kg Body Weight per Min. at Cont. Infusion*	*Casting Dose in Mg per Kg Body Weight*
Horse	0.6	6–7	0.015	0.17
Cow	0.04	10–12	0.0017	0.02
Pig	0.4	6–7	0.014	—
Dog	0.07	8–9	0.004	—

Comparisons between minimal blocking dose, the duration of the succinylcholine iodide (SCh) effect at this dose, the tolerance for succinylcholine iodide in mg per kg body weight per minute at continuous infusion, and the dose in mg per kg body weight that is used in casting large animals.

(From Hansson, C.H.: Studies on the Effect of Succinylcholine in Domestic Animals. Nord. Vet. Med., 10:201, 1958.)

ing the respiratory failure level, parasympathomimetic action is observed (intestinal hypermotility, micturition, and salivation). Sialism is an indication of subsequent respiratory paralysis. Salivation can be corrected by administration of atropine, and its use is advisable. In dogs, prolonged apnea may follow administration of three or more doses (Hall, 1959). Many dogs exhibit depression after recovery, lasting in some instances as long as 18 hours.

When given intravenously, effective doses produce muscular relaxation within 15 seconds. The mean effective dose of succinylcholine *chloride* intravenously for *unanesthetized* dogs is 18 to 26 mcg/lb of body weight; it is suggested that 22 mcg/lb be the initial dosage and further amounts be given to effect (Knill, 1956). In dogs anesthetized with thiopental-trichloroethylene, the minimum relaxing dose of succinylcholine *iodide* is 0.067 mg/kg of body weight (Table 14–4). The use of succinylcholine in thoracic operations is of particular value because paralysis of the diaphragm can easily be produced. The usual dose of succinylcholine *iodide* for this purpose is about 0.15 mg/kg of body weight. The intraperitoneal and subcutaneous routes of administration are ineffective, probably owing to the rate of absorption; consequently, these are not suitable for clinical use.

TABLE 14–4. Effect of Succinylcholine Iodide on Neuromuscular Transmission, Ventilation, and Blood Pressure on Intravenous Injection in the Dog

Experiment (No.)	*Succinylcholine Iodide (Celocurin) (mg/kg)*	*Max. Degree of Relaxation* (%)*	*Duration of Effect (min)*	*Ventilation† (%)*	*Duration of Respiratory Arrest*	*Variation in Blood Pressure (mm Hg)*
I	0.022	25	2–3	100	0	− 1
II	0.045	50	5–7	75	0	+ 4
III	0.060	50	6–11.5	50	0	+ 8
IV	0.066	>50	11–14	50	0	+15
V	0.085	>50	8–11	0	45 sec	− 8
VI	0.11	>50	18–21	0	10 min	− 6
VII	0.22	>50	23–27	0	10 min	− 9

*The degree of relaxation denotes the ratio of the amplitude of contraction of the normal muscle to that of the "curarized" muscle. A degree of relaxation of 50% usually suffices for clinical purposes.

†Ventilation denotes the difference between expiratory and inspiratory pressure in the trachea as a percentage of the basic value of the difference.

(From Hansson, C.H.: Succinylcholine Iodide as a Muscular Relaxant in Veterinary Surgery. J.A.V.M.A., 128:288, 1956.)

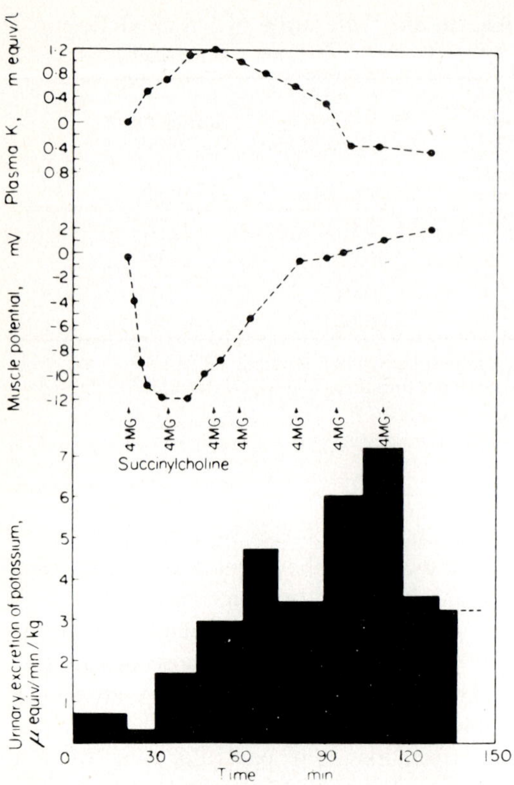

Figure 14–4. The effect of succinylcholine on the plasma potassium concentration, muscle polarization, and urinary excretion of potassium of a 15-kg dog anesthetized with thiopental and nitrous oxide. (From Stevenson, D.E.: A Review of Some Side Effects of Muscle Relaxants in Small Animals. J. Small Anim. Pract., 1:77, 1960. Reprinted with permission from the author and Pergamon Press.)

In miniature swine, the dose of succinylcholine chloride necessary to produce muscle relaxation of sufficient duration for intubation and induction of halothane anesthesia is 1.1 mg/kg (0.50 mg/lb) intravenously (DeYoung et al., 1970). An acute, usually fatal, familial hyperpyrexic syndrome has been observed to result in swine and man from administration of succinylcholine and certain anesthetic drugs (Harrison et al., 1969).

In the past, intravenous succinylcholine has been used extensively without anesthesia for casting and restraining horses during short operations such as castration. This practice should be discontinued for several reasons:

1. It causes extreme fright, and no anesthesia is afforded for painful operations.
2. The resulting apnea produces hypoxia, possible brain damage, and occasional fatalities.
3. Systolic blood pressure has been shown to rise to as high as 400 mm Hg, resulting in vascular damage and even rupture of the aorta (Schleiter and Schneider, 1964). The tachycardia and marked hypertension probably result from stimulation of the autonomic ganglia. Hansson (1958) observed that hypertension did not occur when artificial respiration was given during administration of succinylcholine (Fig. 14–5).
4. ECG changes produced include bradycardia followed by tachycardia, atrioventricular block with extrasystoles, and inversion of the T-wave. These changes occur when succinylcholine is used both alone and in conjunction with thiopental sodium. The disturbances of ventricular rhythm and tachycardia are effectively antagonized by intravenous injection of 0.1 mg/kg of propranolol hydrochloride (Tavernor and Lees, 1970).
5. Acute myocardial hemorrhages have been reported by Larsen et al. (1959). They believe that this strain on the cardiovascular system, even though recovery occurs, may affect the future performance of race horses.

When succinylcholine chloride is used alone, the generally accepted dose for the horse is 4 mg/100 lbs. Higher doses have been recommended abroad.

The following suggestions for use of succinylcholine chloride in horses were made in 1970 by the Research Subcommittee of the Professional Liability Insurance Committee, American Association of Equine Practitioners.

Suggestions for the Use of Succinylcholine Chloride

Although succinylcholine chloride has been used successfully by a large number of veterinarians, complications may occur following the use of this and many other drugs, even under the best of circumstances. Therefore, discreet medical judgment should be exercised in selecting this method of restraint and provision

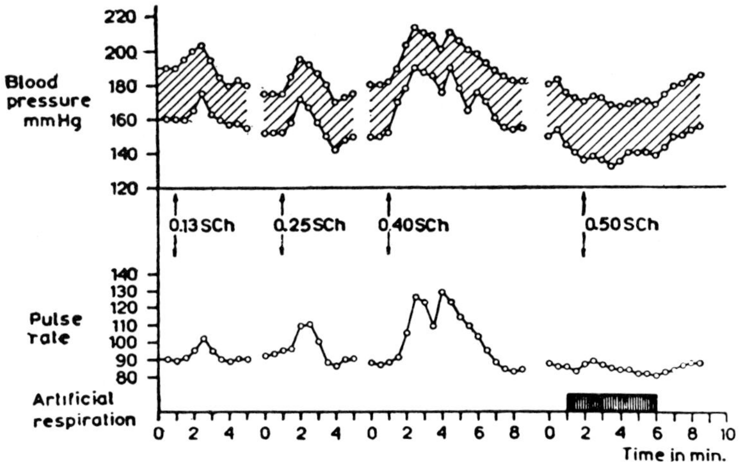

Figure 14–5. Effect of succinylcholine iodide on pulse rate and blood pressure in the horse. Horse—490 kg, 8 years, female, sodium pentobarbital anesthesia.
Upper curve: systolic and diastolic pressure measured in the carotid artery.
Lower curve: pulse frequency.
Intravenous injection of succinylcholine iodide, expressed in mg per kg body weight. Artificial respiration was performed by rhythmical compression of a rubber bladder. (From Hansson, C.H.: Studies on the Effect of Succinylcholine in Domestic Animals. Nord. Vet. Med., 10:201, 1958.)

should be made to handle whatever emergencies arise. The suggestions below may be helpful.

1. Vials of succinylcholine chloride should be held under refrigeration.
2. It is good practice to inform the owner or agent that succinylcholine chloride is to be used as a restraining agent, not as an anesthetic, and that there is always some risk to life involved with any type of restraint, be it physical or chemical.
3. Before using the drug, obtain a thorough history of previous sickness or drug administration. Use of the drug is contraindicated if any of the following have been administered or applied within 30 days:
   a. Any organic phosphate anthelmintic.
   b. Any antibiotic the name of which ends in "mycin."
   c. Any organic phosphate insecticide.
   d. Any other cholinesterase inhibitor.
   e. Procaine.
4. The drug should not be given to debilitated horses.
5. The drug should not be given to excited or exhausted horses.
6. When possible, food should be withheld for 4 to 6 hours prior to administration of the drug.
7. Dosage: The average, normal, healthy horse will be effectively restrained with 0.04 mg of succinylcholine chloride per pound of body weight given intravenously. The objective should be paralysis of skeletal musculature without depression of the respiratory pattern. Overdosing, with paralysis of thoracic musculature, is certain to produce apnea.

   The dosage can usually be reduced if the drug is used in conjunction with preanesthetic agents such as tranquilizers. Such combinations are especially indicated in horses that tend to be unruly or excitable.
8. Some suggested precautions to be taken following the administration of succinylcholine chloride:
   a. Have the horse held by someone familiar with reaction to the drug so as to prevent the horse from falling forward on his nose, causing damage to mouth and hyperflexion of the occipitoatlantal articulation. The latter may result in rupture of the intervertebral artery, with death ensuing shortly thereafter. The horse should also be prevented from falling over backward or in any other way that might result in injury. Turning the horse slowly at the time of collapse should be conducive to a safe fall.
   b. Be prepared with oxygen and the expertise to give artificial respiration if apnea occurs.
9. If death follows the administration of succinylcholine chloride, a necropsy should be performed, because death may well be due

> to some cause unrelated to the drug. Death may result from any form of restraint, chemical or physical, and may be caused indirectly by some physical problem, such as chronic diaphragmatic defect or a verminous aneurysm.

Benson et al. (1979) found that continuous infusion of succinylcholine can be used to induce prolonged muscle relaxation in mechanically ventilated horses anesthetized with halothane. They administered succinylcholine either as a bolus or as a continuous infusion. The bolus dose was 0.33 mg/kg at 15, 45, and 75 minutes; the continuous infusion was 2.2 mg/kg/hr for 1.5 hours, preceded by a loading bolus of 0.33 mg/kg. Each bolus produced paralysis of 3 minutes duration while infusion caused a continuous paralysis.

Transient increases in heart rate and arterial blood pressure were observed after each bolus. Cardiac dysrhythmias did not occur. Serum potassium concentration increased in horses receiving either boluses or continuous infusion; however, there was no electrocardiographic evidence of K^+ intoxication. Serum chloride also increased significantly. Standard bicarbonate was significantly decreased, probably due to increased lactic acid produced during periods of muscle fasciculation with each dose of succinylcholine.

Because they experienced a fatality in a horse using the technique of Benson et al. (1979), Manley and Howitt (1982) tested it in ponies. After thiamylal induction and initiation of halothane maintenance, they gave a bolus of succinylcholine (0.1 mg/kg) followed by continuous infusion of 2.2 mg/kg/hr. Temperature became dramatically elevated in some ponies, with respiratory and metabolic acidosis. For this reason, they advised that this technique should be used with caution. Using essentially the same technique, Hildebrand and Howitt (1983) had severe responses in four of six ponies. These responses were characterized by hyperthermia, hypercapnia, tachycardia, increased pulse pressure, and metabolic acidosis. Two of the six showed signs of phase II block.

Neostigmine, edrophonium, and other anticholinesterases do not antagonize succinylcholine; instead, they prolong its action, except in phase II block. Since prolonged administration or repeated exposure to succinylcholine decreases depolarization despite persistent neuromuscular blockade (phase II block), the interaction of drugs with depolarizing agents varies with the degree of desensitization (Waud, 1981). Except in this situation, no specific pharmacologic antagonist is available. However, in patients showing little recovery, infusion of fresh plasma or whole blood restores plasma cholinesterase activity and thus hydrolyzes the drug.

Succinylcholine is contraindicated in animals suffering from respiratory or liver disease. Lincoff et al. (1957) found that succinylcholine increases intraocular pressure in cats due to contracture of extraocular muscles. For this reason, its use in intraocular operations or glaucoma patients is contraindicated.

Equipment and methods for using succinylcholine in capture and restraint of wild animals are described in Chapters 3 and 18.

AGENTS PRODUCING NONDEPOLARIZATION BLOCK

Agents that act by nondepolarization (competitive blockers, or "true curarizing drugs") produce the following effects:

1. Transmission of the motor nerve impulse across the myoneural junction is prevented, and thus voluntary striated muscle is paralyzed.
2. On direct stimulation, both the nerve and muscle fiber remain excitable throughout the block.
3. During the block, acetylcholine is produced in normal quantities at the end-plate region by stimulation of the motor nerve.
4. Anticholinesterases (neostigmine, pyridostigmine, edrophonium) are antagonistic to these blocking agents.
5. Nondepolarization block is also antagonized by depolarizing relaxants, potassium ions, and cold.

Drugs of clinical importance in this group are:

1. The curare alkaloids, tubocurarine, and

the dimethyl ether of tubocurarine (Metocurine).

2. Synthetic compounds such as gallamine (Flaxedil) and pancuronium (Pavulon).

Tubocurarine Chloride, U.S.P.

Tubocurarine chloride is a white or yellowish-white crystalline solid that forms aqueous solutions with a pH of approximately 3. Tubocurarine is obtained from the plant *Chondodendron tomentosum* and is standardized by biological assay. It is marketed as sterile solution containing 3 mg (20 units/ml). The drug is quite stable, and aqueous solutions can be stored for long periods or even autoclaved without serious decomposition.

There are no significant differences in the pharmacokinetic parameters of tubocurarine, pancuronium, and metocurine (Ham, 1980). These parameters may, however, be altered by disease, drug therapy, and anesthesia. Table 14–5 indicates the effect of changes in acid-base balance. In man, hepatic insufficiency increased the volume of distribution, prolonged the half-life of the elimination phase, and reduced the serum clearance rates; the dose required was thus increased and the duration of effect prolonged. Elimination is likewise delayed in renal disease. Serum and renal clearance have also been shown to be reduced in cats by hypothermia (temperature reduction from 34° to 28° C). The effects of potassium, sodium, and calcium concentrations appear unpredictable, although calcium seems to antagonize neuromuscular blockade; magnesium increases the action of nondepolarizing muscle relaxants. In cats, antagonism of tubocurarine and pancuronium-induced blockade is opposed by respiratory acidosis and metabolic alkalosis. Both amide and ester types of local anesthetics enhance the effects of tubocurarine. Interaction with other drugs is discussed elsewhere in this chapter.

A wide species variation in response to tubocurarine has been observed. Commercial solutions of curare are too concentrated for safe administration to small animals. For this reason, they are diluted with physiologic saline so that each ml contains 2 units. Curare, like pentobarbital, should be given "to effect" and a full 2 minutes should be taken for the injection. Rapid injection may produce bradycardia, tachycardia, or even cardiac collapse.

The use of curare with general anesthetics permits the use of less anesthetic, and good muscular relaxation is still obtained.

When administration with thiopental is desired, the anesthetic is diluted so that each ml contains one-half gr (32 mg), and the dose is calculated at one-sixth to one-eighth gr/lb. Tubocurarine is mixed with the anesthetic at a rate of 1 ml (3 mg) for each 40 lbs of body weight. Injection is made intravenously over 3 to 5 minutes.

Wright and Hall (1961) state that the effective dose for dogs is 0.2 mg/lb and that at this level a fall in blood pressure due to blocking of autonomic ganglia and histamine release occurs. Its use in this species, therefore, is somewhat risky. Similar hypotension occurs on intravenous administration to cats. The dose for pigs is 0.14 mg/lb, and doses up to 0.03 mg/lb have been

TABLE 14–5. Changes in Duration and Magnitude of Tubocurarine- and Pancuronium-Induced Neuromuscular Blockades with Alterations of Acid-Base Balance

Acid-Base Status	*Tubocurarine*	*Pancuronium*
Respiratory acidosis ($P_{CO_2} > 60$ mm Hg)	Increased	Increased or no change
Respiratory alkalosis ($P_{CO_2} < 30$ mm Hg)	Decreased or no change	Decreased or no change
Metabolic acidosis (pH < 7.20)	Increased or no change	Increased or no change
Metabolic alkalosis (pH > 7.60)	Increased or decreased	Increased

(From Ham, J.: Factors Affecting Administration of Nondepolarizing Neuromuscular Blocking Agents. In Volume 8, *ASA Refresher Courses in Anesthesiology.* Edited by S.G. Hershey. J.B. Lippincott Co., Philadelphia, 1980.)

used in young calves and lambs (Hall, 1966). According to Booth (1963), because ether has a curariform action, only one-third the dose of curare should be used. Interaction with anesthetics is also discussed elsewhere in this chapter. Most commonly used antiarrhythmic drugs enhance tubocurarine neuromuscular blockade. In cats, lidocaine, phenytoin, propranolol, and quinidine have been shown to increase the duration and intensity of blockade. Ketamine has a similar action in cats, while experimentally, furosemide also appears to enhance blockade (Ham, 1980).

Injecting tubocurarine-H_3 into dogs, Cohen et al. (1967) found that combined renal and hepatic elimination accounted for 85% of the injected dose within 24 hours. Approximately 75% was recovered in urine and 11% in the bile. When the renal pedicles were ligated, 39% was found in the bile after 24 hours. No significant biotransformation could be determined.

Neostigmine methylsulfate (1:2000), given in 0.5- and 2-ml doses, is a limited antagonist for curare and is effective only against minimal paralytic doses. It is ineffective against larger doses and may actually prolong curarization.

Metocurine Iodide Injection, U.S.P. (Metubine Iodide)

The iodide of dimethyl tubocurarine, Metocurine, is an odorless, pale yellow, crystalline powder. It is slightly soluble in water, forming aqueous solutions with a pH of about 6.1. It is prepared from tubocurarine by substituting two hydroxyl groups with OCH_3 groups. The substitution is accompanied by an increase in potency. Each milliliter of solution contains 2 mg of Metocurine. The pH is adjusted to 4 to 4.3.

In dogs, dimethyl tubocurarine is two to three times more potent than tubocurarine chloride. It is similar in action to tubocurarine, but the duration of neuromuscular block is slightly shorter. It is claimed to have less effect on autonomic ganglia and to produce less histamine release. According to Wright and Hall (1961), equipotent doses of dimethyl tubocurarine and tubocurarine produce comparable depression of blood pressure.

TABLE 14–6. Duration of Paralysis of Dogs Given Gallamine Triethiodide or Succinylcholine Chloride (0.4 mg/kg)

	Return to 1/10 Twitch (min)	*Return to Complete Twitch (min)*
Gallamine	26 ± 7	40 ± 11
Succinylcholine	22 ± 12	37 ± 19

Mean and standard deviation values for two groups of eight dogs.

(From Evans, A.T., Anderson, L.K., Eyster, G.E., and Sawyer, D.C.: Cardiovascular Effects of Gallamine Triethiodide and Succinylcholine Chloride During Halothane Anesthesia in the Dog. Am. J. Vet. Res., 38:329, 1977.)

Gallamine Triethiodide (Flaxedil)

Gallamine triethiodide is a white, odorless, crystalline solid which is soluble in water. The commercially available solution has a pH of about 3.2; it is marketed in 10 ml multiple-dose vials, each ml containing 20 mg. It has three quaternary ammonium groups which form salts with acids and dissolve to produce weak acid solutions. In general, gallamine is nonreactive and stable in solution. Seven milligrams of gallamine are approximately equivalent in action to 1 mg of tubocurarine chloride.

Gallamine produces a nondepolarization block at the neuromuscular junction. In addition, it produces some vagal block, and tachycardia occurs quickly after intravenous injection in the dog. Like pancuronium, it appears to have indirect sympathomimetic activity (Lebowitz and Savarese, 1980). It does not produce histamine release in the dog. There is no indication that clinical doses cause any action on the liver or kidneys. Gallamine does affect amphibian and mammalian myelinated nerve fibers, blocking K^+ and Na^+ channels (Smith and Schauf, 1981). In cats, a transient fall in blood pressure occurs on intravenous injection, and this has been attributed by Wright and Hall (1961) to its inhibitory effect on cholinesterase produced by the liver.

Gallamine is slowly detoxified in the body, and most is excreted unchanged in the urine. Thirty to 100% of the total dose injected into cats can be recovered from the urine within 2 hours (Mushin et al., 1949). Feldman (1969) found that 84% of ^{3}H-gallamine was excreted in the urine of dogs in 24 hours. For this reason, it is contraindicated in animals suffering from renal failure, but may be used in animals with compensated chronic nephritis.

For complete paralysis in dogs, 0.4 mg/kg should be given intravenously. Apnea lasts for approximately 15 to 25 minutes (Table 14–6). Similar doses in cats produce 10 to 20 minutes of apnea. No adverse side effects occur in either species though, as previously mentioned, a transient hypotension may occur in the cat.

DeJong et al. (1968) state that the average dose of gallamine that effectively blocks neuromuscular transmission in the cat is 1 to 2 mg/kg. Using 12.5 mg/kg, they concluded that gallamine has essentially no effect on impulse transmission in the cat's spinal cord.

In cats, 0.03 to 0.07 mg/kg of succinylcholine increased the mean intraocular pressure from 9.1 to 20.4 mm Hg. Prior administration of gallamine prevented the rise in intraocular pressure, following succinylcholine injection (Miller et al., 1968).

In the horse, 0.3 mg/lb of gallamine does not ordinarily cause respiratory arrest, whereas 0.5 mg/lb does so for 10 to 20 minutes. Hall (1966) reports that 0.4 mg/kg of gallamine is effective in young lambs and calves but produces prolonged apnea; 0.5 mg/kg has been reported for the cow. In contrast, 0.2 mg/kg may not always produce apnea in pigs.

Gallamine has been used extensively as an immobilizing agent for wild animals and, when neostigmine is used as an antidote, has proved to be effective (see Chap. 18).

Pancuronium Bromide (Pavulon)

Pancuronium bromide is a nondepolarizing aminosteroid neuromuscular blocking agent, which is free from hormonal action. It is packaged in 2-ml ampules containing 4 mg of the drug and also in 10-ml vials containing 1 mg/ml.

Pancuronium has a more rapid onset of action than other nondepolarizing agents, and its duration is similar to or less than that of tubocurarine. Reversal is accomplished with neostigmine or pyridostigmine and atropine. There is lack of histamine release and associated bronchospasm, ganglionic blockade, and hypotension. Fialho and Lumb (1980) found that pancuronium (0.055 mg/kg) had little effect on blood pressure or heart rate when administered intravenously to dogs with spinal trauma.

Up to 25,000 times the neuromuscular blocking dose can be given to cats without mortality, provided artificial ventilation is maintained. Doses of pancuronium vary somewhat with species. In general, the dose for dogs, cats, swine, and goats is 0.01 to 0.05 mg/lb. Fialho and Lumb (1980) have used 0.11 mg/kg for intubating the dog without anesthesia. For intubating the pig, 0.02 mg/lb gives 6 to 10 minutes of relaxation. In goats, 0.025 mg/kg was used by Parvongnukul and Lumb (1978) to provide relaxation during insertion of total hip prostheses. This dose produced 45 minutes of relaxation. Weaver (1970) reported using 0.1 mg/kg in horses and 0.005 mg/kg in sheep.

As much as 20 to 30% of injected pancuronium is metabolized primarily to 3-hydroxypancuronium and smaller amounts to 17- and 3,17-hydroxypancuronium. In man, pancuronium is 2, 50, and 52 times as potent as these metabolites. Booij et al. (1979) found that, although more neostigmine is required to antagonize 17- or 3, 17-hydroxypancuronium, there is no problem with reversal since these two metabolites are not potent muscle relaxants and do not appear in large amounts. Since pancuronium can be easily reversed, has no histaminic effect, and is longer acting than gallamine, it is probably the relaxant of choice.

MISCELLANEOUS RELAXANTS

Guaifenesin (Gecolate; Glycodex)

Guaifenesin (glyceryl guaiacolate), a common decongestant and antitussive, has been used extensively in horses as a muscle relaxant. According to Roberts (1968), its unique advantage is that it produces muscle relaxation with little effect on respiration.

Guaifenesin, which chemically is similar to mephenesin, blocks impulse transmission at connecting neurons in the spinal cord and brain stem. While relaxation of the skeletal muscles is produced, the diaphragm continues to function and there is no respiratory paralysis. The respiratory rate may be increased while the tidal volume decreases. The minute volume is unchanged. The pharyngeal and laryngeal muscles are relaxed, facilitating intubation. A state of drowsiness and partial analgesia is also produced. Preanesthetic and anesthetic agents are potentiated.

Guaifenesin is available commercially in two forms: powder and 5% solution. The powder is prepared for injection by dissolving it under aseptic conditions in warm (not to exceed 100° F) sterile water. The pH, osmolality, stability, and bacteriostatic characteristics of 5, 10, and 15% solutions of guaifenesin were studied by Grady and McDonell (1980). They found that a 10% solution of guaifenesin in sterile distilled water was more suitable for equine anesthesia than solutions in 0.9% saline or 5% dextrose. The commercially available 5% guaifenesin solution contains dextrose (50 mg), propylene glycol (20.7 mg), edetate disodium (0.75 mg), 0.5% formalin, and distilled water.

Recumbency can be produced in the horse by intravenous administration of 160 mg/kg of guaifenesin (Tavernor, 1970). The lethal dose in horses is at least three times the calculated dose (Gertsen and Tillotson, 1968).

Guaifenesin (5% in 5% dextrose) given alone intravenously produces gentle, excitement-free relaxation and recumbency in horses. This technique can be used for intubation and induction of gas anesthesia. The duration of recumbency when given at the rate of 1 ml/lb is approximately 9 minutes. The blood pressure during this period is stable, in contrast to the use of succinylcholine, which causes a drastic increase (425/320 mm Hg), and barbiturates, which produce a marked decrease (45/20 mm Hg) (Heath, 1970). Tavernor (1970) has likewise indicated that the cardiovascular and respiratory effects of guaifenesin, either alone or in combination with pentothal sodium, are relatively benign when compared with the effects of succinylcholine on these systems.

Gertsen and Tillotson (1968) suggested addition of either 40 gr of pentobarbital sodium or 2.0 g of thiamylal per liter of 5% solution. The dose of either mixture is calculated at 1 ml/lb of body weight. Roberts (1968) suggested that 0.25 g of thiopental sodium or methitural sodium/50 kg of body weight be added. These solutions are given intravenously at the rate of 5 g of guaifenesin/50 kg.

Wright et al. (1979) gave horses acepromazine (0.6 to 0.8 mg/kg IV), followed by 5% guaifenesin IV and thiamylal (5 mg/kg IV) to produce recumbency. Halothane was then given via a semiclosed system. In the immediate post-induction period, they found large decreases in systolic blood pressure (62 ± 19 mm Hg), which gradually rose toward normal. They warned against using this technique when hypotension is a potential problem.

The cardiopulmonary effects of guaifenesin and xylazine-guaifenesin have been examined in horses by Hubbell et al. (1980). They found that heart rate, respiratory rate, right atrial pressure, pulmonary artery pressure, and cardiac output were essentially unchanged when guaifenesin alone was given. Systolic, diastolic, and mean arterial pressures were decreased. PaO_2 was transiently reduced.

Intravenous xylazine (1.1 mg/kg) prior to guaifenesin administration reduced the dose necessary for lateral recumbency (88 ± 10 mg/kg). There were significant transient decreases in heart and respiratory rates, cardiac output, and PaO_2. Systolic, diastolic, and mean arterial blood pressures were decreased and central venous pressure increased.

As other drugs in the mephenesin group, guaifenesin in high concentration produces hemolysis and hemoglobinuria if given intravenously. The drug is conjugated to glucuronide in the liver and largely excreted in the urine. The exact mechanism of inactivation in the body is poorly understood. Significant amounts of guaifenesin pass the placental barrier in the mare (Hubbell et al., 1980).

Davis and Wolff (1970) found a pronounced sex difference in duration of action, stallions, requiring longer to recover than mares. This was attributed to slower disappearance of the drug from the plasma. There is no antagonist for guaifenesin. Concurrent administration of physostigmine is contraindicated.

Although it is used in the horse, guaifenesin is not of value in the dog, because of the large volume of solution necessary and the brief, shallow muscular relaxation produced (Tavernor and Jones, 1970).

ANTICURARIFORM AGENTS

Antagonists to the muscle relaxants are at present limited to those effective against the antidepolarizing drugs. These include edrophonium, neostigmine, and pyridostigmine, all of which are anticholinesterases. The neuromuscular action of these drugs is due to their inhibitory effect on acetylcholine hydrolysis, thus intensifying acetylcholine effects.

Complications and side effects caused by these agents are due chiefly to an excess of acetylcholine acting on the postganglionic parasympathetic fibers. These are more pronounced with neostigmine than with edrophonium or pyridostigmine and include salivation, bronchial secretion, intestinal hypermotility, and bradycardia.

The use of antagonists should seldom be necessary if proper care is exerted in administration of muscle relaxants. When respiratory exchange is inadequate, it is recommended that artificial respiration be administered until spontaneous respiration resumes. If an antagonist is needed, the initial dose should be small, and atropine should be given concurrently to prevent side effects.

Edrophonium Chloride (Tensilon)

Edrophonium is the most rapid acting of the three anticurariform agents, requiring 30 to 60 seconds. Temporary improvement of neuromuscular activity followed by recurarization may occur. For this reason, recovered patients should never be left unobserved. Recent evidence indicates that edrophonium has not been administered in adequate doses (0.5 to 1.0 mg/kg), but when they are used, edrophonium is a safe and effective antagonist.

Adverse reactions include salivation, bronchial secretion, intestinal hypermotility, and bradycardia. These reactions are due to an excess of acetylcholine acting on postganglionic parasympathetic fibers. Atropine should be given concurrently to prevent these from occurring.

Because of its relatively short action, edrophonium has been used as a test agent to determine if apnea following use of a depolarizing agent is due to phase I or phase II block.

Edrophonium chloride is available in multiple-dose vials containing 10 mg/ml. The dose is listed in Table 14–7.

Neostigmine Methylsulfate (Prostigmine)

The action of neostigmine is of longer duration than that of edrophonium. Side effects are similiar but more pronounced. The onset of action is 120 to 240 seconds. The duration of action is longer, and for this reason neostigmine is more frequently used as an antagonist, since recurarization is less apt to occur than with edrophonium. Neostigmine may also be used for definitive antagonism following a test dose of edrophonium. As with the latter, the dose should be preceded by administration of atropine.

Neostigmine methylsulfate is available in multiple-dose vials containing 1 mg/ml. The dose is listed in Table 14–7.

Pyridostigmine Bromide (Regonol; Mestinon)

Pyridostigmine bromide is an analogue of neostigmine, but differs from it clinically by having fewer side effects, such as bradycardia, salivation, and gastrointestinal stimulation. It is a cholinesterase inhibitor. Each ml contains 5 mg of pyridostigmine bromide with 0.2% parabens and 0.02% sodium citrate. The pH is adjusted to approximately 5.0.

In animal studies, pyridostigmine has a slower onset and longer duration of action than does neostigmine. It is contraindicated in mechanical, intestinal, and urinary tract obstructions. When pyridostigmine is used, the muscarinic side effects should be prevented by administration of atropine or glycopyrrolate immediately prior to pyridostigmine. A suggested initial dose of pyridostigmine is 0.2 mg/kg.

When one is using muscle relaxant antagonists, several points should be considered if antagonism is inadequate (Cronnelly, 1980).

TABLE 14–7. Recommended Dose of Antagonists for Nondepolarizing Muscle Relaxants

Agent	Initial Dose		Onset of Action in Minutes	Repeat Dose of Antagonist*	Minutes Between Doses
	Antagonist	Atropine			
Neostigmine (Prostigmine)	0.03–0.10 mg/10 lbs	0.02 mg/lb	2–4	0.015–0.05 mg/10 lbs	5–8
Edrophonium (Tensilon)	0.5–1.0 mg/10 lb	0.02 mg/lb	0.5–1	0.25 mg/10 lbs	2–4

*If initial dose does not produce desired effect.

(After Foldes, F.F.: *Muscle Relaxants in Anesthesiology.* Charles C Thomas, Springfield, Illinois, 1957.)

Enough time must be allowed for antagonism to occur. In speed of onset, the antagonistic drugs rank as follows: edrophonium, neostigmine, pyridostigmine. In significant respiratory acidosis ($Paco_2 > 50$ mm Hg), it may not be possible to anatagonize a nondepolarizing blockade. This is not the case with metabolic acidosis; rather, metabolic alkalosis prevents antagonism.

Other drugs, such as antibiotics, may inhibit antagonism. Antibiotic blockade most often cannot be satisfactorily antagonized (see Table 14–2).

Elevated serum magnesium or low potassium or calcium may augment blockade. Renal failure should also be considered with gallamine and decamethonium, which depend on the kidney for excretion. A more detailed discussion of relaxant/drug interactions is given by Miller (1981).

HYPOTENSIVE AGENTS

Control of blood loss during surgery has always presented a problem. A number of solutions have been advanced, including deliberate withdrawal of blood and subsequent reinfusion. The development of sympathetic blocking agents has led to their trial in deliberate induction of hypotension. They have been found particularly valuable in brain surgery on man. Among the agents that have been used are quaternary ammonium compounds, such as pentamethonium and hexamethonium, thiophanium derivatives, such as trimethaphan and, more recently, sodium nitroprusside. Outwardly it would appear that this technique produces shock. Paradoxically, however, it has been pointed out by Boba and Converse (1957) that there is good evidence to indicate lowered blood pressure with prevention of vasoconstriction, such as occurs with these agents, prevents or prolongs the onset of irreversible shock.

Blood pressure in the surgical wound can be estimated where the patient's position is other than parallel to the floor. Blood pressure generally is 1 mm Hg less than at heart level for every 1.5 cm the wound is above the heart. When the wound is below the heart, the arterial pressure is 1 mm Hg/1.5 cm more than at heart level. With a mean blood pressure below 60 mm Hg, the femoral pulse in the dog can hardly be felt. For patient safety, arterial blood pressure should be monitored continuously, either indirectly by Doppler apparatus, or directly by an intra-arterial catheter and pressure transducer (see Chap. 19 for monitoring techniques).

Tilting the operating table supplements the action of hypotensive agents. A high positive pressure in the airway does this also. Excessive bleeding may be managed by more tilt, deeper anesthesia, or increased pressure in the airway. Excessive hypotension can be treated effectively by infusion of lactated Ringer's solution or, with excessive blood loss, by rapid blood transfusion.

For neurosurgery, deliberate hypotension plus mild hypothermia may be combined effectively.

Trimethaphan Camsylate (Arfonad)

Trimethaphan is a thiophanium derivative that has the characteristic ganglionic blocking and hypotensive effects of tetraethylammonium bromide (TEA). Intravenous doses ranging from

0.015 to 0.25 mg/kg show an average of 30 times the potency and twice the duration of circulatory depressor effects of TEA in the dog, cat, and monkey. About 20 times the intravenous dose is required intramuscularly in the dog and cat to cause an equal vasodepression. Oral administration produces erratic results.

There is wide species variation in the acute toxicity of the thiophanium compounds. On intravenous injection, trimethaphan is 2 to 4 times as toxic as TEA in mice, rats, and rabbits, and 75 times as toxic in dogs (Randall et al., 1949). In all species except the dog, toxic doses of TEA and trimethaphan produce death by respiratory failure. In the dog, death appears due to hemorrhagic shock, apparently from profound fall in blood pressure, with hemorrhage into the gastrointestinal tract and petechia in the internal organs. This state of hemorrhagic shock in dogs appears to be accompanied by release of histamine and heparin since administration of antihistamine and antiheparin agents modifies the lethal effect. A prolonged clotting time is also found in dogs after intravenous doses of trimethaphan ranging from 0.25 to 1.0 mg/kg. Because of these effects, the drug is contraindicated in the dog; they have not been demonstrated in other species.

Trimethaphan has been shown to have chiefly a direct vasodilator action with little effect produced by ganglionic blockade (McCubbin and Page, 1952). In dogs, a dose of 0.05 mg/kg depresses the blood pressure from 20 to 50 mm Hg for 2 to 8 minutes. Longer periods of hypotension can be produced by intravenous infusion of 0.02 mg/kg/min.

The LD_{50} of trimethaphan is quite high in monkeys. According to Aguilar and Boldrey (1960), 50 mg/kg produces respiratory failure or may, as the result of persistent hypotension, cause circulatory failure, poikilothermy, and necrosis of the proximal convoluted tubules of the kidney with hematuria and uremia. The clinical dose for monkeys is 2 to 4 mg/kg and in dogs 0.03 to 0.05 mg/kg. The drug appears to be excreted rapidly in the urine after intravenous injection, and this may be the cause of renal toxicity (Gertner et al., 1955). Approximately 33% is excreted in the first 3 hours after administration, but no drug is found thereafter in a biologically active form in the urine. The mechanism of inactivation of the remainder is unknown.

Neostigmine in large doses and ephedrine in doses of 1 mg/kg intravenously will abolish the depressor and ganglionic blocking effects of both TEA and trimethaphan.

Sodium Nitroprusside (Nipride)

Sodium nitroprusside (SNP) is a potent hypotensive agent for intravenous administration. Its effect is almost immediate and ends when infusion is stopped. Its action is probably due to the nitroso (NO) group. The hypotensive effects are caused by peripheral vasodilatation as a result of direct action on the blood vessels, independent of autonomic intervention. No relaxation is produced in smooth muscle elsewhere in the body. The brief duration of action is due to rapid conversion to thiocyanate. The hypotensive effect is increased by ganglionic blocking agents, volatile liquid anesthetics, such as halothane and enflurane, and by most other circulatory depressants.

In man, SNP has been used extensively to reduce hemorrhage during surgery of the hip, breast, and brain. SNP is now used in operations for pheochromocytoma instead of alpha blockers.

When used for hypotension during anesthesia, SNP is administered as an infusion mixed with 5% dextrose in water. Because of its rapid onset of action and potency, it should always be administered by means of an infusion pump or micro-drip regulator to provide precise measurement of the flow rate. *It should never be given by direct injection.* When it is given acutely, doses exceeding 1.0 to 1.5 mg/kg cause toxicity in dogs (Michenfelder, 1977); in baboons the dose is over 4.0 mg/kg (MacDowall et al., 1974).

Sodium nitroprusside is metabolized to cyanide and then to thiocyanate (Vessey et al., 1979). If excessive amounts are used, thiocyanate toxicity may occur. Gross overdosage may cause cyanide intoxication. Since cyanide is converted into thiocyanate by an hepatic enzyme, rhodanese, SNP should probably not be used in patients with hepatic insufficiency. Thiocyanate inhibits uptake and binding of iodine and should be used with caution in hypothyroidism or in severe renal disease.

SNP in dextrose solution tends to deteriorate in the presence of light. Solutions should not be kept or used longer than 4 hours. For small animals, 50 mg of sodium nitroprusside should be diluted in 1000 ml of 5% dextrose in water and the bottle and administration tubing promptly wrapped in aluminum foil to protect from light. Freshly prepared solutions have a faint brownish tint, and unused portions and solutions that are highly colored should be discarded. No other drugs should be administered in the same solution or through the same intravenous tubing.

The concentration and rate of administration must be adjusted for various species. The average dose of SNP in humans is 3 μg/kg/minute (range 0.5 to 10 μg/kg/minute); rates greater than 10 μg/kg/minute are rarely used. If at this rate reduction of blood pressure is not attained within 10 minutes, administration should be stopped.

Arterial blood pressure should be monitored directly in all patients (Cole, 1978). The first sign of SNP overdosage is profound hypotension. Metabolic acidosis may precede this dosage. Massive overdosage may produce signs similar to those for cyanide poisoning with imperceptible pulse, reduced heart sounds, hypotension, shallow breathing, widely dilated pupils, and pink color. Oxygen alone does not provide relief. In dogs subjected to one hour of SNP-induced hypotension (mean arterial pressure of 50 mm Hg), minimal metabolic disturbances were seen. Dogs subjected to 40 mm Hg for one hour exhibited changes indicating cerebral and systemic hypoxia. These were in dogs given over 1.0 mg/kg of SNP and were presumably due to cyanide toxicity (Michelfelder and Theye, 1977). Renal blood flow in dogs given SNP is maintained (Wang et al., 1977).

When signs of overdosage occur, SNP administration should be stopped *immediately.* A bolus of thiosulfate (30 mg/kg) plus constant infusion of 60 mg/kg/hr is the most effective and safest prophylactic agent against cyanide toxicity in the dog (Ivankovich et al., 1980).

Cole (1978) points out that the two most common problems with SNP are reflex tachycardia and gross overdose with resultant cyanide poisoning. Tachycardia is due to stimulation of the baroreceptor mechanism. This causes an increase in cardiac output and peripheral resistance, which tend to return the arterial pressure to its normal level. A temptation is to increase the dose of SNP because of the rising blood pressure. Reflex tachycardia is best treated with small doses of a beta-adrenergic blocker such as propranolol. Although reflex tachycardia does occur with SNP, it is less troublesome than with a ganglionic blocker such as trimethaphan. Patients given too much SNP develop metabolic acidosis from acute cyanide poisoning. Cyanide acts through inhibition of tissue oxidative processes, by blocking the action of cytochrome oxidase and producing histotoxic hypoxia. Normal metabolism of pyruvate is inhibited, and it is converted to lactate. Metabolic acidosis then develops.

REFERENCES

Adams, H.R., Teske, R.H., and Mercer, H.D.: Anesthetic-Antibiotic Interrelationships. J.A.V.M.A., 168:409, 1976.

Aguilar, J.A., and Boldrey, E.B.: The Effect of Arfonad on the Monkey. Anesthesiology, 21:3, 1960.

Benson, G.J., Hartsfield, S.M., Smetzer, D.L., and Thurmon, J.C.: Physiologic Effects of Succinylcholine Chloride in Mechanically Ventilated Horses Anesthetized with Halothane in Oxygen. Am. J. Vet. Res., 40:1411, 1979.

Boba, A., and Converse, J.G.: Ganglionic Blockade and Its Protective Action in Hemorrhage: A Review. Anesthesiology, 18:559, 1957.

Booij, L.H.D.J., Miller, R.D., Jones, M.J.W., and Stanski, D.R.: Antagonism of Pancuronium and Its Metabolites by Neostigmine in Cats. Anesth. Analg., 58:483, 1979.

Booth, N.H.: Personal communication. Colorado State University, Fort Collins, Colorado, 1963.

Clitherow, J.W., Mitchard, M., and Harper, N.J.: The Possible Biological Function of Pseudocholinesterase. Nature, 199:1000, 1963.

Cohen, E.N., Brewer, H.W., and Smith, D.: The Metabolism and Elimination of d-Tubocurarine-H_2. Anesthesiology, 28:309, 1967.

Cole, P.: The Safe Use of Sodium Nitroprusside. Anaesthesia, 33:473, 1978.

Croft, P.G.: The Photomotor Reflex as an Indicator of Consciousness in the Immobilized Dog. J. Small Anim. Pract., 2:206, 1961.

Cronnelly, R.: Update on Muscle Relaxants and Their Antagonists. Am. Soc. Anesth. 1980 Annual Refresher Course Lectures, St. Louis, Missouri.

Davis, L.E., and Wolff, W.A.: Pharmacokinetics and Metabolism of Glyceryl Guaiacolate in Ponies. Am. J. Vet. Res., 31:469, 1970.

DeJong, R.H., Robles, R., and Morikawa, K.I.: Gallamine (Flaxedil) and Synaptic Transmission in the Spinal Cord. Science, 160:768, 1968.

DeYoung, D.W., Lumb, W.V., and Chase, P.: Succinylcholine Chloride Dosage in Miniature Swine. Lab. Anim. Care, 20:998, 1970.

Dowdy, E.G., Duggar, P.N., and Fabian, L.W.: Effect of Neuromuscular Blocking Agents on Isolated Digitalized Mammalian Hearts. Anesth. Analg., 44:608, 1965.

Feldman, S.A.: The Excretion of Gallamine in the Dog. Anesthesiology, 30:593, 1969.

Fialho, S.A.G., and Lumb, W.V.: Anesthesia for Spinal Trauma and Recording Somatosensory Evoked Potentials. Vet. Anesth., 8:18, 1980.

Gertner, S.B., Little, D.M., and Bonycastle, D.D.: Urinary Excretion of Arfonad by Patients Undergoing "Controlled Hypotension" during Surgery. Anesthesiology, 16:495, 1955.

Gertsen, K.E., and Tillotson, P.J.: Clinical Use of Glyceryl Guaiacolate in the Horse. Vet. Med./Small Anim. Clin., 63:1062, 1968.

Grady, J.L., and McDonell, W.N.: Evaluation of Concentrated Solutions of Guaifenesin for Equine Anesthesia. J.A.V.M.A., 176: 619, 1980.

Hall, L.W.: Accidents and Emergencies in Anesthesia. Mod. Vet. Pract., 40:28, 1959.

Hall, L.W. (Ed.): *Wright's Veterinary Anaesthesia and Analgesia,* 6th ed., Bailliere, Tindall and Cassell, London, 1966.

Hall, L.W., Lehman, H., and Silk, E.: Response in Dogs to Relaxants Derived from Succinic Acid Choline. Br. Med. J., 1:134, 1953.

Ham, J.: Factors Affecting Administration of Nondepolarizing Neuromuscular Blocking Agents. ASA Refresher Courses in Anesthesiology, 8:61, 1980.

Hansson, C.H.: Studies on the Effect of Succinylcholine in Domestic Animals. Nord. Vet. Med., 10:201, 1958.

Harrison, G.G., Saunders, S.J., Biebuyck, J.F., Hickman, R., Dent, D.M., Weaver, V., and Terblanche, J.: Anaesthetic-Induced Malignant Hyperpyrexia and a Method for its Prediction. Br. J. Anaesth., 41:844, 1969.

Hazelwood, J.C., and Heath, G.E.: A Comparison of Cholinesterase Activity of Plasma Erythrocytes, and Cerebrospinal Fluid of Sheep, Calves, Dogs, Swine, and Rabbits. Am. J. Vet. Res., 37:741, 1976.

Heath, R.B.: Personal communication. Colorado State University, Fort Collins, Colorado, 1970.

Hildebrand, S.V., and Howitt, G.A.: Succinylcholine Infusion Associated with Hyperthermia in Ponies Anesthetized with Halothane. Am. J. Vet. Res., 44:2280, 1983.

Himes, J.A., Edds, G.T., Kirkham, W.W., and Neal, F.C.: Potentiation of Succinylcholine by Organophosphate Compounds in Horses. J.A.V.M.A., 151:54, 1967.

Hubbell, J.A.E., Muir, W.W., and Sams, R.A.: Guaifenesin: Cardiopulmonary Effects and Plasma Concentrations in Horses. Am. J. Vet. Res., 41:1751, 1980.

Irwin, R.L., Wells, J.B., and Whitehead, R.W.: Effect of Calcium on the Duration of Apnea Induced by Succinylcholine. Anesthesiology, 17:759, 1956.

Ivankovich, A.D., Braverman, B., Kanuru, R.P., Heyman, H.J., and Paulissian, R.: Cyanide Antidotes and Methods of Their Administration in Dogs: A Comparative Study. Anesthesiology, 52:210, 1980.

Katz, R.L.: A Nerve Stimulator for the Continuous Monitoring of Muscle Relaxant Action. Anesthesiology, 26:832, 1965.

Kivisselgaard, N., and Moya, F.: Investigation of Placental Thresholds to Succinylcholine. Anesthesiology, 22:7, 1961.

Knill, L.M.: Pharmacodynamics of Succinylcholine Chloride in the Dog. Master's Thesis, Colorado State University, Fort Collins, Colorado, 1956.

Larsen, L.H., Loomis, L.N., and Steel, J.D.: Muscular Relaxants and Cardiovascular Damage: With Special Reference to Succinylcholine Chloride. Aust. Vet. J., 35:269, 1959.

Lebowitz, P.W., and Savarese, J.J.: Cardiovascular and Autonomic Effects of Neuromuscular Blockers. ASA Refresher Courses in Anesthesiology, 8:103, 1980.

Lincoff, H.A., Breinin, G.M., and DeVoe, A.G.: The Effect of Succinylcholine on the Extraocular Muscles. Am. J. Ophthalmol., 43:440, 1957.

Manley, S.V., and Howitt, G.: Hyperthermia in Halothane Anesthetized Ponies Administered Succinylcholine by Infusion. Proc. Am. Coll. Vet. Anesth., Scientific Mtg., Las Vegas, 1982.

McCubbin, J.W., and Page, I.H.: Nature of the Hypotensive Action of a Thiophanium Derivative (RO 2-2222) in Dogs. J. Pharmacol. Exper. Ther., 105:437, 1952.

McDowall, D.G., Keaney, N.P., Turner, J.M., Lane, J.R., and Okuda, Y.: The Toxicity of Sodium Nitroprusside. Br. J. Anaesth., 46:327, 1974.

Michenfelder, J.D.: Cyanide Release from Sodium Nitroprusside in the Dog. Anesthesiology, 46:196, 1977.

Michenfelder, J.D., and Theye, R.A.: Canine Systemic and Cerebral Effects of Hypotension Induced by Hemorrhage, Trimethaphan, Halothane, or Nitroprusside. Anesthesiology, 46:188, 1977.

Miller, R.D.: Neuromuscular Blocking Agents. In *Drug Interactions in Anesthesia*. Edited by N.T. Smith, R.D. Miller, and A.N. Corbascio. Lea & Febiger, Philadelphia, 1981.

Miller, R.D., Way, W.L., and Hickey, R.F.: Inhibition of Succinylcholine-Induced Increased Intraocular Pressure by Non-Depolarizing Muscle Relaxants. Anesthesiology, 29:123, 1968.

Mushin, W.W., Wien, R., Mason, D.F.J., and Langston, G.T.: Curare-like Actions of Tri-(Diethylaminoethyoxy)-Benzene Triethyliodide. Lancet, 1:726, 1949.

Palmer, J.S., Jackson, J.B., Younger, R.L., Hunt, L.M., Danz, J.W., and Wunderlich, B.W.: Normal Cholinesterase Activity of the Whole Blood of the Horse and Angora Goat. Vet. Med., 58:885, 1965.

Parvongnukul, K., and Lumb, W.V.: Evaluation of Polytetrafluoroethylene-Graphite-Coated Total Hip Prostheses in Goats. Am. J. Vet. Res., 39:221, 1978.

Pittinger, C.B., and Morris, L.E.: Placental Transmission of d-Tubocurarine Chloride from Maternal to Fetal Circulation in Dogs. Anesthesiology, 14:238, 1953.

Pittinger, C.B., and Morris, L.E.: Observations of the Placental Transmission of Gallamine Triethiodide (Flaxedil), Succinylcholine Chloride (Anectine) and Decamethonium Bromide (Syncurine) in Dogs. Anesth. Analg., 34:107, 1955.

Radeleff, R.D., and Woodard, C.T.: Cholinesterase Activity of Normal Blood of Cattle and Sheep. Vet. Med., 51:512, 1956.

Randall, L.O., Peterson, W.G., and Lehman, G.: The Ganglionic Blocking Action of Thiophanium Derivatives. J. Pharmacol. Exp. Ther., 97:48, 1949.

Roberts, D.: The Role of Glyceryl Guaiacolate in a Balanced Equine Anesthetic. Vet. Med./Small Anim. Clin., 63:157, 1968.

Robertson, G.S.: Serum Cholinesterase Deficiency I: Disease and Inheritance. Br. J. Anaesth., 38:355, 1966.

Savarese, J.J., and Kitz, R.J.: Pharmacology of Relaxants. ASA Refresher Courses in Anesthesiology, 3:153, 1975.

Schleiter, H., and Schneider, J.: Effect of Intramuscular Injection of Succinylcholine Chloride and Hyaluronidase in the Horse. Wien. tierarzl. Monatsschr., 51:381, 1964.

Short, C.E., Cuneio, J., and Cupp, D.: Organophosphate-Induced Complications During Anesthetic Management in the Horse. J.A.V.M.A., 159:1319, 1971.

Smith, K.J., and Schauf, C.L.: Gallamine Triethiodide (Flaxedil): Tetraethylammonium- and Pancuronium-Like Effects in Myelinated Nerve Fibers. Science, 212:1170, 1981.

Standaert, F.G.: Neuromuscular Transmission—What Is A Cholinergic Receptor? Annual Refresher Course Lectures. Am. Soc. Anesthesiologists, 1980.

Stevenson, D.E.: A Review of Some Side-Effects of Muscle Relaxants in Small Animals. J. Small Anim. Pract., 1:77, 1960.

Stowe, C.M.: The Curariform Effect of Succinylcholine in the Equine and Bovine Species: A Preliminary Report. Cornell Vet., 45:193, 1955.

Stowe, C.M., Bieter, R.N., and Roepke, M.H.: The Relationship Between Cholinesterase Activity and the Effects of Succinylcholine Chloride in the Horse and Cow. Cornell Vet., 48:241, 1958.

Strelitz, F.: Studies on Cholinesterase. Purification of Pseudo-Cholinesterase from Horse Serum. Biochem. J., 38:86, 1944.

Tavernor, W.D.: The Influence of Guaiacol Glycerol Ether on Cardiovascular and Respiratory Function in the Horse. Res. Vet. Sci., 11:91, 1970.

Tavernor, W.D., and Jones, E.W.: Observations on the Cardiovascular and Respiratory Effects of Guaiacol Glycerol Ether in Conscious and Anaesthetized Dogs. J. Small Anim. Pract., 11:177, 1970.

Tavernor, W.D., and Lees, P.: The Influence of Thiopentone and Suxamethonium on Cardiovascular and Respiratory Function in the Horse. Res. Vet. Sci., 11:45, 1970.

Vessey, C.J., Simpson, P.J., Adams, L., and Cole, P.V.: Metabolism of Sodium Nitroprusside and Cyanide in the Dog. Br. J. Anaesth., 51:89, 1979.

Wang, H.H., Liu, L.M.P., and Katz, R.L.: A Comparison of the Cardiovascular Effects of Sodium Nitroprusside and Trimethaphan. Anesthesiology, 46:40, 1977.

Ward, F.P., and Glicksberg, C.L.: Effects of Dichlorvos on Blood Cholinesterase Activity in Dogs. J.A.V.M.A., 158:457, 1971.

Waud, B.E.: Interaction of Muscle Relaxants and Other Drugs, ASA Refresher Courses in Anesthesiology, 9:213, 1981.

Waud, B.D., and Waud, D.R.: The Margin of Safety of Neuromuscular Transmission in the Muscle of the Diaphragm. Anesthesiology, 37:417, 1972.

Weaver, B.M.Q.: Personal communication. Department of Veterinary Surgery, University of Bristol, Bristol, England, 1970.

Winnie, A.P., and Collins, V.J.: The Doxapram Test: A New Technique for the Differential Diagnosis of Apnea. Anesthesiology, 26:265, 1965.

Woodward, G.T.: The Treatment of Organic Phosphate Insecticide Poisoning with Atropine Sulfate and 2-PAM (2-Pyridine Aldoxime Methiodide). Vet. Med., 52:471, 1957.

Wright, J.G., and Hall, L.W.: *Veterinary Anesthesia and Analgesia,* 5th ed. Williams & Wilkins, Baltimore, 1961.

Wright, M., McGrath, D.J., and Raffe, M.: Indirect Blood Pressure Readings in Horses Before and After Induction of General Anesthesia with Acetylpromazine, Glyceryl Guaiacolate and Sodium Thiamylal. Vet. Anesth., 6:41, 1979.

CHAPTER 15

Local Anesthetic Agents

DESIRABLE CHARACTERISTICS OF LOCAL ANESTHETIC AGENTS

A number of characteristics are desirable in a local anesthetic agent. They include: 1) good penetrating qualities in body tissues, 2) high potency so that low concentrations can be used, 3) rapid onset, 4) long duration of action, 5) low systemic toxicity, 6) no irritation to nerve and other body tissues, 7) reversible action, and 8) availability in sterile solution or ease of sterilization. Unfortunately, no agent possesses all of these characteristics. Tables 15–1 and 15–2 summarize the characteristics of some local anesthetics employed today.

Mechanism of Action

Local anesthetics are reversible in their action in contrast to substances such as phenol or alcohol that also block impulse conduction in nerve fibers. Pure local anesthetic is a weak base. Salts of this base are readily soluble in water and stable in solution, in which case the local anesthetic cation is in dissociation equilibrium with the uncharged local anesthetic base. Relative concentrations of cation and base vary with hydrogen ion concentration of the solution. The lipid solubility of the local anesthetic determines drug penetration and diffusion. The cation binds to the anionic receptors of the nerve membrane to plug the internal pore of the sodium channels. Sodium entrance into the axon is prevented, and depolarization cannot occur. Local anesthetic block is thus a nondepolarized block, and the effects are influenced by the pK_a of the anesthetic (de Jong, 1979). The molecular mechanisms of local anesthetic action have been reviewed by Strichartz (1976).

Since the myelin sheath of nerves is both an electrical and a pharmacologic insulator, access of local anesthetic to the myelinated nerve membrane is limited to the nodes of Ranvier. Therefore, a higher concentration of local anesthetic is necessary to induce anesthesia of myelinated in contrast to nonmyelinated fibers. The C_m is the minimum concentration of local anesthetic that will block impulse conduction within a specified time. The smaller the C_m, the more potent the anesthetic. It is comparable to MAC for an inhalation anesthetic.

Because the local anesthetic is thought to attach to the internal opening of the sodium channel in the membrane, it must diffuse through the nerve membrane. Diameter of the nerve fiber is thought to influence anesthetic action directly, perhaps due to changes in surface area to volume relationships, and to the greater internodal distance of thick nerve fibers. Gissen et al. (1980) challenged the traditional concept of sequential

TABLE 15–1. Data Concerning Local Anesthetic Agents

Agent—Ester-Type (Generic Name)	*Cocaine*	*Procaine*	*Chloroprocaine*	*Tetracaine*	*Hexylcaine*
Trade Name		*Novacain Winthrop Laboratories*	*Nesacaine Pennwalt Inc.*	*Pontocaine Breon Laboratories Inc.*	*Cyclaine Merck and Company, Inc.*
pK_a		8.9	8.7	8.5	
Molecular Weight	339.81	272.77	307.2	300.6	297.85
Potency (Procaine = 1)	4	1	2.4	10–20	4
Toxicity (Procaine = 1)	4	1	0.5	8	4
Onset		Slow	Fast	Slow	
Duration	20–30 min	30–90 min	up to 60 min	3–10 hrs	3–6 hrs
Use Topical	3–10%	—		0.5–2.0%	2.5–5%
Infiltration	*	0.5%	102%	0.1%	0.5%
Nerve Block	*	2%	2%	0.5–0.2%	0.5–1%
Epidural	*	2–4%	2–3%	0.2%	1.0–1.5%
Spinal	*	2–5%		0.2–0.5%	1.5–2%

*Not recommended for use.

Agent—Amide-Type (Generic Name)	*Lidocaine*	*Prilocaine*	*Mepivacaine*	*Bupivacaine*	*Etidocaine*
Trade Name	*Xylocaine Astra Pharma-ceutical Products*	*Citanest Astra Pharma-ceutical Products*	*Carbocaine Breon Laboratories Inc.*	*Marcaine Breon Laboratories Inc.*	*Duranest Astra Pharma-ceutical Products*
pk_a	7.9	7.9	7.6	8.1	7.7
% of Protein Binding (mg/ml plasma)	64	55	77	95	95
Molecular Weight	234	257	246	288	276
Potency (Procaine = 1)	1.5–2.0 Varies with conc.	1.5–2.0 As lidocaine IV	2.0	8	
Toxicity (Procaine = 1)	1.0–1.4	S.C. 50% less than lidocaine	1.5	Greater margin of safety than lidocaine	As bupivacaine IV, SC half as toxic as bupivacaine
Onset	Fast	Fast	Fast	Intermediate	Fast
Duration	.75–3 hrs	.75–4 hrs		3–10 hrs	3–10 hrs
Use Topical	2–4%				
Infiltration	0.5–1%	1%	1%	0.25%	0.5%
Nerve Block	1–2%	1–2%	1–2%	0.25–0.75%	0.5–1.0%
Epidural	1–2%	1–3%	1–2%	0.25–0.75%	0.5–1.5%

TABLE 15–2. Suggested Toxic Arterial Blood Levels and Doses of Local Anesthetics

	Seizure Activity-Threshold					Preseizure Activity	
	Cat	Dog		Monkey		Man	
	Dose (mg/kg)	Arterial Blood Level (μg/ml)	Dose (mg/kg)	Arterial Blood Level (μg/ml)	Dose (mg/kg)	Arterial Blood Level (μg/ml)	Dose (mg/kg)
Mepivacaine	22	9–20		22	18–21	5–6 20.5 (convulsions)	5
Lidocaine	8–22		27	23–26	14–23	5–8 19.6 (convulsions)	6–7 >55 μg/kg/ min (convulsions)
Bupivacaine	3–6	2–8		6	4–5	>4	
Tetracaine							2.5
Procaine	45		100			13	18–20
Chloroprocaine							23
Prilocaine	35			21	18		

(From Steen, P.A., and Michenfelder, J.D.: Neurotoxicity of Anesthetics—Review. Anesthesiology, 50:437, 1979.)

nerve blocking action by local anesthetics, which held that the larger the diameter of an axon, the more resistant it is to local anesthetic. Although B fibers are more sensitive to local anesthetics than pain-conducting C or delta fibers, it was still held that B fibers were an exception and that large-diameter A fibers were more resistant to local anesthetics than were nonmyelinated C fibers. Gissen et al. (1980) proposed that the larger the diameter of an axon, the more susceptible it may be to conduction block by local anesthetics. They indicated that large-diameter fibers with longer internodal distance should be blocked at lower concentrations of local anesthetics than should small-diameter fibers. Their studies were, however, conducted at room temperature and not body temperature.

When one is anesthetizing a peripheral nerve, differential blockade may occur. Pain may be overcome completely (i.e., the delta and the C fibers blocked), but motor function and touch (alpha and beta fibers) remain unaffected. A more concentrated anesthetic solution is necessary to achieve motor block in addition to sensory block. Once the local anesthetic has been deposited about the nerve, it diffuses from the outside toward the nerve center. The outer parts of the nerve, the mantle fibers, are thus anesthetized first and the core fibers last. The latter fibers in a nerve supplying a limb, for instance, are those that innervate the distal limb; thus, anesthesia spreads in a distal direction. The process is reversed during recovery. The opposite occurs during intravenous regional anesthesia. Anesthetic is delivered to the nerve via centrally located vessels, and a core-to-mantle diffusion gradient is established (de Jong, 1979). Sensations disappear in the following order: pain, cold, warmth, light touch, joint, proprioception, and deep pressure. They return in approximately the reverse order. This is most dramatically experienced in spinal or epidural procedures.

Pharmacology

Local anesthetic agents fall into two categories: 1) agents with an ester link between the aromatic end of the molecule and the intermediate chain; these are similar to procaine, and 2) agents with an amide-link; these are similar to lidocaine. Pharmacologic activity is influenced primarily by lipid solubility, protein binding, pK_a, and vasodilator activity. Increased protein binding is believed responsible for increased duration of action. Since the base form is responsible for diffusion across the nerve sheath and the charged form causes conduction blockade, agents with a lower pK_a, such as lidocaine, possess a more rapid onset of action than agents such as bupivacaine, tetracaine, and procaine (Covino, 1979). All local anesthetics except cocaine cause peripheral vasodilation, thereby enhancing vascular absorption. Absorption also varies with site of injection, dosage, concurrent use of a vasoconstrictor, and the specific agent employed. The blood level of locally administered anesthetic agents is related to the total dose of drug administered rather than volume or concentration.

Following absorption, local anesthetics distribute in total body water. There is initial rapid clearance from the blood related to uptake by vessel-rich tissues, and a slower disappearance rate due to distribution to more slowly perfused tissues, metabolism, and excretion. Ester or procaine-like agents are hydrolyzed in plasma by the enzyme pseudocholinesterase. These same procaine-like anesthetics, which are derivatives of p-aminobenzoic acid, have an antisulfonamide action. They are thus contraindicated during sulfonamide therapy which impedes the utilization of p-aminobenzoic acid in organisms sensitive to sulfonamide. The amide or lidocaine-like agents undergo enzymatic degradation and conjugation primarily in the liver. Less than 5% of unchanged amide drugs are excreted in the urine (Covino, 1979).

When one is considering duration of action, local anesthetics are categorized into three groups: 1) Procaine and 2-chloroprocaine have a relatively short duration of action (30 to 60 minutes). 2) Mepivacaine, lidocaine, and prilocaine have an intermediate duration (90 to 240 minutes). 3) Tetracaine, bupivacaine, and etidocaine are agents with longer duration (180 to 600 minutes). There remains a need for a drug with ultralong duration of analgesia, preferably for several days with no effect on motor function. Efforts to delay release of anesthetic have been unsuccessful. Recently, the epidural or intrathecal use of opiates for pain relief has shown promise. Duration of postoperative pain relief, up to 72 hours, has been reported following a single epidural injection of 2 to 10 mg of morphine in man. This is believed to be related to activation of opiate receptors in the spinal cord (Covino, 1981). Delayed respiratory depression has, however, been reported. Scurlock and Curtis (1981) have synthesized ultralong-acting analgesic agents that are derivatives of tetraethylammonium. Average duration of analgesia was approximately 16 days with nerve blocks in rats. These were reversible, and no toxicity was observed. These agents are thought to act at the potassium channels in the nerve membranes in addition to initially acting at the sodium channels.

VASOCONSTRICTORS

In 1903 H. Braun discovered that when epinephrine hydrochloride was added to local anesthetic solutions, anesthesia was greatly prolonged. This prolongation occurs with all injectable local anesthetics in use at present. The effect of epinephrine is to produce a marked vasoconstriction; hence, the anesthetic is removed from the site of injection more slowly. Uptake of lidocaine is reduced more than other amide-linked agents (Atkinson et al., 1977). This results in longer anesthetic action and decreases the toxicity of the anesthetic, since it can be detoxified over a longer period of time. The maximum safe concentration of epinephrine with a local anesthetic agent is 1:50,000; greater concentration may cause local tissue necrosis. An exception to this rule is in epidural anesthesia where concentrations up to 1:10,000 may be safely used. It is probably unnecessary to use a strength greater than 1:200,000. Intrathecal epinephrine is avoided by some because of the danger of neural ischemia (Atkinson et al., 1977). Other vasoconstrictors employed less frequently are phenylephrine hydrochloride and cobefrin hydrochloride. They do not have any real advantage over epinephrine (Tainter et al., 1938).

Vasoconstrictors are contraindicated in extremities because the ischemia produced may cause gangrene. If volatile anesthetics (especially halothane) are administered concurrently with a local anesthetic containing epinephrine, beta-blocking agents should be available and hypoxia and hypercarbia avoided because of possible ventricular fibrillation.

HYALURONIDASE

Hyaluronidase is a mucolytic enzyme that hydrolyzes hyaluronic acid, the ground substance preventing diffusion of foreign materials in the tissues. When hyaluronidase is added to solutions of local anesthetics, it promotes diffusion and absorption. In therapeutic doses it is nontoxic, the ratio of toxic to therapeutic dose being 200:1 (Seifter, 1950).

For infiltration anesthesia, hyaluronidase is used in a concentration of 100 to 150 TRU (turbidity reducing units) per 100 ml of anesthetic solution. The efficiency of a local anesthetic is increased since the area affected is enlarged. Outwardly, it would seem to be of particular value in nerve blocks, in that the anesthetic would not have to be deposited so accurately. However, Moore (1950) and Eckenhoff and Kirby (1951) found that hyaluronidase did not increase the incidence of successful blocks. On the other hand, the duration of anesthesia is decreased and the toxicity increased due to more rapid absorption. This can be counteracted by addition of epinephrine to the solution. When such a combination is used for infiltration anesthesia, the area of skin anesthetized is roughly doubled (Booth, 1977). Hyaluronidase does not increase the efficiency of solutions used for epidural or spinal anesthesia. Because of its cost, it is seldom used with local anesthetic agents in animals.

TOXICITY OF LOCAL ANESTHETICS

With respect to the use of local anesthetic agents in humans, Adriani (1956) has said:

> Few potentially hazardous drugs are used as thoughtlessly, as indiscriminately, and with less knowledge of their applied pharmacology, as are

the local anesthetics. The number of fatalities and near catastrophes from the misuse of these drugs is difficult to estimate because statistics are not accurate. The number of fatalities and various types of untoward responses is higher than one surmises.

Fortunately, with the exception of primates, the problem of toxicity from local anesthetics is not as great in animals as it is in man. Documented deaths in animals from injection of local anesthetics are uncommon and usually confined to very small or young animals.

Toxic symptoms produced by all local anesthetic agents are similar, though toxic and lethal doses vary widely (Tables 15–2, 15–3, and 15–4). Untoward responses are of two types: local and systemic. Local damage consists of transient or permanent injury to the tissues. The accepted drugs currently in use do not generally produce this difficulty. An example of local tissue damage is in equine lameness blocks where bandaging is necessary to reduce inflammatory swelling. Nerves may be damaged from direct intraneural injection or from extended exposure to concentrated anesthetic solutions. Single and especially repeated exposures are detrimental to wound healing, an observation supported by cytotoxic studies (Sturrock and Nunn, 1979). In isolated nerve trunks, irreversible block can be produced (Steen and Michenfelder, 1979).

Anesthetic toxicity is usually due to inadvertent rapid intravenous injection or extravascular administration of an excessive dose. Toxicity is influenced by such factors as route of administration, acid-base status, absorption, tissue distribution, metabolism, and species. Prilocaine and lidocaine are similar in terms of anesthetic potency and rapid IV toxicity. Prilocaine is approximately 60% less toxic than lidocaine following subcutaneous administration because of its slower absorption and more rapid clearance. There is an inverse relationship between P_{CO_2} level and convulsive threshold of local anesthetic agents. The convulsive threshold of procaine in cats decreases from 35 mg/kg to 15 mg/kg when Pa_{CO_2} is elevated from 25 to 40 mm Hg to 65 to 81 mm Hg. Susceptibility to convulsions is related to the degree of development of the CNS, primates being the most susceptible (Booth, 1977).

In regional block procedures, the anesthetic is deposited near a nerve or spinal root. Much of the perineurally injected anesthetic is absorbed into the blood. The concentration in the blood reaches a peak in as little as 5 minutes or as long as 60 minutes after injection depending upon vascularity and absorption, then falls as the drug is eliminated, redistributed, and biotransformed. Systemic reactions occur when local anesthetics are absorbed into the general circulation in toxic levels. Although all are ultimately absorbed, under ordinary circumstances a toxic level is not attained and no systemic effects occur.

In general, reactions are avoided by: 1) limiting the total quantity of drug used, 2) using dilute solutions, 3) retarding absorption by addition of a vasoconstrictor, and 4) administering

TABLE 15–3. The Intravenous Toxicity of a Series of Local Anesthetic Agents to Mice, Guinea Pigs, and Rabbits (Results Are Expressed as LD_{50}, in Terms of Mg of Base/Kg of Body Weight)

Agents	*Mice*	*No. of Animals*	*Guinea Pigs*	*No. of Animals*	*Rabbits*	*No. of Animals*
Procaine	78 ± 5	60	56 ± 4	25	41 ± 2	25
Neothesin	32 ± 4	40	16 ± 2	30	18 ± 6	35
Hexylcaine	24 ± 2	60	17 ± 2	25	14 ± 2	20
Cocaine	25 ± 4	40	13 ± 2	20	11 ± 1	15
Butacaine	19 ± 2	40	10 ± 2	25	10 ± 1	25
Tetracaine	9 ± 1	40	4 ± 0.25	50	4.5 ± 1	25
Dibucaine	6.5 ± 0.7	40	2.8 ± 0.2	40	2.8 ± 0.5	25

(From Beyer, K.H., Latven, A.R., Freyburger, W.A., and Parker, M.P.: A Comparative Study of the Activity and Toxicity of Hexylcaine (1-Cyclohexylamino-2-Propylbenzoate): A New Local Anesthetic Agent. J. Pharmacol. Exp. Ther., 388:93, 1948.)

TABLE 15–4. The Subcutaneous Toxicity of Local Anesthetic Agents Dissolved in Aqueous Solution and (for Guinea Pigs) in 1:50,000 Solution of Epinephrine Hydrochloride (Results Are Expressed as LD_{50}, in Terms of Mg of Base/Kg of Body Weight)

	Mice		Guinea Pigs				Rabbits	
Agent	Aqueous Soln.	No. of Animals	Aqueous Soln.	No. of Animals	Epinephrine Soln.	No. of Animals	Aqueous Soln.	No. of Animals
Procaine	720 ± 64	70	353 ± 18	25	500 ± 146	25	595 ± 56	20
Neothesin	1140 ± 96	50	255 ± 33	20	305 ± 98	20	385 ± 45	25
Hexylcaine	1080 ± 213	60	146 ± 15	25	385 ± 40	25	164 ± 31	25
Cocaine	140 ± 21	40	27 ± 3	25	87 ± 7	25	70 ± 2	25
Butacaine	110 ± 12	70	39 ± 8	25	71 ± 7	20	30 ± 8	30
Tetracaine	64 ± 8	70	19 ± 6	20	78 ± 11	20	13 ± 2	20
Dibucaine	32 ± 3	90	18 ± 2	20	35 ± 4	30	7 ± 1	25

(From Beyer, K.H., Latven, A.R., Freyburger, W.A., and Parker, M.P.: A Comparative Study of the Activity and Toxicity of Hexylcaine (1-Cyclohexylamino-2-Propylbenzoate): A New Local Anesthetic Agent. J. Pharmacol. Exp. Ther., 388:93, 1948.)

a central nervous system depressant prior to anesthesia.

When the concentration of local anesthetic in the general circulation reaches the toxic level, two types of symptoms may be seen either singly or together. These are 1) cardiovascular and 2) central nervous types.

The cardiovascular type of reaction is caused by decreased cardiac output due to depression of the myocardium, bradycardia, direct local vasodilation, and indirect conduction blockade of autonomic nerve fibers. Thus, there is peripheral vasodilation with profound hypotension and circulatory collapse. Severe hypotension is also a complication of subarachnoid or high epidural anesthesia with attendant thoracolumbar preganglionic blockade. Vasopressors administered intravenously will overcome the hypotension.

The central nervous type is characterized by initial excitation followed by CNS depression due to inhibition of cortical neurons. Apprehension, excitement, and nausea or vomiting usually are seen before convulsions occur. Additional anesthetic may cause cessation of convulsions, respiratory arrest, and flattening of the brain wave pattern (Covino, 1979). Bupivacaine, tetracaine, and etidocaine are the most toxic in terms of convulsive activity. Benzodiazepines or short-acting barbiturates are used to counteract the convulsive action of local anesthetics. Care should be exercised in their use, since depression, coma, and respiratory and circulatory failure follow the convulsive seizures. Barbiturates counteract the central nervous system stimulation, but do not neutralize local anesthetics or hasten their detoxification and elimination.

Recently diazepam has gained favor for either prevention or therapy of the convulsive action of local anesthetics. Studies using this drug in cats, mice, and monkeys have demonstrated an increase in seizure threshold to as much as double the toxic dose of local anesthetic (Steen and Michenfelder, 1979).

Respiratory stimulants (analeptics) are contraindicated for treatment of the apnea. Local anesthetics depress the central nervous system, which does not respond to these stimulants. Controlled respiration and oxygen should be administered.

Although local anesthetics cross the placenta rapidly, probably by simple diffusion, drug concentrations in the fetus and neonate are generally low and do not cause significant clinical depression. Large doses may produce excessive fetal and neonatal blood levels with cardiovascular and central nervous system toxicity. Thus, small doses of local anesthetics that are rapidly metabolized, such as procaine or 2-chloroprocaine, and highly protein-bound, such as bupivacaine and etidocaine, may offer further protection. When lidocaine is infused intravenously into lambs, the onset of seizure activity occurs when fetal arterial blood levels reach 6.9 to 40.0 μg/ml of lidocaine. Susceptibility to such seizures increases with gestational age; susceptibility of the ewe and term fetus is similar. Bradycardia has been reported in sheep fetuses with high levels of mepivacaine and within 60 seconds of a single intravenous injection of 14 to 37 μg/kg of lidocaine. Since uterine blood flow is crucial to the evironment of the fetus, it is pertinent that local anesthetics at toxic blood levels constrict uterine vessels. This constriction may also be increased in ewes by the injection of 0.10 to 1.00 μg/kg/min of epinephrine. When uterine blood flow is reduced sufficiently, fetal asphyxia results. Fetal monkeys have tolerated a reduction in mean maternal arterial pressure to 50 mm Hg but not to 40 mm Hg or lower (Ralston and Shnider, 1978).

COCAINE HYDROCHLORIDE, U.S.P.

From a practical standpoint, the significance of cocaine to veterinary anesthesiology is historical. Cocaine has the disadvantage of being toxic to the tissues when injected; therefore, newer less toxic, nonaddictive, synthetic "caines" have supplanted its use.

Cocaine in 2 to 4% aqueous solution produces good surface anesthesia of the cornea and conjunctiva. In addition, it causes a vasoconstriction of superficial vessels and mydriasis. Occasionally, it may produce corneal irritation with cloudiness and even ulceration. For this reason, proparacaine, lidocaine, or tetracaine are more generally used. Five to 10% cocaine hydrochloride solutions have also been used for topical anesthesia of the equine larynx. Since cocaine and its derivatives are habit-forming, they are subject to the federal narcotic laws and may be purchased only by individuals possessing a narcotic license.

PROCAINE HYDROCHLORIDE, U.S.P. (NOVOCAIN)

Procaine hydrochloride was first synthesized by Einhorn in 1905. Because procaine was the first of the synthetic local anesthetics to be used clinically, it has served as a criterion for newer local anesthetic drugs. It is an ester-linked local anesthetic. Procaine is not as active as cocaine but is only about one-fourth as toxic.

TABLE 15–5. Average Minimal Lethal Dose of Procaine Hydrochloride (in g/kg)

	Route of Administration	
Species	*Subcutaneous*	*Intravenous*
Guinea Pig	0.43	0.05
Rabbit	0.46	0.055
Cat	0.45	0.045
Dog	0.25	—

(Graubard, D.J., and Peterson, M.C.: *Clinical Uses of Intravenous Procaine.* Courtesy of Charles C Thomas, Publisher, Springfield, Illinois, 1950.)

Procaine hydrochloride is a white, crystalline, water-soluble powder. Solutions are relatively stable, can be sterilized repeatedly by boiling without loss of potency, but should be refrigerated to retard hydrolysis. Solutions containing epinephrine are sensitive to heat, air, and sunlight. Those that have begun to deteriorate have a yellowish tint and should be discarded. Procaine hydrochloride solutions have a pH of approximately 6.0 when fresh; on standing they become more acid.

Lethal doses of procaine for four species are listed in Table 15–5.

Intravenous procaine hydrochloride has been used in man for treatment of spastic muscles, inflammatory conditions, and cardiac arrhythmia. In dogs, Jones (1951) found that up to 6 mg/kg could be safely injected intravenously in a 20-minute period without disturbing the animals. However, this dose did not produce analgesia, and convulsive muscular contractions were seen at levels producing analgesic effect. The heart rate was increased and became regular. For dogs, the minimum lethal dose of intravenous procaine hydrochloride injected within 5 seconds was approximately 100 mg/kg of body weight. At necropsy, an enlarged liver and engorged spleen were found along with a variable hyperemia of the lungs and kidneys. A rapid intravenous injection of procaine in dogs produces respiratory failure (Hulpieu and Cole, 1951). Oxygen and controlled respiration are often life-saving.

The pharmacokinetics and behavioral effects of procaine given intravenously and intramuscularly to horses have been studied by Tobin et al. (1976, 1977). Rapid intravenous injection of 1 g of procaine hydrochloride in a Thoroughbred mare produces excitement for as long as 4 minutes. Initial blood concentrations range from 0.5 to 1.0 μg/ml. Horses proved to be at least 20 times more sensitive to the central stimulant action of procaine than are humans.

Procaine is hydrolyzed to para-aminobenzoic acid (PABA) and diethylaminoethanol (Fig. 15–1). In the dog, procaine is converted rapidly into these end products which are then eliminated by the kidneys; the procaine blood level itself is not significantly lowered by the kidneys. According to Dunlop (1935), in nephrectomized dogs the end products may be found in the blood as long as the animal survives. The liver is not essential for the detoxification of procaine since other tissues are able to convert it into these end products. However, the liver detoxifies procaine more rapidly and efficiently than other tissues.

Procaine is used for infiltration, conduction, and spinal anesthesia in animals. Without added vasoconstrictor, the duration is relatively brief because of rapid absorption and destruction by the tissues. One or two percent solutions are generally employed; 4% solutions are more commonly used in large animals. One ml of epinephrine hydrochloride solution, U.S.P. (1:1,000), added to each 99 ml of anesthetic solution will give a concentration of 1:100,000. Procaine is sometimes combined with tetracaine hydrochloride to increase potency and duration of action. Procaine is not an effective surface anesthetic, and therefore is seldom used for this purpose. It is contraindicated during sulfonamide therapy because of its relationship to p-aminobenzoic acid, and is lethal in the parakeet.

LIDOCAINE HYDROCHLORIDE (XYLOCAINE; LIGNOCAINE)

Lidocaine is an amide-linked local anesthetic and is chemically unrelated to cocaine, procaine, or derivatives of these substances. It is quite stable, even when boiled with strong acids or alkalies, and solutions may be autoclaved repeatedly if necessary. Goldberg (1947) found the absolute toxicity was greater than that of procaine but the security coefficient, which takes into account the therapeutic efficiency of both drugs, was 2 to 4 times greater than that of procaine. Bremer et al. (1948) have indicated that the onset of anesthesia is twice as rapid as that attained with procaine, and the duration exceeds that of procaine by 50% or more. The elimination half-life of intraveous lidocaine in the blood of adult, neonatal, and fetal sheep has been reported to be 31, 51, and 33 minutes respectively (Morishima et al., 1981). Metabolic clearance was the same in both adult and fetal sheep and approximated hepatic blood flow. It is biodegraded in the liver, diethylaminoacetic acid being the chief metabolite. As in the case of prilocaine, its metabolism can give rise to methemoglobin (Atkinson et al., 1977).

Use of 7.0 ml of 2% lidocaine for plantar nerve block in the horse has been shown to produce detectable saliva levels in 30 minutes. Values peaked at 20 to 24 hours and were not detectable at 48 hours. Urinary elimination occurred 7 to 48 hours after injection. A similar saliva and urine profile was observed after topical application. Lidocaine was not detectable in urine and saliva more than 72 hours after administration (Courtot, 1979). In dogs, the dose for epidural anesthesia is 1 ml/10 lb of 2% solution with epinephrine 1:100,000. In adult horses and cattle, up to 10 to 12 ml of 2%

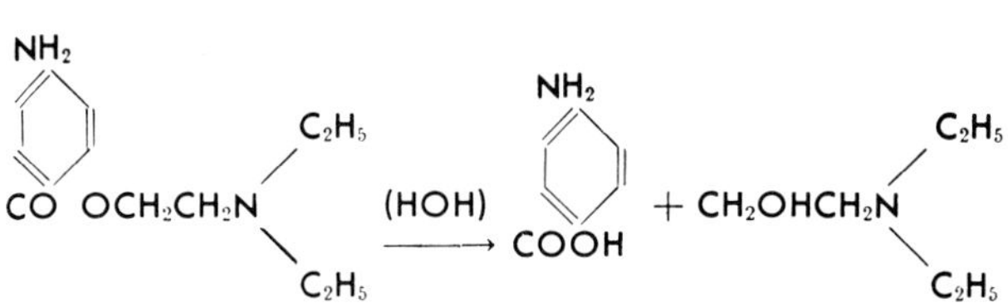

Procaine PABA Diethylaminoethanol

Figure 15–1. Procaine is hydrolized to para-aminobenzoic acid and diethylaminoethanol.

lidocaine hydrochloride can be used without the onset of incoordination of the rear limbs. For infiltration, 0.5% without epinephrine is suggested. In cats, for epidural anesthesia 2 ml of 2% solution with 1:100,000 epinephrine is the average dose. Four percent lidocaine is used for surface anesthesia of mucous membranes, particularly those of the throat and larynx, prior to endotracheal intubation. It is too concentrated to be used for injection, but may be used in the eye.

Lidocaine may also be given intravenously prior to intubation. It suppresses the cough reflex and mitigates the arterial hypertension and tachycardia seen with endotracheal intubation. Since a 10 to 28% reduction in halothane MAC has been observed in dogs with blood lidocaine levels between 3 and 10 μg/ml, prevention of cardiovascular stimulation by lidocaine may in part be due to an increase in the depth of anesthesia (Hamill et al., 1981). Combination of lidocaine (4 mg/lb) with sodium pentothal for induction of anesthesia in dogs has been found to provide similar benefits (Rawlings and Kolata, 1983). Use of lidocaine as an antiarrhythmic agent is discussed in Chapters 20 and 21.

The LD_{50} of lidocaine for mice is 48, 170, and 360 mg/kg of body weight when administered subcutaneously, intraperitoneally, and intravenously (Truant and Wiedling, 1958). When lidocaine was administered at the rate of 2 mg/kg/min, 5.8 ± 1.8 mg/kg intravenously were required to induce convulsions in sheep (blood concentration was 11.7 ± 2.0 μg/ml). Hypotension was induced with 31.2 mg/kg, respiratory arrest with 32.4 ± 2.8 mg/kg, and circulatory collapse with 36.7 ± 3.3 mg/kg (Morishima et al., 1981).

PRILOCAINE HYDROCHLORIDE (CITANEST)

Prilocaine hydrochloride is closely related chemically to lidocaine, is amide-linked, but derived from toluidine instead of xylidine. In animals, it has been shown that prilocaine possesses local anesthetic activity comparable to that of lidocaine but has a more prolonged action and induces less systemic toxicity (Wiedling, 1960; Astrom and Persson, 1961*a, b*). Lund and Cwik (1965*a*) found that lidocaine probably has greater penetration powers or diffusion capacity than prilocaine when used for epidural anesthesia in man. Prilocaine has a longer duration of action when injected either epidurally or intrathecally. Epidural prilocaine anesthesia in sheep is of similar duration to lidocaine anesthesia. Duration is longer following intrathecal use (Booth, 1977).

Large doses of prilocaine may cause stimulation and depression of the central nervous system along with depression of cardiovascular function; however, the amount required for equivalent effects is much greater than that of lidocaine (Wiedling, 1960; Sadove et al., 1964). Convulsions and cardiovascular depression are of shorter duration than those following lidocaine. The toxicity of prilocaine in several species of animals was determined to be from 20 to 50% less than that of lidocaine (Richter, 1958; Wiedling, 1960). Death following massive doses of prilocaine is due primarily to respiratory arrest rather than to cardiovascular depression, suggesting that death can be prevented by adequate resuscitation.

Lund and Cwik (1965*b*) investigated the methemoglobinemia associated with administration of large doses of prilocaine to man. They stated that this condition is not accompanied by dyspnea, tachycardia, or hypotension and does not respond to administration of oxygen. The maximum amount of methemoglobin forms within 1½ to 2½ hours after administration. It appears that methemoglobinemia is due to a metabolic breakdown product of prilocaine, o-toluidine, rather than to the drug itself (Fujimori and Nishimura, 1964; Onji and Tyuma, 1965).

In addition to interfering with direct transport of oxygen, methemoglobin also causes a left shift in the oxyhemoglobin dissociation curve. This can become clinically significant in extreme cases.

Methemoglobinemia can be treated with methylene blue. A 1% solution is given intravenously at a dose of 1 to 2 mg/kg of body weight over a 5-minute period. Methemoglobinemia occurs in cats with doses of 7.5 mg/kg of prilocaine and presumably with all other animal species. The advantages of prilocaine, such as high potency, prolonged action, and low relative systemic toxicity, must therefore be weighed against the potential hazards of an occasional methemoglobinemia (Onji and Tyuma, 1965). It is most useful in man when a high dosage and strong concentration are required of an analgesic drug, when injection is into a vascular area, or for local intravenous analgesia (Atkinson et al., 1977).

Prilocaine hydrochloride is supplied in 30-ml vials of 1 or 2% solution and ampules containing 1, 2, or 3% solution. All solutions contain sodium chloride, 6 mg/ml, and are adjusted to a pH of 6.0 to 7.0 with sodium hydroxide.

MEPIVACAINE HYDROCHLORIDE, U.S.P. (CARBOCAINE)

Mepivacaine is an amide-linked local anesthetic that was synthesized in 1956; it is soluble in water and 70% becomes protein-bound (slightly more than lidocaine). It is clinically comparable to lidocaine, 2 to 2.5 times as potent an analgesic as procaine with approximately 1 to 1.5 times its toxicity. It is slightly less toxic than lidocaine; its onset is slightly slower but its action is longer even without epinephrine. It is used for infiltration, intra-articular anesthesia, nerve block, and epidural anesthesia, a 2% solution having been found especially useful for equine nerve blocks, because there is less post-injection edema than with lidocaine. A 1% solution with epinephrine has been recommended for canine epidural anesthesia at a dose of 0.5 ml each 30 seconds until caudal digital reflexes are lost; surgical analgesia to T_5 is thus induced (Perrson, 1970). Mepivacaine has also been used for topical anesthesia of the equine larynx.

BUPIVACAINE HYDROCHLORIDE U.S.P. (MARCAINE)

Bupivacaine is an amide-linked local anesthetic, a homologue of mepivacaine that was synthesized in 1957. It is of high potency, has a long duration of action, and is stable. Onset of action is rapid and anesthesia lasts several hours (5 to 16 hours in man). It is four times more potent than mepivacaine and lidocaine (Atkinson et al., 1977). Bupivacaine hydrochloride is supplied in 0.25%, 0.5%, and 0.75% solutions and is used in man for infiltration, nerve block, and epidural block.

ETIDOCAINE HYDROCHLORIDE (DURANEST)

Etidocaine is a local anesthetic of the amide type. Compared to lidocaine, it has greater lipid solubility and protein binding capacity. It has a rapid onset (3 to 5 minutes) and prolonged duration (5 to 10 hours) in laboratory animals. Etidocaine is metabolized by the liver and its metabolites are excreted via the kidney. It is indicated for infiltration, nerve block, and epidural anesthesia, and provides especially strong motor blockage (Booth, 1977; Covino, 1979).

HEXYLCAINE HYDROCHLORIDE (CYCLAINE)

Hexylcaine hydrochloride is soluble to a concentration of 12% in water; 1% solution is stable on boiling, autoclaving, and storage at room temperature. One percent solution has a pH of 3.9.

Hexylcaine hydrochloride is an ester-linked anesthetic, is 4 to 8 times more active than procaine, and produces anesthesia of longer duration probably because it is more slowly hydrolyzed. Experimental and clinical investigations have shown it to have a comparatively low order of toxicity (Beyer et al., 1948).

One percent solution is suggested for infiltration and nerve blocks; a 2% solution may be used in large animals. For topical anesthesia of the eye, 1 or 2% solutions are recommended. Five percent hexylcaine is used in the ear for removal of grass awns and in the vagina for catheterization.

For epidural anesthesia in cattle, horses, and dogs, 0.2 to 0.6, 0.2 to 0.4, and 0.5 to 1.0 mg/lb have been recommended, respectively.

BUTACAINE SULFATE. U.S.P. (BUTYN)

Butacaine sulfate is a white, crystalline, water-soluble powder that is ester-linked and closely related chemically to procaine. Solutions are used for surface anesthesia of mucous membranes and the cornea. It has a rapid onset of action, penetrates well, and has a fairly long duration of anesthesia. It does not cause mydriasis or damage to the cornea, as is sometimes produced by cocaine, but does slow corneal healing. It is no longer widely used. Because it is approximately 9 times more toxic than procaine, it is never used for infiltration anesthesia.

Butacaine sulfate is usually used as a 2% solution that is instilled in the eye or applied on any mucous membrane. When it is applied in the eye once, minor anesthesia is produced. If it is instilled four times at 1-minute intervals, surgical anesthesia is produced.

Solutions must be stored in brown bottles to prevent deterioration.

Butacaine sulfate ointment, N.N.R. for local use, contains 1% of the anesthetic.

TETRACAINE HYDROCHLORIDE, U.S.P. (PONTOCAINE)

Tetracaine hydrochloride, an ester-linked anesthetic, is a white crystalline substance easily precipitated from solution by bases. Crystals or solutions should not be autoclaved.

Although it has been employed as an all-purpose anesthetic, its systemic toxicity is 12 to 20 times that of procaine, and its anesthetic potency is no more than 10 times the latter. For this reason, its use is confined chiefly to topical application. As a surface anesthetic, its potency is 10 times greater than that of cocaine. Along with its potency, the toxicity is also high, but tetracaine gives the most profound topical anesthesia of the commonly used agents. For anesthesia of the cornea and of mucous membranes, a 0.5% solution is adequate. It should not be used in conjunction with sulfonamides.

PROPARACAINE HYDROCHLORIDE (OPHTHAINE)

Proparacaine hydrochloride, an ester-linked topical anesthetic, has a potency similar to or slightly greater than that of tetracaine, and is available as a 0.5% solution. It induces little or no local irritation, its action is rapid, and its effect lasts approximately 15 minutes. Some local irritation may occur several hours after instillation. Surface analgesia develops in less than 1 minute. In man, it has been used for cataract surgery, in which case a longer induction period is required. One drop of a 0.5% solution is recommended at 5- to 10-minute intervals for 5 to 7 times. It has also been used for topical analgesia of the nose and ear, for wounds, and prior to catheterization. Softening and erosion of corneal epithelium and conjunctival congestion have been observed after its use in man. Allergic reactions are rare. Proparacaine is currently the topical agent of choice for corneal anesthesia.

ETHYL ALCOHOL

When injected into soft tissue, 5 ml of absolute alcohol causes an area of necrosis 1 cm in diameter. When it is injected around a nerve, neuritis and degeneration occur, followed by sclerosis. Thirty percent alcohol temporarily destroys sensory nerves which regenerate in time. The duration of block depends on the size of the nerve and degree of destruction.

According to Adriani (1947), destruction of nerve tissue with alcohol is similar to that obtained by sectioning a nerve and is typical of wallerian degeneration. Small unsheathed nerves may be permanently destroyed, whereas large heavily sheathed nerves are only temporarily affected. Since nerves regenerate, after a variable period of time function may return. Fibrosis that accompanies the injection may predispose to neuritis.

ETHYL CHLORIDE, U.S.P.

Ethyl chloride is occasionally used as a local anesthetic. For this purpose, it is marketed under pressure in containers equipped with a fine capillary nozzle and a control valve that allows the liquid to be sprayed from the container (Fig. 15–2). As it is sprayed on the skin, it evaporates instantly, removing heat in the process and caus-

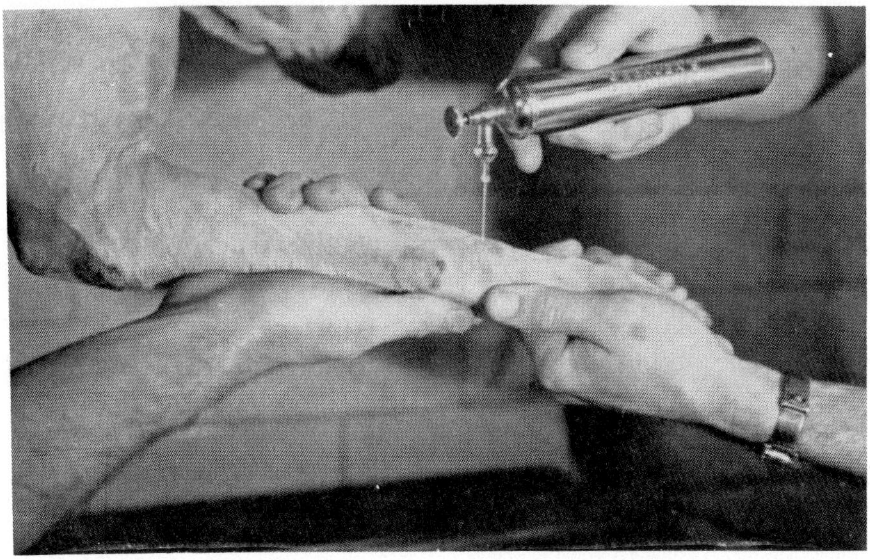

Figure 15–2. Ethyl chloride is sprayed on the skin to produce surface anesthesia.

ing an area of skin to freeze. Surface anesthesia lasting from 30 to 60 seconds is produced. Overzealous administration produces frostbite. Because the anesthesia is superficial and of short duration, and because frozen tissue is not easily dissected, its use is confined to simple incisions or punctures such as the drainage of abscesses. Healing may be delayed and tissues damaged.

REFERENCES

Adriani, J.: *Local Anesthetics*. Merck, Sharp & Dohme Seminar Report, Fall, 1956.

Adriani, J.: *Techniques and Procedures of Anesthesia*. Charles C Thomas, Springfield, Illinois, 1947.

Astrom, A., and Persson, N.H.: The Toxicity of Some Local Anesthetics after Application on Different Mucous Membranes and Its Relation to Anesthetic Action on the Nasal Mucosa of the Rabbit. J. Pharmacol. Exp. Ther., 132:87, 1961*a*.

Astrom, A., and Persson, N.H.: Some Pharmacological Properties of O-Methyl-a-Propylamino-propionanilide; A New Local Anaesthetic. Br. J. Pharmacol., 16:32, 1961*b*.

Atkinson, R.S., Rushman, G.B., and Lee, J.A.: *A Synopsis of Anaesthesia*, 8th ed. Year Book Medical Publishers, Chicago, 1977.

Beyer, K.H., Latven, A.R., Freyburger, W.A., and Parker, M.P.: A Comparative Study of the Activity and Toxicity of Hexylcaine (1-Cyclohexylamino-2-Propylbenzoate): A New Local Anesthetic Agent. J. Pharmacol. Exp. Ther., 93:388, 1948.

Booth, N.H.: Local Anesthetics. In *Veterinary Pharmacology and Therapeutics*, 4th ed. Edited by L.M. Jones, N.H. Booth, and L.E. McDonald. Iowa State University Press, Ames, 1977.

Bremer, G., Ekmanner, S., Persson, H., and Standberg, N.: Xylocaine: A New Local Anesthetic. Br. Dent. J., 85:278, 1948.

Courtot, D.: Elimination of Lignocaine in the Horse. Ir. Vet. J., 33:205, 1979.

Covino, B.G.: Pharmacology of Local Anesthetics, Lecture #208, Annual Refresher Course Lectures, Am. Soc. Anesthesiol., 1979.

Covino, B.G.: Editorial Views: Ultra-Long Acting Anesthetic Agents. Anesthesiology, 54:263, 1981.

de Jong, R.H.: Physiology of Local Anesthesia. Lecture #207, Annual Refresher Course Lectures, Am. Soc. Anesthesiol., 1979.

Dunlop, J.G.: The Fate of Procaine in the Dog. J. Pharmacol. Exp. Ther., 55:464, 1935.

Eckenhoff, J.E., and Kirby, C.K.: The Use of Hyaluronidase in Regional Nerve Blocks. Anesthesiology, 12:27, 1951.

Fujimori, M., and Nishimura, K.: Methemoglobin Due to Local Anesthetics (A Preliminary Report). Far East J. Anesth., 4:4, 1964.

Gissen, A.J., Covino, B.G., and Grequs, J.: Differential Sensitivities of Mammalian Nerve Fibers to Local Anesthetic Agents. Anesthesiology, 53:467, 1980.

Goldberg, L.: Pharmacological Properties of Xylocaine. Svensk. Tandl.-Tidskr., 40:819, 1947.

Hamill, J.F., Bedford, R.F., Weaver, D.C., and Colohan, A.R.: Lidocaine before Endotracheal Intubation: Intravenous or Laryngotracheal? Anesthesiology, 55:578, 1981.

Hulpieu, H.R., and Cole, V.V.: Effects of Oxygen Analeptics and Artificial Respiration on the Toxicity of Procaine. Proc. Soc. Exp. Biol. Med., 76:62, 1951.

Jones, L.M.: The Toxic and Analgesic Effects of Procaine Hydrochloride Administered Intravenously in the Dog. Vet. Med., 46:93, 1951.

Lund, P.C., and Cwik, J.C.: Citanest: A Clinical and Laboratory Study. Part 1. Anesth. Analg., 44:623, 1965*a*.
Lund, P.C., and Cwik, J.C.: Methemoglobinemia: A Clinical and Laboratory Study. Part 2. Anesth. Analg., 44:712, 1965*b*.
Moore, D.C.: An Evaluation of Hyaluronidase in Local and Nerve Block Analgesia: A Review of 519 Cases. Anesthesiology, 11:470, 1950.
Morishima, H.O., Pedersen, H., Finster, M., Sakuma, K., Bruce, S.L., Gutsche, B.B., Stark, R.I., and Covino, B.G.: Toxicity of Lidocaine in Adult, Newborn, and Fetal Sheep. Anesthesiology, 55:57, 1981.
Onji, Y., and Tyuma, I.: Methemoglobin Formation by a Local Anesthetic and Some Related Compounds. Acta Anaesthesiol. Scand., 16:151, 1965.
Perrson, F.: Epidural Analgesia in Dogs with Special Reference to Intra-Arterial Blood Pressure. Acta Vet. Scand., 11:186, 1970.
Ralston, D.H., and Shnider, S.M.: The Fetal and Neonatal Effects of Regional Anesthesia in Obstetrics. Review Article. Anesthesiology, 48:34, 1978.
Rawlings, C.A., and Kolata, R.J.: Cardiopulmonary Effects of Thiopental/Lidocaine Combination during Anesthetic Induction in the Dog. Am. J. Vet. Res., 44:144, 1983.
Richter, A.W.: Estimation of the I.V. Mean Lethal Dose for Mice by a Constant Infusion Titration. Acta Pharmacol., 15:37, 1958.
Sadove, M.S., Rosenberg, R., Heller, F.N., Stortz, M.J., and Albrecht, R.F.: Citanest, A New Local Anesthetic Agent. Anesth. Analg., 43:527, 1964.
Scurlock, J.E., and Curtis, B.M.: Tetraethylammonium Derivatives: Ultralong-acting Local Anesthetics? Anesthesiology, 54:265, 1981.
Seifter, J.: Studies on the Pharmacology and Toxicology of Testicular Hyaluronidase. Ann. N.Y. Acad. Sci., 52:1141, 1950.
Steen, P.A., and Michenfelder, J.D.: Neurotoxicity of Anesthetics—Review. Anesthesiology, 50:437, 1979.
Strichartz, G.: Molecular Mechanisms of Nerve Block by Local Anesthetics. Anesthesiology, 45:421, 1976.
Sturrock, J.E., and Nunn, J.F.: Cytotoxic Effects of Procaine, Lignocaine and Bupivacaine. Br. J. Anaesth., 51:273, 1979.
Tainter, M.L., Throndson, A.H., and Moore, S.M.: Vasoconstrictors on the Clinical Effectiveness and Toxicity of Procaine Anesthetic Solutions. J. Am. Dent. Assoc., 25:1321, 1938.
Tobin, T., Blake, J.W., Sturma, L., Arnett, S., and Truelove, J.: Pharmacology of Procaine in the Horse. Pharmacokinetics and Behavioral Effects. Am. J. Vet. Res., 38:637, 1977.
Tobin, T., Blake, J.W., Tai, C.Y., Sturma, L., and Arnett, S.: Pharmacology of Procaine in the Horse: Procaine Esterase Properties of Equine Plasma and Synovial Fluid. Am. J. Vet. Res., 37:1165, 1976.
Truant, A.P., and Wiedling, S.: A Contribution to the Pharmacological and Toxicological Evaluation of a New Local Anesthetic, dl-*N*-Methylpipecolyl-2-6-Xylidide. Acta Chir. Scand., 116:351, 1958.
Wiedling, S.: Studies on *a*-*N*-Propylamino-2-Methylpropionanilide: New Local Anaesthetic. Acta Pharmacol., 17:233, 1960.

CHAPTER 16

Local Anesthesia and Nerve Blocks

TOPICAL ANESTHESIA

Local anesthetic agents applied to the unabraded skin surface have no effect, and even when applied to raw skin surfaces of animals, these agents are often of dubious value. This is due, in part, to the natural tendency of animals to lick wounds and keep them clean.

Nevertheless, local anesthetics frequently are used in combination with other therapeutic agents in a cream or jelly to produce surface anesthesia and thus prevent scratching, licking, chewing, and rubbing of inflammatory conditions such as dermatitis, otitis externa, conjunctivitis, and granulating wounds. On mucous surfaces, the anesthetic effect is good. For example, anesthetic ointments are generally quite effective in treatment of pruritus ani. Jellies are useful in lubricating endotracheal catheters, as they help prevent laryngospasm and postintubation cough. When instilled in the eye, local anesthetics produce good surface anesthesia and suppress blepharospasm.

Topical anesthesia is employed to produce surface anesthesia of the conjunctiva and cornea for minor surgical procedures, tonometry, and beta ray therapy. When one is using anesthetics in the eye, it is important to consider that some, especially tetracaine, may cause sensitization, and that butacaine, cocaine, dibucaine, phenacaine, and proparacaine delay corneal epithelialization, whereas 2% piperocaine and 2% lidocaine cause no delay. Proparacaine (0.5%) is considered the corneal anesthetic of choice and 4% lidocaine is probably second (Severin, 1976). Because proparacaine causes a transient corneal roughening (30 to 60 minutes), ophthalmoscopy should be performed before its use. For research purposes, Nixon et al. (1977) monitored anesthesia of the eye by electroencephalography. Test agents were instilled into the eye via an indwelling subpalpebral lavage apparatus.

Local anesthetics are frequently used topically to lubricate and anesthetize mucous surfaces for procedures such as nasal, lacrimal, endotracheal, and urethral catheterization, and for otic examination.

Solutions may be injected into the urethra of animals suffering from obstruction due to calculi with good results. Anesthetizing the mucous membrane relieves spasm and facilitates passage of stones. Solutions may be injected into joint cavities or bursae to aid in the diagnosis of lameness. Injection sites are those used for intrasynovial injection of other medication. In addition to these applications, topical anesthetics are commonly used for laryngeal and teat surgery in large animals.

INFILTRATION AND FIELD BLOCK

Infiltration and field block anesthesia are used chiefly for removal of small superficial tumors, débridement and suturing of wounds, laparotomy, cesarean section, tail amputation, vulval suturing, teat surgery, diagnostic and surgical procedures of the lower limb of the horse, and realignment of fractures.

Tumors, Wounds, and Cutaneous Biopsies

The surgical site should be clipped and washed, and a suitable antiseptic applied to the skin. Injection of local anesthetic is made with a syringe to which a fine caliber needle is attached. In most small animal patients, a 1- or 1½-inch, 22-gauge needle is suitable, while in large animals 1½- to 8-inch, 20- to 16-gauge needles are commonly used. The needle is held with the bevel against the skin and the shank at an acute angle as it is inserted. An intradermal wheal can be raised prior to insertion of the needle into the subcutaneous tissue. Such wheals are not usually used in large animals. When injections are made with the needle in a fixed position, aspiration should be performed to determine that the point is not within a blood vessel. If, on aspiration, blood returns to the syringe, the point of the needle must be repositioned. Infiltration of subcutaneous tissue may be continuous if the needle is kept constantly in motion.

When removing a small tumor or similar lesion, the anesthesiologist makes a diamond-shaped block by linear infiltration of anesthetic agent as shown in Figure 16–1. This is accomplished by holding the needle practically parallel to the skin surface and injecting anesthetic as the needle is advanced its full length. The deep tissues are infiltrated by injections around the periphery so that they form a cone, the apex of which is directly beneath the lesion. Time required for development of anesthesia varies according to the local anesthetic selected. The block should be tested prior to surgery.

Infiltration anesthesia is contraindicated in malignant tumors since the infiltration procedure may transplant tumor cells to otherwise normal tissues. Results are poor when anesthetic is infiltrated into inflamed tissues because of acidic conditions with impaired dissociation of the anesthetic.

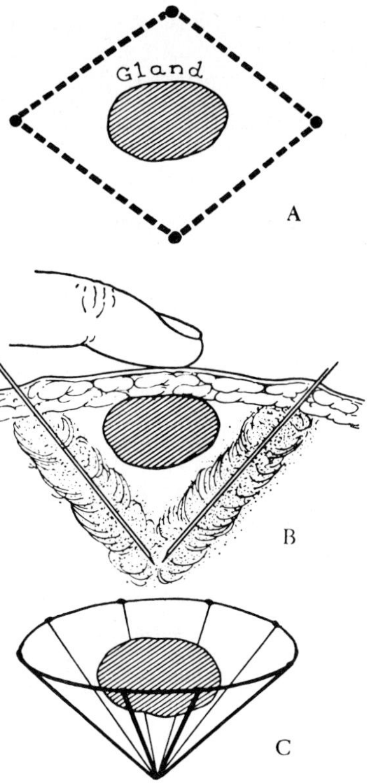

Figure 16–1. Field block for biopsy of lymph node (or for equivalent operation). *A*, Outline on cutaneous surface of diamond-shaped field block. *B*, Node is continuously palpated throughout the injection to avoid losing it. *C*, A cone of anesthetic is deposited around the node. (From Lundy, J.S.: *Clinical Anesthesia*. W.B. Saunders Co., Philadelphia, 1942.)

Laparotomy (Celiotomy)

Local infiltration or field block anesthesia in conjunction with preanesthetic sedation is used for cesarean section in the dog. When the dog appears tranquilized, lidocaine or other appropriate local anesthetic is injected at three levels along the incision line using a 1-inch 22-gauge needle. The first level is in the deep layer of the skin and produces a skin bleb. The second is in the deep subcutaneous tissue, and the third in the muscle. The injection is fanned out at the ends of the incision. Approximately 3 ml of 2% lidocaine are used for a 20-pound dog. Others use 0.5 to 1% lidocaine or 0.5 to 2% procaine. In the event anesthesia of relatively long duration is required, epinephrine may be incorporated in the anesthetic and/or the upper range of anesthetic concentration used.

A profoundly tranquilized bitch should be removed from the puppies for 3 to 4 hours postoperatively, since she may chew and kill them before tranquilization subsides.

In large animals, especially cattle, infiltration of the abdominal wall with 1 to 2% lidocaine or 1 to 4% procaine is commonly used for cesarean section and laparotomy. As in cesarean section of the bitch, it is necessary to infiltrate the various layers of the abdominal wall. When anesthetizing the bovine flank, one commonly employs a field block. The line of infiltration is shaped like an inverted "L," horizontally beneath the lumbar transverse processes, and vertically behind the last rib. Although sensation to the flank region is thus blocked (field block), the anesthetic is not injected directly into the tissues to be incised. Impaired wound healing is thus less likely.

Advantages claimed for the use of local infiltration are reduced risk for patients having a poor prognosis, and simplicity with minimal risk of recumbency in the bovine.

Disadvantages of local infiltration and field block for laparotomy both in large and small animals include incomplete anesthesia, especially of the peritoneum, and unsatisfactory muscle relaxation. Optimal conditions for surgery are thus reduced, and the potential for such complications as hemorrhage and contamination is increased.

Ring Block

A ring block is a field block in which the soft tissues around an extremity are infiltrated to induce anesthesia distally.

A use for ring block is in amputation of puppies' tails. This is performed by depositing a ring of anesthetic around the tail proximal to the amputation site. Two precautions should be observed if this procedure is used. First, the small size of most puppies precludes the use of large quantities of local anesthetic agent. Toxic symptoms and even death occur with large doses. Second, vasoconstrictors should not be used in the anesthetic solution, since it is possible to compromise the blood supply of the tail close to the site of infiltration with resulting necrosis of tissue proximal to the amputation site.

A ring block using 1 to 2% lidocaine, or 1 to 2% mepivacaine is commonly used for surgery of the equine and bovine limbs. A tourniquet applied proximal to the site of injection enhances the efficiency of the block.

INTRAVENOUS REGIONAL ANESTHESIA OF THE LIMB

Despite description of this technique as early as 1908, intravenous anesthesia of the limb was not widely used. Only since the introduction of lidocaine has it been reassessed and its use become commonplace. After adequate sedation, a tourniquet is applied to the limb. A sphygmomanometer cuff is appropriate. In the bovine, in which this technique has become popular, the tourniquet may be applied above (Prentice et al., 1974) or just below the carpus and hock (Knight, 1980). After appropriate preparation of the site, 10 to 30 ml of 2% lidocaine or mepivacaine are injected into an accessible vein (e.g., radial, metatarsal). Complete anesthesia occurs in the distal limb in approximately 5 to 10 minutes in more than 80% of cases. Speed of onset of anesthesia is related to the volume injected. After completion of the operation, the tourniquet is released and sensation returns in 3 to 5 minutes, but evidence of partial anesthesia may persist for 30 minutes. In man, peak plasma levels after cuff release are 20 to 80% lower than when the same dose is given directly into a vein, and are inversely proportional to tourniquet time (Atkinson et al., 1977). Similar low peak plasma levels have been observed after tourniquet release in calves (Bogan and Weaver, 1978). Knight (1980) indicated that the tourniquet should not be left on cattle longer than 60 minutes; Prentice et al. (1974) found tourniquet application safe for 75 minutes. No toxic signs were observed. The technique has also been used in sheep, goats, and pigs (Knight, 1980) and dogs (Hall, 1971). Donchin et al. (1980) indicated that the procedure induced acidosis of the occluded limb, which was corrected by injection of sodium bicarbonate into the same vein. Sodium bicarbonate also suppressed the rate at which the concentration of anesthetic (bupivacaine) decreased after tourniquet release; this decrease may prolong residual analgesia.

CONDUCTION ANESTHESIA

Nerve blocks in small animals have never been popular among veterinarians because, although good anesthesia of an area is achieved, restraint is often a problem. Since more satisfactory anesthetic techniques are available, dental nerve blocks have largely been abandoned. In large animals, however, conduction anesthesia is used not only for surgery but also for diagnosis, prognosis, and even therapy. Paravertebral and ophthalmic blocks are commonly used in cattle, whereas in the horse nerve blocks of the limbs are used most frequently.

Conduction Anesthesia of the Head

Infraorbital Nerve

Dog. The infraorbital nerve supplies all upper teeth on its respective side. It can be blocked at two sites:

1. The first site is in the pterygopalatine fossa at its point of entry into the infraorbital canal (maxillary foramen). In the average dog, a 2-inch 20-gauge needle is inserted about 1 inch below the lateral canthus of the eye with the point directed medially, between the malar bone anteriorly and the coronoid process of the mandible posteriorly, until the border of the malar bone has been passed. Then the needle is pointed anteriorly toward the gingival border of the upper incisor teeth (Fig. 16–2). The maxillary foramen is encountered at a depth of 1 to 1½ inches (Frank, 1928). Two ml of 2% procaine or its equivalent are injected. All of the upper teeth on that side of the head will be desensitized.

Lacroix (1957) has described an alternative method in which the needle is inserted from within the mouth.

> "The syringe is introduced just posterior to and parallel with the long axis of the last molar tooth. The solution is injected slowly as the needle is

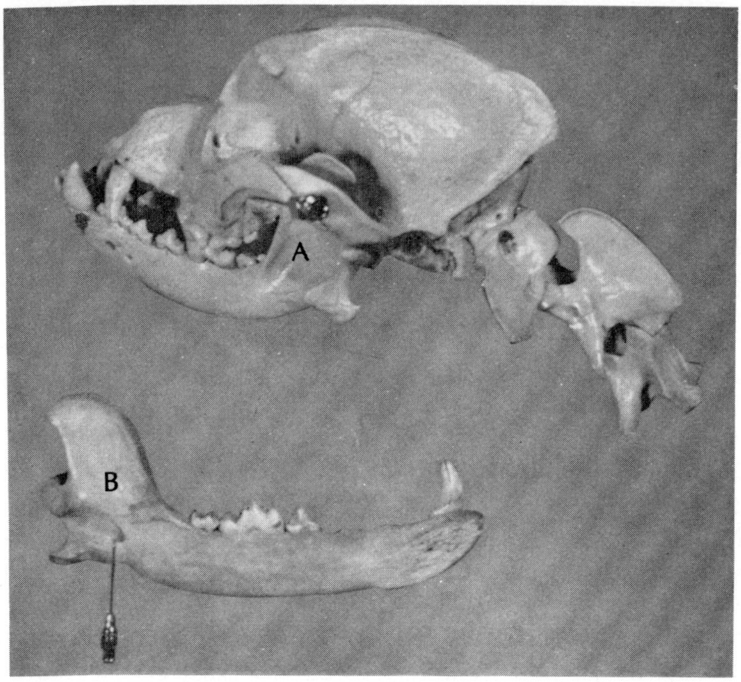

Figure 16–2. Locations for blocking the maxillary (A) and mandibular (B) nerves in the dog. Medial aspect of mandible is shown.

pushed into the tissues. The depth of penetration varies with the size of the subject. A needle one inch in length is sufficient for the largest dog. . . ."

2. The infraorbital nerve can also be blocked in the lower part of the infraorbital canal. The upper lip is retracted and the infraorbital foramen is located by palpation of its border, dorsal to the third premolar, where the mucous membrane of the lip reflects on the gum. After preparation of the gum, the needle is inserted into the canal about one-half inch, and 1 ml of 2% procaine or its equivalent is injected. The incisors, canine, and first two premolars of that side are desensitized.

Horse. The infraorbital nerve of the horse may be blocked at three sites: 1) at the infraorbital foramen, 2) within the infraorbital canal, and 3) within the pterygopalatine fossa at its point of entry (maxillary foramen) into the infraorbital canal.

1. Blockade at the infraorbital foramen anesthetizes the skin of the lip, nostril, and face to the level of the foramen. The foramen lies approximately 1 to 2 cm superior to the midpoint of an imaginary line between the anterior extremity of the facial crest and the nasomaxillary notch. The lip of the foramen can usually be palpated beneath the levator nasolabialis muscle. After suitable preparation of the site, a 20-gauge 2.5- to 5.0-cm needle is inserted to the lip of the foramen and 5 to 10 ml of 2% mepivacaine or equivalent are injected.

2. If the needle is inserted into the canal, the canine and incisor teeth, with associated alveoli and gum, and the skin below the medial canthus of the eye are anesthetized. For this procedure a 5- to 8-cm 18- to 20-gauge needle is inserted 1 to 3 cm anterior to the foramen and threaded into the infraorbital canal, and 5 to 10 ml of 2% mepivacaine or equivalent are injected.

3. To anesthetize the skin of the nose and upper lip and the osseous part of the upper jaw with teeth and gums, the infraorbital nerve is blocked as it enters the canal. Prior to entering the infraorbital canal, it is termed the maxillary nerve. After preparation of the site, a 10-cm 18- or 20-gauge needle is inserted 2 to 3 cm below

the lateral canthus of the eye (just ventral to the facial crest) in a medial slightly dorsoanterior direction. The needle is passed along the posterior surface of the maxillary tuberosity to the maxillary foramen, and penetrates 6 to 8 cm. Injection of 10 ml of 2% mepivacaine or equivalent is adequate. If the needle is ventrally located, the maxillary artery may be punctured, and blood will flow from the needle.

Cow. See the discussion of ophthalmic nerve block.

Mandibular Nerve

Dog. This nerve supplies the teeth of the lower jaw and can be blocked at two sites:

1. The first site is at the mandibular foramen. The depression just in front of the angular process of the mandible is palpated. A 1-inch 22-gauge needle is inserted at right angles to the ventral border of the jaw just medial to the bone, for a distance of one-half to three-fourths inch (Frank, 1928). Two ml of mepivacaine or equivalent are deposited at this site. All the teeth on that side of the lower jaw are desensitized.

Lacroix (1957) has described an alternative approach from within the mouth. The needle is inserted medial and parallel to the long axis of the sixth molar with the point inclined toward the mandible. The anesthetic is deposited in the tissues around the nerve by gauging the relative positions of the needle and nerve.

2. The second site is through the mental foramen. There are three mental foramina: anterior, middle, and caudal. The middle one is used for this procedure. The foramen is situated immediately beneath the anterior root of the second lower premolar, about one-half the distance between the dorsal and ventral borders of the mandible. The opening cannot be felt with the finger, and a search must be made with the needle point. The needle is inserted about three-eighths inch into the foramen, and 1 ml of 2% lidocaine solution or equivalent is injected into the mandibular canal. The incisors, canine, and first two premolars on that side are desensitized.

The position of the various foramina in the three head shapes observed in dogs varies considerably. In addition, there are anastomoses between sides so that complete block of the incisors on a given side may not occur.

Horse. As in the dog, the mandibular nerve is blocked at either the mandibular or mental foramen. Blockade at the former anesthetizes the lower jaw, lip, and teeth. The foramen lies at the intersection of two imaginary lines: continuation of the anterior border of the supraorbital process and continuation of the inferolateral border of the upper molars. A 10- to 15-cm 18-gauge needle is inserted at the ventromedial border of the mandible and directed along its medial border of the mandible until the foramen is reached. Ten to 15 ml of 2% mepivacaine or other suitable anesthetic are deposited about this location.

Should anesthesia of the lower lip only be required, this can be accomplished by blockade at the mental foramen. If anesthesia of the lower incisors is necessary, anesthetic can be injected via this foramen into the mandibular foramen. Hall (1971) states that this is difficult, and failure may result. The lateral border of the foramen can be palpated beneath the depressor labii inferioris of the lower lip and on the lateral border of the ramus below the middle of the interdental space. The nerve is anesthetized at the foramen with 5 ml of 2% mepivacaine or equivalent.

Cornual Nerve Block

Cow The cornual nerve is a terminal branch of the ophthalmic division of the trigeminal nerve. Blockade, which is indicated for dehorning in ruminants, was first described by Emmerson (1933) and later modified by Browne (1938).

The site of injection lies midway along a line joining the center of the orbit and the base of the horn (Fig. 16–3). The lateral border (frontal crest) of the frontal bone is palpated and a 20-gauge 3- to 4-cm needle is inserted in a downward and inward direction keeping as close to the frontal crest as possible. Since the nerve is more superficially located close to the horn, Browne (1938) suggested that the injection should be made at the facial crest but only 2 to 3 cm anterior to the base of the horn. At this location the nerve is 0.5 to 1 cm below the skin, and the needle should only penetrate skin and

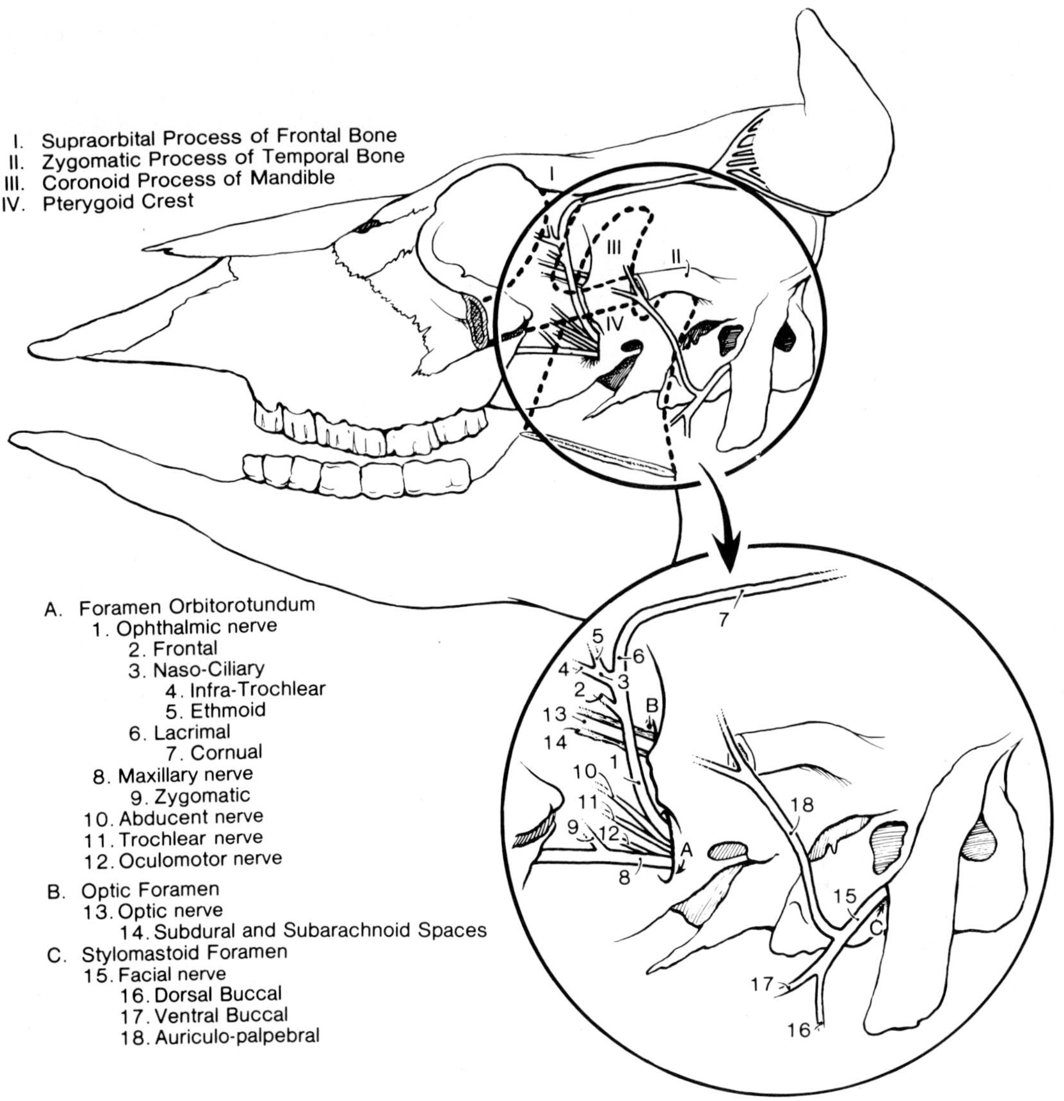

Figure 16–3. Innervation of the eye and eyelid.

cutaneous muscle. Five ml of 2% lidocaine or equivalent are usually adequate for this nerve block. In large cattle, a second injection 1 cm behind the first to block the posterior division of the nerve is indicated.

Goat. The horns of the goat are innervated by cornual branches of the lacrimal and infratrochlear nerves (Fig. 16–4). The former is blocked behind the root of the supraorbital process and as close as possible to the caudal ridge of the root of this process. The latter is blocked as close as possible to the dorsomedial margin of the orbit where the nerve is sometimes palpable (Vitums, 1954).

Conduction Anesthesia of the Eye and Associated Structures

Cow. A nerve block for surgery of the bovine eye, including enucleation, was described by Peterson (1951), who has subsequently modified this slightly (Peterson, 1966). The nerves blocked (Fig. 16–3) are:

1. Auriculopalpebral branch (motor) of the facial nerve.

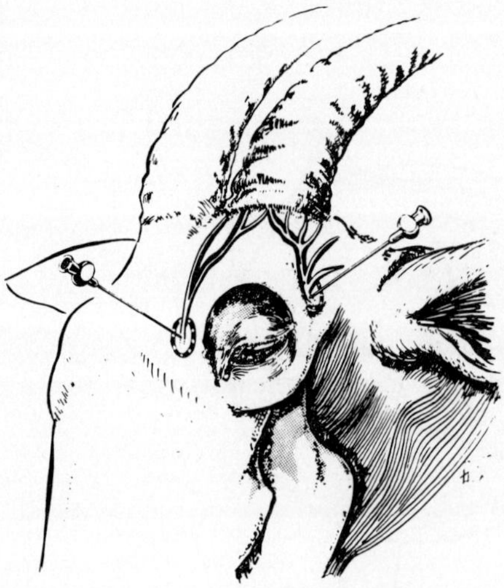

Figure 16–4. Nerve blocks for dehorning goats. The cornual branches of both the lacrimal and infratrochlear nerves must be blocked. (From Hall, L.W., and Clarke, K.W.: *Veterinary Anaesthesia,* 8th ed. Baillière Tindall, London, 1983.)

2. Maxillary branch of trigeminal nerve (sensory) innervating the lower eyelid, soft and hard palate, the nasal cavity, maxilla and adjoining bones, the maxillary sinus, and the region supplied by the infraorbital nerve.
3. Ophthalmic branch of the trigeminal nerve (sensory) innervating the horn (cornual), the upper eyelid, third eyelid, medial canthus, caudal part of nasal septum, cornea, sclera, and frontal sinus.
4. Oculomotor, trochlear, and abducens nerves, which provide motor innervation to the ocular muscles.

Since these nerves, with the exception of the auriculopalpebral, pass through the foramen orbito rotundum, anesthetic is deposited just anterior to this foramen (Peterson, 1951). A slightly curved 12- to 15-cm 16- or 18-gauge needle is inserted in the caudal angle formed by the supraorbital process and the zygomatic arch, and is directed horizontally for 7 to 11 cm until it strikes the floor of the pterygopalatine fossa just anterior to the foramen orbito rotundum. Maintaining the horizontal plane prevents puncture of the subarachnoid space surrounding the optic nerve. Should the needle strike the pterygoid crest at a depth of 5 to 7 cm, it is redirected slightly craniad. Since the bony floor of the pterygopalatine fossa is quite thin, care should be taken to avoid perforation and deposition of anesthetic into the pharynx. Once the needle contracts this bony plate, it is retracted approximately 1.0 cm, since the lateral pterygoid muscle separates the nerve from the bony plate. Ten to 15 ml of 2% lidocaine or equivalent are injected.

After emerging from the foramen orbito rotundum, the nerves pass in a more craniodorsad direction into the orbital cavity. The needle is partially withdrawn and redirected at about a 15° angle caudally and a 15° angle dorsally. It is inserted until the tip reaches the bony shelf separating the temporal fossa and orbital cavity. At this point, the tip is manipulated craniad until it slips off the shelf and penetrates an additional 0.7 to 1.5 cm. An additional 15 ml of 2% lidocaine or equivalent are injected. Upon withdrawal of the needle until the point is subcutaneous, it is redirected posteriorly along the zygomatic arch for 2 to 3 cm to block the auriculopalpebral nerve. Dilatation of the pupil is indicative of a satisfactory retrobulbar block. An alternate method of retrobulbar block is to insert a similarly curved needle through the upper or lower lid midway between the lateral and medial canthi. The needle is pushed dorsally or ventrally around the eyeball (Elmore, 1980).

When this procedure is performed for reasons other than enucleation of the eye, an ophthalmic ointment should be applied to prevent drying of the cornea.

Auriculopalpebral Nerve Block

This block is used to cause partial paralysis of the muscles of the eyelids, thereby facilitating examination and therapy, especially in large adult cattle. Immobilization of the lids may be incomplete owing to innervation of the upper and lower lid by branches of the oculomotor and buccal nerves.

Dog (Palpebral Nerve). The palpebral nerve is a branch of the auriculopalpebral which, in turn, is a branch of the facial nerve. It can be anesthetized by subcutaneous injection of 1 ml of a local anesthetic approximately 1 cm dorsal to the zygomatic arch at its most lateral projection. Anesthesia of all the muscles of the eyelids except the levator palpebrae will be produced. This is helpful in application of beta ray therapy to the cornea or in ocular surgery. Unless general anesthesia is also used, the animal is unable to close the eyelids but can still rotate and retract the eyeball. Ophthalmic ointment should be used to protect the cornea from drying.

Horse. The site of injection is situated 3 cm below the highest point of the dorsal border of the zygomatic arch. A 5-cm 20-gauge needle is inserted obliquely upward and inward to the dorsal border of the zygomatic arch and approximately 5 ml of 2% mepivacaine or equivalent are injected.

Cow. The superficial temporal vessels are palpated as they pass dorsally over the zygomatic arch, approximately halfway between the base of the ear and the angle between the supraorbital and zygomatic arches. The nerve is slightly superficial and caudad to these vessels. A 3- to 5-cm 18-gauge needle is inserted at this location to the zygomatic arch, and 5 ml of 2% mepivacaine or equivalent are injected as the needle is slowly withdrawn.

Conduction Anesthesia of the Forelimb

Dog

Block of the Brachial Plexus. Anesthesia of the brachial plexus in the dog has been described by Tufvesson (1951) who states that it is indicated for operative interference of the foreleg at, or below, the elbow joint. He indicates that luxations and fractures are easily reduced because of complete muscular relaxation.

With the skin prepared, a 3-inch 18-gauge needle is inserted in the triangular depression bounded by the anterior border of the supraspinatus muscle, the thoracic wall, and the dorsal border of the brachiocephalicus muscle. The needle is directed caudally, lateral to the thoracic wall and medial to the subscapularis muscle, until the point is even with the spine of the scapula. After aspirating to prevent intravascular injection, 10 ml of 2% lidocaine are deposited around the brachial plexus. In puppies and toy breeds, the dose is reduced accordingly. Paralysis is the first sign of anesthesia; full anesthesia requires 18 minutes and lasts 1 to 2 hours.

Radial Nerve. The radial nerve can be blocked where it spirals around the humerus from the medial to the lateral surface. In some dogs, the nerve can be palpated at this site, which is one-half the distance from the olecranon to the acromion. This is distal to the branches to the triceps brachii and produces paralysis of the extensors of the carpus and digits with anesthesia of the dorsal and lateral aspect of the forearm and the dorsal aspect of the paw.

Median, Ulnar, and Musculocutaneous Nerves. Together, the median and ulnar nerves supply all flexors of the carpus and digits and are sensory to the carpal, metacarpal, and digital pads. The ulnar nerve supplies sensation to the caudal surface of the forearm and lateral side of the fifth digit. The musculocutaneous nerve supplies the biceps brachii and brachialis muscles and is sensory to the medial aspect of the forearm. In the middle of the humerus, all three nerves lie around the brachial vessels, the median and ulnar posterior to the brachial artery, and the musculocutaneous anterior.

For complete loss of sensation in areas supplied by the median and ulnar nerves, it is necessary to block both plus the musculocutaneous nerve, which supplies a branch to the median at the elbow. This is best accomplished by injecting the three nerves on the medial aspect of the humerus as they course distally accompanied by the brachial artery. Pulsation of the artery may serve as a guide. At least 2 ml of 2% lidocaine or equivalent solution should be infiltrated around the vessel, care being taken to prevent intravascular injection.

Horse

Block of the median, ulnar, and musculocutaneous nerves anesthetizes the forelimb distal to the carpus. The areas anesthetized are illustrated in Figure 16–5.

Median Nerve. This nerve is anesthetized 5 cm below the medial aspect of the elbow joint at the distal edge of the posterior superficial flexor muscle. The nerve accompanied by the median vessels is usually 1.5 to 3 cm deep at this point. A 3- to 5-cm 20-gauge needle is

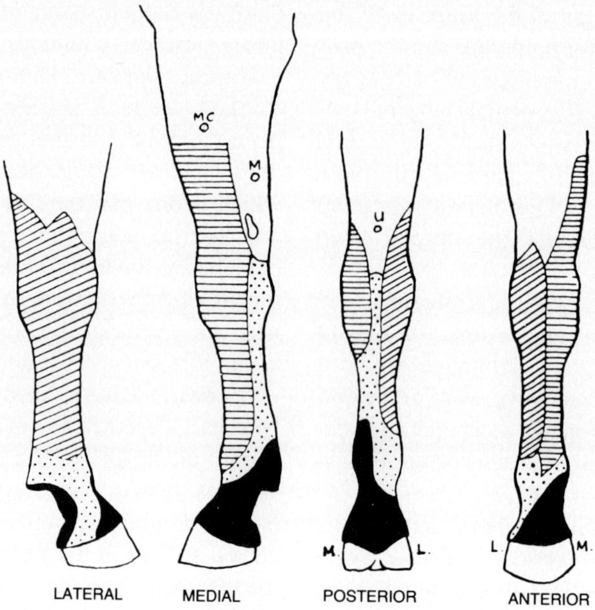

Figure 16–5. Desensitization of the forelimb of the horse by perineural injection (after W. Bolz). Median nerve (black); ulnar nerve (oblique lines); musculocutaneous nerve (transverse lines); and additional area desensitized when the three nerves are blocked simultaneously (spotted). (From Hall, L.W., and Clarke, K.W.: *Veterinary Anaesthesia*, 8th ed. Baillière Tindall, London, 1983.)

inserted in the groove between the posterior border of the radius and the anterior edge of the flexors of the carpus, in a slightly upward direction. The point of the needle should be kept close to the posterior border of the radius.

If the median vein is punctured, the needle should be withdrawn until it is just outside the vein before injection of 5 to 10 ml of 2% mepivacaine or equivalent.

Musculocutaneous Nerve. The site for injection is on the anteromedial aspect of the proximal antebrachial region. The main trunk of the nerve lies superficially over the radius and extensor carpi radialis muscle and in the angle between the cephalic and accessory cephalic veins. Mepivacaine (5 to 10 ml of 2%) is infiltrated subcutaneously between the two veins and just anterior to the accessory cephalic vein (Peterson, 1966).

Ulnar Nerve. Much of the area innervated by the ulnar nerve is also innervated by the median nerve. Ulnar nerve block is thus used in conjunction with median and musculocutaneous nerve blocks. To block this nerve, 5 to 10 ml of 2% mepivacaine or equivalent are injected one hand's-breadth above the accessory carpal bone and slightly lateral to it, in the depression between the ulnaris lateralis and the flexor carpi ulnaris. At this location, the nerve lies at a depth of 1.0 to 2.0 cm.

Anterior, Lateral, and Posterior Cutaneous Antebrachial Nerves. Peterson (1966) recommends concurrent blockade of these nerves, since the proximal areas of the carpus are not fully anesthetized by block of the musculocutaneous, median, and ulnar nerves. Mepivacaine (5 to 10 ml of 2%) is the anesthetic of choice.

The anterior cutaneous antebrachial nerve innervates the skin of the anterior forearm. The nerve is blocked subcutaneously over the deltoid process of the humerus and in the angle between the biceps brachii and the lateral head of the triceps.

The lateral cutaneous antebrachial nerve lies subcutaneously and is anesthetized just below the lateral head of the triceps and halfway between the deltoid tuberosity and the lateral epicondyle of the humerus. The resulting block denervates the skin of the lateral forearm and carpus.

The posterior cutaneous antebrachial nerve supplies sensation to the posterior aspect of the forearm. The nerve is blocked by the subcutaneous injection of anesthetic one hand's-breadth below the olecranon.

Volar (Metacarpal) and Plantar (Metatarsal) Nerves. These nerves supply sensation to the pastern, hoof, and most of the fetlock. They may be blocked either at the lateral and medial aspect of the fetlock joint where they can be palpated, or in the groove between the suspensory ligament and the deep flexor tendon. In the latter location, the nerves are blocked in the proximal or distal fourth of the metacarpus. The needle is inserted with the limb held up, or bearing weight. To avoid breaking the needle in the event of sudden movement, it is desirable to direct the needle proximally. Injection in the midmetacarpal region is contraindicated, because an anastomosing branch from medial to lateral volar nerve crosses the limb at this site and may escape blockade. Since the nerve lies beneath the deep fascia at a depth of 1.0 to 2.0 cm, appearance of a subcutaneous bleb during injection suggests that the needle point is too superficial. Although the nerve block may be performed from both lateral and medial approaches, some prefer to block both nerves via a lateral approach (Peterson, 1966). The lateral nerve is blocked with the aid of a 5- to 7-cm

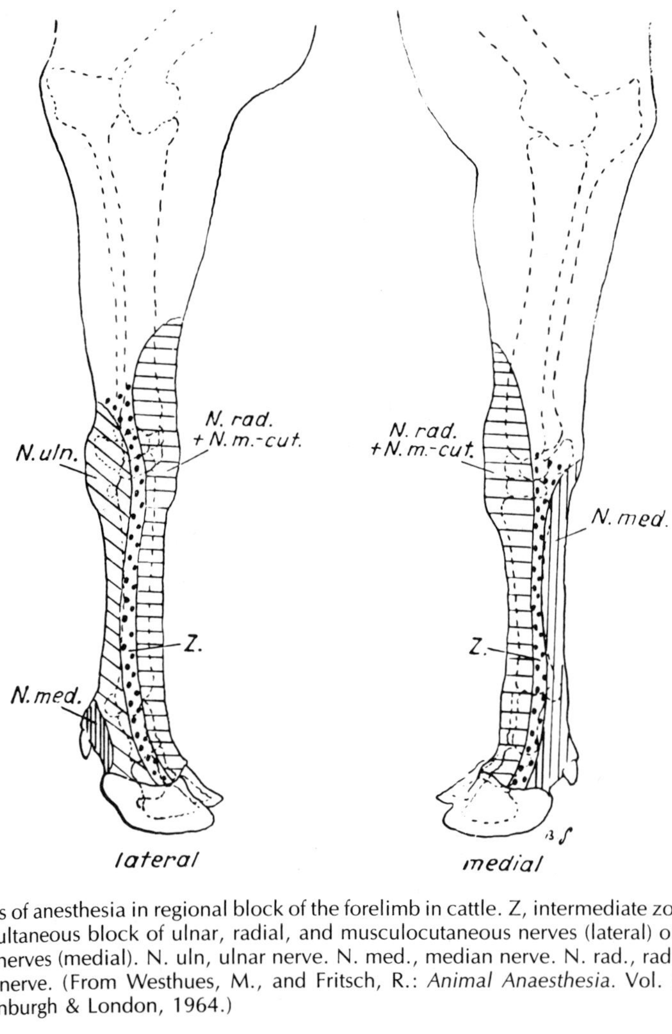

Figure 16–6. Areas of anesthesia in regional block of the forelimb in cattle. Z, intermediate zone, only anesthetized respectively by simultaneous block of ulnar, radial, and musculocutaneous nerves (lateral) or median, radial, and musculocutaneous nerves (medial). N. uln, ulnar nerve. N. med., median nerve. N. rad., radial nerve. N. m.-cut., musculocutaneous nerve. (From Westhues, M., and Fritsch, R.: *Animal Anaesthesia.* Vol. I. Local Anaesthesia. Oliver & Boyd, Edinburgh & London, 1964.)

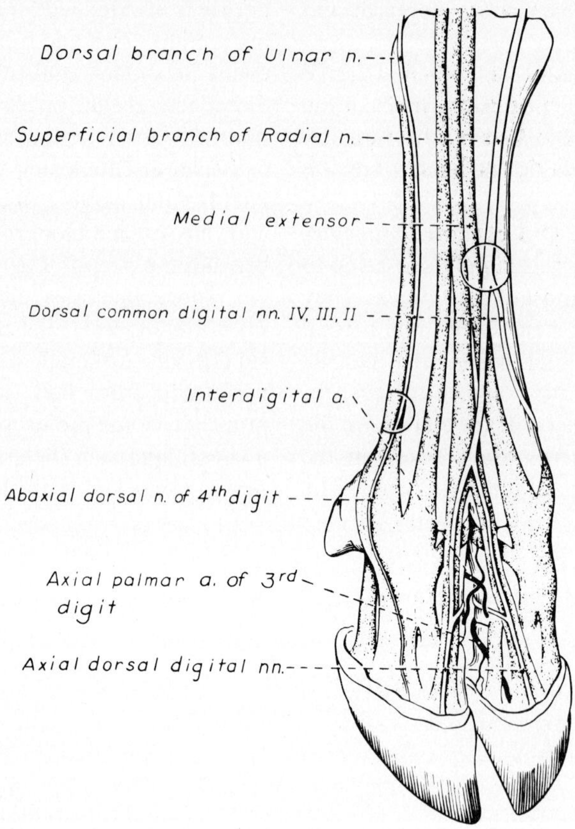

Figure 16–7. Right forefoot of the cow, dorsolateral aspect. (From Habel, R.E.: Guide to the Dissection of Domestic Ruminants, 2nd ed. Habel, Ithaca, N.Y., 1970.)

20-gauge needle that is then pushed straight through the space between the suspensory ligament and the deep flexor tendon until the point of the needle can be felt lightly on the medial side of the limb. After one has aspirated to ensure that the volar vessels have not been punctured, 5 to 10 ml of 2% mepivacaine are injected over the medial nerve. A branch supplying the anterior fetlock region passes just distal to the button of the splint bone and may be blocked at this location.

Digital (Posterior Digital) Nerve. This block is used to exclude sensation from the heels and the posterior two-thirds of the hoof. The nerve is anesthetized midway between the fetlock joint and the coronary band in the groove between the first phalanx and the deep flexor tendon. The nerve lies just posterior to the digital artery at a depth of 1.0 to 1.5 cm. At this location, the nerve lies in the superficial fascia but deep to the ligament of the ergot (Peterson, 1966). Mepivacaine (5 ml of 2%) is injected.

Cow

Brachial Plexus. Loss of sensation distal to the elbow joint may be induced by injection of local anesthetic over the ventral roots of the sixth to eighth cervical and first and second thoracic nerves as they pass over the lateral aspect of the middle third of the first rib (Westhues and Fritsch, 1964). An 18-gauge 16-cm needle is inserted at the level of the acromion of the scapula and 12 to 14 cm anterior to it. The needle is directed posteriorly and horizontally until it contacts the lateral aspect of the first rib, where 10 to 15 ml of 1 or 2% lidocaine or equivalent are injected. The needle is then withdrawn and redirected so that similar amounts are injected

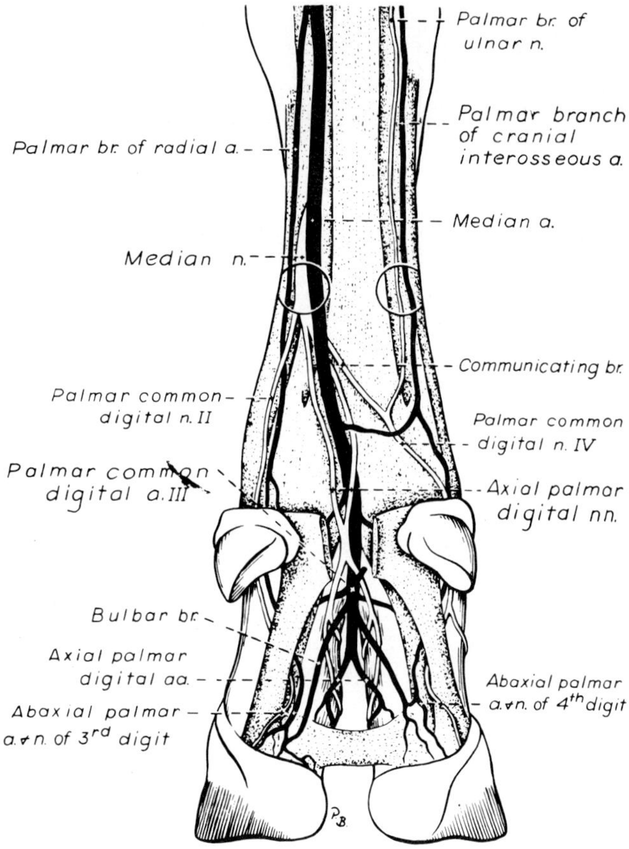

Figure 16–8. Right forefoot of the cow, palmar aspect. (From Habel, R.E.: uide to the Dissection of Domestic Ruminants, 2nd ed. Habel, Ithaca, N.Y., 1970.)

until a band of anesthetic 6 to 8 cm long has been injected along the rib and below the initial site. Care should be taken to preclude injection into one of the brachial vessels located adjacent to the distal third of the first rib.

Median and Ulnar Nerves. The median and ulnar nerves are palpated respectively just anterior and posterior to the medial epicondyle of the humerus at the elbow joint and beneath the superficial fascia. Lidocaine solution (25 to 35 ml of 2%) is injected beneath the fascia and over the nerves at these sites. The resulting nerve blocks anesthetize the posteromedial (volar-medial) surface of the metacarpus and the posterior (volar) surface of the digits (Westhues and Fritsch, 1964).

The ulnar nerve may also be blocked a hand's-breadth above the accessory carpal bone in a location similar to that used for ulnar block in the horse.

Cutaneous Medial and Dorsal Antebrachial Nerves. The medial nerve is a branch of the musculocutaneous, while the dorsal nerve is a cutaneous branch of the radial nerve. Together these nerves innervate the medial and dorsal surfaces of the carpus and, in conjunction with the median and ulnar nerves, the limb distal to the carpus (Fig. 16–6). These nerves are blocked anteriorly a hand's breadth above the carpus by injection of 20 ml of 2% lidocaine in a band 4 to 6 cm wide adjacent to the radius. Alternatively, 10 ml of anesthetic are injected adjacent to the radius and medial to the tendon sheath of the extensor carpi radialis 6 to 8 cm above the radiocarpal joint. The needle is then directed medially around the radius for 4 to 5 cm and an additional 10 ml of anesthetic are injected (Westhues and Fritsch, 1964).

Digital Regions. Unlike the horse, blockade of the volar nerves is insufficient for induction

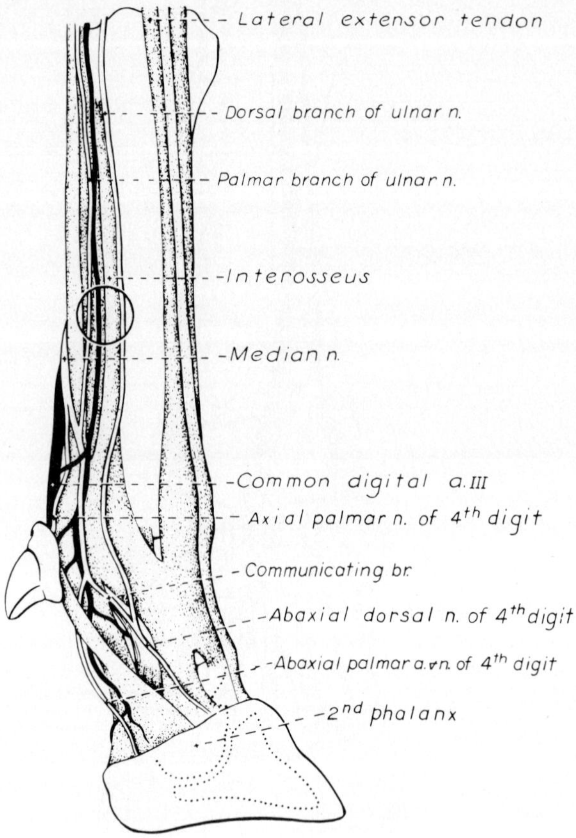

Figure 16–9. Right forefoot of the cow, lateral aspect. (From Habel, R.E.: Guide to the Dissection of Domestic Ruminants, 2nd ed. Habel, Ithaca, N.Y., 1970.)

of regional anesthesia of the digit, and it is necessary to block also the dorsal metacarpal branches of the radial, musculocutaneous, and ulnar nerves.

Dorsal Metacarpal Nerve (Superficial Branch of the Radial). This is a continuation of the radial nerve and is joined in the distal third of the forearm by the cutaneous branch of the musculocutaneous nerve. Alternatively, the cutaneous branch of the musculocutaneous may descend independently, adjacent to the superficial branch of the radial nerve. Below the midmetacarpal region the dorsal metacarpal nerve (superficial radial) can be palpated medial to the tendon of the medial digital extensor (Fig. 16–7), where it can be blocked by the injection of 10 to 15 ml of 2% lidocaine or equivalent beneath the fascia.

Medial Volar (Palmar) Nerve. This is a continuation of the median nerve (Fig. 16–8), which in the midmetacarpal region divides in a variable manner into three volar (palmar) digital nerves and part of a fourth (Habel, 1970). The nerve is blocked approximately one hand's-breadth below the carpus at the medial aspect of the superficial flexor tendon. A 5- to 7-cm 18-gauge needle is inserted dorsad and at right angles to the metacarpus, through skin and regional fascia to the medial border of the interosseous muscle (Westhues and Fritsch, 1964). Ten to 15 ml of 2% lidocaine solution are injected as the needle is slowly withdrawn.

Lateral Volar (Palmar) and Dorsal Ulnar Nerves. These nerves are blocked by the subfascial injection of 10 ml of 2% lidocaine or other appropriate local anesthetic both anterior and posterior to the interosseous muscle in the midmetacarpal region (Figs. 16–8 and 16–9).

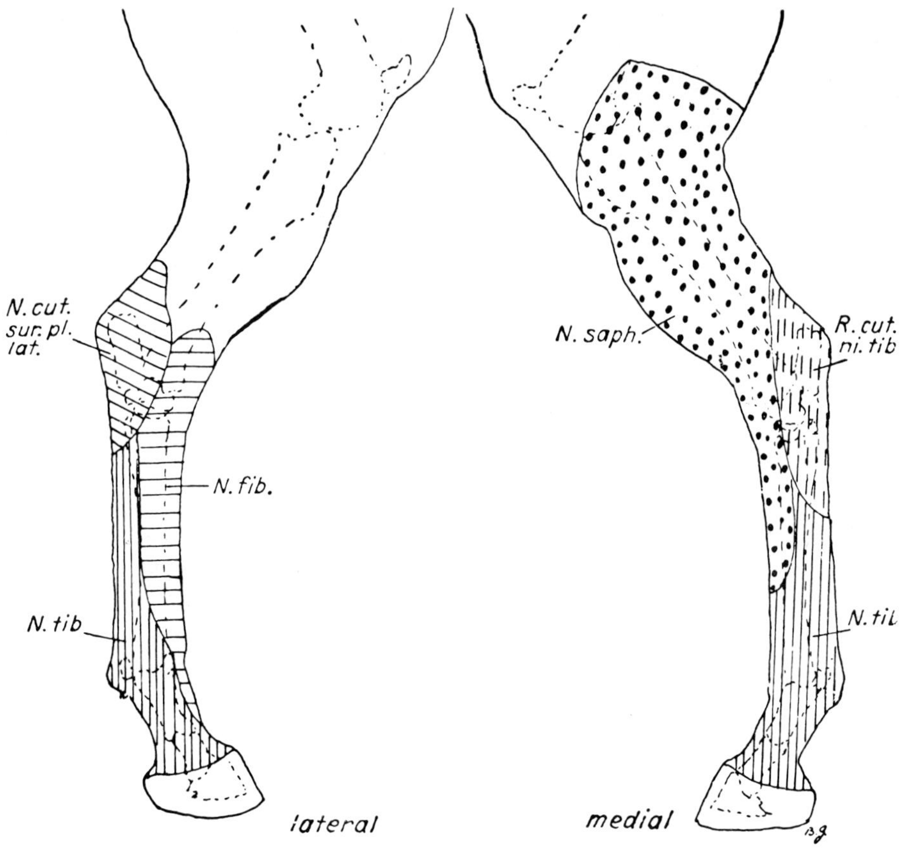

Figure 16–10. Areas of anesthesia in regional block of the hindlimb in the horse. N. cut. sur. pl. lat., posterior cutaneous nerve. N. tib., tibial nerve. N. fib., fibular (peroneal) nerve. N. saph., saphenous nerve. R. cut. ni. tib., cutaneous branch of tibial nerve. (From Westhues, M., and Fritsch, R.: *Animal Anaesthesia*. Vol. I. Local Anaesthesia. Oliver & Boyd, Edinburgh & London, 1964.)

Interdigital Block. For interdigital surgery, Elmore (1981) blocks branches of the medial dorsal and plantar or palmar nerves. Using a 5-cm, 16- or 18-gauge needle, 10 ml of 2% lidocaine are injected into the soft area proximal to the junction of the claws on both the dorsal and volar surfaces of the pastern. The soft area is immediately proximal to the fibrous tissue band connecting the claws. The needle is inserted proximal to this band in a slightly downward direction toward the middle of the interdigital space to a depth of 5 cm.

Conduction Anesthesia of the Hindlimb

Dog

Saphenous Nerve. This is a branch of the femoral nerve and is motor to the sartorius muscle and sensory to the medial surface of the thigh, stifle, and leg. It can be reached in the femoral triangle as it runs distally just cranial to the femoral artery. Using the arterial pulse as a landmark, one makes an injection of 2 ml of 1 or 2% lidocaine anterior to the artery, being careful to prevent intravascular injection.

Peroneal (Fibular) Nerve. The peroneal nerve, a terminal branch of the sciatic nerve, supplies the flexors of the hock and extensors of the digits. It is sensory to the dorsal aspect of the tibial region, hock, and paw. It passes laterally, under cover of the biceps femoris, around the fibula just below its head. It can be infiltrated by injecting 2 ml of 1 or 2% lidocaine just posterior and dorsal to the head of the fibula.

Tibial Nerve. The tibial nerve is the other terminal branch of the sciatic. It is motor to the

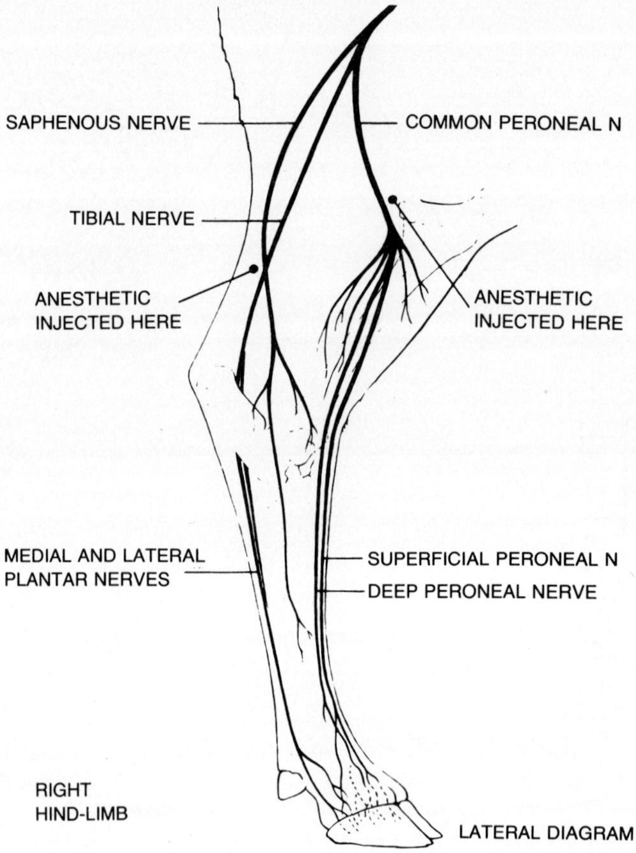

Figure 16–11. Innervation of the bovine hindlimb. The sites for peroneal and tibial nerve blocks are indicated. (From Collin, C.W.: A Technique to Produce Analgesia of the Hind Digits of Cattle. Vet. Rec., 75:833, 1963.)

extensors of the hock and flexors of the digits and supplies sensation to the plantar surface of the paw. It can be blocked just above the stifle joint by inserting the needle from behind into the popliteal space between the two heads of the gastrocnemius muscle; 2 ml of 1 or 2% lidocaine are injected.

Sciatic Nerve. The terminal branches of the sciatic nerve have been described. It supplies the caudal thigh muscles, which extend the hip and flex the stifle. Sensory branches innervate the skin on the caudal and lateral aspect of the true leg. The nerve can be blocked most easily where it passes over the lesser sciatic notch. The needle is inserted at a right angle posterior to the femur for a variable depth depending upon the size of the animal; 2 ml of 1 or 2% lidocaine are injected.

Horse

Techniques for regional anesthesia of the hind-limb have not been fully developed; therefore, it is not surprising that, with the exception of the plantar and digital nerves, they are used less frequently.

The areas supplied by the tibial and peroneal (fibular) nerves are illustrated in Figure 16–10. Complete anesthesia distal to the hock necessitates block not only of these two nerves but also of the saphenous, the superficial peroneal, and the posterior cutaneous branch of the tibial nerve (Hall, 1971).

Tibial Nerve. This nerve is blocked by the injection of 15 to 20 ml of 2% mepivacaine or equivalent one hand's-breadth above the point of the hock. If the limb is flexed slightly, it is generally possible to palpate the nerve between

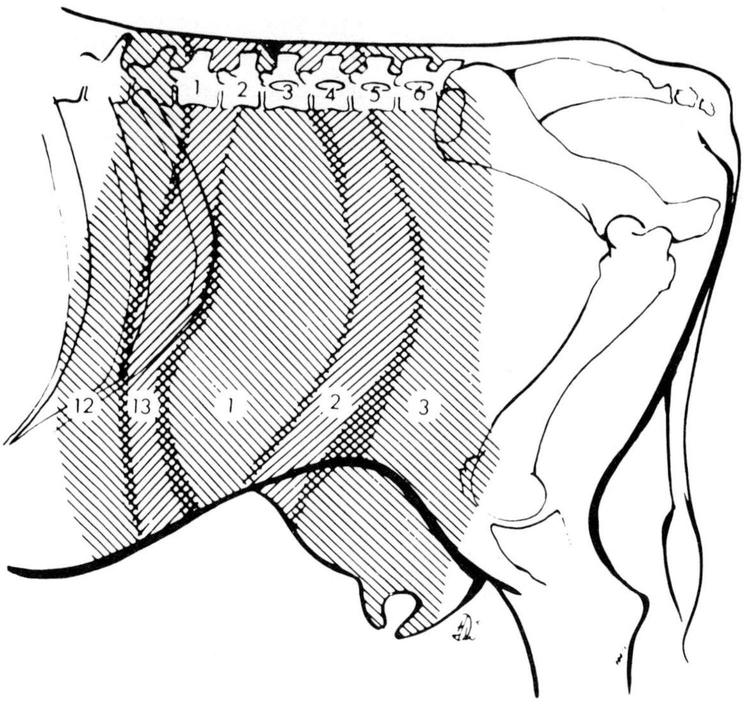

Figure 16–12. Dermatomes supplied by spinal nerves T12, T13, and S1, S2, S3 are indicated by shaded areas. Lumbar paravertebral block will anesthetize these areas. (From Hall, L.W., and Clarke, K.W.: *Veterinary Anaesthesia*, 8th ed. Baillière Tindall, London, 1983.)

the Achilles tendon and long digital extensor. A 5-cm 20-gauge needle is inserted from the medial aspect of the limb and should penetrate the subcutaneous fascia. If blockade of the cutaneous branch of the tibial nerve is required, 5 to 10 ml of anesthetic are injected between the fascia and skin as the needle is withdrawn. Block of this nerve desensitizes the posteromedial aspect of the hock (Westhues and Fritsch, 1964).

Peroneal (Fibular) Nerve. The site of injection is located in the flexed limb just above the lateral malleolus of the fibula and between the long and lateral extensors. The needle should be introduced through the deep fascia to a depth of 2 cm, and 10 ml of 2% mepivacaine are injected. Anesthesia of the superficial peroneal is accomplished by subcutaneous injection of additional anesthetic solution during withdrawal of the needle (Westhues and Fritsch, 1964). The peroneal nerve may also be blocked beneath the fascia and against the head of the fibula.

Saphenous Nerve. This nerve is blocked on the medial aspect of the limb where it emerges from the femoral canal between the sartorius and gracilis and perforates the deep fascia. The injection should be made between the saphenous vein and the aponeurosis of the sartorius; 10 ml of 2% mepivacaine are used.

Metatarsal and Digital Nerves. These nerves are anesthetized in a manner comparable to that used for the metacarpal and digital nerves of the forelimb.

Cow

Since epidural injections may be conveniently used for anesthesia of the hindlegs, there has been little emphasis upon nerve blocks of this region. Collin (1963) reviewed methods for the induction of regional anesthesia of the digits of the hindlimb and reported a method by which this could be produced by two injections (Fig. 16–11).

Peroneal Nerve. This nerve is blocked immediately behind the posterior edge of the lateral condyle of the tibia (see Fig. 16–10). The lateral

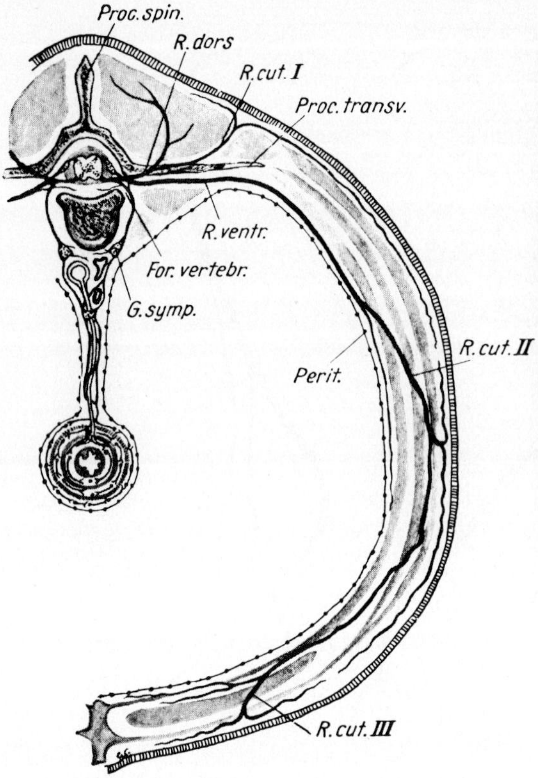

Figure 16–13. Division of lumbar nerves innervating abdominal wall of cattle. Proc. spin., spinal process. Proc. transv., transverse process. For. vertebr., intervertebral foramen. G. symp., sympathetic ganglia. Perit., peritoneum. R. dors., dorsal branch (lumbar nerve). R. ventr., ventral branch (lumbar nerve). R. cut. I, cutaneous branch, dorsal spinal (lumbar nerve). R. cut. II and III, cutaneous branches, ventral spinal nerve (lumbar nerve). (From Westhues, M., and Fritsch, R.: *Animal Anaesthesia*. Vol. I. Local Anaesthesia. Oliver & Boyd, Edinburgh & London, 1964.)

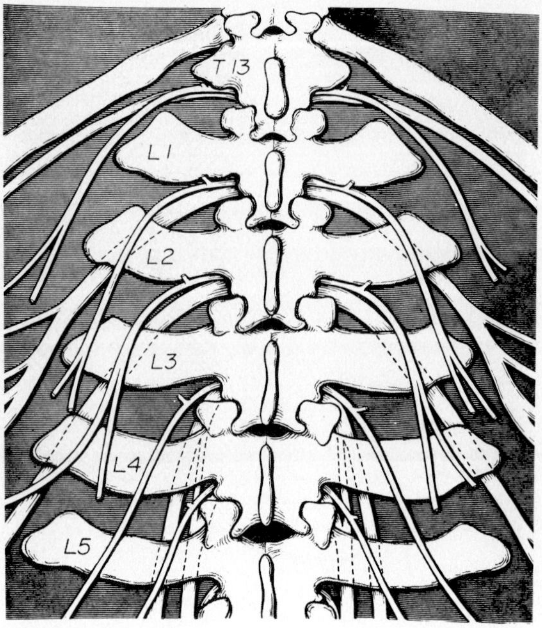

Figure 16–14. Lumbar nerves of the cow, dorsal aspect. (From Habel, R.E.: *Guide to the Dissection of Domestic Ruminants*, 2nd ed. Habel, Ithaca, N.Y., 1970.)

condyle is palpated, and a 3- to 5-cm 18-gauge needle is inserted through the skin and aponeurotic sheath of the biceps femoris until the point just touches the posterior edge of the condyle (Collin, 1963). Anesthesia results 5 to 20 minutes after 20 ml of 2% lidocaine solution are injected.

Alternatively, Raker (1956) has suggested that the superficial peroneal be blocked subcutaneously in the proximal third of the metatarsus and in the dorsal midline. The deep peroneal nerve is anesthetized in the midmetatarsal region beneath the extensor tendons.

Tibial Nerve. This nerve is blocked approximately 10 cm above the tuber calcis on the medial aspect of the limb and immediately in front of the Achilles tendon (see Fig. 16–11). Fifteen to 20 ml of 2% lidocaine are injected. Loss of sensation results in 15 minutes (Collin, 1963).

The tibial nerve divides into lateral and medial plantar metatarsal nerves. Raker (1956) recommends that these nerves be blocked 5 cm above the fetlock in the groove between the suspensory and flexor tendons.

Conduction Anesthesia of the Trunk

Paravertebral Anesthesia

Cow. Paravertebral anesthesia was introduced by Sellheim in 1906 and developed by Lawen in 1911. The technique constitutes block of the spinal nerves as they emerge from the intervertebral foramina. The technique of lumbar paravertebral anesthesia was introduced in cattle by Farquharson (1940) in order to induce anesthesia of the lateral abdominal wall. This region is innervated by the dorsal and ventral branches of the thirteenth thoracic (T13) and

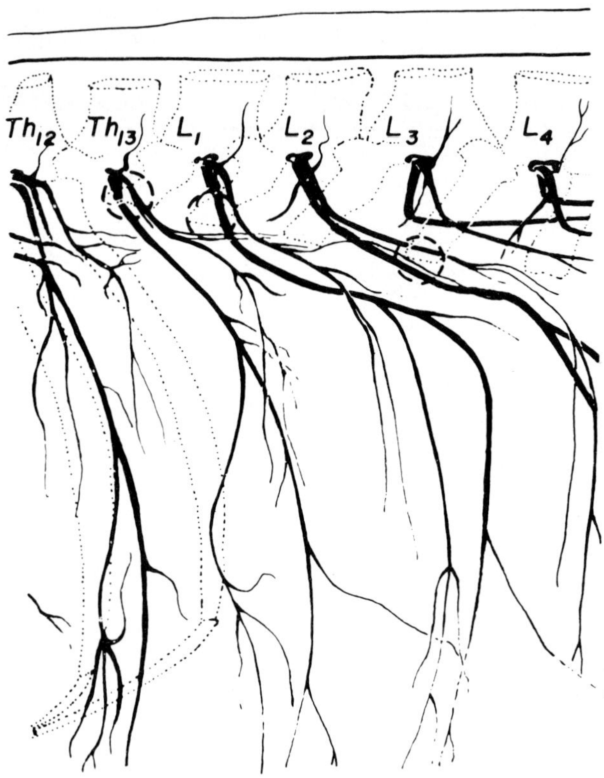

Figure 16–15. The emergence and distribution of nerve trunks of the twelfth and thirteenth thoracic and first and second lumbar vertebrae, on the left side in the cow (after Schreiber). The three areas infiltrated with an anesthetic at the ends of the first, second, and fourth transverse processes are marked with a broken line. (From Cakala, S.: A Technic for the Paravertebral Lumbar Block in Cattle. Cornell Vet., 51:5, 1961.)

first and second lumbar (L1 and L2) nerves (Fig. 16–12).

The dorsal branch divides into medial and lateral cutaneous branches. The latter supplies much of the upper paralumbar fossa while the remainder of this region is innervated by the ventral branch (Fig. 16–13). Since L3 provides some motor function to the hindlimb, it is preferable to avoid anesthesia of this nerve.

Although varying techniques are used, the nerves are usually blocked as they leave the intervertebral foramina or as the dorsal and ventral branches pass respectively above and below the transverse processes. A technique based upon that originally recommended by Formston in 1945 (cited by Hall, 1971) has been found satisfactory. The transverse processes of L1, L2, and L3 are palpated and the injection site located between the end of the transverse process and the midline at 5, 6.5, and 8 cm, respectively, from the midline (Peterson, 1966). A small amount of local anesthetic may be injected subcutaneously if desired, after which a 10-cm 18-gauge needle is inserted downward until it reaches the anterior border of the lumbar transverse process. At this point 5 ml of 2% lidocaine or equivalent are injected to anesthetize the dorsal branch of the spinal nerve. The needle is then advanced so that it penetrates the intertransverse ligament and passes over the anterior border of the lumbar transverse process to a depth of not more than 0.5 cm. Additional anesthetic is injected immediately beneath the intertransverse ligament, thereby anesthetizing the ventral branch. Since the spinal nerves concerned pass laterally in an oblique manner (Fig. 16–14), it is a useful practice to withdraw the needle until the border of the transverse process is once again detected and to redirect it both 1 cm medial and 1 cm lateral to the original in-

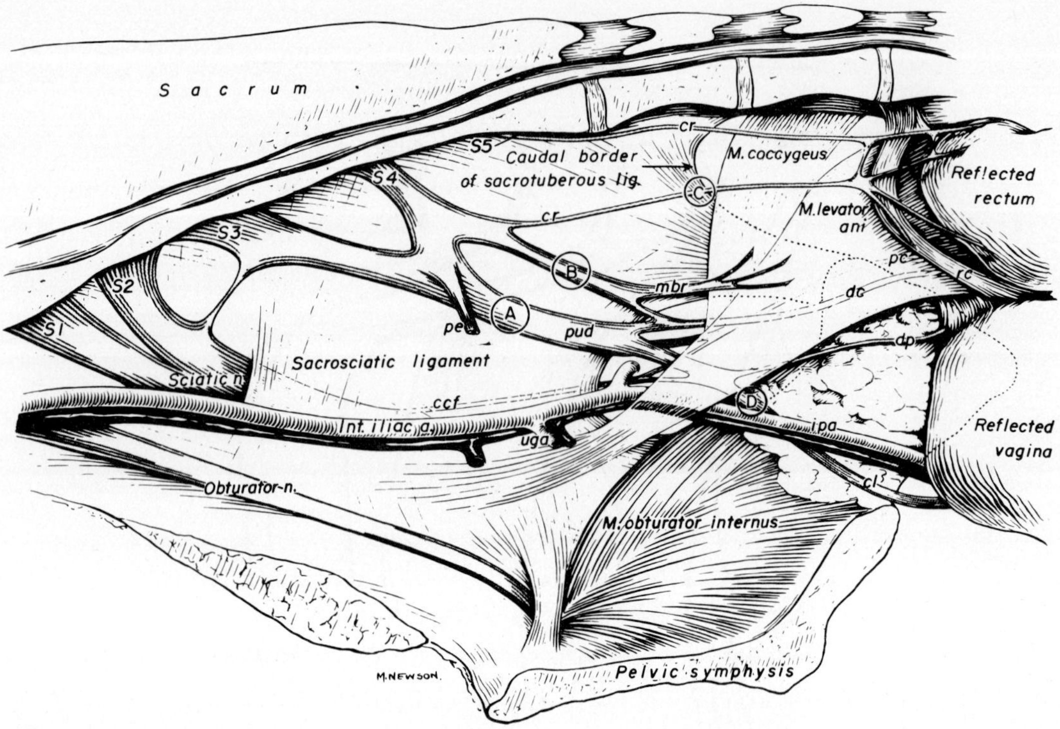

Figure 16–16. Diagram of the nerves on the medial surface of the right pelvic wall of a cow, with the pelvic viscera drawn caudad: *A, B, C,* Points of injection recommended by Larson; *D,* additional point recommended by Habel; *ccf,* anastomosis between sciatic and pudendal nerves; *cl,* nerve to clitoris; *dc,* distal cutaneous branch of pudendal n.; *ipa,* internal pudendal artery; *mbr,* muscular branch of coccygeus and levator ani; *pc,* proximal cutaneous branch of pudendal n.; *pe,* pelvic n.; *pud,* pudendal n.; *rc,* m. retractor clitoridis; *S 1–5,* sacral nerves; *uga,* urogenital artery. (From Habel, R.E.: A Source of Error in the Bovine Pudendal Nerve Block. J.A.V.M.A., 128:16, 1956.)

jection site. In this way, it is unlikely that the nerve will be missed by injecting too close or too far from the midline.

Cakala (1961) has recommended a more lateral approach. A 6-cm 18-gauge needle is inserted horizontally and anesthetic is injected above and below the ends of the transverse processes of L1, L2, and L4, thereby blocking spinal nerves T13, L1, and L2 (Figs. 16–14 and 16–15).

In the original report by Farquharson (1940), a more medial approach was utilized, and the appropriate nerves were blocked posterior to the mamillary process of the vertebra. This location is often more difficult to detect and results in greater spinal curvature, since blockade of the dorsal branches is such that relaxation of the dorsal lumbar muscles is more complete.

Small Ruminant. In sheep and goats, a technique similar to that of Formston's in cattle is satisfactory. The injection site is approximately 3 cm from the midline.

Pudendal Nerve Block (Ruminant)

This nerve is derived from the ventral branches of spinal nerves S3, S4, and occasionally S2 and passes caudoventrad on the medial surface of the sacrosciatic ligament. It receives an anastomosing branch from the sciatic nerve at the lesser sciatic foramen.

The pudendal nerve gives off a proximal and a distal cutaneous branch to the caudal femoral region, branches to the skin and muscles of the labia of the cow or the skin and muscle derivatives of the embryonal cloacal sphincter of the bull, and supplies a superficial perineal or a mammary branch to the upper caudal part of the scrotum. It terminates as the nervus clitoridis in the female and the nervus dorsalis penis in the bull. The latter innervates the retractor penis muscle, the glans penis region, and part of the prepuce. The hemorrhoidal nerves (S4 and S5) supply the skin and muscles (medial and lateral coccygeal) of the anus and perineum (Peterson, 1966). This nerve block is indicated for examination, treatment, and surgery of the penis. Caudal epidural anesthesia is preferable for surgery of the vulvar and perineal regions.

The technique for pudendal nerve block was originally reported by Larson (1953). After appropriate skin preparation, anesthetic is injected subcutaneously beside the anus at the deepest point of the ischiorectal fossa, and a 1- to 2-cm 13- or 14-gauge needle is inserted through the skin. With the hand in the rectum, a 12- to 25-cm 18-gauge needle is passed through the larger needle, guided to the pudendal and hemorrhoidal nerves, and 25 ml of 2% lidocaine or equivalent are injected at the sites indicated in Figure 16–16. The contralateral pudendal and hemorrhoidal nerves are blocked in a similar manner.

The pudendal nerve is located by palpation in the following manner (Peterson, 1966):

1. Locate the lesser sciatic notch and foramen.
2. Locate the internal iliac (pudendal) artery at the cranial angle of this notch.
3. Move the hand craniad and locate the superior ischiatic spine.
4. Palpate the pudendal nerve just caudodorsad to the internal iliac artery.
5. After injection of anesthetic over the pudendal nerve, additional anesthetic is injected caudodorsad to anesthetize the hemorrhoidal nerves.

The pudendal nerve may also be blocked in sheep using digital palpation of the lesser sacrosciatic foramen as a guide (McFarlane, 1963).

REFERENCES

Atkinson, R.S., Rushman, G.B., and Lee, J.A.: *A Synopsis of Anaesthesia*, 8th ed. Year Book Medical Publishers Inc., Chicago, 1977.

Bogan, J.A., and Weaver, A.D.: Lidocaine Concentrations Associated with Intravenous Regional Anesthesia of the Distal Limb of Cattle. Am. J. Vet. Res., 39:1672, 1978.

Browne, T.G.: The Technique of Nerve-Blocking for Dehorning Cattle. Vet. Rec., 50:1336, 1938.

Cakala, S.: A Technic for the Paravertebral Lumbar Block in Cattle. Cornell Vet., 51:5, 1961.

Collin, C.W.: A Technique to Produce Analgesia of the Hind Digits of Cattle. Vet. Rec., 75:833, 1963.

Donchin, Y., Ramu, A., Olshwang, D., Neiman, Z., and Magora, F.: Effect of Sodium Bicarbonate on the Kinetics of Bupivacaine in I.V. Regional Anaesthesia in Dogs. Br. J. Anaesth., 52:969, 1980.

Elmore, R.G.: Food-Animal Regional Anesthesia. Bovine Blocks: Ocular. Vet. Med. Small Anim. Clin., 75:1760, 1980.

Elmore, R.G.: Food-Animal Regional Anesthesia. Bovine Blocks: Interdigital Nerve Block. Vet. Med. Small Anim. Clin., 76:82, 1981.

Emmerson, M.A.: Nerve Blocking in the Dehorning of Cattle. University of Pennsylvania Veterinary Extension Quarterly, 34:5, 1933.

Farquharson, J.: Paravertebral Lumbar Anesthesia in the Bovine Species. J.A.V.M.A., 97:54, 1940.

Frank, E.R.: Dental Anesthesia in the Dog. J.A.V.M.A., 73:232, 1928.

Habel, R.E.: *Guide to the Dissection of Domestic Ruminants*, 2nd ed. Habel, Ithaca, N.Y., 1970.

Hall, L.W., Ed.: *Wright's Veterinary Anaesthesia and Analgesia*. 7th ed. Baillière Tindall, London, 1971.

Knight, A.P.: Intravenous Regional Anesthesia of the Bovine Foot. Bovine Pract., 11:14, 1980.

Lacroix, J.V.: Chapter 13, Dental Nerve Blocking. In *Canine Surgery*, 4th ed. Edited by K. Mayer, J.V. Lacroix, and H.P. Hoskins. American Veterinary Publications, Inc., Evanston, Illinois, 1957.

Larson, L.L.: The Internal Pudendal (Pubic) Nerve Block for Anesthesia of the Penis and Relaxation of the Retractor Penis Muscle. J.A.V.M.A., 123:18, 1953.

McFarlane, I.S.: The Lateral Approach to Pudendal Nerve Block in the Bovine and Ovine. J. S. Afr. Vet. Med. Assoc., 34:73, 1963.

Nixon, G.A., Bond, G.G., Reer, P.J., and Cloyd, G.G.: New Method for Determining Eye Anesthesia. Am. J. Vet. Res., 38:281, 1977.

Peterson, D.R.: Nerve Block of the Eye and Associated Structures. J.A.V.M.A., 68:145, 1951.

Peterson, D.R.: Anatomy Lecture Notes. Oklahoma State University, 1966.

Prentice, D.E., Wyn-Jones, G., Jones, R.S., and Jagger, D.W.: Intravenous Regional Anaesthesia of the Bovine Foot. Vet. Rec., 94:293, 1974.

Raker, C.W.: Regional Anesthesia of the Bovine Foot. J. Am. Vet. Med. Assoc., 128:238, 1956.

Severin, G.A.: *Veterinary Ophthalmology Notes*, 2nd ed. Colorado State University Printing Service, Fort Collins, Colorado, 1976.

Tufvesson, G.: Anestesi av Plexus Brachialis. Nord. Vet. Med., 3:183, 1951.

Vitums, A.: Nerve and Arterial Blood Supply to the Horns of the Goat with Reference to the Sites of Anesthesia for Dehorning. J.A.V.M.A., 125:284, 1954.

Westhues, M., and Fritsch, R.: *Animal Anaesthesia. I. Local Anaesthesia*. Oliver & Boyd, Edinburgh, 1964.

CHAPTER 17

Spinal Anesthesia

Spinal anesthesia is the induction of regional anesthesia by injection of local anesthetic solutions into the spinal canal. Injection of anesthetic within the canal but outside the dura mater is termed *epidural (extradural) anesthesia;* injection into the cerebrospinal fluid is termed *subarachnoid (subdural) anesthesia*. The terms *spinal anesthesia* or *spinal analgesia* in human literature refer to subarachnoid anesthesia. *Epidural anesthesia* is also classified according to the site at which the injection is made (i.e., caudal, lumbosacral, and lumbar), or according to the extent of the block (i.e., anterior [high] and posterior [low]).

HISTORY OF SPINAL ANESTHESIA

Spinal anesthesia was first reported by J. Leonard Corning in 1885. He accidentally punctured the dura while experimenting with the action of cocaine on the spinal nerves of the dog, and later intentionally repeated the procedure. After the initial clinical application of subarachnoid anesthesia in man by Bier in 1898, this technique was first used in animals by Cuillé and Sendrail in 1901 (Brook, 1935). During this same year, epidural anesthesia was first reported in dogs by Cathelin. Owing, however, to the larger quantities of anesthetic required and to the toxicity of cocaine, it was not until 1921 that it was used clinically in man by Labat (Atkinson et al., 1977). Subsequently, the technique was reported extensively in animals, first in 1925 by Pape and Pitzschki in horses, in 1926 by Benesch in cattle, and in 1927 by Frank in the dog and cat (cited by Westhues and Fritsch, 1964). Because of the greater ease of administration and the reduced tendency for neurologic complications, epidural anesthesia has largely replaced subarachnoid anesthesia in animals.

APPLIED ANATOMY

Although the anatomy of the nervous system in relation to anesthesia is discussed in Chapter 4, it is pertinent to review significant features of the epidural space. This space lies within the vertebral canal and surrounds the spinal cord and its enveloping membranes (spinal pia mater, arachnoid, and dura mater). It is bounded internally by the dura mater (a continuation of the meningeal layer of the dura mater of the brain). Externally, it is limited by vertebral bodies and arches, intervertebral discs, and associated ligaments. The periosteum of the vertebrae is a continuation of the outer layer of the cerebral dura and joins with the internal meningeal layer of the dura mater at the foramen magnum. The epidural space terminates at this point. The space contains spinal nerve roots, blood vessels, spinal membranes within which are the cord and associated spinal fluid, and fat and areolar tissue in which the cord is suspended. The dorsal (posterior) sensory and ventral (anterior) motor roots of the spinal nerves usually penetrate the dura separately and unite within the epidural space. The roots of the posterior lumbar nerves of the horse are reported to unite within the dura (Dellmann and McClure, 1975).

The distribution of spinal nerves that may be anesthetized during epidural anesthesia is shown in Table 17–1. It is important to appreciate that these nerves include vasoconstrictor fibers of the sympathetic nervous system. Major blood vessels of significance within the spinal canal are the paired vertebral venous sinuses, which extend longitudinally along the floor of the vertebral canal. Since they anastomose freely with other veins draining the trunk and with the azygos vein, they provide an alternative route for venous return which bypasses the caval system. They may be inadvertently punctured during spinal injections and provide a route by which spinal anesthetics rapidly enter the systemic circulation. In addition to these vessels, branches of cervical, intercostal, lumbar, and iliolumbar arteries enter the canal via intervertebral foramina.

Since the epidural space communicates with surrounding tissues via the intervertebral foramina, and indirectly via ramifications of the venous sinuses, the pressure within this space is directly related to that of the thoracic and abdominal cavities. Pressure in the thoracic and lumbar epidural space thus reflects that in the posterior (inferior) vena cava.

SITE OF ACTION AND SPREAD OF ANESTHETIC

Until recently the mechanisms of subarachnoid and epidural anesthesia were considered to be different. Such clear-cut compartmentalization is not now tenable. Investigations that imposed a revised viewpoint have been summarized by Bromage (1979) and include the following: 1) spinal meninges are permeable to local anesthetics, especially at the arachnoid villi surrounding the dorsal root cuffs; 2) labeled local anesthetics have been shown to pass quite rapidly from the epidural space into the cerebrospinal fluid (Table 17–2), concentrations greater than the minimum effective concentration being found in the pia mater, spinal roots, and periphery of the spinal cord; 3) subarachnoid local anesthetics act on the cord as well as the spinal roots; and 4) within limits, the spread of epidural local anesthetics is contingent upon the mass of drug injected, and pharmacologic blockade may spread farther than the solution within the epidural space. It is thus apparent that subarachnoid local anesthetics act at the periphery of the spinal cord as well as on the spinal roots, and that epidural local anesthetics act at multiple sites. These sites include: 1) mixed spinal nerves, 2) spinal roots (probably not in the dorsal root ganglia), 3) the perimeter of the spinal cord, with the depth of penetration of the spinal being contingent upon dose, concentration, and lipid solubility of the anesthetic (Bromage, 1979).

In contrast to these observations, Skarda et al. (1981*a,b*) were unable to detect analgesic levels of procaine in the subarachnoid fluid of cattle after the single epidural injection of 400 mg (8 ml) or 500 mg (10 ml) at L1/L2; nor were they able to detect a relationship between total mass of procaine injected and the number of spinal segments anesthetized. The peak average subarachnoid concentration of procaine was 160.7 ± 63.7 μg/ml at 25.0 ± 6.7 minutes after injection. These investigators conjectured that analgesia was induced after the anesthetic had diffused through the intervertebral foramina, thereby blocking the nerves at a paravertebral site. They indicated that unilateral or bilateral blockade can be achieved by appropriate placement of the needle in the epidural space.

From the preceding discussion, it is apparent that the action of epidural anesthetic depends in

TABLE 17–1. Distribution of the Sensory and Motor Fibers of the Spinal Nerves*

Spinal Region	*No. of Nerve*	*Structures Supplied* — *Sensory*	*Structures Supplied* — *Motor*
Coccygeal	All	Greater part of tail	Coccygeal muscles
Sacral	5 and 4	Croup, base of tail; anus, vulva, perineum and adjacent parts	Anus, terminal part of rectum, vagina, penis, bladder, urethra
Sacral	3, 2 and 1	Dorsal branches—sensory to region of croup	
Lumbar	6, 5 and 4	Ventral branches—enter into the formation of the lumbosacral plexus	
Lumbosacral plexus	Posterior gluteal nerve (1 and 2 S.)	Lateral and posterior parts of hip and thigh	Extensors of hip (in part)
	Great sciatic nerve (5 and 6 L., 1 S.)	Middle of tibial region to foot	Flexors of the stifle (in part); flexors and extensors of hock and digit
	Anterior gluteal nerve (5 and 6 L., 1 S.)	Lateral aspect of thigh	Flexors and abductors of hip
	Obturator nerve (4 and 5 L.)	Mesial aspect of thigh	Adductors of hip
	Femoral nerve (4 and 5 L.)	Anterior and mesial aspects of limb as low as hock	Flexors of hip (in part), extensors of stifle
Lumbar	3	Loins and croup, anterior aspect of stifle, scrotum, prepuce, and inguinal region; mammary gland	Sublumbar group (in part), posterior parts of abdominal muscles
	2	Loins, flank, anterior and lateral aspect of thigh, scrotum, prepuce, mammary gland	Sublumbar group (in part), posterior parts of abdominal muscles
	1	Loins, posterior abdominal region, lateral aspect of thigh	Posterior parts of abdominal muscles
Thoracic	Last two	Abdominal wall and flank	Abdominal muscles
	Midthoracic region to last pair	Anterior and ventral parts of abdominal wall	Intercostal muscles, anterior parts of abdominal muscles

*Some variation occurs among species.
(From Hall, L.W., Ed.: *Wright's Veterinary Anaesthesia, and Analgesia,* 7th ed. Baillière Tindall, London, 1971.)

part upon spread of the solution. Segmental spread, for instance in lumbar epidural, occurs at sites other than the epidural space, possibly to the subarachnoid or subpial space (Bromage, 1979). While it would seem that the degree to which the anesthetic spreads depends largely upon the relation of volume of solution injected to size of the epidural space, clinical observations have shown that, within certain limits, the extent of blockade is mainly determined by the mass of solute (drug) injected (Fig. 17–1). At low concentrations, however, less drug is required to block a spinal segment. Beyond a certain point, high concentrations do not shorten the time required for the onset of anesthesia, nor do they improve the quality of the blockade by transforaminal leakage and additional paravertebral block.

Spread of anesthetic within the epidural space is also influenced by gravity and epidural pressure. Gravity favors downward flow and can thus be used to influence the direction of spread. Since the greatest negative pressure is in the thoracic epidural space, anterior lumbar injections of anesthetic tend, other factors being equal, to spread anteriorly. Whatever the pattern

TABLE 17–2. Diffusion of Local Anesthetics from Epidural Space to Subarachnoid Space

			Epidural Dosage		Cerebrospinal Fluid (CSF)				
							Total Clearance into Perfused Subarachnoid Space		
Authors	*Analgesic Drug*	*Animal Species*	*Concn. (%)*	*Dose (mg)*	*Time of Peak Concn. (min)*	*Peak Concn. (mg/ml)*	*mg*	*% of Epidural Dose*	*Site of Sampling CSF*
Numans and Havinga (1943)	Procaine	Calf	1.5	120–150	10	0.2–0.4			Lumbar
Numans and Havinga (1943)	Procaine	Cow	1.5	1,500–2,100	10	0.5			Lumbar
Rudin et al. (1951)	Procaine	Dog	2	200	4–8	0.8	8–24	3–10	Cisterna magna
Kronke (1951)	Tetracaine	Man	0.3	50	30–40	0.2–0.5			Lumbar
Buchholz and Korner (1952)	Tetracaine	Man	0.3	60	30–40	0.01–0.02			Lumbar
Frey and Soehring (1954)	Procaine	Dog	2		10	1.0–1.2			Lumbar
Foldes and Davis (1954)	2-Chloroprocaine	Man	3	1,000	30	0.23			Lumbar
Frumin et al. (1953)	Procaine	Man	2	400	20	0.15–0.2			Lumbar
Onchi et al. (1956)	Lidocaine	Man	0.8–2.0	280–400	15	0.1–0.25			Lumbar
Krumperman et al. (1960)	2-Chloroprocaine	Man	3	Varied	—	0.25			Lumbar
Usubiaga et al. (1964)	Procaine	Dog	2	5 mg/kg	5–25 (av. 15)	0.2–0.5 0.5–0.7+		7.3	Lumbar
Bromage and Burfoot (1964)	^{14}C-Lidocaine	Dog	2	100–200	5–10	1.4 2.2+			Lumbar via cisterna magna
Lund et al. (1965)	Lidocaine Prilocaine	Man	2 and 3	600–900	30–45	0.09–0.27			Lumbar

+ = After second injection.
(From Bromage, P.R.: Physiology and Pharmacology of Epidural Analgesia. Anesthesiology, 28:592, 1967.)

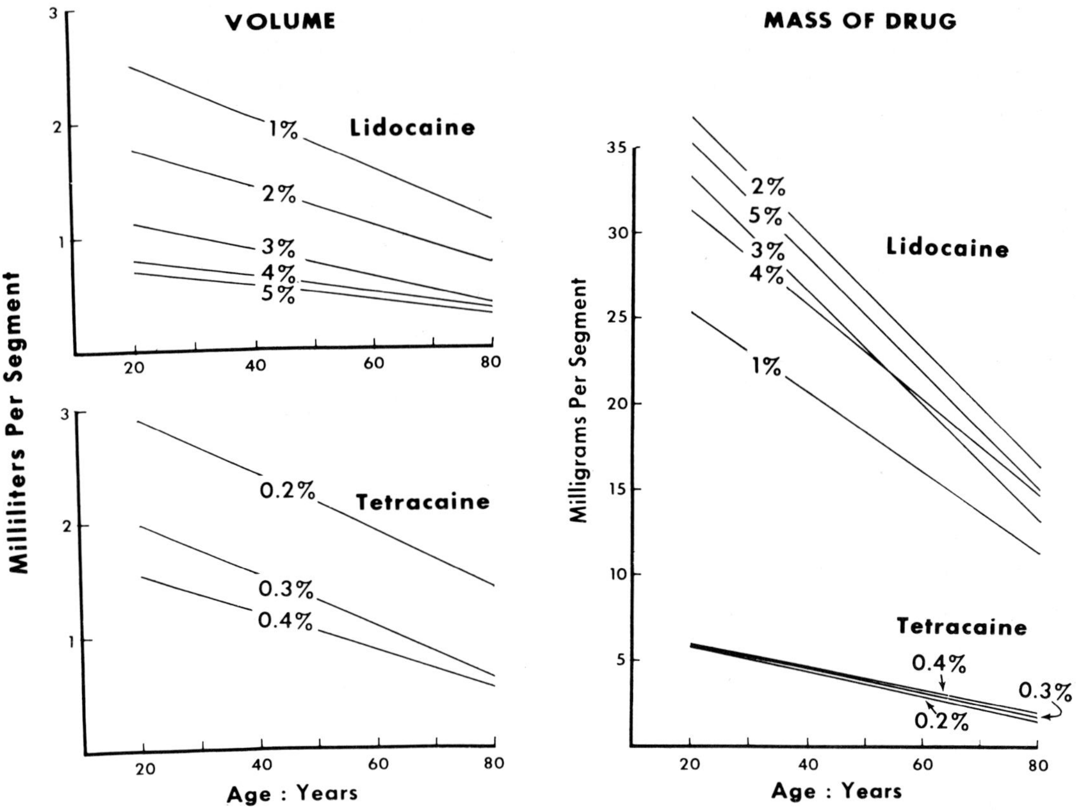

Figure 17–1. Epidural dose requirements in man for lidocaine (lignocaine, xylocaine) and tetracaine (pontocaine) in relation to age, expressed as volume of solution and mass of solute (drug) needed to block one spinal segment. Note that above a certain concentration the mass of drug required is virtually constant at any given age. In weak solution (e.g., 1% lidocaine) 20 to 40% less drug is needed. (From Bromage, P.R.: Physiology and Pharmacology of Epidural Analgesia. Anesthesiology, 28:592, 1967.)

of spread, however, the blockade occurs earliest and is most intense at the site of injection (Bromage, 1967). Spread of anesthetic is also probably increased by rapid injection, but at the cost of a higher degree of incomplete analgesia (Erdemir et al., 1965).

In women, advanced pregnancy reduces the amount of epidural anesthetic required by one-third to one-half at term. It has been suggested that this is due to vertebral plexus distension resulting from partial occlusion of the inferior vena cava by the pregnant uterus. This venous engorgement restricts the epidural space and limits the necessary dose (Bromage, 1967). The effect of pregnancy on epidural anesthesia of animals has not been elucidated.

MODIFICATION OF EPIDURAL ANESTHETIC SOLUTIONS

The intensity and duration of epidural blockade, including the associated sympathetic blockade, are markedly enhanced by 1:300,000 to 1:100,000 dilutions of epinephrine. The intensity of motor block, for instance, is increased 50 to 100% by use of 1:200,000 epinephrine, and the duration of action is likewise extended. A 1% solution of epinephrine will permanently damage the canine spinal cord (Bromage, 1967). Since tissue penetration is improved at a high pH and stability of epinephrine in anesthetic solutions requires a low pH, the addition of epinephrine of relatively high pH just prior to use is preferred (Bonica et al., 1957). In contrast to tissue penetrance, optimal anesthetic uptake and activity require a relatively low pH. Combination of high pH at the injection site and low intracellular pH at the site of action can be achieved to some extent by modification of the local P_{CO_2} of the tissues. Local anesthetic salts of carbonic acid with a high P_{CO_2} should therefore be more efficient than the traditional hydrochloride. The improved quality of blockade when carbonated salts of lidocaine and prilocaine are used would seem to confirm this.

Attempts to localize and prolong the epidural effect of local anesthetics by increasing their viscosity have been disappointing (Bromage, 1967).

EFFECTS OF EPIDURAL ANESTHESIA

Prior to considering the effects of epidural anesthesia upon the various body systems, one must appreciate that they result from both local and systemic actions. The influence of vascular absorption has often been ignored, yet one quarter of an epidural anesthetic has been recovered from the azygos vein of the dog within 40 minutes after injection. This amount is halved by adding epinephrine (1:200,000) to the anesthetic solution (Bromage, 1967). The hazards of vascular uptake are also reduced by using no more anesthetic than is necessary and by selecting anesthetics that are highly protein-bound.

Neurologic Effects

Locally, nerve fibers are blocked in the following order in man (Atkinson et al., 1977): 1) autonomic preganglionic β fibers with consequent sympathetic blockade (Greene, 1958), 2) temperature fibers, 3) pain fibers, 4) touch fibers, 5) deep pressure fibers, 6) somatic motor fibers, 7) fibers conveying vibratory sense and proprioceptive impulses. Return of sensation occurs in the reverse order. Large motor fibers may, due to their size and covering, be unaffected by epidural anesthesia (Landau et al., 1960; Atkinson et al., 1977). The largest such nerves are those that innervate the limbs.

In addition to local effects, convulsions may result from absorption of toxic concentrations into the circulation. Electroencephalographic changes may also result, when severe hypotension (less than 60 mm Hg systolic pressure) results.

Cardiovascular Effects

Blockade of the sympathetic efferents in the affected spinal segments and the effects of local anesthetic and/or epinephrine absorbed from the epidural space produce cardiovascular changes. These include 1) dilatation of resistance and capacitance vessels, 2) paralysis of cardiac sympathetic fibers in anterior thoracic blockade, 3) reduced cardiac output from beta-receptor blockade and smooth muscle depression from circulating local anesthetic, and 4) beta-receptor stimulation with increased cardiac output and decreased peripheral resistance due to absorption of epinephrine (Bromage, 1967). The overall effect is likely to be a greater fall in mean arterial pressure than if epinephrine had not been used. In the dog, it would appear that the majority of the myocardial depression resulting from a 5 mg/kg epidural injection of lidocaine is due to circulating anesthetic (Galindo and Sprouse, 1962).

Respiratory Effects

In thoracic blockade, there is intercostal paralysis which is compensated by increased diaphragmatic activity unless phrenic blockade is also induced. Decreases in mean expiratory reserve volume up to 21% have been reported in man, while mean inspiratory capacity was little affected (Atkinson et al., 1977). Lumbar blockade, on the other hand, may improve effective ventilation when this is impaired by abdominal pain.

Visceral Effects

Since sympathetic stimulation reduces hepatic blood flow and depletes hepatic glycogen and norepinephrine, splanchnic blockade protects against this. However, hepatic blood flow is markedly diminished should epidural blockade cause systolic pressure to fall to below 60 or 70 mm Hg. Although it has been shown that epidural analgesia inhibits the hyperglycemic response to surgical stress, this could not be correlated with plasma insulin, glucagon, cortisol, growth hormone, or prolactin levels (Brandt et al., 1976).

Although spinal denervation does not affect uterine motility, accompanying hypotension, circulating local anesthetics, or epinephrine may do so. The fetus may be similarly affected by hypotension and absorbed drugs.

In sacral blockade, parasympathetic control of the smooth muscle of the rectum, bladder, vagina, retractor penis, and the constrictor of the vulva is lost. Consequently, the rectum dilates, the vagina is often ballooned, and there is relaxation of the bladder and retractor penis (Westhues and Fritsch, 1964). Any effects on renal function result from hypotension.

Effects on body temperature are variable; vasodilatation favors heat loss; absence of sweating, where this is relevant, favors hyperpyrexia in hot environments. Catecholamine secretion is depressed and less heat is produced (Atkinson et al., 1977).

METHOD OF EPIDURAL INJECTION

The anatomic location for injection depends upon the type of block desired, the species, and individual preference. Once selected, the site should be clipped, cleansed, and disinfected. Depending upon the species and animal, it may be necessary to inject a small amount of local anesthetic solution subcutaneously to minimize movement during insertion of the spinal needle. The needle selected will likewise vary with the anesthesiologist, the species, and the size of animal to be injected; it should have a short bevel and preferably be fitted with a stylet. If injection is to be performed in the laterally recumbent animal, spinal flexion is advantageous. A midline approach is generally used, and every effort should be made to insert the needle in the median plane. If the needle is carefully inserted, it can usually be felt penetrating the interarcuate ligament prior to entering the epidural space. Location of the needle in the epidural space is indicated by the following: 1) sudden reduced resistance to insertion of the needle; 2) ease of injection of a small amount of air, local anesthetic, or saline; and 3) in the anterior lumbar or thoracic region, the drawing in of a small amount of anesthetic on the needle hub into the lumen of the needle by negative epidural pressure. In caudal locations, the needle may penetrate the floor of the vertebral canal, in which case there is marked resistance to injection. Prior to injection of anesthetic, an aspiration test for blood or cerebrospinal fluid should be made. If blood is aspirated, the needle point should be relocated. If cerebrospinal fluid is aspirated, an alternative site or anesthetic procedure should be used.

Although the amount of anesthetic injected varies with the size of animal and type of block desired, it is important to recall that old animals and those at parturition may require less. The extent and intensity of the blockade can be extended by additional injections 10 to 20 minutes after the first. If motor blockade is not required, weaker anesthetic concentrations should be used. Whatever the amount and concentration of anesthetic solution, it should be injected slowly. Rapidly injected anesthetic extends farther, but the intensity of the block may be impaired.

COMPLICATIONS AND SEQUELAE OF EPIDURAL ANESTHESIA

Inadequate blockade may result from insufficient or too dilute anesthetic solution, from faulty injection technique, or from inadequate dispersal of anesthetic. Bradley et al. (1980) reported inadequate blockade in 9 of 54 canine patients; 5 of these were believed to be due to faulty technique. The most common cause of improper administration was obesity. These authors also reported transient Schiff-Sherrington reaction in 2 dogs. Incomplete or patchy blocks are sometimes encountered in animals, especially horses, which have had previous epidural injections. Severe hypotension may occur, especially in ruminants, when sympathetic vasoconstrictor fibers to the abdominal viscera are blocked. Appropriate therapy should include vasopressors having both alpha- and beta-receptor effects (e.g., metaraminol bitartrate).

Epidural solutions that inadvertently enter the

subarachnoid space or spread too far anteriorly may induce total subarachnoid or epidural anesthesia. In such cases, there is not only marked hypotension but also severe respiratory depression or even apnea. Controlled or assisted ventilation together with intravenous injection of pressor drugs is essential. Should convulsions occur from absorption of toxic anesthetic concentrations, diazepam or an intravenous thiobarbiturate is indicated.

Although unusual, occasional cases of paresis and meningitis have been attributed to epidural injections.

ADVANTAGES AND DISADVANTAGES OF EPIDURAL ANESTHESIA

In contrast to general anesthesia, the fetus is not depressed by epidural anesthesia, respiration does not usually require assistance, and a single injection provides excellent analgesia, relaxation, and reduced bleeding during operation. The technique has wide application beyond the usual indication of cesarean section (Bone and Peck, 1956; Bradley et al., 1980). Meningitis and neurologic sequelae are less common than when subarachnoid injections are used.

In comparison with intravenous anesthesia, there is considerable delay before epidural anesthesia is achieved. In large animals, loss of control of the limbs may result in excitement and injury. Restraint is required in all species during epidural anesthesia. Since relatively large doses (5- to 10-fold or more) of anesthetic are required in comparison with subarachnoid anesthesia, systemic and toxic effects may occur. In some species, especially swine, placement of the needle in the epidural space may be difficult. In lumbosacral or more anterior injections, relatively large volumes of anesthetic solution may be inadvertently injected into the cerebrospinal fluid.

CAUDAL EPIDURAL ANESTHESIA

Horses

Lumbar, lumbosacral, or even anterior caudal epidural anesthesia is rarely used because of the temperament of horses, the possibility of injury during recovery, and the difficulties of prolonged restraint. The amount of anesthetic injected is small, so that only posterior blockade is induced, and the animal remains standing, with appropriate restraint such as stocks. Chemical sedation such as xylazine may also be needed. The technique is thus used for obstetrical manipulations and for surgical procedures of the tail, perineum, vulva, vagina, rectum, and bladder.

Since the first coccygeal vertebra is usually fused with the sacrum, the injection is usually made through the first or second intercoccygeal space. This space, which is easily palpated when the tail is raised, is often 1 to 2 inches craniad to the most proximal long hairs of the tail and approximates the level of the caudal fold when the tail is raised. The exact site should, however, always be determined by palpation. The site is clipped and washed, and skin disinfectant is applied. Injection of a small subcutaneous wheal of anesthetic over the site is often advantageous to minimize movement during insertion of the large epidural needle. A sterile 2- to 3-inch, 18-gauge needle (short bevel) is inserted perpendicular to the skin (Fig. 17–2) in the middle of the space and in a median plane. Just prior to entry into the epidural space, the needle can be felt to penetrate the interarcuate ligament. Location of the needle in the epidural space (at a depth of 1 to 2 inches) is confirmed by the methods previously mentioned. Penetration of the intervertebral disc or the ligamentous floor of the vertebral canal is less likely if the bevel of the needle is ventrally located during insertion.

In an alternative method of epidural injection, a 3- to 4-inch, 18-gauge needle is inserted just posterior to the first intercoccygeal space and directed forward at an angle of 30° with horizontal (see Fig. 17–2). The needle may thus be threaded into the vertebral canal.

Depending upon the procedure and the size of the animal, 3 to 25 ml of 1.5 to 2.5% procaine, or equivalent, are injected epidurally. It should be recalled that the total mass of solute is more important than volume or concentration of solution in determining the extent of the

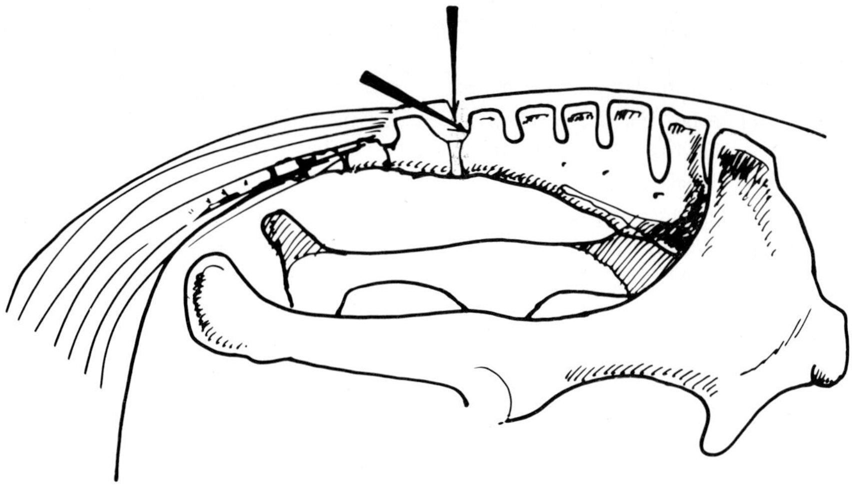

Figure 17–2. Epidural injection in the horse. Arrows indicate two directions (perpendicular to the skin or at an angle of 30° from horizontal) for injection in the first intercoccygeal space.

block. Alternative solutions include 1 to 2% lidocaine, 1% hexylcaine, and 1 to 2% mepivacaine. Ten to 12 ml of 2% lidocaine can be injected in large horses without danger of ataxia (Tufvesson, 1963). Maximal blockade generally requires 10 to 20 minutes to develop. If doubt exists regarding the dose to be used, it is preferable to underdose, leaving the needle in situ for additional anesthetic should this be needed. If repeated injections are anticipated, use of an indwelling catheter is preferable. Some recommended dosages are illustrated in Table 17–3. The quality and duration of the blockade are improved by inclusion of 1:100,000 to 1:200,000 epinephrine in the anesthetic solution. Inadequate epidural anesthesia can result from faulty placement of the needle, inadequate dosage, inadequate dispersal of anesthetic, and from variations in conformation. Inadequate dispersal with asymmetric and incomplete desensitization may occur in horses that have had previous epidural injections, or that have a septum within the epidural space. Variations in conformation and slope of the croup may facilitate or impede forward dispersal of the local anesthetic in the epidural space. For prolonged epi-

TABLE 17–3. Dosages Recommended for Caudal Analgesia in the Adult Standing Horse

Local Anesthetic	*Solution (%)*	*Volume (ml)*	*Duration of Analgesia (hr)*
Procaine	3	3–10	2
	6	5	½–1
Procaine	1	30–40	1–2
Procaine with epinephrine 1:1000		less than 20	½–2
Procaine	1	up to 25	1
Procaine	—	up to 25	—
Procaine	1–2	10	—
Lidocaine	1		
Procaine	2–2½	up to 25	
Lidocaine	2	up to 12	
Lidocaine	2	1 ml/150 lb	
Lidocaine	2	6–10	

(From Skarda, R.T.: Practical Regional Anesthesia. In *Equine Medicine and Surgery*, 3rd ed. Edited by R.A. Mansmann, E.S. McAllister, and P.W. Pratt. American Veterinary Publications, Santa Barbara, California, 1982.)

dural anesthesia in man (5 to 16 hours), 0.5% bupivacaine with epinephrine is used.

Anterior epidural anesthesia is not recommended. If it is employed, the horse should be recumbent prior to injection and must be restrained until limb coordination is fully regained. Fifty to 120 ml of 1% procaine via the first intercoccygeal space are recommended for severe obstetrical manipulations and 30 to 80 ml of 2% procaine for surgical procedures (Hall, 1971). Tufvesson (1963) has indicated that 100 to 150 ml of 2% lidocaine induces anesthesia to the level of the costal arch.

Cattle

Both posterior and anterior epidural anesthesia may be induced in cattle. Unlike the horse, cattle do not become excited and struggle while recumbent, although loose hobbling of the hind legs to prevent excessive abduction is indicated. Since the ruminant has a large abdominal mass, it is important to appreciate that vasomotor paralysis during anterior epidural anesthesia may cause severe hypotension. The indications for posterior anesthesia are similar to those in the horse. Anterior epidural together with preanesthetic sedation is satisfactory for surgery of the hindquarters, udder, uterus, penis, scrotum, and abdomen.

As in the horse, the site of injection is commonly the first intercoccygeal space, although the sacrococcygeal or second and third intercoccygeal spaces may also be used. A suitable space is easily located by palpation. Dorsoventral manipulation of the tail may be necessary in beef breeds. The site is clipped, cleansed, and disinfected. A subcutaneous wheal of anesthetic over the site is usually unnecessary. For epidural injection, a 1½- to 3-inch, 18-gauge needle with short bevel is directed in a manner similar to that described for the horse (see Fig. 17–2). Elmore (1980) recommends the use of a Tuohy or Hustead epidural needle. If threading of the needle along the canal is preferred, a 3-inch needle is used via the second or third intercoccygeal space. If repeated injections are required, use of an indwelling catheter is preferable. Normally the distance from the skin to the floor of the canal is three-fourths to two inches. The needle is inserted to the floor of the canal and is then withdrawn slightly. As in the horse, it is important to keep the needle in the median plane. Location of the needle in the epidural space is confirmed by methods described previously. Onset of the block is evidenced by flaccidity of the tail and failure of the anal sphincter to contract when touched. Although commencing relaxation of the tail can be detected quite quickly, maximal action requires 10 to 20 minutes and with most anesthetics persists for 60 to 90 minutes.

Local anesthetics commonly used for this purpose include 1.5 to 5% procaine, 1 to 2% lidocaine, and 1 to 2% mepivacaine. Depending on the size of the animal and the concentration of anesthetic, 3 to 20 ml may be used. If the animal is to remain standing, the initial dose should not exceed (depending on size) 10 to 15 ml of 2% procaine, 5 to 10 ml of 2% lidocaine, or equivalent. For continuous posterior epidural, Elmore (1980) has recommended 5 to 6 ml of 2% lidocaine every 4 to 6 hours. This is sufficient to control straining due to acute vulvovaginitis. In posterior anesthesia, the region innervated is that supplied by sacral nerves 3, 4, and 5 and the coccygeal nerves (see Table 17–1).

If sufficient anesthetic is administered to induce blockade of the anterior sacral region, control of the hindlimbs is affected, and the animal is unable to stand. Since in this anterior sacral region the epidural space is considerably enlarged, the amount of anesthetic necessary to extend the blockade craniad a small distance may be considerable. For adult cattle, 100 to 150 ml of 2% procaine (depending upon size) are considered adequate for amputation of the udder or digit, and for cesarean section (Hall, 1971). To avoid undesirable spread cranially with consequent respiratory embarrassment, the chest should be elevated slightly. When one is positioning the animal, it should be recalled that if the animal is in lateral recumbency, blockade is most efficient on the down side.

In anterior epidural anesthesia, especially when the blockade includes all lumbar segments, severe hypotension may occur. Clinical signs include a weak, rapid pulse and rapid, shallow respirations. During recovery, injury to the hip joints or pelvis may result from severe abduction of the limbs unless this is prevented by tying the legs loosely together. Rarely, epidural anesthesia may be followed by some loss of coordination of the tail. This presumably results from introduction of infection at the time of injection.

Despite the possible hazards of hypotension or, in the event of severe overdosage, total epidural blockade with respiratory failure, anterior epidural anesthesia has certain advantages over general anesthesia. Aspiration of rumen contents is not a hazard, and the method is simple, inexpensive, and requires minimal equipment.

Sheep and Goats

The indications and technique in sheep and goats are similar to those for bovine caudal epidural anesthesia, injection being made via the sacrococcygeal space. Sheep have been recommended as a laboratory animal for testing spinal and epidural anesthetics (Lebeaux, 1975). For adults, 3 to 5 ml of 2 or 3% procaine, or 2 to 5 ml of 1 or 2% lidocaine or equivalent induces posterior anesthesia, while it is not advisable to exceed 10 ml of 3% procaine for anterior anesthesia. Animals should be so positioned that spread into the thoracic epidural space is unlikely.

LUMBOSACRAL EPIDURAL ANESTHESIA

Lumbosacral epidural anesthesia is used in preference to caudal epidural in dogs, cats, swine, and small ruminants. The lumbosacral space, with the exception of large and fat swine, is easily located in these species, but is rarely used in horses and cattle. Since blockade is most intense at the site of injection, this site is preferred where anesthesia of the anterior sacral and lumbar nerves is desired. Disadvantages include the possibility that the dura may be penetrated (for the dural sac usually terminates in the anterior sacral region) and the need for more precise restraint during lumbosacral injection.

Small Ruminants

Indications for administration via this route are similar to those for induction of anesthesia by the caudal route in larger animals. The sheep or goat is restrained in lateral recumbency, the back is flexed, and the hind legs are held forward. The site of injection is immediately posterior to the last lumbar vertebral spine, which lies along an imaginary line joining the anterior border of each ilium. After preparation of the site, a 3-inch, 18-gauge needle with stylet is inserted immediately behind the last lumbar spine. The needle should not deviate from the midline and is directed in a slightly posterior direction (10 to 15% from vertical). If the needle is advanced slowly, it can usually be felt to penetrate the interarcuate ligament. Methods by which epidural placement of the needle is confirmed have been described previously. Penetration of the dura should be avoided. Should this happen, it is preferable either to proceed with subarachnoid injection or to terminate the procedure. Epidural injection after puncture of the dura may result in dangerous subarachnoid concentrations of anesthetic. Depending upon the size of the animal, 5 to 12 ml of 4% procaine, 2% lidocaine, or equivalent are injected epidurally.

For unilateral anesthesia, the animal is restrained on the side to be anesthetized until blockade occurs; for bilateral anesthesia, the animal is restrained in sternal recumbency. With lidocaine and 1:100,000 epinephrine, induction requires 10 to 15 minutes and lasts from 2 to 3 hours. The areas of anesthesia resulting from sacrococcygeal, lumbosacral, and lumbar epidural injections of 1.5% lidocaine solution in goats have been reported by Linzell (1964) and are illustrated in Figure 17–3. In some goats that had been previously sedated with chlorpromazine, he observed transient mild convulsions 1 to 2 minutes after lumbosacral epidural injection of 8 to 10 ml of 1.5% lidocaine with epinephrine. The use of 10 ml of 0.25% bupivacaine epidurally in sheep has been shown to produce analgesia for 365 ± 57 minutes (Lebeaux, 1975). He also observed transient signs of central nervous system irritation for 1 to 2 minutes after epidural injection.

Pigs

Since in larger pigs anatomic landmarks are sometimes difficult to locate, it is fortunate that

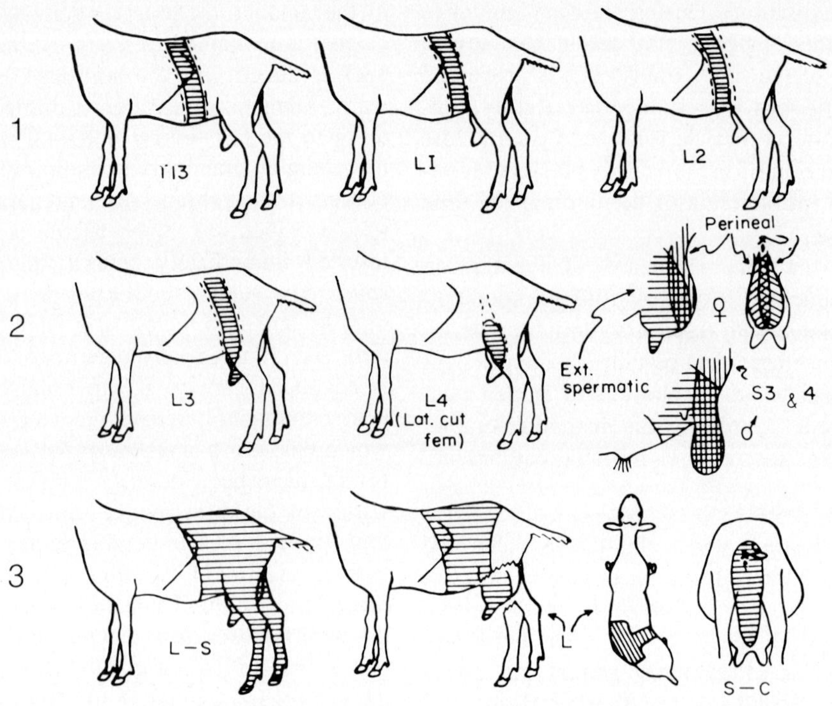

Figure 17–3. *Rows 1 and 2,* Dermatomes of some lumbar and sacral nerves plotted by recording mixed action potentials, L4 lateral cutaneous femoral branch only. *Row 3,* Areas of anesthesia after epidural injections: L–S Lumbosacral 8 to 10 ml; L Lumbar 1 to 2.5 ml on left, S–C Sacrococcygeal 2 ml. (From Linzell, J.L.: Some Observations on General and Regional Anaesthesia in Goats. In *Small Animal Anaesthesia.* Edited by O. Graham-Jones. Proceedings of a Symposium Organized by the British Small Animal Veterinary Association. Pergamon Press Limited, Oxford, England, 1964.)

the lumbosacral space is relatively large. In adult swine, it is approximately 1.5 cm long and 2.5 cm across (Hall, 1971). Epidural anesthesia is used in swine for abdominal surgery, for castration of larger animals, and for obstetrical manipulations. After suitable sedation, the hog is restrained, depending upon size, in a lateral recumbent or standing position; the latter is preferable. The site is located in the midline, just posterior (usually 1 to 2 inches) to a line joining the anterior borders of the ilia (Elmore, 1981). This line bisects the spine of the last lumbar vertebra. The injection site is prepared as previously described and a 3- to 6-inch, 18-gauge needle is inserted just behind the last lumbar spine in a median and posterior direction. Hall (1971) recommends an angle of 20° with vertical. Elmore (1980), using a more posterior site, suggests passing the needle downward in a slightly cranial direction. The needle must penetrate to a depth of 2 to 4 inches according to the size of the animal. Libera (cited by Westhues and Fritsch, 1964) locates the lumbosacral space by relating the crown-rump length to its distance anterior to the base of the tail (Table 17–4). Trim (1980) considers the patella to be a reliable landmark in large swine in which it is not possible to palpate the iliac crest. With the animal standing in a normal position, the crest of the ilium is directly vertical to the patella.

Once the needle is inserted, the usual precautions are taken, although penetration of the dural sac is usually not a problem due to its small size at this location in swine. The dura is more likely to be penetrated if the needle is mistakenly inserted into the last lumbar interspace. The dose of anesthetic recommended is 1 ml of 2% procaine solution or equivalent with epinephrine per 10 lb of body weight, with a

TABLE 17–4. Location of Lumbosacral Space in the Pig by Relating the Crown-Rump Length to the Distance from the Base of the Tail to the Injection Site

Crown-Rump Length	*Tail Base-Lumbosacral Space*
80– 90	14–16
90–100	16–18
100–117	17–19
118–126	19–21
127–130	21–23
131–140	24–26
140+	26–28+

All distances in centimeters

(From Westhues, M., and Fritsch, R.: *Animal Anaesthesia—Local Anaesthesia*. Oliver & Boyd, Ltd., Edinburgh, 1964.)

maximum of 20 ml (Hall, 1971). Getty (1966) recommends a similar volume of 4% procaine solution or 1 ml per 20 lb of 2% lidocaine solution. Such a dose of the latter produces complete loss of sensation of the paralumbar fossa, testicles, and scrotum within 10 minutes. Trim (1980) recommends 1 ml of 2% lidocaine per 7.5 kg for pigs weighing up to 50 kg, and thereafter 1 ml per 10 kg up to a maximum of 20 ml. This dose produces analgesia as far forward as L1. It should be remembered that epidural injection in lateral recumbency induces anesthesia predominantly of the lower side. Appropriate positioning of the animal during induction is therefore necessary.

In view of possible complicating hypotension, Booth (1969) recommends premedication with an intramuscular injection of ephedrine (25 to 40 mg/70 kg) 5 to 10 minutes prior to epidural injection.

Dogs

Early workers injected the dog at the sacrococcygeal space (Fig. 17–4) but abandoned this technique since it was difficult. Brook (1935) has pointed out that the dimensions of the sacral meningeal cul-de-sac are so small that a needle penetration at this point is highly improbable and thus the injection is extradural. In the dog, the greater splanchnic nerve arises from the twelfth thoracic sympathetic ganglion. If anesthetic solution passes cranially past the first lumbar segment, a serious fall in blood pressure may occur. Brook has suggested that the animal be restrained on its back immediately following injection so that the sensory dorsal spinal nerve roots are more profoundly affected than the ventral roots containing the vasomotor fibers.

Bone and Peck (1956) have listed indications for epidural anesthesia in dogs as follows:

1. Cesarean section
2. Ovariohysterectomy
3. Castration
4. Reduction of rectal prolapse
5. Caudectomy
6. Mammectomy
7. Excision of skin tumors of the hindquarters
8. Fracture repair, especially pelvic
9. Relaxation of the abdomen to facilitate palpation
10. Repair of wounds of the hindquarters

Preanesthetic administration of a narcotic or tranquilizer aids in restraint during injection but is not essential, and hypotensive agents should be avoided. The area over the lumbosacral space is clipped and scrubbed with a suitable antiseptic. Table 17–5 gives a dose schedule for three commonly used agents.

For abdominal operations, Frey and Volker (cited by Westhues and Fritsch, 1964) relate the required dose to the crown-rump measurement (Table 17–6). For operations on the hindquarters and perineal regions, this dose is reduced by 20 to 50%. Muir (1981) uses 1 ml of 2% lidocaine/10 lb to produce analgesia up to L2; 1 ml/7.5 lb produces analgesia up to T5.

Two techniques may be used for restraining dogs during the injection procedure. In the first, an assistant places the dog's head under one arm and grasps a hind leg in the stifle area with each hand (Fig. 17–5). With the second technique, the dog is held by an assistant with the hindquarters bent over the edge of a table. Bradley et al. (1980) recommend a sternal position with rear legs rotated cranially, a lateral flexed position, or a standing position. The injection site is located with the left hand by placing the thumb and second finger on the ilial crests while the index finger palpates and marks the lumbosacral space immediately posterior to the spi-

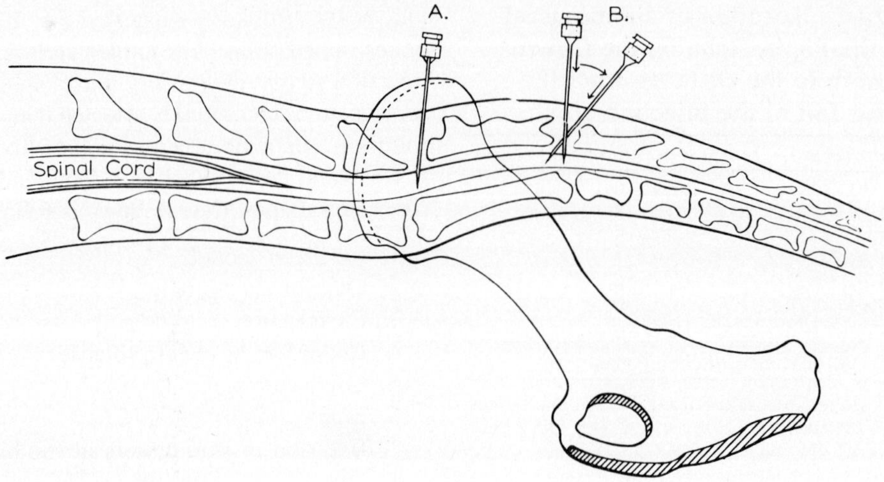

Figure 17–4. Sites for epidural injection in the dog: at the lumbosacral space, *(A)* and at the sacrococcygeal space *(B)*. The latter is not used clinically.

nous process of L7. Grafe and Schulze (1949) have reported underdevelopment or absence of the lumbosacral space in some dogs.

A three-quarter inch, 24-gauge needle is used for puppies, a 1½-inch, 20-gauge needle for medium-sized dogs, and a 3-inch, 20-gauge needle for large or obese dogs. A short bevelled spinal needle with stylet is preferred. The needle is slanted forward at a slight angle. A subcutaneous wheal of anesthetic at the injection site is optional.

As the needle is inserted through the intervertebral ligament, a distinct popping sensation is felt. The needle is introduced further until it touches the floor of the spinal canal and is then withdrawn approximately one-eighth inch. The usual precautions are taken to assure correct location of the needle, and the injection is then made slowly over a 15- to 30-second period; otherwise, vomiting and convulsions may result. *There should be no resistance* to the injection; if it occurs, the needle must be repositioned.

When injection is properly performed, anesthesia begins almost immediately. The tail relaxes, followed by the anal sphincter, and soon the rear quarters collapse. With the loss of pudendal nerve activity, the patient may pass flatus

TABLE 17–5. Dosage for Epidural Anesthesia in the Dog and Cat

Agent	*Percent Solution*	*Epinephrine*	*Dog*	*Cat*	*Duration*
Procaine	1	None	1 ml/5 lbs	1 ml/5 lbs	15–20 minutes
	2	None	1 ml/5 lbs	1 ml/5 lbs	20–25 minutes
	2.5	1:10,000	1 ml/5 lbs Reduce as weight increases over 20 lbs	1 ml/5 lbs	25–35 minutes
Hexylcaine (Cyclaine)	1	None	1 ml (puppies)		
	2	None	1 ml/12.5 lbs		30–60 minutes
	5*	None	0.5 to 2.0 ml (Approximately 1 ml/25 lbs)		6–12 hours
Lidocaine (Xylocaine)	2	1:100,000	2 to 10 ml	2 ml	

*Not recommended because prolonged paralysis may occur.

TABLE 17–6. Relation of Crown-Rump Length (Occiput-Base of Tail) of the Dog to the Desirable Dose of Epidural Anesthetic

Crown-Rump Length (cm)	*1–2% Procaine (ml)*
Up to 40	Up to 2.0
45	3.0
50	3.5
55	4.25
60	5.0
65	5.5
70	6.5
75	7.0
80	8.0
85	8.5
90	9.25
95	10.0
100	10.75

(From Westhues, M., and Fritsch, R.: *Animal Anaesthesia—Local Anaesthesia*. Oliver & Boyd, Ltd., Edinburgh, 1964.)

and have loss of urinary bladder control. Injection in an improper location results in:

1. Delay in onset of anesthesia;
2. Unilateral hindlimb paresis due to anesthesia of one sciatic nerve, at or near the sciatic foramen;
3. Partial anesthesia of tail or perineal region due to injection of dorsal branches of sacral nerves;
4. Shock and/or death from injecting subarachnoid space.

If analgesia is incomplete on one side, the patient should be placed in a lateral position for 5 minutes with the desired side down. Reinjection after 1, 2, and 3 above can be performed without adverse results. Should hypotension occur, treatment with pressor drugs is indicated.

Klide and Soma (1968) describe a technique for continuous epidural anesthesia. A 17-gauge, 3-inch Tuohy needle is inserted in the lumbosacral space, and a sterile vinyl catheter is passed through it for a distance of one-half to one inch. The needle is then carefully withdrawn to prevent cutting the catheter. Once epidural anesthesia is established, more anesthetic is injected as needed at about half the original dose per hour.

Cats

Epidural anesthesia in the cat has been described by Garcia (1953). The patient is restrained on the operating table with tapes, the head facing toward the anesthesiologist's right (Fig. 17–6). Preanesthetic sedation is advisable. The crest of the ilium on either side is used as a landmark. The thumb and second finger of the left hand are placed on the two crests, and the left index finger is used to palpate the depression of the lumbosacral fossa in the median line.

Following preparation of the area, a 1-inch, 22-gauge needle held in the right hand is introduced into the fossa, leaving the left index finger in position to serve as a guide. The needle is inserted in a vertical position just behind the anterior boundary of the fossa. As the needle passes through the fibrous intervertebral ligament, a definite pop is usually felt and resistance to passage of the needle ceases. In an adult cat, about one-third of the needle shank is visible above the skin surface. Back pressure is applied on the plunger of the syringe to insure against an intravenous tap. The dose of mepivacaine or bupivacaine is calculated on the basis of 0.5 ml/5 lb of body weight. Muir (1981) recommends the same dose of lidocaine as for the dog, but cautions that the spinal cord does not terminate until S1 in the cat. The injection should be made very slowly. When the needle is correctly placed and injection commenced, the cat's tail usually fibrillates. This is indicative of proper positioning of the needle. Relaxation begins almost immediately, reaches its full effect in 5 to 10 minutes, and lasts from 20 to 30 minutes. Again, improper injection may result in unilateral hindlimb paresis or partial anesthesia of the tail or perineal region. In the event poor anesthesia is obtained, the patient can be reinjected.

Garcia (1953) states that he has never experienced a fatality with epidural anesthesia in cats and recommends it for orchiectomy, hysterectomy, hysterotomy, and treatment of urolithiasis.

Others have found that this type of anesthesia leaves much to be desired. Even when it is done well, the restraint problem still exists. When this procedure has been performed by veterinary stu-

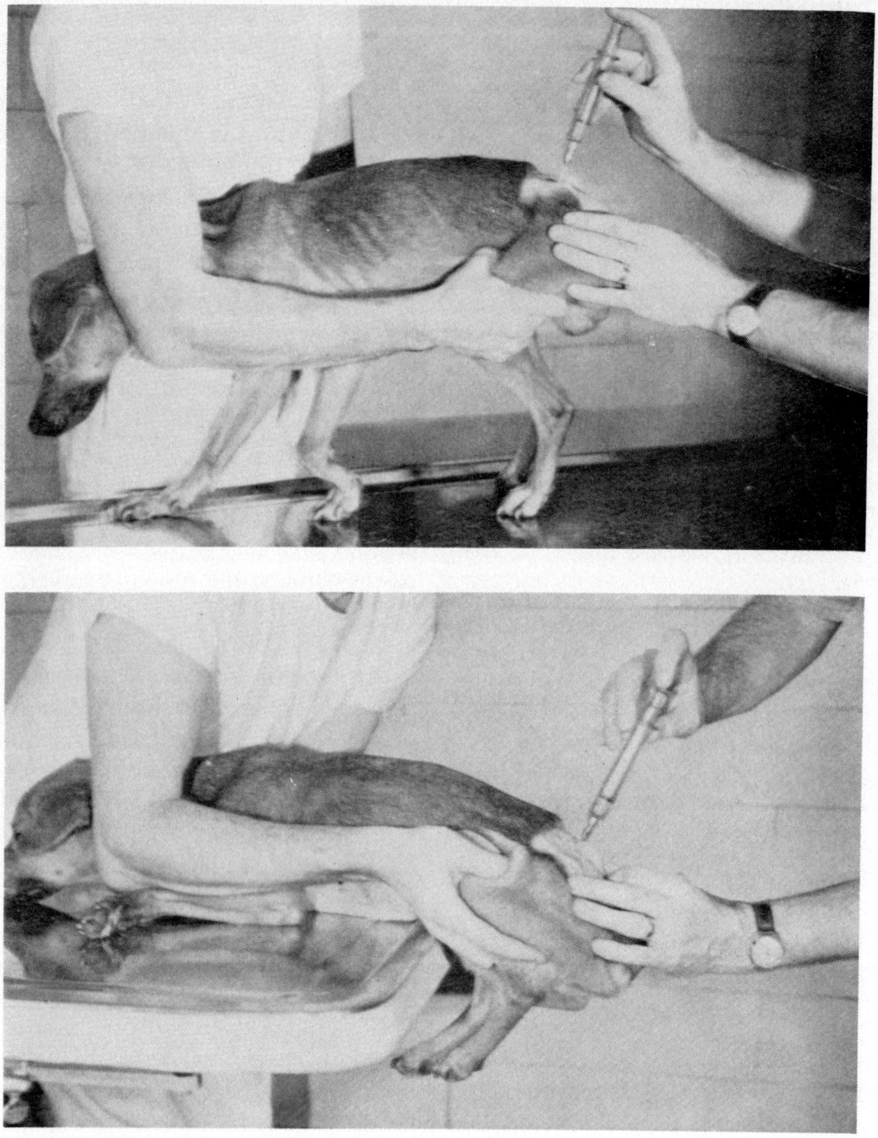

Figure 17–5. Positions for inducing epidural anesthesia in the dog.

dents, several fatalities have occurred. Unfortunately, no records exist to indicate the mortality associated with this technique.

Epidural anesthesia of cats has also been used to study the relative effectiveness of local anesthetic agents (Duce et al., 1969). Typical responses were flaccid paralysis of the hindlimbs and block of the flexion reflex. Using 2.5 ml of 1.5% lidocaine caused paralysis to become apparent in 2.4 ± 0.6 minutes; block of the hindlimb flexion reflex occurred in 79% of cases. Paralysis persisted for 44 ± 9 minutes. No systemic effects were noted when the aforementioned dose of lidocaine was used. Severe depression mydriasis, tonic convulsions, and salivation were noted when 1% tetracaine (1.5 ml) was used.

LUMBAR (SEGMENTAL) EPIDURAL ANESTHESIA IN RUMINANTS

Epidural blockade is most effective in the region of the injection. Injection in the anterior

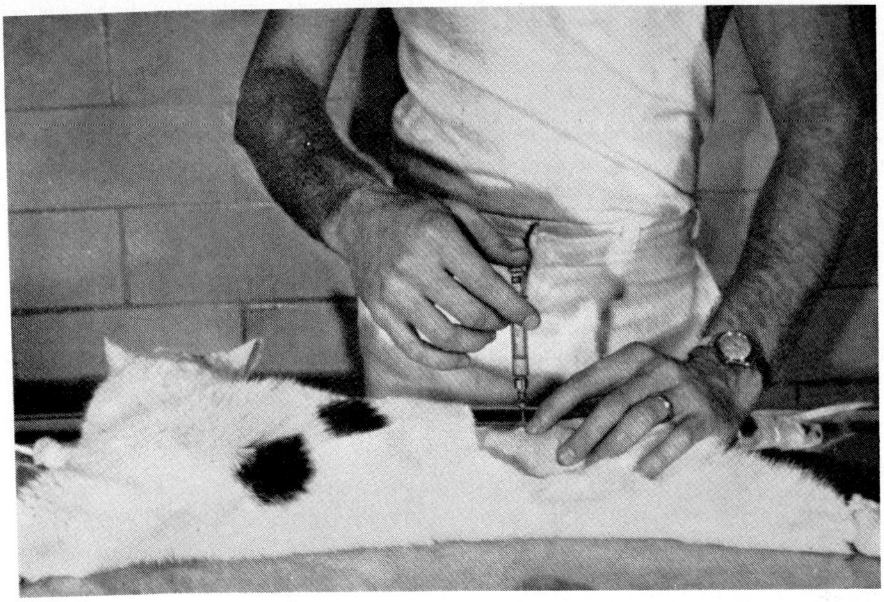

Figure 17–6. Position for epidural anesthesia in the cat. The cat is spread-eagled on the table with gauze tapes.

lumbar region is therefore most effective for desensitization of the paralumbar fossa. Injection at this site provides anesthesia of the abdominal wall without loss of locomotor control, and with much less anesthetic than that required to induce similar desensitization via the caudal or lumbosacral route. By varying the placement of the epidural needle, one can induce unilateral or bilateral blockade (Skarda and Muir, 1979). It is thus possible to achieve selective segmental anesthesia for abdominal surgery in the standing animal with a single injection of a relatively small amount of anesthetic solution. Alternatively the technique may be used for recumbent procedures, including correction of displaced abomasum.

Although caudal epidural anesthesia has been used in clinical veterinary medicine for as long as 35 years, it was not until 1948 that Buchholz described lumbar segmental epidural anesthesia in cattle, goats, and dogs. Practicality of the procedure in the horse has been confirmed subsequently by Magda et al. (1952), Arthur (1956), St. Clair and Hardenbrook (1956), and by Skarda and Muir (1979) in cattle and by Linzell (1964) in goats. Since this technique permits abdominal surgery in the standing animal, it is not surprising that its use has been confined largely to the ruminant.

Although any intervertebral space may be used, the preferred site is that closest to the spinal nerves to be anesthetized. The interspaces most commonly used are the thoracolumbar or first interlumbar. While Buchholz (1948) originally used a midline approach, a paramedian is now preferred (Fig. 17–7). This approach avoids the dense ligaments above and between the vertebral spines. Movement of the animal may, however, bend the needle. For anesthesia of the last thoracic and first lumbar nerves, the site is one-half to three-quarters inch on the opposite side of the midline from that which is to be anesthetized, and the same distance posterior to a line connecting the anterior border of transverse processes of the second lumbar vertebra.

The site is suitably prepared, and a small amount of anesthetic is injected subcutaneously. A one-half-inch 14-gauge needle is inserted through the skin at this location. Through this needle an 18-gauge, 5- or 6-inch spinal needle is passed downward and medially at an angle of 10 to 15° for 3 to 4 inches. Needle placement closer to the midline provides bilateral analgesia (Skarda and Muir, 1979). Direction of the bevel of the needle cranially and laterally limits the caudal flow of anesthetic and thereby the caudal extent of the blockade. The needle should ultimately enter the epidural space via the dorsal intervertebral space between the base of the vertebral spines. Since this space is actually a short canal (1 cm deep, 0.8 cm wide, and 0.5 cm long in the adult Jersey cow), the needle point may engage in the wall of the canal unless properly inclined (Arthur, 1956). Passage of the needle through the interarcuate ligament is characterized by increased resistance. Entry into the epidural space is indicated by termination of this resistance and by evidence of subatmospheric pressure within the epidural space. A small drop of saline applied to the hub of the needle is aspirated into its lumen, and there is no resistance to injection of air or fluid. Penetration of the subarachnoid space is indicated by aspiration of cerebrospinal fluid. Under such circumstances the procedure is preferably terminated, although Arthur (1956) reports successful completion of lumbar epidural injection after relocation of the needle. Depending upon animal size and the extent of anesthesia required, 6 to 15 ml of 4% procaine, 2% lidocaine solution, or equivalent have been found satisfactory. Beef cattle generally require slightly more anesthetic than dairy cattle. Greater amounts desensitize the fourth lumbar nerve and impair movement of the pelvic limb. Small amounts tend to induce unilateral anesthesia with sometimes undesirable lateral spinal curvature (Arthur, 1956). In average-size cows (500 kg), 8 ml of 5% procaine was sufficient to anesthetize the dorsal and ventral roots of the last thoracic and first two lumbar nerves (Skarda and Muir, 1979). Analgesia of udder and teats was also produced in 70% of such cases. When udder and teats were affected, there was some weakness of the pelvic limbs. For anesthesia of the teats, blockade of the second, third, and fourth lumbar nerves is required. In this instance, epidural injection between the second and third lumbar vertebrae is preferred. Satisfactory anesthesia usually develops within 10 to 15 minutes. Since vasomotor nerves are also desensitized, the skin temperature of the affected segment is increased. Skarda and Muir (1979) only detected minor changes in heart and respiratory rates, rectal temperature, rate of ruminal contraction, arterial blood pH, and gas tensions in cows undergoing unilateral or bilateral blockade.

Using 5 ml of 1.5% lidocaine solution, Linzell (1964) has reported satisfactory segmental anesthesia in the goat by injection at the first lumbar interspace (see Fig. 17–3).

SUBARACHNOID (SPINAL) ANESTHESIA

Although commonly used in man, subarachnoid anesthesia is rarely used in animals. Successful use of this technique has been reported in horses and cattle (Westhues and Fritsch, 1964), sheep (Hall, 1971; Lebeaux, 1975), and dogs. Restraint and aseptic technique are more demanding when one is using this procedure. Spread of anesthetic in this space is readily influenced by such physical factors as gravity and, therefore, by the position of the patient, specific gravity of the anesthetic solution, convection forces in the spinal fluid, and the force and rate of injection (Atkinson et al., 1977). Hall (1971) has indicated that it is more likely than epidural anesthesia to be complicated by meningitis, postoperative malaise, and severe hypotension. Smaller amounts of anesthetic are required than for epidural anesthesia, and toxic reactions are thus less likely to occur. Occasionally, in the dog, the subarachnoid space may be penetrated at the lumbosacral space. If this occurs, a different anesthetic technique may be used or only one-half of the dose injected.

In horses and cattle, subarachnoid anesthesia is induced with 2 to 4 ml of 5% procaine solution or equivalent via the lumbosacral space. Hall (1971) uses 1.5 to 2 ml of 0.5% dibucaine in 6% dextrose. This solution is heavier than cerebrospinal fluid (hyperbaric) and flows to the most dependent part of the subarachnoid space. Positioning of the animal is used to influence the location of the block. When 2 to 3% lidocaine is used, the spread is not as easily controlled and the duration of anesthesia is less.

In sheep, 1 ml of 0.25% tetracaine in 5% dextrose solution injected at the lumbosacral space produced analgesia in all spinal segments posterior to S1. Onset of anesthesia was com-

Figure 17–7. Transverse section through the joints between the articular processes of the first and second lumbar vertebrae. The body of the first lumbar segment is viewed from its posterior aspect. *1,* Needle in position. *2,* Spinal cord surrounded by meninges. *3,* Left first lumbar nerve. *4,* Body of first lumbar vertebra. *5,* Spinous process. *6,* Transverse process. *7,* Sectioned interlocking articular processes. (From Hall, L.W., Ed.: *Wright's Veterinary Anaesthesia and Analgesia,* 8th ed. Baillière Tindall, London, 1983.)

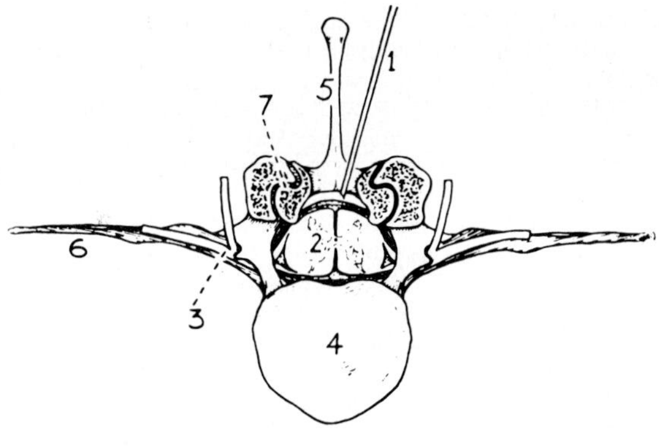

plete in 8 minutes and lasted approximately 3 hours. Sheep were tilted 10° caudad after subarachnoid injection (Lebeaux, 1975). Mennerat (cited by O'Connor, 1931) claimed to have used subarachnoid anesthesia in the dog with complete success; however, this procedure has never gained popularity in small animal practice.

Skarda and Muir (1981*a*) have reported effective segmental thoracolumbar subarachnoid analgesia in cattle. A 17-gauge Huber-point needle was used to place a catheter with stylet into the subarachnoid space at the lumbosacral intervertebral space. The tip of the spinal needle was positioned about 10° cranially from perpendicular, so that the bevel of the needle was located under the arch of the sixth lumbar vertebra. After removal of the stylet, an 80- to 100-cm polyethylene catheter (0.95 mm OD, 0.625 mm ID) with a stainless steel reinforced spring guide (0.52 mm OD) was passed through the needle and advanced for approximately 60 cm to the thoracolumbar intervertebral space. The Huber-point needle and spring guide were removed. The position of the catheter was confirmed radiographically. Procaine hydrochloride (1.5 to 2.0 ml of 5% solution) was injected at a rate of 0.5 ml/30 seconds. Segmental anesthesia from T9 to L4 on one or both sides was achieved in 7 to 10 minutes and lasted 43.7 ± 17.6 minutes. Although a significant increase in heart rate and decrease in respiratory rate were observed, there was no effect upon mean arterial blood pressures, $Paco_2$, Pao_2, and pHa (Skarda and Muir, 1981*b*). The technique permits repeated small maintenance doses to be administered, requires minimal doses of anesthetic agent, and produces minimal physiologic disturbance. It does, however, require an exacting and sterile technique and, in the event of overdosage, may produce loss of motor control of the pelvic limbs.

Skarda and Muir (1982) have also employed this technique in adult horses. They used 1.5 ml of 2.0% mepivacaine hydrochloride at the rate of 0.5 ml/minute. Bilateral segmental analgesia from T12 to L3 was induced in 5 to 10 minutes and lasted 42.4 ± 15 minutes. A significant increase in heart rate and decrease in respiratory rate were observed.

REFERENCES

Arthur, G.H.: Some Notes on a Preliminary Trial of Segmental Epidural Anaesthesia of Cattle. Vet. Rec., 68:254, 1956.

Atkinson, R.S., Rushman, G.B., and Lee, J.A.: *A Synopsis of Anaesthesia,* 8th ed. Williams & Wilkins, Baltimore, 1977.

Bone, J.K., and Peck, J.G.: Epidural Anesthesia in Dogs. J.A.V.M.A., 128:236, 1956.

Bonica, J.J., Backup, P.H., Anderson, C.E., Hadfield, D., Crepps, W.F., and Monk, B.F.: Peridural Block: Analysis of 3,637 Cases and A Review. Anesthesiology, 18:723, 1957.

Booth, N.H.: Anesthesia in the Pig. Fed. Proc., 28(4):1547, 1969.

Bradley, R.L., Withrow, S.J., Heath, R.B., Perkins, D., Kirkwood, M., and Mergler, R.: Epidural Analgesia in the Dog. Vet. Surg., 9:153, 1980.

Brandt, M., Kehlet, H., Binder, C., Hagen, C., and McNeilly, A.S.: Effect of Epidural Analgesia on the Glycoregulatory Endocrine Response to Surgery. Clin. Endocrinol., 5:107, 1976.

Bromage, P.R.: A Comparison of the Hydrochloride and Carbon Dioxide Salts of Lidocaine and Prilocaine in Epidural Anesthesia. Acta Anaesth. Scand. (Suppl.), 16:55, 1965.

Bromage, P.R.: Physiology and Pharmacology of Epidural Analgesia. Anesthesiology, 28:592, 1967.

Bromage, P.R.: Subarachnoid and Peridural Anesthesia. Annual Refresher Course Lectures, Lecture #209, Am. Soc. of Anesthes., 1979.

Brook, G.B.: Spinal (Epidural) Anaesthesia in the Domestic Animals. Vet. Rec., 15:549, 1935.

Buchholz, J.: Beitrog zur Extraduralen Anästhesie unter Besondue Berucksichtigung der Frage, ob die Injecktionsstelle fur die Extradurale Anästhesie beim Rind Kranialwarts vershoben werden Kann. Diss. Giessen Tierarzt. Umschau, 3:149, 1948.

Dellmann, H.D., and McClure, R.C.: The Central Nervous System. In Sisson and Grossman's *The Anatomy of The Domestic Animals*, 5th ed. Edited by R. Getty. W.B. Saunders Co., Philadelphia, 1975.

Duce, B.R., Zelechowski, K., Camougis, G., and Smith, E.R.: Experimental Epidural Anaesthesia in the Cat with Lignocaine and Amethocaine. Br. J. Anaesth., 41:579, 1969.

Elmore, R.G.: Food Animal Regional Anesthesia. Vet. Med. Small Anim. Clin., 75:1017, 1980.

Elmore, R.G.: Food Animal Regional Anesthesia. Porcine Blocks: Lumbosacral (Epidural). Vet. Med. Small Anim. Clin., 76:387, 1981.

Erdemir, H.A., Soper, L.E., and Sweet, R.B.: Studies of Factors Affecting Peridural Anesthesia. Anesth. Analg., 44:400, 1965.

Galindo, A.H., and Sprouse, J.H.: The Effect of Anesthesia on Cardiac Excitability Produced by Single Pulse Electrical Stimulation. Anesth. Analg., 41:659, 1962.

Garcia, J.G.: Epidural Anesthesia in the Cat. The Allied Vet., July–August, 20, 1953.

Getty, R.: Epidural Anesthesia in the Hog: Its Technique and Applications. In Scientific Proceedings, 100th Annual Meeting, Am. Vet. Med. Assoc., 1966.

Grafe, W., and Schulze, W.: Zur Technik der Lumbo-sacren Extradural-anäesthesie beim Hund. Berl. Munch. Tierarzt. Wehnschr., 10:140, 1949.

Greene, N.M.: Area of Differential Block in Spinal Anesthesia with Hyperbaric Tetracaine. Anesthesiology, 19:45, 1958.

Hall, L.W., Ed.: *Wright's Veterinary Anaesthesia and Analgesia,* 7th ed. Baillière Tindall, London, 1971.

Klide, A.M., and Soma, L.R.: Epidural Analgesia in the Dog and Cat. J.A.V.M.A., 153:165, 1968.

Laundau, W.M., Weaver, R.M., and Hornbien, T.F.: Sudimotor Nerve Functions in Man. Differential Nerve Block Studies in Normal Subjects and in Spasticity and Rigidity. Arch. Neurol., 3:10, 1960.

Lebeaux, M.: Sheep: A Model for Testing Spinal and Epidural Anesthetic Agents. Lab. Anim. Sci., 25:629, 1975.

Linzell, J.L.: Some Observations on General and Regional Anaesthesia in Goats. In *Small Animal Anaesthesia.* Proceedings of a Symposium Organized by The British Small Animal Veterinary Association. Pergamon Press, London, 1964.

Magda, I.I., Shalduga, N.E., and Voskovoinikor, M.: Einige Bemerkungen in Verbindung mit Pansenschnitt (Lumbale Epidural—Anasthesie). Veterinariya, 29:47, 1952.

Muir, W.W.: *An Outline of Veterinary Anesthesia.* Author, Columbus, Ohio, 1981.

O'Connor, J.J.: *Dollar's Veterinary Surgery,* 2nd ed. Alexander Eger, Chicago, 1931.

Skarda, R.T., and Muir, W.W.: Segmental Lumbar Epidural Analgesia in Cattle. Am. J. Vet. Res., 40:52, 1979.

Skarda, R.T., and Muir, W.W.: Segmental Thoracolumbar Subarachnoid Analgesia in Cows. Am. J. Vet. Res., 42:632, 1981*a*.

Skarda, R.T., and Muir, W.W.: Effects of Segmental Subarachnoid Analgesia on Arterial Blood Pressure, Gas Tensions, and pH in Adult Conscious Cows. Am. J. Vet. Res., 42:1747, 1981*b*.

Skarda, R.T., and Muir, W.W.: Segmental Thoracolumbar Spinal (Subarachnoid) Analgesia in Conscious Horses. Am. J. Vet. Res., 43:2121, 1982.

St. Clair, L.E., and Hardenbrook, H.J.: Lumbar Epidural Anesthesia in Cattle. J.A.V.M.A., 129:405, 1956.

Trim, C.M.: Epidural Analgesia in Swine. Vet. Anesth., 8:23, 1980.

Tufvesson, G.: Local Anaesthesia in Veterinary Medicine. Astra, Ltd., Stockholm, 1963.

Westhues, M., and Fritsch, R.: *Animal Anaesthesia—Local Anaesthesia.* Oliver & Boyd, Edinburgh, 1964.

CHAPTER 18

Anesthesia of Laboratory and Zoo Animals

Veterinarians are frequently called upon to anesthetize a wide variety of mammals, birds, reptiles, and fish. Some of the lower species of mammals, such as rabbits, rats, and mice, have been used through the years to assess anesthetic agents, and a mass of data is available concerning these species. Others have been anesthetized rarely if at all, and little specific information is available; that which follows may serve as a basis for further investigations. For additional information on anesthesia, restraint, and handling of wild animals, the reader is referred to the texts by Fowler (1978*a,b*), Green (1979), and Nielson et al. (1983).

CRUSTACEANS

The optimal effective concentration of tricaine methanesulfonate for two species of amphipods is 0.5 g/L (Gamble, 1969). Induction requires 25 minutes; duration of anesthesia up to 2 hours does not influence the recovery period. In gravid females, there is premature release of eggs or young from the brood pouch. This dose is quite high when compared with that for fish (see the following section). A similar decreased sensitivity of crustacea has been observed when quinaldine is used as an anesthetic.

Isobutyl alcohol is nontoxic to lobsters *(Hom-*

arus americanus) in concentrations ranging up to 14.4 ml/L in aerated seawater at 10° C (Foley et al., 1966). It is effective at doses as small as 0.5 ml/L, but induction is slowed. Recovery from anesthesia, however, is little different than with higher concentrations. For routine use, concentrations between 1.5 and 7.0 ml/L are recommended.

On immersion in the anesthetic solution, the lobster becomes agitated and gradually loses control of its chelae and walking legs, which then become tangled and stiffened in an upright position. Once anesthetized, lobsters can be exposed to air and manipulated for at least 10 minutes before any response is noted. They can be exposed for periods of 1 hour after treatment without fatality if then returned to seawater.

FISH

A large number of agents have been used to anesthetize fish; a partial listing is shown in Table 18–1. Fish are affected by abrupt variations in water temperature, pH, and mineral content. Therefore, water in which the fish is living is preferable for making anesthetic solutions. The degree of sedation and anesthesia is judged according to the criteria in Table 18–2. Squeezing the muscle at the base of the tail is a good test for anesthesia. The response should be diminished but not absent.

For handling fingerling trout for fin-clipping, ether anesthesia was found to increase efficiency markedly. A 1% aqueous solution was placed in a basin and additional ether was added as required; thus, the concentration varied considerably after the initial fish were anesthetized (Eschmeyer, 1953).

Amobarbital (0.5 gr/gal) can be used to anesthetize fish for transportation. With this method only one-third to one-fourth the water normally required is needed, since the fish become calm and use less oxygen. The small water volume facilitates transplanting operations by airplane. Because of its slow action, sodium amytal has no practical value in spawning or fin-clipping operations.

Methyl pentynol is a liquid with an acrid odor. It is dissolved in water at the rate of 0.5 to 0.9 ml/L of water. Induction requires 2 to 3 minutes and recovery 5 to 20 minutes. Respiratory arrest tends to develop in deep anesthesia making maintenance difficult. According to McFarland and Klontz (1969), this is one of the more popular anesthetics for fish.

Quinaldine is a water-insoluble, colorless, oily liquid that turns reddish brown when exposed to air. It can be dissolved in acetone for

TABLE 18–1. Recommended Concentrations and Qualities of Agents for Anesthetizing Fish

		Anesthetic Qualities		
Anesthetic	*Concentration**	*Induction Time, min*	*Maintenance*	*Recovery Time, min*
Carbon dioxide	200 ppm	1–2	Good	5–10
Electricity		Immediate	Poor	5–30
Diethyl ether	10–50 ml	2–3	Fair	5–30
Secobarbital	35 mg	30–60	Good	60+
Amobarbital	7–10 mg	30–60	Good	60+
Urethan	5–40 mg	2–3	Good	10–15
Chloral hydrate	0.8–0.9 g	8–10	Poor	20–30
Tertitary amyl alcohol	0.5–1.25 ml	10–20	Fair	20–90
Tribromoethanol	4–6 mg	5–10	Fair	20–40
Chlorobutanol	8–10 mg	2–3	Good	30–60
2-Phenoxyethanol	0.1–0.5 ml	10–30	Fair	5–15
4-Styrylpyridine	20–50 mg	1–5	Good	20–30
Methyl pentynol	0.5–0.9 ml	2–3	Fair	5–20
Quinaldine	0.01–0.03 ml	1–3	Fair	5–20
Tricaine methanesulfonate (MS-222)	25–100 mg	1–3	Excellent	3–15

*Expressed as milligram or milliter per liter of water unless otherwise noted.
(From McFarland, W.N., and Klontz, G.W.: Anesthesia in Fishes. Fed. Proc., 28:1535, 1969.)

TABLE 18–2. Behavioral Changes in Fish at Various Levels of Anesthesia

	Stage	
Normal		Reactive to external stimuli; muscle tone normal
Light sedation	1	Slight loss of reactivity to external visual and tactile stimuli; equilibrium normal
Deep sedation	2	Total loss of reactivity to external stimuli except strong pressure; slight decrease in opercular rate; equilibrium normal
Partial loss of equilibrium	3	Partial loss of muscle tone; swimming erratic; increased opercular rate; reactive only to strong tactile and vibrational stimuli
Total loss of equilibrium	4	Total loss of muscle tone and equilibrium; rapid opercular rate (slow with some agents), reactivity only to deep pressure stimuli
Loss of reflex reactivity	5	Total loss of reactivity; opercular movements very shallow; heart rate very slow
Medullary collapse	6	Opercular movements cease immediately after gasping, followed by cardiac arrest

(From McFarland, W.N., and Klontz, G.W.: Anesthesia in Fishes. Fed. Proc., 28:4, 1969.)

subsequent addition to water. The dose is 0.01 to 0.03 ml/L of water. Induction requires 1 to 3 minutes with recovery in 5 to 20 minutes. It may be used over a wide range of temperatures.

4-Styrylpyridine is a fine white powder freely soluble in water. The dose for fish is 20 to 25 mg/L of water. This is one of the few fish anesthetics that has been found on toxicity testing to be safe for handling by humans. Induction with this agent requires 1 to 5 minutes with recovery in 20 to 30 minutes.

2-Phenoxyethanol is an oily liquid with both anesthetic capability and chemotherapeutic properties against bacterial infections in fish. The dose is 0.1 to 0.5 ml/L of water. Induction requires 10 to 30 minutes with recovery in 5 to 10 minutes.

Tricaine methanesulfonate (MS-222) has been approved by the Food and Drug Administration as a sedative for fish, providing they are not used as food for 21 days. The drug does not affect the palatability. In anesthetizing most common fishes (teleosts), concentrations of 0.5 to 1.0 g/gal of fresh water are used, and the temperature is maintained at 40 to 60° F. Induction time varies depending on concentration and the period of exposure to the solution. The fish is immersed until it becomes immobilized, at which time it can be removed for examination, treatment, or surgery. While the fish is exposed to the air, provision should be made to keep it wet. For longer anesthesia, the fish can be reimmersed or the gills sprayed with solution. Repeated use tends to reduce the concentration; for best results, therefore, fresh solutions should be used. Bluegills, bass, trout, and salmon have been anesthetized in concentrations of 1:3000 to 1:25,000 for weighing, tagging, and spawn collection, with anesthesia varying in duration from 3 minutes to several hours depending again on concentration and immersion time. For large numbers of fish, a closed recirculating system may be advantageous (Hublou, 1957).

Tricaine methanesulfonate can be used for transporting fish without water (Martin and Scott, 1959). A dilution of 0.25 g/gal with water temperature of 5° C is used. When the fish turn over in the water, they are allowed to remain 8 minutes, following which they are transferred to tanks containing layers of moss and chipped ice. Fish so anesthetized can be held for 4 to 4½ hours with a mortality of approximately 10%.

Treatment of fungal infections and other localized diseases in pet or ornamental fish can be performed with tricaine methanesulfonate anesthesia. For "tranquilization" of pet or ornamental fish for transportation, low concentrations are used. Gossington (1957) employs 0.14 to 0.32 g/gal depending upon the species of fish, size of container, and presence or absence of oxygen (Table 18–3).

Large fish, such as sharks and rays, cannot be conveniently immersed in a solution. Therefore, Gilbert and Wood (1957) developed a method by which these fish can be anesthetized while struggling behind a boat on either a hook

TABLE 18–3. Dose of Tricaine Methanesulfonate for Ornamental Fish

Variety of Fish	Concentration	Anesthesia Time
Tropicals at 75 to 80° F:		
Live bearers	0.32 g per gal	to 12 hrs, uncrowded
Egglayers	0.24 g per gal	to 12 hrs, uncrowded
For uncrowded shipment of pugnacious species, without oxygen:		
Bettas, piranhas	0.25 g per gal	to 48 hr
For goldfish, with oxygen:		
Goldfish variety	0.14 g per gal	to 48 hrs

(From Gossington, R.E.: An Aid to Fish Handling—Tricaine. Aquarium J., 28:318, 1957.)

or a harpoon. Tricaine in a concentration of 1:1000 (1/g/L of seawater) is used. The head of the fish is held above the water level by means of a gaff or leader; small fish may be temporarily removed from the water. By means of a water pistol, rubber bulb syringe, or small hand pump, the solution is introduced into the mouths of fish or the spiracles of rays and sprayed over the gill exits of the pharynx. Small species require approximately 100 ml and larger fish up to 1 L of solution. The action of the drug is quite rapid, 15 seconds being required for a visible effect to take place. A 400-pound shark may be anesthetized in 1 minute or less. The fish may then be manipulated either in or out of the water until recovery begins to take place. If additional anesthesia is required, it may be given, or recovery may be hastened by washing the gills with fresh seawater. This can be accomplished with large fish by ''walking'' the fish in a pool with its mouth open or by spraying a stream of fresh seawater into the mouth. Recovery usually begins to take place within 5 to 30 minutes after the fish is returned to the water.

The time elapsing before loss of muscular activity appears to be directly proportional to the concentration of drug that is used. Figure 18–1 shows the suggested dose for sharks. The effect of a given concentration varies inversely with the size of the fish. An increase in toxicity has been observed and correlated with a marked rise in temperature of the immersing solution.

Benzocaine (ethyl ester of paraminobenzoic acid) is insoluble in water and is dissolved in acetone (40 mg/ml) to prepare an anesthetic for fish. Sufficient anesthesia for tagging, marking, and measuring is produced by 20 to 30 ppm (5 ml in 8 L of salt or fresh water); 50 ppm pro-

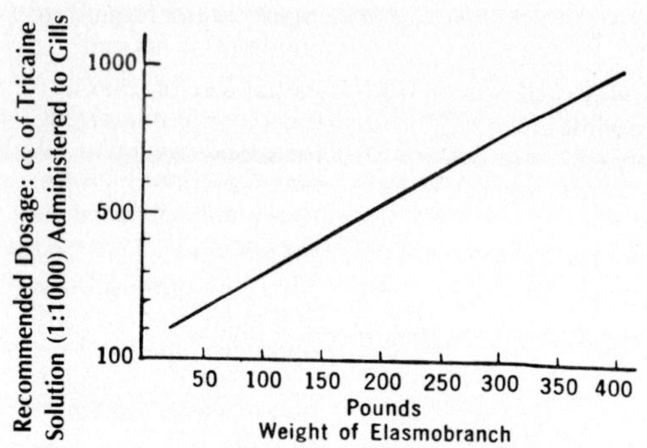

Figure 18–1. Dose of tricaine solution (1:1000 concentration) recommended to anesthetize a shark or ray in 60 seconds or less. The solution should be sprayed over the gill exits of the pharynx while the head of the elasmobranch is held above the water level. If the head remains under water, proportionally stronger concentrations must be utilized. (From Gilbert, P.W., and Wood, F.G., Jr.: Method of Anesthetizing Large Sharks and Rays Safely and Rapidly. Science, 126:212, 1957.)

duces surgical anesthesia. According to Green (1979), it is possibly the agent of choice for fish.

Propoxate hydrochloride (R 7464) is one of several 1-substituted imidazole-5-carboxylic acid esters having hypnotic activity, and it is a safe anesthetic for cold-blooded vertebrates including fish (Green, 1979). Tranquilization for up to 16 hours results from 0.25 ppm in salt or fresh water, while light surgical anesthesia requires 4 ppm.

Metomidate (see Chap. 13) in aqueous solution has been used on a variety of fish, ranging from trout and salmon to goldfish (Scordelis, 1977). The optimal dose ranged from 7.5 (salmonids) to 15 ppm (goldfish). The onset of anesthesia was 2 to 5 minutes, and recovery lasted 6 to 12 minutes.

An inexpensive method for anesthetizing

large fish in tank trucks or other large volumes of water is by the use of carbon dioxide (Fish, 1942). This is produced by addition of calculated amounts of technical-grade sodium bicarbonate and sulfuric acid to water with a temperature between 45 and 60° F. The carbon dioxide content of the water is determined by titration with N/44 sodium hydroxide. Some type of recirculating equipment must be available to disperse the reagents when added. Care must be taken in the storage and handling of sulfuric acid.

Carbon dioxide concentrations of 400 ppm for as long as 20 minutes of anesthesia appear to cause no permanent ill effect. The optimum carbon dioxide concentration for anesthetizing salmon and steelhead trout is 200 ppm. At this concentration, the fish gradually lose consciousness, turn over, and sink to the bottom of the tank within 90 seconds after the solution reaches full strength. The depth of respiration is used as a measure of the approaching lethal end point. Respiratory movement gradually lessens and finally ceases, at which time the fish will not revive when placed in fresh water.

After the period of exposure during which the fish are sorted or otherwise handled (which should not exceed 5 minutes), the carbon dioxide is neutralized by addition of the proper quantity of sodium carbonate. This quickly restores the original carbon dioxide concentration. Following neutralization with sodium carbonate, the fish remain anesthetized for an additional 5 to 10 minutes.

A tumor operation on a 500-pound jewfish, performed while submerged 16 feet under water in a 500,000-gallon tank, has been reported (Anonymous, 1958). By feeding it small fish containing tranquilizers and then injecting it with a local anesthetic, workers prepared the fish for operation.

Intracranial injection of procaine for anesthesia of fish has been described by Kisch (1947). With the fish on its stomach, a 20-gauge needle is inserted through the skull on the midline slightly posterior to a line connecting both eyes. One-fourth to 1 ml of 5% procaine is injected intracranially. Within a few minutes the fish becomes immobilized, and anesthesia lasts for one-half to one hour. The fish continues to breathe, and the head should be kept submerged for proper oxygenation. This type of anesthesia has been used in laboratories studying the fish heart.

FROGS, TOADS, NEWTS, SALAMANDERS, AND MUD PUPPIES

There are wide interspecies differences in the reaction of frogs to anesthetic agents (Kaplan et al., 1962). No preanesthetic preparation is necessary.

Three sites for intravascular injection are the dorsal lymph sacs, ventral lymph sacs, and ventral abdominal vein. The dorsal lymph sacs are paired organs located on either side of the last vertebra. The location of these paired lymph hearts can be determined by observation of their rhythmic beating. One can inject 2 to 3 ml of solution at one time by this route.

Leopard frogs *(Rana pipiens)* can be anesthetized with either hexobarbital (120 mg/kg) or pentobarbital (60 mg/kg) in the dorsal lymph sac (Kaplan et al., 1962). With the former, induction occurs in roughly 22 minutes, and surgical anesthesia lasts for about 3 hours. With the latter, induction averages 31 minutes, and anesthesia is maintained for approximately 9 hours. Neither anesthetic provides complete muscular relaxation. Intramuscular chlorpromazine followed by pentobarbital in the dorsal lymph sac is highly fatal to *R. pipiens*. Leopard frogs can be anesthetized by administration of 60 mg/kg of pentobarbital intraperitoneally. Induction averages 18 minutes, and deep anesthesia persists for an average of 9.5 hours.

Paraldehyde (4.2 g/kg) injected into the ventral lymph sac produces narcosis in approximately 15 minutes (Blume and Sroka, 1943). Chloral hydrate may be injected into the dorsal lymph sac at a rate of 1 to 2 ml of a 10% solution (Tanner, 1954). Injection of ketamine (55 to 210 mg/kg) into the dorsal lymph sac causes severe depression of pulse and respiration and is not recommended (Wass and Kaplan, 1974).

The frog breathes mainly through its skin, and inhalation anesthetics may be introduced by this route. The frog may be placed in a bell jar, or

TABLE 18–4. Data for Methoxyflurane Anesthesia in *Rana pipiens* (Acclimatized to 21°C)*

Number Frogs (and Sex)	*Body Weight (g)*	*Induction Time (min) for Deep Anesthesia (mean ± SD)*	*Duration (min) of Deep Anesthesia (mean ± SD)*	*Time (hr) for Full Recovery† (mean ± SD)*
15 (male)	48–98	2.0 ± 0.1	37.9 ± 21.1	7 ± 0.5
15 (female)	69–101	2.0 ± 0.2	38.7 ± 20.5	7 ± 0.4

*All data are bound to the ambient temperature, in frogs as in other ectotherms.

†Recovery time is the time from the end of the period of deep anesthesia to the time that such processes as righting reflexes, sensation, and locomotion are reestablished.

(From Wass, J.A., and Kaplan, H.M.: Methoxyflurane Anesthesia for *Rana pipiens*. Lab. Anim. Sci., 24:669, 1974.)

other closed container, along with ether-soaked cotton. An alternative is to wrap the frog in ether-soaked cotton without placing it in a container. Deep ether anesthesia is prolonged and characterized by very slow shallow respirations.

Methoxyflurane-soaked cotton in a semiclosed jar produces a period of excitement followed by deep anesthesia in approximately 2 minutes (Table 18–4) (Wass and Kaplan, 1974).

Intracranial procaine anesthesia has been described in frogs (Kisch, 1947). In bullfrogs weighing 250 to 500 g, 0.4 to 0.6 ml of 3 to 5% procaine hydrochloride solution is injected with a 20-gauge needle just caudal to the midpoint between the eyes. Anesthesia develops after a few minutes of excitement and persists for about 1 hour. No lasting side effects have been reported. Spinal anesthesia has been described in *R. pipiens* by Bieter et al (1932). Injection is made at the urostyle with a tuberculin syringe and 26-gauge needle. Procaine (0.21 mg/g) produces 90 to 125 minutes of anesthesia.

Parker (1939) has reported the use of hypothermia in frogs. Immersion in a cracked ice-water mixture for 10 to 15 minutes produces anesthesia.

A number of agents have been used to produce anesthesia of amphibians by immersion. Among them are chlorobutanol, alcohol, propoxate, and tricaine methanesulfonate. It should be emphasized that this type of anesthesia is dependent upon several factors, including size, physical condition, and environmental temperature. Frogs may be immersed from 4 to 8 minutes in 0.2% chlorobutanol, following which they may be kept in chlorobutanol-soaked cotton to extend the duration of anesthesia. Recovery from immersion takes place in 3 to 6 hours. Frog tadpoles immersed in 0.03% chlorobutanol frequently die (Witschi, 1927). Ten percent ethyl alcohol can be used to anesthetize frogs, since it is absorbed through their intact skin (Kaplan and Kaplan, 1961; Fankhauser, 1945). Three-inch frogs *(R. pipiens)* are placed in a container filled with alcohol to a depth of 8 to 10 mm. When deep anesthesia is reached, the frog is washed with tap water and placed in water 8 to 10 mm deep to recover. About 10 minutes are required to induce surgical anesthesia, which lasts about 20 minutes. Variations in induction and duration of anesthesia occur, depending upon the frog's size and the ambient temperature, but the total duration is about 41 minutes. Higher concentrations of alcohol or a longer immersion time may prove fatal.

Sixteen ppm of propoxate will cause loss of righting reflex in frogs (Green, 1979). Propoxate (4 ppm) has also been used to anesthetize adult salamanders without mortality (Thienpont and Niemegeers, 1965).

Adult frogs *(R. pipiens)* may be anesthetized by immersion in 0.1% (1:1,000) tricaine methanesulfonate (Yankow, 1962). A 1:3,000 solution is recommended for tadpoles and adults of *R. pipiens* (McGovern and Rugh, 1944). It has no effect on frog spermatozoa and is satisfactory for amphibian embryos at all stages of development. Larvae of the spotted salamander *(Ambystoma punctatum)* may be placed in 1:7,500 solution, the induction period varying with the age and size of the larvae. When body length was 10 mm, narcosis occurred in 2 hours, whereas at 33 mm it developed in 5 to 10 minutes (Karczmar and Koppanyi, 1948).

The red spotted newt *(Diemictylus triturus viridescens)* has been anesthetized in the aquatic adult stage by immersion in 0.2% chlorobutanol. Larvae may be anesthetized in 1:3,000 to 1:5,000 solutions (Fankhauser, 1945).

Tricaine methanesulfonate (1:3,000) has been used for *Ambystoma maculatum* embryos, larvae, and adults (Copenhaver, 1939). It has also been used in 1:2,000 solution for the larvae of *Triturus torosus,* the California newt, and for the mud puppy.

Propoxate (4 ppm) has been used successfully to anesthetize adult salamanders (Thienpont and Niemegeers, 1965).

During anesthesia and the recovery period, amphibians must be kept moist over the entire body, but care should be taken that they do not become immersed since they may drown. They should be kept at room temperature during the recovery period. Postoperative complications experienced in other animals, such as vomiting, are not a problem.

SNAKES AND LIZARDS

Rather obvious differences exist in the respiratory system of the snake when compared to other reptiles. The single lung consists of an elongated, thin-walled, hollow, tubular organ. The trachea is unusual in that it is open along the side within the lung. The lung terminates in an indistinguishable air sac (similar to that seen in birds) which may continue almost to the cloaca. Without a diaphragm, an inspired breath can inflate the snake for almost its entire length. This is especially obvious in certain species such as the hognose snake. Calderwood (1971) has suggested that these features predispose to respiratory arrest. The basal metabolic rate of snakes is low and related to the environmental temperature. Snakes are also resistant to hypoxia and can hold their breath for several minutes.

Intramuscular althesin is an effective anesthetic in lizards and chelonians, but the effect varies in snakes (Lawrence and Jackson, 1983). Induction and recovery times are slow. The optimum dose in lizards and chelonians is 15 mg total steroid/kg; surgical anesthesia for 15 to 30 minutes will be produced.

Small snakes and almost all poisonous varieties are placed in a glass aquarium fitted with an airtight sliding glass or plastic lid (Fig. 18–2). Methoxyflurane is dispensed by means of cotton wrapped in gauze and taped to the aquarium wall. Contact of the snake's skin with the anesthetic should be avoided since it may produce a premature partial shed. In most cases, a short period of excitement precedes the anesthetic state. The snake is left in the chamber, which is turned so that the snake is on its back. When respiration continues at a regular rate but the inverted snake is unable to right itself, it can safely be removed from the chamber for examination. The total time elapsing after the snake is placed in the chamber until the desired anesthetic state has been reached varies between 15 and 25 minutes in snakes of 0.5 to 10 lbs when the room temperature is between 75 and 78° F. (Soifer, 1969). Variations in room temperature affect the rate of vaporization of methoxyflurane.

When ether-soaked cotton is used, anesthesia usually develops in about 3 minutes. There is a wide margin of safety, approximately 1 hour being required to kill a snake in a closed jar containing ether vapor. Three minutes within the jar will produce roughly 15 minutes of anesthesia. The ambient temperature is important since snakes are poikilothermic, and anesthesia should be induced at room temperature. In no instance should this procedure be done at high temperatures. Anesthesia is not accompanied by muscle relaxation; hypertonicity usually results (Van Stee, 1960).

Although placement of anesthetic in a closed chamber is commonly used for induction, the method does have certain disadvantages. The concentration of anesthetic depends upon box size and temperature, and hypoxia may develop unless supplemental oxygen is provided.

Methods commonly used to determine depth of anesthesia are useless in this species. There are no toes to pinch or eyelids to blink. Touching the muscles firmly along the vertebral column

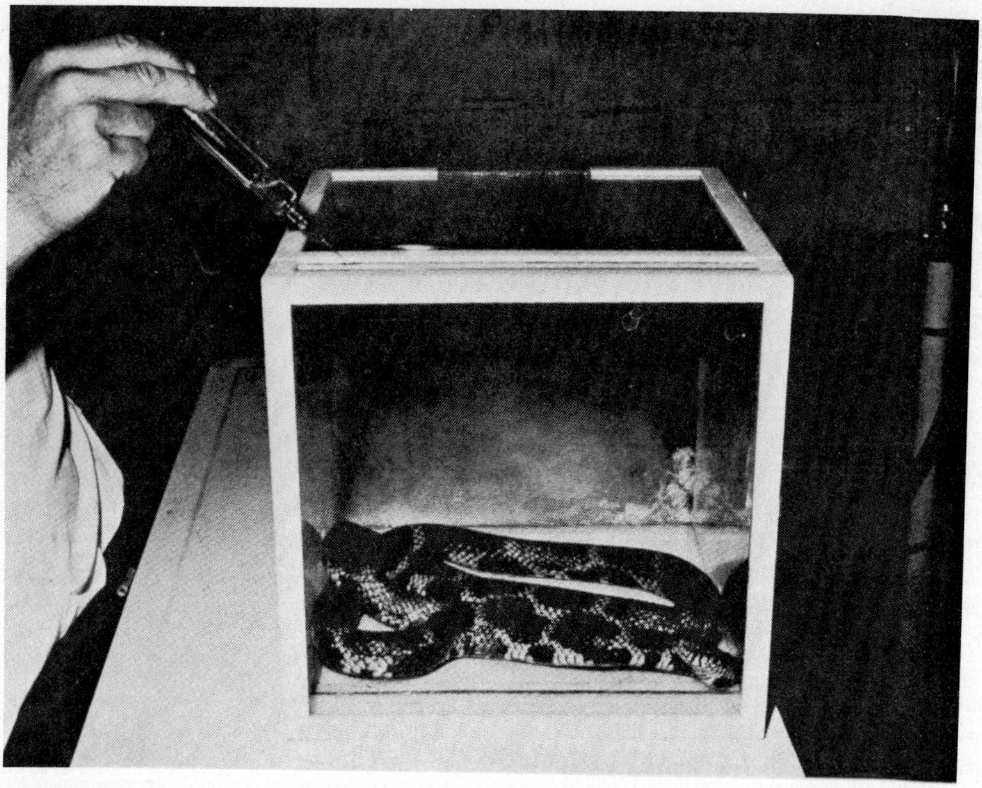

Figure 18–2. Anesthetic chamber for snakes. At least one side must be transparent for close observation during induction. (From Gandal, C.P.: A Practical Anesthetic Technique in Snakes, Utilizing Methoxyflurane. Anim. Hosp., 4:258, 1968.)

produces a spastic reaction in a snake not fully under the effects of the anesthetic. A more accurate method of determining depth is to check the tonus of the forked tongue. The tip of the tongue is gently grasped with tongue forceps, and an attempt is made to withdraw it from its sheath. Marked resistance is met unless the snake is properly anesthetized. During surgical anesthesia, the tongue may be fully withdrawn and should remain extruded. There is an obvious dilatation of the pupils when surgical anesthesia has been reached.

The snake lacks an epiglottis, and the marked anterior position of the glottis makes it possible to place an endotracheal catheter in the unanesthetized animal (Fig. 18–3). A strip of adhesive tape is placed around the tube, tracheal opening, and lower jaw to fix it in position. This method can be utilized for anesthetizing large snakes. By means of a closed system, the snake

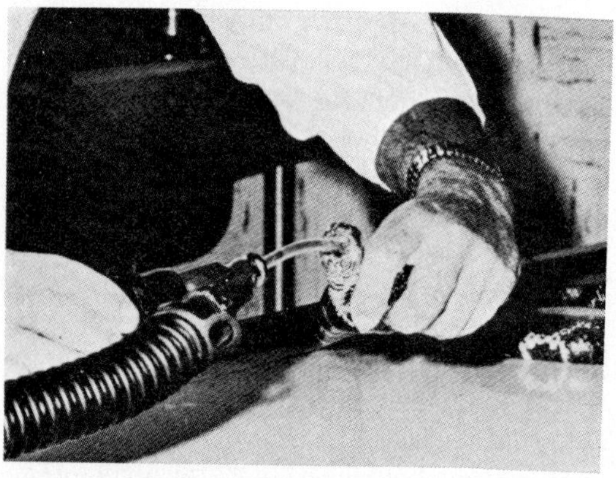

Figure 18–3. For longer procedures, snakes may be intubated and connected to an anesthetic machine. (From Gandal, C.P.: A Practical Anesthetic Technique in Snakes, Utilizing Methoxyflurane. Anim. Hosp., 4:258, 1968.)

is carefully "bagged" until relaxation occurs. Additional anesthetic is administered via mask since the respiratory action of the snake is not forceful and will not drive the gases through the anesthesia machine. For this reason, administration via a T-piece type system is preferable. Gas flows from 50 to 500 ml/min are used, depending upon the size of the snake. Recovery may be hastened by gentle evacuation of the lungs. This is accomplished by a milking action of the hand drawn from the cloacal end of the snake toward the head (Soifer, 1969).

Halothane, with or without nitrous oxide, is a satisfactory anesthetic for snakes. Bullsnakes *(Pituophis catenifer)* and chicken snakes *(Elaphe quadrivittata)* ranging from 4 to 6 feet long can be placed in a clear plastic bag, the air expressed, and a gaseous mixture consisting of 4% halothane, 72% nitrous oxide, and 24% oxygen introduced (Kramer et al., 1965*a*). Induction requires 20 to 30 minutes. Once relaxation has occurred, the snake is removed from the bag and intubated. Anesthesia can be maintained with a mixture of 3% halothane, 48% oxygen, and 49% nitrous oxide. The depth of anesthesia can be readily altered by a few compressions of the rebreathing bag, a pressure of 10 to 12 mm Hg being required to expand the snake's thorax. Observation of the snake prior to anesthetization allows determination of its respiratory rate at the ambient temperature. To terminate anesthesia, the snake can be ventilated with oxygen.

Other inhalation anesthetics may be used. Although Gandal (1968) considered methoxyflurane to be the safest, deaths have been reported in cobras (Burke and Wall, 1970). Prior to extubation, the snake should be ventilated with oxygen. If the agent employed has a high solubility coefficient, such as methoxyflurane or ether, the period of ventilation should be prolonged.

Ketamine may be administered subcutaneously or intramuscularly to snakes (Glenn et al., 1972; Cooper, 1974*a*). The dose is approximately 40 to 60 mg/kg. The depth of anesthesia is indicated by squeezing the tail and testing the righting reflex. A wide dose range of ketamine is effective in venomous snakes when injected intramuscularly, depending upon the effect desired (Glenn et al., 1972) (Table 18–5). Snakes receiving 60 to 80 mg/kg were tranquil for 48 to 96 hours; after 132 mg/kg or more they remained tranquil for 5 to 7 days.

TABLE 18–5. Recommended Doses of Ketamine HCl for Tranquilizing and Anesthetizing Snakes

Doses (mg/kg)	*Remarks*
(A) 22 to 44	Dosage usually effective for tranquilizing effect; used mainly in small (<2 kg) snakes and as the initial injection to test response to anesthesia; slight mobility is retained.
(B) 55 to 88	Dosage required for most surgical procedures; effects last 1 to 3 days.
(C) 99 to 132	Total accumulative dose (mg/kg) recommended for snakes that do not reach depth of anesthesia required from doses (A) or (B). Effects last 2 to 6 days; at 132-mg/kg dose levels, respiratory-support measures may be required.

(From Glenn, J.L., Straight, R., and Snyder, C.C.: Clinical Use of Ketamine Hydrochloride as an Anesthetic Agent for Snakes. Am. J. Vet. Res., 33:1901, 1972.)

Snakes become sluggish at low temperatures, and Vierheller (1959) has reported an instance in which advantage was taken of this fact to facilitate radiography of a Pacific rattler. The snake was placed in a refrigerator at about 45° F for 1 hour following which it was transported in a sack containing ice cubes from the owner's home to a veterinary hospital. Though tractable, the snake was still able to coil and raise its head. Three weeks following hypothermia the snake gave birth to eight living young.

Mosby and Cantner (1955) have administered tribromoethanol orally with a syringe to snakes and turtles (Table 18–6). These responded quickly and remained narcotized longer than warm-blooded animals.

Several agents can be injected into the pleuroperitoneal cavity of snakes in the posterior third of the body on the ventral midline (Wallach, 1969). Etorphine hydrochloride (2.0 to 15.0 mg), thiopental sodium (0.016 to 0.025 mg/g), and pentobarbital sodium (0.015 to 0.050 mg/g) have all been used. Kramer et al. (1965*a*) found that thiopental and thiamylal ad-

TABLE 18–6. Reactions of Various Forms of Wildlife to Orally Administered Tribromoethanol

Type of Specimen	*Dosage in g/lb*	*Time Required to Anesthetize in Minutes*	*Time Required to Recover In Hours*	*Remarks*
Turtle, snapper	0.08	5	48	Still drowsy 3.5 days later
Snake, copperhead	0.05	3	6+	
Snake, coachwhip	0.08	3–5	6+	
Blackbird, rusty	0.15	7	1.5	
Starling	0.12	1	3+	
Chipmunk	0.02	1	3.5	Resp. rate changes 132-34-60
Opossum	0.11	6	10+	Still drowsy after 24 hrs
Woodchuck	0.09	2	0.5	Easily handled for 1 hr
Cat, domestic	0.09	4	24	Resp. rate changes 35-14-20
Skunk, striped	0.06	3	2.5	

(From Mosby, H.S., and Cantner, D.E.: The Use of Avertin in Capturing Wild Turkeys and as an Oral-Basal Anesthetic for Other Wild Animals. Southwest Vet., 9:132, 1955.)

ministered intraperitoneally at levels of 2 to 6 mg/kg of body weight produced a high mortality rate with very slow recovery, requiring 48 to 72 hours. Cooper (1974*a*) has also reported fatalities with pentobarbital, phencyclidine, and metomidate.

Procaine hydrochloride has been used as a euthanatizing agent for reptiles. A 10% solution is injected into the pleuroperitoneal cavity a short distance behind the heart at the rate of 0.05 ml (0.47 mg)/g of body weight. Death occurs in 5 to 15 minutes (Livezey, 1957).

Lizards of various species may be anesthetized by the same methods used for snakes.

TURTLES

Most turtles are easily handled. Box turtles must have their shells forced apart if an injection is to be made. Soft-shelled aquatic turtles, which move quickly and can bite and scratch, should be handled with tongs and tied with ropes to a fixed support (Kaplan, 1969). No special preoperative preparation is necessary for these species.

Intramuscular injections can be made in the gluteal muscles of the hind leg. Intracardial injections are made by angling a long needle between the neck and one forelimb. Intravenous injections can be made by drilling the plastron with a drill press and a 1½" diameter bit to expose the ventral abdominal vein.

The respiratory movements of turtles are produced chiefly by muscles at each leg pocket and beneath the viscera (Betz, 1962). With deep anesthesia, these muscles may become paralyzed, and artificial respiration may be needed. It is usually not necessary, however. Induction of inhalation anesthesia may be complicated by the ability of turtles to switch to anaerobic respiration. To obviate this, 5 to 10% CO_2 may be added to the inspired mixture (Stunkard and Miller, 1974).

Only a few anesthetic drugs have been used on turtles, and little is known about their relative advantages. Intramuscular althesin (15 mg total steroid/kg) is effective for 15 to 30 minutes of surgical anesthesia (Lawrence and Jackson, 1983). Ether can be administered with a nasal cone. Induction of deep anesthesia requires about 37 minutes for species of Pseudemys and may last for as much as 10 hours in 25% of the turtles. There is adequate muscular relaxation with a fall in rectal temperature and a marked drop in the pulse rate after several hours.

Ensley (1981) anesthetized a Galapagos 151-kg tortoise with 500 mg of ketamine IM, followed by halothane-N_2O via mask and endotracheal tube.

Adult Pseudemys turtles can be effectively anesthetized by intramuscular administration of 10 mg/kg of chlorpromazine followed by an intracardiac injection, between neck and forelimb, of 10 mg/kg of pentobarbital (Young and Kaplan, 1960). Deep anesthesia develops 15 minutes after injection, with surgical anesthesia lasting approximately 3 hours. In most turtles, muscular relaxation is fully attained in 1 hour. Chlorpromazine reduces the induction time needed with pentobarbital alone and produces a more predictable response.

Etorphine (0.5 to 5 mg IM) has been reported to produce analgesia and ataxia in red-eared turtles; in Galapagos tortoises 10 to 15 mg produced analgesia adequate for minor surgery (Wallach et al., 1967).

Pseudemys may be anesthetized with 16 mg/kg of pentobarbital intraperitoneally. Deep anesthesia develops in about 65 minutes and lasts roughly 3 hours. Poor muscular relaxation is common. Vos-Maas and Zwart (1976) reported an unpredictable response with pentobarbital (50 mg/kg) in red-eared turtles, but produced satisfactory relaxation and analgesia with chloral hydrate-pentobarbital-magnesium sulfate (2.5 ml/kg, IM).

Wood et al. (1982) anesthetized the green sea turtle *(Chelonia mydas)* with pentobarbital, thiopental, or ketamine (Table 18–7). They found that pentobarbital was satisfactory, but produced prolonged recovery times. Recovery from thiopental was rapid, but the anesthesia produced was somewhat erratic. Ketamine was satisfactory when given intraperitoneally, though the dose required proved expensive.

Soifer (1969) believes that methoxyflurane is the safest anesthetic for turtles. Small species can be placed in any container that is reasonably airtight such as a glass jar, plastic sack, or covered aquarium. A reservoir for anesthetic is produced with several cotton balls wrapped in a 3″ by 3″ gauze sponge and taped to the wall of the chamber. Cooper (1976) reported that induction of inhalation anesthesia can be facilitated by turning the animal on its back, which increases respiration. Tonus of the head, neck, and limbs can be used to judge the depth of anesthesia. Respiratory movements can be observed as alternating concavity and convexity of the skin adjacent to the limbs and tail. With such rudimentary methods to determine depth of anesthesia, close and frequent examination of the subject is necessary.

When the desired state has been reached, the animal is removed from the chamber and additional anesthetic is administered with a face mask. Suitable masks can be made from various sizes of glass vials or from plastic containers in which disposable syringes are packaged. These are fitted with cotton balls soaked in the anesthetic agent.

It is possible to anesthetize the turtle or tortoise using the face mask as the sole means of administration. The difficulty comes in the animal's ability to withdraw its head into the safety of its shell. Box turtles and several other varieties are capable of enclosing the soft portions of their bodies within the carapace and plastron (top and bottom shells) making the mask method unusable. Cooper (1976) suggests 60 to 80 mg/kg IM of ketamine to facilitate administration of halothane-N_2O. Another alternative is to open the mouth manually and spray the larynx with topical anesthetic, after which a wooden dowel with a hole through it is positioned crosswise in the mouth and an endotracheal tube is inserted.

Soifer (1968) has reported anesthetizing a 500-pound 60-year-old Galapagos tortoise. Methoxyflurane, administered from an anesthetic

TABLE 18–7. Summary of Anesthetic Parameters for Drugs used to Anesthetize Green Sea Turtles

No. of Turtles	*Drug*	*Dosage (mg/kg)*	*Route*	*Induction Time (min)*	*Duration of Anesthesia (min)*	*Recovery Time (hr)*
8	Sodium pentobarbital	10.0–25.0	IV	14–120	40–240	4–24
11	Ketamine hydrochloride	38.0–71.0	IP	2–10	2–10	<4
26	Sodium thiopental	18.8–31.4	IV	5–10	5–120	<6

(From Wood, F.E., Critchley, K.H., and Wood, J.R.: Anesthesia in the Green Sea Turtle, *Chelonia mydas*. Am. J. Vet. Res., 43:1882, 1982.)

machine with a mask, was continued for over 1 hour.

Turtles, like other ectotherms, should be held postoperatively at a moderate relative humidity and room temperature.

ALLIGATORS AND CROCODILES

These species are seldom anesthetized. The sense of pain in alligators does not appear to be highly developed, but they resent restraint (O'Connor, 1981). Both alligators and crocodiles detoxify drugs slowly, resulting in prolonged recovery from anesthesia.

Pleuger (1950) administered pentobarbital orally and intraperitoneally to alligators and crocodiles. Alligators weighing 5 lbs or less given 1.5 gr orally were profoundly anesthetized in a few hours. A 300-lb crocodile was given 30 gr of pentobarbital orally by means of a balling gun on a 10-foot pole. This produced slight sedation for 24 hours.

American alligators weighing 2 to 5 kg can be given pentobarbital intramuscularly in the base of the tail at a rate of 3.5 to 4.0 mg/lb. Recovery occurs in 2 to 3 hours (Brisbin, 1966). Alligators given tricaine methanesulfonate intramuscularly at the rate of 40.0 to 45.0 mg/lb are completely relaxed in 10 minutes with recovery in 9 to 10 hours. Intramuscular succinylcholine chloride causes skeletal muscle relaxation in 4 minutes when given to alligators at a rate of 1.35 to 2.25 mg/lb. Recovery occurs in 7 to 9 hours.

Ketamine partially immobilizes alligators and crocodiles in doses of 12 to 15 mg/kg IM. Immobilization is adequate to allow maintenance of anesthesia with 2% halothane plus N_2O-O_2.

Wallach (1969) and Wallach and Hoessle (1970) reported use of etorphine in alligators and crocodiles ranging in weight from 0.25 to 150 lbs. Intraperitoneal injection shortened the induction time but did not alter the general effect. The dose ranged from 0.5 to 20 mg.

Generalized hypothermia has also been utilized with these species (Griner, 1969). Small subjects can be placed in a refrigerator and larger ones in a walk-in cooler until sedated.

The immobility reflex (see Chap. 13) can be used to induce an hypnotic state in young alligators (O'Connor, 1981). They are turned on their backs and the abdomen is stroked. Recalcitrant individuals can be strapped to a long three-inch-thick board to prevent them from moving their powerful tails.

CAGED BIRDS

Veterinarians are frequently confronted with the necessity for administration of anesthesia to various avian species. Agents that have been employed include methoxyflurane, halothane, ether, ethyl chloride, pentobarbital, chloral hydrate, ketamine, metomidate, and tribromoethanol. For an extensive review of drugs used in avian anesthesia, the reader is referred to Fedde (1978). Table 18–8 outlines the progression of signs of surgical anesthesia in birds.

With the high basal metabolic rate of birds, there is increased risk of hypoglycemia from food deprivation. The rapid heart rate changes drastically in response to fear or physical exertion, and there is increased potential for temperature loss due to the differential between the bird's body, the environment, and/or an inhaled gas. Thermal regulation is less efficient and less adaptable in birds than in mammals. Prevention of heat loss is critical, especially in the young. Temperature monitoring and a controlled source of heat are necessary for even the shortest procedures. Use of heating pads during surgery and heated recovery cages is essential. Acute cardiovascular failure may result from restraint, and hypotension may develop due to sudden changes in posture during anesthesia. Trauma in handling and anesthesia should be avoided by securing the wings to the back and fastening the legs together with adhesive tape. Preanesthetic tranquilization is also indicated.

Volatile anesthetics have proved satisfactory, but must be given with caution because of the bird's air sac system, which may allow a dangerous overconcentration of the anesthetic before the anesthesiologist realizes this has occurred. Poorly ventilated air sacs may be a source of high concentrations of inhalation anesthetic agents that may subsequently be released into the circulation. Postanesthetic

TABLE 18–8. Progression of Signs of Surgical Anesthesia in Birds

	Stages of Anesthesia			
	Induction and Narcosis	*Light*	*Medium*	*Deep*
Signs	Eyelids closing, wings starting to droop, head lowered			
Voluntary movement	Can be aroused and is sensitive to pain	Absent	Absent	Absent
Respirations	Deep, rapid, and regular without stimulation	Deep and rapid	Slow, deep, and regular	Slow, regular, and shallow
Corneal reflexes	Present	Present	Slow or intermittent	Absent
Pedal reflexes	Present	Present	Slow or intermittent	Absent
Palpebral reflexes	Present	Present	Absent	Absent
Cere reflexes	Present	Present	Absent	Absent

(From Arnall, L.: Anesthesia and Surgery in Cage and Aviary Birds. Vet. Rec., 73:139, 1961.)

administration of oxygen for five minutes or longer is therefore important.

Boever and Wright (1975) have pointed out that because there are over 850 species of birds, varying in size, behavior, and feeding habits, it is impossible to determine a dosage of ketamine applicable to all (Tables 18–9, 18–10, 18–11, 18–12). They recommend the following doses as guidelines.

1. Birds weighing less than 100 g (canaries, finches, parakeets, and small birds) 0.1 to 0.2 mg/g.
2. Birds weighing between 250 and 500 g (parrots, pigeons, and other medium-sized birds) 0.05 to 0.1 mg/g.
3. Birds weighing between 500 and 3000 g (chickens, owls, hawks, and other larger birds) 0.02 to 0.1 mg/g.
4. Birds weighing more than 300 g (ducks, swans, and larger birds) 0.02 to 0.05 mg/g.

TABLE 18–9. Ketamine in Birds Weighing Less than 100 G

Species	*Weight (g)*	*Dose (mg/g)*	*Induction Time (min)*	*Duration (min)*	*Comments*
Java rice bird	24	0.11	1	10	Immobilized
Java rice bird	25	0.11	1	15	Immobilized
Java rice bird	23	0.17	2	25	Immobilized
Java rice bird	26	0.17	1	30	Immobilized
Java rice bird	26	0.22	2	40	Immobilized; skin biopsy taken
Lady gouldian finch	15	0.22	3	75	Immobilized
Sora rail	82	0.22	1	15	Immobilized
Java rice bird	26	0.33	1	20	Anesthetized
Java rice bird	24	0.33	1	40	Immobilized; wing amputation
Java rice bird	27	0.33	1	35	Immobilized; leg amputation
Java rice bird	23	0.33	1	—	Respiratory failure and death
Java rice bird	26	0.33	1	—	Respiratory failure and death
Java rice bird	25	0.33	1	—	Respiratory failure and death

(From Boever, W.J., and Wright, W.: Use of Ketamine for Restraint and Anesthesia of Birds. Vet. Med./Small Anim. Clin. 70:86, 1975.)

TABLE 18–10. Ketamine in Birds Weighing 250 to 500 G

Species	*Weight (g)*	*Dose (mg/g)*	*Induction Time (min)*	*Duration (min)*	*Comments*
Pigeon	300	0.04	3	20	Immobilized
Pigeon	360	0.04	2	25	Immobilized
Pigeon	300	0.08	2	20	Immobilized
Pigeon	390	0.09	2	120	Immobilized
Pigeon	390	0.10	3	10	Immobilized
Double yellow-head parrot	500	0.10	3	40	Immobilized; set broken leg
Pigeon	480	0.11	2	35	Anesthetized
Pigeon	420	0.11	2	—	Respiratory failure and death
Laughing gull	330	0.11	2	5	Immobilized
Sea gull	420	0.11	3	20	Immobilized
Pigeon	360	0.13	1	—	Respiratory failure and death
Sea gull	420	0.13	2	60	Anesthetized
Sea gull	390	0.13	2	15	Immobilized
Sea gull	300	0.13	1	40	Anesthetized; wing amputation
Sea gull	360	0.13	1	50	Anesthetized; skin biopsy removed
Sea gull	300	0.15	2	90	Anesthetized
Pigeon	360	0.17	1	—	Respiratory failure and death
Sea gull	300	0.18	2	80	Anesthetized
Sea gull	390	0.19	2	30	Anesthetized
Sea gull	420	0.20	2	80	Anesthetized
Sea gull	360	0.22	1	—	Respiratory failure and death

(From Boever, W.J., and Wright, W.: Use of Ketamine for Restraint and Anesthesia of Birds. Vet. Med./Small Anim. Clin., 70:86, 1975.)

TABLE 18–11. Ketamine in Birds Weighing 500 to 2,000 G (0.5 to 2 Kg)

Species	*Weight (g)*	*Dose (mg/g)*	*Induction Time (min)*	*Duration (min)*	*Comments*
Eared owl	800	0.02	2	40	Immobilized
Barred owl	1,200	0.04	2	45	Anesthetized
Domestic chicken	1,800	0.04	3	10	Immobilized
Eared owl	800	0.09	1	70	Anesthetized
Eared owl	800	0.11	2	35	Anesthetized; pinioned left wing
Domestic chicken	1,700	0.11	3	30	Immobilized
Barred owl	1,200	0.13	1.5	90	Anesthetized
Domestic chicken	1,500	0.13	2	60	Immobilized
Sea gull	500	0.13	2	60	Anesthetized
Sea gull	600	0.15	2	55	Anesthesized
Domestic chicken	1,700	0.17	3	75	Immobilized
Sea gull	800	0.17	2	60	Anesthetized

(From Boever, W.J., and Wright, W.: Use of Ketamine for Restraint and Anesthesia of Birds. Vet. Med. Small Anim. Clin., 70:86, 1975.)

TABLE 18–12. Ketamine in Birds Weighing More than 3,000 G (3 Kg)

Species	*Weight (g)*	*Dose (mg/g)*	*Induction Time (min)*	*Duration (min)*	*Comments*
Double-wattled cassowary	45,000	0.02	4	90	Immobilized. Examined bumblefoot lesions. Dose delivered via carbon dioxide-powered dart.
Black swan	3,500	0.06	2.5	45	Immobilized; pinioned left wing
Black swan	3,500	0.06	2		Immobilized; pinioned left wing. Died of trauma to head during recovery thrashing.

(From Boever, W.J., and Wright, W.: Use of Ketamine for Restraint and Anesthesia of Birds. Vet. Med. Small Anim. Clin., 70:86, 1975.)

During recovery from ketamine excitement is common, with wing-flapping and head-shaking. Therefore, the bird must be protected in a well-padded area. Birds with long necks are particularly at risk during this period.

Harcourt-Brown (1978) has used althesin as an induction agent or as the sole anesthetic in a wide range of avian species. The intramuscular dose was 36 mg/kg and the intravenous dose was 10 mg/kg. Supplementary halothane was administered in some instances.

Methoxyflurane is probably the safest volatile agent for use in birds. Small birds may be anesthetized by placing the bird in a closed container, such as a 1-quart instant coffee jar, into which 0.1 ml of methoxyflurane is injected (Gandal, 1967). Induction requires 30 to 45 seconds following which the bird may be removed from the jar and anesthesia maintained with a methoxyflurane-soaked cotton pledget held at the bird's nostrils. A mask for small birds can be made from a plastic disposable syringe container into which cotton is inserted.

With larger birds the coffee jar can be used as a mask, the bird's head being inserted and a towel wrapped around the opening. Following induction, use of the mask may be continued, or the bird may be intubated and connected to an anesthesia machine.

Hoge (1966) has described the use of a modified coffee can for induction of anesthesia (Fig. 18–4).

An effective semiopen system can be devised from a Simplex intravenous set. The bell, which conventionally fits over the bottle, is used as a mask. The fluid administration tube is shortened and attached to an anesthetic vaporizer. The air intake tube, attached to the bell, is shortened to approximately 1½ times the bird's tidal volume, producing a modified Ayre's T-system.

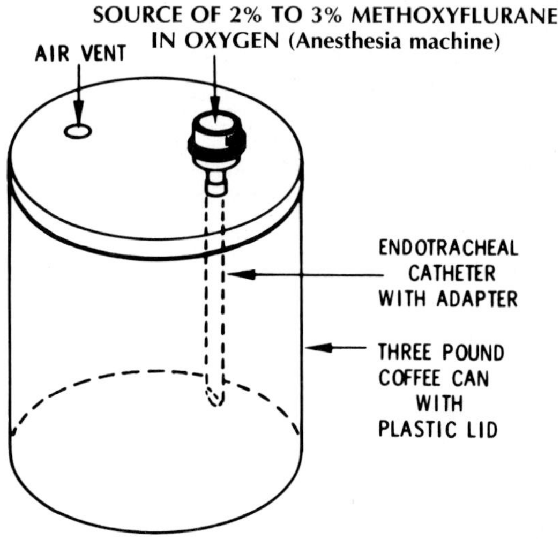

Figure 18–4. An anesthesia canister for anesthetizing birds or small rodents. (After Hoge, R.S.: Anesthesia and Surgery for Egg Bound Parakeets. Anim. Hosp., 2:46, 1966.)

Ether can be used for brief anesthesia, the bird being held in a recumbent position and ether sprayed from a 2-ml syringe, equipped with a 26-gauge, one-quarter-inch needle, into a nostril from a distance of about 1 inch. Administration must be discontinued as soon as struggling ceases and should be resumed at intervals as the bird begins to regain consciousness (Friedberg,

1961). Ethyl chloride also can be administered in much the same fashion from a dispenser. Its safety margin is greater than that of ether when used on birds. Ferguson (1961) has recommended the use of preanesthetics plus ethyl chloride for parakeets. A tablet containing ¼ gr of morphine sulfate and $\frac{1}{150}$ gr of atropine sulfate is diluted in 3 ml of sterile water, and 0.1 ml is given subcutaneously. After 30 minutes the bird is anesthetized with ethyl chloride sprayed on cotton and held over the nostrils.

It is difficult to administer anesthetics intravenously to small birds (Gandal, 1956). In addition to the small caliber of the accessible veins, restraint of a bird in an unnatural position is likely to induce shock, which is frequently fatal. Because the wing must be held extended, sudden movements by the bird may result in fracture or luxation of the wing bones. Even when venipuncture is accomplished, bird veins are so thin-walled that any struggling during injection is likely to cause their rupture.

If intramuscular pentobarbital sodium is used (Table 18–13), it should be diluted so that 1 ml is added to 8 ml of sterile water. This gives a concentration of approximately 7 mg/ml. A 35-g bird requires 0.2 ml of this diluted solution, which is injected into the pectoral muscle or the abdominal cavity with a 25-gauge needle. This dose is approximately 1.5 mg of the drug. The anesthetic stage is reached in 2 to 3 minutes and persists for about 30 minutes.

For administration of anesthetic to small species, a microliter or 1-ml glass tuberculin syringe and 25-gauge needle are recommended. Larger needles and syringes are used with correspondingly larger birds. Small birds, such as canaries and parakeets, may be weighed on a small two-pan scale by placing the bird head first in a cone made of paper toweling or in a small cardboard box or ice cream carton (Fig. 18–5). If a container is used frequently, time will be saved by marking the weight on the outside to avoid repeated weighing.

Following injection of anesthetic, the bird should be released in a small well-ventilated confined area. Small caged birds can be returned to the cage. As anesthesia develops, these birds will become unable to maintain themselves in an upright position and, if sitting on perches, will rotate and become suspended head down until deeper anesthesia causes them to fall to the floor of the cage.

Leonard (1960) believes oral pentobarbital is safer for parakeets and canaries than that given parenterally. He suggests that birds fasted for 24 hours be given 2.0 mg of pentobarbital sodium diluted in 0.25 ml of water orally. A second dose may be given in 15 minutes if necessary.

During the recovery period it is important that birds be kept warm; a temperature of 85 to 90° F is optimum. A simple incubator can be made from heating tape and an inexpensive chicken brooder thermostat (Lynn, 1967). A commercially made unit that provides oxygen, carbon dioxide absorption, nebulization, and high humidity is also available.*

Occasionally, small birds will evidence handling shock. If this develops, a heat lamp should be judiciously applied until arousal occurs. Oxygen administration may also be of value.

Procaine is toxic for parakeets and should *never* be used in this species. Procaine penicillin is also contraindicated.

*See Appendix A for manufacturer.

TABLE 18–13. Sodium Pentobarbital Dosages for Parakeets

Bird's Wt (g)	30	32	34	36	38	40	42	44	46	48	50	52
Site of injection					I.M.—pectoral region							
Volume of injection (ml)	.025	.026	.028	.03	.031	.033	.035	.036	.038	.039	.041	.048
Amount of active ingredient (mg)	1.50	1.60	1.70	1.80	1.90	2.00	2.10	2.20	2.30	2.40	2.50	2.60
Strength: 60 mg per ml												

(Adapted from AAHA Bulletin, 29th Annual Committee Reports, 1962, and Donovan, C.A.: Restraint and Anesthesia of Caged Birds. Vet. Med., 53:541, 1958.)

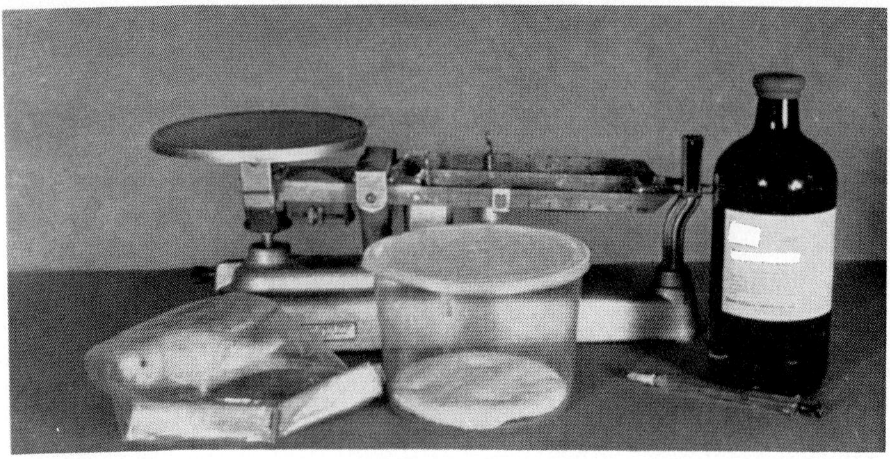

Figure 18–5. Equipment for anesthetizing small birds. The bird is placed in a plastic bag or container for weighing.

POULTRY

Medium-sized and large birds can easily be intubated, even without preanesthetic agents. With the bird's mouth held open, the larynx is observed behind the base of the tongue. Once it is intubated, a closed-system anesthetic machine can be used for induction and maintenance (Bennett, 1968). An alternative method is to direct the flow of anesthetic gas into the mouth until the bird relaxes, at which time it can be intubated (Anderson, 1967).

Intraperitoneal injection is accomplished in the midline, halfway between the cloaca and sternum, by directing the needle cranially almost parallel to the abdominal wall (Graham-Jones, 1966).

In medium- and large-sized birds, the carotid vessels in the neck can be palpated to determine the heart rate.

The use of halothane anesthesia in turkeys has been described by Jones (1966). It is not necessary to take them off feed and water prior to anesthesia, nor is premedication necessary. The bird is held by an assistant with the body under the left arm and the head held with the right hand. The anesthesiologist delivers the anesthetic to the bird by means of a suitable face mask using a concentration of 2 to 4% halothane with a flow rate of 1 to 2 L/min of oxygen. Surgical anesthesia is determined by pinching the pericloacal skin, comb, or wattles. The corneal reflex, with movement of the membrana nictitans, persists throughout anesthesia. Recovery is uneventful and occurs within 5 to 20 minutes.

A unique method for anesthetizing birds weighing over 50 g has been described by Whittow and Ossorio (1970). With this method, halothane or methoxyflurane vapor is administered directly into the intraclavicular air sac by means of a special apparatus. The bird is lightly restrained on its back and a 2-in, 16-gauge thin-walled needle is inserted at an angle of approximately 40° to the horizontal, 3 to 4 cm rostral to the angle of the furcula. Penetration of the air sac is indicated by lack of resistance to the needle and by the ease with which air can be introduced or removed with a syringe. A PE-90 polyethylene catheter is passed through the needle into the sac, and the needle is withdrawn. Oxygen is first administered to determine the rate at which gas can be given without over-expanding the air sac of the bird. For rapid induction of anesthesia, halothane is administered. Halothane has proved to be the best agent for induction, whereas methoxyflurane has provided better maintenance of anesthesia. This method has been used successfully on white Leghorn chickens, turkeys, ducks, pigeons, quail, grackles, and sparrows.

This technique also provides a highly effective means of resuscitation following an overdose of anesthetic.

TABLE 18–14. Number of Chicks Responding to Varying Dosages of 0.5% Pentobarbital Sodium

	Dosage in ml							
	0.50	*0.40*	*0.35*	*0.30*	*0.25*	*0.20*	*0.15*	*0.10*
Single Comb White Leghorn								
Dead	6	3	0	0	0	0	0	0
Unconscious	4	7	10	10	10	10	10	2
Lethargic	0	0	0	0	0	0	0	8
Commercial Hybrid No. A								
Dead	4	2	0	0	0	0	0	0
Unconscious	6	8	10	10	10	10	10	1
Lethargic	0	0	0	0	0	0	0	9
White Plymouth Rock								
Dead	4	0	0	0	0	0	0	0
Unconscious	6	10	10	9	7	2	2	0
Lethargic	0	0	0	1	3	8	8	10
New Hampshire								
Dead	5	1	0	0	0	0	0	0
Unconscious	0	4	5	5	4	3	0	0
Lethargic	0	0	0	0	1	2	5	5

(From Morgan, W.: Effective Anesthesia for Chicks. Proc. S.D. Acad. Sci., 36:105, 1957.)

Morgan (1957) found a breed variation in susceptibility of chicks to 0.5% pentobarbital sodium (Tables 18–14 and 18–15).

Metomidate has been given to chickens in doses of 10, 15, and 20 mg/kg (Jones, 1972). They were not anesthetized, but exhibited sedation and hypnosis for up to 30 minutes. Turkeys receiving 10, 15, 20, and 30 mg/kg showed evidence of sedation and hypnosis and were anesthetized for 15 minutes with the highest dose. Excitement during recovery has been reported in storks and cranes by Jones (1977).

Gallamine has been used as an immobilizing agent in pigeons at the rate of 5 to 10 mg/bird (Desmedt and Delwaide, 1966). They state that depolarizing muscle relaxants readily produce contracture of avian muscle and for this reason are not very useful.

Young (1948), in describing wing amputation in birds, suggests the use of local anesthesia. The feathers are removed over a 2-inch area around the outer joint of the wing. With a 1-inch, 20-gauge needle, 2% procaine is injected on the upper and lower surfaces of the wing medial to the joint. The needle is pointed toward the body and nearly parallel to the wing as it is inserted. One milliliter divided into equal parts on the upper and lower surfaces of the wing is usually sufficient for small birds such as ducks. Two milliliters are required for a bird the size of a pelican.

Procaine hydrochloride has also been used in chickens and quail for gastrointestinal surgery with good results (Hollingsworth and Howes, 1965).

Friedberg (1962) has stated that a spray con-

TABLE 18–15. Average Time (in Minutes) Required for Chicks to Recover from 0.5% Pentobarbital Anesthesia

	Dosage in ml						
	0.50	*0.40*	*0.35*	*0.30*	*0.25*	*0.20*	*0.15*
Single Comb White Leghorn	172	220	117	110	114	95	66
Commercial Hybrid No. A	215	200	122	107	91	80	48
White Plymouth Rock	219	175	93	112	85	86	33
New Hamsphire	—	119	142	115	72	40	—
Overall Average	202	179	119	111	91	75	49

(From Morgan, W.: Effective Anesthesia for Chicks. Proc. S.D. Acad. Sci., 36:105, 1957.)

taining ethyl aminobenzoate, butyl aminobenzoate, and tetracaine hydrochloride* is a good topical anesthetic for birds and superior to ethyl chloride for local anesthesia. It has antiseptic properties and also penetrates the tissues well.

Geese are extremely sensitive to reserpine, 0.5 g per ton of growing ration causing excessive tranquilization, reduced feed intake, and loss of weight (Wilgus, 1960). Even as little as 0.0625 g per ton of feed for a period of 7 days causes inanition. This level for 3 or 4 days at 6 weeks of age results in a lasting degree of tranquilization.

For handling wild pheasants on game farms, reserpine can be added to the feed at a ratio of 8 g/30 lbs. This amount is sufficient for approximately 200 birds (40 mg/bird) and, if fed in the afternoon, will be consumed by the following morning. When fed on the day prior to handling, it will increase efficiency and reduce injuries to birds and handlers (Hewitt, 1959).

Flocks of pullets affected with hysteria have been successfully treated with a tranquilizer, metoserpate hydrochloride (Reynolds and Maplesden, 1977). It can also be used when birds are handled, debeaked, or transported. Because of residues, it cannot be used in chickens over 16 weeks of age.

CAPTURE OF FERAL BIRDS

Tribromoethanol was used by Mosby and Cantner (1955) in capturing wild turkeys. The dose of undiluted tribromoethanol was 0.75 ml on approximately 60 kernels of whole corn. Since the amount taken by an individual bird could not be controlled, an estimate was first made of the number of feeding birds and the amount of bait required was then determined. The area was inspected 5 to 10 minutes after the turkeys had eaten and, following collection of anesthetized birds, their crops were irrigated as quickly as possible.

The oral dose of tribromoethanol for turkeys, administered with a hypodermic syringe, is 60 to 90 mg/lb.

Metomidate is highly water-soluble and has an astringent taste. Acceptance of metomidate-treated bait varies markedly among species of birds. Common crows *(Corvus brachyrhynchos)* rarely eat a kernel of treated bait, whereas mourning doves *(Zenaidura macroura)* are not adversely affected by the taste when the bait is dry.

In capturing wild mourning doves, Martin (1967) has found metomidate or methohexital most effective. A mixture of wheat and cracked corn is used as bait, a solution of drug being thoroughly mixed with it. With metomidate, 1.5 to 2 g of drug per cup of bait produces a mortality rate of less than 6%, with an onset of capture time of roughly 10 minutes and recovery time of 5 hours. With methohexital sodium, 1.25 g of drug per cup of bait produces a mortality rate of less than 8% with a 12-minute capture time and 3½-hour recovery time. Secobarbital sodium and alpha chloralose are less effective and produce higher mortality rates.

Williams (1967) has used metomidate stirred thoroughly into containers of dampened whole or cracked yellow corn to capture wild turkeys. Because metomidate on moist bait is distasteful to turkeys, the bait is usually permitted to dry about 24 hours before use. Methocel* may be used along with metomidate to prevent it from "flaking off" of the bait. In turkeys, metomidate produces narcosis, starting in about 3 minutes and becoming complete in 15 minutes. It is superior to alpha chloralose for capturing wild turkeys because the rate of induction is rapid and the mortality rate low (less than 3% at minimum effective dosage levels).

Williams et al. (1966) have developed a technique for capturing wild turkeys *(Meleagris gallopava)* with alpha chloralose administered on bait. The recommended dose is 2 g of alpha chloralose per cup of coarse cracked yellow corn. The corn is lightly wet with water to make the drug adhere to it. The first signs of narcosis occur in about 30 minutes. Deep narcosis occurs about 2 hours after feeding, at which time the bird may be captured with a long-handled dip net or by hand. The mortality rate using alpha chloralose on bait was 11.5% of a total of 592

*Cetacaine; see Appendix A.

*See Appendix A for manufacturer.

birds captured. This compares favorably with a cannon net technique.

Ducks, such as mallards, teal, widgeon, and pintails, can also be captured with this technique using a dose of 0.16 to 0.25 g per cup of bait.

Wild geese may be attracted to a site by baiting with whole-ear corn followed by shelled corn (Crider and McDaniel, 1967). Corn for baiting is usually soaked in water for 2 to 3 hours, the excess drained, and alpha chloralose powder thoroughly stirred into it with a spatula. The bait is mixed not more than 3 hours before use, to avoid drying and flaking of the powder. The optimum dose of alpha chloralose is 0.25 g per cup of corn. The mortality, including those birds that drown, is 2.5%. Recovery occurs in approximately 6 to 8 hours. Approximately 1 hour after feeding, the geese become narcotized and can be captured by hand.

RAPTORS

Reserpine has been found by Dodge (1963) to be useful in taming and training falcons. Newly caught haggard prairie falcons *(Falco mexicanus)* are given 1 to 2 mg/lb orally in meat the first day, and a second dose of 0.5 mg/lb is given the following day. Vomiting may reduce the effectiveness of the first dose. The birds become progressively relaxed, and in about 8 hours a hypnotic state develops from which they can be aroused. Their temperatures drop from approximately 108° F to below 100° F. During the period of tranquilization, which lasts 5 to 6 days, the birds will not eat and must be force-fed daily. After effects of the drug have ceased, most birds remain tame and tractable.

When meprobamate was used for the same purpose, some muscular relaxation was produced and the wings of the bird drooped. This has not been observed with reserpine. Phenothiazine derivatives have produced excitement.

Because the breast muscles are so important in flying, falcons should never be injected in the breast, but rather in the leg muscles if intramuscular injection is to be performed. The femoral and jugular veins are readily accessible in falcons for intravenous injection.

Intravenous ketamine (35 mg/kg) and diazepam (1 to 1.5 mg/kg) have been used successfully for 45 minutes of anesthesia, in various raptors (Table 18–16). Owls required smaller doses than other species, perhaps because of their abundant body fat. In 40 birds, there were 6 adverse reactions, including 5 deaths (Redig and Duke, 1976). More recently, Redig (1983) has indicated a preference for ketamine-xylazine (Table 18–17).

Althesin has been used in several species of birds. Holt (1977) successfully administered 6 mg of total steroid/kg plus halothane to a long-eared owl for wing amputation. Adverse reactions have been reported by others in red-tailed hawks, mallards, and geese.

Old World vultures of several species have been given metomidate at 3 to 4 mg/kg for immobilization and light anesthesia. These conditions persist for about 30 minutes at this dose level (Houston and Cooper, 1973). Doses of 10 mg/kg or more have been given intramuscularly to eagles, hawks, vultures, and owls for laparoscopy (Cooper, 1974*b*).

PENGUINS

The administration of 2.5% thiamylal intravenously in a penguin has been reported by Dilebone (1965). Injection was made into a vein on the posteromedial aspect of one flipper. Additional increments were given as needed to allow removal of tumors about the head.

BATS

Bats should be handled with thick leather gloves to prevent one from being bitten (Church and Noronha, 1965). Fruit bats (*Eidolon helvum* Kerr) can be relaxed with chlorpromazine injected intramuscularly (2.5 mg/100 g). After the tranquilizer has taken effect, they can be mounted on a restraining board with wings extended and ether administered with a face mask (Ladhani and Thies, 1968). There is no reason to believe that halothane or methoxyflurane could not be administered in this fashion also.

Henson (1969) has used intraperitoneal pentobarbital injections of 0.05 mg/g in a number of genera *(Rhinolophus, Hipposideros, Tadar-*

TABLE 18–16. Intravenous Doses of Ketamine HCl and Diazepam That Induced Satisfactory Anesthesia in Raptors*

Procedure	Species	No. of Subjects	Weight (kg)		Ketamine Dosage (mg/kg)		Diazepam Dosage (mg/kg)		Duration (min)	
			$\bar{x}$	Range	$\bar{x}$	Range	$\bar{x}$	Range	$\bar{x}$	Range
Reduction of long bone fractures	Red-tailed hawk *(Buteo jamaicensis)*	9	0.942	0.675 to 1.35	35.30	29.6 to 39.60	1.50	0.74 to 2.00	114	60 to 150
	Broad-winged hawk *(Buteo platypterus)*	3	0.37	0.29 to 0.46	46.30	43.50 to 51.80	1.21	0.72 to 1.45	120	60 to 180
	Rough-legged hawk *(Buteo lagopus)*	1	0.720	—	30.00	—	1.25	—	40	—
	Turkey vulture *(Cathartes aura)*	1	2.12	—	35	—	0.71	—	30	—
	Kestrel *(Falco sparvarius)*	1	0.115	—	35	—	2.17	—	40	—
	Great-horned owl *(Bubo virginianus)*	3	1.27	1.14 to 1.40	26	15.93 to 37.12†	1.20	1.10 to 1.25	120	50 to 240
	Snowy owl *(Nyctea scandiaca)*	2	1.96	1.80 to 2.12	17.85	17.00 to 18.70	1.18	1.1 to 1.25	420	360 to 480
	Barred owl *(Strix varia)*	2	0.72	0.56 to 0.88	9.45	8.90 to 10.00	0.87	0.74 to 1.00	270	—
Amputation of a limb	Broad-winged hawk	1	0.610							
	Rough-legged hawk	2	0.85	0.73 to 0.98	32.82	27.4 to 30	1.00	1.00 to 1.50	50	
	Great-horned owl	1	1.140		28.70		1.25		47.5	40 to 55
Laparotomy and gonad inspection	Red-tailed hawk	2	1.30	1.20 to 1.40	26.30		1.15		50	
					20.75	20.0 to 21.50	1.25	—	75	60 to 90
Minor procedures	Prairie falcon *(Falco mexicanus)*	1	0.450	—	22.50	—	1.00	—	45	—
	Peregrine falcon *(Falco peregrinus)*	3	0.908	0.660 to 1.080	30	—	1.20	—	100	90 to 110
	Gyrfalcon *(Falco rusticolus)*	2	1.490	1.420 to 1.560	20	—	1.20	—	47.5	30 to 65

*Atropine sulfate was also administered at the rate of 0.05 mg/kg.
†This high value is a cumulative dosage administered by slow intravenous infusion over a 4-hour period.
(From Redig, P.T., and Duke, G.E.: Intravenously Administered Ketamine HCl and Diazepam for Anesthesia of Raptors. J.A.V.M.A., 169:886, 1976.)

TABLE 18–17. Intravenous Ketamine-Xylazine Doses for Adult Raptors

Species	*Amount of Ketamine (ml)**
Kestrel, saw-whet owl	0.03
Screech owl, boreal owl	0.05
Short-eared, long-eared, and broad-wing owl	0.06
Merlin, sharp-shinned hawk	0.06
Cooper's hawk, barred owl	0.10
Goshawk—male	0.10
female	0.15
Great-gray owl	0.10
Great-horned owl, snowy owl	0.15 to 0.25 (marginal)†
Bald eagle, golden eagle	0.15–0.20
Gyrfalcon	0.15
Red-tailed, Swainson's, rough-leg, and ferruginous hawks	0.10–0.15
Turkey vulture	0.15

*Solution containing 100 mg/ml; mix with an equal volume of xylazine (20 mg/ml).

†For great-horned owls and snowy owls, use sodium pentobarbital IV: for owls between 1100 and 1400 g, give 35 to 40 mg (0.6 ml); for larger owls up to 2200 g, give 50 to 55 mg (0.8 ml). Pentobarbital solution contains 1 gr (60 mg)/ml.

(From Redig, P.T.: Personal communication. Department of Veterinary Biology, College of Veterinary Medicine, University of Minnesota, St. Paul, 1983.)

ida, Molussus, Eptesicus, Chilonycteris, Artibeus) in order to implant electrodes on the round window of the cochlea or in the brain. Grinnell (1963) and Suga (1964) have used smaller doses (0.03 to 0.045 mg/g) for *Myotis lucifugus* and *Pleocotus townsendii*.

ARMADILLOS

There are ten living genera of armadillos. *Dasypus novemcinctus*, the most common, weighs 4 to 5 kg as an adult. Armadillos should be caught close to the base of the tail to avoid the hind claws. The armadillo may lie completely still without breathing for long periods, because it can incur a large oxygen debt. It also has the ability to recover spontaneously from repeated episodes of ventricular fibrillation (Hoff et al., 1982).

Injections may be given into the subcarapal tissues or the spinal muscles by inserting a needle between two bands slightly to one side of the midline. The site should be thoroughly cleansed to avoid danger of abscess formation.

Fentanyl-droperidol (0.20 to 0.25 ml/kg intramuscularly) produces sufficient depression and analgesia for surgery (Szabuniewicz and McCrady, 1969).

Premedication with intramuscular atropine sulfate (1/500 gr) is used before semi-open ether anesthesia to diminish the profuse secretions induced. Short procedures may be done with open ether alone under close supervision, although this is hazardous because of the breath-holding habit (Anderson and Benirschke, 1966). After the excitement phase there is a period when bouts of apnea alternate with rapid respirations. If ether administration is continued during apnea, heavy concentrations are inspired leading to fatal respiratory arrest. A soft polyethylene endotracheal tube .25 to .50 inch in external diameter is easily placed after grasping the epiglottis with long narrow forceps. Following intubation, anesthesia may be administered with an anesthetic machine.

Long procedures can be performed with slow intravenous infusion of thiopental (Anderson and Benirschke, 1966). Five ml of 0.5% solution infused over a period of 1 hour are adequate and safe for most adults. The usual dosage is 5 to 6 mg/kg/hr. Wampler (1969) has given pentobarbital, 25 mg/kg, via the superficial femoral vein. Half the dose is given rapidly followed by the remainder "to effect." Apnea and breath-holding do not occur. Midline cesarean section can be performed with local infiltration of lidocaine solution.

Blood specimens are readily obtained by car-

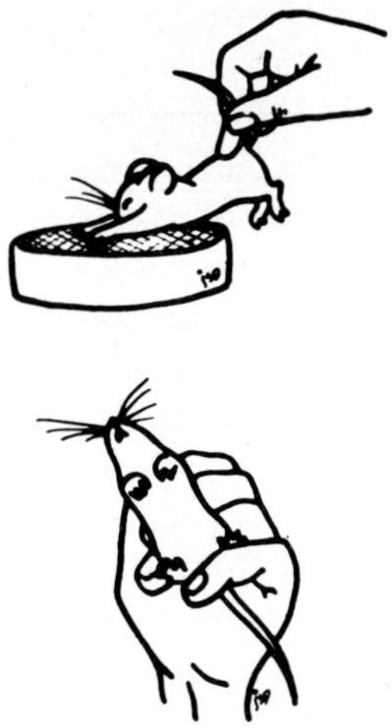

Figure 18–6. Handling mice for injections. The upper figure illustrates the proper positioning of the animal. The lower figure shows its proper restraint. (From Taber, R., and Irwin, S.: Anesthesia in the Mouse. Fed. Proc., 28:1528, 1969.)

diac puncture or from the two prominent superficial femoral veins. These are the only accessible superficial veins and can be easily catheterized.

MICE

Mice may be lifted by the tail for handling, but should be supported after lifting lest they climb their tail and bite the handler. Methods for restraining and holding mice are illustrated in Figure 18–6.

It is possible to inject mice in the lateral vein of the tail, though extensive practice is necessary for proficiency (Croft, 1960). The dorsal metatarsal vein may also be used after the hair

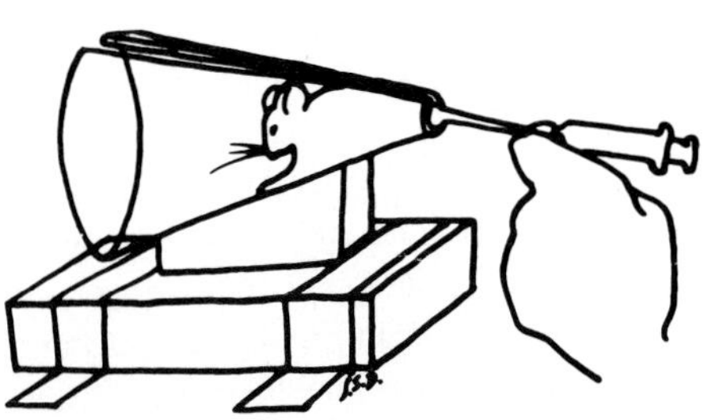

Figure 18–7. Device for intravenous injection in mice. (From Taber, R., and Irwin, S.: Anesthesia in the Mouse. Fed. Proc., 28:1528, 1969.)

TABLE 18–18. Duration of Anesthesia and Recovery in Mice Given a Combination of Ketamine and Xylazine (50 mg/kg Each Drug)

Mouse Strain	Sex	No. Mice	Duration of Anesthesia* (minutes)	Recovery Time† (minutes)
C57BL	M	25	98(20–163)‡	18(7–40)
C57BL	F	25	106(23–153)	16(5–35)
DBA	M	25	64(25–125)	18(10–35)
DBA	F	25	86(20–145)	15(5 –35)

*Time from loss of reflexes until return of reflexes.
†Time from return of reflexes until ambulation.
‡Mean (range).

(From Mulder, K.J., and Mulder, J.B.: Ketamine and Xylazine Anesthesia in the Mouse. Vet. Med. Small Anim. Clin., 74:569, 1979.)

has been clipped. A 27- or 28-gauge needle is used for injection (Fig. 18–7).

Intraperitoneal or intramuscular injections of ketamine, diluted in saline-dextrose to give 20 mg/ml, may be used in mice. The dose for abdominal surgery is 200 mg/kg. Smoother anesthesia can be achieved by adding xylazine (7 mg xylazine to 35 mg ketamine). The dose of this mixture is 70 to 80 mg (based on ketamine content) intramuscularly, and produces approximately 20 minutes of anesthesia. Another combination of ketamine and xylazine has been used in mice by Mulder and Mulder (1979): 100 mg (1 ml) of ketamine is mixed with 100 mg of xylazine (large animal concentration) and diluted with 4.6 ml of sterile water. One-tenth ml of the mixture is given per 30 g of body weight. This provides 50 mg/kg of each drug. Induction time is 5 minutes; duration and recovery times are shown in Table 18–18.

Ether, methoxyflurane, and halothane have been employed to anesthetize mice. The animal is usually placed in a bell jar or other container with a pledget of anesthetic-soaked cotton and is removed when anesthetized. Additional anesthesia may be provided by means of a small nose cone (Fig. 18–8).

Anesthetic chambers have been developed for mice and other small laboratory animals that enable anesthetization of several animals simultaneously (Fig. 18–9). These chambers produce better control of anesthetic concentrations and carbon dioxide levels.

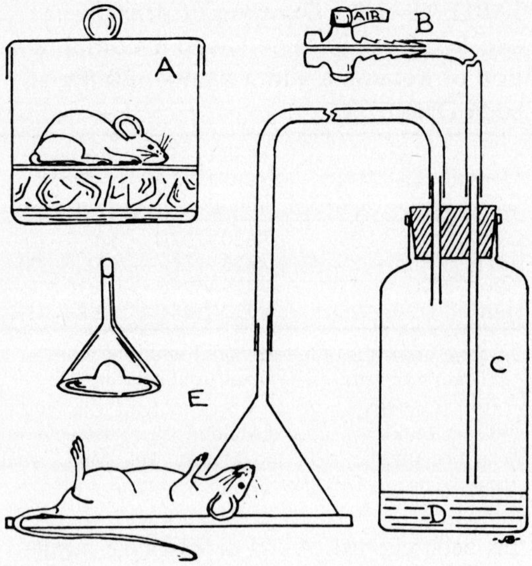

Figure 18–8. *A*, glass jar for induction; *B*, piped air inlet; *C*, glass rod to surface of *D*, anesthetic agent; *E*, mouse operating table. (From Hagen, E.O., and Hagen, J.M.: A Method of Inhalation Anesthesia for Laboratory Mice. Lab. Anim. Care, 14:13, 1964.)

For brief periods of anesthesia (1 minute or less), carbon dioxide may be used (see section on guinea pigs).

Intravenous or intraperitoneal pentobarbital sodium can be used in mice. The intraperitoneal dose is 90 mg/kg and is administered using a tuberculin syringe and 24-gauge needle. A mortality of approximately 20% will occur since the response of mice to pentobarbital varies widely (Table 18–19). Males require less pentobarbital than females. Dolowy et al. (1960) have advocated use of preanesthetic chlorpromazine to increase the duration of surgical anesthesia and to lower the mortality rate (Table 18–20).

Other barbiturates that have been used in mice include hexobarbital (100 mg/kg IP) and thiopental (25 to 50 mg/kg IV).

Anesthetized mice are particularly susceptible to cold, and therefore should be kept in a warm draft-free location until fully conscious.

RATS

Rats that are not tame are difficult to manage without experience. Although gloves may be worn, it is preferable to avoid their use since they impede the fingers, and there is a tendency to crush the animals rather than to grasp them securely. Using the thumb and forefingers of the left hand, the anesthesiologist grasps the tail, lifts the animal out of the cage quickly, and places it head-down on the upper surface of the right thigh. With the thumb and forefinger of the right hand, he then quickly grasps the animal by the scruff of the neck and, without the left hand releasing its hold on the tail, turns it on its back. The rat, when placed on the thigh, will strain to pull away from the hand grasping the tail. If, however, the animal is not caught immediately in the right hand, it cannot be carried by the tail any length of time, as it will turn and climb its own tail far enough to bite the hand restraining it. A second method, which utilizes gloves, is to grasp the animal with the palm of the hand over the back and, with the thumb and forefinger, to fold the forelegs across each other under the animal's chin. With the legs held correctly, the animal cannot depress its chin to bite.

A Turkish towel may be used for restraint while making intravenous injections into the tail veins or obtaining blood samples from them. The unanesthetized rat is rolled in the towel as shown in Figure 18–10. The towel is folded over the rat, rolled, and pinned with safety pins, making sure the legs are secure. Rats may be left so restrained for hours without harm. A commercial rat restraining cage is shown in Figure 18–11.

The dorsal metatarsal vein is suitable for intravenous injection of rats and mice after the hair has been clipped with scissors. A 27- or 28-gauge needle is optimal. For intravenous injection of anesthetized rats, the lingual vein can be used. A small suture can be passed through the tip of the tongue for traction and aids in exposure.

There are age and sex differences in the response of rats to ketamine (Waterman and Livingston, 1978). Sleeping time decreases as young rats mature from 1 to 3 weeks. After three weeks, females sleep longer than males. Ketamine potentiates the production of restraint-induced stress ulcers in the stomachs of rats. This effect is presumably due to splanchnic vaso-

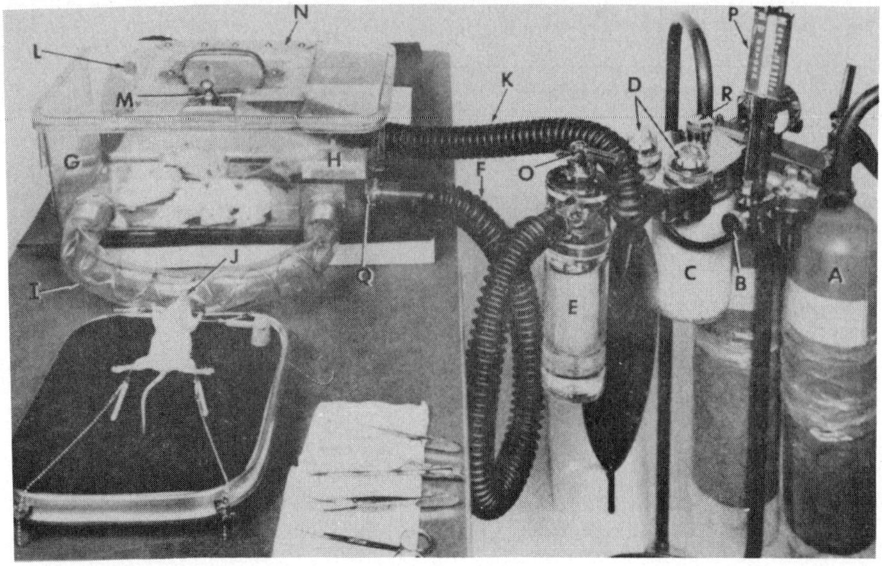

Figure 18–9. Anesthetic unit for small mammals. *A*, O_2 tank; *B*, O_2 control valve; *C*, soda lime container; *D*, check valve; *E*, anesthetic container and vaporizer; *F*, inlet tube; *G*, polycarbonate chamber (converted mouse cage), 5 inches high, 13 inches long, 8½ inches deep; top is ¼-inch Lucite screwed into cage top edge; cutout in top is 4 × 5 inches covered by a 6 × 7-inch hinged piece of Lucite with self-sealing sponge gasket. Volume of chamber plus external circuit *(I)* is about 8,000 ml. *H*,, screen-covered curved metal sheet for diverting a portion of the mixture into external circuit. *I*, external circuit; 1¼-inch Tygon tubing containing no. 10 stainless steel coil to maintain patency and rigidity of tubing. Connector fittings are 1-inch stainless steel threaded pipe with internal and external threaded retaining collars. *J*, hole in external circuit for animal's muzzle, stoppered when not in use; *K*, outlet tube; *L*, exit port for anesthetic and gases, ⅝-inch stainless steel threaded pipe with internal and external threaded retaining collars; *M*, cover latch; *N*, cover hinge; *O*, vaporizer control valve; *P*, O_2 flow rate indicator; *Q*, entry port (as in *L*); *R*, relief valve. (From Simmons, M.L., and Smith, L.H.: An Anesthetic Unit for Small Laboratory Animals. J. Appl. Physiol., 25:324, 1968.)

TABLE 18–19. Duration of Surgical Anesthesia and Survival Rates in Female Albino Mice (Harlan) after Intraperitoneal Injection of 0.5% Pentobarbital Sodium

*Group**	*Pentobarbital Na (mg/kg)*	*Animals in Surgical Anesthesia (%)*	*Survivors (%) 1 day*	*Survivors (%) 1 week*	*Av. Duration and Range of Surgical Anesthesia in Survivors (min)*
1	65	20	90	90	3.6 (0–8)
2	80	30	100	80	3.6 (0–19)
3	90	80	80	80	6.0 (0–20)
4	100	100	70	70	111.0 (109–115)
5	110	100	40	40	124.0 (84–168)
6	120	100	20	20	127.0 (123–132)

*Ten animals were used per group.

(From Dolowy, W.C., Mombelloni, P., and Hesse, A.L.: Chlorpromazine Premedication with Pentobarbital Anesthesia in a Mouse. Am. J. Vet. Res., 21:156, 1960.)

TABLE 18–20. Duration of Surgical Anesthesia and Survival Rates in Female Albino Mice (Harlan) after Injection of 0.5% Chlorpromazine Hydrochloride Intramuscularly, Followed by 0.5% Pentobarbital Sodium Intraperitoneally 30 Minutes Later

Group	No. of Animals	Chlorpromazine Hydrochloride (mg/kg)	Pentobarbital Na (mg/kg)	Animals in Surgical Anesthesia (%)	Survivors (%)		Av. Duration and Range of Surgical Anesthesia in Survivors (min)
					1 day	1 week	
1	5	25	40	40	80	80	82 (0–95)
2	5	50	40	20	80	80	95 (0–95)
3	30	50	50	80	87	87	22 (0–51)
4	10	60	50	50	100	80	17 (0–56)
5	10	60	60	100	80	60	78 (67–99)

(From Dolowy, W.C., Mombelloni, P., and Hesse, A.L.: Chlorpromazine Premedication with Pentobarbital Anesthesia in a Mouse. Am. J. Vet. Res., 21:156, 1960.)

constriction. Ketamine does not produce ulcers in unstressed rats (Cheney et al., 1974).

Neither ketamine nor xylazine when given alone will produce satisfactory surgical anesthesia in rats. When combined, however, they are satisfactory (Van Pelt, 1977). The mixture is made by adding 0.15 ml of xylazine (100 mg/ml stock solution) to each ml of ketamine (100 mg/ml stock solution). The intramuscular dose is 0.87 to 1.3 ml/kg.

For prolonged anesthesia in rats, pentobarbital sodium may be used. The animal's weight in grams is determined. For convenience, pentobarbital solution should be diluted so that each ml contains 30 mg (3% solution). A 0.25-ml syringe with a scale of 0.01 ml should be used. The dose on the scale is then the same as the animal's weight in grams divided by 10. For light anesthesia, 3 mg/100 g are sufficient; 4 to 5 mg/100 g will produce deep surgical anesthesia. The solution is given intraperitoneally just lateral to the umbilicus. Complete anesthesia will develop in 5 to 15 minutes and will be effective for approximately 45 minutes. Injection can be made subcutaneously, but the effect develops more slowly and is of longer duration. If anesthesia lightens before the desired time has elapsed, a second dose approximately one-quarter of the first can be given after 45 minutes.

Albino strains of rats have a significantly lower LD_{50} for intraperitoneally injected pento-

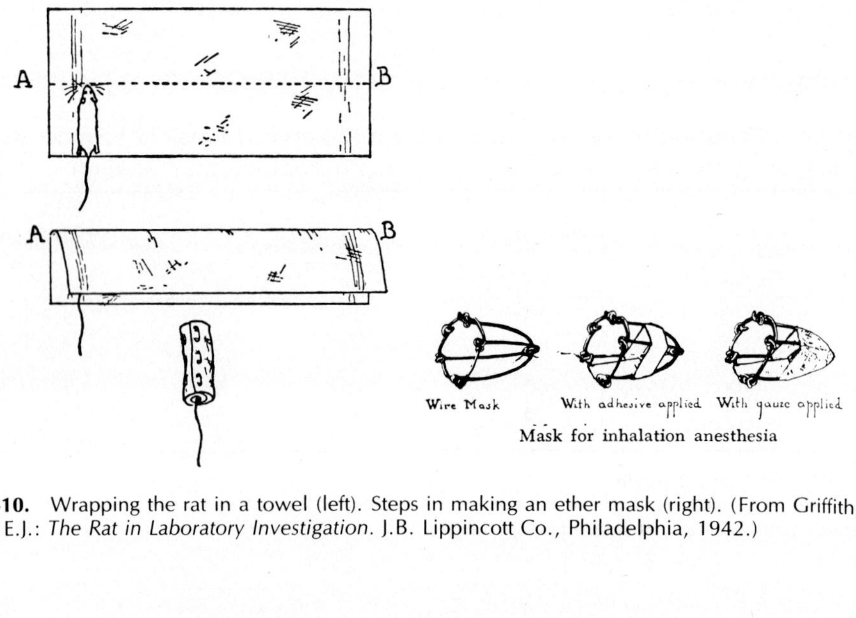

Figure 18–10. Wrapping the rat in a towel (left). Steps in making an ether mask (right). (From Griffith, J.Q., Jr., and Farris, E.J.: *The Rat in Laboratory Investigation*. J.B. Lippincott Co., Philadelphia, 1942.)

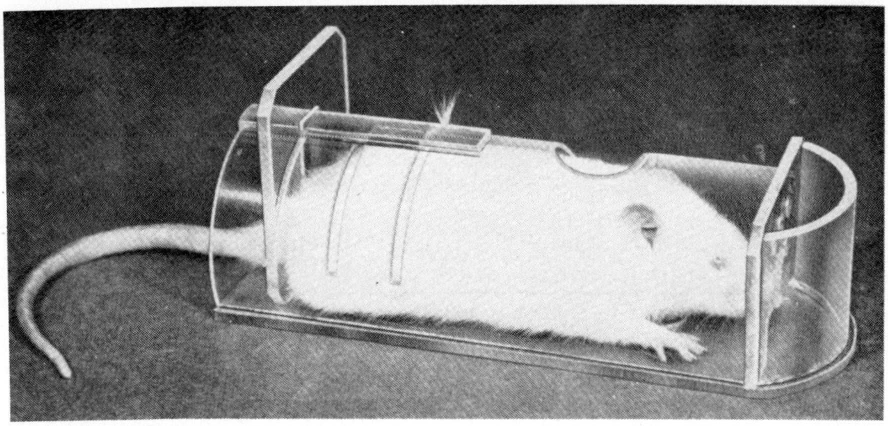

Figure 18–11. A plastic restrainer for rats. Ether-soaked cotton can be placed in the well at right to anesthetize the animal. (Courtesy of Fisher Scientific Company, Pittsburgh, Pennsylvania.)

barbital than do pigmented strains. This may be due to inability of the albino strains to metabolize the drug effectively (Shearer et al., 1973). On the other hand, Westenberg and Bolam (1981) could find no difference in the LD_{100} for pentobarbital in albino and pigmented rats of the same strain.

When carbon dioxide was compared with ether as anesthetics for removing blood samples from rats, Fowler et al. (1980) found little difference in their effects on blood values.

In rats, intraperitoneal injection of 3.5% chloral hydrate solution at the rate of 1 ml/100 g of body weight produces adynamic ileus, and its use by this route is contraindicated (Leary and Manning, 1981*a*,*b*).

Freshly distilled ethanol, given intraperitoneally as a 20% solution in saline (20 ml/kg), gives about 1 hour of complete relaxation suitable for producing CNS lesions or thyroidectomies. It is not recommended for hepatectomy or hypophysectomy. For placing lesions in the anterior hypothalamus of the rat, 3 mg/kg of phenoxybenzamine are added to minimize bleeding (Florsheim, 1968).

Fentanyl-droperidol has been used by Jones and Simmons (1968) as a neuroleptanalgesic for splenectomy of rats (Table 18–21). The induction time for rats receiving 0.02 to 0.03 ml/100 g is 8.5 minutes ± 1.5 minutes as measured by loss of righting reflex. The drug mixture is diluted with physiologic saline to make a 10% solution and is injected into the posterior thigh muscles. A dose of 0.02 ml per 100 g is optimal. Recovery occurs in 1 to 2 hours with complete immobility from 30 minutes to 1 hour.

Of the inhalation agents, methoxyflurane, halothane, and ether are most commonly used. Chloroform is not a satisfactory anesthetic for rats because of the high mortality rate. Rats may be placed in a bell jar containing a pledget of anesthetic-soaked cotton. If longer anesthesia is desired, a mask, such as shown in Figure 18–10, may be used after the animal is removed from the bell jar. Anesthesia may be induced using only the mask if the animal is held as shown in Figure 18–12. To prevent excessive mucus formation in the respiratory tree, atropine may be given with ether, but it is not essential.

There is a difference in the ability of various rat strains to respond to the nephrotoxic effects of inorganic fluoride, a metabolic end product of methoxyflurane. Fischer 344 rats are particularly susceptible, whereas Long-Evans and Sprague-Dawley strains are not (Cousins et al., 1973). Conversely, Van Dyke and Wood (1973) could find no difference in the ability of hepatic microsomes of three strains to enzymatically release inorganic fluoride from methoxyflurane.

The effects of thiopental or halothane on the acid-base status of rats have been investigated by Kaczmarczyk and Reinhardt (1975). They found marked respiratory depression with thiopental (100 mg/kg IP), and 36% of the rats died.

TABLE 18–21. Dose Range and Survival Rate of Rats Receiving Fentanyl-Droperidol*

Stock	*Dose Rate/ 100 Grams*	*No. Animals Used*	*Splenec-tomy*	*Survival*
Long-Evans	.01 ml	6	3/6	6/6
Long-Evans	.02 ml	6	4/6	6/6
Sprague-Dawley	.02 ml	6	6/6	6/6
Long-Evans	.03 ml	3	2/3	2/3
Sprague-Dawley	.03 ml	9	4/9	9/9
Totals		30	19/30	29/30

*Innovar-Vet. Each ml contains 0..4 mg of fentanyl and 20 mg of droperidol.

(From Jones, J.B., and Simmons, M.L.: Innovar-Vet as an Intramuscular Anesthetic for Rats. Lab. Anim. Care, 18:642, 1968.)

With 1% halothane in oxygen, acid-base parameters remained essentially normal for 6 hours and no rats died.

An endotracheal insufflation technique can be used in rats. Anesthesia is first induced by means of the bell jar or mask, following which a midline longitudinal cervical incision is made exposing the trachea. A small hole is clipped between two cartilage rings, and a glass tube drawn to a diameter of 1 mm at one end is then introduced into the lumen of the trachea. The other end is connected to an apparatus shown in Figure 18–13. By raising tube A, one decreases pressure in the tracheal tube; by lowering tube A, one increases it. The percentage of anesthetic in the mixture can also be varied by raising or lowering tube B. A water pressure of 1 cm and a distance of 4 cm between the surface of the ether and tube B are optimal. With this method, anesthesia may be maintained for periods of two hours or longer. If open chest surgery is to be performed, curare at a dose of 0.1 mg/100 g may be used to prevent respiratory movements.

Molello and Hawkins (1968) have described a simple multicompartment anesthetic chamber for rats and other small laboratory animals (Fig. 18–14).

Carbon dioxide anesthesia is effective for short procedures in rats. It may be administered into a chamber from a cylinder mixed with oxygen (1:1 or 3:2), or by evaporation of dry ice (see section on Guinea Pigs). Fowler et al. (1980) could find little effect on hematologic

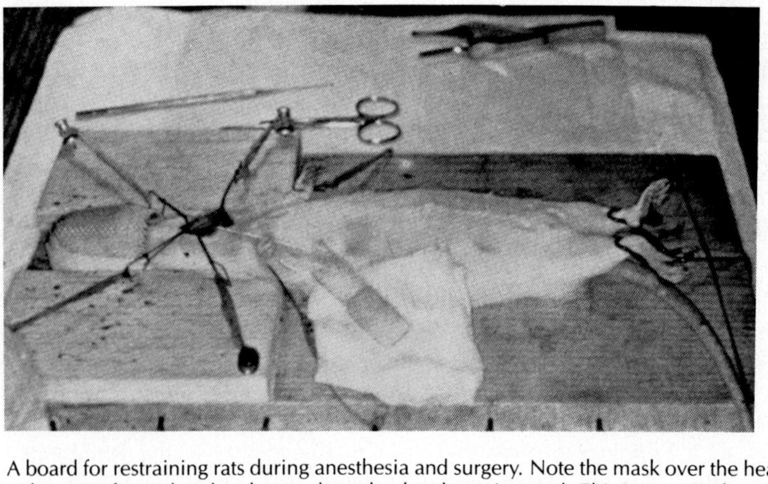

Figure 18–12. A board for restraining rats during anesthesia and surgery. Note the mask over the head. In addition, a tracheotomy has been performed and a glass endotracheal catheter inserted. This in turn is placed in a small vial that contains anesthetic-soaked cotton. Maintenance of anesthesia may be performed by either of these two methods.

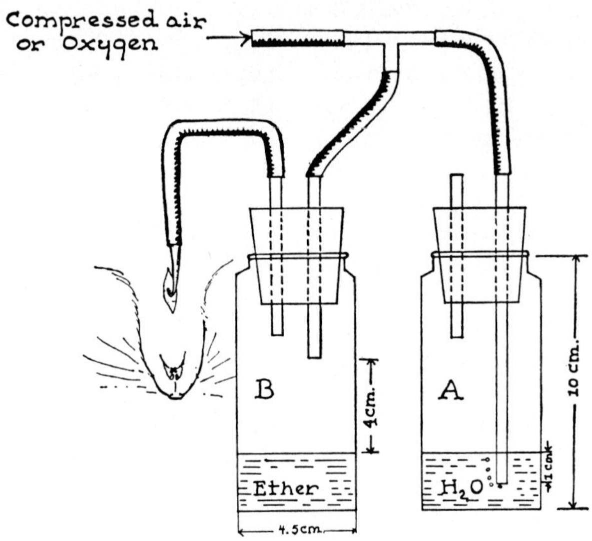

Figure 18–13. Sketch of apparatus for endotracheal ether anesthesia. (From Griffith, J.Q., Jr., and Farris, E.J.: *The Rat in Laboratory Investigation.* J.B. Lippincott Co., Philadelphia, 1942.)

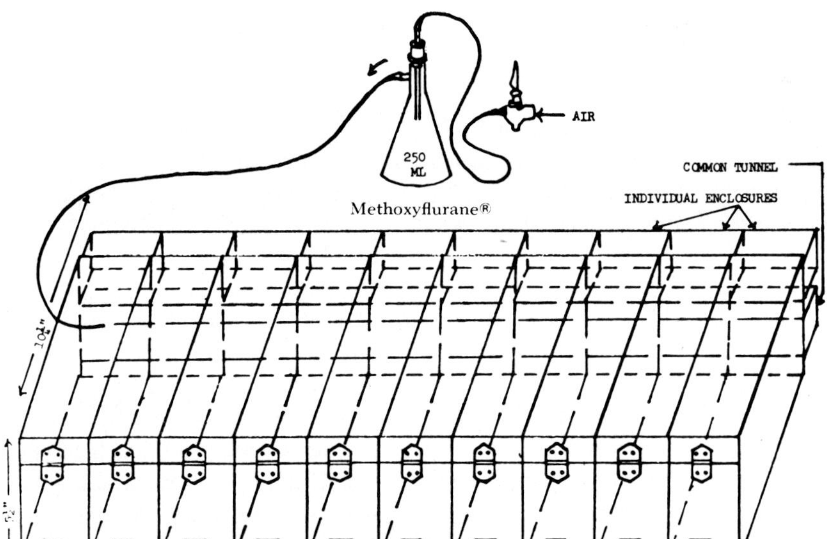

Figure 18–14. The anesthetic apparatus contains 10 units, each accessible through a swinging door. Anesthesia is provided through a common tunnel that opens into the individual enclosures by means of a control valve. The anesthetic then flows from the individual enclosures into the units through an opening on each rear panel. (From Molello, J.A., and Hawkins, K.: Methoxyflurane Anesthesia of Laboratory Rats. Lab. Anim. Care, 18:581, 1968.)

parameters, except blood glucose, when this technique was used for orbital blood collection.

Weisner (1934) has used hypothermia for castration of 12-hour-old rats. He states that it is practical only for operations on the newborn. The rat is wrapped in filter paper, placed in a test tube, and immersed in a thermos bottle filled with ice. The test tube must be dry or the rat will freeze to it. The rat is cooled until its body temperature falls to about 2° C, at which temperature it is immobile and shows no reaction to stimuli. Anesthesia lasts for 3 to 10 minutes after the rat is removed from the thermos, and the operation is performed during this period. Gradual rewarming is then allowed by placing the animal in a cool place for 10 to 30 minutes followed by warming in the palm of the hand for 20 minutes. When the animal has recovered, it is cleaned and returned to its mother. At least one young should be left in the nest with the mother during the procedure, and the operated animal should be returned in front of the nest rather than placed in it. The mother then retrieves it.

Libbin and Person (1979) have used a cold room at 7° C to induce hypothermia in neonatal rats for short periods (5 to 7 min) of surgery.

MONGOLIAN GERBILS

The Mongolian gerbil is grasped by the base of the tail during handling since it is agile and may easily wriggle free and escape. For intraperitoneal injection it can be restrained similarly to mice.

The dose of ketamine for the gerbil is approximately 44 mg/kg, IM (Lightfoot and Molinari, 1978).

Satisfactory general anesthesia lasting for 2 to 3 hours can be obtained by using standard pentobarbital sodium (60 mg/ml) solution at a rate of 0.01 ml per 10 g of body weight, up to a total dose of not more than 0.10 ml. The anesthetic is injected subcutaneously at the back of the neck in order to delay the rate of absorption. This is also the most convenient way of injecting gerbils. Two of more than 80 animals died using this method (Marston and Chang, 1965).

Ether or methoxyflurane may be administered in a closed chamber and subsequently maintained with a mask. According to Marston and Chang (1965) the gerbil is not a good subject for ether anesthesia.

GUINEA PIGS

Methoxyflurane, halothane, and ether are commonly employed for inhalation anesthesia of guinea pigs. Nitrous oxide-oxygen (1:1 or 2:1) may be employed as carrier gases for these volatile agents. Because guinea pigs produce copious secretions in the respiratory tract when exposed to inhalant agents, atropine administration and periodic endotracheal aspiration are indicated.

Methoxyflurane produces less salivation or secretion in the respiratory tract and for this reason is the inhalation agent of choice (Hoar, 1964) (Table 18–22). It may be administered by spraying 1 or 2 ml in a simple mask. Chambers or closed-circuit equipment may also be employed. Ketamine (44 mg/kg IM) will produce a tractable animal for maintenance with methoxyflurane.

Because halothane concentrations must be carefully controlled, use of a precision vaporizer is essential. When ether is used, the animal should be fasted for 12 hours and given 0.5 mg of atropine sulfate subcutaneously approximately 15 minutes prior to anesthesia. Induction is usually performed in a bell jar or other closed container with ether-soaked cotton. Maintenance can be performed with a mask.

A peculiar sign exhibited by anesthetized guinea pigs occurs when the induction stage is complete. An extensive squirming movement, which develops in one hind leg and frequently spreads over the entire body, may occur once or twice. Croft (1960) has stated that this movement does not indicate returning consciousness; rather, if anesthesia is deepened at this point the animal may die. If this phenomenon occurs during laparotomy, the intestines are extruded; therefore, it may be preferable to wait until it has occurred before opening the peritoneal cavity.

When pentobarbital sodium is given by in-

TABLE 18–22. Induction and Recovery Times Displayed by Guinea Pigs Subjected to Long-Term Anesthesia with Methoxyflurane

Number of Animals	*Average Induction Time* (min.)*	*Period under Anesthesia (hours)*	*Average Recovery Time* (min.)*
3	7 (6–8)	1	30 (24–36)
3	5 (3–7)	1½	35 (29–41)
4	6 (4–8)	2	38 (30–46)

*Figures in parentheses indicate the range of time encountered.
(From Hoar, R.M.: The Use of Metofane (Methoxyflurane) Anesthetic in Guinea Pigs. Allied Vet., 36:131, 1964.)

traperitoneal injection, anesthesia requires approximately 15 minutes to develop and lasts 1 to 2 hours. The recommended dose is 28 mg/kg; the fatal dose is 56 mg/kg (Croft, 1960). Complete recovery may require as long as 12 hours, and supplementary heat should be provided during this period.

Intravenous injection is difficult to accomplish and is seldom used. When necessary, the marginal vein of the ear, the lingual vein, or the pudic vein in the male are possible sites. The caudal auricular vein can be used for IV injections in the ketamine-sedated (44 mg/kg) guinea pig.

For short periods of anesthesia, such as those needed for inoculation or cardiac puncture, carbon dioxide can be used effectively. Approximately 2 pounds of dry ice are broken into pieces 1 to 2 inches square and placed in the bottom of an open metal container, measuring 18 × 12 × 14 inches deep. The guinea pig is placed on a removable wire platform 5 inches above the bottom of the container. Carbon dioxide liberated from the dry ice produces general anesthesia in 10 to 15 seconds, following which the animal should be removed promptly. Anesthesia lasts approximately 45 seconds and recovery occurs in about 1 minute. In a group of 1460 guinea pigs anesthetized by this method, one death occurred (Hyde, 1962). There is no excitement during induction, and no adverse side effects are seen. The respiration is increased temporarily. Chinchillas, rabbits, rats, mice, and other small species also respond in a similar fashion to this method of anesthesia.

Fentanyl-droperidol (0.88 ml/kg IM) produces excellent anesthesia in guinea pigs. However, treated animals develop swelling and lameness in the injected limb accompanied by self-mutilation (Leash et al., 1973; Newton et al., 1975). Therefore, this anesthetic should be used only for acute studies in this species.

A method for epidural anesthesia in the guinea pig has been developed by Hopcroft (1966) for use in bilateral removal of the adrenal glands. Chlorpromazine (5 to 10 ml) is given in the axillary fold at the rate of approximately 2 mg/100 g. The guinea pig is held on its side with the back flexed to facilitate introduction of the needle into the lumbosacral space. A 23-gauge, 1-inch needle is directed at a 30° angle anteriorly through the skin and into the space until it strikes the floor of the vertebral canal. If no blood or cerebrospinal fluid can be withdrawn, 0.2 to 0.25 ml of warm 1% lidocaine is slowly injected into the epidural space. Successful injection is indicated by a twitching of the hind limbs followed by relaxation of the posterior half of the guinea pig. Guinea pigs under 500 g are given 0.2 ml of lidocaine; those over 550 g are given 0.25 to 0.3 ml. Anesthesia lasts for 45 minutes.

This technique has been modified for continuous epidural administration by Tan and Snow (1968). Propiopromazine is administered subcutaneously as a preanesthetic, at the rate of 5 mg for guinea pigs weighing less than 300 g, 7.5 mg for those weighing 300 to 500 g, and 10 mg for those over 500 g. The guinea pig is restrained in lateral recumbency with the vertebral column flexed to enlarge the intervertebral space at the lumbosacral junction. After skin preparation, the lumbosacral joint is palpated one vertebral space caudal to the iliac crests. A 19-gauge needle with intravenous catheter attached is inserted, with the needle slanted forward at a 30° angle. The site of insertion is approximately 1.5 cm caudal to the lumbosacral fossa and just lateral to the spinous processes of the sacral vertebrae. As the needle point is felt piercing the intervertebral ligament, it is slipped forward into the vertebral canal for approximately 1 cm. The catheter is then introduced through the needle into the epidural space for about 1 cm. No resistance should be felt. Fibrillation of the muscles of the hind limbs may occur indicating the catheter is positioned properly. A 1% lidocaine solution with 1:100,000 epinephrine is warmed to body temperature and injected slowly over a period of 1 to 2 minutes. Guinea pigs weighing less than 500 g may be given up to 0.2 ml, and those weighing more, 0.25 ml. The effect is prompt and lasts 40 to 50 minutes. Repeated injections may be made, subsequent doses usually being smaller than the initial dose and varying between 0.15 and 0.20 ml.

RABBITS

Rabbits may be intubated using a laryngoscope with a Moore or Miller premature infant blade or a canine otoscope. Following induction, the mouth is opened by squeezing the cheeks between the upper and lower teeth with the thumb and index finger. The tongue is grasped with a 4 × 4 sponge, the laryngoscope blade introduced, and the endotracheal catheter inserted into the trachea. With rabbits between 4 and 7 lbs, a larger straight pediatric blade with the terminal end slightly bent is used. A special mouth speculum for use during intubation has been described by Hoge et al. (1969). Endotracheal catheters with an internal bore of 3.0 or 3.5 mm or Cole tubes are generally used.

Both acepromazine and chlorpromazine have been given to rabbits as preanesthetic agents. McCormick and Ashworth (1971) have recommended that 1.0 mg/kg of acepromazine be given intramuscularly prior to methoxyflurane anesthesia. Bree et al. (1971) have shown that large doses (25 to 100 mg/kg) of chlorpromazine given intramuscularly in the thigh cause severe necrotic lesions. They suggest that, if chlorpromazine is used, it be given intravenously at a rate of 7.5 mg/kg.

In rabbits, ketamine alone (44 mg/kg) does not produce adequate analgesia or muscle relaxation. When combined with acepromazine (5 mg/kg) or xylazine (5 mg/kg), it produces good analgesia and relaxation, longer duration (20 to 75 minutes), and smooth recovery. The advantage of this combination is that no special equipment is required (White and Holmes, 1976).

The optimum dose of fentanyl-droperidol* for rabbits is 0.22 ml/kg (1 ml/10 lb) (Strack and Kaplan, 1968). At this rate, it can be used as the sole anesthetic agent or supplemented with inhalant agents such as ether. Naloxone and doxapram will partially antagonize the combination (Khanna and Pleuvry, 1978).

The use of paraldehyde as an anesthetic agent for albino rabbits has been compared with pentobarbital sodium (Pandeya and Lemon, 1965). Intravenous injections of pentobarbital sodium (30 mg/kg) resulted in 12 deaths out of 68 rabbits. When paraldehyde was used at a rate of 1 ml/kg, the onset of anesthesia following deep intramuscular or intraperitoneal injection was between 20 and 30 minutes. There were only 2 deaths out of 173 applications. Repeated daily injections of paraldehyde did not decrease the dosage necessary. Unless paraldehyde injections were deep intramuscular or intraperitoneal, ulcers and skin sloughing resulted at the injection site.

Supplementary inhalation anesthesia is necessary with either paraldehyde or pentobarbital for abdominal surgery. A combination of paraldehyde (0.5 ml/kg) and ketamine (50 mg/kg) has been recommended by Kisloff (1975) for this procedure.

Hodesson et al. (1965) found that the optimal doses of diazepam or propiopromazine as preanesthetics are between 5 and 10 mg/kg of body weight. The optimal preanesthetic dose of paraldehyde is 0.3 ml/kg of body weight. The action of either propiopromazine or diazepam is enhanced by simultaneous administration of paraldehyde. The combinations of diazepam-paraldehyde or propiopromazine-paraldehyde

*See Appendix A for manufacturer.

are drawn into the same syringe and given simultaneously in the dorsal aspect of the thigh.

Methoxyflurane provides good relaxation and analgesia and is nonirritating (Hodesson et al, 1969). It may be administered either by means of a small canine face mask or endotracheal catheter attached to an anesthetic machine, or by a mask containing a 4 × 4 sponge onto which the anesthetic is sprayed from a syringe (Sawyer, 1965*a*). Ketamine (44 to 55 mg/kg IM) given as a preanesthetic produces a smoother induction (Wass et al., 1974). During anesthesia, a respiratory rate of 18 to 24 per minute is desirable.

Sherrard (1966) has used halothane-nitrous oxide for anesthesia of rabbits. Induction is done in a plexiglas box (18″ × 10″ × 8″) connected to an anesthetic machine and fitted with adjustable air vents. Induction is with nitrous oxide-oxygen (2.5:1) followed by halothane. A foam-lined face mask is then applied. The rebreathing bag is flushed every 10 minutes. Recovery requires 10 to 30 minutes.

A simple closed-circuit anesthetic apparatus has been used for administration of cyclopropane or halothane to rabbits (Watson and Cowie, 1966). It can be made of standard laboratory glassware (Fig. 18–15). Anesthesia is induced by intravenous methohexital and an endotracheal catheter inserted.

Wright (1957) has described ether anesthesia in the rabbit administered by a semiclosed technique. The respirations and degree of muscular relaxation are used to determine the depth of anesthesia. When it is becoming dangerously deep, the eyeball becomes unusually prominent giving a "pop-eyed" appearance. Ether is not used for initial induction of anesthesia in rabbits because they evidence considerable laryngospasm. However, it may be used following induction.

The dose of pentobarbital usually recommended for rabbits is 30 mg/kg, but there is wide variation in response. A dose of 15 mg/kg may be sufficient for one, whereas another may require 50 mg/kg. Intravenous injection of 30 to 50 mg/kg of pentobarbital sodium satisfactorily anesthetizes cottontail rabbits *(Sylvilagus floridanus)* according to Casteel and Edwards (1965). The arousal time also varies widely, ranging from 1 to 10 hours. The depth of respiration is the best sign of anesthesia; it should be regular, deep, and slower than in the unanesthetized animal.

Thiopental is also used in rabbits. The average dose is about 50 mg/kg; if a 2.5% solution is used, the dose is 2 ml/kg. Recovery from thiopental anesthesia is rapid.

One percent thiamylal given intravenously was found to be the most adaptable anesthetic for surgical procedures in albino rabbits according to Gardner (1964). It required the least attention to anesthetic problems and complications. The mean dose is 31 mg/kg with an induction time of 3 minutes. Rapid administration may cause respiratory paralysis, which can be counteracted by light, continuous pressure over the cardiac area.

The méan duration of anesthesia with 1% thiamylal is 8.61 minutes with a range from 5 to 10 minutes. The mean recovery time is 10 minutes with a range from 5 to 15 minutes.

When barbiturates are administered to rabbits, they are usually given intravenously in the marginal vein of the ear. The animal is weighed and prepared by plucking or clipping the hair over the vein. If rabbits are anesthetized only occasionally, it is recommended that the animal be wrapped in a towel with the four legs securely included.

With practice, use of a towel becomes unnecessary. An assistant stands behind the animal and puts both hands over its eyes, directing the ear toward the anesthesiologist with his thumbs. The animal's rear is placed against the chest of the assistant, who leans forward with his forearms lightly restraining the animal on either side. The assistant can compress the marginal ear vein at the base of the ear. The anesthesiologist grasps the ear between thumb and second finger at its distal end, holding the index finger extended under the ear for support. The injection should be made toward the distal end of the ear so that if the first attempt is unsuccessful another may be made more proximal. A 24- or 25-gauge needle is inserted with the bevel upward and is threaded up the vein for 4 or 5 mm. In laboratories where anesthetization of

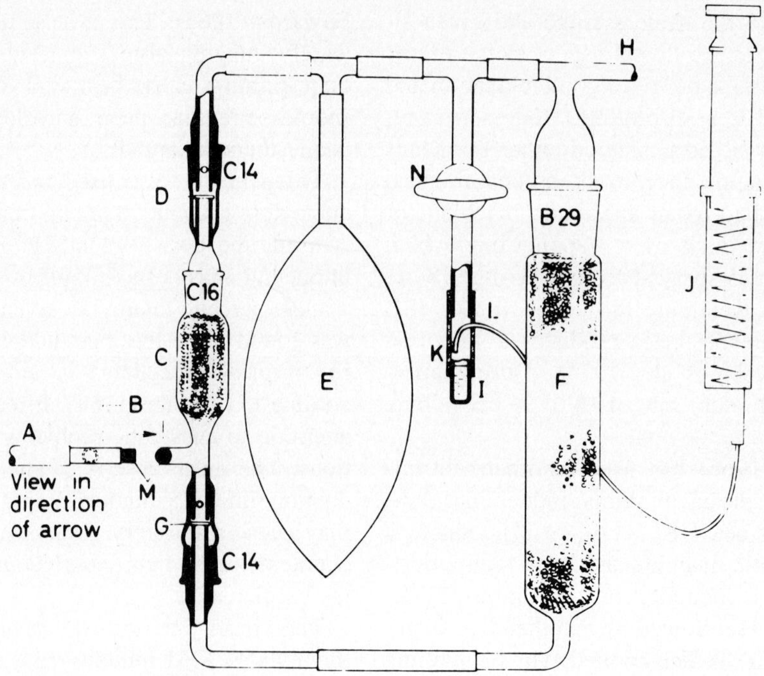

Figure 18–15. Diagram of anesthetic apparatus. The sizes of the standard glass joints are indicated—B29, C14, C16. *A*, Endotracheal tube. *B*, Side-arm tube. *C*, Container for calcium chloride. *D*, Expiratory valve. *E*, Rebreathing bag (capacity about 700 ml). *F*, Container for soda lime. *G*, Inspiratory valve. *H*, Side tube for addition of cyclopropane and oxygen. *I*, Vial of halothane. *J*, 20 ml nylon syringe with spring-return piston. *K*, Polyvinyl chloride tube for holding vial of halothane. *L*, Polyethylene tube from syringe. *M*, Stopper in side-arm tube. *N*, Tap for entry of halothane vapor. (From Watson, S.C., and Cowie, A.T.: A Simple Closed-Circuit Apparatus for Cyclopropane and Halothane Anesthesia of the Rabbit. Lab. Anim. Care, 16:515, 1966.)

rabbits is carried out frequently, a restraining box will facilitate injection and will allow this procedure to be done by one person (Fig. 18–16).

The anesthetic is injected slowly. Often air bubbles may be seen traveling up the vein as injection is started. This assures that the needle is in the lumen and is not of any particular danger to the animal. During injection, the respirations should be carefully observed. After the rabbit gives a deep sigh, about 0.75 ml is injected slowly. The anesthesiologist should then pause, leaving the syringe and needle in place gripped firmly between the thumb and forefinger of the left hand, and test the animal's reflexes. While the anesthesiologist holds the rabbit's head with his right hand, the assistant lightly pinches the Achilles tendon at the heel. If anesthesia is not deep, the animal may give a forcible jerk; for this reason, the head should be held firmly. Further injection of anesthetic is made until the Achilles tendon reflex produces only a moderate withdrawal response or tensing of the leg muscles. At this stage the animal is in surgical anesthesia, but the corneal reflex is still present and the pupil moderately dilated. In the rabbit, loss of the corneal reflex is a sign of dangerously deep anesthesia. With surgical anesthesia, the respirations are regular. When the needle is withdrawn, a cotton pledget can be held over the insertion site with slight compression between the thumb and forefinger for a minute or two. Should the need arise for supplementary anesthesia, the assistant should hold the head firmly when the ear is punctured since the rabbit may otherwise jerk violently at this time.

According to Field (1957), albino rabbits are difficult to anesthetize to a satisfactory depth of anesthesia with intravenous pentobarbital. This

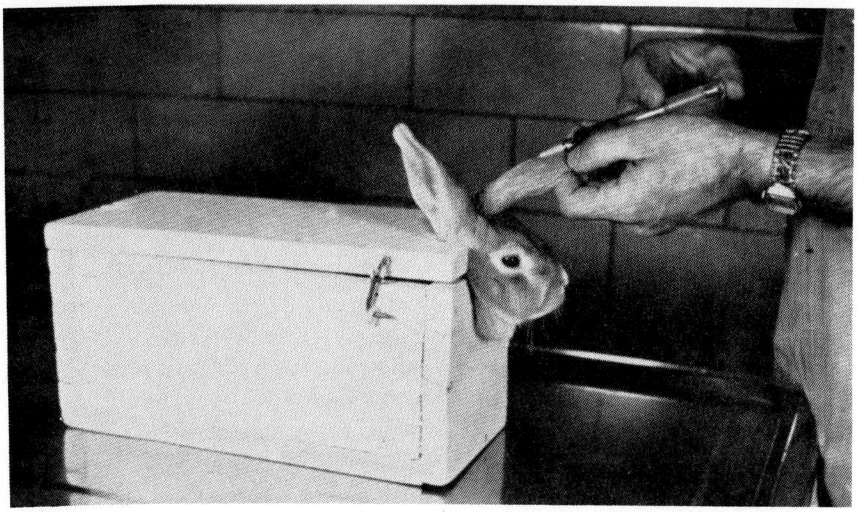

Figure 18–16. Injection of the marginal ear vein of a rabbit using a restraining box.

is because there is a small margin of safety between the surgical anesthetic dose and one causing respiratory arrest. He recommends that albino rabbits, and to a lesser extent "fancy breeds," should not be used for recovery experiments, and indicates that mixed breed animals give most satisfactory results.

When respiratory arrest does occur, it is usually caused by too rapid administration of anesthetic. If one holds the rabbit's chest in the hand to compress it *lightly,* the animal will resume respiration. Because this continues only as long as the chest is squeezed and stops when pressure is removed, it is only a temporary measure. To obtain more prolonged effect, a piece of rubber tubing can be placed around the chest to give moderate compression and can be held in position with forceps. Artificial respiration can be performed by rocking the animal alternately head-down and head-up. This can be continued gently and is usually effective. Oxygen administration and other resuscitative measures should also be undertaken if necessary.

The rabbit is routinely placed on a heating pad while on the operating table, and following surgery is placed in a baby incubator at 95° F until completely recovered from the anesthetic.

The domestic rabbit may be placed in a somnolent state of hypnosis by a manipulative and vocal procedure. The rabbit is grasped firmly but gently by the skin over the withers with the left hand, its hind quarters supported with the right hand, and placed on a table. The right hand is placed on the chest of the rabbit, and it is gently forced onto its back with the right hand on the chest. Support of the back is important since the rabbit can break its vertebral column by violent kicking with both hind legs.

At the same time a soothing monotone is started with a low voice, using a rhythmic cadence and reassuring words (their content is not essential). "E-A-S-Y" repeated slowly and monotonously is quite effective. The abdomen is repeatedly stroked, in the direction of the hair, using the broad surface of four fingers of the right hand. This rhythmic stroking and low monotone are continued slowly, while the left hand grasps the ears close to the head in order to hold it close to the table.

The animal quickly begins to relax, and its breathing becomes less rapid and deeper. The pupils contract, but the eyelids remain open. Respiration becomes slow and deep, and the animal remains relaxed and motionless even though the stroking and monotone are stopped. It is advisable, however, to continue these during any operative procedures. If breathing starts to accelerate (indicated by quivering of the nostrils) or if other evidence of restlessness or agitation appears, the operation must be instantly stopped until stroking and monotone restore hypnosis. Care must be taken to avoid anything that will destroy the mood and hypnotic effect, such as loud noises, sudden moves, or accidental blows to the animal's legs or body. The operator should work slowly and gently when grasping the skin or legs of the animal.

It is possible to hypnotize rabbits regardless of age or sex upon the first attempt, although more time is usually required to induce hypnosis upon the first occasion. The state is more quickly reached after the procedure has been done a few times. This apparently is a conditioning process that makes subsequent attempts easier.

According to Rapson and Jones (1964), this method has been used successfully in several routine procedures, including injections of up to 5 ml of liquid into the gluteal muscles, intraperitoneal injections, heart puncture, and catheterization of the femoral vein with withdrawal of 40 ml of blood. The latter involves incising the skin, catheterizing the vein, and suturing the skin after withdrawal of blood. The procedures by these workers required 15 to 30 minutes of hypnosis. On two occasions the animals suddenly "awoke," but in 20 to 30 seconds were quickly restored to the somnolent state and the operation was completed. In no case was manifestation of pain elicited.

HAMSTERS

Methoxyflurane, ether, halothane, and pentobarbital sodium are the anesthetics commonly employed in hamsters. The procedures for induction and administration of anesthesia are similar to those for the guinea pig, though fasting and atropine administration are not essential.

Pentobarbital is given intraperitoneally approximately one-quarter-inch lateral to the umbilicus. Intravenous injection is extremely difficult.

Methohexital (7.5 mg/ml) and diazepam (1.25 mg/ml) can be mixed in the same syringe in a ratio of 3:1 (Ferguson, 1979). The mixture turns white, but does not precipitate. It is administered intraperitoneally at the rate of 4.0 ml/kg. Onset of anesthesia is rapid, and it lasts approximately 20 to 25 minutes. Further increments of 1.5 mg/kg can be given to prolong anesthesia.

Althesin (150 mg/kg IP) produces deep sedation with analgesia for 20 to 60 minutes.

CHINCHILLAS

Chinchillas are easily removed from their cages by grasping them by the base of the tail and lifting them off their feet. Methoxyflurane-N_2O is satisfactory for anesthesia in chinchillas; halothane or halothane-N_2O may also be used.

Ether has been employed extensively as an inhalant anesthetic. Slow recovery with pulmonary complications has been the rule rather than the exception. The chinchilla apparently does not tolerate ether as well as other domestic animals do.

For cesarean section in chinchillas, Hayes (1955) has advocated intramuscular administration of 15 mg of meperidine approximately 30 minutes prior to operation, followed by 1% hexylcaine solution injected subcutaneously along the proposed line of incision. This produces sedation along with good local anesthesia. Recovery is almost immediate; the young will nurse within minutes, and the mother will often eat within an hour.

Diazepam (5 mg/kg) plus ketamine (15 to 20 mg/kg) intramuscularly or intraperitoneally will produce relaxation and analgesia for 1 to 2 hours.

Riddell (1952) has used epidural anesthesia for cesarean section and states that the landmarks are easily located since the lumbosacral fossa is comparatively large. He reports one fatality in six cases.

Thiopental sodium in dilute solution has been given intravenously "to effect" for dental procedures (Boothe, 1953).

SQUIRRELS

Methoxyflurane, halothane, and ether by inhalation are suitable for squirrels. Tribromoethanol has also been given orally in doses of 0.06 to 0.08 g/lb (Mosby and Cantner, 1955).

Ketamine (10 to 20 mg/kg) can be used to immobilize squirrels.

PRAIRIE DOGS

Combined ketamine (100 to 150 mg/kg) and xylazine (20 mg/kg) intramuscularly produce 1.5 to 2 hours of satisfactory surgical anesthesia in prairie dogs (Roslyn et al., 1979). Xylazine is administered 10 minutes prior to ketamine or may be given in the same syringe. For longer anesthesia, additional ketamine may be given. Ether or other inhalant anesthetics can then be administered via mask.

AGOUTIS

Agoutis are large, excitable, agile rodents. They can injure themselves or handlers if not carefully restrained. Bacher et al. (1976) found that ketamine (25 to 35 mg/kg) was the preferred immobilizing agent in agoutis. Higher doses (63 to 83 mg/kg) were required for painful procedures. Xylazine, phenothiazine tranquilizers, and fentanyl-droperidol were not effective. Halothane produced good surgical anesthesia following ketamine administration.

COYPU (NUTRIA)

The coypu is difficult to restrain, and intravenous injections are difficult because of a lack of readily accessible superficial veins. Endotracheal intubation can be performed in anesthetized animals with a slightly flexible tube containing a curved stylet. Intubation is performed blindly. Animals weighing 3 to 5 kg require a 5-mm endotracheal catheter. On insertion, apnea usually occurs.

Cambridge (1962) has described various anesthetic techniques for the coypu. He states that ether is unsatisfactory for long anesthetic periods because it causes pulmonary edema, whereas halothane and cyclopropane are suitable. Halothane-nitrous oxide-oxygen has also been used. Halothane produces hypotension, which in long experiments (6 to 8 hours) can be maintained at 50 mm Hg. Chloralose at the rate of 80 mg/kg intraperitoneally produces sedation but no anesthesia.

Pentobarbital (40 mg/kg) intraperitoneally does not give adequate surgical anesthesia, and at 80 mg/kg its duration of action is too short to be effective.

Van Foreest (1980) used ketamine (10 to 20 mg/kg) plus 2 mg of xylazine in 4 to 5 kg nutria for tail amputation. The high dose of ketamine produced prolonged anesthesia, whereas the low dose was insufficient except for handling. Atropine (0.1 mg/kg) was given as a preanesthetic.

Succinylcholine bromide at the rate of 2 mg/kg intramuscularly causes profound relaxation for 15 minutes without apnea.

MARMOTS

Intramuscular pentobarbital, ketamine, and droperidol-fentanyl have been tried in wild marmots for intraoral examinations by Noyes and Siekierski (1975). Of these agents, the droperidol (20 mg/ml) and fentanyl (0.4 mg/ml) combination* gave best results. Anesthesia for 30 to 60 minutes was produced by 0.3 to 0.4 ml/kg.

MINK

For restraint and anesthesia of mink, a metal tube such as described by Hummon (1945) is convenient. The dimensions vary according to the size of the mink being restrained. One end is covered with hardware cloth, the other remaining open (Fig. 18–17). The mink is inserted headfirst into the tube. Vaccinations or other injections can be given subcutaneously or intramuscularly on the inner surface of the hind leg while the animal is thus restrained. To anesthetize the animal, a pad of ether-soaked cotton is held over the screened end while the opposite open end is tightly covered. Anesthesia may also be induced with CO_2:O_2 (1:1) or with halothane or methoxyflurane. Maintenance with these agents by means of a nonrebreathing system is satisfactory.

Mink can be rendered less nervous and excitable by administration of 0.036 to 0.05 mg

*See Appendix A for manufacturer.

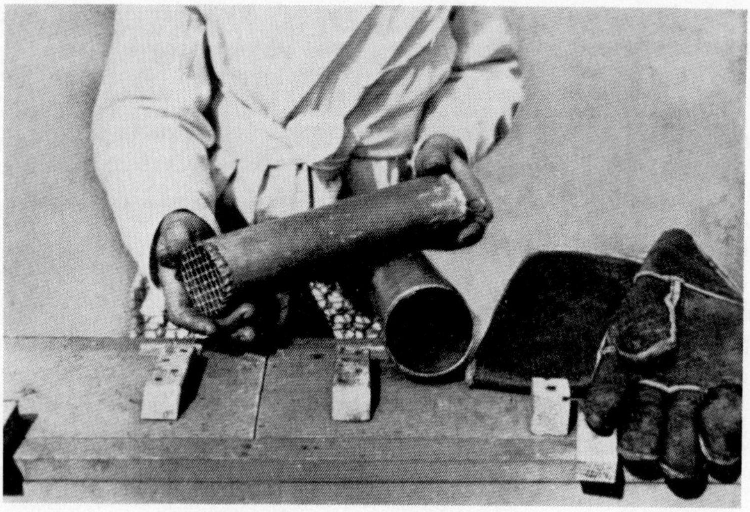

Figure 18–17. A holding tube for mink closed at one end with hardware cloth and reinforced at the open end with a heavy wire. Heavy leather gloves (right) are used in handling the animals. (From Hummon, O.J.: A Device for the Restraint of Mink during Certain Experimental Procedures. J.A.V.M.A., 106:104, 1945.)

of reserpine orally in the feed (Lafortune and Rheault, 1960). There is a wide margin of safety with no cumulative effect.

The average mink (5 lbs) can be given 0.2 ml of propiopromazine followed by 0.2 ml (12 mg) of pentobarbital intraperitoneally to produce 5 to 6 hours of anesthesia (Padgett, 1964). For continuing anesthesia, 0.1 ml of pentobarbital can be given.

Graham et al. (1967) found that the anesthetic dose of pentobarbital given intraperitoneally to mink was 40 mg/kg. This produced deep anesthesia in 75% of the animals.

FERRETS

When one is anesthetizing ferrets, food should be withheld for 12 hours. Atropine (0.04 mg/kg) is given subcutaneously or intramuscularly. Anesthesia is easily induced with methoxyflurane-oxygen in an anesthesia chamber. It may be maintained with a mask or endotracheal tube (Creed and Kainer, 1981). Halothane is also satisfactory, induction being accomplished with a mask. An alternate method for general anesthesia is the use of ketamine (26 mg/kg) and acepromazine (1.1 mg/kg) intramuscularly.

Ketamine (20 to 30 mg/kg IM) produces light surgical anesthesia for 40 to 60 minutes. Althesin (12 to 15 mg of total steroid/kg IM) produces 15 to 30 minutes of light anesthesia.

SKUNKS

Veterinarians are occasionally asked to descent skunks. Usually this operation is performed in young kittens. In general, either a volatile anesthetic, such as ether or methoxyflurane, or pentobarbital sodium are used.

For small skunks, a transparent plastic disposable bag is an ideal container for induction of methoxyflurane or ether anesthesia. The skunk is placed in the bag with anesthetic-soaked cotton and, after induction, the surgery is done through a small opening cut in the bag. On conclusion, the skunk is removed and the bag discarded, eliminating the problem of an odoriferous container.

According to Barry (1958) the best age for removal of the scent glands in skunks is between 5 and 6 weeks when the skunk's weight is about 2 pounds. The sacs may be emptied by turning the animal's hindquarters away from the operator and pulling the tail up and forward, forcing out their contents. Pentobarbital is given intraperitoneally using a 2-ml syringe and 25-gauge needle; the usual dose is from 15 to 30 mg.

Intrathoracic injection of pentobarbital at the rate of 1 ml (60 mg)/5 lbs has been advocated by Taylor (1961), who states induction requires 2 to 4 minutes and recovery occurs in approximately 4 hours.

A device for anesthetizing wild skunks caught in traps has been described by Verts (1960). It consists of a 9-foot pole containing a pentobarbital-loaded syringe, the plunger of which can be pushed by the operator from the handle on the opposite end. This allows the operator to stand about 9 feet from the animal to make an intraperitoneal injection and thus facilitates handling the skunk without exposure to musk or the possibility of being bitten. Pentobarbital solution is given at the rate of 1 ml (60 mg)/6 lbs of body weight. Of over 50 striped skunks *(Mephitis mephitis)* given pentobarbital in this fashion, only one died. With this device, skunks are less likely to expel musk if the operator is slow and deliberate and if the needle is inserted into the abdomen by pushing steadily. Skunks that expel musk usually direct it at the syringe end of the device.

VOLES

Methoxyflurane and halothane, either alone or with N_2O, are probably the best anesthetics for voles.

According to Richmond and Conaway (1969), both ether and pentobarbital can be used for the vole *(Microtus ochrogaster)*. Of the two, pentobarbital is more satisfactory, 0.06 mg/g of body weight intraperitoneally producing 3 hours of surgical anesthesia. Animals to be adrenalectomized were considered to be in a satisfactory state if they shivered violently when the skin was dampened with an alcohol swab. Anesthetized animals that did not shiver usually died following surgery.

The use of pentobarbital for anesthesia of meadow voles has been reported by Lee (1969). For 15 to 20 minutes of surgical anesthesia, 0.06 to 0.09 mg/g is injected intramuscularly. The postoperative use of penicillin-streptomycin appears contraindicated in this species.

STOATS AND WEASELS

Healey (1967) has described a method for anesthetizing the stoat *(Mustela erminea)* and weasel *(Mustela nivalis)*.

These species are extremely fierce and difficult to handle. They will bite through thick leather gloves and if held tightly may be asphyxiated.

A much more satisfactory and less traumatic method is to use a plexiglas transfer box (10″ × 4″ × 4″) attached to the end of the cage by means of a removable slide (Fig. 18–18). A 2½″ diameter hole connects the box to the cage. The animal is easily coaxed into this box, after which it is removed from the cage. Halothane-soaked cotton is then introduced into the box. The animal is usually anesthetized within 30 to 60 seconds, anesthesia lasting about 2 minutes. If further anesthesia is desired, it can be continued by means of a face mask or other inhalation methods.

RACCOONS

The dose of ketamine for raccoons is 20 mg/kg IM (Gregg and Olson, 1975).

Clayton et al. (1966) have reported a method for anesthesia of wild raccoons employing methohexital. Captured wild raccoons are placed in individual burlap bags and weighed, following which a 2.5% solution of methohexital is injected through the bag into the thoracic cavity at the rate of 1 ml/5 lb. The raccoon can be removed from the bag and safely handled in approximately 3 minutes. Recovery requires 12 to 15 minutes. One death occurred in 120 raccoons anesthetized by this method. This probably was due to cardiac tamponade from an intracardial puncture. In a second study, each of 15 captive raccoons was anesthetized from 9 to 52 times for a total of 460 intrathoracic injections with 1 fatality.

Raccoons weighing 15 to 25 lb are immobilized with capture equipment for approximately 7 minutes by 10 mg of succinylcholine chloride (Farrell, 1963). Recovery is complete in 10 minutes. The intramuscular dose of ketamine for the raccoon is 10 mg/lb.

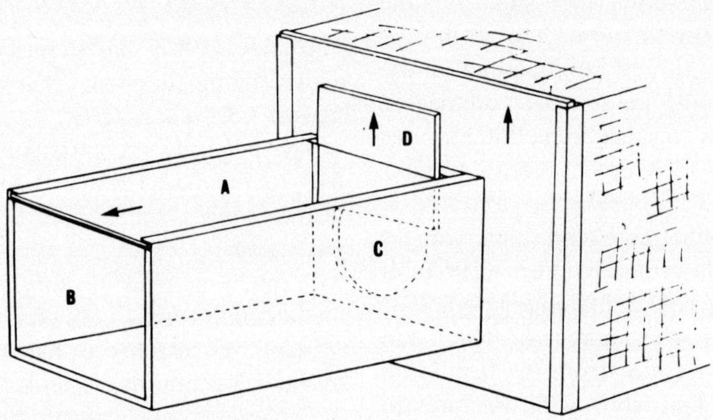

Figure 18–18. Transfer box for anesthetizing small carnivores. Plexiglas sliding top *(A)* and end *(B)* allow visualization of animal. Access hole *(C)* can be blocked by sliding door *(D)* to prevent animal from returning to cage. (From Healey, P.: A Simple Method for Anaesthetizing and Handling Small Carnivores. J. Inst. Anim. Tech., 18:37, 1967.)

OPOSSUMS

Opossums are readily carried by the tail, with precaution taken to prevent the animal from crawling up its own tail and attacking the handler. When removing an animal from a cage, it is wise to distract or immobilize the head while grasping the tail (Krupp and Quillin, 1964).

Ketamine (20 to 25 mg/kg IM) or fentanyl-droperidol (0.75 to 1.0 ml/kg) are satisfactory for restraint (Feldman and Self, 1971).

Halothane, methoxyflurane, ether, and pentobarbital sodium have been used as anesthetics. Halothane may be given by means of a closed system and mask (Luschei and Mehaffey, 1967). Ether is given in a closed box or jar until the animal is unconscious. Atropine should be given prior to use of ether. For prolonged procedures, thiopental may be given to allow intubation, followed by administration of halothane or methoxyflurane from an anesthetic machine. Pentobarbital at a dose of 36 mg/kg produces satisfactory anesthesia when given intravenously. Intraperitoneal injection is less reliable and provides a narrow margin of safety.

Alpha-chloralose gives satisfactory anesthesia for long experiments with a wide margin of safety. Induction is performed with 4% thiopental solution given intravenously. Alpha-chloralose, approximately 12 mg every 2 hours, can then be given to maintain anesthesia.

BADGERS

Badgers are difficult to handle because they bite and scratch.

Phencyclidine, acepromazine, chlorpromazine, and succinylcholine have been successfully used intramuscularly for immobilizing badgers *(Taxidea taxus)* (Table 18–23). Succinylcholine provides the most rapid recovery.

Ketamine was found to be the most satisfactory agent for immobilizing the European badger, *Meles meles* (Mackintosh et al., 1976). The average dose was 19.25 mg/kg, and repeated smaller doses were sometimes administered. Complete recovery occurred in 90 to 180 minutes.

Diethyl ether (and probably other inhalants) can be administered by mask or endotracheal catheter once the animal has been immobilized, or pentobarbital may be administered intraperitoneally (Lechleitner, 1969).

FERAL DOGS, FOXES, COYOTES, JACKALS, HYENAS

Capture of these species has been performed with dart guns and such drugs as nicotine, phencyclidine, etorphine, and succinylcholine. A combination of ketamine and xylazine (5.5 mg/kg of each drug IM) has been found to be effective for anesthesia of adult coyotes (Mulder, 1978). Induction time averages 10 minutes,

TABLE 18–23. Dosages and Effects of Four Drugs Used on Captured Badgers

	Drug			
	Phencyclidine hydrochloride	*Acepromazine maleate*	*Chlorpromazine hydrochloride*	*Succinylcholine chloride*
Number	6	5	5	17
Average dose and range (mg/lb)	1.6(1.2–1.9)	1.2(1.0–1.4)	2.2(1.9–2.7)	0.16(0.12–0.26)*
Immobilization time (minutes after injection until animal was safe to handle)	6(3–9)	22.5(21–25)	14(9–20)	5.5(2–8)
Recovery time (minutes)	348(270–450)	252(220–270)†	312(280–340)†	47(20–68)

*Fifteen animals.
†Three animals.
(From Fitzgerald, J.P.: Four Immobilizing Agents Used on Badgers Under Field Conditions. J. Wildl. Manag., 37:418, 1973. Copyright The Wildlife Society.)

anesthesia 50 minutes, and recovery approximately 30 minutes.

These species are anesthetized with other agents in the same manner as domesticated dogs. Induction is commonly performed in a squeeze cage. An injectable tranquilizer, narcotic, and/or ketamine is administered, followed by an inhalant such as halothane or methoxyflurane.

Coyotes and other carnivores caught in steel traps often injure themselves struggling and, by self-mutilation, may escape. Balser (1965) has developed a cloth-covered diazepam tablet to be attached to the trap. The tablet is ingested by the animal after capture. This not only aids in capture but also helps to prevent harm to the animal.

PRIMATES

In anesthetizing primates, the chief problem lies in restraint of the animals during induction because of their agility and often vicious nature. Gauntlets and a net are essential pieces of equipment. Larger species, such as chimpanzees weighing over 30 pounds, have tremendous strength coupled with a nasty disposition and are often extremely dangerous. For this reason, they should never be handled by persons working alone. If large numbers are to be anesthetized, a squeeze cage is effective and time-saving (Fig. 18–19). See also Figure 3–14.

The use of phencyclidine for restraint, as a preanesthetic, and as the sole agent for anesthesia of primates revolutionized the handling of these species. Because of its addictive properties in humans, its manufacture has been discontinued, and it has been replaced by ketamine. By using squeeze cages, which allow easy intramuscular injection of this agent, one individual can immobilize many animals in a short time.

Ketamine at doses of 10 to 15 mg/kg intramuscularly in chimpanzees results in anesthesia that is adequate for examination, urethral and cardiac catheterization, blood collection, treatment of wounds, tattooing, and tuberculosis testing. To improve muscular relaxation, ketamine can be followed by inhalant anesthetics or pentobarbital sodium intravenously. These combinations produce surgical anesthesia and prevent the involuntary movements observed with ketamine alone.

Chimpanzees have been anesthetized repeatedly with ketamine by Kuhn and Arko (1974) (Table 18–24). They found that tolerance did not develop when injections were made as often as three times a week. Chimoskey et al. (1975) studied the effects of 5 mg/kg of ketamine IM on cardiovascular parameters in baboons *(Papio cynocephalus)*. Cardiac output, peak aortic flow velocity, and peak aortic flow acceleration were all depressed; heart rate and stroke volume were slightly decreased. Primates immobilized with ketamine have near-normal acid-base balance (Bush et al., 1977).

The effects of ketamine:xylazine ratios in monkeys *(Macaca mulatta)* have been studied

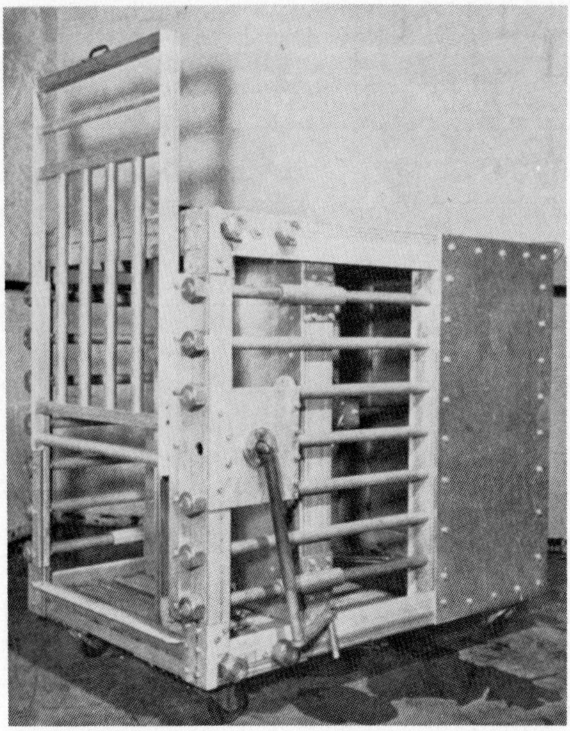

Figure 18–19. Squeeze cage for chimpanzees. (Courtesy of Captain W.E. Britz, Jr., and the U.S.A.F. School of Aerospace Medicine, Brooks AFB, Texas.)

by Naccarato and Hunter (1979). Ketamine alone (2.5 mg/kg) did not produce anesthesia. Xylazine alone at less than 2 mg/kg did not produce anesthesia; 2 mg/kg produced pronounced sedation. Addition of xylazine to ketamine increased the anesthetic duration as a logarithmic function of the xylazine dose (Fig. 18–20).

In baboons, the route of injection is usually intramuscular or into the posterior "pad."

Neuroleptanalgesia in a wide variety of primates ranging from squirrel monkeys to a gorilla has been reported by Marsboom et al. (1963), using droperidol and fentanyl. The mixture may be given intramuscularly or orally in milk or fruit juice.

Intramuscular Technique:

Droperidol	1 mg/kg
Fentanyl	0.020 mg/kg (anthropoids) 0.040 mg/kg (monkeys)

TABLE 18–24. Mean Induction, Anesthetic, and Recovery Times (Minutes) in Chimpanzees Anesthetized with Ketamine

Injections	*Mean Dosage (mg/kg of body weight)*	*Induction Time (min)*	*Anesthetic Time (min)*	*Recovery Time (min)*
902 single	9.2	4.9 (1–20)*	26.1 (5–89)	57.6 (25–148)
73 multiple	13.2	4.9 (1–20)	37.6 (6–142)	74.9 (40–205)

*Range of values.

(From Kuhn, U.S.G., III, and Arko, R.J.: Repeated Ketamine Anesthesia in the Chimpanzee. J.A.V.M.A., 165:838, 1974.)

TABLE 18–25. Immobilization Results of Etorphine in Primates

Species	*Sex*	*Est. Wt. (lb)*	*Etorphine mg*	*Ap mg*	*S mg*	*Imm. Time (min)*	*Nal mg*	*Lag Time (sec)*	*Remarks*
Woolly monkey	F	15	0.03	. .	. .	4.0	. .	. .	Recovered in 1 hour, without nalorphine; dilated pupils
Woolly monkey	M	15	0.06	. .	. .	4.0	50	60	Salivated, muscle tremors
Woolly monkey	F	15	0.03	. .	. .	5.0	. .	. .	Recovered in 45 minutes without nalorphine; tractable, not dilated
Woolly monkey	M	18	0.1	. .	. .	5.0	. .	. .	Reduced effect 3-day-old solution
Spider monkey	F	4	0.03	. .	. .	4.0	. .	. .	Recovered in 3 hours without nalorphine; analgesia in 5 minutes
Spider monkey	F	6	0.03	. .	1.0	4.0	. .	. .	Recovered in 3 hours without nalorphine; analgesia in 5 minutes
Spider monkey	M	5	0.03	1.0	1.0	4.0	. .	. .	Required additional 0.01 mg etorphine
Chimpanzee	F	35	0.06	. .	. .	10.0	. .	. .	Additional 0.04 mg etorphine; good immobility; recovered in 1 hour without nalorphine
Chimpanzee	M	55	0.05	1.0	1.0	5.0	50	300	Sternal recumbency, visual reflex
Chimpanzee	M	65	0.1	1.0	1.0	4.0	75	15	Good immobility, deep analgesia
Orangutan	M	50	0.25	. .	. .	7.0	125	. .	Cardiac arrest, cardiac massage effected recovery

Ap = acepromazine; S = scopolamine; Nal = nalorphine hydrochloride; Lag time = time elapsed from administration of nalorphine to animal standing; . . = drug not used; Imm. time = time elapsed from administration of drug to immobilization.

(From Wallach, J.D., Frueh, R., and Lentz, M.: The Use of M.99 as an Immobilizing and Analgesic Agent in Captive Wild Animals. J.A.V.M.A., 151:870, 1967.)

Oral Technique:

Droperidol	1 mg/kg
Fentanyl	0.040 mg/kg

Sufficient analgesia for 30 to 60 minutes of surgery is produced with either technique.

Administration of etorphine to several species of primates has been reported by Wallach et al. (1967) and is summarized in Table 18–25. When ketamine or fentanyl-droperidol are not available or for some reason cannot be used, promazine at the rate of 1 mg/lb or meperidine at the rate of 5 mg/lb will produce satisfactory results (Table 18–26). Caged monkeys that are hard to manage can sometimes be enticed to reach for fruit held close to the cage bars. Intramuscular injection of these agents can be accomplished by grasping the hand or forearm.

Tranquilizers can be administered to chimpanzees by dissolving the drug in canned pineapple juice. Other tantalizing vehicles for drug administration include maple syrup and peanut butter.

After preanesthetics have taken effect, thiopental, thiamylal, or pentobarbital can be administered intravenously using veins of either the forearm or hind limb. Restraint for this procedure is necessary in most instances despite preanesthetic medication. The assistant can best hold small primates by grasping their arms and holding them behind the animal's back.

Newsome and Robinson (1957) reported trial

TABLE 18–26. Promazine in Captive Wild Animals

Species	*Common Name*	*Weight in lb*	*Dose and Route of Administration*	*Reason for Administration*	*Effect*
Vulpes lagopus	Arctic fox	15	75 mg IM	Apply cast to leg	Sleepy and gentle
Felis concolor	Puma	50	100 mg IM	Postsurgical sedation	Quieted but active if approached
Macaca nigra	Crested ape	30	75 mg IM	Aggressive with mate	Drowsy
Felis leo	African lion	360	180 mg IM	Venipuncture, caudal vein	Calm
Pan troglodytes	Chimpanzee	30	75 mg IM	ECG	Calm
Strepsiceros strepsiceros	Greater kudu antelope	700	1000 mg IM	Hoof trimming	Calm
Papio papio	Guinea baboon	25	50 mg IM	Venipuncture	Tranquil
Odocoileus hemionus	Mule deer	50	100 mg IV	X-ray leg	Calm
Protemnodon ruficollis bennetti	Bennette's wallaby	25	50 mg IV	Treat abscess	Quiet but required restraint

(Data from Heuschele, W.P.: Experiences with Promazine in Captive Wild Animals. Biochemic Rev., 29:3, 1959.)

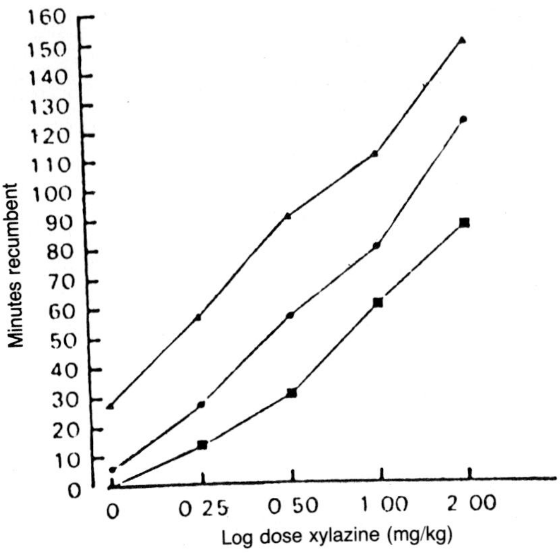

Figure 18–20. Time recumbent as a function of increasing xylazine dose superimposed on ketamine dose. Ketamine: 2.5 mg/kg ■; 5 mg/kg ●; 10 mg/kg ▲. Each point represents a mean of 5 or 6 trials (1 trial per animal). (From Naccarato, E.F., and Hunter, W.S.: Anaesthetic Effects of Various Ratios of Ketamine and Xylazine in Rhesus Monkeys [*Macaca mulatta*]. Lab. Anim., 13:317, 1979.)

of a wide variety of agents for sedation and anesthesia of baboons. Among those used were morphine, methadone, chloral hydrate, chloralose, pentobarbital, hexobarbital, amobarbital, paraldehyde, chlorpromazine, ether, chloroform, and nitrous oxide.

Morphine administered orally or by injection in doses up to 1 gr caused severe skin irritation of the palms and soles with loss of appetite. Sedation was not produced. Amidone was not particularly effective in doses of 80 mg intramuscularly.

Pentobarbital sodium given by intramuscular injection was unpredictable, with animals reacting differently to equal doses on different days. After several hundred injections, it was deemed unsuitable.

Chlorpromazine proved the most valuable sedative, but the response of baboons varied widely. Doses of up to 3.5 mg/kg made the animals apathetic and slow, but they could not be easily handled. When doses were given intramuscularly, the action was slow, maximum effect occurring at 2½ to 6 hours after injection. to 0.03 ml/L of water. Induction requires 1 to

McGill forceps and a laryngoscope are useful in intubating monkeys such as rhesus. Endotracheal catheters in 14 or 16 French sizes are appropriate.

Aronson et al. (1965) have used 1.5 to 2.0 mg/kg of suxamethonium intravenously for intubation of baboons (*Papio* sp.). Only one-half to one minute of relaxation was produced.

The use of halothane in various species of primates has been reported by several investigators (Graham-Jones, 1962; Day, 1965; Aronson et al., 1965).

Steffey et al. (1974) investigated the effects of halothane in stump-tailed macaques *(Macaca actoides)* during spontaneous and controlled ventilation. They found that the dose-dependent depression of cardiovascular function was greater than that observed in dogs and suggested that there was a lesser margin of safety.

Ritzman et al. (1976) found that both halothane and enflurane produced dose-related decreases in heart rate, mean arterial pressure, and peak left ventricular dp/dt in rhesus monkeys. Central venous pressure was increased by both agents. At equal MAC levels, no significant differences in anesthetic effects were noted between the two agents.

Administration of halothane-nitrous oxide has been reported by Day (1965). For chimpanzees weighing 23 kg or more, a mixture of 50% oxygen and 50% nitrous oxide is used in a semiclosed system with a flow rate totaling 4 L/min. With smaller animals, the rate is reduced accordingly. Following administration of 0.2 to 0.5 mg of scopolamine and 10 mg/kg of meperidine, anesthesia may be induced with thiopental (8 to 10 mg/kg). An alternative for larger animals is induction with ketamine. Either method produces a light stage of anesthesia so that the animal will accept a face mask. Human face masks are suitable for use with chimpanzees. Once induction is accomplished, an endotracheal catheter is passed.

The use of methoxyflurane in primates has been reported by Sawyer (1965*b*) and Bennett (1969). It has proved to be a safe and effective agent. Clark et al. (1979) in a comparison of chronic exposure to halothane and enflurane in Cynomolgus monkeys found halothane more

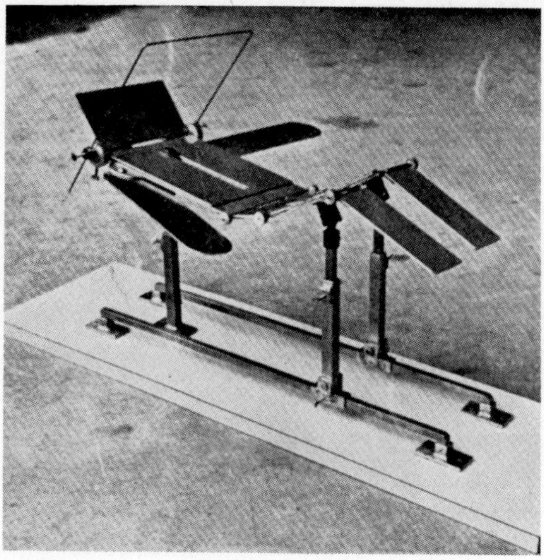

Figure 18–21. This primate operating table can accommodate an animal ranging in size from an adolescent monkey to a young chimpanzee. It can be adjusted to hold the entire animal or any of its extremities in many different positions. The metallic table is easily cleaned and sterilized. (From: Equipment for Primate Studies Custom Made at Delta Center (Editorial). J.A.V.M.A., 152:1467, 1968.)

toxic. Enflurane produced no measurable effects on clinical chemistry parameters measured, when given repeatedly at 1/100 MAC or 1.5 MAC.

During surgery requiring any period of time, small primates should be positioned on a heating pad to maintain body heat. Following removal from the operating table (Fig. 18–21), they should be allowed to recover in an infant incubator maintained at 95° F. Supplemental oxygen should be supplied by flowing it through a nebulizer to maintain the humidity within the incubator. These support procedures shorten the recovery time of primates by approximately 50% (Sawyer, 1965*b*).

Spinal anesthesia is impossible to perform safely in primates without prior anesthesia. Denson et al. (1981) have developed a nonhuman model for spinal anesthesia in the rhesus monkey utilizing lidocaine.

A survey of drug effects on the central nervous system of primates has been compiled by Reynolds (1969).

SWINE

In recent years the pig has been used extensively as a laboratory animal. In the laboratory, different anesthetic techniques are employed than those used "in the field." Poland China, Landrace, Pietrain, Duroc, and possibly other breeds of swine are suceptible to malignant hyperthermia triggered by succinylcholine, halothane, chloroform, and perhaps other inhalant anesthetics, and by exercise-induced stress (Jones et al., 1972).

According to Hall (1971), the pig is easily restrained for 45 to 60 minutes following an intramuscular injection of 0.5 mg/lb of chlorpromazine. Intravenous doses of 75 to 100 mg have been recommended in sows weighing 275 to 300 pounds (Hibbs, 1958). Booth (1963) has suggested preanesthetic administration of atropine sulfate (0.03 to 0.04 mg/lb), meperidine hydrochloride (0.5 to 1.0 mg/lb), and promazine hydrochloride (1.0 mg/lb). These drugs are injected intramuscularly in separate sites 45 to 60 minutes prior to anesthesia. The most predictable phenothiazine tranquilizer for swine is probably acepromazine (0.5 to 1.0 mg/lb, IM) (Benson and Thurmon, 1979). Azaperone, which is not available in the United States, is used extensively as a tranquilizer for swine in other countries (see Chap. 8). Xylazine is not effective; diazepam may be used at the rate of 2.5 to 3.8 mg/lb. Fentanyl-droperidol has been injected intramuscularly as a preanesthetic at a rate of 1 ml/30 lbs (Lumb, 1972).

Ketamine alone produces a cataleptic state in swine that allows minor surgery, but is without sufficient immobilization for major surgical procedures. It is, therefore, combined with other agents such as halothane, methoxyflurane, and nitrous oxide. Swine recovering from ketamine often exhibit excitement. This can be controlled with barbiturates or diazepam. Ketamine should be used cautiously in older swine and in those over 100 lbs, since a phenomenon similar to porcine stress syndrome may occur (Benson and Thurmon, 1979).

For pigs weighing 100 lb or less, atropine (0.02 mg/lb) is given, followed by fentanyl-droperidol (1 ml/30 lb) intramuscularly. When sedation occurs (10 to 15 minutes), ketamine is administered intramuscularly at 5 mg/lb. Surgical anesthesia develops in 5 to 10 minutes and lasts 30 to 45 minutes. Additional increments of ketamine may be given intravenously or intramuscularly to produce a longer effect.

For brief periods of immobilization, acepromazine (0.5 mg/kg IM) followed in 30 minutes by ketamine (15 mg/kg IM) is sufficient. Intramuscular atropine (0.044 mg/kg) will reduce salivation and bronchial secretions. Animals can stand in 65 to 80 minutes postinjection (Gray et al., 1978). Intramuscular ketamine (20 mg/kg) plus xylazine (2 mg/kg) will produce anesthesia in swine in 7 to 10 minutes (Kyle et al., 1979). Additional increments may be given when needed.

For minor surgery in swine, Breese and Dodman (1984) have recommended xylazine (2 mg/kg), ketamine (2 mg/kg), and oxymorphone (0.075 mg/kg) mixed in the same syringe and given intravenously. The dose is doubled for intramuscular administration. Recumbency with narcosis, analgesia, and muscle relaxation are produced for 20 to 30 minutes.

The pig should be fasted 12 to 24 hours prior to general anesthesia. Water should not be withheld for longer than 6 hours. If the animal is not properly fasted, gaseous distension of the digestive tract may develop and cause death by interfering with ventilation and venous return to the heart. Magnesium sulfate or sodium sulfate (25 to 125 g) can be administered orally to assure complete evacuation of the gastrointestinal tract, if abdominal surgery is to be performed.

Because respiratory depression or paralysis can readily occur in swine following induction of general anesthesia, an endotracheal catheter should be routinely inserted to establish an airway (see Chap. 7). Intravenous succinylcholine (0.5 mg/lb) facilitates the procedure. The traditional clinical method of estimating tidal volume by observing chest wall excursions is useless in swine, because of the relative thick, inelastic chest wall. For this reason the tendency is to overventilate this species, with resultant cardiovascular embarrassment. Ventilation with oxygen at a rate of 12 cycles/min with pressures of +12 to +15 and −4 to −6 cm of water is adequate. In swine ranging from 20 to 200 lbs, tidal volumes of 200 to 1000 ml and minute volumes of 3 to 20 L per minute have been found to be satisfactory.

An intravenous anesthetic can be administered by way of the marginal ear vein, recurrent tarsal vein, or anterior vena cava. For prolonged administration, an indwelling catheter should be inserted. To cannulate the anterior vena cava, a 14- to 18-gauge thin-walled medium-beveled 3-in needle is used in swine weighing 20 to 100 lbs. With the animal restrained in dorsal recumbency, the needle is inserted about 2 cm to one side of the cariniform cartilage on a line from the point of the cartilage to the base of the ear. The needle is pushed inward, downward, and backward until its point enters the anterior vena cava (Carle and Dewhirst, 1942). A polyethylene catheter is then threaded through the needle into the vein. If overinserted, the catheter tip will enter the right side of the heart. The needle is withdrawn by sliding it over the catheter. To prevent its accidental withdrawal from the vein, the catheter can be taped or sutured to the animal's skin. An 18-gauge blunted needle is inserted into the lumen of the catheter, and a two-or three-way valve is attached so that injections can be readily made. Commercially available catheters may also be used.

General anesthesia can be induced with intravenous thiopental, thiamylal, or methohexital. The intravenous dose of 5% thiopental solution varies considerably; swine weighing 10 to 50 and 50 to 100 lbs usually require 5.0 and 4.5 mg/lb respectively. Miller and Gudmundson (1964) anesthetized swine with thiamylal at a rate of 2 ml of 10% solution/100 lbs up to 400 lbs, and 0.5 ml for each 100 lbs up to a maximum of 10 ml. Additional doses were administered for prolonged anesthesia. Sawyer et al. (1971) maintained thiamylal anesthesia in swine for 3 hours. Recovery was slow when compared with halothane or methoxyflurane anesthesia. Cardiac output stroke volume and stroke work were depressed (see Table 5–5).

In contrast to the dog, the pig requires extremely deep pentobarbital anesthesia to abolish reflex activity. Moreover, recovery from a single anesthetic dose of pentobarbital is remarkably rapid. It is not uncommon to observe the return of violent motor activity within 10 to 15 minutes. According to Jones (1957), pentobarbital provides a considerable margin of safety in pigs weighing 25 to 30 lbs. An intravenous dose of 11 mg/lb is sufficient to induce general anesthesia. Pentobarbital and atropine can be given intraperitoneally followed by an inhalant anesthetic, such as ether, to maintain surgical anesthesia. This method has been used by Wesolowski (1962) for experimental vascular surgery involving the thoracic vessels of the pig. Sawyer et al. (1971) found that 3 hours of pentobarbital anesthesia in miniature swine produced excessively prolonged recovery periods. Cardiac output, stroke volume, and stroke work were depressed, whereas peripheral vascular resistance was increased.

Halothane or methoxyflurane can be administered for maintenance of anesthesia. Both reduce cardiac output, stroke volume, and stroke work, halothane producing a slightly greater decrease than methoxyflurane. Methoxyflurane has a significantly longer recovery period (Sawyer et al., 1971). Piermattei and Swan (1970) believe that halothane plus equal parts of nitrous oxide and oxygen provide the anesthetic method of choice in pigs subjected to heart-lung bypass.

Following premedication with a small dose of morphine (0.3 to 0.9 mg/kg), the intravenous dose of chloralose necessary to produce hypnotic action in the pig is 55 to 86 mg/kg of body weight (Booth et al., 1960). Paddling movements of the limbs are seen in the pig similar to those reported in sheep by Phillipson and Barnett (1939). Pentobarbital can be administered intravenously in small doses to prevent these movements without interfering greatly with baroreceptor activity. Epidural anesthesia in swine is described in Chapter 17.

Wild hogs may be captured by placing alpha chloralose on corn or in mixtures of flour, peanut butter, sardines, and syrup (Austin and Peoples, 1967). The feeding site should be baited for several days prior to using the drugged bait. One teaspoonful of methocel* per cup added to dampened shelled corn causes the relatively insoluble alpha chloralose to adhere to the corn. The maximum safe dosage for feral hogs is about 1 g/10 lbs; the minimum effective dose is about 1 g/40 lbs. Two grams of alpha chloralose per cup of bait appear to be effective. No bait should be allowed to remain after the trapping operation since it is dangerous for other wildlife.

*See Appendix A for manufacturer.

JAVELINAS

Schilling and Stone (1969) have anesthetized javelinas with thiopental (10 mg/kg) intravenously. The animals were then intubated, and anesthesia was maintained with methoxyflurane.

For additional techniques that may be used, see the section on swine in this chapter.

KANGAROOS AND OTHER MARSUPIALS

Care should be used when catching and restraining kangaroos, since the claws on the hind limbs are well developed and may cause severe lacerations. Occasionally, a kangaroo will bite or claw with its forepaws also.

For capture of macropods, ketamine (3.0 mg/kg) combined with etorphine (0.005 mg/kg) is most successful (Keep, 1978). The induction period is 3 to 4 minutes. Ketamine combined with xylazine (8 mg/kg of each) is also satisfactory (Wilson, 1976).

Althesin at the rate of 15 mg of total steroid/kg intramuscularly produces a flaccid animal in a state of surgical anesthesia.

Phenothiazine tranquilizers may be slow in onset in marsupials, and effects may last for 2 to 3 days. Diazepam is the best drug for tranquilization (Keep, 1978).

Red and gray kangaroos can be anesthetized by intravenous administration of thiopental (1 gr/ml) in the recurrent tarsal vein (Larsen, 1963). Small kangaroos (tammar wallabies and quokkas) may be anesthetized with thiopental intravenously (~28 mg/kg), intubated, and maintained on halothane-oxygen (Richardson and Cullen, 1981).

Inhalation anesthesia in a kangaroo belonging to the Berlin Zoo has been described by Henschel (1958). Following administration of a phenothiazine-type tranquilizer, the animal was intubated, the catheter being brought through the interdental space to avoid the large incisor teeth. A mixture of ether-nitrous oxide-oxygen was administered by means of a closed-circle machine for 4 hours. Recovery was uneventful.

The rat kangaroo (*Potorous tridactylus* Kerr), or potoroo, is a small species that can be picked up by the tail. It will bite, kick, and scratch if not handled carefully. A large plastic tube (6″ diameter × 13″ long) with a slot in the endgate allows access to the tail for venipuncture (Cisar, 1969). The vein, located at the lateral aspect of the base of the tail, can be distended with a tourniquet. In some cases, application of xylene to the skin is necessary to raise the vein. Rat kangaroos have a low tolerance to thiopental, pentobarbital, and ether according to Cisar (1969). A variety of anesthetic agents with the dosages for marsupials are shown in Table 18–27.

ANTELOPE AND GAZELLE

Pronghorn antelope may be immobilized using capture equipment and 6.05 to 9.93 mg/100 lbs of succinylcholine chloride (Beale and Smith, 1967). Gauckler and Kraus (1970) found xylazine (1.0 to 3.0 mg/kg) to be effective for sedation and capture of 17 different species and types of antelope and wild ruminants.

Roan antelope may be immobilized with 11.3 to 13.4 μg/kg of carfentanil plus 755 to 778 μg/kg of azaperone (Hofmyer, 1978). Various anesthetic agents that can be employed in African antelopes and other species are shown in Table 18–28.

TABLE 18–27. Anesthesia in Marsupials

Agent	*Dose and Route*	*Species and Comments*
Azaperone 40 mg/ml	2–4 mg/kg by IM injection	Tranquilization in large macropods
Diazepam 5 mg/ml	2–4 mg/kg IM or IV	All marsupials; tranquilization or anticonvulsant
Diazepam	oral (in feed) 2 mg/kg	Tranquilization in all marsupials
Acepromazine	0.1 mg/kg IM	Indications of some delayed effect (lasts some days); needs quiet and dark for some hours to have maximum effect
Ketamine HCl	20 mg/kg IM	Monotremes for light surgical anesthesia
	25 mg/kg IM	Anesthesia (light) in dasyurids macropods, wombat, koala
	30–50 mg/kg IM	Phalangers for light anesthesia; variable; give 30 mg/kg first, then if insufficient give additional 20 mg/kg
Thiopental	20 mg/kg as 5 or 2.5% sol. (exactly as small animals) by IV injection	All marsupials (tail veins usually easy to use)
Alphaxolone 9 mg/ml Alphadolone 3 mg/ml	0.25–0.5 ml/kg IV to effect	Macropods and phalangers; short duration, can top up; recover fast
Halothane	Inhalation to effect	Bell jar for tiny dasyurids; anesthetic machine and mask or tube in larger species
Etorphine and combinations	0.5 ml of "large animal immobilon" per large kangaroo by IM projectile	Only for capture; restricted availability; can cause excitement and self-injury
Ketamine and xylazine	5 mg/kg ketamine; 2 mg/kg xylazine in same projectile	Capture of macropods

(Adapted from Reddacliff, G.: Therapeutic Index—Marsupials. Proc. Postgrad. Committee Vet. Sci., Univ. of Sidney, 39:1037, 1978.)

TABLE 18–28. Immobilizing Doses of Various Agents in African Wildlife

				Immobilized		Effective Doses of Drugs in Mg				Analgesic Antagonists	
							Immobilon LA				
Species	Age	Sex	Approx. Body Wt (kg)	Total times	No. of animals	Fentanyl	Etorphine +	Acepromazine	Xylazine	Nalorphine	Diprenorphine
Bongo *Boocercus eurycerus*	A	M	300	5	2	70	4.4–4.9	18–20	75	200	6.0
	A	F	220	12	5	40	2.45–2.94	10–20	50	120	3.6
	Imm.	M	{ 50	2 }	1	10	—	—	10	30	—
			80	2 }		15	—	—	10	45	—
Zebra duiker *Cephalophus zebra*	A	M/F	15	18	4	3.0	—	—	2.5–6.0	10	—
	2 wks.	M	1.0	1	1	1.0	—	—	—	2.5	—
Red flanked duiker *Cephalophus rufilatus*	A	M/F	9	9	4	2.0	—	—	2.0	6.0	—
	Imm.	M	5	3	1	1.0	—	—	1.0	2.5	—
Jentink's duiker *Cephalophus jentinkii*	A	M	80	5	1	15	—	—	10	50	—
Maxwell's duiker *Cephalophus maxwellii*	A	M/F	5.0	11	4	1.0–1.5	—	—	1.0–1.5	3–4	—
Yellow-back duiker *Cephalophus sylviculator*	A	M/F	65	11	4	15–20	—	—	10–20	50	—
Black duiker *Cephalophus niger*	A	M	15	3	1	3	—	—	3	10	—
Eland *Taurotragus oryx*	A	F	300	4	1	—	2.94	12	50	—	3.6
	Imm.	M/F	150–200	14	6	—	1.96	8	40–50	—	2.4
	Imm.	M	120	4	2	15–20	1.47	6	20–40	50	2.0
	Imm.	F	60	1	1	12	—	—	12	30	—
Beisa oryx *Oryx beisa*	Imm.	M/F	150	16	5	30	1.96–2.45	8–10	20–30	80	2.4–3.0
Harnessed antelope *Tragelaphus scriptus*	A	M/F	20		3	4.0	—	—	4	10	—
Coke's hartebeeste *Alcelaphus buselaphus cokei*	A	M/F	180	5	3	—	1.47	6	20–30	—	2.0
Impala *Aepyceros melampus*	A } Imm. }	M/F	30–50	8	5	10	—	—	10	25	—
Wildebeeste *Connochaetes tourinus*	A	M/F	180–200	17	5	—	1.47–1.96	6–8	20–30	—	2.0–2.5
	Imm.	F	70	3	1	—	0.49	2	10	—	0.6
Defassa waterbuck *Kobus defassa*	A	M	320	5	2	50	1.96–2.94	8–12	40–50	125	2.4–3.6
Thomson's gazelle *Gazella thomsonii*	A	M/F	18	5	3	5.0	—	—	5.0	12.5	—
Buffalo *Syncerus caffer*	Near A	F	375	3	1	—	2.45	10	25	—	3.0

A = adult

(From Haigh, J.C.: The Immobilisation of Bongo *(Boocercus eurycus)* and Other African Antelopes in Captivity. Vet. Rec., 98:237, 1976.)

Captive Dorcas gazelles have been immobilized for electroejaculation with xylazine (0.23 mg/kg) and ketamine (11.54 mg/kg) (Howard et al, 1981).

Capture myopathy, a potentially fatal condition, has been reported in pronghorns *(Antilocapra americana)* subjected to capture and transport (Chalmers and Barrett, 1977). Affected animals usually have been subjected to strenuous exercise prior to onset of the disease (see Chap. 21).

SHEEP AND GOATS

Sheep and goats are occasionally used as laboratory animals. The chief difficulties experienced during general anesthesia with these species are excessive salivation, tympanites, and regurgitation. The latter two can be eliminated to a great extent by fasting the animal for at least 24 hours and by oral administration of an antiferment one-half hour prior to induction.

Excessive salivation is controlled by intramuscular injection of atropine (15 mg/50 lbs) 15 minutes before induction. To maintain control, it should be given intravenously at 15-minute intervals. According to Booth (1963), a maintenance dose of 3 to 6 mg will accomplish this in animals weighing 65 to 85 lbs.

Triflupromazine (0.5 to 1 mg/lb intravenously) is a satisfactory preanesthetic for goats when combined with either local or general anesthesia (Jha et al., 1961*a*, *b*; Tyagi and Lumb, 1961).

Thurmon et al. (1973) used ketamine alone and in combination with atropine and acepromazine for surgical anesthesia in sheep. Administration of atropine and acepromazine reduced salivation and improved muscle relaxation. Acepromazine reduced the amount of ketamine required and increased recovery time.

Ketamine (11 mg/kg) combined with xylazine (0.22 mg/kg) will induce 40 to 45 minutes of anesthesia in goats. Xylazine administration should precede ketamine administration if one is given separately. The mixture of agents is miscible in the same syringe. Additional increments of ketamine may be used to produce up to 3 hours of anesthesia. The effects of ketamine (25 mg/kg IV) on hematologic and biochemical parameters in goats have been studied by Kumar et al. (1974). They found significant increases in blood glucose during anesthesia and in serum glutamic oxalacetic transaminase at 24 hours postanesthesia.

Etorphine (0.07 mg/kg) with triflupromazine (1.98 mg/kg) has been employed by Thurmon et al. (1974) for surgical anesthesia of goats. Immobilization occurred in approximately 3 minutes and lasted for 60 to 120 minutes. Intravenous injection of diprenorphine produced reversal of immobilization in approximately 13 minutes.

Both thiamylal (4%) and thiopental (5%) have been used satisfactorily in sheep and goats. Since these anesthetics are detoxified at a rapid rate, the dose required for anesthesia varies greatly. An initial intravenous dose of 9 to 10 mg/lb of body weight is usually effective.

Immediately following induction of anesthesia, a cuffed endotracheal catheter is inserted into the trachea to prevent aspiration of regurgitated ruminal contents.

Maintenance of anesthesia can be achieved by repeated injections of anesthetic through an indwelling catheter in the external jugular vein. An alternative is administration of halothane or methoxyflurane by means of an anesthetic machine. Recovery from these volatile liquid anesthetics is rapid and uneventful (Kramer et al., 1965*b*; Dhindsa et al., 1970).

Allam and Churchill (1946) used pentobarbital sodium intravenously in average-sized mature goats. They found that a total dose of 10 gr given in the jugular vein was sufficient to produce general anesthesia. The animals were able to stand in 2 or 3 hours. The anesthetic dose and duration of anesthesia of pentobarbital vary widely in sheep (Phillipson and Barnett, 1939). Approximately 30 mg/kg will produce a short period of surgical anesthesia (15 to 30 minutes) in adult sheep; in lambs the duration is longer.

Regional anesthesia, including paravertebral, epidural, and subarachnoid techniques, is discussed in Chapters 16 and 17.

BIGHORN SHEEP

The effects of several drugs on bighorn sheep have been observed by Logsdon (1969). For tranquilization of penned animals, diazepam can be mixed with feed at the rate of 5.9 mg/lb. Succinylcholine (0.34 to 0.37 mg/lb) injected with capture equipment causes immobilization in approximately 8 minutes and recumbency for approximately 20 minutes.

Etorphine can also be used to capture bighorn sheep (Logsdon, 1969). The dose is approximately 10 μg/lb when given intramuscularly. The additional injection of acepromazine (15 mg) after capture prolongs the effect and facilitates handling. Injection of cyprenorphine produces rapid recovery from the effects of etorphine. It is recommended that cyprenorphine be given in a dose 2½ times the amount of etorphine and that one-half be given intravenously and one-half intramuscularly to produce smooth recovery.

DEER

Kloppel (1969), Hime and Jones (1970), and Hönich (1970) used intramuscular injections of 0.3 to 9 mg/kg of xylazine in red, fallow, and spotted deer. The onset of sedation occurred within 3 to 10 minutes and usually lasted 1 to 2 hours. Hime and Jones (1970) noted that a degree of analgesia was produced, but that supplementation with a local or regional anesthetic was always required for surgery. During onset of sedation there was some salivation, but in no instance did regurgitation of ruminal contents or ruminal tympany occur. An alteration in respiratory rhythm, ranging from transient apnea to a Cheyne-Stokes respiration, was observed most frequently in red deer, moose, sitatunga, and Barbary sheep. Kloppel (1969) indicated that xylazine produced good sedation and analgesia in wild ruminants, but that immobilization and muscle relaxation were sometimes insufficient.

Xylazine at dosages of 0.89 to 8.0 mg/kg was used to immobilize captive white-tailed deer (Roughton, 1975). Induction times were shorter in fawns and freshly trapped deer. Mean induction time was 5.15 ± 4.08 minutes. Immobilization was prolonged with doses above 3 mg/kg.

The intramuscular dose of ketamine for most deer is 10 to 20 mg/kg IM. Ketamine-xylazine, as described for goats, can be used for North American mule deer (Richter, 1977).

Wallach et al. (1967) have used etorphine to immobilize deer and other ruminants (Table 18–29). For fallow deer, Harrington (1974) recommends a mixture of etorphine (2 mg/100 kg) and xylazine (30 mg/100 kg) administered via a syringe weapon. In the same species, Haigh et al. (1977) has used fentanyl (0.3 to 0.66 mg/kg) plus xylazine (0.46 to 1.3 mg/kg). Acepromazine has proved unsuitable for this species.

Père David's deer *(Elaphurus davidianus)* have been successfully darted with a mixture of etorphine (0.012 to 0.021 mg/kg) and xylazine (0.23 to 0.56 mg/kg). Succinylcholine alone proved unsatisfactory (Smeller et al., 1976).

Succinylcholine has been used by Thomas (1961) to immobilize several species of deer (Table 18–30). Boyd (1962) injected succinylcholine chloride intrathoracically and intravenously into trapped Colorado mule deer with a conventional syringe. By the former route, the effective dose was found to be 0.052 mg/lb for adults and 0.078 mg/lb for fawns. Intravenous administration caused severe respiratory paralysis and some deaths. The margin between a safe dose and a lethal one was found to be quite small with both methods.

Blood values for captive white-tailed deer physically restrained or chemically immobilized have been reported by Kocan et al. (1981). Succinylcholine chloride, etorphine, xylazine, and fentanyl were used. Significantly increased body temperatures were found in etorphine and fentanyl groups. They concluded that there were only minor changes in hematologic and serum chemical values with all four agents, provided the conditions caused minimal excitement.

Davis (1963) has anesthetized Colorado mule deer. For tranquilization during transportation, chlorpromazine at a rate of 2 mg/lb is given intramuscularly. Good results have also been obtained in elk with this dose. The effect requires about an hour to reach its height and lasts 16 to 24 hours. If used as a preanesthetic prior to pentobarbital, it is injected intramuscularly at least 1 hour in advance. Deer given perphena-

TABLE 18–29. Results of Etorphine Immobilization in Ruminants

Species	*Sex*	*Est. Wt. (lb)*	*Etorphine (mg)*	*Ap (mg)*	*S (mg)*	*Imm. Time (min)*	*Nal (mg)*	*Lag Time (sec)*	*Remarks*
Aoudad	M	275	1.0	5.0	5.0	13.0	100	15	Good state of immobility
Aoudad	M	200	1.0	5.0	5.0	8.0	200	I	Good state of immobility
Aoudad	F	150	1.0	5.0	5.0	3.0	100	I	Required additional 0.5 mg etorphine to trim
Aoudad	F	150	1.0	2.0	5.0	4.0	100	30	Required additional 0.4 mg etorphine to trim
Aoudad	F	150	2.0	2.0	5.0	3.5	100	I	Teeth grinding, twitching
Aoudad	F	150	2.0	2.0	5.0	6.0	100	I	Teeth grinding, twitching
Eland	F	650	2.0	10.0	25.0	11.0	250	60	Vomiting, pushing wall after nalorphine
Eland	F	650	2.0	10.0	25.0	9.0	250	120	Salivated, pushing wall after nalorphine
Reindeer	M	200	1.0	5.0	4.0	4.0	50	90	In rut, excellent results
Reindeer	M	200	1.0	5.0	4.0	6.0	100	45	Same animal as above, dehorned
Fallow deer	M	90	1.0	3.0	2.0	4.0	50	I	Good immobility, dehorned
Fallow deer	M	100	1.0	3.0	2.0	—	—	—	Dart bounced off; caught by hand 20 min
Fallow deer	M	100	0.5	2.0	2.0	4.0	100	30	Good state of immobility
Fallow deer	M	150	0.5	7.5	1.5	7.0	—	—	Up when approached; 120 min normal
Fallow deer	M	150	1.0	5.0	3.0	8.0	100	—	Free-ranging, died during manual restraint
Fallow deer	M	150	1.0	5.0	3.0	6.0	100	—	Free-ranging, died during manual restraint
Bison	M	250	1.0	5.0	2.0	7.0	100	—	Required minimal restraint
Bison	M	500	1.0	5.0	2.0	—	100	—	Required additional 0.5 mg etorphine, 2 mg Ap, 2 mg S
Bison	M	700	2.0	5.0	5.0	10.0	100	60	Required minimal restraint
Bison	M	1,200	2.5	5.0	25.0	9.0	125	240	Died in 2 hours—pulmonary emphysema
Lesser kudu	F	100	0.5	4.0	4.0	13.0	50	30	Required manual restraint
Greater kudu	M	450	2.5	5.0	5.0	15.0	100	60	Required manual restraint to cast leg
Black buck	M	60	0.5	10.0	10.0	—	50	—	Required additional 1 mg etorphine, 10 mg Ap, 10 mg S, deep analgesia
Giraffe	F	2,500	2.5	30.0	10.0	5.0	160	—	Five small doses of etorphine down 6 minutes after last injection; died following day from dystocia

Ap = acepromazine; S = scopolamine; Nal = nalorphine hydrochloride; Lag time = time elapsed from administration of nalorphine to animal standing; I = immediate recovery; — = drug not used; Imm. time. = time elapsed from administration of drug to immobilization.

(From Wallach, J.D., Frueh, R., and Lentz, M.: The Use of M.99 as an Immobilizing and Analgesic Agent in Captive Wild Animals. J.A.V.M.A., 151:870, 1967.)

TABLE 18–30. Paralyzing Doses of Succinylcholine Chloride and Duration of Paralysis in Wild Animals

Animal	*Scientific Name*	*Sex*	*No.*	*Age*	*Estimated Weight (lb)*	*Dose (mg)*	*Av. Latent Period (min)*	*Maximum Latent Period (min)*	*Minimum Latent Period (min)*	*Duration Paralysis (min)*
Deer, fallow	*Dama dama*	M	7	Adult	135	10	11½	17	7	13
Deer, axis	*Axis axis*	M	1	Adult	120	7	10	—	—	17
Deer, axis	*Axis axis*	F	1	Adult	120	7	8	—	—	19
Deer, sika	*Cervus nippon*	M	2	Adult	170	7	7	7	7	14
Deer, sika	*Cervus nippon*	F	4	Adult	130	7	7	7	7	14
Deer, barasingha	*Cervus dubauceli*	M	5	Adult	450	13	9½	11	7	15 7/10
Deer, barasingha	*Cervus dubauceli*	M	1	Adult	375	13	8½	—	—	20
Deer, barasingha	*Cervus dubauceli*	F	16	Adult	(170–360) Av. 227	6–10 7.2	8	12½	5	(10–30) 17½
Deer, barasingha	*Cervus dubauceli*	M	1	Adult	Emaciated 400	7	9½	—	—	20
Deer, barasingha	*Cervus dubauceli*	M	1	Adult	Emaciated 325	6	9	—	—	30
Wapiti (elk)	*Cervus canadensis*	M	1	Adult	1,100	23	6	6	6	18
Wapiti (elk)	*Cervus canadensis*	F	4	Adult	550	15	5–3/10	7½	3½	(18–25) 2½
Wapiti (elk)	*Cervus canadensis*	M	1	Adult	450	15	5–3/10	7½	3½	21½
Deer, red	*Cervus elaphus*	M	5	Adult	260	15	7½	9½	(16–23) 6½	(14–18) 16
Bison	*Bison bison*	F	1	Adult	700	25	7	7	7	10
Antelope (eland)	*Taurotragus oryx*	F	1	Adult	250	6	9	—	—	14
Monkey, spider	*Ateles geoffroyi*	F	1	Adult	5	5	4½	—	—	20
Monkey, spider	*Ateles geoffroyi*	F	1	Adult	5	10	50 sec.	—	—	30
Monkey, spider	*Ateles geoffroyi*	F	1	Adult	5	20	½	—	—	45
Lion, African	*Panthera leo*	F	1	Adult	275	60	6	—	—	11
Lion, African	*Panthera leo*	F	1	Adult	275	120	2½	—	—	60
Goat, domestic	*Capra prisca*	M	1	Adult	110	70	6½	—	—	60
Goat, domestic	*Capra prisca*	M	1	Adult	110	40	9	—	—	30
Goat, domestic	*Capra prisca*	M	1	Adult	110	20	14	—	—	15
Goat, domestic	*Capra prisca*	F	3	Adult	50—80	20	11	14	9	15
Goat, domestic	*Capra prisca*	F	3	Adult	60	15	11	11	11	17
Goat (Tahr), Himalayan	*Hemitragus jemiahious*	M	2	Adult	165	17½	6	—	—	21½
Goat (Tahr), Himalayan	*Hemitragus jemiahious*	F	2	Adult	115	15	6	—	—	20
Sheep, Barbary	*Ammotragus lervia*	M	2	Adult	200	20	15	17	12	7
Antelope, pronghorn	*Antelope Capra americana*	M	2	1 year	50	5	8	10	6	15

(From Thomas, W.D.: Chemical Immobilization of Wild Animals. J.A.V.M.A., 138:264, 1961.)

zine as a tranquilizer have a tendency to chew on rocks during the recovery period.

The reaction of deer to intravenous pentobarbital varies greatly, and they must be watched closely during the recovery period, which is relatively long. Salivation and bloating are constant problems. If pentobarbital is to be used, it should be preceded by atropine and chlorpromazine, and the animal should be deprived of feed and water for 24 hours prior to induction. The dose of atropine is large, at least one-fourth gr is given initially, and additional increments up to 1 gr may be necessary. In a series of approximately 50 deer, Davis (1963) reported one death and several cases of post-operative pneumonia due to regurgitation of rumen contents. As in other ruminants, endotracheal intubation is mandatory during general anesthesia to obviate such complications.

For short periods of anesthesia (30 minutes), a 7% solution of chloral hydrate can be given intravenously "to effect." The last part of the injection is made slowly. In a series of approximately 25 animals, no deaths occurred, though no attempt was made to starve the animals and no preanesthetic agents were used.

Combined chloral hydrate, halothane, and nitrous oxide anesthesia has been used in mule deer by Wolff et al. (1965). Food and water were withheld for 24 hours prior to anesthesia. Seven percent chloral hydrate was administered intravenously until most voluntary movement ceased. The average dose was 210 ml for a 200-lb deer. Atropine (30 to 45 mg) was administered to prevent excessive salivation. Following intubation, anesthesia was induced with 3 to 5% halothane. The flow of halothane was maintained at approximately 1%, and nitrous oxide was administered in 1:1 ratio with oxygen. Regurgitation was the most frequent complication.

Diazepam has been used to capture 5 species of wild deer by Thomas et al. (1967). The dose ranges from 125 to 250 g/25 lbs of feed. The effects vary depending upon the amount ingested but may persist for several days. Baiting should be done in troughs or other containers and all bait should be removed, since it presents a hazard to other wildlife. Maximum effect occurs 4 to 8 hours after ingestion. Drugged animals should be separated from those untranquilized since the latter may cause injury. As tranquilization occurs, drugged animals eat less so the technique is self-limiting.

ELK, CARIBOU, AND MOOSE

Haigh (1978) has darted caribou with several agents: fentanyl (0.3 to 0.6 mg/kg), xylazine (0.25 to 0.5 mg/kg), and azaperone (0.5 to 1.2 mg/kg). Etorphine (0.02 to 0.1 mg/kg) with hyoscine hydrobromide (0.04 to 0.07 mg/kg) and acepromazine (0.02 to 0.1 mg/kg) have also been used.

Succinylcholine chloride can be used in capture equipment to immobilize Roosevelt elk *(Cervus canadensis roosevelti)*. Best results are obtained using a concentration of 50 mg/ml. Syringes fired into the hip, shoulder, or back muscles produce the most consistent results. Neither the latent period of the drug nor the duration of paralysis is affected by the sex, size, or age of the animals. The average latent period for immobilized animals is 6 minutes. The duration of paralysis varies with the physical condition. The mean dose for cows, bulls, and calves 7 months or older is approximately 14 mg (Harper, 1965).

North American elk *(Cervus canadensis)* can be immobilized using succinylcholine chloride and capture equipment (Flook et al., 1962). Some elk bloat rapidly when down; therefore, all should be rolled onto their briskets and, if necessary, trocarized. Dosage requirements and lethal limits appear to be lower in late winter and early spring than at other times of the year. Total doses recommended are as follows: 15 to 20 mg for calves 4 to 11 months of age; 20 to 25 mg for females 12 months and older; and 25 to 35 mg for males 12 months and older. Of 100 elk, 91 were immobilized and recovered, 7 died, and 2 were not affected.

Gallamine has been used in a limited number of elk to facilitate collection of blood samples (Wolff and Boyd, 1963). The average dose, 60 to 80 mg, was shot intramuscularly with capture equipment. The shortest time for an elk to go down was approximately 80 seconds and the longest 150. Trembling and anxiety preceded collapse of the animals. After struggling ceased, they were securely tied and edrophonium was given intravenously at a rate of 1.0 mg for each 2.0 mg of gallamine administered. The severe respiratory distress produced by gallamine was immediately relieved.

After blood collection, injected elk appeared dull and quiet, and some remained in sternal recumbency for as long as 1½ hours. No deaths occurred in a series of nine animals.

With the use of succinylcholine chloride in capture equipment, 31 moose and 112 Newfoundland caribou were captured successfully (Bergerud et al, 1964). The effective dose for wild moose is 0.020 to 0.030 mg/lb and for caribou 0.45 to 0.65 mg/lb. Captive caribou require smaller doses (0.025 to 0.040 mg/lb).

Xylazine alone produces long-lasting immobility in moose, and treated animals require constant supervision. Xylazine (0.15 to 0.53 mg/kg) plus fentanyl (0.14 to 0.53 mg/kg) was effective in helicopter-assisted capture of moose (Haigh et al., 1977). Hyaluronidase (150 to 300 N.F. units) added to the mixture decreased the induction times 36 to 45%.

CAMELS

Hime and Jones (1970) indicated that large camelidae were especially sensitive to xylazine as a sedative. Intramuscular doses used in Arabian and Bactrian camels ranged from 0.43 to 0.88 mg/kg. In most instances there was no resistance to positioning and manipulation of feet. Onset of sedation usually occurred within 10 minutes and lasted from 45 minutes to 5 hours. Larger doses produced sedation for up to 24 hours. Regurgitation of rumen contents and ruminal tympany were not observed in camelidae or bovidae, and recovery was not accompanied by struggling and excitement.

Custer et al. (1977) used xylazine doses of 0.27 to 0.51 mg/kg IM for restraint of Bactrian camels. Injected camels had significantly lower values for red blood cell counts, hemoglobin, and packed cell volume, and higher blood glucose values than camels that were manually restrained. Doxapram (0.05 to 0.13 mg/kg) was injected intravenously and produced rapid arousal.

Use of chloral hydrate and chloral hydrate-magnesium sulfate solutions intravenously in camels has been described by Singh et al. (1962). They believe that the combination (chloral hydrate, 2 oz, magnesium sulfate, 2 oz; and distilled water, 16 oz) is safer than 10% chloral hydrate solution alone.

Said (1964) has studied several anesthetic combinations in camels. Premedication with intramuscular chlorpromazine (1 mg/kg) reduced the amount of chloral hydrate or pentobarbital sodium necessary for general anesthesia and prolonged the duration. A satisfactory method of general anesthesia for the camel was found to be 0.5 mg/kg of chlorpromazine plus 2.5 g/50 kg of chloral hydrate intravenously, followed by an average of 2.33 g of pentobarbital sodium given intravenously "to effect." This mixture produced surgical anesthesia for about one hour (Fig. 18–22).

For laparotomy and rumenotomy, local anesthesia can be obtained by infiltration of 2% procaine or lidocaine. Epidural anesthesia can be accomplished with the animal fastened in the sitting position. Injection is made with a 5-cm needle at the sacrococcygeal or first coccygeal space, slanting the needle forward about 45° from vertical. Two percent lidocaine is injected; 12 to 16 ml produces analgesia of the anus, udder, vagina, scrotum, and hind limbs; 50 ml produces anesthesia of the hindquarters posterior to the umbilicus.

Guaifenesin (110 mg/kg) and thiopental (4.4 mg/kg) have been used for induction of anesthesia in a bull dromedary. For continuation of general anesthesia, guaifenesin (5% in 5% dextrose) plus thiopental (0.2%) in the same solution was given along with nitrous oxide-oxygen. Halothane-nitrous oxide-oxygen may also be employed (Geddes et al., 1974).

GIRAFFE

Bush et al. (1976) found that xylazine alone was unsuitable for restraint of giraffes. When it was combined with etorphine, satisfactory results were obtained. Doses for Masai and retic-

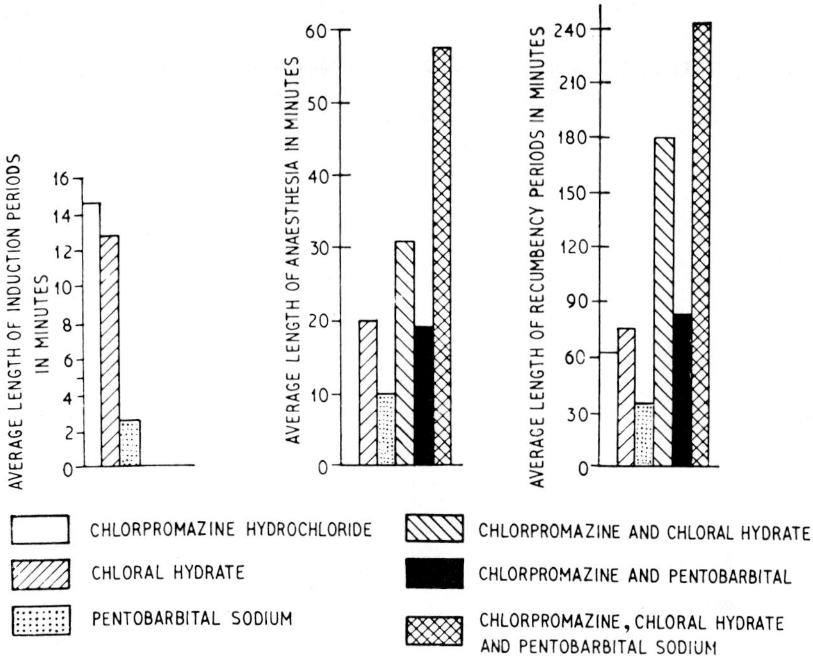

Figure 18–22. Average lengths of induction periods, anesthesia, and recumbency periods following the administration of various drugs in the camel. (From Said, A.H.: Some Aspects of Anaesthesia in the Camel. Vet. Rec., 76:550, 1964.)

ulated giraffes ranged from 20 to 70 mg/kg of xylazine plus 0.8 to 1.5 mg of etorphine.

The dose of succinylcholine chloride for Masai giraffe (*Giraffa camelopardalis tipelskirchi*, Matschie) is 0.024 mg/lb and is rather critical (Talbot and Lamprey, 1961). This differs considerably from the dose for Rothschild's giraffe *(Giraffa camelopardalis rothschildii)* of 0.08 mg/lb (Buechner et al., 1960).

Etorphine has been used for surgical analgesia and restraint in an adult reticulated giraffe *(Giraffa camelopardalis reticulata)* by Williamson and Wallach (1968). They injected 2.5 mg intramuscularly along with 30 mg of acepromazine and 10 mg of scopolamine. This produced recumbency but was supplemented with an additional 1 mg of etorphine to produce surgical analgesia. Nalorphine (250 mg intramuscularly and 250 mg intravenously) quickly counteracted the etorphine.

UNDOMESTICATED CATS

Hime (1974) has given ketamine to a wide variety of undomesticated cats (Table 18–31).

Etorphine has been used successfully by Wallach et al. (1967) to immobilize African lions (Table 18–32). Göltenboth (1968) and Göltenboth and Klös (1970) reported good immobilization and sedation of large feral cats, hyenas, and wolves with 6 to 8 mg/kg of xylazine.

Doses of succinylcholine chloride for African lions are given in Table 18–30. Succinylcholine is highly effective for immobilizing mountain lions *(Felis concolor)* but should not be administered to treed animals that may be subjected to injurious or fatal falls (Hornocker et al., 1965). For adult lions, the dose is 1 mg/14.2 lbs of body weight. Slightly less (1 mg/17.4 lbs) is used for juveniles. An average of 4.05 minutes is required for immobilization with recovery time of approximately 23 minutes. Intraperitoneal pentobarbital (1 ml or 60 mg/5.25 to 5.75 lbs) can be given while the animal is immobilized; however, it produces prolonged anesthesia and is not considered suitable for field use.

Clifford (1958; et al., 1961) has used combined meperidine and promazine as preanes-

TABLE 18–31. Results of the Use of Ketamine in Nondomesticated Cats on 38 Occasions

Species	*Sex*	*Age in years M = months*	*Weight (kg)*	*Dose of Ketamine (mg/kg)*	*Onset Time (min)*
Ocelot (*Felis pardalis*)	F	12	8	5.0	NM
Ocelot	F	12	8	6.0	NM
Ocelot	F	14	8	14.0	10
Serval (*Felis serval*)	M	8M	11	9.0	10
Serval	F	4	9	15.0	NM
Leopard cat (*Felis bengalensis*)	M	10M	3	14.0	NM
Leopard cat	M	10M	3	8.0	U
Leopard cat	F	10M	2	11.6	U
Leopard cat	F	10M	1	15.0	10
Leopard cat	M	10M	2	25.0	8
Clouded leopard (*Neofelis nebulosa*)	M	15	18	8.6	U
Chinese leopard (*Panthera pardus Japonensis*)	F	3.5	38	15.0	7 (C)
Black leopard (*Panthera pardus*)	F	13	54	15.0	19
Margay (*Felis wiedii*)	F	7	3	15.0	NM
Jaguar (*Panthera onca*)	F	14	60	13.0	10
Jaguar	M	5	83	18.0	U
Cheetah (*Acinonyx jubatus*)	M	7	34	8.0	U
Cheetah	M	7	33	11.0	NM
Cheetah	M	7	34	12.0	U
Cheetah	M	7	34	11.5	8 (C)
Cheetah	M	10	42	9.5	6
Cheetah	M	12	30.5	10.0	6
Puma (*Felis concolor*)	F	12	24	11.0	7
Puma	F	12	24	11.0	14
Puma	M	8M	27	15.0	U
Puma	M	8M	27	18.0	U
Puma	F	6	23	22.0	3
Puma	M	14	50	18.0	8
Puma	M	2	30	15.0	7
Puma	M	2	58	20.0	13
Puma	M	2.3	45	18.0	U
Puma	M	2.5	56	25.0	8
Lion (*Panthera leo*)	F	12	150	10.0	U
Lion	M	2	140	18.0	6
Lion	M	3	163	14.0	U (C)
Lion	F	2	95	20.0	5 (C)
Tiger (*Panthera tigris*)	M	15	130	7.0	7
Tiger	F	7	110	14.0	9

NM = not measured
U = never safe to handle
C = convulsions occurred

(From Hime, J.M.: Use of Ketamine in Non-Domesticated Cats. Vet. Rec., 95:193, 1974.)

TABLE 18–32. Results of Etorphine Immobilization of Lions

Species	Sex	Est. Wt. (lb)	Etorphine (mg)	Ap (mg)	S (mg)	Imm. Time (min)	Nal (mg)	Lag Time (sec)	Remarks
African	F	220	0.5	. .	. .	3.0	. .	. .	20 sec. convulsion, required 10 mg Ap
African	F	220	0.5	33.0	30.0	5.0	125	. .	Required additional dose same as first

Ap = acepromazine; S = scopolamine; Nal = nalorphine hydrochloride; Lag time = time elapsed from administration of nalorphine to animal standing; . . = drug not used; Imm. time = time elapsed from administration of drug to immobilization.

(From Wallach, J.D., Frueh, R., and Lentz, M.: The Use of M.99 as an Immobilizing and Analgesic Agent in Captive Wild Animals. J.A.V.M.A., 151:870, 1967.)

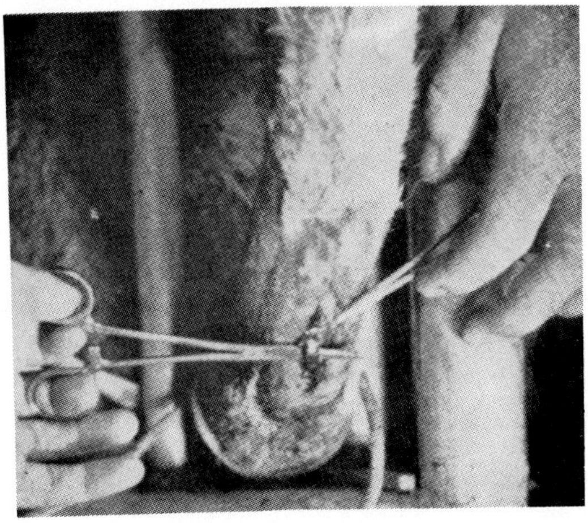

Figure 18–23. Following infiltration with a local anesthetic, the lateral caudal vein of a lion can be exposed for intravenous injection. (Clifford, D.H., Stowe, C.M., Jr., and Good, A.L.: Pentobarbital Anesthesia in Lions with Special Reference to Preanesthetic Medication. J.A.V.M.A., 139:111, 1961.)

thetic agents in an ocelot, a leopard, and in lions. In the latter, 11 mg/kg of meperidine and 4.4 to 9 mg/kg of promazine are recommended. Subcutaneous administration is facilitated by use of a squeeze-cage. After these take effect, pentobarbital is given intraperitoneally, intrathoracically, or intravenously. To accomplish the latter, a tourniquet is applied to the tail and the anesthetic is injected into the caudal vein (Fig. 18–23).

According to Clifford, big cats require less anesthetic to produce surgical anesthesia, certain reflexes may persist longer, and the postanesthetic recovery period is longer. Pentobarbital is a dangerous anesthetic if used to abolish all reflexes in lions. The number and character of the respirations are important criteria with which to evaluate depth of anesthesia. Fewer than 10 respirations per minute should be cause for grave concern. It is suggested that local anesthetics be employed, whenever possible, to avoid large doses of general anesthetic in undomesticated cats.

Halothane or halothane-N_2O is recommended for general anesthesia in feral cats because they provide rapid induction. After preanesthesia, these may be given by mask until the animal is relaxed. Endotracheal intubation is then indicated if anesthesia is to be of considerable duration.

BEARS

Several anesthetic techniques have been used in capturing, immobilizing, and anesthetizing bears.

Alpha-chloralose has been used on bait to capture black bears *(Ursus americanus)*. When chloralose was mixed with honey, 9 of 17 wild bears were captured in the field, a trail hound being used to follow the bears once they had taken the bait. The effective dose for wild bears was 1 g/3 to 8 lb. Recovery occurred in 8 to 10 hours (Stafford and Williams, 1968).

Ketamine and xylazine combined in a ratio of approximately 2:1 produces good anesthesia in captive and wild black bears *(Ursus americanus)*. The optimum dose range is 4.5 to 9.0 mg/kg of ketamine and 2.0 to 4.5 mg/kg of xylazine. There is no difference in sex response, but smaller bears are induced more quickly. Supplemental injections have been used to maintain tractability for as long as 31 hours (Addison and Kolenosky, 1979). Free-ranging polar bears *(Ursus maritinus)* can be immobilized with a specially prepared, concentrated solution containing 200 mg of ketamine and 200 mg of xylazine/ml. Cubs require 2.8 mg/kg of each drug, whereas adults require 6.8 mg/kg (Lee et al., 1981).

Wallach et al. (1967) have used etorphine in immobilization of bears (Table 18–33).

Small bears can be anesthetized with intravenous thiopental, thiamylal, or pentobarbital sodium given in the cephalic or saphenous vein. A squeeze-cage facilitates the procedure. If this is not available, the caged animal is offered a favorite food; when it reaches for it, the paw is grasped by an assistant wearing gloves. A rope is tied around the limb to act as a tourniquet and to distend the vein. Fowler (1960) has described this procedure in a 75-pound Malayan sun bear. Seven hundred fifteen mg of pentobarbital produced surgical anesthesia for two hours. An average of 13.5 mg/kg of pentobarbital intravenously permitted safe handling and minor surgery of American black bears and Himalayan black bears (Clarke et al., 1963). Following induction with an intravenous thiobarbiturate, bears can be given halothane or halothane-N_2O via mask and/or endotracheal catheter. This provides good relaxation for long procedures.

Troyer (1960), in trapping and tagging Kodiak bears, has devised an efficient method for their management. Once the bear is caught by the foot in a special trap, succinylcholine is given intramuscularly in the hind leg by means of a syringe on a long aluminum pole. As soon as it takes effect, and the bear is tied in spread-eagle fashion, a concentrated pentobarbital solution is injected intraperitoneally. Succinylcholine alone is less satisfactory. No deaths occurred in a series of 32 bears. Table 18–34 gives figures representative of effects obtained with this procedure.

FERAL EQUIDAE

Howard et al. (1981) have used etorphine (0.017 mg/kg) for restraint of captive onagers during electroejaculation. The drug was antagonized by diprenorphine following the procedure.

TABLE 18–33. Results of Etorphine Immobilization in Bears

Species	*Sex*	*Est. Wt. (lb)*	*Etorphine (mg)*	*Ap (mg)*	*S (mg)*	*Imm. Time (min)*	*Nal (mg)*	*Lag Time (sec)*	*Remarks*
Spectacled	M	300	1.0	5.0	4.0	3.0	250	300	Good immobility, deep analgesia
Black	F	110	0.5	5.0	5.0	12.0	100	200	Good immobility, deep analgesia
Black	F	110	0.5	5.0	2.0	10.0	50	. .	Same animal as above
Black	M	125	0.1	1.0	1.0	. .	. .	. .	Tranquil, required additional 0.5 mg etorphine to immobilize
Black	M	125	0.5	2.0	2.0	15.0	50	30	Excellent stage of immobility, deep analgesia
Black	M	140	0.5	5.0	5.0	. .	. .	. .	Tranquil, dart bounced off, hand caught
Black	M	140	0.5	5.0	5.0	. .	. .	. .	Tranquil, dart bounced off, additional 0.25 mg etorphine, good immobility

Ap = acepromazine; S = scopolamine; Nal = nalorphine hydrochloride; Lag time = time elapsed from administration of nalorphine to animal standing; . . = drug not used; Imm. time = time elapsed from administration of drug to immobilization.

(From Wallach, J.D., Frueh, R., and Lentz, M.: The Use of M.99 as an Immobilizing and Analgesic Agent in Captive Wild Animals. J.A.V.M.A., 151:870, 1967.)

TABLE 18–34. Effect of Succinylcholine-Pentobarbital Anesthesia on Bears

Sex	Est. Age	Wt.	Succinylcholine* Used (ml)	Effective Time (min)	Recovery Time (min)	Pentobarbital§ Used (ml)	Effective Time (min)	Remarks
M	2½	200	2½	2	7	20	—	
F	3½	305	4	5	§	20	9½	Never went completely down with succinylcholine
F	1½	166	1¾	1⅙	3	7	12	Succinylcholine, 1 ml had no effect
F	1½	157	2	1¾	§	10	6	8 ml pentobarbital not enough so gave 2 ml more
F	3½	292	3	2	3	12	13½	Recovered in 1½ hrs
M	6+	680	7	4	§	8	—	Initial dose of 40 ml had no effect; kept adding at 15-min intervals 10–15 ml until anesthetized
F	1½	146	2	2½	§	10	12	Did not completely relax under succinylcholine
M	1½	158	2¼	2½	§	10	7½	Not out well with succinylcholine, but was under with pentobarbital
M	2½	245	3	3	8	12	13	
F	3½	350	3½	2½	9	31	—	Gave 16 ml pentobarbital; after 15 min gave 15 ml more

*Contains 30 mg/ml of succinylcholine chloride. §Contains 2.75 gr of pentobarbital sodium/ml and in conventional use is given for euthanasia of small animals.

Recovery time was not always known because pentobarbital took effect before recovery from succinylcholine. Effective time of pentobarbital was not always known because bear had not recovered from succinylcholine when pentobarbital became effective.

(Adapted from Troyer, W.: Out for Bear, Jen-Sal J., 43:32, 1960.)

Combined acepromazine (0.04 mg/kg) and etorphine (0.01 mg/kg) have been used in capture equipment for immobilization of kiang (Seidel et al., 1982). Reversal was performed with diprenorphine and nalorphine.

Once restrained, feral equidae may be given both injectable and inhalant general anesthetics in the same manner as domesticated species (see Chaps. 10, 12).

WATER BUFFALO

The domestic buffalo *(Bubalus bubalis)* is raised mainly in Asia as a producer of meat and milk. It has only distant relationship to the American bison *(Bison bison)* discussed in the following section. Most anesthetic techniques for the buffalo have been inferred from work with cattle. Recent studies have shown considerable species variation.

The effects of xylazine on buffalo calves have been studied by Peshin et al. (1978) and Peshin and Kumar (1979). Doses of 0.22 and 0.44 mg/kg IV, and 0.44 mg/kg IM were used. Recovery times were dose-related and varied from 65 to 130 minutes for the intravenous doses. The intramuscular dose lasted 150 minutes until standing. Administration of 0.04 mg/kg of atropine IM reduced salivary secretions and cardiac changes observed with xylazine alone.

Pathak et al. (1982) have given ketamine (2.0 mg/kg, IV) alone and with chlorpromazine (2.0 mg/kg, IM) to buffalo calves. Pretreatment with chlorpromazine increased the duration of analgesia and recovery time. Short-term surgical procedures (5 to 10 minutes) could be performed in animals given the mixture.

Although there are no reports on inhalation general anesthesia in buffaloes, halothane or isoflurane should prove satisfactory if delivered via endotracheal catheter with a semiclosed circuit technique.

Intravenous retrograde regional anesthesia of the forelimb (see Chap. 16) in buffalo has been described by Manohar et al. (1971).

Use of guaifenesin (165 mg/kg, IV) in buffalo calves caused significant hypotension, plus other cardiovascular and respiratory effects deemed undesirable (Singh et al., 1981).

Chloral hydrate proved more satisfactory than hexobarbital or thiopental in buffaloes according to Gadzhiev (1955). It was administered intravenously at the rate of 0.13 to 0.18 g/kg.

For buffalo calves, Johari and Sharma (1962) used a mixture of chloral hydrate (30 g), magnesium sulfate (15 g), and thiopental (2.5 g) in 1000 ml of distilled water. Thirty minutes following subcutaneous administration of .05 to .20 gr of atropine, the mixture was given intravenously at approximately 0.9 ml/lb. Anesthesia is obtained for 15 to 25 minutes and may be prolonged by additional injections.

BISON

Bison are generally dangerous and difficult to handle, and mature animals require heavy equipment for restraint. Capture equipment is necessary to catch free-roaming animals.

Lasater et al. (1965) anesthetized bison *(Bison bison)* with chloral hydrate (250 mg/kg) to achieve deep surgical anesthesia. After anesthesia was induced, 0.02 mg/kg of succinylcholine intravenously produced approximately 12 minutes of muscle relaxation with apnea. The susceptibility to succinylcholine parallels the degree and duration of neuromuscular paralysis seen in cattle following comparable doses of succinylcholine. Tubocurarine chloride given intravenously at the rate of 0.03 mg/kg produced 20 minutes of relaxation and reduced respiratory movements without apnea.

Once bison are restrained, intravenous and inhalant agents may be used as in cattle.

RHINOCEROS

Several agents have been used successfully for immobilizing rhinoceros. Harthoorn and Player (1964) reported narcotizing a series of 18 white rhinoceros *(Ceratotherium simum simum)* with a mixture of morphine or diethylthiambutene plus chlorpromazine. The dose used was approximately 1.5 g of morphine, 175 mg scopolamine, and 725 mg chlorpromazine. Immobilization required 30 to 45 minutes for a 3500-lb animal. A variation of this mixture was the substitution of diethylthiambutene for morphine, the dose of the former for a 3000-lb animal being approximately 3.0 g. These mixtures have also been used successfully on black rhinoceros. Nalorphine can be used to reverse the action of either of the aforementioned narcotic agents.

Denney (1969) has immobilized black rhinoceros with combinations of etorphine and acepromazine, etorphine, acepromazine, and azaperone, or etorphine and azaperone (Table 18–35).

Hofmyer (1978) has used carfentanil in capture equipment on black rhinos. Doses ranged from 1.0 to 1.5 mg in juveniles to 2.5 to 3.0 mg in adults. Deep narcosis was obtained, which could be antagonized with diprenorphine or cyprenorphine

DeVos (1978) has also used carfentanil on this species (Table 18–36).

ELEPHANTS

Several agents have been used to immobilize and anesthetize elephants. Meperidine hydrochloride has been administered at the rate of 1 mg/lb of body weight to allow manipulation of a painful fracture (Counsilman, 1954). Repeated doses of pentobarbital have been given in the middle auricular vein of Indian elephants for treatment of convulsions due to poisoning (Anderson, 1968).

Gray (1969) has immobilized Ceylon elephants with etorphine and found the dose to be approximately twice that for the African elephant, Ceylon elephants requiring about 1 mg/1000 lb.

To sedate adult Asian elephants for air transport, Bongso (1980) used xylazine (100 to 175 mg of 10% solution). The animals remained standing in cages but were somnolent. Injections

TABLE 18–35. Drug Immobilization Data on 11 Black Rhinoceros in East Africa

Sex	Weight (kg) A-actual E-estimated	Doses of Drugs in mg (and μg/kg): Analgesic		Neuroleptic		Antidote		Elapsed Time (Min) from Injection to:				
		Etorphine	Fentanyl	Ace-promazine	Azaperone	Nalorphine	Route	Ataxia	Immob.	Down	Antidote	Up
Female	818 E	2.0 (2.44)		25.0 (30.56)		200.0 (244.50)	IM	7	10	15	118	126
Male	1185 A	2.0 (1.69)		20.0 (16.87)	250.0 (210.97)	200.0 (168.78)	IM	5	21	25	258	270
Male	1085 A		20.0* (18.43)	10.0 (9.27)	300.0 (276.50)			7				
		2.0† (1.84)		20.0 (18.43)		300.0 (276.50)	IM		5	7	63	81
Male	1196 A	2.0 (1.76)		25.0 (21.74)		300.0 (250.84)	IM	5	20	25	170	177
Male	955 E	2.0 (2.09)		25.0 (26.18)	200.0 (209.53)			8	13	18	Drowned in lake	
Male	1033 A	2.0 (1.93)		25.0 (24.20)	200.0 (193.61)	300.0 (290.42)	IM	7	—	42	74	77
Male	700 E	2.0 (2.86)		25.0 (35.71)	200.0 (285.71)	250.0 (357.14)	IM	5	—	12	66	79
Female	400 E	1.0 (2.50)		20.0 (25.00)	200.0 (250.00)	200.0 (250.00)	IM	7	10	12	46	55
Male	600 E	2.0 (3.33)			350.0 (583.33)	200.0 (333.33)	IM	7	—	13	60	65
Male	750 E	2.5 (3.33)			400.0 (533.33)	250.0 (333.33)	IM	4	7	9	51	63
Female	820 E	2.25 (2.74)			400.0 (487.80)	180.0 (219.51)	IM	5	6	10	65	77

*First syringe, little effect other than slight ataxia after 28 minutes.
†Second syringe.
(From Denney, R.N.: Black Rhinoceros Immobilization Utilizing a New Tranquillizing Agent. East Afr. Wildl. J., 7:159, 1969.)

TABLE 18–36. Recommended Optimal Dosage Regime of Carfentanil (R33799) and Additives for the Immobilization of 19 Free-Ranging Wild Animal Species

		Analgesic (Narcotic)		Additive				Analgesic Antagonist			
		Carfentanil		Xylazine		Azaperone		Naloxone		Cyprenophine	
	Adult Body Weight (kg)	Dosage Rate (μg per kg)	Total Dose* (mg)	Dosage Rate (μg per kg)	Total Dose* (mg)	Dosage Rate (μg per kg)	Total Dose* (mg)	Multi-plication Factor	Total Dose† (mg)	Multi-plication Factor	Total Dose† (mg)
African elephant	5000	1	5	—	—	—	—	6–10	40	10–12	50
Square-lipped rhinoceros	2000	1	2	—	—	100	200	6–10	16	10–12	20
Black rhinoceros	1000	1.5	1.5	—	—	150	150	8–10	10	10–12	12
Giraffe	1000	3(1.5)§	3(1.5)§	40	40	100	100	3–4	12	4–5	15
African buffalo	700	5	3.5	50	35	150	105	2–3	10	3–4	12.5
Eland	800	8	6.4	200	160	300	240	2–3	15	3–4	20
Roan antelope	250	10	2.5	100	25	300	75	2–3	7	3–4	10
Blue wildebeest	220	8	1.75	80	17.5	240	52.5	2–3	5	3–4	6
Black wildebeest	150	8	1.2	80	12	240	36	2–3	3.5	3–4	5
Red hartebeest	140	10	1.4	100	14	300	42	2–3	4	3–4	5
Tsessebe	140	10	1.4	100	14	300	42	2–3	4	3–4	5
Blesbok	90	10	0.9	100	9	300	27	2–3	2.5	3–4	3.5
Common waterbuck	240	10	2.4	100	24	300	72	2–3	7	3–4	8
Greater kudu	260	10	2.6	100	26	300	78	2–3	7	3–4	8
Gemsbok	180	10	1.8	100	18	300	54	2–3	5	3–4	7
Impala	50	7	0.35	100	5	300	15	3–4	1.4	4–5	1.7
Springbok	35	10	0.35	100	3.5	300	10.5	3–4	1.4	4–5	1.7
Steenbok	12	10	0.12	100	1.2	300	3.6	3–4	0.4	4–5	0.5
Warthog	80	12.5	1	100	8	300	24	3–4	4	4–5	5
Burchell's zebra‡											

*Analgesic or additive total dose = Analgesic rate x body weight.
†Analgesic antagonist total dose = Analgesic total dose x multiplication factor.
‡R33799 is not recommended for the zebra. Etorphine is recommended as the principal immobilizing agent.
§Figures in parentheses denote noncasting dosage levels for giraffe.
The dosages listed are for free-ranging wild animals. Wild animals adapted to captive conditions usually require lower dosages.
When a short induction period is required, the R33799 dosage rate can be drastically increased.
R33799 can be used without an additive. In cases of excitable species and warthog, a mixture or "cocktail" is recommended. Xylazine is preferred.
Although diprenorphine is not listed as an antagonist, it can be used with equal success in dosages slightly less than cited for cyprenorphine.
Nalorphine hydrobromide can also be used as an antagonist.

(From DeVos, V.: Immobilisation of Free-Ranging Wild Animals Using a New Drug. Vet. Rec., 103:64, 1978.)

TABLE 18–37. Optimum Dosage Rates of Etorphine and M-183 (in Mg/Kg) in Neuroleptanalgesic Mixtures for 16 Species of Wild-Hoofed Animals in South African National Parks

Species	Sex	Range Adult Body Weight in kg	Dosage Rates in μg/kg	
			Etorphine	M-183*
Elephant	M	5443–6804	1.03– 1.47	
	M	3175–5443	0.91– 1.89	
	F	3175–5443	0.91– 1.89	
Square-lipped rhinoceros	M	1361–2268	0.88– 2.2	
	M or F	1134–1814	0.82– 2.2	
Hippopotamus	M	1588–2041	2.45– 3.15	
	F	1361–1724	2.32– 2.93	
Giraffe	M & F	907–1361		2.94– 5.51
	Young M & F	272– 544		3.68– 7.35
Warthog	M & F	64– 100	10.00–23.44	
Zebra	M & F	249– 340	5.88– 8.03	5.88– 8.03
	Young M & F	113– 159	6.29– 8.85	6.29– 8.85
Impala	M & F	45– 75	5.55–11.11	5.55–11.11
Blue wildebeest	M & F	204– 295	6.77– 9.80	
	Young M & F	91– 204	4.90–10.99	
Red hartebeest	M	158– 204	4.90– 6.32	
	F	127– 172	4.36– 5.91	
Tsessebe	M & F	113– 158	4.75– 8.85	
Buffalo	M	590– 907	4.41–10.17	
	F	454– 680	4.41– 8.81	
Waterbuck	M	215– 272	11.02–16.28	
	F	158– 227	8.81–15.82	
Kudu	M	249– 295	13.56–16.06	
	F	127– 181	13.81–23.62	
Eland	M	544– 907	5.51–11.03	
	F	227– 386	10.36–17.62	
Sable antelope	M & F	204– 249	8.03– 9.80	8.03– 9.80
Roan antelope	M & F	204– 272+	7.35–14.71	7.35–14.71

*M-183 is the acetyl ether of etorphine (M-99) and is not commercially available.

(From Pienaar, U.D., Van Niekerk, J.W., Young, E., and Van Wyk, P.: Neuroleptic Narcosis of Large Wild Herbivores in South African National Parks with the New Potent Morphine Analogues M-99 and M-183. J. S. Afr. Vet. Med., 37:277, 1966.)

were repeated at the same dose rate at approximately three-hour intervals.

Bongso and Perera (1978) have used a commercial mixture of etorphine-acepromazine (2.45 mg/ml of etorphine and 10 mg/ml of acepromazine—see Chap. 8) in control of adult male Asian elephants. The dose was 1 ml/4 ft of shoulder height and was given via capture equipment. The mixture was believed to be more effective than etorphine alone.

The dose of etorphine for the African elephant varies from 4 to 8 mg or an effective dose of 0.67 mg/1000 lb. A resuscitating dose of cyprenorphine for an elephant is about 60 mg (Harthoorn, 1967).

Wallach and Anderson (1968) have reported the use of etorphine in 21 African elephants *(Loxodanta africana africana)*. Six elephants ranging from 6,000 to 13,000 lbs were given etorphine at the rate of 4 to 6 mg. All were

TABLE 18–38. Dosage Rates of Drugs Used for Neuroleptic Narcosis in Species of Hoofed

Species	No. of Successful Cases	Mortality	Sex	Range Adult Body Weight (lbs)	Neuroleptic (Major Tranquilizer) Phencyclidine (mg)	Fluanisone† (mg)
Elephant (*Loxodonia africana africana*)	34	2	M M F	12,000–15,000 7,000–12,000 7,000–12,000		
Square-lipped Rhinoceros (*Ceratotherium simum simum*)	3	1	M M & F	3,000– 5,000 2,500– 4,000		
Hippopotamus (*Hippopotamus amphibius capensis*) (on land)	2	1	M F	3,500– 4,500 3,000– 3,800		
Giraffe (*Giraffa camelopardalis giraffa*)	73	8	M & F M & F	2,00– 3,000 Young 600– 1,200		
Warthog (*Phacochoerus aethiopicus sundevalli*)	2	—	M & F	140–220		10
Zebra (*Equus burchelli antiquorum*)	106	7	M & F M & F	550–750 Young 250–350		20 10
Impala (*Aepyceros melampus melampus*)	47	2	M & F	100–165		
Blue wildebeest (*Connochaetes (Gorgon) taurinus taurinus*)	124	8	M & F M & F	450–650 Young 200–450		20 (or 10 + 10 Ac. prom.§) 10
Red hartebeest (*Acelaphus buselaphus caama*)	5	—	M F	350–450 280–380		10 10
Tsessebe (*Damaliscus lunatus lunatus*)	1	—	M & F	250–350		10 (or 5 + 5 Ac. prom.)
Buffalo (*Syncerus caffer caffer*)	19	—	M F	1,300–2,000 1,000–1,500		40 (or 30 + 20 Ac. prom.) 30 (or 20 + 15 Ac. pr.)
Waterbuck (*Kobus ellipsiprymnus ellipsiprymnus*)	5	—	M F	475–600 350–500		Preferable to Ac. prom. alone. *20 + 10 Ac. prom. *20 + 10 Ac. prom.
Kudu (*Trogelaphus strepsiceros strepsiceros*)	13	1	M F	550–650 280–400	75–100 50	Alternative to Sernylan‖ *50 *40
Eland (*Taurotragus oryx oryx*)	2	—	M F	1,200–2,000 500–850	100–150 75–100	Alternative to Sernylan. 50–60 *50
Sable antelope (*Hippotragus niger niger*)	2	1	M & F	450–550		*20 (or 10) + 20 Trifluopromazine
Roan antelope (*Hippotragus equinus equinus*)	1	—	M & F	450–600 +		*20–30 (or 15 + 20 Trifluopromazine)

*The dosages marked with an * are subject to further confirmation.
†Fluanisone (R2028) is a neuroleptic of the butyrophenone series.
‡M-183 is the acetyl ether of etorphine (M-99) and is not commercially available.
§Ac. prom. = acepromazine
‖Sernylan (phencyclidine) is not available commercially.

(From Pienaar, U.D., Van Niekerk, J.W., Young, E., and Van Wyk, P.: Neuroleptic Narcosis of Large Wild Herbivores in South African National Parks with the New Potent Morphine Analogues M-99 and M-183. J.S. Afr. Vet. Med., 37:277, 1966.)

Wild Animals in South African National Parks

Dosages (total average dose for adult animals)

Ataractic (Tranquilizer)			*Narcotic*		*Parasympatholytic*	*Morphine Antagonist*	
Acepromazine (mg)	*Trifluopromazine (mg)*	*Chlorpromazine (mg)*	*Etorphine (mg)*	*M-183‡ (mg)*	*Hyoscine Hydrobr. (mg)*	*Cyprenorphine (mg)*	*Nalorphine Hydrobr. (mg)*
50–60 40–60 40–50			7–8 5–6 5–6			60 40 40	1500–4000 (Not recommended)
40 (optional) 40 (optional)			2–3 1.5–2.5		100 (optional) 75 (optional)		250–500 250–500
40 (optional) 40 (optional)			5 4		100 (optional) 100 optional)		250–500 250–500
40 20				4–5 2	100 50		250–500 100–200
20			1.0–1.5		5–10		50–100
Alternative to Fluanisone 20 10			2 1	Alternative 2 1	20 20	5	100 50–100
5			0.25–0.5	Alternative 0.25–0.5	5		10 (immediately) +40
20			2 1		20 (optional) 10 (optional)		100 50–100
15 10			1.0 0.75		10 (optional) 10 (optional)		100 75–100
10			0.75–1.0		10 (optional)		100
20 20			4–6 3–4		75–100 (optional) 50–100 (optional)		200–400 200
20 20 Not recommended			*3.0–3.5 *2.0–2.5		20–30 (optional) 20–30 (optional)		200 100–200
Not recommended	50 50	Alternative to trifluopromazine. 1.5–2.0 mg/lb body weight	4 2.5–3		50 (optional) 30 (optional)		200 100–200
Not recommended	50–100 50		5–6 4		100 (optional) 50 (optional)		200–400 200
Not recommended	20–30		2	Alternative 2	20 (optional)		200
Not recommended	20–30		2–3	Alternative 2–3	20 (optional)		200–300

immobilized and went down in sternal or lateral recumbency. The latter is preferred because sternal recumbency places great pressure on the diaphragm. One 8500-lb animal given 4 mg was immobilized in the standing position. Seven elephants were given etorphine plus acepromazine. Five were given etorphine plus scopolamine, and three were given a mixture of all three drugs.

Etorphine alone immobilizes adult African elephants satisfactorily with a dose of 6 mg in elephants ranging from 4,000 to 15,000 lbs. The addition of acepromazine (25 to 50 mg) prolongs the tranquil state. The inclusion of scopolamine is deemed of little value. When the three drugs are combined, a prolonged state of depression occurs.

For inhalation anesthesia, halothane-N_2O via a mask over the trunk, following suitable preanesthetic medication, is suggested. Because of the animal's enormous size, high flows from a 10% halothane vaporizer should be used.

Data on immobilization of elephants and many other species with several agents are shown in Tables 18–37, 18–38, 18–39, and 18–40.

SEALS AND SEA LIONS

A restraining cage designed for pinnipeds has been described by Ridgway and Simpson (1969) (Fig. 18–24).

Phenothiazine-derived tranquilizers are ineffective or fatal to seals and sea lions (Hubbard and Poulter, 1968). Chlordiazepoxide produces a true ataractic effect in the California sea lion but has no effect on harbor seals. Diazepam produces an ataractic effect on harbor seals but has no effect on California sea lions.

For spaying Northern fur seals, propriopromazine (4 mg/kg) followed in 30 minutes with ketamine (11 mg/kg) intramuscularly has been found satisfactory (Keyes, 1971). Geraci (1973) has used 4.5 to 11.0 mg/kg of ketamine in ringed seals and sea lions. Atropine (0.3 to 0.6 mg) was given concurrently to some to prevent salivation. Animals with respiratory problems should not be given ketamine. Geraci et al. (1981) immobilized phocid seals repeatedly with a combination of ketamine (1.5 mg/kg) and diazepam (0.05 mg/kg) IM or IV. They preferred the combination over ketamine alone, because induction and recovery were smoother. Weddell seals have been sedated with intramuscular ketamine (2 mg/kg) followed by administration of halothane (Hochachka et al., 1977).

Ling et al. (1967) found that 2.5 mg/kg of succinylcholine was effective in immobilizing Southern elephant seals *(Mirounga leonina)*. These seals are generally so lethargic that they can be injected at close range with a pole syringe. Needles up to 4 inches × 14 gauge are necessary to penetrate the skin and underlying blubber.

For intravenous injections, sea lions are best restrained in a squeeze-cage to allow access to a protruding flipper (Eiseman et al., 1965). A vein on the ventral aspect of the flipper, approximately 3 cm anterior to its posterior edge, can be used for intravenous administration. Thiamylal can be given at the rate of 1 mg/lb to produce anesthesia. It should be given rapidly to minimize struggling and to produce relaxation. Methoxyflurane can be administered by means of a face mask. Sea lions may hold their breath for as much as 5 minutes. When they do breathe, their air intake is enormous and rapid. For this reason, the respiratory pattern is not an accurate gauge of the depth of anesthesia. Once the sea lion is anesthetized, it is relatively easy to insert an endotracheal catheter for administration of anesthetic or oxygen.

Ridgway and Simpson (1969) have used halothane given by means of a mask as the principal agent for sea lions. About $\frac{1}{60}$ gr of atropine is given to a 50-kg sea lion subcutaneously with the animal strapped to a restraining board. Once the animal is induced, the trachea is intubated for further halothane administration. Concentrations of 0.75 to 1.5% are administered for prolonged anesthesia. Recovery from halothane alone is rapid.

PORPOISES

Porpoises breathe through a modified nasal orifice, called the blowhole, located on the dor-

TABLE 18–39. Data on Immobilization of African Animals with a Projectile Syringe

Species	*Drug*	*Dose*	*Mortality**	*Remarks*
Kob antelope *(Adenota kob thomasi)*	Succinylcholine chloride	Approx. 0.15 mg/lb in adult males	Approx. 10%	Add 5 mg atropine per 100 lb if pregnant
Hartebeest *(Alcelaphus lelwel jacksonii)*	Succinylcholine chloride		None	
	Gallamine triethiodide		None	Slower reaction than succinylcholine
Waterbuck *(Kobus defassa ugandae)*	Succinylcholine chloride		None	
	Gallamine triethiodide		None	Slower reaction than succinylcholine
Hippopotamus *(Hippopotamus amphibius)*	Succinylcholine chloride	0.08 mg/lb	2/23	Avoid immobilizing in water, if possible, since animal may drown
	Gallamine triethiodide	1.8 mg/lb	0/2	May be safer than succinylcholine
Buffalo *(Syncerus caffer)*	Gallamine triethiodide	1.2–1.3 mg/lb	0/6	Average time to go down was 11 minutes
	d-tubocurarine		1/4	Add atropine to solution
Giraffe *(Giraffa camelopardalis)*	Gallamine triethiodide	1.7 mg/lb	0/8	Wide variation in time required to go down
Rhinoceros *(Diceros bicornis)*	Gallamine triethiodide	0.8–0.9 mg/lb	2/10	Animals run long distances before going down
Elephant *(Loxodonta africana)*	Gallamine triethiodide	1.2 mg/lb	1/7	Appears quite effective

*Fractions indicate number of deaths/number injected. Neostigmine methylsulphate was generally used as an antidote. (From Harthoorn, A.M., and Lock, J.A.: Advances in the Use of Muscle Relaxing Drugs for Immobilization and Handling of Larger Land Mammals. J. Small Anim. Pract., 2:163, 1961; Buechner, H.K., Harthoorn, A.M., and Lock, J.A.: Immobilizing Uganda Kob with Succinylcholine Chloride. Can. J. Comp. Med., 24:317, 1960.)

TABLE 18–40. Chemical Restraint of Large, Feral Animals Kept in Captivity

Family Groups	*Suggested Drugs and Dosage*	*Comments on Other Drugs*	*Other Comments*
Kangaroos and wallabies	Etorphine—0.1 mg per 20 lb body wt.	Phenothiazine-derivative tranquilizers are not effective for restraint.	
	Etorphine—1 mg per 200 lb	Succinylcholine is effective, but hazardous.	
Elephants	Etorphine—1 mg per 2000 lb body wt. given intramuscularly		If this dosage is ineffective, further attempts for restraint should not be made for 24 hours; then the dosage can be increased by half the original dosage.
Zebras and other wild equines	Etorphine—1 mg per 200 lb body wt. Can be mixed with acepromazine—2 mg per 100 lb body wt.	Phenothiazine tranquilizers are ineffective as sole restraint agents.	Care must be exercised not to cause severe exertion and excitement in these animals. A tie-up syndrome has been seen in sedentary individuals that were exerted.
Camels and llamas	Etorphine—2 mg per 500 lb body wt.		Emprosthotonic reflexes have occurred.
Tapir	Etorphine—1 mg per 100 lb body wt.		
Elk and large deer	Etorphine—1 mg per 100 lb body wt.		This drug is not very effective in small deer.
Giraffes	Etorphine—3 mg per 400 lb body wt.		Etorphine has variable effect on giraffes. A relatively high dosage is suggested because of the effectiveness of the antagonist, cyprenorphine.
American bison	Etorphine—1 mg per 200 lb body wt.		Great care must be taken with herds because of their tendency to charge a single downed animal and human handlers.

(From Sedgwick, C.J., and Acosta, A.L.: Capture Drugs. Mod. Vet. Pract., 50:32, 1969.)

sum of the head just anterior to the cranial vault. It appears on the surface as a single, transversely crescentic opening with a forward-facing concavity. It is closed by a muscular nasal plug and opens through the action of forehead muscles. Normally, it remains closed. Ventral to the blowhole are vestibular and tubular air sacs connected to the paired nares, which begin a few centimeters down the respiratory passage. A septum divides the nares for 10 to 12 cm, after which the respiratory passage becomes single again just above the glottis. The larynx forms an arytenoepiglottal tube giving a direct opening from the internal nares to the lungs, thus allowing the animal to breathe only through the blowhole (Fig. 18–25).

Approximately 10 cm from the base of the larynx the trachea gives off a separate right bronchus, and at about 15 cm it bifurcates into two main bronchi. It is important, when the animal is intubated, that the endotracheal tube extend only about 20 cm past the proximal tip of the glottis so that all of the lungs will be ventilated.

Porpoises can take one full respiration in 0.3 seconds. With a tidal volume of 5 to 10 L, the flow rates through the air passages range from 30 to 70 L/second during expiration and inspiration. Porpoises breathe 2 to 3 times each minute. Each breath is deep (approximately 80% tidal air). After inspiration, the animal holds an apneustic plateau for 20 to 30 seconds followed by rapid exhalation.

The central nervous control of respiration in the porpoise is not fully understood.

To produce a calming effect, paraldehyde in

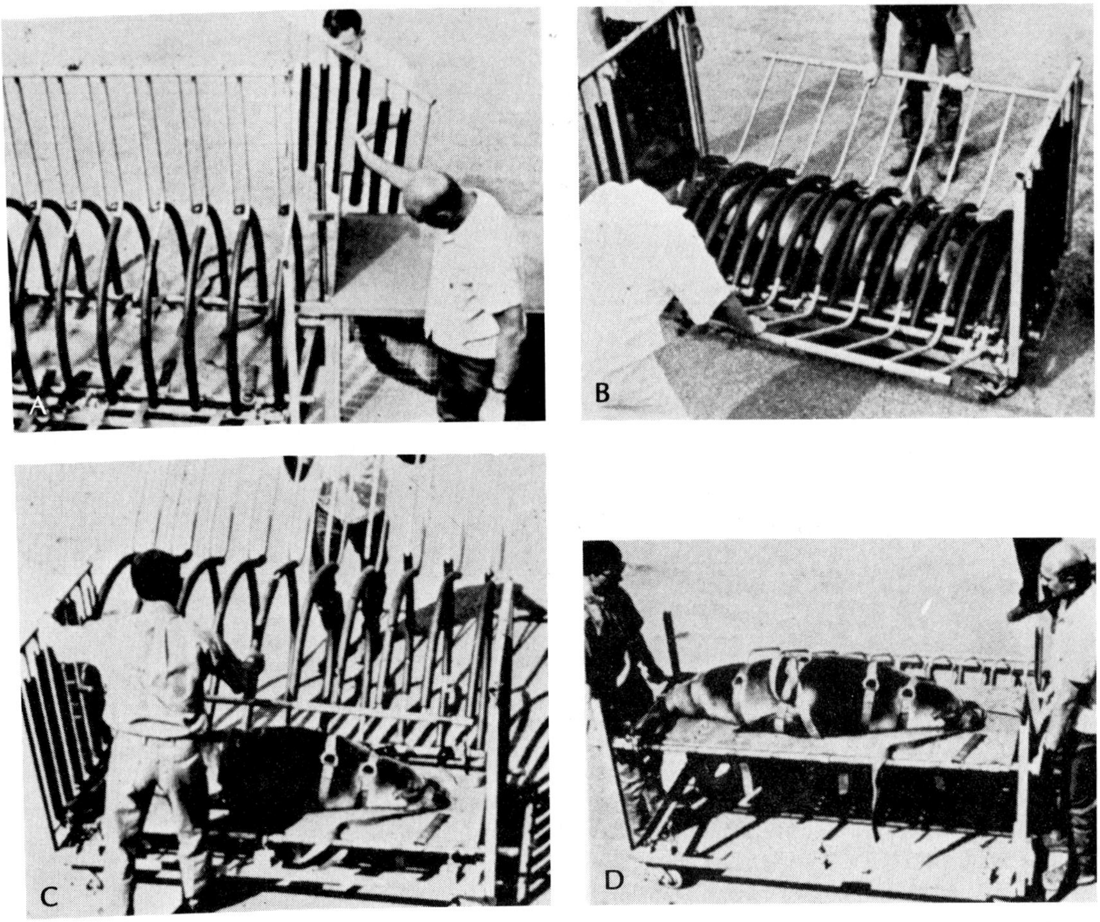

Figure 18–24. *A*, Sea lion being driven from transport cage to restraining cage. *B*, The animal is completely restrained by the cage bars. *C*, The side bars and end of the cage are removed. *D*, The animal, securely restrained on the bottom of the cage, may be carried to an examining or operating room. Slots in the cage bottom allow adaptation for animals of various sizes. (From Ridgway, S.H., and Simpson, J.G.: Anesthesia and Restraint of the California Sea Lion, *Zalophus californianus*. J.A.V.M.A., 155:1059, 1969.)

fish can be administered orally to porpoises (McBride and Kritzler, 1951).

Thiopental-halothane anesthesia in the porpoise has been described by Ridgway and McCormick (1967). The awake porpoise can be intubated; however, intubation is facilitated by injection of 10 mg/kg of thiopental into one of the tail fluke veins.

A 24- to 30-mm modified equine endotracheal tube with inflatable cuff is used. The mouth is held open with towels by assistants. The hand inserted into the pharynx grasps the larynx, pulls it from its intranarial position and, with two fingers inserted into the glottis, guides the tube in along the palm of the hand. In *Delphinus delphis* and *Stenella styx*, Rieu and Gautheron (1968) have described a method of introducing the tube through the blowhole.

For induction without thiopental, 3.5% halothane is administered for 5 to 15 minutes, after which 0.75 to 1.0% is used to maintain surgical anesthesia. If thiopental is used for intubation, 2.0% halothane is sufficient followed by 0.75 to 1.0%. Loss of swimming movements of the tail flukes indicates surgical anesthesia and occurs after loss of strong corneal and eyelid reflexes. The swimming reflex is considered the best criterion for assessing the depth of anesthesia.

During the recovery period, the animal is

1. *Blowhole*
2. *Cranium*
3. *Cerebral hemisphere*
4. *Cerebellum*
5. *Bony nares*
6. *Nasal cavity*
7. *Glottis*
8. *Nasopharyngeal sphincter*
9. *Esophagus*
10. *Arytenoid cartilage*
11. *Cricoid cartilage*
12. *Trachea*
13. *Eparterial bronchus*
14. *Tracheal cartilages*
15. *Thyroid cartilage*
16. *Epiglottic cartilage*
17. *Hyoid bone*
18. *Tongue*
19. *Oral cavity*
20. *Palate*
21. *Oropharyngeal sphincter*

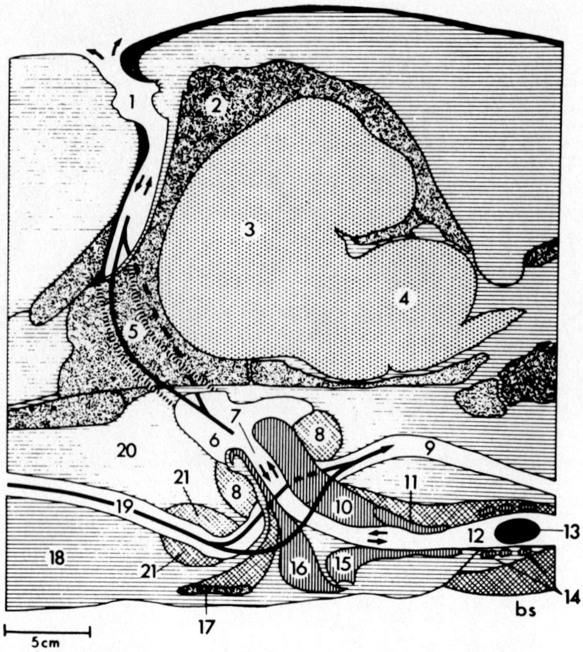

Figure 18–25. Sagittal view of the head and neck of the bottlenose dolphin. (From Nagel, E.L., Morgane, P.J., and McFarland, W.L.: Anesthesia for the Bottlenose Dolphin. Vet. Med./Small Anim. Clin. 61:230, 1966.)

placed on 60% ambient air and 40% oxygen, and the endotracheal catheter is kept in position until the blowhole reflex returns. This requires 15 to 45 minutes following cessation of anesthetic administration. Anesthesia with halothane has been maintained for periods up to 21 hours.

The heart rate under anesthesia is generally 100 to 120/minute. Arterial pH averages 7.35, Po_2 is maintained at 100 to 200 mm Hg, and Pco_2 is 35 to 50 mm Hg. In unanesthetized animals, arterial Po_2 is 65 to 98 mm, and Pco_2 is 40 to 60 mm.

Thiopental (10 mg/kg) produces 10 to 15 minutes of light anesthesia and 45 minutes of respiratory paralysis during which the animal must be artificially ventilated. A dose of 15 to 25 mg/kg produces surgical anesthesia for 10 to 25 minutes, with respiratory paralysis lasting 1 to 2½ hours.

Lilly (1961) gave pentobarbital intraperitoneally to 5 *Tursiops truncatus* in doses from 10 mg/kg to 30 mg/kg. All died, apparently from respiratory failure.

Bird (1964) developed an apneustic plateau control unit for use with the Bird Mark 9 respirator. This unit, which was designed to imitate the natural respiration of the porpoise, inflates the lungs rapidly, holds an apneustic plateau for a variable period, and then deflates the lungs.

Nagel et al. (1964) found that plasma cholinesterase is not present in *Tursiops truncatus*. Injection of 1 mg/kg of succinylcholine produces muscle relaxation of 30 to 60 minutes duration.

Reflexes that may be observed for depth of anesthesia in the porpoise include: 1) contraction of the eyelid on tapping the inner canthus of the eye, 2) contraction of the eye muscles when the cornea is touched, 3) contraction of the throat muscles when the hand is inserted into the pharnyx, 4) retraction of the tongue on being pulled, 5) reflex movements of the body when the anus is distended, 6) tail movements, 7) movements of the pectoral flippers in response to scratch or pinprick of the chest or axillary region, 8) movement of the blowhole on insertion of the finger into the nares or vestibular sacs, and 9) vaginal or penile movements when the vagina or prepuce is distended by insertion of the fingers or instruments.

Timing of removal of the endotracheal tube is critical. The correct time is when the animal is completely capable of breathing on its own, as manifested by movements of the blowhole and thorax, and by struggling and "bucking." At this time, the endotracheal tube is removed, and the larynx is placed into its normal intranarial position. If the animal does not blow within 3 minutes or if the heart rate falls below 60, the tube must be reinserted and the animal ventilated for a few more minutes.

Porpoises in water are near neutral in buoyancy. Out of water, there are abnormal stresses that must be overcome in breathing and maintaining circulation. For this reason, the animal should be returned to water as soon as possible.

REFERENCES

Addison, E.M., and Kolenosky, G.B.: Use of Ketamine Hydrochloride and Xylazine Hydrochloride to Immobilize Black Bears *(Ursus americanus)*. J. Wildl. Dis., 15:253, 1979.

Allam, M.W., and Churchill, E.A.: Pentobarbital Sodium Anesthesia in Swine and Goats. J.A.V.M.A., 109:355, 1946.

Anderson, I.L.: Tutu Poisoning in Two Circus Elephants. N.Z. Vet. J., 16:146, 1968.

Anderson, J.C.: A Simple Method of Anesthesia in the Fowl. Vet. Rec., 81:130, 1967.

Anderson, J.M., and Benirschke, K.: The Armadillo in Experimental Biology. Lab. Anim. Care, 16:202, 1966.

Anonymous: Dr. Bob Knowles Operates on Giant Fish and Makes News Headlines and T.V. Mod. Vet. Pract., 39:17, 1958.

Aronson, H.B., Robin, G.C., Weinberg, H., and Nathan, H.: Some Observations on General Anesthesia in the Baboon. Anesth. Analg., 44:289, 1965.

Austin, D.H., and Peoples, J.H.: Capturing Hogs with Alpha Chloralose. Proc. 21st Ann. Conf., Southeast Assoc. Game and Fish Comm., New Orleans, Louisiana, 1967.

Bacher, J.D., Potkay, S., and Baas, J.E.: An Evaluation of Sedatives and Anesthetics in the Agouti *(Dasyprocta sp.)*. Lab. Anim. Sci., 26:195, 1976.

Balser, D.S.: Tranquilizer Tabs for Capturing Wild Carnivores. J. Wildl. Man., 29:438, 1965.

Barry, J.A.: Removal of Scent Glands in Skunk. M. S. U. Vet., 19:77, 1958.

Beale, D.M., and Smith, A.D.: Immobilization of Pronghorn Antelopes with Succinylcholine Chloride. J. Wildl. Man., 31:840, 1967.

Bennett, R.R.: Methoxyflurane Anesthesia in the Sub-Human Primate. Pract. Vet., 41:20, 1969.

Bennett, R.R.: The Use of Metofane in Experimental Laboratory Birds. Pract. Vet., 6:184, 1968.

Benson, G.J., and Thurmon, J.C.: Anesthesia of Swine Under Field Conditions. J.A.V.M.A., 174:594, 1979.

Bergerud, A.T., Butt, A., Russel, H.L., and Whalen, H.: Immobilization of Newfoundland Caribou and Moose with Succinylcholine Chloride and Cap-Chur Equipment. J. Wildl. Man., 28:49, 1964.

Betz, T.W.: Surgical Anesthesia in Reptiles, with Special Reference to the Water Snake, *Natrix rhombifera*. Copeia, 2:284, 1962.

Bieter, R.N., Harvey, A.M., and Burgess, W.W.: Spinal Anesthesia in Summer Frogs. J. Pharmacol. Exp. Ther., 45:291, 1932.

Bird, F.M.: Personal communication. Palm Springs, California, 1964.

Blume, W., and Sroka, K.: Comparative Studies on the Action of Paraldehyde and Methaldehyde on Frogs, Fishes and Leeches. Arch. Exp. Pathol. Pharmacol., 202:1, 1943.

Boever, W.J., and Wright, W.: Use of Ketamine for Restraint and Anesthesia of Birds. Vet. Med., 70:86, 1975.

Bongso, T.A.: Use of Xylazine for the Transport of Elephants by Air. Vet. Rec., 107:492, 1980.

Bongso, T.A., and Perera, B.M.A.O.: Observations on the Use of Etorphine Alone and in Combination with Acepromazine Maleate for Immobilisation of Aggressive Asian Elephants *(Elephas maximus)*. Vet. Rec., 102:339, 1978.

Booth, N.H.: Personal Communication. Colorado State University, Fort Collins, 1963.

Booth, N.H., Bredeck, H.E., and Herin, R.A.: Baroceptor Reflex Mechanisms in Swine. Am. J. Physiol., 199:1189, 1960.

Boothe, H.W.: Diseases of the Chinchilla. Proc., A.V.M.A., 19th Annual Meeting, 1953.

Boyd, R.J.: Succinylcholine Chloride for Immobilization of Colorado Mule Deer. J. Wildl. Man., 26:332, 1962.

Bree, M.M., Cohen, B.J., and Abrams, G.D.: Injection Lesions Following Intramuscular Administration of Chlorpromazine in Rabbits. J.A.V.M.A., 159:1598, 1971.

Breese, C.E., and Dodman, N.H.: Xylazine-Ketamine-Oxymorphone: An Injectable Anesthetic Combination in Swine. J.A.V.M.A., 184:182, 1984.

Brisbin, I.L.: Reactions of the American Alligator to Several Immobilizing Drugs. Copeia, 1:129, 1966.

Buechner, H.K., Harthoorn, A.M., and Lock, J.A.: Control of African Wild Animals. Nature, 185:47, 1960.

Burke, T.J., and Wall, B.E.: Anesthetic Deaths in Cobras *(Naja naja* and *Ophiagus hannah)*. J.A.V.M.A., 157:620, 1970.

Bush, M., Custer, R., Smeller, J., and Bush, L.M.: Physiologic Measures of Nonhuman Primates During Physical Restraint and Chemical Immobilization. J.A.V.M.A., 171:866, 1977.

Bush, M., Ensley, P.K., Mehren, K., and Rapley, W.: Immobilization of Giraffes with Xylazine and Etorphine Hydrochloride. J.A.V.M.A., 169:884, 1976.

Calderwood, H.W.: Anesthesia for Reptiles. J.A.V.M.A., 159:1618, 1971.

Cambridge, G.W.: Anaesthetic Procedures Suitable for the Coypu. J. Physiol. Proc., 162:48P, 1962.

Carle, B.N., and Dewhirst, W.H., Jr.: A Method for Bleeding Swine. J.A.V.M.A., 101:495, 1942.

Casteel, D.A., and Edwards, W.R.: Surgical Anesthesia for Cottontails. J. Wildl. Man., 29:196, 1965.

Chalmers, G.A., and Barrett, M.W.: Capture Myopathy in

Pronghorns in Alberta, Canada. J.A.V.M.A., 171:918, 1977.

Cheney, D.H., Slogoff, S., and Allen, G.W.: Ketamine-Induced Stress Ulcers in the Rat. Anesthesiology, 40:531, 1974.

Chimoskey, J.E., Huntsman, L.L., Gams, E., and Flanagan, W.J.: Effect of Ketamine on Ventricular Dynamics of Unanesthetized Baboons. Cardiovasc. Res. Cent. Bull., 14:53, 1975.

Church, J.C.T., and Noronha, R.F.X.: The Use of the Fruit Bat in Surgical Research. E. Afr. Med. J., 42:348, 1965.

Cisar, C.F.: The Rat Kangaroo *(Potorous tridactylus)*. Handling and Husbandry Practices in a Research Facility. Lab. Anim. Care., 19:55, 1969.

Clark, G.C., Kesterson, J.W., Coombs, D.W., Cherry, C.P., Prentice, D.E., and Kohn, F.E.: Comparative Effects of Repeated and Prolonged Inhalation Exposure of Beagle Dogs and Cynomolgus Monkeys to Anaesthetic and Subanaesthetic Concentrations of Enflurane and Halothane. Anaesth. Scand. (Suppl.), 71:1, 1979.

Clarke, N.P., Huheey, M.J., and Martin, W.M.: Pentobarbital Anesthesia in Bears. J.A.V.M.A., 143:47, 1963.

Clayton, F.W., Bauman, T.E., and Kintner, L.D.: Successful Use of Intrathoracic Anesthesia in Wild Raccoons. Vet. Med./Small Anim. Clin., 61:44, 1966.

Clifford, D.H.: Observations on Effect of Preanesthetic Medication with Meperidine and Promazine on Barbiturate Anesthesia in an Ocelot and a Leopard. J.A.V.M.A., 133:459, 1958.

Clifford, D.H., Stowe, C.M., Jr., and Good, A.L.: Pentobarbital Anesthesia in Lions with Special Reference to Preanesthetic Medication. J.A.V.M.A., 139:111, 1961.

Cooper, J.E.: *Anesthesia and Surgery in Reptiles*. Cotswold Herpetological Soc. 2nd Symp., Cocklands Press, Burford, England, 1976, p. 16.

Cooper, J.E.: Ketamine Hydrochloride as an Anaesthetic for East African Reptiles. Vet. Rec., 95:37, 1974*a*.

Cooper, J.E.: Metomidate Anaesthesia of Some Birds of Prey for Laparotomy and Sexing. Vet. Rec., 94:437, 1974*b*.

Copenhaver, W.M.: Initiation of Beat and Intrinsic Contraction Rates in the Different Parts of the Ambystoma Heart. J. Exp. Zool., 80:193, 1939.

Counsilman, J.W.: Demerol Hydrochloride as an Anaesthetic for an Elephant. N. Am. Vet., 35:835, 1954.

Cousins, M.J., Mazze, R.I., Barr, G.A., and Kosek, J.C.: A Comparison of the Renal Effects of Isoflurane and Methoxyflurane in Fischer 344 Rats. Anesthesiology, 38:55, 1973.

Creed, J.E., and Kainer, R.A.: Surgical Extirpation and Related Anatomy of Anal Sacs of the Ferret. J.A.V.M.A., 179:575, 1981.

Crider, E.D., and McDaniel, J.C.: Alpha-Chloralose Used to Capture Canada Geese. J. Wildl. Man., 31:258, 1967.

Croft, P.G.: *An Introduction to the Anaesthesia of Laboratory Animals*. The Universities Federation for Animal Welfare, London, 1960.

Custer, R., Kramer, L., Kennedy, S., and Bush, M.: Hematologic Effects of Xylazine When Used for Restraint of Bactrian Camels. J.A.V.M.A., 171:899, 1977.

Davis, R.W.: Personal Communication. Colorado State University, Fort Collins, 1963.

Day, P.W.: Anesthetic Techniques for the Chimpanzee. In *Experimental Animal Anesthesiology*. Edited by D.C. Sawyer. U.S.A.F. School of Aerospace Medicine, Brooks Air Force Base, Texas, 1965.

Denney, R.N.: Black Rhinoceros Immobilization Utilizing a New Tranquillizing Agent. E. Afr. Wildl. J., 7:159, 1969.

Denson, D.D., Bridenbaugh, P.O., Phero, J.C., Raj, P.P., Turner, P.A., and Ohlweiler, D.F.: Evaluation of Lidocaine Spinal Anesthesia in the Rhesus Monkey. Anesth. Analg., 60:756, 1981.

Desmedt, J.E., and Delwaide, P.J.: Physiological Experimentation on the Pigeon. Lab. Anim. Care, 16:191, 1966.

DeVos, V.: Immobilisation of Free-Ranging Wild Animals Using a New Drug. Vet. Rec., 103:64, 1978.

Dhindsa, D.S., Hoversland, A.S., and Kluempke, R.: Halothane Semiclosed-Circuit Anesthesia in Pygmy and Large Goats. Am. J. Vet. Res., 31:1897, 1970.

Dilebone, R.P.: Thiamylal Anesthesia in a Penguin. J.A.V.M.A., 147:1076, 1965.

Dodge, A.B.: Personal Communication. Fort Collins, Colorado., 1963.

Dolowy, W.C., Mombelloni, P., and Hesse, A.L.: Chlorpromazine Premedication with Pentobarbital Anesthesia in a Mouse. Am. J. Vet. Res., 21:156, 1960.

Eiseman, B., Dilbone, R., and Slater, A.B.: Devocalizing Sea Lions. J.A.V.M.A., 147:1086, 1965.

Ensley, P.K.: Electrosurgical Excision of a Mass in the Cloacal Region of a Male Galapagos Tortoise. J.A.V.M.A., 179:1289, 1981.

Eschmeyer, P.H.: The Effect of Ether Anesthesia on Fin-Clipping Rate. Progressive Fish Culturist, 15:80, 1953.

Fankhauser, G.: The Effects of Changes in Chromosome Number on Amphibian Development. Q. Rev. Biol., 20:20, 1945.

Farrell, R.K.: Personal Communication. Washington State University, Pullman, 1963.

Fedde, M.R.: Drugs Used for Avian Anesthesia: A Review. Poult. Sci., 57:1376, 1978.

Feldman, D.B., and Self, J.L.: Sedation and Anesthesia of the Virginia Opossum. Lab. Anim. Sci., 21:717, 1971.

Ferguson, B.R.: Personal Communication. Denver, Colorado, 1961.

Ferguson, J.W.: Anaesthesia in the Hamster Using a Combination of Methohexitone and Diazepam. Lab. Anim., 13:305, 1979.

Field, E.J.: Anaesthesia in Rabbits. J. Anim. Tech. Assoc., 8:47, 1957.

Fish, F.F.: The Anaesthesia of Fish by High Carbon Dioxide Concentrations. Trans. Am. Fisheries Soc., 72:25, 1942.

Flook, D.R., Robertson, J.R., Hermanrude, O.R., and Buechner, H.K.: Succinylcholine Chloride for Immobilization of North American Elk. J. Wildl. Man., 26:334, 1962.

Florsheim, W.H.: Personal Communication. Veterans Administration Hospital, Long Beach, California, 1968.

Foley, D.M., Stewart, J.E., and Holley, R.A.: Isobutyl Alcohol and Methyl Pentynol as General Anesthetics for the Lobster, *Homarus americanus* Milne-Edwards. Can. J. Zool., 44:141, 1966.

Fowler, M.E.: Extracting Canine Teeth of a Bear. J.A.V.M.A., 137:60, 1960.
Fowler, M.E.: *Restraint and Handling of Wild and Domestic Animals*. Iowa State Univ. Press, Ames, 1978*a*.
Fowler, M.E.: *Zoo and Wild Animal Medicine*. W.B. Saunders Co., Philadelphia, 1978*b*.
Fowler, S.L., Brown, J.S., and Flower, E.W.: Comparison between Ether and Carbon Dioxide Anaesthesia for Removal of Blood Samples from Rats. Lab. Anim., 14:275, 1980.
Friedberg, K.M.: Anesthesia of Parakeets and Canaries. J.A.V.M.A., 141:1157, 1962.
Friedberg, K.M.: Problems Encountered in Pet Bird Practice. Vet. Med., 56:157, 1961.
Gadzhiev, M.A.: Non-inhalation Narcosis in Buffaloes. Trud. Mosk. Vet. Akad., 9:236, 1955.
Gamble, J.C.: An Anaesthetic for *Corophium volutater* (Pallas) and *Marinogammarus obtusatus* (Dahl), Crustacea, Amphipoda. Experientia, 25:539, 1969.
Gandal, C.P.: Satisfactory General Anesthesia in Birds. J.A.V.M.A., 128:332, 1956.
Gandal, C.P.: Synopsis—Avian Anesthesia and Surgery. Proc. Am. Anim. Hosp. Assoc. 1967, p. 22.
Gandal, C.P.: A Practical Anesthetic Technique in Snakes Utilizing Methoxyflurane. Anim. Hosp., 4:258, 1968.
Gardner, A.F.: The Development of General Anesthesia in the Albino Rabbit for Surgical Procedures. Lab. Anim. Care, 14:214, 1964.
Gauckler, V.A., and Kraus, M.: Zur Immobilisierung von Wildwiederkauern mit Xylazin (Bay Va 1470). Der Zoologische Garten, 38:1, 1970.
Geddes, L.A., Tacker, W.A., Jr., and Rosborough, J.P.: Cardiac Output in an Anesthetized Dromedary. Am. J. Vet. Res., 35:131, 1974.
Geraci, J.R.: An Appraisal of Ketamine as an Immobilizing Agent in Wild and Captive Pinnipeds. J.A.V.M.A., 163:574, 1973.
Geraci, J.R., Skirnisson, K., and St. Aubin, D.J.: A Safe Method for Repeatedly Immobilizing Seals. J.A.V.M.A., 179:1192, 1981.
Gilbert, P.W., and Wood, F.G., Jr.: Method of Anesthetizing Large Sharks and Rays Safely and Rapidly. Science, 126:212, 1957.
Glenn, J.L., Straight, R., and Snyder, C.C.: Clinical Use of Ketamine Hydrochloride as an Anesthetic Agent for Snakes. Am. J. Vet. Res., 33:1902, 1972.
Göltenboth, R.: Aus der Arbeit des Zootierarztes. Dtsch. Tieraerztl. Wschr., 75:337, 1968.
Göltenboth, R., and Klös, H.G.: Erfahrungen mit BAY Va 1470 vei der Ruhigstellung von Zootieren. Berlin. Munchen. Tieraerztl. Wschr., 83:147, 1970.
Gossington, R.E.: An Aid to Fish Handling—Tricaine. Aquarium J., 28:318, 1957.
Graham, D.L., Dunlop, R.H., and Travis, H.F.: Barbiturate Anesthesia in Ranch Mink *(Mustela vison)*. Am. J. Vet. Res., 28:293, 1967.
Graham-Jones, O.: The Clinical Approach to Tumours in Cage Birds. III. Restraint and Anaesthesia of Small Cage Birds. J. Small Anim. Pract., 7:231, 1966.
Graham-Jones, O.: Notes on the Restraint and Anaesthesia of Primates. Nord. Vet.-Med., 14:76, 1962.
Gray, C.W.: Personal Communication. National Zoological Park, Washington, D.C., 1969.
Gray, K.N., Raulston, G.L., Flow, B.L., Jardine, J.H., and Huchton, J.I.: Repeated Immobilization of Miniature Swine with an Acepromazine-Ketamine Combination. Southwest Vet., 31:27, 1978.
Green, C.J.: *Animal Anaesthesia*. Laboratory Animals Ltd., London, 1979.
Gregg, D.A., and Olson, L.D.: The Use of Ketamine Hydrochloride as an Anesthetic for Raccoons. J. Wildl. Dis., 11:335, 1975.
Griner, L.A.: Personal Communication. San Diego Zoological Garden, San Diego, California, 1969.
Grinnell, A.D.: The Neurophysiology of Audition in Bats: Intensity and Frequency Parameters. J. Physiol., 167:38, 1963.
Haigh, J.C.: Capture of Woodland Caribou in Canada. Proc. Am. Assoc. Zoo Vet., Knoxville, Tennessee, 1978, p. 110.
Haigh, J.C., Stewart, R.R., Frokjer, R., and Hauge, T.: Capture of Moose with Fentanyl and Xylazine. J. Zoo Anim. Med., 8:22, 1977.
Hall, L.W.: *Wright's Veterinary Anaesthesia and Analgesia*, 7th ed. Baillière Tindall, London, 1971.
Harcourt-Brown, N.H.: Avian Anaesthesia in General Practice. J. Small Anim. Pract., 19:573, 1978.
Harper, J.A.: Immobilization of Roosevelt Elk by Succinylcholine Chloride. J. Wildl. Man., 29:339, 1965.
Harrington, R.: Immobilon-Rompun in Deer. Vet. Rec., 94:362, 1974.
Harthoorn, A.M.: Comparative Pharmacological Reactions of Certain Wild and Domestic Mammals to Thebaine Derivatives in the M-series of Compounds. Fed. Proc., 26:1251, 1967.
Harthoorn, A.M., and Player, I.C.: The Narcosis of the White Rhinoceros: A Series of Eighteen Case Histories. Tijkschr. Diergeneesk, 89:225, 1964.
Hayes, F.A.: Modifications for Cesarian Section in Chinchillas. Vet. Med., 50:367, 1955.
Healey, P.: A Simple Method for Anaesthetizing and Handling Small Carnivores. J. Inst. Anim. Tech., 18:37, 1967.
Henschel, V.E.: Intubations-Narkose biem Kanguruh. Berliner and Muncheur Fierarztlicke Wochenschrift, 71:225, 1958.
Henson, O.W.: Personal Communication. Yale University, New Haven, Connecticut, 1969.
Hewitt, O.H.: The Use of Serpasil in the Rearing and Handling of Pheasants. Conference on the Use of the Tranquilizing and Antihypertensive Agent Serpasil in Animal and Poultry Production. Rutgers, The State University, New Brunswick, New Jersey, 1959.
Hibbs, C.M.: Use of Chlorpromazine in Swine. Vet. Med., 53:571, 1958.
Hime, J.M.: Use of Ketamine Hydrochloride in Non-Domesticated Cats. Vet. Rec., 95:193, 1974.
Hime, J.M., and Jones, D.M.: The Use of Xylazine in Captive Wild Animals. Zoological Society of London; Sonderdruck aus Verhandlungsbericht des XI. Internationalen Symposiums uber die Erkrankugen der Zootiere, Budapest, 1970.
Hoar, R.M.: The Use of Metofane (Methoxyflurane) Anesthetic in Guinea Pigs. Allied Vet., 36:131, 1964.
Hochachka, P.W., Liggins, G.C., Quist, J., Schneider, R., Snider, M.Y., Wonders, T.R., and Zapol, W.M.: Pulmonary Metabolism During Diving: Conditioning Blood for the Brain. Science, 198:831, 1977.
Hodesson, S., Rich, S.T., Washington, J.O., and Apt, L.: Anesthesia of the Rabbit with Equithesin Following the

Administration of Preanesthetics. Lab. Anim. Care, 15:336, 1965.
Hodesson, S., Snow, I.B., and Wood, A.I.: Intubation Technique and Methoxyflurane Administration in Rabbits. Lab. Anim. Care, 19:593, 1969.
Hoff, H.E., Coles, S.K., Szabuniewicz, M., and McCrady, J.D.: The Respiratory Heart Rate Relationship in the Armadillo. Cardiovasc. Res. Cent. Bull., 21:37, 1982.
Hofmyer, J.M.: Immobilization of Black Rhinos, Eland and Roan Antelope with R33799. Report, Etosha Ecological Institute, South-West Africa, October, 1978.
Hoge, R.J.: Anesthesia and Surgery for Egg Bound Parakeets. Anim. Hosp., 2:46, 1966.
Hoge, R.S., Hodesson, S., Snow, I.B., and Wood, A.I.: Intubation Technique and Methoxyflurane Administration in Rabbits. Lab. Anim. Care, 19:593, 1969.
Hollingsworth, H., and Howes, J.R.: A Comparison of Some New Anesthetics for Avian Surgery. Poultry Sci., 44:1380, 1965.
Holt, P.E.: The Use of a Steroid Anaesthetic in a Long-Eared Owl *(Asio otus)*. Vet. Rec., 101:118, 1977.
Hönich, M.: Untersuchungen uber wirtung von BAY Va 1470 biem wild. From the Laboratory for Game Diseases, Ministry of Agriculture, Budakeszi, Hungary. Presented at the 12th International Symposium on Diseases of Zoo Animals, Budapest, 1970.
Hopcroft, S.C.: A Technique for the Simultaneous Bilateral Removal of the Adrenal Glands in Guinea Pigs, Using a New Type of Safe Anesthetic. Exp. Med. Surg., 24:12, 1966.
Hornocker, M.G., Craighead, J.J., and Pfeiffer, E.W.: Immbolizing Mountain Lions with Succinylcholine Chloride and Pentobarbital Sodium. J. Wildl. Man., 29:880, 1965.
Houston, D.C., and Cooper, J.E.: Use of the Drug Metomidate to Facilitate the Handling of Vultures. Internat. Zoo Yearbook, 13:269, 1973.
Howard, J.G., Pursel, V.G., Wildt, D.E., and Bush, M.: Comparison of Various Extenders for Freeze-Preservation of Semen from Selective Captive Wild Ungulates. J.A.V.M.A., 179:1157, 1981.
Hubbard, R.C., and Poulter. T.C.: Seals and Sea Lions as Models for Studies in Comparative Biology. Lab. Anim. Care, 18:249, 1968.
Hublou, W.F.: A Method of Using an Anesthetic in Marking Fins. Progressive Fish Culturist, 19:40, 1957.
Hummon, O.J.: A Device for the Restraint of Mink During Certain Experimental Procedures. J.A.V.M.A., 106:104, 1945.
Hyde, J.L.: The Use of Solid Carbon Dioxide for Producing Short Periods of Anesthesia in Guinea Pigs. Am. J. Vet. Res., 23:684, 1962.
Jha, S.K., Lumb, W.V., and Johnston, R.F.: Some Effects of Triflupromazine Hydrochloride on Goats. Am. J. Vet. Res., 22:915, 1961*a*.
Jha, S.K., Lumb, W.V., and Johnston, R.F.: Establishment of Permanent Carotid Loops in Goats. Am. J. Vet. Res., 22:948, 1961*b*.
Johari, M.P., and Sharma, S.P.: General Anaesthesia in Buffaloes by Intravenous Use of Chloral-Thiopentone Sodium Mixture. Indian J. Vet. Sci., 32:235, 1962.
Jones, D.M.: The Sedation and Anaesthesia of Birds and Reptiles. Vet. Rec., 101:340, 1977.
Jones, E.W., Nelson, T.E., Anderson, I.L., Kerr, D.D., and Burnap, T.K.: Malignant Hyperthermia of Swine. Anesthesiology, 36:42, 1972.
Jones, J.B., and Simmons, M.L.: Innovar-Vet as an Intramuscular Anesthetic for Rats. Lab. Anim. Care, 18:642, 1968.
Jones, L.M.: *Veterinary Pharmacology and Therapeutics,* 2nd ed. Iowa State College Press, Ames, 1957.
Jones, R.S.: Anaesthesia in Poultry. Proc. Assoc. Vet. Anaes., 3:91, 1972.
Jones, R.S.: Halothane Anaesthesia in Turkeys. Br. J. Anaesth., 38:656, 1966.
Kaczmarczyk, G., and Reinhart, H.W.: Arterial Blood Gas Tensions and Acid-Base Status of Wistar Rats During Thiopental and Halothane Anesthesia. Lab. Anim. Sci., 25:184, 1975.
Kaplan, H.M.: Anesthesia in Amphibians and Reptiles. Fed. Proc., 28:1541, 1969.
Kaplan, H.M., and Kaplan, M.: Anesthesia of Frogs with Ethyl Alcohol. Proc. Anim. Care Panel, 11:31, 1961.
Kaplan, H.M., Brewer, N.R., and Kaplan, M.R.: Comparative Value of Some Barbiturates for Anesthesia in the Frog. Proc. Anim. Care Panel, 12:141, 1962.
Karczmar, A.C., and Koppanyi, T.: Action of Central Nervous System Depressants at Different Growth Periods of Salamander *(Ambystoma punctatum)* Larvae. Fed. Proc., 7:231, 1948.
Keep, J.M.: Marsupial Anaesthesia. Proc. Postgrad. Committee Vet. Sci., Univ. of Sidney, 36:123, 1978.
Keyes, M.C.: Personal Communication. National Marine Fisheries Service, St. Paul Island, Alaska, 1971.
Khanna, V.K., and Pleuvry, B.J.: A Study of Naloxone and Doxapram as Agents for the Reversal of Neuroleptanalgesic Respiratory Depression in the Conscious Rabbit. Br. J. Anaesth., 50:905, 1978.
Kisch, B.: A Method to Immobilize Fish for Cardiac and Other Experiments with Procaine. Biol. Bull., 93:208, 1947.
Kisloff, B.: Ketamine-Paraldehyde Anesthesia for Rabbits. Am. J. Vet. Res., 36:1033, 1975.
Kloppel, G.: Zur Immobilisation von Zoo- und Wiltieren. Kleintier-Praxis, 14:203, 1969.
Kocan, A.A., Glenn, B.L., Thedford, T.R., Doyle, R., Waldrup, K., Kubat, G., and Shaw, M.G.: Effects of Chemical Immobilization on Hematologic and Serum Chemical Values in Captive White-Tailed Deer. J.A.V.M.A., 179:1153, 1981.
Kramer, K.L., Silverstein, A.M., and Parshall, C.J., Jr.: Surgical Anesthesia in Snakes. In *Experimental Animal Anesthesiology.* Edited by D.C. Sawyer. U.S.A.F. School of Aerospace Medicine, Brooks Air Force Base, Texas, 1965*a*.
Kramer, K.L., Silverstein, A.M., and Parshall, C.J., Jr.: Surgical Anesthesia in Sheep. In *Experimental Animal Anesthesiology.* Edited by D.C. Sawyer. U.S.A.F. School of Aerospace Medicine, Brooks Air Force Base, Texas, 1965*b*.
Krupp, J.H., and Quillin, R.: A Review of the Use of the Opossum for Research: Husbandry, Experimental Techniques and Routine Health Measures. Lab. Anim. Care, 14:189, 1964.
Kuhn, U.S.G., III, and Arko, R.J.: Repeated Ketamine Anesthesia in the Chimpanzee. J.A.V.M.A., 165:838, 1974.
Kumar, A., Thurmon, J.C., Dorner, J.L.: Hematologic and

Biochemical Findings in Sheep given Ketamine Hydrochloride. J.A.V.M.A., 165:284, 1974.
Kyle, O.C., Novak, S., and Bolooki, H.: General Anesthesia in Pigs. Lab. Anim. Sci., 29:123, 1979.
Ladhani, F.W., and Thies, R.E.: Fiber Lengths and End-Plate Locations in Fruit Bat Web Muscles. Proc. Soc. Exp. Biol. Med., 127:787, 1968.
Lafortune, J.G., and Rheault, J.P.E.: Essai d'Evaluation Clinique de la Reserpine (Serpasil) *Chex le Vison*. Can. J. Comp. Med. Vet. Sci., 24:243, 1960.
Larsen, L.H.: Restraint and Anaesthesia of Wild Animals in Captivity. Aust. Vet. J., 39:73, 1963.
Lasater, G.M., Stowe, C.M., Good, A.L., Short, E.C., and Pacheco-Perez, D.: Some Effects of Autonomic and Curariform Drugs in Bison. Cornell Vet., 55:309, 1965.
Lawrence, K., and Jackson, O.F.: Alphaxalone/Alphadolone Anaesthesia in Reptiles. Vet. Rec., 112:26, 1983.
Leary, S.L., and Manning, P.J.: Adynamic Ileus in Rats after Intraperitoneal Chloral Hydrate Anesthesia. Abstract 83, Publication 81-3, Am. Assoc. Lab. Anim. Sci., 1981*a*.
Leary, S.L., and Manning, P.J.: Fat Rats. Lab. Anim., 11:17, 1981*b*.
Leash, A.M., Beye, R.D., and Wilber, R.G.: Self-Mutilation Following Innovar-Vet Injection in the Guinea Pig. Lab. Anim. Sci., 23:720, 1973.
Lechleitner, R.J.: Personal Communication. Colorado State University, Fort Collins, Colorado, 1969.
Lee, C.: Personal Communication. Albany Medical College, Albany, New York, 1969.
Lee, J., Schweinsburg, R., Kernan, F., and Haigh, J.: Immobilization of Polar Bears (*Ursus maritinus*, Phipps) with Ketamine Hydrochloride and Xylazine Hydrochloride. J. Wildl. Dis., 17:331, 1981.
Leonard, R.H.: Parakeet and Canary Practice. J.A.V.M.A., 136:378, 1960.
Libbin, R.M., and Person, P.: Neonatal Rat Surgery: Avoiding Maternal Cannibalism. Science, 206:66, 1979.
Lightfoot, W.E., and Molinari, G.F.: Comparison of Ketamine and Pentobarbital Anesthesia in the Mongolian Gerbil. Am. J. Vet. Res., 39:1061, 1978.
Lilly, J.C.: *Man and Dolphin*. Doubleday, New York, 1961.
Ling, J.K., Nicholls, D.G., and Thomas, C.D.B.: Immobilization of Southern Elephant Seals with Succinylcholine Chloride. J. Wildl. Man., 37:468, 1967.
Livezey, R.L.: Procaine Hydrochloride as a Killing Agent for Reptiles and Amphibians. Herpetologica, 13:280, 1957.
Logsdon, H.S.: Use of Drugs as a Capture Technique for Desert Bighorn Sheep. Thesis, Colorado State University, Fort Collins, 1969.
Lumb, W.V.: Unpublished Data. Colorado State University, Fort Collins, 1972.
Luschei, E.S., and Mehaffey, J.J.: Small Animal Anesthesia with Halothane. J. Appl. Physiol., 22:595, 1967.
Lynn, R.: Incubators for Parakeets. Anim. Hosp., 3:126, 1967.
Mackintosh, C.G., MacArthur, J.A., Little, T.W.A., and Stuart, P.: The Immobilization of the Badger. Br. Vet. J., 132:609, 1976.
Marsboom, R., Mortelmans, J., and Vercruysse, J.: Neuroleptanalgesia in Monkeys. Vet. Rec. 75:132, 1963.
Marston, J.H., and Chang, M.C.: The Breeding, Management and Reproductive Physiology of the Mongolian Gerbil *(Meriones unguiculatus)*. Lab. Anim. Care, 15:34, 1965.
Martin, L.L.: Comparison of Methoxymol, Alpha-chloralose and Two Barbiturates for Capturing Doves. 21st Annual Conference, Southeastern Association of Game and Fish Commissioners, New Orleans, 1967.
Martin, N.V., and Scott, D.C.: Use of Tricaine Methanesulfonate (M.S. 222) in the Transport of Live Fish without Water. Progressive Fish Culturist, 27:183, 1959.
Manohar, M., Kumar, R., and Tyagi, R.P.S.: Studies on Intravenous Retrograde Regional Anaesthesia of the Forelimb in Buffalo Calves. Br. Vet. J., 127:401, 1971.
McBride, A.F., and Kritzler, H.: Observations on Pregnancy, Parturition, and Postnatal Behavior in the Bottlenose Dolphin. J. Mamml., 32:251, 1951.
McCormick, M.J., and Ashworth, M.A.: Acepromazine and Methoxyflurane Anesthesia of Immature New Zealand White Rabbits. Lab. Anim. Sci., 21:220, 1971.
McFarland, W.N., and Klontz, G.W.: Anesthesia in Fishes. Fed. Proc., 28:1535, 1969.
McGovern, S.H., and Rugh, H.: Efficacy of M-Amine Ethyl Benzoate as an Anesthetic for Amphibian Embryos. Proc. Soc. Exp. Biol. Med., 57:127, 1944.
Miller, A.E., and Gudmundson, J.: Use of Thiamylal in Mature Swine. Can. Vet. J., 5:217, 1964.
Molello, J.A., and Hawkins, K.: Methoxyflurane Anesthesia of Laboratory Rats. Lab. Anim. Care, 18:581, 1968.
Morgan, W.: Effective Anesthesia for Chicks. Proc. S.D. Acad. Sci., 36:105, 1957.
Mosby, H.S., and Cantner, D.E.: The Use of Avertin in Capturing Wild Turkeys and as an Oral Basal Anesthetic for Other Wild Animals. Southwest Vet., 9:132, 1955.
Mulder, J.B.: Anesthesia in the Coyote Using a Combination of Ketamine and Xylazine. J. Wildl. Dis., 14:501, 1978.
Mulder, K.J., and Mulder, J.B.: Ketamine and Xylazine Anesthesia in the Mouse. Vet. Med. Small Anim. Clin., 74:569, 1979.
Naccarato, E.F., and Hunter, W.S.: Anaesthetic Effects of Various Ratios of Ketamine and Xylazine in Rhesus Monkeys *(Macaca mulatta)*. Lab. Anim., 13:317, 1979.
Nagel, E.L., Morgane, P.J., and McFarland, W.L.: Anesthesia for the Bottlenose Dolphin, *Tursiops truncatus*. Science, 146:1591, 1964.
Newsome, J., and Robinson, D.L.H.: Sedatives and Anaesthetics for Baboons. Br. Vet. J., 113:163, 1957.
Newton, W.M., Cusick, P.K., and Raffe, M.R.: Innovar-Vet-Induced Pathologic Changes in the Guinea Pig. Lab. Anim. Sci., 25:597, 1975.
Nielson, L., Haigh, J.C., and Fowler, M.E.: *Chemical Immobilization of North American Wildlife*. IR Publications Ltd., New York, 1983.
Noyes, D.H., and Siekierski, D.M.: Anesthesia of Marmots with Sodium Pentobarbital, Ketamine Hydrochloride, and a Combination of Droperidol and Fentanyl. Lab. Anim. Sci., 25:557, 1975.
O'Connor, P.: Personal Communication. Halloran Veterinary Hospital, Staten Island, New York, 1981.
Padgett, G.A.: Personal Communication. Washington State University, Pullman, Washington, 1964.

Pandeya, N.K., and Lemon, H.M.: Paraldehyde: An Anesthesia for Recovery Experiments in Albino Rabbits. Lab. Anim. Care, 15:304, 1965.

Parker, G.H.: General Anesthesia by Cooling. Proc. Soc. Exp. Biol. Med., 42:186, 1939.

Pathak, S.C., Nigam, J.M., Peshin, P.K., and Singh, A.P.: Anesthetic and Hemodynamic Effects of Ketamine Hydrochloride in Buffalo Calves *(Bubalis bubalis)*. Am. J. Vet. Res., 43:875, 1982.

Peshin, P.K., and Kumar, A.: Physiologic and Sedative Effects of Xylazine in Buffaloes. Indian Vet. J., 56:864, 1979.

Peshin, P.K., Kumar, A., and Singh, H.: Xylazine in Buffaloes I: Cardiovascular, Respiratory and Sedative Effects. Pantnagar J. Res., 3:245, 1978.

Phillipson, A.T., and Barnett, S.F.: Anaesthesia in Sheep. Vet. Rec., 51:869, 1939.

Piermattei, D.L., and Swan, H.: Techniques for General Anesthesia in Miniature Pigs. J. Surg. Res., 10:587, 1970.

Pleuger, C.A.: Gastrotomy in a Crocodile: A Case Report. J.A.V.M.A., 117:297, 1950.

Rapson, W.S., and Jones, T.C.: Restraint of Rabbits by Hypnosis. Lab. Anim. Care, 14:131, 1964.

Redig, P.T.: Personal Communication. Univ. Minnesota, St. Paul, 1983.

Redig, P.T., and Duke, G.E.: Intravenously Administered Ketamine HCl and Diazepam for Anesthesia of Raptors. J.A.V.M.A., 169:886, 1976.

Reynolds, H.H.: Nonhuman Primates in the Study of Toxicological Effects on the Central Nervous System: A Review. Ann. N.Y. Acad. Sci., 162:617, 1969.

Reynolds, W.A., and Maplesden, D.C.: Metoserpate Hydrochloride for the Treatment of Hysteria in Replacement Pullets. Avian Dis., 21:720, 1977.

Richardson, K.C., and Cullen, L.K.: Anesthesia of Small Kangaroos. J.A.V.M.A., 179:1162, 1981.

Richmond, M., and Conaway, C.H.: Management, Breeding, and Reproductive Performance of Vole, *Microtus ochrogaster*, in a Laboratory Colony. Lab. Anim. Care, 19:80, 1969.

Richter, A.G.: Ketamine-Xylazine Immobilization of a Mule Deer. J.A.V.M.A., 171:987, 1977.

Riddell, W.K.: Caudal Anesthesia in Canine Surgery. J. Small Anim. Med., 1:159, 1952.

Ridgway, S.H., and McCormick, J.G.: Anesthetization of Porpoises for Major Surgery. Science, 158:510, 1967.

Ridgway, S.H., and Simpson, J.G.: Anesthesia and Restraint for the California Sea Lion. *Zalophus californianus*. J.A.V.M.A., 155:1059, 1969.

Rieu, M., and Gautheron, B.: Preliminary Observations Concerning a Method for Introduction of a Tube for Anesthesia in Small Delphinids. Laboratorie d' Acoustique Animals. Lab. Pub. Jouy-en-Josas, France, 78, 1968.

Ritzman, J.R., Erickson, H.H., and Miller, E.D.: Cardiovascular Effects of Enflurane and Halothane on the Rhesus Monkey. Anesth. Analg., 55:85, 1976.

Roslyn, J., Thompson, J.E., Jr., and DenBesten, L.: Anesthesia in Prairie Dogs. Lab. Anim. Sci., 29:542, 1979.

Roughton, R.D.: Xylazine as an Immobilizing Agent for Captive White-Tailed Deer. J.A.V.M.A., 167:574, 1975.

Said, A.H.: Some Aspects of Anaesthesia in the Camel. Vet. Rec., 76:550, 1964.

Sawyer, D.C.: Anesthetic Techniques of Rabbits and Mice. In *Experimental Animal Anesthesiology.* Edited by D.C. Sawyer. U.S.A.F. School of Aerospace Medicine, Brooks Air Force Base, Texas, 1965*a*.

Sawyer, D.C.: Anesthetic Techniques of the *Macaca Mulatta.* In *Experimental Animal Anesthesiology.* Edited by D.C. Sawyer. U.S.A.F. School of Aerospace Medicine, Brooks Air Force Base, Texas, 1965*b*.

Sawyer, D.C., Lumb, W.V., and Stone, H.L.: Cardiovascular Effects of Halothane, Methoxyflurane, Pentobarbital and Thiamylal. J. Appl. Physiol., 30:36, 1971.

Schilling, T.W., and Stone, H.L.: Comparative Cardiovascular Measurements in the Javelina *(Tayassu tajacu)*. Lab. Anim. Care, 19:331, 1969.

Scordelis, P.: Internal Communication. Tavolek Inc., Redmond, Washington, 1977.

Sedgwick, C.J., and Acosta, A.L.: Capture Drugs. Mod. Vet. Pract., 50:32, 1969.

Seidel, V.B., Straub, G., Carlo, W.-R., and Effert, W.: Anästhesie, Hämatologie und Biochemie beim Kiang (Equus hemionus kiang, Moorcroft, 1981). Sonderdruck aus Verhandlungsbericht des XXIV. Internationalen Symposiums über die Erkrankungen der Zootiere, Veszprém, 1982.

Shearer, D., Creel, D., and Wilson, C.E.: Strain Differences in the Response of Rats to Repeated Injections of Pentobarbital Sodium. Lab. Anim. Sci., 23:662, 1973.

Sherrard, E.: Anaesthesia of Rabbits. Vet. Rec., 78:253, 1966.

Singh, J., Sobti, V.K., Kohli, R.N., Kumar, V.R., and Khanna, A.K.: Evaluation of Glyceryl Guaiacolate as a Muscle Relaxant in Buffalo Calves. Zbl. Vet. Med. A, 28:60, 1981.

Singh, R., Rathor, S.S., and Kohli, R.N.: A Note on Preliminary Observations on the Use of Some General Anaesthetics in the Camel. Indian Vet. J., 39:614, 1962.

Smeller, J., Bush, M., and Seal, U.S.: Observations on Immobilization of Père David's Deer. J.A.V.M.A., 169:890, 1976.

Soifer, F.K.: Personal Communication. Bellaire Boulevard Animal Clinic, Houston, Texas, 1969.

Soifer, F.K.: Surgery Successful on 500-lb. Tortoise. J.A.V.M.A., 152:418, 1968.

Stafford, S.K., and Williams, L.E., Jr.: Data on Capturing Black Bears with Alpha-chloralose. Proc. 22nd Annual Conference Southeastern Assoc. of Game and Fish Commissioners, Baltimore, Maryland, 1968.

Steffey, E.P., Gillespie, J.R., Berry, J.D., Eger, E.I., and Rhode, R.A.: The Cardiovascular Effects of Halothane in the Stumptail Monkey During Spontaneous and Controlled Ventilation. Am. J. Vet. Res., 35:1315, 1974.

Strack, L.E., and Kaplan, H.M.: Fentanyl and Droperidol for Surgical Anesthesia of Rabbits. J.A.V.M.A., 153:822, 1968.

Stunkard, J.A., and Miller, J.C.: An Outline Guide to General Anesthesia in Exotic Species. Vet. Med. Small Anim. Clin., 69:1181, 1974.

Suga, N.: Single Unit Activity in Cochlear Nucleus and Inferior Colliculus of Echolocating Bats. J. Physiol., 172:449, 1964.

Szabuniewicz, M., and McCrady, J.D.: Some Aspects of the Anatomy and Physiology of the Armadillo. Lab. Anim. Care, 19:843, 1969.

Taber, R., and Irwin, S.: Anesthesia in the Mouse. Fed. Proc., 28:1528, 1969.

Talbot, L.M., and Lamprey, H.F.: Immobilization of Free-Ranging East African Ungulates with Succinylcholine Chloride. J. Wildl. Man., 25:303, 1961.

Tan, E., and Snow, H.D.: Continuous Epidural Anesthesia in the Guinea Pig. Am. J. Vet. Res., 29:487, 1968.

Tanner, J.T.: Some Useful Demonstrations in Teaching Zoology. Turtox News, 32:2, 1954.

Taylor, M.E.: Personal Communication. Show Low, Arizona, 1961.

Thienpont, D., and Niemegeers, C.J.E.: Propoxate (R7464): A New Potent Anesthetic Agent in Cold Blooded Vertebrates. Nature (London), 205:1018, 1965.

Thomas, J.W., Robinson, R.M., and Marburger, R.G.: Use of Diazepam in the Capture and Handling of Cervids. J. Wildl. Man., 31:686, 1967.

Thomas, W.D.: Chemical Immobilization of Wild Animals. J.A.V.M.A., 138:263, 1961.

Thurmon, J.C., Kumar, A., and Link, R.P.: Evaluation of Ketamine Hydrochloride as an Anesthetic in Sheep. J.A.V.M.A., 162:293, 1973.

Thurmon, J.C., Nelson, D.R., and Kumar, A.: Etorphine and Triflupromazine as Immobilizing Agents in the Goat. J.A.V.M.A., 165:168, 1974.

Troyer, W.: Out for Bear. Jen-Sal J., 43:32, 1960.

Tyagi, R.P.S., and Lumb, W.V.: Uterine Healing after Cesarotomy in Goats. Am. J. Vet. Res., 22:1097, 1961.

Van Dyke, R.A., and Wood, C.L.: Metabolism of Methoxyflurane: Release of Inorganic Fluoride in Human and Rat Hepatic Microsomes. Anesthesiology, 39:613, 1973.

Van Foreest, A.: Use of Ketamine/Xylazine Combination for Tail Amputation in Nutria. J. Zoo Anim. Med., 11:19, 1980.

Van Pelt, L.F.: Ketamine and Xylazine for Surgical Anesthesia in Rats. J.A.V.M.A., 171:842, 1977.

Van Stee, E.W.: Personal Communication. Michigan State University, East Lansing, Michigan., 1960.

Verts, B.J.: A Device for Anesthetizing Skunks. J. Wildl. Man., 24:344, 1960.

Vierheller, R.C.: What is Your Diagnosis? J.A.V.M.A., 134:9, 1959.

Vos-Maas, M.G., and Zwart, P.: A Technique for Intravenous Injection in the Red-Eared Turtle *(Pseudemys scriptor elegans)*. Lab. Anim., 10:399, 1976.

Wallach, J.D.: Medical Care of Reptiles. J.A.V.M.A., 155:1017, 1969.

Wallach, J.D., and Anderson, J.L.: Oripavine (M.99) Combinations and Solvents for Immobilization of the African Elephant. J.A.V.M.A., 153:793, 1968.

Wallach, J.D., Frueh, R., and Lentz, M.: The Use of M.99 as an Immobilizing and Analgesic Agent in Captive Wild Animals. J.A.V.M.A., 151:870, 1967.

Wallach, J.D., and Hoessle, C.: M-99 as an Immobilizing Agent in Poikilotherms. Vet. Med. Small Anim. Clin., 65:165, 1970.

Wampler, S.N.: Husbandry and Health Problems of Armadillos, *Dasypus novemcinctus*. Lab. Anim. Care, 19:391, 1969.

Wass, J.A., and Kaplan, H.M.: Methoxyflurane Anesthesia for *Rana Pipiens*. Lab. Anim. Sci., 24:669, 1974.

Wass, J.A., Keene, J.R., and Kaplan, H.M.: Ketamine-Methoxyflurane Anesthesia for Rabbits. Am. J. Vet. Res., 135:317, 1974.

Waterman, A.E., and Livingston, A.: Effects of Age and Sex on Ketamine Anesthesia in the Rat. Br. J. Anesth., 50:885, 1978.

Watson, S.C., and Cowie, A.T.: A Simple Closed-Circuit Apparatus for Cyclopropane and Halothane Anesthesia of the Rabbit. Lab. Anim. Care, 16:515, 1966.

Weisner, B.P.: The Post-Natal Development of the Genital Organs of the Albino Rat. J. Obstet. Gynecol., British Empire, 41:867, 1934.

Wesolowski, S.A.: *Evaluation of Tissue and Prosthetic Vascular Grafts*. Charles C Thomas, Springfield, Illinois, 1962.

Westenberg, I.S., and Bolam, J.M.: Lethal Doses of Pentobarbital Sodium in Albino Versus Pigmented Rats: A Within Strain Comparison. Lab. Anim. Sci., 31:360, 1981.

White, G.L., and Holmes, D.D.: A Comparison of Ketamine and the Combination Ketamine-Xylazine for Effective Surgical Anesthesia in the Rabbit. Lab. Anim. Sci., 26:804, 1976.

Whittow, G.C., and Ossorio, N.: A New Technique for Anesthetizing Birds. Lab. Anim. Care, 20:651, 1970.

Wilgus, H.S.: Reserpine for Tranquilizing Geese. The Second Conference on the Use of Reserpine in Poultry Production. The Institute of Agriculture, University of Minnesota, St. Paul, Minnesota, 1960.

Williams, L.E., Austin, D.H., and Peoples, J.: Progress in Capturing Turkeys with Drugs Applied to Baits. Proc., 20th Annual Conference, Southeastern Association of Game and Fish Commissioners, New Orleans, 1966.

Williams, L.E., Jr.: Preliminary Report of Methoxymol to Capture Turkeys. Proc., 21st Annual Conference, Southeastern Association of Game and Fish Commissioners, New Orleans, 1967.

Williamson, W.M., and Wallach, J.D.: M.99-Induced Recumbency and Analgesia in a Giraffe. J.A.V.M.A., 153:816, 1968.

Wilson, G.R.: Intramuscular Anaesthesia in the Red Kangaroo. Aust. Vet. Pract., 6:51, 1976.

Witschi, E.: Testis Grafting in Tadpoles of *Rana temporaria* and Its Bearing on the Hormone Theory of Sex Determination. J. Exp. Zool., 47:269, 1927.

Wolff, W.A., and Boyd, R.J.: Personal Communication. Colorado State University, Fort Collins, 1963.

Wolff, W.A., Davis, R.W., and Lumb, W.V.: Chloral Hydrate-Halothane-Nitrous Oxide Anesthesia in Deer. J.A.V.M.A., 147:1099, 1965.

Wood, F.E., Critchley, K.H., and Wood, J.R.: Anesthesia in the Green Sea Turtle, *Chelonia mydas*. Am. J. Vet. Res., 43:1882, 1982.

Wright, J.G.: *Veterinary Anaesthesia*, 4th ed. Williams & Wilkins, Baltimore, 1957.

Yankow, M.: An Unusual Case of Limb Regeneration. Turtox News, 40:146, 1962.

Young, R., and Kaplan M.: Anesthesia of Turtles with Chlorpromazine and Sodium Pentobarbital. Proc. Anim. Care Panel., 10:57, 1960.

Young, W.A.: Wing Amputation of Birds in Lieu of Pinioning. J.A.V.M.A., 112:224, 1948.

CHAPTER 19

Monitoring Anesthesia

INTRODUCTION

In the past, response of the patient to an anesthetic has been assessed in large part by the senses of the anesthesiologist. As a result, anesthesia has been more an art than a science.

The veterinarian in practice may serve as both anesthesiologist and surgeon, and while operating may be the only person available to observe the anesthetized patient. Under these circumstances, he develops a "sixth sense" concerning the patient's status. By observing respiratory movements, the color of the tissues, pulsation of blood vessels, and the color of blood in the operative field, he continuously assesses cardiac and respiratory function.

Many types of monitoring equipment have become available to furnish objective data concerning the state of the patient. Some of these devices have practical use in clinical practice, whereas others, because of cost or the limited value of the information obtained, are restricted to the research laboratory.

Cullen (1961) has wisely pointed out that monitors are *not* a substitute for clinical observation and good judgment on the part of the anesthesiologist and surgeon.

> . . . information provided by the instruments should be considered to be a portion, and most likely a small portion, of the data necessary for critical evaluation of the patient's condition. Unwarranted reliance on gadgetry can result only in restricted information, misleading information (at times), and deterioration of clinical acuity.

RESPIRATION

Respiratory rate and tidal and minute volume may be monitored.

Respiratory Rate

Excursions of the rebreathing bag on an anesthetic machine indicate respiratory rate, but do *not* indicate tidal volume.

A simple respiratory rate monitor may be attached as an accessory to the exhalation valve of an anesthetic circuit that whistles with each exhalation. Its chief disadvantage is that it increases resistance to expiration. Respiratory rate may also be monitored by inserting a thermistor probe into the airway or by attaching it to the external nares. The temperature fluctuations may be converted to an audible signal, traced on appropriate recorder, or exhibited on an oscilloscope.

Beven (1980) monitored respiratory patterns in rats by detecting the changes in light intensity

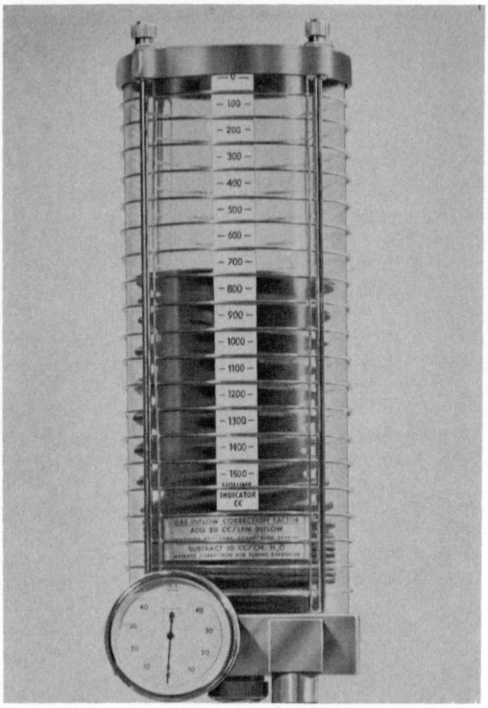

Figure 19–1. The ventimeter, a tidal volume indicating device for use in anesthetic breathing circuits. (Courtesy of Air-Shields, Inc., Hatboro, PA.)

caused by respiratory movements. A fixed source of incident light was used, and a photodiode was positioned to measure reflected light. The paratracheal placement of a carbon button microphone element with amplifier and earphones has also been recommended (Skaredoff and Viquera, 1979).

Tidal and Minute Volume

In addition to the respiratory rate monitors described in the preceding section, tidal and minute volume are commonly monitored with devices such as the ventimeter (displacement), rotor (inferential) flowmeters, the pneumotachograph, or electronic flowmeters.

The ventimeter is a tidal volume indicating device for use in breathing circuits (Fig. 19–1). The volume, pressure, and pattern of each inspiration and expiration are directly visible in the movement of a volumetrically calibrated bellows and an aneroid manometer. The breathing bag is not replaced by the bellows, the patient's respirations moving both reservoirs simultaneously. Little expiratory impedance is added by the ventimeter. The patient's tidal volumes are monitored continuously during spontaneous respiration, during positive pressure breathing produced by compression of the rebreathing bag, or during mechanical ventilation. Inadequate or excessive ventilation can be quickly recognized during inhalation anesthesia with closed, semiclosed, or nonrebreathing systems. The ventimeter incorporates a phased "pop-off" valve which, in all of these techniques, remains closed during inspiration; conventional "pop-off" valves are kept closed. Overflow of gas from the system occurs at low back pressure and is limited to a short interval immediately after expiration. Even when flows of 50 to 75 L per minute are suddenly introduced (by an oxygen flush valve) into the circuit, total pressure never exceeds 3 cm of water during expiration. Leaks in the system are indicated by a falling end-expiratory rest position of the ventimeter bellows. In addition, the need for adjustment of gas flow is obvious if the bellows either falls or remains fully extended.

Tidal volume can be read directly from the instrument. The ventimeter does not interfere with customary use of the rebreathing bag. By compressing the bag according to observed tidal volumes, one can maintain the patient's ventilation within any desired limits (for example, within ± 5% of the measured tidal volume during a control or induction period).

To assist ventilation manually, the ventimeter is watched, and the bag is compressed synchronously with the inspiratory excursion of the bellows. With a closed system, the start of an active inspiration can be detected with the first 10 ml inspired. Cardiac pulsations, which are sometimes transmitted to the bellows, are of lesser magnitude.

The ventimeter is made for routine use without removal from the anesthetic machine. The anesthesiologist can thus detect hypoventilation, which is less obvious with the rebreathing bag alone. Hypoventilation is corrected in the conventional manner by squeezing the rebreathing bag, and the ventimeter serves as continual objective evidence of performance.

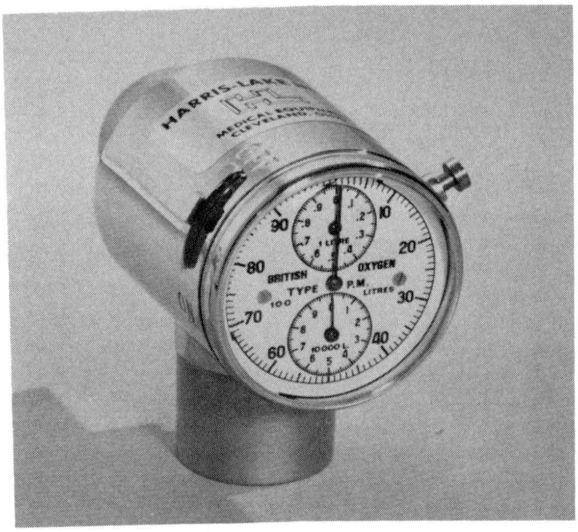

Figure 19–2. The Wright respirometer. (Courtesy of Harris Calorific Co., Cleveland, Ohio.)

In rotor or inferential meters, volume is inferred from the number of revolutions of a vane that is rotated by the gas stream (Atkinson et al., 1977). Meters of this type include the Wright respirometer, the Dräger volumeter, and the Monaghan (Bennett) ventilation meter.

Basically, the Wright instrument consists of a rotor running on jeweled bearings. It is connected by a watch-type movement to hands on the dial (Fig. 19–2). Air passing through the inlet turns the rotor at a rate approximately proportional to the volumetric air flow through the instrument (Fig. 19–3). Two scales indicate volume up to 100 L with a minimum of 0.01 L. A physiologic model is available that has a third small scale indicating volumes up to 10,000 L. An on-off switch enables air to bypass the rotor when measurements are not desired. A reset button positions the hands at zero.

The Wright respirometer has virtually no resistance to flow, can be inserted into an anesthetic circuit with proper adapters, and is sensitive to flow in only one direction. Its chief disadvantages are its inaccuracy, especially with low flows, and its delicacy, which subjects it to damage.

In the Monaghan ventilation meter, air passes between the teeth of two interlocking rotors and turns the rotors in so doing (see Fig. 19–3). To avoid friction, there is clearance between the rotors and the housing. This clearance is responsible for negative error at low flow rates; nevertheless, this meter was found to be more accurate than other gas volume meters (Wright, Dräger, and Parkinson and Cowan) tested (Byles, 1960). It does, however, have greater resistance to flow and larger dead space than the Wright respirometer, and is unsuitable for measurement in a to-and-fro system (Cooper, 1969).

The Dräger volumeter operates in a similar manner to the Monaghan (Byles, 1960), but is slightly less accurate.

The capacity of the aforementioned and similar respirometers is too small for large animals. A bell spirometer for use in horses has been described (McDonell, 1974).

Poiseuille's law states that, under capillary conditions in a rigid straight tube, delivery is proportional to pressure loss per unit of length. The continuous measurement of pressure loss (pressure difference between two points on the tube) gives a differential curve whose ordinates represent the velocity of the air current. A proportional relationship exists between the velocity of the air current and the volume of air delivered. Integration of the pressure changes permits display of individual tidal volumes or minute volume. This principle forms the basis for the pneumotachograph.*

The instrument (Fig. 19–4) consists of a large outer tube containing many small ducts (0.8 mm × 32 mm) through which the air passes. These small capillary-type ducts prevent turbulence.

Two ducts on the large tube lead to a differential pressure transducer and communicate pressure differences from the two positions on the tube. If the velocity of the air current does not exceed a certain value, the air particles move through the pneumotachograph under capillary conditions, ensuring a strict proportion between velocity and transducer deflection. Once this limit is exceeded, turbulences appear that can be detected as oscillations on the recording.

To prevent water vapor condensation within

*See Appendix A for manufacturer.

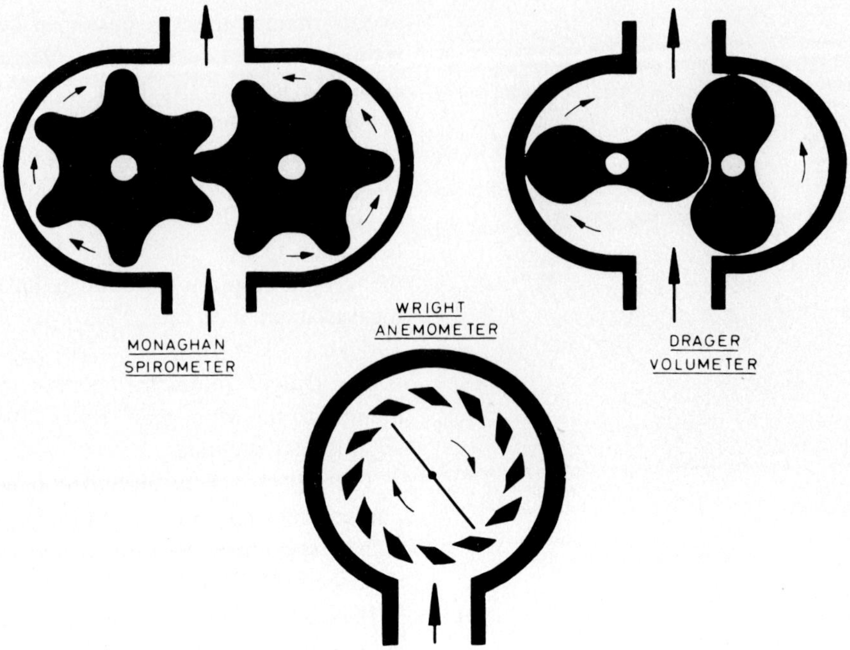

Figure 19–3. Mechanism of rotary respirometers (diagrammatic and not to scale.) (From Byles, P.H.: Observations on Some Continuously-Acting Spirometers. Br. J. Anaesth., 32:470, 1960.)

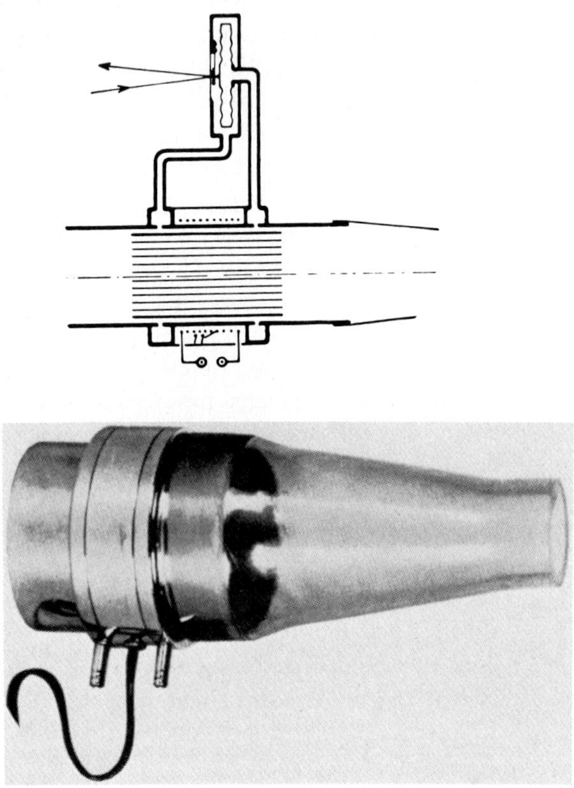

Figure 19–4. The pneumotachograph. The schematic drawing illustrates the principles involved. See text for explanation. (Courtesy of Dr. A. Fleisch.)

the capillary ducts, the apparatus has a built-in heating element.

Six sizes of pneumotachograph are available to accommodate a wide range of tidal volumes (0.1 to 14 L/sec).

Electronic respiratory monitors that continuously display the respirations per minute, tidal volume, and minute volume have been introduced. An alarm may be activated if either the minute volume or the respiratory rate changes to a degree exceeding upper and lower limits previously set by the operator. A transducer is inserted into the airway to sense the gas flow. The sensing element is an electrically heated platinum wire that responds to temperature fluctuations related to flow. Like other monitors, the range at which they operate limits their use to animals weighing less than 200 lbs.

Pulmonary ventilation may also be measured by classic recording spirometers. Most such systems, however, are difficult to adapt to inhalation anesthetic techniques (Cooper, 1969). To obviate problems associated with anesthetic circuits and the uptake and elimination of anesthetics, Nunn (1956) recorded respiratory activity during anesthesia by means of volume changes in a rigid container surrounding the reservoir bag.

Respiration may also be measured by recording chest movements. The chest may be surrounded by a lightly inflated rubber tube, which measures the pressure changes induced by respiration, or a mercury-in-rubber strain gauge may be placed about the chest (Cooper, 1969).

The electrical impedance between two electrodes placed across the chest has also been used to measure pulmonary ventilation (Baker and Hill, 1969; Freundlich and Erickson, 1974). The latter authors found useful correlation ($r = 0.89$) between impedance waveform amplitude and tidal volume; artifacts were easily detected, and electrocardiographs could be attained via the same electrodes.

Kerfoot and Domeier (1972) modified a capacitance respirometer to record pulmonary function values in large animals such as hogs. Respiratory volumes and flow rates were measured by means of surface area changes of the abdomen and rib cage during the respiratory cycle. Data were obtained without the inconvenience and discomfort of airway intubation and without tight-fitting neck collars or mouthpieces. With the simultaneous recording of esophageal pressure, compliance was also monitored.

A new fluidic device, with no moving parts, has been reported (Hedenstierna et al., 1976). Normal minute volumes were accurate to within $\pm$ 5%. The instrument tended to underrate at low volumes and to overrate at high volumes. Various sizes can be made to adapt to various gas flow rates.

Functional Residual Capacity

Functional residual capacity (FRC) is especially important to the anesthesiologist; it has a significant impact on induction and recovery and varies considerably according to body position, especially in the large animal. It is, however, difficult to monitor. Compliance and resistance are also influenced by lung volume. To measure lung volume, gas dilution methods or a whole-body plethysmograph are required.

Rosenthal (1981) has indicated that compliance is probably the most suitable parameter to follow the FRC, since deviations of FRC from normal result in alterations in compliance (volume change/pressure change). Volume change can be based upon expired tidal volume, whereas pressure change may be measured with an esophageal balloon to measure transthoracic pressure. Others use airway pressure; if this is used, it is preferable to measure the plateau pressure attained during peak inspiratory hold, rather than peak inspiratory pressure. The latter is influenced by airway pressure.

Respiratory and Anesthetic Gases

Gas analyzers have been devised to measure continuously such gases as carbon dioxide and various inhalant anesthetics during anesthesia. These operate on the principle of infrared absorption and measure any one gas in the anesthetic mixture. Infrared analyzers have a short response time and are fairly accurate.

The detection unit contains two identical infrared sources that emit parallel beams of radiation, pulsed by a chopper (Fig. 19–5). One

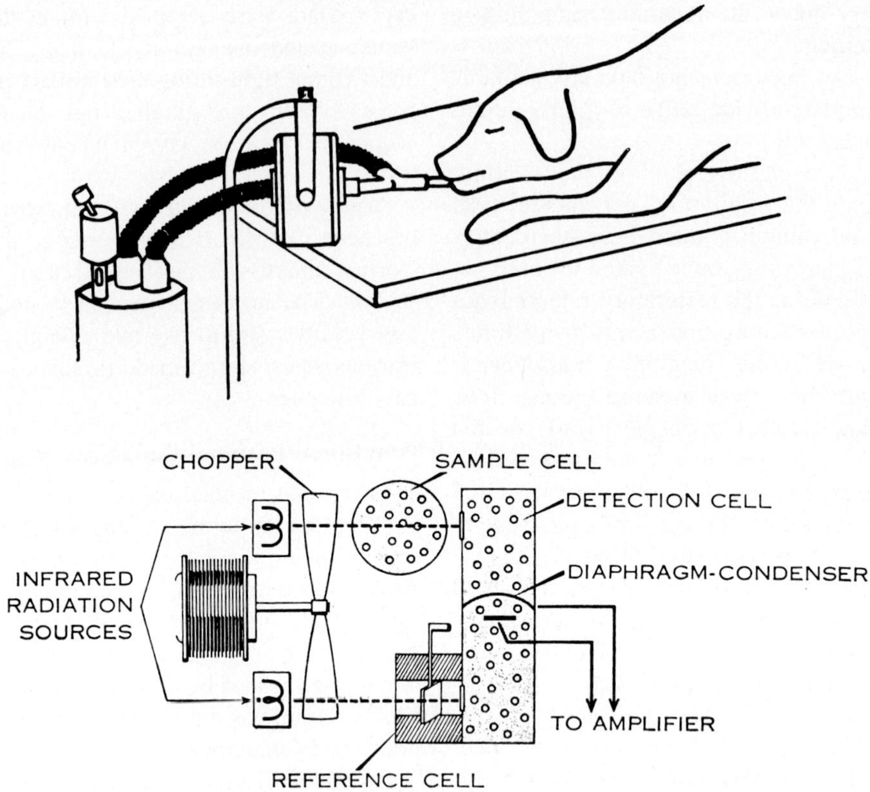

Figure 19–5. Breathe-through sampling cell, for measuring concentrations of respiratory and anesthetic gases, connected in a circle system. A schematic diagram of the apparatus is shown below. (Courtesy of Spinco Division, Beckman Instruments, Inc., Palo Alto, California.)

beam passes through the sample cell, the other through a reference cell. Both beams then pass into a detection cell, consisting of two rigid chambers divided by a diaphragm. Both chambers of the detection cell are charged to equal pressure with the gas being measured.

When the gas being measured enters the sample cell, it absorbs infrared radiation at the same wavelengths as gas in the detection cell. This reduces the amount of radiation reaching one side of the detection cell and produces a lower pressure in that side. The diaphragm moves toward the side of lower pressure, and this is translated into electrical impulses that actuate the indicating meter and recorder.

A breathe-through sampling cell is used in anesthetic circuits, the patient's exhaled breath passing through the cell.

Alternatively, samples are aspirated continuously (0.5 to 1.5 L/min) (Burton, 1969) from the trachea or from the top of the endotracheal tube. The former is preferred when tidal volumes are low and dead space washout may be incomplete.

Oxygen concentrations of inhaled or exhaled gases may be made paramagnetically as with the Pauling oxygen meter, or polarographically by means of a modified Clark-type electrode (Burton, 1969). These devices can be placed in the anesthesia circuit to give a continuous analog readout of the percentage of O_2 in the circuit. This is especially valuable in preventing anoxia when high concentrations of N_2O are used. The devices are equipped with a high/low alarm that can be preset to the desired O_2 level.

In-circuit monitoring of halothane concentrations has been made possible by the introduction of a monitor (Fig. 19–6) in which the measuring

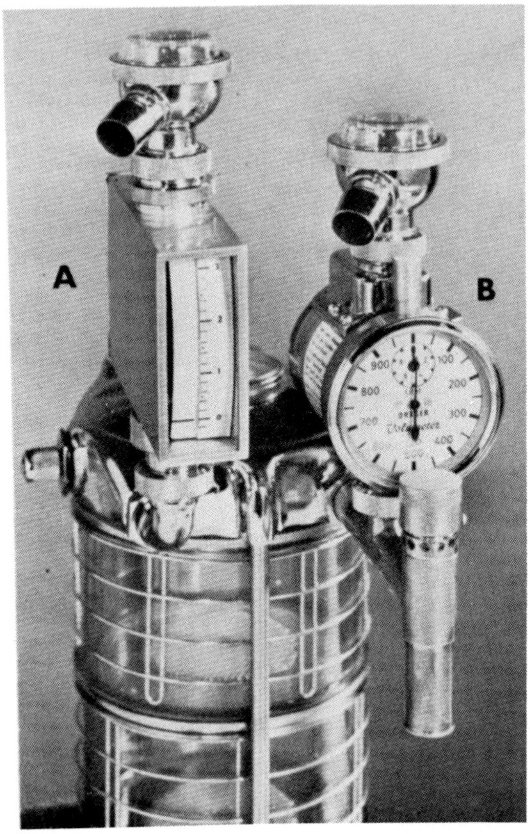

Figure 19–6. *A,* The Narkotest-M, an instrument for measuring halothane concentrations in the inhaled gas during anesthesia. *B,* The Dräger Volumeter for measuring tidal and minute volume. (Courtesy of North American Dräger, Inc., Telford, Pennsylvania.)

principle is based on the solubility of halothane in silicone elastomers.* Accuracy is reduced by concurrent use of nitrous oxide.

Monitoring the concentration of inhaled anesthetics and oxygen assures the delivery of desired concentrations. End-tidal concentrations of anesthetics provide MAC values. MAC correlated with arterial PO_2 values and the end-tidal oxygen concentrations indicate the alveolar-arterial oxygen difference.

End-tidal PCO_2 determinations indicate the effectiveness of ventilation. When ventilation remains constant, rapid changes in end-tidal PCO_2 indicate a change in either total pulmonary capillary blood flow or distribution (Burton, 1969).

During anesthesia, the end-tidal PCO_2 provides a relatively constant relationship to the arterial PCO_2, although an average difference of 4.6 to 5.0 mm Hg occurs between the two. Differences may be accentuated by hyperventilation in patients with lung disease and in patients in a lateral position. Nonperfusion of ventilated alveoli has been considered the principal cause of increased physiologic dead space with variable arterial to end-tidal PCO_2 differences (Takki et al., 1972). Using an infrared CO_2 analyzer and tracheal gas aspirated at the rate of 280 ml per minute via an endotracheal tube adapter, Hightower et al. (1980) found a strong correlation between the end-tidal CO_2 values and arterial CO_2 values ($r = 0.8$) in anesthetized dogs. This correlation was highly significant for CO_2 values between 31.3 and 61 mm Hg.

In 14 resting conscious horses, no difference was noted between tracheal end-tidal PCO_2 and carotid arterial PCO_2 values. Similar tracheal PO_2 samples were significantly higher than carotid arterial PO_2 values (Littlejohn, 1969).

Blood Oxygen

Gross arterial hypoxemia is readily recognized by cyanosis of visible mucous membranes, unpigmented skin, and exposed tissues. In man, the degree of hypoxemia is best judged by observation of the lips and buccal mucosa; the conjunctiva, nail bed, and earlobe are less satisfactory (Nunn, 1966). In anemic animals, color changes may not occur until arterial oxygen saturation has fallen as low as 55%.

Blood oxygen is measured by a polarographic technique using a modified Clark electrode, or by direct measurement of color change (oximetry). Arterial oxygen determinations are commonly used to assess the adequacy of oxygenation during anesthesia or artificial respiration and to determine the alveolar-arterial PO_2 gradient ($A\text{-}aPO_2$) as an index of venous admixture. Samples are drawn from the femoral, carotid, or lingual arteries in the small animal, and from the coccygeal, mandibular, radial, saphenous, brachial, caudal auricular, digital, carotid arteries or aorta in large animals. Oxygen values for blood samples taken from the caudal auricular artery are consistently lower than those from the brachial artery (Fisher et al., 1980).

*See Appendix A for manufacturer.

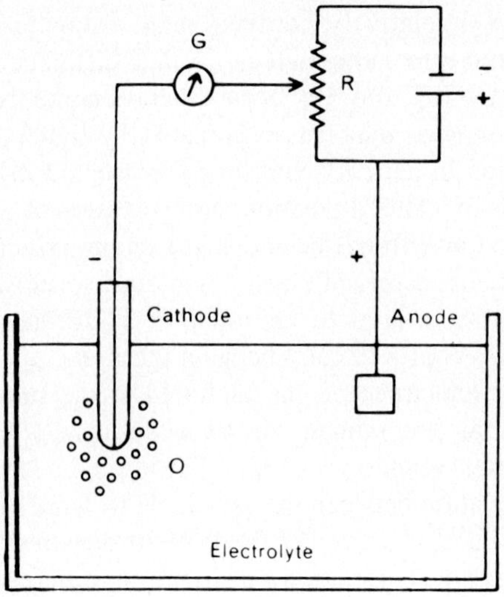

Figure 19–7. Basic arrangement of a simple oxygen polarographic cell. (From Smith, A.C., and Hahn, C.E.W.: Electrodes for the Measurement of Oxygen and Carbon Dioxide Tensions. Br. J. Anaesth., 41:731, 1969.)

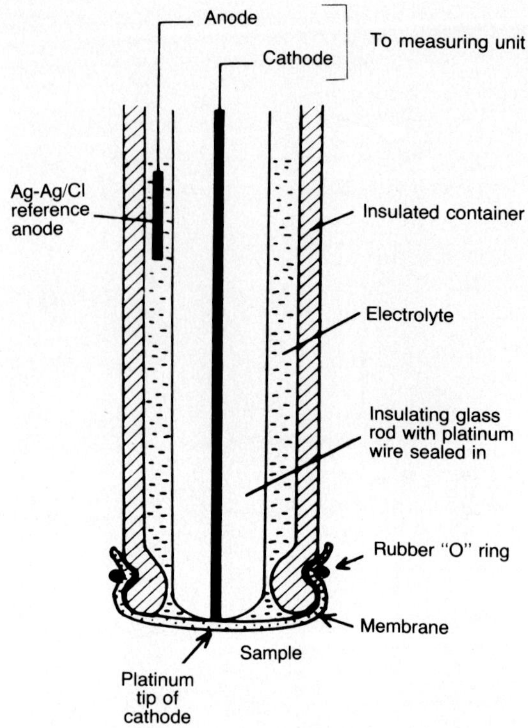

Figure 19–8. Clarke-type oxygen electrode. (From Smith, A.C., and Hahn, C.E.W.: Electrodes for the Measurement of Oxygen and Carbon Dioxide Tensions. Br. J. Anaesth., 41:731, 1969.)

Rose and Rossdale (1981) indicate that the carotid arteries of the horse are most superficial in the caudal half of the neck. Puncture requires a 21-gauge 3.75-cm needle inserted slightly above the jugular vein. Alternative sites in the conscious horse are the palmar (digital) arteries or the median artery. Arterial puncture may cause vessel spasm, intraluminal clotting, hemorrhage and, rarely, necrosis and infection. Previously cannulated vessels have a significant incidence of diminished or absent flow for limited periods of time (Shapiro et al., 1977). Cannulation is, however, necessary if repeated or continuous sampling is performed. Indwelling Po_2 electrodes mounted in the catheter tip facilitate continuous monitoring.

When the cathode of a simple polarographic cell (Fig. 19–7) is made slightly negative with reference to the anode, oxygen molecules at the cathode are electrolyzed, and the resulting current is measured by a galvanometer. The pattern of this response (polarogram) is indicative of the type and amount of substance dissolved in the electrolyte (Smith and Hahn, 1969). Because blood proteins quickly interfere with the action of a simple cathode, it is protected by a membrane (polyethylene, polypropylene, Teflon, or Mylar) permeable to oxygen but not to ionized contaminants of the blood. Such a closed electrode, the basis for current oxygen electrodes, was reported by Clarke in 1956 (Fig. 19–8). To relate measurements to body temperature, the system has been enclosed in a water bath at 37° C (Laver and Seifen, 1965).

Equipment of this type* is currently used for determining blood oxygen. Samples are collected in syringes from which the air has been expelled and in which dead space is filled with heparin solution; oxylates, EDTA, and citrates are unacceptable anticoagulants for blood gas samples. Glass syringes are advantageous owing to less friction and to greater ease in expelling air bubbles. In plastic syringes, Po_2 values in excess of 400 mm Hg drop more rapidly than in glass syringes (Shapiro et al., 1977). The syringe tip must be closed after sampling.

*See Appendix A for manufacturer.

Since blood consumes oxygen, the Po_2 is preferably measured immediately after collection; should this be impossible, the blood should be stored at 0 to 4° C and the determination made within 1 hour. Because of drift of blood gas and pH electrodes, calibration and quality assurance, at least at 4-hour intervals, are essential for accurate results (Shapiro et al., 1977). When it is necessary to use capillary blood, or small amounts of blood, the sample is collected in a heparinized capillary tube that is immediately sealed. Arterial blood is normally used for determination of the oxygen tension and, consequently, the sufficiency of the supply of oxygen to all cells of the body. Full significance is, of course, contingent upon regional perfusion, the rate at which oxygen is extracted, the susceptibility of pertinent tissues to hypoxia, hemoglobin concentration, and arterial and mean capillary pH and Pco_2 (Brewis, 1969).

In dogs, toenail blood can be used for estimating arterial blood pH, Pco_2, and standard bicarbonate level when arterial blood samples cannot be obtained. Estimation of the acid-base status of arterial blood by measuring pH, Pco_2, and standard bicarbonate in toenail blood is more accurate when systolic blood pressure is greater than 80 mm Hg (Sharpe et al., 1968). Changes in pulse pressure or subcutaneous temperature (31.8 to 38.0 C) have no significant effect on the readings. Rodkey et al. (1978) have also found arterialized capillary blood from the punctured posterior medial margin of the shaved ear to be satisfactory for determination of acid-base and blood gas status.

Determination of the mixed venous oxygen tension per se is of little significance, for the resulting value is contingent upon both the arterial tension and the efficiency and results of tissue perfusion. Abnormal lowering of the mixed venous oxygen tension relative to arterial tension does, however, imply circulatory impairment (Brewis, 1969).

Multiple sampling of the oxygen content of venous blood from individual organs may overcome many objections to the use of mixed venous blood (Brewis, 1969). In man, earlobe capillary blood has been found to correlate closely with arterial blood (Langhands and Wallace, 1965). Large discrepancies may, however, occur when capillary samples are taken from patients with autonomic upset, such as that due to cold, pain, or surgical stimulation (Adams et al., 1967). Jugular venous Po_2 levels below 30 mm Hg have been shown to reflect impaired cerebral function in man (Brewis, 1969).

An oximeter composed of an earpiece, amplifier with power supply, and recording device can measure the oxygen saturation of blood circulating through the ear of man. When blood flow is reduced, the efficiency of the unit is limited. This instrument operates on the principle that oxygenated hemoglobin transmits 70% of incident red light with a wavelength of 6400 Angstrom units, while transmission by reduced hemoglobin is negligible. This or similar devices may be used on relatively translucent appendages of animals.

Huch and Huch (1976) report that under normal conditions the Po_2 at the skin surface in man is close to 0, mainly because skin blood flow is so regulated that it supplies just the amount of oxygen needed for consumption by the skin. Thus, to monitor arterial Po_2, transcutaneous Po_2 measurements require hyperperfusion in the region being measured. The Po_2 electrode is heated to provide the required local hyperemia; the instrument reads oxygen tension in torr. It maintains the local temperature at any desired level and also measures the rate of skin cooling by capillary blood flow, which has been found to be a sensitive indicator of relative perfusion in the area. The instrument is attached to the skin by a self-adhesive ring after hair has been removed by shaving. Transcutaneous Po_2 readings and arterial Po_2 readings are not identical but correlate closely. Differences are consistent in each individual so that the instrument can be calibrated with one arterial Po_2 assay. This same apparatus can also be adapted to measure blood Pco_2 levels.

Both arterial oxygen and carbon dioxide tensions have been continuously recorded in vivo in the cat by mass spectrography. Samples were obtained via a polyethylene catheter inserted in the aorta (Woldring et al., 1966).

Other measurements used to assess oxygenation are the ventilatory parameters, the inspired oxygen concentration, the alveolar/arterial oxygen tension difference or alveolar/arterial oxygen tension ratio, total oxygen uptake, the metabolic effects of hypoxia (lactate/pyruvate, acid-base, and hepatic enzyme values), and the cardiovascular and cerebral responses.

Pulmonary evaluation and monitoring also involve the lung tissues themselves and require consideration of radiographs, physical examination, bronchoscopy, and biopsy. It is difficult to monitor pulmonary extravascular water or pulmonary edema, although it is important to do so. There are advocates for monitoring colloidal osmotic pressure as an indicator of changes in the pulmonary extravascular water (Rosenthal, 1981).

Arterial Carbon Dioxide

Arterial carbon dioxide tension is used 1) to determine the efficiency of pulmonary ventilation; 2) to calculate the dead space to expired tidal volume ratio (VD/VT); and 3) with the pH, to determine metabolic and respiratory compensation. Arterial carbon dioxide tension is commonly measured either by a Severinghaus-type electrode* or by interpolation from the acid-base state with the aid of a Siggaard-Andersen nomogram (Fig. 19–9).

The CO_2 electrode is basically a pH electrode enclosed in a bicarbonate solution by means of a membrane permeable to carbon dioxide (Figs. 19–10, 19–11).

The P_{CO_2} of the blood sample changes that of the bicarbonate solution in the electrode and, consequently, the hydrogen ion concentration of the solution. The potential across the pH-sensitive glass of the electrode likewise changes and is measured in mV. The change of pH is governed by the equation:

$$pH = constant - S \log P_{CO_2}$$

The relationship between the change of pH in the bicarbonate solution and the change in P_{CO_2} of the bicarbonate solution has been defined as the sensitivity factor (S) for the electrode. For the perfect electrode, S is equal to -1; the sensitivity of many CO_2 electrodes is close to this degree of perfection (Smith and Hahn, 1969).

*See Appendix A for manufacturer.

Blood samples are collected by direct arterial puncture, or arterialized capillary blood from a vasodilated region is an acceptable alternative. Limitations to the use of venous or capillary blood samples are similar to those described previously. When comparing the use of arterial and capillary blood samples from the horse, Littlejohn and Mitchell (1969) found that the accuracy of capillary samples was acceptable for clinical investigation of pH, but not for P_{CO_2} or HCO_3^- (Table 19–1).

Blood pH

Measurement of blood pH (arterial or capillary samples) is accomplished by means of a glass electrode similar to that incorporated in the P_{CO_2} electrode (see Figs. 19–10, 19–11). The active element within the electrode is a glass membrane, consisting of a three-dimensional lattice of silicon and oxygen atoms that hold cations of alkali metals within the mesh (Adams et al., 1967). Hydrogen ions from a sample pass into the lattice, displace the metallic cations, and set up an electromotive force across the glass membrane, which is compared with a mercury calomel reference electrode. Connection of the glass and reference electrodes is usually via a salt bridge solution of potassium chloride (Adams et al., 1968). The conventional glass electrode has been modified to permit development of the microelectrode.

Since variations may result from a number of sources, including accumulation of proteins and colloids on the electrode, and since the electrodes are temperature-sensitive, determinations should be made at 37° C and the system should be tested periodically.

Plotting of pH against log P_{CO_2} allows, with the aid of a nomogram, determination of the acid-base status (see Fig. 19–9). The CO_2-bicarbonate diagram (Campbell et al., 1968) also provides a useful means for visualizing the acid-base status of a patient (Fig. 19–12). For additional information regarding blood gases, pH, and acid-base status, reference should be made to Chapter 6 and reviews by Adams et al. (1967;

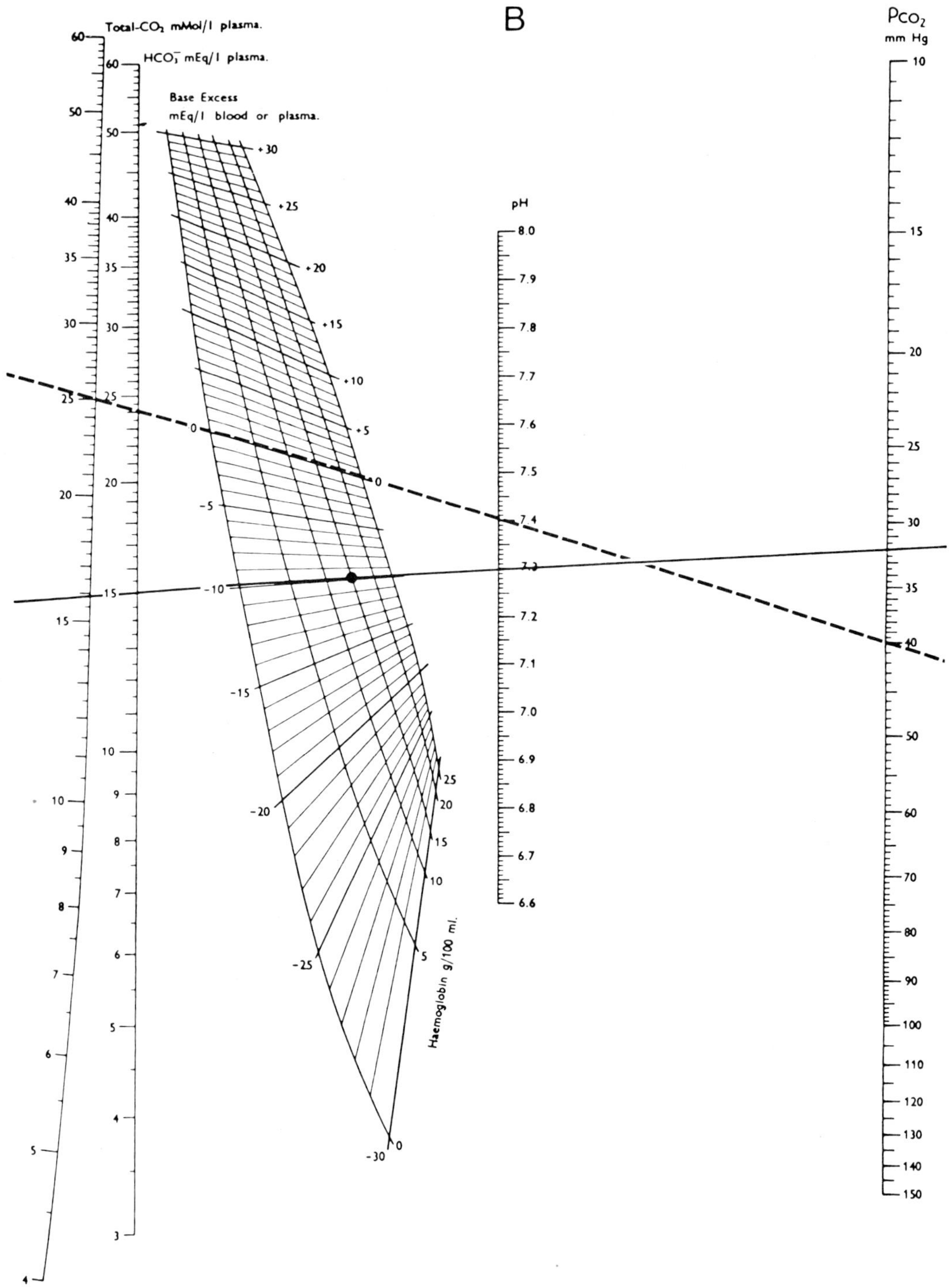

Figure 19–9. Alignment nomogram. Dotted line is normal acid-base balance. Continuous line is an example of a calculation. If determined $Paco_2$ = 32, pH = 7.29, and hemoglobin = 15, base excess would be −10 mEq/L. If the formulas described under Alkalinizing Agents, Chapter 20, are used, the amount of bicarbonate or tromethamine needed to correct the imbalance can be calculated. (From Siggaard-Andersen, O.: Blood Acid-Base Alignment Nomogram. Scandinav. J. Clin. Lab. Invest., 15:211, 1963.)

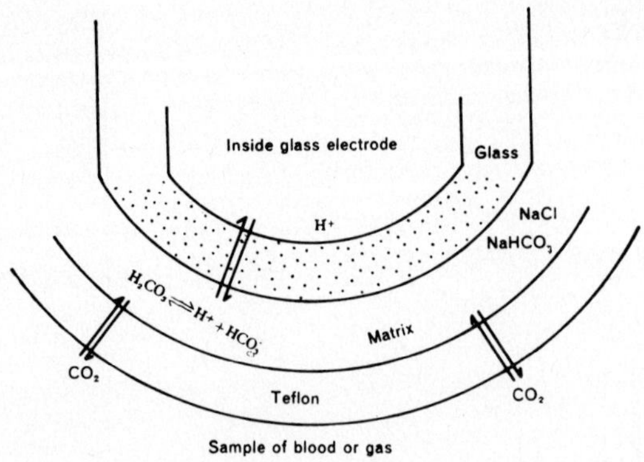

Figure 19–10. Diagram of tip of carbon dioxide electrode. (From Smith, A.C., and Hahn, C.E.W.: Electrodes for the Measurement of Oxygen and Carbon Dioxide Tensions. Br. J. Anaesth., 41:731, 1969.)

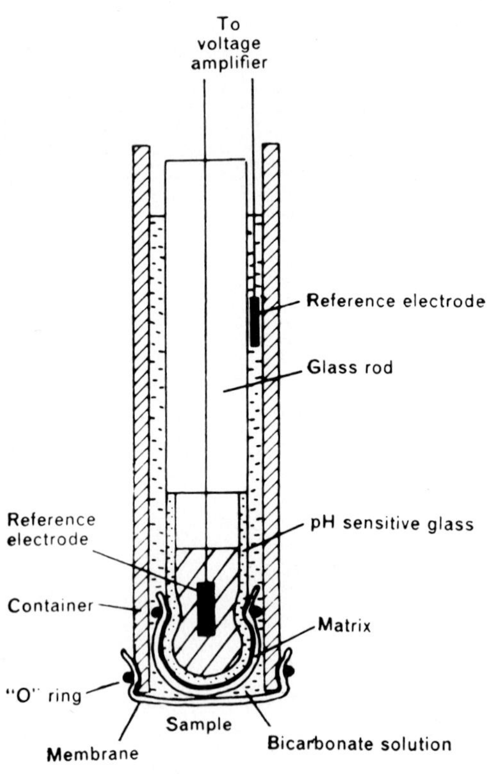

Figure 19–11. Diagram of carbon dioxide electrode. (From Smith, A.C., and Hahn, C.E.W.: Electrodes for the Measurement of Oxygen and Carbon Dioxide Tensions. Br. J Anaesth., 41:731, 1969.)

1968), Smith and Hahn (1969), Bear and Gribik (1974) and Cornelius (1981).

CIRCULATION

Pulse

The rate and force of the pulse have long been used as an indication of the state of the cardiovascular system. A fast, weak pulse is present in shock and is a sign of impending vascular collapse.

The pulse in most animals can be felt, depending on the species, in one or more of the following arteries: mandibular, radial, carotid, digital, femoral, and coccygeal. Electronic pulse detection is discussed in the section on blood pressure. Variations of the pulse or heart rate provide useful information regarding the status and safety of surgical anesthesia (see Chap. 5).

Monitoring the pulse pressure contour as an indication of cardiac output and stroke volume has been reviewed by Prys-Roberts (1969).

Heart Rate

The heart rate can be obtained by means of a stethoscope taped to the patient's chest in the area of the apex beat. A more reliable method is to insert an esophageal stethoscope in the esophageal lumen to the cardiac region (Fig. 19–13). It should be pointed out that heart and pulse rates are not always the same, since a pulse deficit may exist.

Cardiac rate meters that can be connected to the patient by conventional electrocardiographic leads are available. The peak of the QRS signal is used to trigger the meter, which indicates the rate. The monitor can be preset to acceptable upper and lower limits of heart rate. If the rate exceeds or declines below these limits, an audible alarm sounds and a flashing red light may be activated.

Electrocardiography

Despite the advent of numerous other monitoring devices, the electrocardiogram remains an important and practical monitor during anesthesia. It provides immediate information re-

TABLE 19–1. Comparison of Arterial and Capillary Sample Results in Horses

	pH			P_{CO_2} mm Hg			(HCO_3^-)		
Condition of Horses	*Art.*	*Cap.*	*A-c*	*Art*	*Cap.*	*A-c*	*Art.*	*Cap.*	*A-c*
Clinically normal	7.390	7.410	−0.020	37.0	41.5	−4.5	21.9	25.6	−3.7
Laryngeal hemiplegia	7.390	7.390	0	48.0	48.0	0	28.4	28.4	0
Clinically normal	7.410	7.410	0	47.0	46.5	+0.5	29.1	28.9	+0.2
Severe wound	7.370	7.350	+0.020	50.0	50.0	0	28.3	27.1	+0.2
Clinically normal	7.400	7.385	+0.015	45.0	47.5	−2.5	27.2	27.7	−0.5
Clinically normal	7.420	7.365	+0.055	43.0	48.0	−5.0	27.3	26.9	+0.4
Laryngeal hemiplegia	7.430	7.420	+0.010	46.5	44.0	+2.5	30.2	27.9	+2.3
Partial posterior paresis	7.400	7.380	+0.020	44.0	45.0	−1.0	26.6	26.0	+0.6
Clinically normal	7.405	7.390	+0.015	45.0	43.0	+2.0	27.6	25.5	+2.1
Severe wound	7.410	7.400	+0.010	51.5	48.5	+3.0	32.0	29.4	+2.6
Clinically normal	7.435	7.430	+0.005	43.5	45.0	−1.5	28.6	29.4	−0.8
Chronic diarrhea	7.285	7.300	−0.015	42.5	38.5	+4.0	19.5	18.4	+1.1
Means	7.395	7.386	+0.009	45.08	45.46	−0.38	27.2	26.76	+0.46
Standard deviations of differences			±0.0194			±2.83			±1.76
Correlation coefficient 'r'	0.85 ($P < 0.001$)			0.694 ($P < 0.02$)			0.870 ($P < 0.001$)		

(From Littlejohn, A., and Mitchell, B.: Acid-Base and Blood Gas Studies in Horses. I. A Comparison of Capillary and Arterial Blood Samples for the Estimation of Acid-Base Values in Horses. Res. Vet. Sci., 10:260, 1969.)

garding cardiac rate and rhythm and myocardial oxygenation, but does not reflect the adequacy of cardiac output (Michenfelder, 1968).

Analysis of the ECG is based on the amplitude and direction of deflection and the duration of components. Normal and abnormal variations occur in the ECG. From the standpoint of anesthesia, the ECG can give useful information in two ways. Electrocardiography should be employed diagnostically in suspected instances of heart disease prior to anesthesia. During the anesthetic period, electrocardiography is a means of monitoring the heart. In this instance, the ECG is usually displayed on an oscilloscope, so that aberrations in the ECG during anesthesia and cardiac manipulation can immediately be detected and corrective steps taken (see Chaps. 20 and 21). A strip chart recorder may be attached to provide permanent records of relevant recordings.

In diagnostic electrocardiography, the electrical flow in the heart is measured from several points or leads on the body. In monitoring anesthesia, only one lead is generally used, the most informative in most species being lead II. This is a bipolar lead between the right forelimb and left hindlimb. With this lead, electric potentials flowing toward the hindlimb produce positive deflections, whereas those flowing toward the right forelimb cause negative deflections. In the dog, Sattler (1965) recommends the electrode placement as indicated in Figure 19–14. In contrast, Hamlin (1976) recommends leads on all four limbs and two positions on the chest monitored separately. He recommends noninvasive contacts rather than hypodermic needles or clips, which may cause artifacts in the recording. They are, however, the only practical contacts in small laboratory animals. Whatever lead is used, an easily recognizable P-wave is necessary to establish the relationship of atrial to ventricular depolarization and thus the origin of arrhythmias that may occur (Michenfelder, 1968).

As an ECG is produced, a repetitive analog recording of cardiac electrical impulses, which is time-related, is formed. At the commonly used paper speed of 25 mm/sec, the distance between two heavy lines represents 1/5 second (0.2 sec). The distance between two closely spaced lines is 1/25 second (0.04 sec.). The background grid printed on the paper contains 1-mm squares. Time intervals are measured by counting millimeter (or 5-mm) squares horizontally and converting into seconds by multiplying by 0.04. Oscilloscopes for monitoring the ECG generally display a direct digital readout of the heart rate.

Voltage measurements are made vertically in millivolts. The electrocardiograph is initially

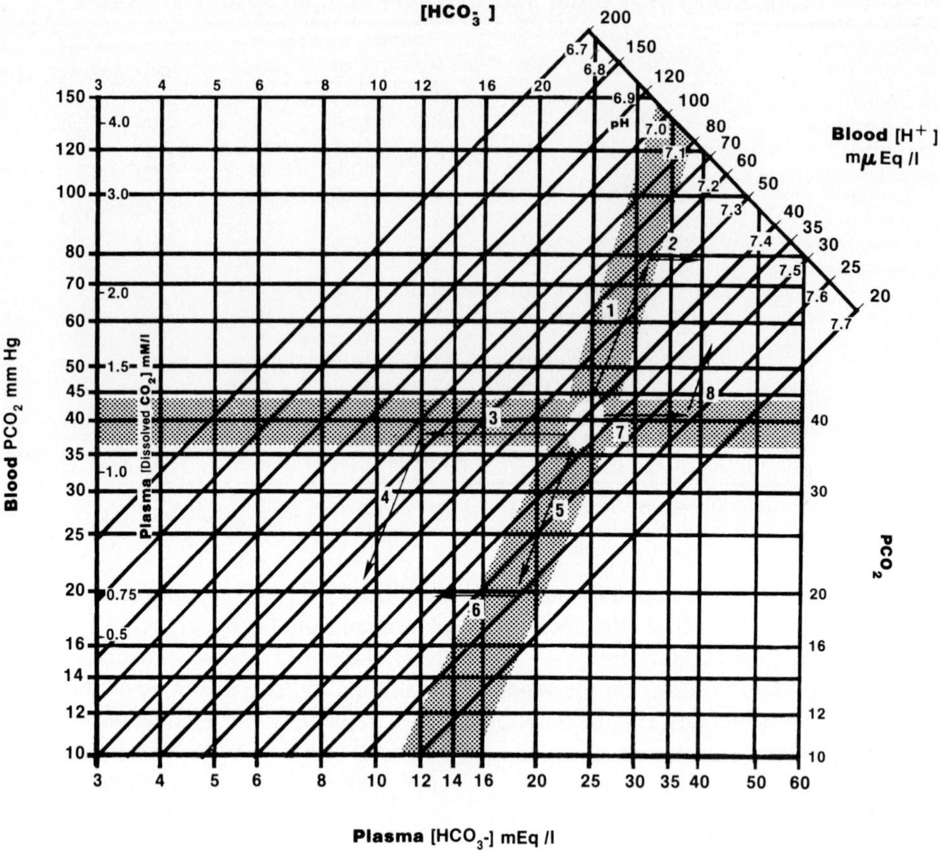

Figure 19–12. The CO_2/bicarbonate diagram. Note the progress of a patient by serial estimations. Arrow 1, Respiratory acidosis. Arrow 2, Compensatory metabolic alkalosis. Arrow 3, Metabolic acidosis. Arrow 4, Compensatory respiratory alkalosis. Arrow 5, Respiratory alkalosis. Arrow 6, Compensatory metabolic acidosis. Arrow 7, Metabolic alkalosis. Arrow 8, Compensatory respiratory acidosis. (From Lee, J.A., and Atkinson, R.S.: *A Synopsis of Anaesthesia,* 6th ed. Williams & Wilkins, Baltimore, 1968.)

calibrated so that each millimeter square represents 0.01 millivolt or 10 squares = 1.0 millivolt.

Normal values for electrocardiograms in various species of animals have been determined by many investigators (Table 19–2). Data are given for the common arrhythmias and conduction disturbances reported in domestic animals by Buchanan (1965). Some are regarded as normal in specific species. Examples are sinus arrhythmia in dogs, and wandering pacemaker, S-A block, and incomplete A-V block with dropped beats in horses. In a survey of dogs, the ratio of one or more spontaneous abnormal arrhythmias and conduction disturbances was 32/1000 in a 3000-dog sample.

Equidae are believed to have a higher incidence of cardiac arrhythmias at rest than any other domestic species (Hilwig, 1977). During anesthesia and surgery, artifacts may arise owing to disconnection of an electrode, superimposition of a potential from personnel, improper grounding, electrocautery, diathermy, and surgical manipulations. Should cardiac arrest occur, the ECG differentiates between asystole and ventricular fibrillation. Intraoperative electrocardiographic tracings obtained during equine monitoring are summarized in Table 19–3. A portable system for monitoring both cardiovascular and respiratory function in large animals has been described by Kvart et al. (1982).

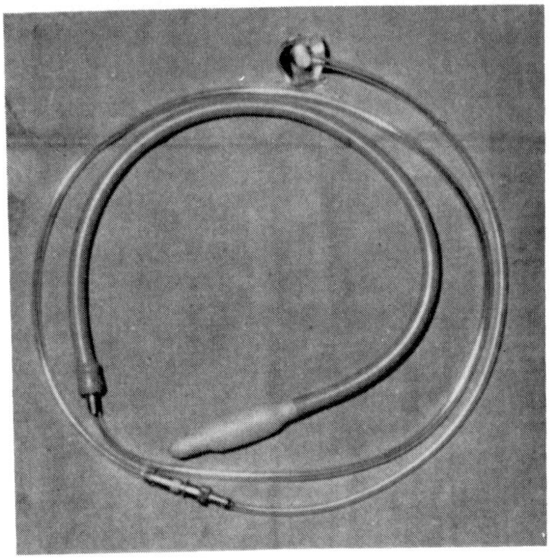

Figure 19–13. The esophageal stethoscope is composed of an acoustical transducer connected to an earpiece. In use, the transducer is inserted in the esophagus to heart level. (Courtesy of Dr. N.R. Cholvin, Iowa State University, Ames, Iowa.)

Diagnoses and treatment of cardiac arrhythmias and arrest are discussed in Chapter 21.

Blood Pressure

One of the most useful determinations made during anesthesia in man is that of arterial blood pressure. Unfortunately, the method of indirect measurement used has not been readily applicable to animals and, until recent years, the determination of blood pressure in anesthetized animals has been largely ignored. The difficulties associated with indirect measurement in animals are those of hearing, feeling, or visualization of vascular changes with traditional methods used in man. Now, however, blood pressure can be measured indirectly with the aid of microphones for sound, pressure transducers for pulse (plethysmograph), ultrasound to detect arterial wall movement, and photoelectric transducers for skin color (Coulter et al., 1981) (Figs. 19–15, 19–16).

Two methods for indirect blood pressure measurement have had application for some time. Both of these utilize a pressure cuff and an electronic pulse detection and indication system. One operates on the principle that the volume of blood in a vessel network fluctuates with each cardiac cycle. This can be detected by observing changes in the transmittance of a beam of light passing through the network (Robinson and Eastwood, 1959). With a sensitive crystal photocell, low-intensity light source, and an amplifier, fluctuations can be detected in any tissue through which light can be transmitted. In operation, a photocell lamp assembly is clipped on a toe or other appendage, and the light intensity and amplifier gain are adjusted until fluctuations are recorded. A blood pressure cuff is then placed around the limb and inflated until fluctuations disappear. Pressure is slowly lowered until fluctuations reappear, at which point cuff pressure approximates systolic blood pressure. By proper connections, the system can be attached to a recorder, oscilloscope, or speaker if so desired.

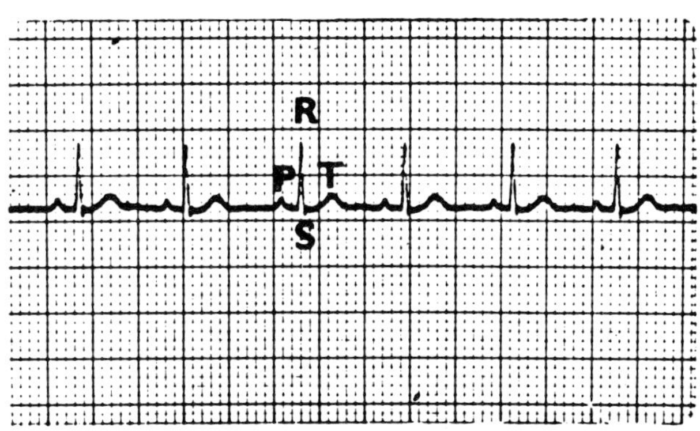

Figure 19–14. Normal monitoring lead QRST complex; active electrode placement mucosa of lip and vulva, ground electrode opposite lip. (From Sattler, F.P.: Monitoring the Canine Electrocardiogram in Clinical Aspects of Canine Cardiology. Am. Anim. Hosp. Assoc., 1965.)

TABLE 19–2. The Electrocardiogram of Various Mammals

Animal	*Rate*	*P-R Interval*	*QRS*	*Q-T Interval*
Mouse	650–900	0.05	0.015	0.06
Rat	380–520	0.05	0.02	0.08
Guinea pig	200–325	0.06–0.07	0.03	0.12
Rabbit	170–280	0.06–0.10	0.03	0.18
Cat	110–130	0.08	0.03	0.18
Goat	70–120	0.12–0.14	0.05	0.26–0.32
Sheep	52–100	0.08	0.04	0.24
Pig	80–90	0.12–0.14	0.06	0.22–0.28
Donkey	60–80	0.20	0.06	0.40–0.44
Cow	60–80	0.16–0.30	0.08–0.12	0.36–0.44
Bull	36–60	0.16–0.20	0.08–0.10	0.36–0.40
Horse	24–50	0.35–0.42	0.08–0.12	0.40–0.60
Elephant	24–53	0.28–0.35	0.12–0.18	0.52–0.70
Dog	70–120	0.06–0.15	0.03–0.07	0.12–0.23

(From Severin, G.A.: Veterinary Cardiology Notes. Colorado State University, Fort Collins, 1971.)

The second method operates on the same principle, except that it picks up the Korotkoff sounds and pulse waves by means of a displacement condenser microphone placed over an artery and held without pressure by tape (Weinreb et al., 1960). If such equipment is not available to detect Korotkoff sounds, the manometer needle may be observed for oscillations. These begin several mm Hg higher than systolic pressure. A general measurement is thus obtained.

More recently, an ultrasonic Doppler sensing device* has been used to detect arterial wall movement. All of these indirect techniques require use of a location adequate for application of an inflatable cuff to occlude a regional artery. Although cuff size may influence such measurements, attention to technique and repeatability are more important and permit detection of relative changes. Use of the ultrasonic Doppler technique has been found reliable in several species (Coulter et al., 1981; Hahn et al., 1973). When one compares ultrasonic and photoelectric* methods in the dog, photoelectric systolic pressures are lower and diastolic pressures higher than respective ultrasonic pressures. Use of a tail-cuff plethysmographic method has been

TABLE 19–3. Intraoperative Electrocardiographic Tracings in the Horse

Normal	*Artifact*	*Abnormal*	*Causes of Abnormalities*
Notched P wave Inverted T wave Rate: 30 to 50 beats per minute	60-Cycle interference Diathermy Baseline changes with respiration Muscle fasciculations Movement of surgical instruments Disconnection of lead	1. Rate; bradycardia, <30 beats per minute; tachycardia, >50 beats per minute 2. Rhythm: sinus dysrhythmia; artrioventricular block; ventricular extrasystole 3. Arrest: asystole; fibrillation	Surgical stimulus Anesthetic agent Myocardial sensitization to catecholamines: endogenous or exogenous Premedication Anesthetic depth Hypoxia Hypercapnia Hypocapnia Hypotension Hypertension Electrolyte abnormalities Acid-base abnormalities Adjunct drugs such as succinylcholine, adrenergic drugs Vagal reflexes Altered body temperature Excessive volume replacement

(From Manley, S.V.: Monitoring the Anesthetized Horse. Vet. Clin. N. Am., 3:115, 1975.)

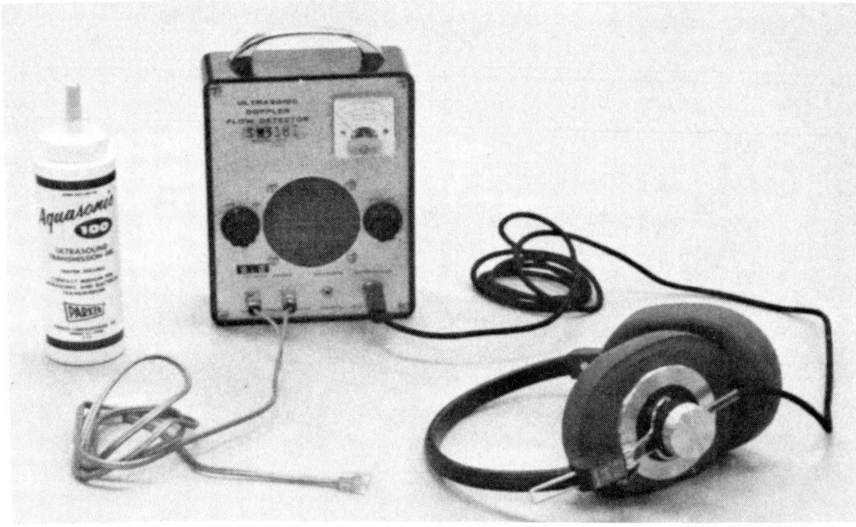

Figure 19–15. Doppler apparatus used for indirect blood pressure measurement. The apparatus consists of battery box, earphones, and small, plastic-covered transducer pickup. The Doppler effect is utilized to determine rate of blood flow by directing a source of ultrasound against the moving bloodstream and measuring the change in frequency of the reflected ultrasound waves that bounce back from the moving column of blood. (Ultrasonic Doppler Flow Detector, Parks Electronics Laboratory, Beaverton, Oregon.) (From Sattler, F.P., Knowles, R.P., and Whittick, W.G.: *Veterinary Critical Care*. Lea & Febiger, Philadelphia, 1981.)

found satisfactory in the rat and cat (Mahoney and Brody, 1978).

Direct measurement of arterial blood pressure is now being used with increasing frequency in animals. It is most easily accomplished by percutaneous insertion of an indwelling catheter.* In large animals, incision of the skin to allow insertion of the catheter may be necessary. Preferred arteries for percutaneous catheterization include the femoral in small animals, the mandibular, carotid, or digital in the horse, the coccygeal in cattle, and the radial in primates. The catheter is filled with sterile heparinized saline and connected via tubing directly to a manometer (Fig. 19–17) or to a pressure transducer and recording or monitoring device. The latter is preferable, often providing immediate display of both blood pressure and ECG, and thus their correlation.

Central Venous Pressure

Determination of the central venous pressure (CVP) provides a valuable indication of the efficacy of cardiac function in relation to the volume of circulating blood. By monitoring CVP, it is possible to determine the adequacy of fluid and blood replacement and to recognize ineffective cardiac pumping. Since the venous system contains 70 to 80% of the blood volume, changes in venous tone significantly affect circulatory hemodynamics. Venous tone is increased by skin stimulation, hypocapnia, intermittent positive-pressure-ventilation, low arterial pressure, catecholamines, cardiac failure, and cold; it is decreased by sleep, hypercapnia, ganglionic blocking drugs, thiopental, histamine, nitrites, and warmth (Atkinson et al., 1977).

CVP is monitored by means of a catheter in the anterior or posterior vena cava, which is attached to a saline manometer* (Fig. 19–18). For accurate CVP measurements, the catheter *must* be located in the cava close to the heart, since smaller veins contain valves that affect the pressure. To avoid errors, the zero point of the manometer *must* be level with the patient's right atrium and *must* be adjusted if the patient moves. An inexpensive line level, available at hardware stores, will aid in accomplishing this.

*See Appendix A for manufacturer.

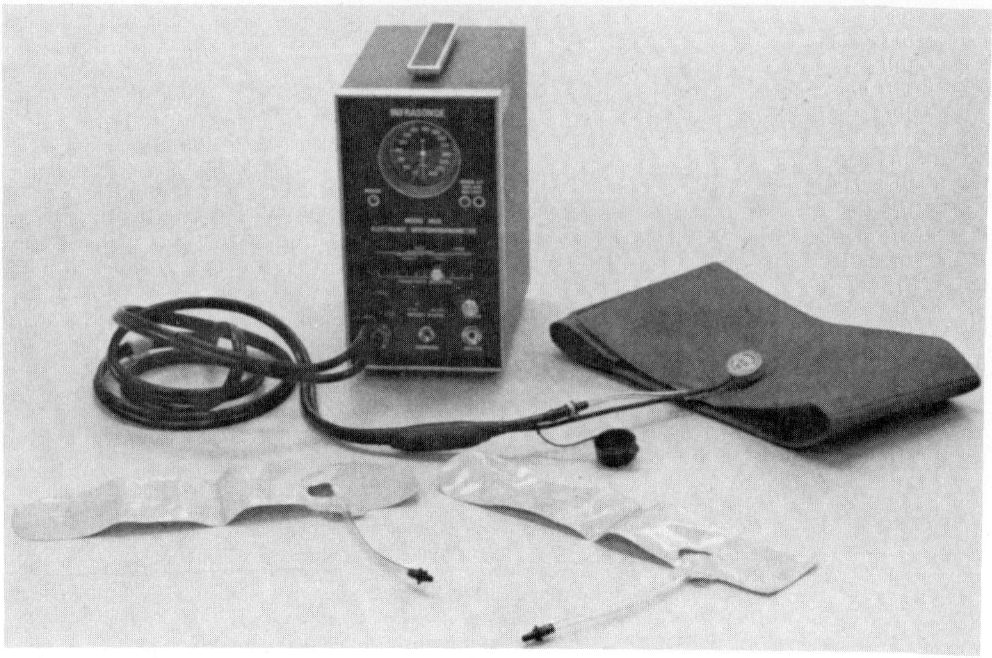

Figure 19–16. An electronic blood pressure monitor (Infrasonde) can be used to monitor blood pressure in animals. The instrument detects arterial wall flutter at subaudible frequencies. The signal is then converted to an AM-FM modulated audio tone for easy systolic determinations. In animals, diastolic determinations are not as reliable. Cuffs of several sizes are available to accommodate various leg sizes. (From Sattler, F.P., Knowles, R.P., and Whittick, W.G.: *Veterinary Critical Care.* Lea & Febiger, Philadelphia, 1981.)

Commercially available CVP sets contain a built-in level. The catheter is inserted percutaneously into the jugular or cephalic vein, and the tip is advanced until it reaches the anterior vena cava. When the catheter enters the thorax, pressure fluctuations occur in relation to respiration. Pressure fluctuations are accentuated when the catheter enters the atrium of the heart, and passage into the ventricle may initiate ventricular arrhythmias.

Pressure readings fluctuate with cardiac and respiratory cycles. In the dog and cat, CVP ranges from 3 to 7.5 cm of H_2O regardless of body position. In the horse there is significant variation because of body position. The normal standing horse and laterally recumbent horse have similar values (12 $\pm$ 6 cm H_2O), whereas values of 25 to 30 cm H_2O are not unusual in dorsal recumbency (Manley, 1981).

Monitoring the central venous pressure is indicated especially in shock, in patients requiring the infusion of large amounts of fluid or blood, and in acute circulatory failure. It indicates the adequacy of fluid replacement, the onset of overloading, and the ability of the right side of the heart to tolerate and eject a fluid load. It does not indicate the functional efficiency of the left side of the heart.

Measurement of pulmonary artery wedge pressure is discussed in the section on cardiac output.

Cardiac Output

Owing to the difficulties involved, measurement of cardiac output is not routinely used to monitor the circulation. Instead, blood pressure and electrocardiographic monitoring are used despite the truth of the statement of Jarisch in 1928 (cited by Prys-Roberts, 1969):

> It is a source of regret that the measurement of flow is so much more difficult than the measurement of pressure. This has led to an undue interest in the blood pressure manom-

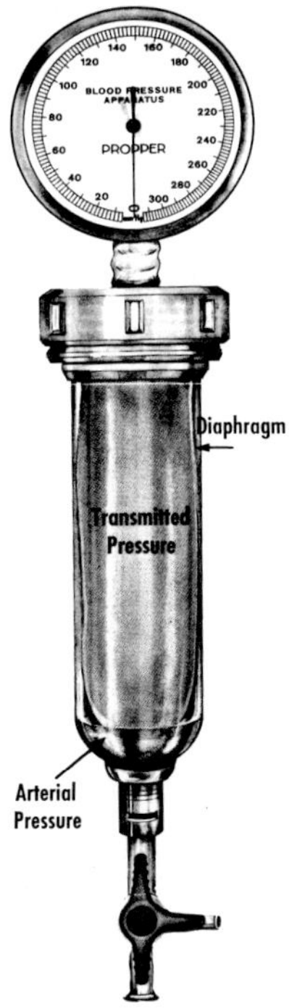

Figure 19–17. An arterial pressure monitor. In use, an arterial cannula filled with heparinized saline is attached to the connector (bottom). Arterial pressure is transmitted through the diaphragm and registers on the dial. (Courtesy of U.S. Catheter and Instrument Corporation, Glens Falls, New York.)

> eter. More organs, however, require flow rather than pressure. . . .

Methods for determination of cardiac output (CO) commonly involve the use of indicator or thermodilution techniques. Use of the Fick principle is not usually practical during anesthesia.

Rosenthal (1981) has briefly summarized the important factors relative to cardiac output monitoring. A balance between intravascular volume, cardiac output, and vascular resistance must be achieved for tissue perfusion sufficient to maintain aerobic metabolism. Adequate cardiac output is vital and is contingent upon preload, contractility, afterload, and heart rate. Preload is the end-diastolic volume (EDV) in either ventricle. The ventricular end-diastolic pressure (EDP) is used as a measure of preload. Monitoring this allows for interpretation of the adequacy of intravascular volume in relation to myocardial performance. Monitoring filling pressure alone is insufficient; the measurement of stroke volume with EDP is also required.

Pulmonary artery wedge pressure (PAWP) is determined by insertion of a catheter, via a peripheral vein, through the right side of the heart and into a branch of the pulmonary artery. It is passed to the point where its circumference exceeds the lumen of the branch and it becomes wedged. It thus measures the back pressure from the left ventricle (left ventricular end-diastolic pressure). This value indicates left ventricular function.

The importance of monitoring PAWP is based on the requirement for adequate left heart output to perfuse the heart, brain, kidney, and splanchnic circulation, and the lack of correlation between the left and right heart preload values in many disease states. The CVP may indicate normovolemia or hypervolemia even though PAWP may be low, necessitating volume therapy to insure adequate stroke volume (SV). It is important to optimize preload relative to stroke volume.

Introduction of the flow-directed thermistor-tipped pulmonary artery catheter (Swan-Ganz) permits pulmonary artery wedge and central venous pressure monitoring and cardiac output measurement by thermodilution. A known amount of sterile cold solution is injected into the right atrium, and the resultant temperature change is detected by the thermistor in the pulmonary artery. This allows calculation of cardiac output. With arterial pressure monitoring, this technique provides for continuous and accurate hemodynamic assessment. Unless there is increased pulmonary vascular resistance or tachycardia, pulmonary artery diastolic pressure (PADP) correlates well with PAWP. Complications of pulmonary artery catheterization include arrhythmias, infection, venous thrombosis, pulmonary infarcts, and perforation.

Afterload is the wall tension in the ventricle at the time of ejection. Monitoring is best accomplished in terms of its major determinant: impedance to ventricular output. In the absence of ventricular outlet obstruction, pulmonary and systemic vascular resistance is monitored as right- or left-side afterload, respectively.

$$\text{PVR} = \frac{\text{PAWP}}{\text{CO}} \times 80 \text{ and SVR} = \text{MAP} - \frac{\text{CVP}}{\text{CO}} \times 80$$

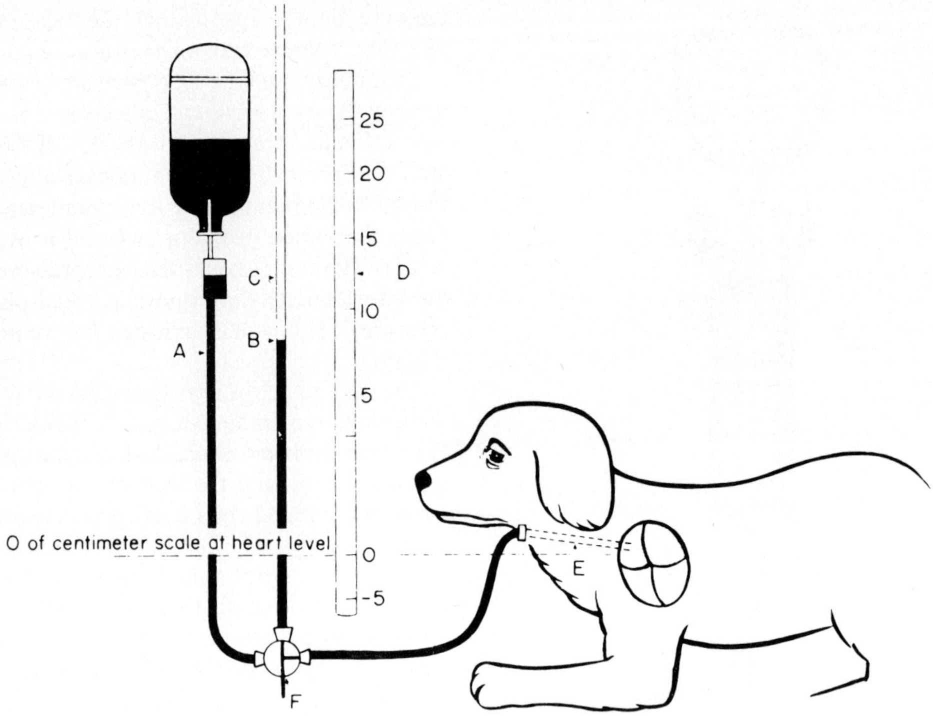

Figure 19–18. Central venous pressure manometer: *A,* standard intravenous infusion tube; *B,* central venous pressure level; *C,* 30-in intravenous extension tube; *D,* centimeter scale; *E,* plastic tube in great veins in thorax or right atrium via jugular vein; *F,* three-way stopcock set in measuring position (open from manometer to catheter). (From Kirk, R.W.: *Current Veterinary Therapy III—Small Animal Practice.* W.B. Saunders Co., Philadelphia, 1968.)

where SVR = systemic vascular resistance, PVR = pulmonary vascular resistance, MAP = mean arterial pressure, and units = dynes per second per centimeter to 5 power.

Preload, contractility, afterload, and heart rate all contribute to myocardial oxygen demand, which must be balanced against oxygen supply. Because 70% of coronary perfusion occurs during diastole, the time for diastole as well as diastolic pressure is indeed important. The diastolic pressure time index (DPTI), the area under the diastolic portion of the arterial pressure waveform, is used as a measurement of myocardial oxygen delivery. The rate pressure product (heart rate × systolic pressure) is used as an indicator of myocardial oxygen demand.

Blood and Extracellular Fluid Volume

In examining the patient prior to anesthesia, one should assess fluid and electrolyte balance. Criteria have been developed, based on physical examination, to aid in quantitating the amount of fluid deficit (Table 19–4). Measurement of serum electrolytes is also needed to determine the type of imbalance that may be present.

Serum sodium determinations give a useful index of extracellular fluid tonicity and volume. A close approximation of total solute concentration of serum (mOsm/L) can be obtained by doubling the serum sodium concentration in milliequivalents per liter. A closer approximation can be obtained with the following formula (Wingfield, 1984):

$$\text{Plasma osmolality (mOsm)} = 1.86\ ((\text{Na}^+ + \text{K}^+)\ (\text{mg/dl})) + \frac{\text{Glucose (mg/dl)}}{18} + \frac{\text{Blood Urea Nitrogen (mg/dl)}}{2.8} + 9$$

Normal values fall between 290 and 310 mOsm; tolerable limits are from 270 to 330 mOsm. Hyponatremia is the only cause of hypo-os-

TABLE 19–4. Estimation of the Degree of Dehydration as a Percentage of Body Weight from Physical Examination

Percentage of Dehydration	*Physical Examination Findings*
<5%	No abnormalities.
5%	Slightly "doughy" inelasticity of skin.
7%	Definite inelasticity of skin; capillary refilling time 2 to 3 seconds*; slight depression of eye into orbit.
10–12%	Severe skin inelasticity; capillary refilling time >3 seconds; markedly sunken eyeballs; shock in debilitated animals; involuntary muscle twitching.
12–15%	Marked shock; imminent death.

*Normal capillary refilling time = 1½ to 2 seconds.
(From Cornelius, L.M.: Fluid, Electrolyte, Acid-Base, and Nutritional Management. In *Pathophysiology in Small Animal Surgery.* Edited by M.J. Bojrab. Lea & Febiger, Philadelphia, 1981.)

molality. Hyperosmolality may be caused by hypernatremia or an increase in concentration of other osmotically active particles (Haskins, 1981). For further information on fluid, electrolyte, and nutritional balance, the reader is referred to Cornelius (1981).

Other laboratory tests that will aid in determining the state of hydration include packed cell volume (PCV) and the total solids (TS) concentration in plasma. Persistently high PCV and TS readings occur with dehydration and inadequate replacement; however, these are tests of the plasma space only and do not reflect the entire extracellular fluid space (EFS). When total plasma protein is below 3.5 g/dl, the colloid oncotic pressure of the vascular compartment may be jeopardized, and further volume therapy should be in the form of plasma or a colloid solution, such as dextran.

Blood Loss

When major blood loss occurs or is anticipated, measurement of the amount lost facilitates accurate replacement. A rough estimate of blood loss can be obtained by counting the sponges used. The average 4 × 4 sponge will contain 10 ml of blood; the average 12 × 12 laparotomy pad will contain 50 to 75 ml.

Determination of blood loss by weighing sponges and drapes before and after surgery, by measuring the amount of blood within the suction bottle, and by estimating that on the floor is relatively efficient when conscientiously performed. The amount of blood in drapes and sponges can also be determined by placing them in electrolyte solutions or in water and by measuring the change in conductance or the amount of hemoglobin by colorimetry. Monitors that automatically determine the amount of blood in sponges and drapes by these techniques are available (Klopstock et al., 1959).

The above techniques compare favorably with determination of blood loss by measurement of the blood volume before and after surgery. The development of rapid techniques utilizing radioactive-iodine-dilution methods and automatic counting of the radioactive blood sample* have made this technique less cumbersome.

Serial hematocrit determinations or weighing the patient before and after surgery have been found inefficient when compared with gravimetric or colorimetric techniques and with determination of the blood volume (Moore et al., 1965). Although the latter techniques may be advantageous where major surgical procedures are frequently performed, sound clinical judgment based on the pulse, the central venous and arterial pressures, and the circulatory response to fluid and blood replacement is preferred.

Blood Anesthetic Levels

Inhalation anesthetics in blood may be determined by chromatographic analysis. Cole et al. (1975) have described a simple heated-precolumn device for such analysis. Whole blood containing an internal standard is directly injected into the device. Results are obtained rapidly and have acceptable accuracy.

URINE OUTPUT

In shock, prolonged anesthesia, or compromised kidney function, monitoring of urine output is indicated. At arterial blood pressures below 60 mm Hg, urine flow ceases. Based

*See Appendix A for manufacturer.

TABLE 19–5. Volumes and Specific Gravities of Urine

Animal	Volume (ml/kg body wt/day)	Specific Gravity Mean and Range
Cat	10–20	1.030 (1.020–1.040)
Cattle	17–45	1.032 (1.030–1.045)
Dog	20–100	1.025 (1.016–1.060)
Goat	10–40	1.030 (1.015–1.045)
Horse	3–18	1.040 (1.025–1.060)
Sheep	10–40	1.030 (1.015–1.045)
Swine	5–30	1.012 (1.010–1.050)
Man	8.6–28.6	1.020 (1.002–1.040)

(From Gans, J.H., and Mercer, P.F.: The Kidneys. In *Dukes' Physiology of Domestic Animals*, 9th ed. Edited by M.J. Swenson. Copyright © 1977 by Cornell University. Used by permission of the publisher, Cornell University Press.)

upon the output, intravenous fluid administration can be adjusted to maintain a proper blood pressure for urine flow.

The patient should be catheterized and the urine collected in a calibrated container. Output determinations should be made at 15-minute intervals or longer, depending upon the need. Specific gravity measurements and urinalyses can also be performed if necessary. Table 19–5 lists urine outputs and specific gravities of common species. In the dog, a flow of 1 to 2 ml/kg/hr is considered adequate.

Urine output is a reflection of cardiovascular and renal homeostasis. A low output may be due to several factors, such as dehydration, premedication or concurrent medication, use of inhalant anesthetics, reduced cardiac output, and renal disease (Bastron, 1981). High output is generally due to overzealous fluid administration, and is an indication to slow the flow rate.

TEMPERATURE

Determination of body temperature may be of interest under many conditions during anesthesia (see Chap. 21) and is essential in hypothermia.

For routine use, a conventional rectal thermometer is adequate. It should be realized, however, that it has certain shortcomings. It is inconvenient to read repeatedly and almost impossible to observe if the patient is draped for surgery. The temperature of the liver and other deep organs is always 1° or 2° C higher than the rectum. In addition, feces in the rectum insulate the thermometer from rapid temperature changes. For these reasons, insertion of a thermistor into the thoracic esophagus is preferred.

Several types of thermistor thermometers are sold commercially. These operate on the principle that electrical resistance of the thermistor changes with variation in temperature, and this change is measured and recorded on a dial. Waterproof probes containing thermistors are available with cables of sufficient length that they can be inserted in the patient and monitored at some distance. Multichannel units are used when the temperature in more than one location is desired.

ELECTROENCEPHALOGRAPHY

Caton (1875) first noted the occurrence of electrical potentials in the brains of animals. Other workers noted that anesthesia produced changes in these potentials, but it was not until 1937 that Gibbs et al. published their work suggesting:

> A practical application of these observations might be the use of the elecroencephalogram as a measure of the depth of anesthesia during surgical operations. The anesthetist and surgeon could have before them on tape or screen a continuous record of the electrical activity of both heart and brain.

Subsequently, EEG patterns associated with specific anesthetics and levels of anesthesia have been described. Despite this, the technique has achieved only limited use owing 1) to the difficulty of immediate interpretation of complex and voluminous data, 2) to the greater precision of anesthesia resulting from development of new agents, new vaporizers, and the derivation of MAC, and 3) to the use of multiple anesthetic agents. Saidman (1979) states that current understanding permits a clinically adequate estimation of anesthetic depth without using the EEG. He does, however, believe it to be beneficial in instances of potential compromise of cerebral perfusion. To facilitate ongoing interpretation of data and the assessment of trends, several data processing procedures have been developed. Compressed spectral array (CSA) provides a frequency power histogram with time compression; density modulated spectral analysis provides a similar display and utilizes more conventional equipment. A single-channel cerebral function monitor (CFM) has also been developed. It compresses time, but also weights frequencies most affected by cerebral hypoxia (Saidman, 1979). Currently, the main application of the EEG in the operating room is to assess the adequacy of cerebral circulation (Atkinson et al., 1977).

A basic pattern of the EEG during anesthesia can be constructed that allows classification (Fig. 19–19). As induction of anesthesia is started, frequency increases to 20 to 30 cycles per sec. The small rapid wave pattern is replaced, as consciousness is lost, by a large slow wave that increases in amplitude as it slows (50 to 300 microvolts, 1 to 5 cycles/sec). As anesthesia deepens, the wave may become regular in form and repetition time, with secondary faster waves superimposed on it. Finally, the amplitude begins to decrease with periods of relative cortical inactivity (burst suppression). These may continue until depression results in the entire loss of cortical activity with a flat tracing (see Fig. 24–1).

Changes seen during anesthesia vary with the anesthetic in use. Electroencephalographic changes during the administration of various anesthetic agents have been described by Faulconer and Bickford (1960).

In addition to anesthetic effects, the EEG is modified by variation in oxygen and carbon dioxide tensions. Hypoxia (40% arterial oxygen saturation or less) causes slowing of the frequency of the waves (Atkinson et al., 1977). Elevated carbon dioxide tensions potentiate the effect of other anesthetic agents.

Considerable work has been done in both dogs and cats to determine the effects of preanesthetic and anesthetic agents, muscle relaxants, anoxia, carbon dioxide, and hypothermia on the electroencephalographic pattern (Martin et al., 1959). Klemm (1968) studied the electroencephalogram of dogs during light and deep sodium pentobarbital anesthesia. Electroencephalograms of deeply anesthetized dogs were similar to those of lightly anesthetized dogs. Deep anesthesia often abolished spindling. "Burst suppression" (see Fig. 19–19) was infrequent, but was more commonly observed as the depth of anesthesia was increased. Hamlin

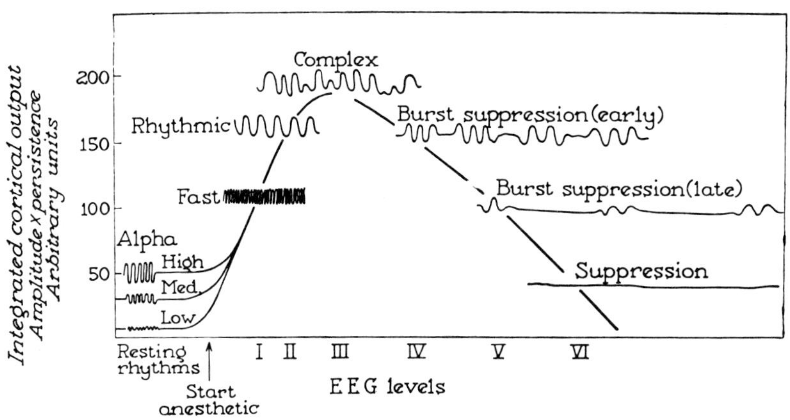

Figure 19–19. Diagram of average changes in the electroencephalographic pattern during anesthesia. (From Martin, J.T., Faulconer, A., Jr., and Bickford, R.G.: Electroencephalography in Anesthesia. Anesthesiology, 20:359, 1959.)

et al. (1965) have reported varying patterns of cortical depression in dogs anesthetized with sodium pentobarbital.

When studying the feline electroencephalogram during thiopental anesthesia, Hatch et al. (1970) were unable to detect clinically useful relationships between EEG pattern, plasma thiopental concentration, and the stage of anesthesia. A review of animal electroencephalography and some anesthetic effects on the encephalogram has been published by Klemm (1969).

MUSCLE RELAXATION

During use of muscle relaxants, greater precision may be achieved by monitoring neuromuscular function. Several techniques may be used (Ali and Savarese, 1976); the peripheral nerve stimulator (Fig. 19–20) is the most commonly used method in man (Savarese and Kitz, 1975). With this equipment, the type and degree of neuromuscular block can be determined. To differentiate the type of block, a sequence of nerve stimulations producing twitch-tetanus-twitch is used (Fig. 19–21). A twitch response is produced by a single stimulus of less than 20 cps; tetanus is caused by repeated stimuli of more than 20/sec. It is estimated that a normal twitch can be elicited when as many as 80% of the receptors are still occupied by a curariform agent. At this point, however, the patient is still in a precarious state, and changes in P_{CO_2}, temperature, or electrolytes could induce return of paralysis. A tetanic response at 100 cps, which indicates at least 50% of the receptors are available, is considered a better indicator of recovery.

When paralysis due to nondepolarizing agents is incomplete, single-twitch (1 to 10/sec) and tetanic (10 to 50/sec) rates of stimulation lead to successive fade in response, a response that may also result from use of volatile anesthetic agents. After a volley of tetanic stimuli, there is an increased response to a single-twitch impulse (post-tetanic facilitation). In contrast to nondepolarizing agents, depolarizing relaxants produce no fade in response to single-twitch and tetanic impulses, and there is no post-tetanic facilitation (Atkinson et al., 1977). When fade or facilitation follow administration of depolar-

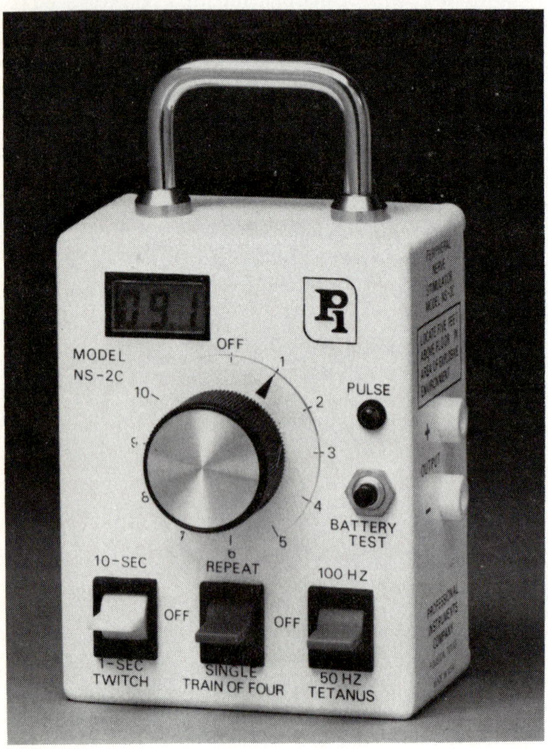

Figure 19–20. Peripheral nerve stimulator. In operation, needle or skin electrodes are connected to output jacks at side of instrument. Twitch, tetanus, and train of four stimuli may be produced. Current delivered to the patient is indicated by digital display at upper left. (Courtesy of Professional Instruments Company, Houston, Texas.)

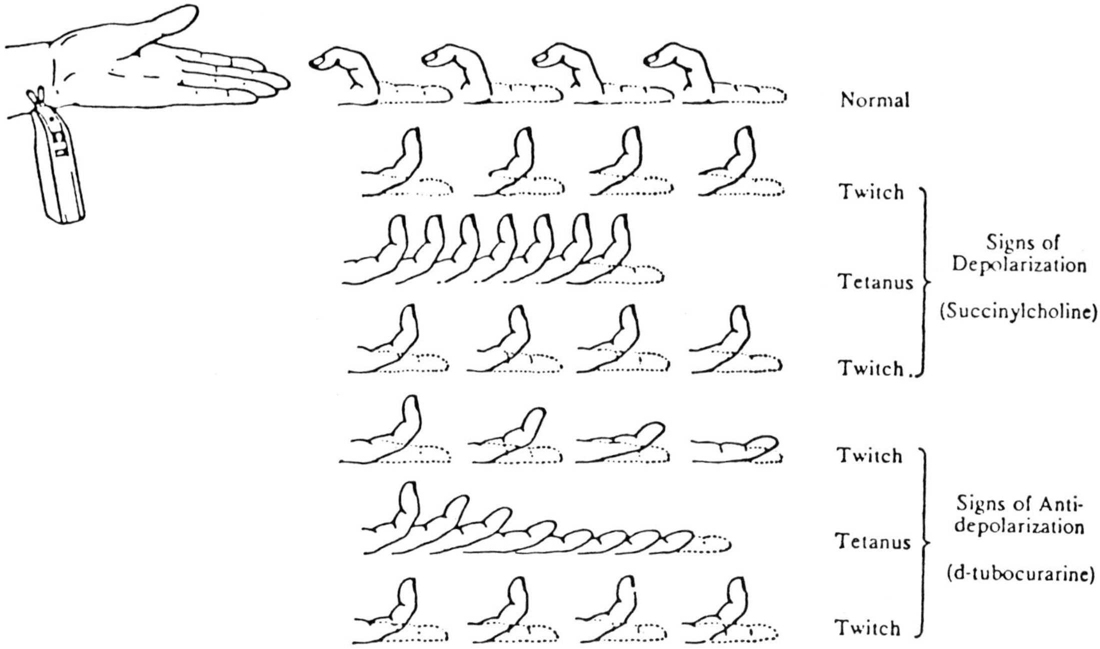

Figure 19–21. The characteristic movements of the fingers in the two classical types of neuromuscular block—depolarization and antidepolarization—upon electrical nerve stimulation. (Churchill-Davidson, H.C.: A Portable Peripheral Nerve–Stimulator. Anesthesiology, 26:224, 1965.)

izing agents, phase II type block has developed (see Chap. 14).

Frequently used sites for nerve stimulation in man are over the ulnar nerve at the wrist or elbow. In animals, the facial, ulnar, radial, and tibial nerves have been used (Jones, 1978; Benson et al., 1979; Manley, 1981). In horses, Benson et al. (1979) used two-needle electrodes inserted subcutaneously near the tibial nerve above the hock. They found maximal twitch response occurred with 200 to 300 V, 1.3 ms duration, at 5-sec intervals.

Manley (1981) recommended a supramaximal stimulus over the facial nerve in the horse every 6 to 10 sec to monitor the effect of a relaxant, thereby evaluating need for additional dosage and progress of recovery. Normal twitches of the nostrils and upper lip were brisk and vigorous, becoming progressively weaker as relaxation was achieved. In man, certain twitch heights (percentage of control height) are considered adequate for specific anesthetic regimens. If any twitch response is visible, overdosage of a nondepolarizing agent has not occurred, and adequate antagonism by anticholinesterase agents should be achieved (Savarese and Kitz, 1975). Train-of-four nerve stimulation (over 2 sec) tests the neuromuscular junction more vigorously than a single twitch. The ratio of the height of the fourth to the first twitch response obviates the use of control heights, correlates well with the adequacy of neuromuscular function, and provides more sensitive and reliable evaluation of respiratory function than that achieved by use of a sustained tetanic stimulus (Savarese and Kitz, 1975). Cullen and Jones (1982) have assessed the extent of neuromuscular block in the dog by this method.

REFERENCES

Adams, A.P., Morgan-Hughes, J.O., and Sykes, M.K.: pH and Blood-Gas Analysis. I. Methods of Measurement and Sources of Error Using Electrode Systems. Anaesthesia, 22:575, 1967.

Adams, A.P., Morgan-Hughes, J.O., and Sykes, M.K.: pH and Blood-Gas Analysis. II. Anaesthesia, 23:47, 1968.

Ali, H.H., and Savarese, J.J.: Monitoring of Neuromuscular Function. Anesthesiology, 45:216, 1976.

Atkinson, R.S., Rushman, G.B., and Lee, J.A.: *A Synopsis of Anaesthesia,* 8th Ed. Year Book Medical Publishers, Chicago, 1977.

Baker, L.E., and Hill, D.W.: The Use of Electrical Impedance Techniques for Monitoring of Respiratory Pattern during Anaesthesia. Br. J. Anaesth., 41:2, 1969.

Bastron, R.D.: Hepatic and Renal Physiology. In *Anesthesia*. Edited by R.D. Miller. Churchill Livingstone, New York, 1981.

Bear, R.A., and Gribik, M.: Assessing Acid-Base Imbalances Through Laboratory Parameters. Hosp. Pract., 9:157, 1974.

Benson, G.J., Hartsfield, S.M., Smetzer, D.L., and Thurmon, J.C.: Physiologic Effects of Succinylcholine Chloride in Mechanically Ventilated Horses Anesthetized with Halothane in Oxygen. Am. J. Vet. Res., 40:1411, 1979.

Beven, J.L.: A New System for Monitoring Respiratory Patterns of Small Laboratory Animals. Lab. Anim. 14:133, 1980.

Brewis, R.A.L.: Clinical Measurements Relevant to the Assessment of Hypoxia. Br. J. Anaesth., 41:742, 1969.

Buchanan, J.W.: Spontaneous Arrhythmias and Conduction Disturbances in Domestic Animals. Ann. N.Y. Acad. Sci., 127:224, 1965.

Burton, G.W.: Measurement of Inspired and Expired Oxygen and Carbon Dioxide. Br. J. Anaesth., 41:723, 1969.

Byles, P.H.: Observations on Some Continuously-Acting Spirometers. Br. J. Anaesth., 32:470, 1960.

Campbell, E.J.M., Dickinson, C.J., and Slater, J.D.H.: *Clinical Physiology*, 3rd ed. Blackwell Scientific Publications, Oxford, 1968.

Caton, R.: Electric Currents of the Brain. Br. Med. J., 2:278, 1875.

Clarke, L.C.: Monitor and Control of Blood and Tissue Oxygen Tensions. Trans. Am. Soc. Art. Intern. Org., 2:41, 1956.

Cole, W.J., Salamonsen, R.F., and Fish, K.J.: A Method for the Gas Chromatographic Analysis of Inhalation Anaesthetics in Whole Blood by Direct Injection into a Simple Precolumn Device. Br. J. Anaesth., 47:1043, 1975.

Cooper, E.A.: The Measurement of Ventilation. Br. J. Anaesth., 41:718, 1969.

Cornelius, L.M.: Fluid, Electrolyte, Acid-Base, and Nutritional Management. In *Pathophysiology in Small Animal Surgery.* Edited by M.J. Bojrab, Lea & Febiger, Philadelphia, 1981.

Coulter, D.B., Whelan, S.C., Wilson, R.C., and Goetsch, D.D.: Determination of Blood Pressure by Indirect Methods in Dogs Given Acetylpromazine Maleate. Cornell Vet., 71:76, 1981.

Cullen, L.K., and Jones, R.S.: Residual Non-Depolarising Neuromuscular Block Assessed by Train-Of-Four Stimulation in the Dog. Res. Vet. Sci., 32:121, 1982.

Cullen, S.C.: Monitors and Clinical Judgment. Am. J. Surg., 102:300, 1961.

Faulconer, A., Jr., and Bickford, R.G.: *Electroencephalography in Anesthesia*. Charles C Thomas, Springfield, Illinois, 1960.

Fisher, E.W., Sibartie, D., and Grimshaw, W.T.R.: A Comparison of the pH, P_{CO_2}, and Total CO_2 Content in Blood from the Brachial and Caudal Auricular Arteries in Normal Cattle. Br. Vet. J., 136:496, 1980.

Freundlich, J.J., and Erickson, J.C.: Electrical Impedance Pneumography for Simple Nonrestrictive Continuous Monitoring of Respiratory Rate, Rhythm and Tidal Volume for Surgical Patients. Chest, 65:181, 1974.

Gibbs, F.A., Gibbs, E.L., and Lennox, W.G.: Effect on Electroencephalogram of Certain Drugs which Influence Nervous Activity. Arch. Intern. Med., 60:154, 1937.

Hahn, A.W., Garner, H.E., Coffman, J.R., and Sanders, C.W.: Indirect Measurement of Arterial Blood Pressure in the Laboratory Pony. Lab. Anim. Sci., 23:889, 1973.

Hamlin, R.L.: Electrocardiography. In *Applied Electronics and Animal Physiology.* Edited by W.R. Klemm. Charles C Thomas, Springfield, Illinois, 1976.

Hamlin, R.L., Redding, R.W., Reiger, J.E., Smith, R.C., and Prynn, R.E.: Insignificance of the "Glucose Effect" in Dogs Anesthetized with Pentobarbital. J.A.V.M.A., 146:238, 1965.

Haskins, S.C.: Personal Communication. School of Veterinary Medicine, University of California, Davis, 1981.

Hatch, R.C., Currie, R.B., and Grieve, G.A.: Feline Electroencephalograms and Plasma Thiopental Concentrations Associated with Clinical States of Anesthesia. Am. J. Vet. Res., 31:291, 1970.

Hedenstierna, G., Lundberg, S., Rawlings, D., and Sedey, H.: Evaluation of a New Spirometer Based on a Fluidistor Technique. Acta Anaesthesiol. Scand., 20:7, 1976.

Hightower, C.E., Kiorpes, A.L., Butler, H.C., and Fedde, M.R.: End-Tidal Partial Pressure of CO_2 During Various Ventilatory Regimens in Halothane-Anesthetized Dogs. Am. J. Vet. Res., 41:610, 1980.

Hilwig, R.W.: Cardiac Arrhythmias in the Horse. J.A.V.M.A., 170:153, 1977.

Huch, A., and Huch, R.: Transcutaneous, Non-invasive Monitoring of P_{CO_2}. Hosp. Pract., 11:43, 1976.

Jones, R.S.: Patient Monitoring During Anaesthesia. J. Small Anim. Pract., 19:373, 1978.

Kerfoot, E., and Domeier, E.: Pulmonary Function Measurements of Large Animals. The Use of Capacitance Respirometer. Lab. Anim. Sci., 22:854, 1972.

Klemm, W.R.: Subjective and Quantitative Analyses of the Electroencephalogram of Anesthetized Normal Dogs: Control Data for Clinical Diagnosis. Am. J. Vet. Res., 29:1267, 1968.

Klemm, W.R.: *Animal Electroencephalography.* Academic Press, New York, 1969.

Klopstock, R., LeVeen, H.H., and Levitan, P.I.: Instantaneous Blood Loss Determination During Thoracic Surgery. J. Thorac. Cardiovasc. Surg., 38:746, 1959.

Kvart, C., Aronsson, T., and Molander, C.: A Portable System for Monitoring Cardiovascular and Respiratory Function in Large Animals. J.A.V.M.A. 180:1227, 1982.

Langhands, J.H.M., and Wallace, W.F.M.: Small Blood Samples from Ear-Lobe Punctures. Lancet, 2:315, 1965.

Laver, M.B., and Seifen, A.: Measurement of Blood Oxygen Tension in Anesthesia. Anesthesiology, 26:73, 1965.

Littlejohn, A.: Acid-Base and Blood Gas Studies in Horses II. Tracheal End-Tidal and Arterial Blood Gas Tensions in Horses. Res. Vet. Sci., 10:263, 1969.

Littlejohn, A., and Mitchell, B.: Acid-Base and Blood Gas

Studies in Horses. I. A Comparison of Capillary and Arterial Blood Samples for Estimation of Acid-Base Values in Horses. Res. Vet. Sci., 10:260, 1969.

Mahoney, L.T., and Brody, M.J.: A Method for Indirect Recording of Arterial Pressure in the Conscious Cat. J. Pharmacol. Methods, 1:61, 1978.

Manley, S.V.: Monitoring the Anesthetized Horse. Vet. Clin. N. Am. Large Anim. Pract., 3:111, 1981.

Martin, J.T., Faulconer, A., Jr., and Bickford, R.G.: Electroencephalography in Anesthesiology. Anesthesiology, 20:359, 1959.

McDonell, W.N.: The Effect of Anaesthesia on Pulmonary Gas Exchange and Arterial Oxygenation in the Horse. Thesis, University of Cambridge, 1974.

Michenfelder, J.D.: Electrocardiography for the Anesthesiologist. 19th Annual Refresher Course Lectures, Annual Meeting, Am. Soc. Anesth., Washington, D.C., 1968.

Moore, R.C., Canizaro, P.C., Sawyer, R.B., Darin, J.C., and Moncrief, J.A.: An Evaluation of Methods for Measuring Operative Blood Loss. Anesth. Analg., 44:130, 1965.

Nunn, J.F.: A New Method of Spirometry Applicable to Routine Anaesthesia. Br. J. Anaesth., 34:422, 1956.

Nunn, J.F.: Oxygen Measurement and Its Significance in Anaesthesia. Proc. R. Soc. Med., 59:905, 1966.

Prys-Roberts, C.: The Measurement of Cardiac Output. Br. J. Anaesth., 41:751, 1969.

Robinson, R.E., and Eastwood, D.W.: Use of a Photo-Sphygmometer in Indirect Blood Pressure Measurements. Anesthesiology, 20:704, 1959.

Rodkey, W.G., Hannon, J.P., Dramise, J.G., White, R.D., S Welsh, D.C., and Persky, B.N.: Arterialized Capillary Blood Used to Determine the Acid-Base and Blood Gas Status of Dogs. Am. J. Vet. Res., 39:459, 1978.

Rose, R.J., and Rossdale, P.D.: Techniques and Clinical Application of Arterial Blood Collection in the Horse. Equine Vet. J., 13:70, 1981.

Rosenthal, M.H.: Monitoring the Critically Ill Patient. ASA Refresher Courses in Anesthesiology, 9:155, 1981.

Saidman, L.J.: Monitoring the Electroencephalogram. Annual Refresher Course Lectures, Lecture #234A, Am. Soc. Anesthesiolgy, 1979.

Sattler, F.P.: Monitoring the Canine Electrocardiogram in Clinical Aspects of Canine Cardiology. Am. Anim. Hosp. Assoc., 1965.

Savarese, J.J., and Kitz, R.J.: Pharmacology of Relaxants. ASA Refresher Courses in Anesthesiology, 3:153, 1975.

Shapiro, B.A., Harrison, R.A., and Walton, J.R.: *Clinical Application of Blood Gases,* 2nd ed. Yearbook Medical Publishers, Inc., Chicago, 1977.

Sharpe, J.J., Nelson, A.W., and Lumb, W.V.: Estimation of Arterial Acid-Base Values from Toenail Blood of the Anesthetized Dog. Am. J. Vet. Res., 29:2365, 1968.

Skaredoff, M.N., and Viquera, M.G.: New Respiratory Monitor. Anesthesiology, 51:570, 1979.

Smith, A.C., and Hahn, C.E.W.: Electrodes for the Measurement of Oxygen and Carbon Dioxide Tensions. Br. J. Anaesth., 41:731, 1969.

Takki, S., Aromaa, U., and Kauste, A.: The Validity and Usefulness of End-Tidal P_{CO_2} during Anesthesia. Ann. Clin. Res., 4:278, 1972.

Weinreb, H.L., Naftchi, N., and Mendlowitz, M.: The Measurement of Digital Arterial Blood Pressure. A.M.A. Arch. Surg., 80:131, 1960.

Wingfield, W.E.: Personal Communication. College of Veterinary Medicine, Colorado State University, Fort Collins, 1984.

Woldring, S., Owens, G., and Woolford, D.C.: Blood Gases: Continuous *in vivo* Recordings of Partial Pressures by Mass Spectrography. Science, 153:885, 1966.

CHAPTER 20

Drugs and Equipment for Anesthetic Emergencies

The wide variety of drugs and equipment used in anesthetic emergencies warrants more detailed description than can be given in a chapter on management of emergencies. For this reason they are discussed first.

BLOOD AND BLOOD SUBSTITUTES

Whole Blood

Use of whole blood in prevention and treatment of shock is commonplace in small animal practice. A canine donor is kept in many hospitals, and blood is withdrawn as needed. From the standpoint of availability in emergency situations, banking of whole blood is more desirable. In addition, plasma from blood that becomes outdated can be collected for storage and future use.

For optimum results, blood should be collected aseptically in sterile plastic storage bags or bottles containing a solution of citric acid, sodium citrate, sodium phosphate, and dextrose

(CPD solution) or citric acid, sodium citrate, and dextrose (ACD solution). These slow hemolysis and delay diffusion of potassium from red cells into the plasma. Stored blood should be maintained at a temperature of 38 to 42° F. If during storage the blood temperature rises to above 60° F, there is rapid destruction of blood cells even though the blood is subsequently cooled.

Feline blood, because of the small volumes involved, is usually drawn in large heparinized plastic syringes (450 μ of heparin/100 ml of blood) and administered to the recipient immediately. Because heparin gradually loses its anticoagulant activity in stored blood, it should be stored at 1 to 6° C and used within 48 hours.

The length of time transfused red cells survive in the recipient is roughly in proportion to the duration of storage. Under optimum conditions, more than 90% of the red cells will survive in the recipient when blood is stored for 1 to 10 days; from 10 to 21 days approximately 70% of the red cells will survive. Even when they are stored for 21 days, under optimum conditions 70 to 80% of transfused red blood cells survive in the recipient at least 5 days.

As described in Chapter 6, 2,3-DPG reduces the oxygen affinity of hemoglobin by a factor of 26. In stored blood there is a rapid decrease in 2,3-DPG, which in turn increases hemoglobin affinity for oxygen. Thus, blood stored for over 24 hours loses much of its ability to release oxygen to the tissues. A specific difference has been found: man, horse, dog, rabbit, guinea pig, and rat are adversely affected by low 2,3-DPG levels, whereas sheep, cow, goat, and cat are affected minimally or not at all (Kaneko, 1980). Canine 2,3-DPG decreases to less than half of normal value with storage in ACD solution for 21 days. CDP anticoagulant maintains 2,3-DPG better, but the difference is not significantly greater.

Smith et al. (1978) found that a mixture of ascorbate phosphate, citric acid, sodium citrate, sodium phosphate, and dextrose (SMB) would extend the shelf life of canine blood for as long as 6 weeks.

When time permits and when valuable animals are transfused, crossmatching of donor and recipient blood is desirable. Severe and even fatal reactions may develop upon administration of subsequent transfusions or in cases of isosensitization due to transplacental immunization (Schalm, 1965). Hemolytic anemia in newborn animals may also be caused by previous transfusion of the dam with incompatible blood.

At least 8 erythrocytic antigens (A, C, D, K, P, Q, T, and U) with corresponding antibodies have been identified in the horse (Stormont, 1982). Successful multiple whole blood transfusions can be performed when group-specific blood is used.

Many erythrocytic antigens have been demonstrated in cattle, sheep, and swine. These fall into 11 systems in cattle, 15 in pigs, and 8 in sheep.

At least 15 different isoantibodies have been demonstrated in the serums of transfused dogs. Only the A factor (subtype A_1) appears to be involved in transfusion reactions. The risk of pairing an A_1 donor with an A-negative recipient to cause a transfusion reaction is about 25%. The ideal canine blood donor is A-negative and Tr-negative.

Cats have two blood factors, A and B. Rarely, a third, AB, is encountered. Based on the incidence of these factors, Auer et al. (1982) have hypothesized that the chance of a transfusion reaction in cats is 3/8. Others have found the incidence much lower (Cotter, 1982; Hayes et al., 1982). The calculated red blood cell mass in normal cats is 17.0 ± 4.07 ml/kg (Breznock and Strack, 1983).

Clark and Woodley (1959) determined that average healthy dogs have a blood volume equal to 8.1% of their body weight. When they injected red blood cells by various routes into dogs, they found that 81.7% of the red blood cells given intraperitoneally were absorbed intact, 48% being absorbed in the first 24 hours. Less than 3% of the red blood cells injected intramuscularly and subcutaneously were absorbed intact, and over 97% were destroyed at the injection site. When intramedullary transfusions were given in the femur, red cells passed rapidly into the circulation, 95.3% being absorbed intact. Jones and Brock (1960) were unable to demonstrate the uptake of more than 5%

of intact red blood cells injected intraperitoneally in cattle.

Under most circumstances, blood is administered intravenously, the rate of injection depending upon the degree of need and size of the animal. Elevation of the central venous or pulmonary wedge pressures indicates that the rate of injection is too rapid, or that overtransfusion has occurred. In the past, too rapid administration was thought to cause right heart embarrassment. However, Firt and Hejhal (1957) demonstrated in dogs that sodium citrate, rather than the rate of administration, is the cause of overloading and failure of the heart. Cardiac failure is produced by vasoconstriction of the pulmonary vascular bed and, in larger doses, depression of the myocardium. In shock, cardiac disease, severe anemia, or liver damage, small intravenous doses of citrate, even the amount contained in a slow transfusion of a small quantity of blood, may be dangerous. Heparinized blood, on the other hand, can be safely transfused at fast rates either intravenously or intra-arterially (over a pint a minute when given simultaneously in both jugular veins). The advantage of intra-arterial transfusion of citrated blood is possibly that citrate filters into the interstitial fluid, and a lower concentration reaches the myocardium and pulmonary vascular circuit.

The toxic effect of citrate during transfusion can be counteracted by simultaneous intravenous administration of calcium and procaine. Calcium cannot be given mixed with the transfusion blood, but should be given intravenously in a different vein than the one used for transfusion because of the danger of clotting.

Ten percent calcium gluconate (0.7 ml/kg) alone reduces the effect of citrate 50 to 60%. For best results in dogs, 10% calcium gluconate (0.6 ml/kg) and 1% procaine hydrochloride (0.5 ml/kg) are given intravenously, starting before and continuing during transfusion (Fig. 20–1).

One should always be aware of the possible bad effects of administering large quantities of banked ACD blood (Howland and Schweizer, 1965). It contains no ionized calcium, is high in potassium, is considerably more acid than normal blood, and is generally very cold (4° C). With massive transfusions in man, it has been shown that the temperature of the heart can be lowered to below 30° C, a level at which fibrillation readily occurs. Malm et al. (1966) determined that transfusion of ACD-preserved blood stimulates catecholamine release with increased peripheral vascular resistance, reduced microcirculation, and increased metabolic acidosis. This response can be eliminated by adjusting the pH of the blood to 7.4 or greater prior to transfusion. If large volumes of blood are given, prophylactic intravenous administering of calcium chloride, procaine, and sodium bicarbonate and warming of the blood will help to avoid complications. Several types of blood-warming devices have been developed (Fig. 20–2).

In contrast, Kahn et al. (1979) studied changes in ionized Ca^{++}, citrate, and H^+ concentrations in humans receiving massive transfusions of CPD-preserved blood. They concluded that, despite depression of Ca^{++}, there were no significant hemodynamic changes. Bicarbonate need be administered only if metabolic acidosis is determined to be present.

The use of blood in cardiopulmonary bypass has focused interest on microaggregates. Many hemodynamic factors have been implicated in the development of post-traumatic pulmonary insufficiency or "shock lung," and various embolic or occlusive states have been attrituted to fat, parenchymatous emboli, or disseminated intravascular coagulation (DIC). In dog studies, McNamara (1972) reinfused autologous stored blood into either pulmonary artery. Infusion consistently produced a significant increase in vascular resistance in the infused lung, which could be prevented by filtration of the blood prior to administration.

In human blood stored in ACD solution, light and electron microscopic observations indicate that the microaggregates that develop consist primarily of degenerated platelets, leukocytes, and strands of fibrin. The most significant factor that determines the volume of microaggregates is the duration of storage. During the first seven days, they consist almost entirely of platelets, and the platelet count drops dramatically. Leukocytes begin to clump at about the eighth day,

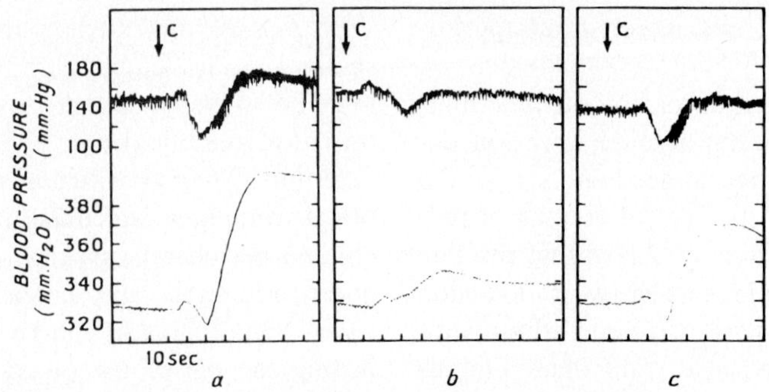

Figure 20–1. The effect of calcium and procaine on pulmonary vasoconstriction and myocardial depression produced by injection of 1.5 mg/kg of 3.8% citrate in a dog: a, the effect of citrate alone; b, the effect of citrate with 10% calcium gluconate 0.8 ml/kg and 1% procaine 0.5 ml/kg; c, the effect of citrate with calcium alone (in the above dosage). Citrate and calcium injected at C. (From Firt, P., and Hejhal, L.: Treatment of Severe Haemorrhage. Lancet, 273:1132, 1957.)

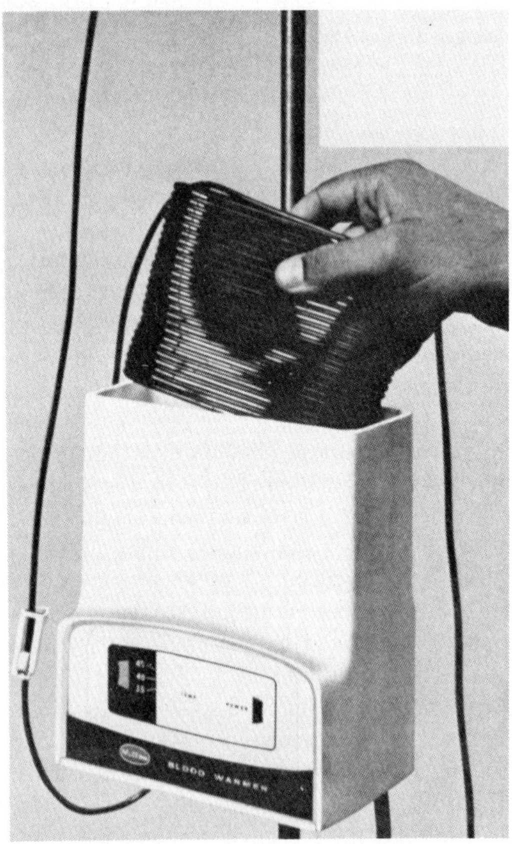

Figure 20–2. Blood warmer. The water bath in this unit is constantly cycled between 39 and 40° C. Blood entering the coil at 2 to 6° C will exit the coil at 35° C ± 2° C. (Courtesy of McGraw Laboratories, Division of American Hospital Supply Corporation, Evanston, Illinois.)

while their number declines steadily in the blood throughout three weeks of storage.

In terms of anticoagulant used, heparin causes a massive and sustained rise in particles during the first 24 hours. After the seventh day, ACD- and CPD-stored blood shows no difference in the extent of microaggregate formation, but during the first week there is a larger volume in CPD than in ACD. Blood stored after arterial donation has fewer microaggregates than after venous donation. There is no difference between storage in plastic bags or storage in glass bottles (Walter, 1978).

Two types of blood filters are available commercially that remove most microaggregates. Screen or surface filters are designed to remove these by simple sieving, while some adsorption of smaller particles occurs. The screen pore diameter determines the size of microaggregates filtered. Screen filters generally have a pore diameter of approximately 40 μm and are protected by a clot screen.

Depth filters present a large foreign surface to the blood and provide filtration by adsorption of particles to various materials (Marshall et al., 1978). The disadvantage of depth filters is that the pressure necessary for filtration increases markedly with repeated units of blood. With continued use, depth filters tend to become less efficient because of channeling. A screen filter, on the other hand, becomes more efficient owing to the increasing adsorption that reduces the pore size. Cellular changes and a decrease in deformability occur during blood storage. Further damage occurs during filtration, particularly with depth filters. Microfiltration appears to have no effect on the coagulation and fibrinolytic mechanisms in either fresh or stored blood, and platelet function is not affected; however, the number of platelets is significantly reduced in either fresh or stored blood by passage through a depth filter. This reduction is not found with a 40-μm screen filter.

The depth filter, then, more completely removes all sizes of microaggregates from transfused blood, but at the cost of a high resistance to flow and possible damage to the red cells. There appears to be no clinical or experimental evidence that the smallest particles are harmful, perhaps because they are too small to lodge in the pulmonary capillaries. Screen filters with 40-μm holes allow the unimpeded passage of 10 or more units of blood without apparent damage to the red cells (Walter, 1978).

The amount of whole blood needed varies widely depending on the circumstances. The average intravenous dose is from 5 to 10 ml per pound of body weight. In acute continuing hemorrhage, however, blood must be given until the hemorrhage stops. Occasionally, because of severe vascular collapse, it is impossible to cannulate a vein for transfusion. In this situation, a direct cut-down on a large vessel should be performed immediately. Hesitation may mean loss of a patient that otherwise could be saved.

In severe exsanguinating hemorrhage, intra-arterial administration of blood has been advocated. With this procedure, it is possible to administer a large quantity of blood rapidly, thus maintaining the arterial pressure without the possibility of overburdening the heart. A simple pressurized transfusion set* has been developed that allows administration of blood under pressure without fear of air embolism (Fig. 20–3).

Zenoble and Stone (1978) have reported autotransfusion of blood into actively bleeding dogs; however, this technique is not widely practiced.

Perfluorochemical Emulsions (Fluosol D-A)

Perfluorochemical whole blood substitutes have been tried on a limited basis in man and

*See Appendix A for manufacturer.

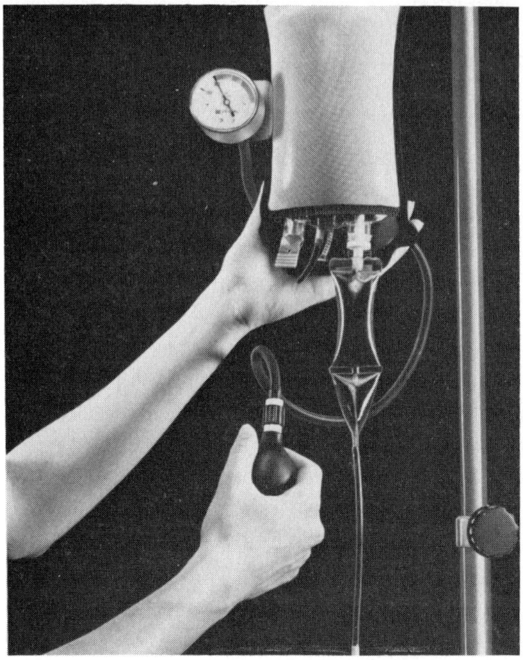

Figure 20–3. Pressure infuser for rapid administration of blood or plasma. Plastic bag containing desired fluid is inserted into the infuser. When the infuser is inflated by pumping the bulb, pressure is exerted on the fluid, which is then forced into the patient. Gauge indicates approximate pressure of administration. Because the two compartments do not communicate, the danger of air embolism is eliminated. (Courtesy of Fenwal Laboratories, Division of Travenol Laboratories, Inc., Deerfield, Illinois.)

probably will become available for veterinary use (Ohyanagi et al., 1979; Lapin et al., 1980). Some can dissolve as much as 60% oxygen by volume, in contrast to whole blood which dissolves about 20%. In dogs, fluorocarbon infusions have been shown to reduce myocardial ischemic damage after coronary occlusion (Glogar et al., 1981).

Plasma

Plasma has all the properties of whole blood except its oxygen-carrying capacity. In shock not accompanied by loss of blood, it is preferred to whole blood, since administration of the latter produces a polycythemia with a disproportionate number of red blood cells in relation to the liquid portion of the circulating blood. On a volume-for-volume basis, plasma contains almost twice as much protein as is found in whole blood, since 40 to 50% of whole blood is red blood corpuscles. Plasma contains 6 to 7% protein, 60% of which is albumin. Because of its small molecular weight, however, albumin exerts 80% of the colloidal osmotic pressure of the blood. One gram of albumin retains 18 ml of water within the circulation. In addition to their osmotic pressure effects, the proteins of plasma can be metabolized by the body.

Plasma is usually obtained from banked whole blood that has become outdated. The supernatant plasma is siphoned into sterile containers and the cellular sediment discarded. Fifty percent dextrose solution is added as a stabilizer to make a final concentration of 5% dextrose. Liquid plasma can be stored at room temperature for as long as 6 months without appreciable deterioration provided bacterial contamination has not occurred. If kept in a liquid state, however, it is more frequently stored under refrigeration at 38 to 40° F. Plasma stored in the liquid state should be filtered prior to use since flocculation rapidly occurs.

Frozen plasma may be kept indefinitely without flocculation or the danger of bacterial growth. When needed, it should be quickly thawed at approximately 100° F. Filtration of frozen plasma generally is not necessary.

A working rule for plasma administration is to give 0.66 ml/lb for each unit the hematocrit reading is over 45. If the hematocrit is 60 in a 35-lb dog:

$$60 - 45 = 15$$

$$15 \times \tfrac{2}{3} \times 35 = \text{ml of plasma}$$

Extra plasma is rapidly removed from the circulation and, from a practical standpoint, excessive amounts are unlikely to be administered.

Dextran (Macrodex; Rheomacrodex)

Dextran, a polymer of glucose, is a water-soluble, high-molecular-weight polysaccharide, obtained by bacterial fermentation of sucrose. Crude dextran is hydrolized and differentially fractionated to obtain dextrans of varying molecular size. Two solutions are used clinically: one with a medium molecular weight of approximately 70,000 (dextran 70), and one with a low molecular weight of 40,000 (dextran 40).

Dextran 70 exerts an "osmotic increment" effect on the circulating blood of about 100%. That is, it draws an equivalent amount of fluid from the tissues into the blood vessels to increase the circulating plasma volume (Fig. 20–4), Table 20–1). At 4 hours, 80% of the dextran is still circulating in the blood; as much as 50% may be excreted in the urine within 24 hours. A small portion that is not excreted is oxidized over a period of weeks.

Dextran is antigenic, and at any sign of reaction the infusion should be stopped. If a reaction is not experienced on the first injection, repeat infusions may usually be given without ill effect. Dextran is not stored in the body and has no harmful effect on renal, hepatic, or other body functions. Mild diuresis follows its injection. It has the advantage that it is not species-specific as are blood and plasma.

Dextran is a useful antithrombotic agent in surgery. Aberg et al. (1979) found that dextran interferes with the metabolism of factor VIII. The antithrombotic effect of dextran may, therefore, be caused by a temporary factor VIII defect influencing platelet function and thrombus stability. There is no evidence that dextran produces proteolysis.

The dose of dextran 70 varies depending upon the need of the animal. A basic dose of 3 ml/lb of body weight is suggested. There is little danger of toxic overdosage. In man, administration of more than 2,000 ml of dextran intravenously may increase the bleeding time (Howard et al., 1959). Because of the expense of dextran solution, its use in animals has been limited.

Dextran 40 has more particles per unit weight than dextran 70 and is more osmotically active. However, its smaller molecules pass through the semipermeable capillaries into the interstitial space and through the glomerular capillaries into the urine. For this reason, its osmotic effect is transient in comparison to dextran 70. Most dextran 40 is excreted within 6 hours, producing some diuresis (Fig. 20–5).

In man, acute oliguric renal failure is an infrequent adverse reaction that occurs following

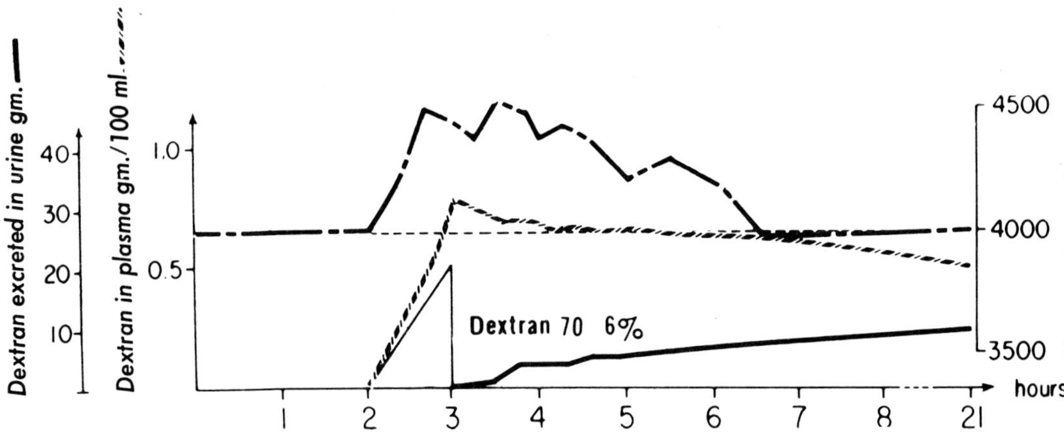

Figure 20–4. Changes in plasma volume, dextran concentration in plasma, and dextran excretion in urine following infusion of 500 ml of 6% solution of dextran 70 (Macrodex). (From Atik, M.: Dextran 40 and Dextran 70. Arch. Surg., 94:664, 1967.)

administration of dextran 40 (Van den Berg and Pineda, 1980). Preexisting renal disease is a predisposing factor. Damage apparently is caused by tubular plugging with urine of high specific gravity.

Dextran 40 is not recommended for replacement of blood volume or extracellular fluid loss, but is used to improve the microcirculation and to prevent erythrocyte aggregation and increased blood viscosity. By so doing, it increases capillary flow and brings noncirculating blood back into active circulation. Both dextran 70 and dextran 40 have antithrombogenic effects.

TABLE 20–1. Comparison between Dextrans

	Dextran 40	*Dextran 70*
Average molecular weight	40,000	70,000
Range, 90% of molecules	10,000 to 80,000	25,000 to 200,000
Volume expansion quality	Fairly good, transient	Good, lasts several hr
Excretion	Rapid	Fairly slow
Relative increase in viscosity of red blood cell (RBC) suspension	Slightly more than albumin or plasma	More
Effect on aggregation	Prevention, deaggregation	Slight, variable
Effect on microcirculation	Appreciable	Slight, variable
Antithrombogenic effect	Appreciable	Appreciable
Dosage	10 to 15 ml/kg/24 hr	10 to 15 ml/kg/24 hr
Speed of infusion	Over 12–24 hr 1) to improve microcirculation 2) for antithrombogenic effect	1) 1 to 2 hr for volume replacement 2) 6 to 8 hr for antithrombogenic effect
Untoward effects		
Anaphylactoid reaction	Not observed	Occasionally seen
Pulmonary edema	May occur if given rapidly	More apt to occur if given rapidly
Increased bleeding	Rarely seen at recommended dose	Occasionally seen
Interference with blood typing	Not significant	Has been reported
Contraindications	Pulmonary edema, thrombocytopenia	Congestive heart failure, coagulation defects

(From Atik, M.: Dextran 40 and Dextran 70. Arch. Surg., 94:664, 1967.)

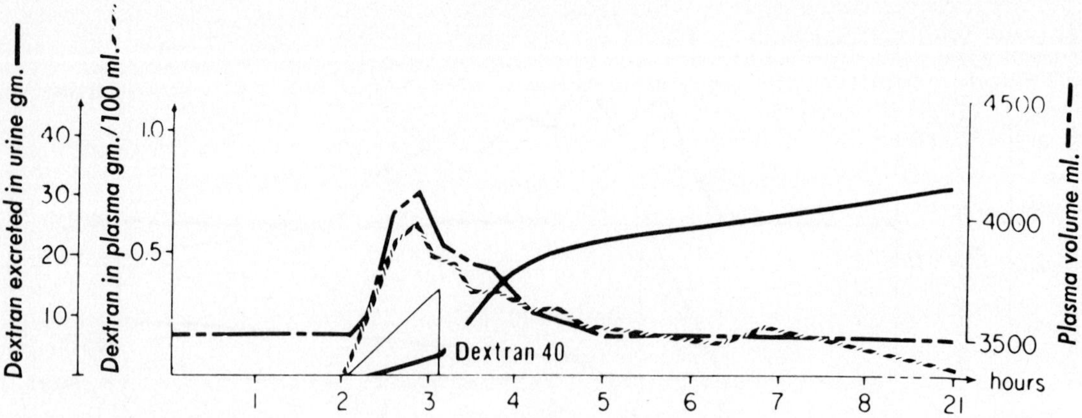

Figure 20–5. Changes in plasma volume, dextran concentration in plasma, and dextran excretion in urine following infusion of 500 ml of 10% solution of dextran 40 (Rheomacrodex). (From Atik, M.: Dextran 40 and Dextran 70. Arch. Surg., 94:664, 1967.)

Dextran 40 is available as a 10% solution in either normal saline or 5% dextrose in water. Studies in animals undergoing long periods of pump-oxygenator perfusion indicate that dextran 40 prevents intravascular hemagglutination (blood sludging), maintains normal distribution of blood flow in the kidney, maintains circulatory volume and flow during hypothermic extracorporeal circulation, reduces the occurrence of microinfarcts in the liver, kidney, and myocardium, and diminishes denaturation of plasma protein at the blood-gas interface in pump oxygenators. Dextran 40 is commonly used as part of the priming fluid for pump oxygenation equipment, but should not be used alone for this purpose. Total dosage during the first 24 hours should not exceed 20 ml/kg. The first 500 ml can be infused rapidly with the remainder given more slowly. Total daily dosage beyond the first 24 hours should not exceed 10 mg/kg.

Even in emergency situations, it is not wise to replace the entire blood loss with dextrans. Lactated Ringer's solution, plasma, or whole blood should be used in conjunction with dextran 70.

Hetastarch (Hespan)

Hetastarch is used for plasma volume expansion in the treatment of shock caused by hemorrhage, burns, surgery, or sepsis. It has also been used as a plasma expander during cardiopulmonary bypass and as a hemodilution agent to prime heart-lung machines (Lee et al., 1975; Mishler et al., 1975).

Hetastarch, also called hydroxyethyl starch, is a branched polymer of glucose partially resistant to enzymatic breakdown. It is marketed as a 6% solution in 0.9% sodium chloride, with a pH of 5.5 and calculated osmolality of approximately 310 mOsm/L. When hetastarch is infused, plasma volume expands slightly more than the volume of the infused material and then decreases over the next 24 to 36 hours. About 40% of the total dose appears in the urine within 24 hours, but a small amount persists for weeks to months after a single dose and accumulates after multiple doses. In animals, after large doses, hetastarch persists in reticuloendothelial cells in the liver and other organs.

This volume expander has been widely used in humans in Europe and other areas, but not in the United States. In a randomized crossover study comparing 500 ml of 5% albumin and 6% hetastarch in 10 hypovolemic postoperative human patients, both caused marked improvement in plasma volume and flow, and small transient increases in arterial and venous pressures and urine output (Lazrove et al., 1980). Results were similar in another randomized trial comparing hetastarch and 5% albumin in 14 human patients in shock due to hemorrhage or sepsis; no significant differences in hemodynamic or respiratory function were found (Munoz et al., 1980).

Persons receiving hetastarch infusions have increased serum alpha-amylase levels because hetastarch binds the enzyme and prevents its normal excretion in the urine (Mishler and Durr, 1979). Large doses of hetastarch given for several days in succession for leukapheresis have increased plasma volume and altered blood coagulation (Rock and Wise, 1979). Hetastarch is contraindicated for patients with severe bleeding disorders, and for those with severe congestive heart failure or renal failure. Other adverse effects include vomiting, chills, peripheral edema, and anaphylactoid reactions. In a large study, severe reactions (shock, cardiac or respiratory arrest, or both) occurred in 0.003% of persons given plasma-protein-solution infusions compared to 0.006% with hetastarch, 0.008% with dextran, and 0.038% with gelatin solutions (Ring and Messmer, 1977).

Hetastarch is administered by intravenous infusion only. Total dosage and rate of infusion depend upon the amount of blood lost and the resultant hemoconcentration. Total dosage does not usually exceed 20 ml/kg of body weight. In acute hemorrhagic shock, 20 ml/kg/hr may be used; in burn or septic shock, it is usually administered at slower rates.

Dextrose

Dextrose, either as a 5% solution or in the form of 5% dextrose in isotonic saline, has been commonly administered by intravenous drip during anesthesia to help maintain blood pressure, produce mild diuresis, and provide a readily accessible route for administration of other drugs. Five percent dextrose is isotonic with blood but contains no ions. When given intravenously, it is rapidly metabolized, leaving free water.

Webb et al. (1950) demonstrated that 5% dextrose in isotonic saline (D5W) given intraperitoneally produced a prolonged tissue dehydration by attracting water (Fig. 20–6). It has also been shown by Zontine and Donovan (1969) that 5% dextrose given subcutaneously to dogs produces a 10 to 20% reduction in total plasma volume and electrolytes within 3 hours after injection. This is sufficient to kill patients in which venous return is already severely diminished. For this reason, 5% dextrose or saline-dextrose should *only* be given intravenously.

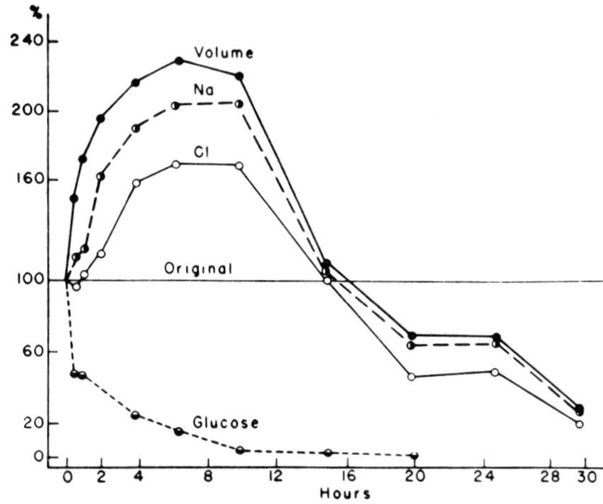

Figure 20–6. Cumulative data showing the increase in volume of intraperitoneal fluid and dissolved electrolytes attracted from the tissues by an intraperitoneal injection of 5% dextrose in isotonic saline. (From Webb, W.R., Lemmer, K.A., and Elman, R.: Absorption Rates, Electrolyte and Volume Changes Following Subcutaneous and Intraperitoneal Injections of Solutions Containing Salt, Glucose, and Amino Acids. Surg. Gynec. Obstet., 91:265, 1950. By permission of Surgery, Gynecology & Obstetrics.)

Lactated Ringer's Solution

Ringer's lactate contains 2.5 g sodium lactate, 6 g sodium chloride, 0.3 g potassium chloride, and 0.2 g calcium chloride/L. The lactate is metabolized by the liver, yielding an excess of sodium. Ringer's lactate is valuable in combating acidosis, provided liver function is not depressed. Commercial solutions have a pH of approximately 6.3. Those containing benzyl alcohol as a preservative are toxic for cats (Cullison, 1983).

Ringer's lactate solution has been used alone as priming solution for cardiopulmonary bypass, as much as 126 ml/kg being used successfully in children (DeBoer, 1969).

Rush et al. (1969) have used Ringer's lactate solution as blood replacement in surgical patients with excellent results. The replacement ratio was 3 or 4:1. Serial hematocrits were determined, and when blood dilution produced an hematocrit below 28%, whole blood was administered to maintain the hematocrit at that level. Replacement of whole blood losses with saline solutions accomplishes the following:

1. The vascular volume is increased in proportion to the extracellular fluid increase, since saline solutions quickly distribute throughout the extracellular fluid space. Both vascular volume and blood pressure can thus be maintained.
2. Hemodilution lowers blood viscosity and produces better tissue perfusion.
3. Compensatory changes in cardiac output maintain the efficiency of oxygen transport with hematocrits between 30 and 50%.
4. Although at low hematocrits cardiac output increases, the work of the heart does not increase proportionately owing to decreased peripheral resistance produced by hemodilution.
5. Diuresis is produced, theoretically insuring patency of the kidneys and decreasing the likelihood of tubular necrosis.
6. Use of whole blood with its inherent dangers is avoided.

According to Moss (1969) vascular reexpansion following graded hemorrhages in splenectomized dogs necessitates the following: 36% hemorrhage requires 5:1 replacement; 60% requires 6:1; and 75% requires 8:1. Urine output is considered the best clinical guide to adequate vascular re-expansion with Ringer's lactate solution.

The exogenous lactate in Ringer's lactate solution is cleared rapidly from the blood after blood volume replacement in animals with hemorrhagic shock (Trinkle et al., 1968).

ALKALINIZING AGENTS

Sodium Bicarbonate Injection, U.S.P.

Sodium bicarbonate solution is a preparation of sodium bicarbonate ($NaHCO_3$) in sterile water for injection.

Solutions contain 7.5% and 8.4% sodium bicarbonate in 50-ml ampules and vials. Each 1 ml of 7.5% $NaHCO_3$ = 75 mg $NaHCO_3$ = 0.893 mEq sodium and 0.893 mEq bicarbonate. Each 1 ml of 8.4% $NaHCO_3$ = 84 mg $NaHCO_3$ = 1.0 mEq sodium and 1.0 mEq bicarbonate. Sodium bicarbonate solution is usually administered intravenously, either in another parenteral solution or undiluted in emergencies. An isotonic solution results when a 50-ml vial of 7.5% sodium bicarbonate is added to 200 ml of water for injection; with a 50-ml vial of 8.5% solution, 224 ml of sterile water are required.

Sodium bicarbonate is indicated in the treatment of metabolic acidosis (Fig. 20–7). Acidosis is caused either from a loss of base or from an excess of hydrogen ions. By administration of additional base, the condition can be ameliorated. Metabolic acidosis may be caused by a variety of clinical conditions including renal disease, diabetes, prolonged anesthesia, extracorporeal circulation, and cardiac arrest. Sodium bicarbonate is also indicated in barbiturate intoxication to facilitate dissociation of barbiturate-protein complex.

Overcorrection of the bicarbonate deficit produces metabolic alkalosis with a rise in blood pH. From a clinical standpoint, alkalosis is seldom encountered. However, administration of sodium bicarbonate is generally contraindicated in patients losing chloride through vomiting or in those with hypokalemia. Because sodium bicarbonate produces sodium retention, it should be used with caution in patients with congestive heart failure or other conditions causing edema.

The dose of sodium bicarbonate is determined by the base deficit of the blood (see Chap. 19) and clinical symptoms of the patient. Quantitative estimation of bicarbonate dose may be calculated from the formula: Base deficit $\times$ 0.3 $\times$ body weight (kg) = mEq of $NaHCO_3$.

The factor 0.3 $\times$ body weight is an approximation of the acute volume of distribution of infused HCO_3^-; 0.3 $\times$ body weight approximates the extracellular fluid compartment. Distribution to interstitial fluid requires approximately 30 min to be 98% complete. Although the factor 0.6 has been utilized in the formula, the use of 0.6 $\times$ body weight assumes that the volume of HCO_3^- distribution is in the total body water. About 18 hrs are required for completion. When

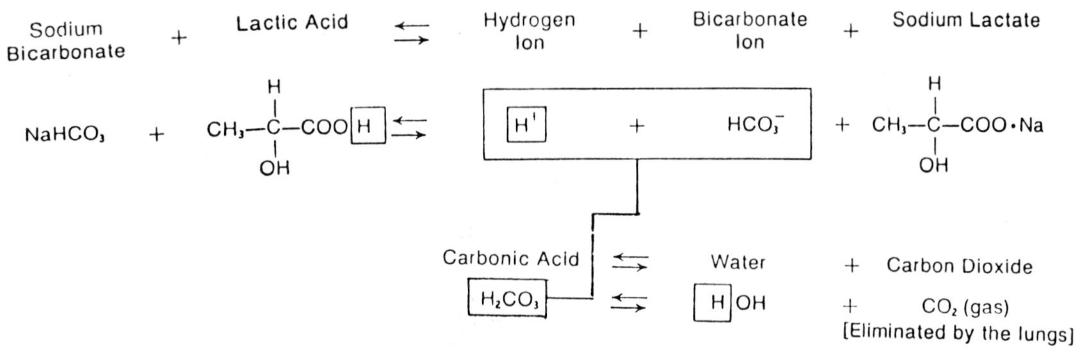

Figure 20–7. When sodium bicarbonate is infused intravenously in lactic acidosis, CO_2 is one of the end products of the reaction.

the 0.6 factor is used, the dose of HCO^-_3 may be too high and, if given, must be administered slowly. The amount of HCO_3^- needed to correct base deficit in metabolic acidosis varies widely depending upon the cause of the acidosis and variations in distribution of HCO^-_3 into intracellular spaces. Overtreatment should be avoided. Acid-base measurements should be made *frequently* since changes with anesthesia and disease processes are dynamic.

Intravenous sodium bicarbonate administration leads to increased CO_2 levels in the blood and cerebrospinal fluid (CSF). Because plasma HCO^-_3 enters the CSF more slowly, a paradoxical acidosis in the brain may result. General depression of the central nervous system, including the medullary centers, may develop, reducing respiratory drive. Adequate ventilation is thus mandatory to prevent ill effects.

Usually half the calculated dose is administered and a second base deficit determination made. When the base deficit of a patient with acidosis is unknown, the safe average dose of sodium bicarbonate is 5.0 mEq (420 mg) per kilogram.

To correct for the acidity inherent in ACD-preserved blood, the contents of 1 ampule added to 250 ml of sterile water for injection may be given for every 2 units (1000 ml) of blood administered.

Hypertonic sodium bicarbonate (7.5% = 1500 mOsm/L) has been shown to cause hyperosmolality of the blood when given in large quantities for acute cardiac resuscitation (Mettar et al., 1974). In man, plasma osmolality levels have exceeded 400 mOsm/kg, and serum sodium concentrations of more than 200 mEq/L have been reported. Experimental and clinical observations indicate that increases in plasma osmolality to levels exceeding 350 mOsm are potentially fatal. Detrimental effects of alkalemia include an increase in the affinity of hemoglobin for oxygen and an unfavorable effect on oxygen release. Routine measurement of plasma osmolality, in addition to acid-base determinations, is recommended prior to administration of additional doses of alkali (see Chap. 19).

Another detrimental effect is prolongation of thrombin clotting and prothrombin times (Wong et al., 1980).

The effect of mild and severe acute alkalosis due to intravenous sodium bicarbonate infusion on glomerular filtration rate, renal plasma flow, and sodium and potassium clearance has been investigated in dogs (Kanter, 1963). The maximum load given was over 50 g of sodium bicarbonate intravenously in 4 hours, at a rate of 2.5 mEq/minute. With maximum sodium bicarbonate loading, plasma potassium fell from 3.8 to 2.7 mEq/L, and plasma sodium increased from 144.4 to 170.8 mEq/L. There was no apparent acute detrimental renal effect. No depression of glomerular filtration rate or of renal plasma flow was seen, although the arterial blood pH increased from 7.32 to 7.61. Similarly, no significant effect was seen on blood pressure, hematocrit, filtration fraction, heart rate, or rectal temperature. Urine flow and urine pH increased significantly.

Rapid infusion of 3 L of 5% sodium bicarbonate in 5% dextrose in normal horses produced a highly significant metabolic alkalosis and, in some animals, muscle spasms or fasciculations, shivering, and hyperactivity (Rumbaugh et al., 1981). Respiratory rates increased transiently. Alterations in pH, P_{CO_2}, plasma bicarbonate, and base balance were significant for 4 hours and, in 4 of 8 horses, had not returned to normal at 8 hours. Plasma Na^+ increased, while K^+ and Cl^- decreased significantly.

Should alkalosis result from sodium bicarbonate administration, the use of bicarbonate should be discontinued, and the patient should be treated according to the degree of alkalosis. Sodium chloride injection (0.9%) intravenously is usually sufficient to correct plasma chloride. If alkalosis is severe enough to be accompanied by hyperirritability or tetany, intravenous ammonium chloride (NH_4Cl) may be given as a 1/6 molar solution (167 mEq/L). Calcium gluconate may also be useful in controlling tetany.

Because of potential hazards associated with indiscriminant administration of sodium bicarbonate, Bishop and Weisfeldt (1976) have advised that 1) it not be administered in cardiac resuscitation without adequate ventilation, 2) it not be given in repeated doses without confirmation of acidosis, and 3) it not be given where cardiac arrest is of brief duration and preexisting acidosis is unlikely.

Tromethamine (THAM)

Tromethamine is an organic amine buffer for correction of severe systemic acidosis, such as that which occurs during shock, cardiac operations with extracorporeal circulation, cardiac arrest, and massive transfusions of ACD blood (Nahas, 1963). Given intravenously, it acts as an amine proton acceptor, attracting hydrogen ions to form salts that are then excreted by the kidneys. There is no increase in CO_2 level as occurs with sodium bicarbonate (Fig. 20–8).

It also acts as an osmotic diuretic, increasing urine flow, urine pH, excretion of electrolytes, fixed acids, and carbon dioxide. Approximately 30% of tromethamine at pH 7.4 is not ionized and is capable of penetrating cells to combine with intracellular acid anions. About 70% is ionized and is effective in the extracellular fluid.

Nahas (1959) found that tromethamine prevented the increase in arterial P_{CO_2}, the drop in arterial pH, the increase in cerebral spinal fluid pressure, and the progressive decrease in arterial oxygen saturation accompanying apneic oxygenation in dogs. Gibson et al. (1979) reported that pretreatment with tromethamine protected mice against the neurochemical and behavioral effects of hypoxia.

Tromethamine appears to exert an inotropic effect that is more evident in ischemic than in normal myocardium (Effron et al., 1978). It has been proposed that this effect results from intracellular buffering that increases the efficiency of energy production and utilization.

Tromethamine is contraindicated in anuria and uremia. Large doses may depress respiration owing to pH change and CO_2 reduction with subsequent increase in blood lactate. Rapid infusion may produce ECG changes similar to those of hyperkalemia (Darby and Anderson, 1966). Hypoglycemia may also occur. For these

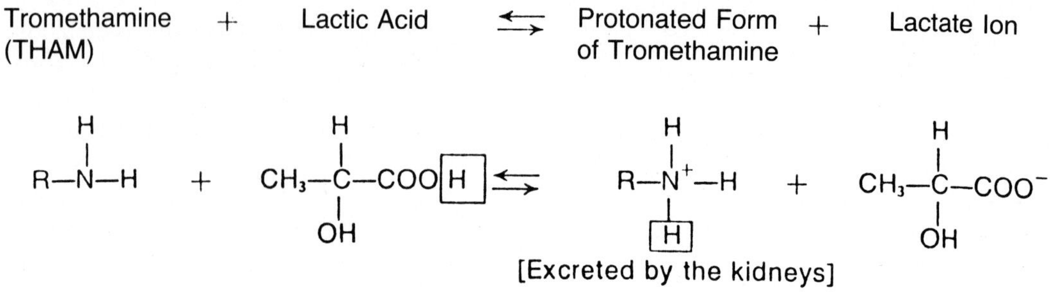

Figure 20–8. Action of tromethamine in removal of hydrogen ions from the blood.

reasons, blood pH, P_{CO_2}, bicarbonate, glucose, and electrolyte determinations should be performed during administration of large quantities. The coagulation time is increased in dogs.

Tromethamine is supplied in 500-ml bottles containing 18 g (150 mEq) of tromethamine and approximately 3 g (50 mEq) of acetic acid. The pH is approximately 8.6. The approximate intravenous dosage may be estimated from the buffer base deficit.

Tromethamine (ml, of 0.3 M) required = body weight (kg) × base deficit (mEq/L) × 1.1.

A 70-kg patient with a buffer base deficit of 5 mEq/L would require 70 × 5 × 1.1 = 385 ml of tromethamine solution containing 13.9 g (115 mEq).

The average single dose in man is 3.8 ml/lb. The total dose should be based on serial determinations of the patient's arterial blood pH (normal 7.35 to 7.45) and base deficit (anything exceeding 5 mEq/L with pH of 7.2 or below.) During cardiac bypass surgery, an average dose of approximately 9.0 ml/kg (324 mg/kg) has been used. This is equivalent to a total dose of 630 ml (189 mEq) for a 70-kg patient. A total single dose of 500 mg (150 mEq) is considered adequate for most adult humans. Larger single doses (up to 1000 ml) may be required in unusually severe cases.

The pH of stored blood ranges from 6.80 to 6.22 depending upon duration of storage. The amount of tromethamine solution needed to correct this acidity ranges from 15 to 77 ml added to each 500 ml of blood. Clinical experience indicates that an average of 60 ml for 500 ml of ACD blood is usually adequate.

In treatment of cardiac arrest, tromethamine solution should be given at the same time that other standard resuscitative measures, including cardiac massage, are being applied. Doses ranging from approximately 3.5 to 6.0 ml/kg have been injected into a peripheral vein. Additional amounts may be required to control systemic acidosis persisting after cardiac arrest is reversed.

The intravenous lethal dose of tromethamine in the dog is 500 mg/kg when given at 50 mg/kg/min.

VASOACTIVE DRUGS

Vasoactive drugs have been used in anesthesia principally for treatment of hypotension and circulatory shock. In this regard, they mimic or antagonize the body's endogenous hormones (Fig. 20–9).

Following Ahlquist's classification of alpha and beta receptors in the cardiovascular system (see Chap. 4), drugs acting upon these receptors can be classified as follows: 1) alpha-adrenergic (alphamimetic), 2) beta-adrenergic (betamimetic), 3) mixed alpha- and beta-adrenergic, 4) alpha blocking (alphalytic), and 5) beta blocking (betalytic).

The spectrum of actions produced by these drugs is illustrated in Figure 20–10. The alphamimetic agents, methoxamine, phenylephrine and, to a lesser degree, levarterenol, metaraminol, and epinephrine, have their primary effects upon the resistance vessels. They produce a rise in arterial blood pressure and an increase in the volume of blood in the capacitance system (Tables 20–2, 20–3). Excessive administration produces a severe rise in peripheral vascular resistance comparable to aortic constriction. Heart rate is reflexly slowed, and venous return is decreased. Levarterenol, metaraminol, and epinephrine also have secondary betamimetic actions producing increased heart rate, reduced arterial pressure, and reduced blood volume in the capacitance vessels.

Mephentermine and isoproterenol have almost pure betamimetic effects, causing increased heart rate and reduced veous pooling with increased venous return to the heart. At the same time, they reduce arteriolar constriction and act as vasodilators.

Alphalytic drugs, such as phentolamine, phenoxybenzamine, and the phenothiazine tranquilizers, block the effects of alphamimetic agents on the vasculature. This results in reduced arterial blood pressure, increase in venous return, and increased cardiac output. Their action thus simulates betamimetic drugs. When a mixed alpha- and betamimetic agent, such as epinephrine, is combined with an alphalytic agent, the betamimetic action becomes apparent.

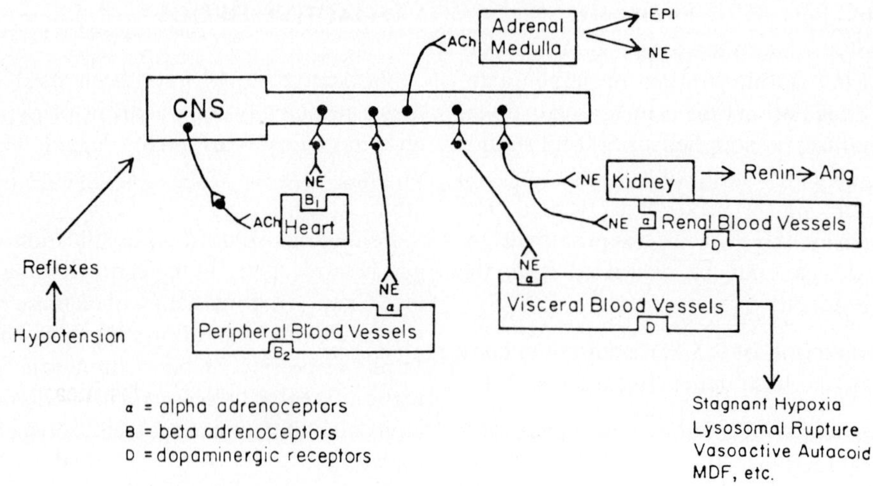

Figure 20–9. Involvement of sympathoadrenal responses in cardiovascular changes associated with hypotension and circulatory shock. Cardiovascular reflexes are activated by hypotension. Increased sympathetic discharge results in increased release of epinephrine *(EPI)* and norepinephrine *(NE)* from the adrenal medulla, and increased release of NE at sympathetic neuroeffector junctions of the heart, kidney, and blood vessels. β_1 receptors of the heart subserve increased myocardial contractility and heart rate; α receptors of blood vessels subserve vasoconstriction. Renin release from the kidney increases formation of angiotensin *(Ang)*. β_2 receptors subserve vasodilatation. Dopamine-responsive, or "dopaminergic," receptors *(D)* seem to be concentrated in the renal and mesenteric arterial beds and subserve vasodilatation. Splanchnic vasoconstriction and resulting visceral hypoxia and ischemia lead to breakdown of lysosomal membranes, release into the circulation of autolytic lysosomal enzymes, formation of endogenous vasoactive substances (such as autacoids), and perhaps a specific myocardial depressant factor *(MDF)*. *ACh* = acetylcholine. (From Adams, H.R., and Parker, J.L.: Pharmacologic Management of Circulatory Shock: Cardiovascular Drugs and Corticosteroids. J.A.V.M.A., 175:86, 1979.)

Combined alpha and beta blockade can be produced by ganglionic-blocking drugs, spinal block, or spinal cord transection.

Betalytic agents, such as propranolol, produce decreased heart rate, increased peripheral vascular resistance, and pooling in the capacitance vessels with reduced venous return.

Current therapy of most types of shock is not directed toward maintenance of arterial blood pressure per se, but rather toward ensuring adequate tissue perfusion. For this reason, the use of alphamimetic agents is decreasing, and betamimetic and alphalytic agents are more commonly used.

ALPHA-ADRENERGIC AGENTS

Methoxamine Hydrochloride, U.S.P. (Vasoxyl)

Methoxamine is a prototype of the alphamimetic drugs. It produces a marked vasopressor response that is due almost completely to increased peripheral resistance without direct myocardial stimulation. Compensatory bradycardia follows the rise in blood pressure. Following intravenous injection, an immediate response occurs that persists for about 1 hour. On intramuscular injection, response occurs within 15 minutes and lasts for approximately 90 minutes. Tachyphylaxis has been observed in experimental animals.

Brill et al. (1959) have shown that methoxamine is capable of suppressing ventricular arrhythmias experimentally produced in dogs by several methods. The dose used was 0.5 to 1 mg/kg of body weight. Arrhythmias were suppressed for periods of 30 to 60 minutes.

In dogs whose hearts were made susceptible to cardiac arrhythmias by administration of cyclopropane, chloroform, the production of myocardial infarcts, or diphtheria toxin myocarditis, methoxamine failed to provoke arrhythmias. Moreover, it prevented epinephrine-cyclopropane or epinephrine-chloroform ventricular tachycardia and fibrillation. Slowing of

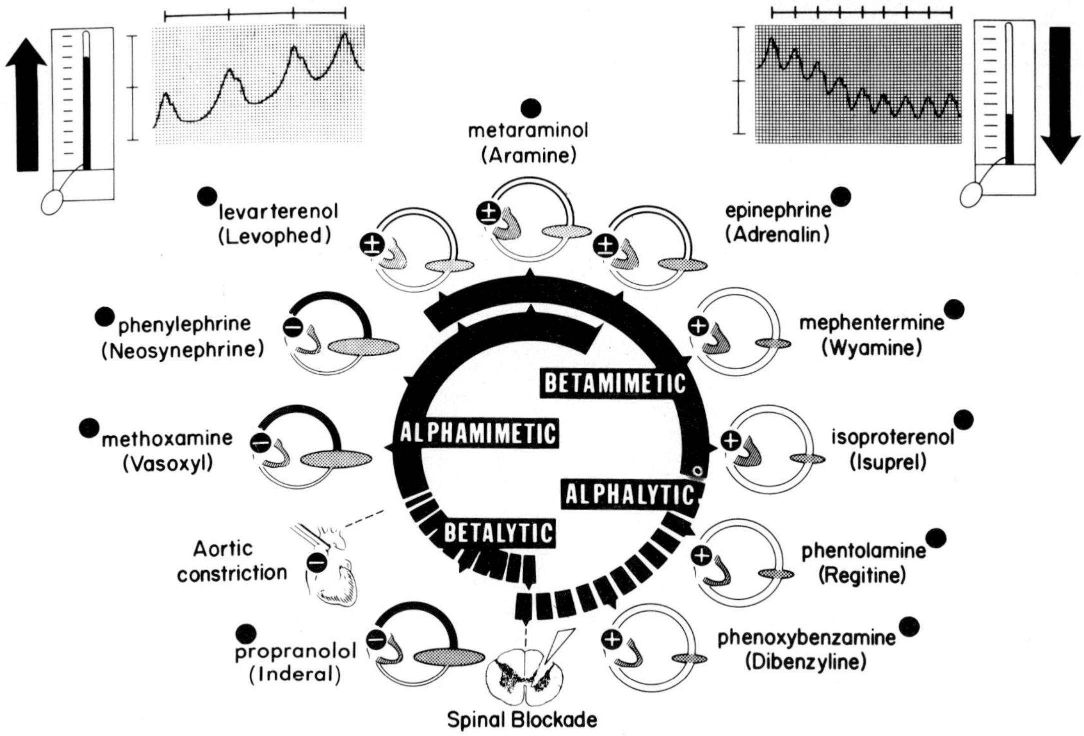

Figure 20–10. Spectrum of hemodynamic actions of vasoactive drugs. The sphygmomanometers and strip charts in upper right and left corners indicate the general actions of the drugs on either side of the circle.

Alphamimetic drugs increase peripheral vascular resistance, arterial blood pressure, and peripheral vascular pooling of blood with reflex slowing of the heart rate. Mixed alpha- and betamimetic drugs increase arterial blood pressure with some stimulation of the heart rate and force of contraction. Alphalytic drugs dilate the peripheral vasculature, and the heart is reflexly stimulated. Betalytic drugs slow the heart and decrease the force of contraction while allowing vasoconstriction to occur unopposed. (From the Shock Research Unit of the University of Southern California School of Medicine. Reproduced by permission from: Weil, M.H., and Bradley, E.C.: Circulatory Effects of Vasoactive Drugs in Current Use for Treatment of Shock. Bull. N.Y. Acad. Med., 42:1023, 1966.)

the heart rate and, on overdose, sinus pauses and brief periods of A-V nodal rhythm are produced by methoxamine. With lethal doses, if death occurs from respiratory arrest, cardiac action continues for some time (Lahti et al., 1955).

DeBeer et al. (1956) studied the effect of methoxamine and found it to be an effective agent for restoration of blood pressure in dogs in hypotensive states produced by hemorrhage, trauma, burns, tourniquet release, histamine, barbiturate overdose, and ganglionic blockade. It proved longer lasting than either ephedrine or d-desoxyephedrine in restoring and maintaining blood pressure. In normotensive dogs and cats, 0.4 mg/kg produced tachyphylaxis when given as a second dose following an initial dose of the same amount of drug. At 0.8 mg/kg, second doses actually produced a depressor effect. In hypotensive animals, doses of 0.4 mg/kg produced effective and prolonged response.

Methoxamine has been advocated in cardiopulmonary resuscitation by Livesay et al. (1978) and Redding et al. (1983). Both of these groups believe that the pure α-adrenergic effect maximizes myocardial oxygen supply/demand balance.

Methoxamine hydrochloride is marketed in 1-ml ampules containing 20 mg of the drug. Its chief advantage over other sympathomimetic amines is its prolonged effect from a single intramuscular injection. (Levarterenol, on the other hand, gives momentary control of blood pressure through adjustment of the rate of infusion, since it is a short-acting drug.)

TABLE 20–2. Effects of Vasoactive Drugs on Mean Arterial Pressure, Heart Rate, and Venous Return

Drug	*No. of Dogs*	*Mean Arterial Pressure mm Hg Control*	*Test*	*Heart Rate Beats/Min Control*	*Test*	*p*	*Change in Venous Return ml*	*p*
Isoproterenol	20	106	70	136	185	<0.001	+109	<0.001
Mephentermine	41	93	91	136	167	<0.001	+ 82	<0.001
Levarterenol	34	93	138	145	164	<0.001	+ 34	NS
Metaraminol	37	88	132	139	151	<0.01	+ 3	NS
Epinephrine	35	95	131	151	165	<0.001	− 21	NS
Angiotensin	36	91	124	143	141	NS	− 51	<0.001
Phenylephrine	37	88	147	149	137	<0.05	− 74	<0.001
Methoxamine	32	88	119	146	140	NS	− 79	<0.001

NS = not significant

(From the Shock Research Unit of the University of Southern California School of Medicine. Reproduced by permission from: Weil, M.H., and Bradley, E.C.: Circulatory Effects of Vasoactive Drugs in Current Use for Treatment of Shock. Bull. N.Y. Acad. Med., 42:1023, 1966.)

TABLE 20–3. Changes in Liver Weight and Portal Vein Pressure Following Administration of Vasoactive Drugs, with Cardiac Output Kept Constant

Drug	*No. of Dogs*	*Change in Liver Weight g*	*Change in Portal Vein Pressure mm Hg*
Isoproterenol	4	−19.4	−2.7
Mephentermine	7	−35.2	−1.6
Levarterenol	5	− 9.7	+0.2
Metaraminol	8	− 4.6	+0.6
Epinephrine	5	−11.9	+4.5
Angiotensin	9	− 8.7	+3.4
Phenylephrine	4	+33	+7
Methoxamine	6	+18	+3.9

(From the Shock Research Unit of the University of Southern California School of Medicine. Reproduced by permission from: Weil, M.H., and Bradley, E.C.: Circulatory Effects of Vasoactive Drugs in Current Use for Treatment of Shock. Bull. N.Y. Acad. Med., 42:1023, 1966.)

Methoxamine can be given either intramuscularly or intravenously. The former does not cause tissue necrosis.

Phenylephrine Hydrochloride, U.S.P. (Neo-Synephrine)

Phenylephrine is a synthetic sympathomimetic amine with alpha-adrenergic action essentially equal to levarterenol. It is less potent than the latter and has a longer duration of action with minimal cardiac effect and little central stimulation. Reflex bradycardia occurs following injection. In cyclopropane-sensitized hearts, ventricular tachycardia or fibrillation is not produced. Phenylephrine has been recommended as a vasopressor for use with halothane or isoflurane, because it produces fewer arrhythmias than epinephrine or metaraminol (Tucker et al., 1974). Phenylephrine hydrochloride is available as a 1.0% sterile solution for injection. The intravenous dose for dogs is 0.04 mg/lb; the subcutaneous or intramuscular dose is approximately 0.08 mg/lb.

Phenylephrine is sometimes added to solutions of local anesthetic agents in a concentration of 1:2500 to produce prolongation of action of the local anesthetic and to reduce its toxicity.

MIXED ALPHA- AND BETA-ADRENERGIC AGENTS

Dopamine Hydrochloride (Inotropin)

Dopamine hydrochloride is the naturally occurring catecholamine precursor of norepinephrine, and stimulates both alpha- and beta-adrenegic receptors (see Fig. 4–14). Each milliliter contains 40 mg of dopamine hydrochloride in water for injection, U.S.P., with 1% sodium bisulfite as a preservative.

Dopamine exerts an inotropic effect on the myocardium, causing increased cardiac output but with less increase in myocardial oxygen consumption than isoproterenol. Its use is usually not associated with tachyarrhythmia. Dopamine increases systolic and pulse pressure with little effect on diastolic pressure. Total peripheral resistance at low and intermediate doses is usually unchanged. In contrast to other vasopressors, blood flow to peripheral vascular beds may decrease while mesenteric and renal flow increases (Robie et al., 1974). Dopamine has been reported to dilate the renal vasculature by activation of a dopaminergic receptor (Dinerstein et al., 1979). This effect is accompanied by an increase in glomerular filtration rate, renal blood flow, and sodium excretion.

Dopamine is used for correction of hemodynamic imbalances present in shock (Reid and Thompson, 1975), trauma, open heart surgery, renal failure, and chronic cardiac decompensation. When indicated, blood volume should be restored with a suitable plasma expander or whole blood prior to administration of dopamine. In man, it is suggested that volume be increased until central venous pressure is 10 to 15 cm H_2O or pulmonary wedge pressure is 14 to 18 mm Hg. At this point, administration of diluted dopamine is instituted at doses of 2.5 mcg/kg/min, and the dosage is increased gradually as needed. Measurement of urine flow is one of the signs by which adequacy of vital organ perfusion can be monitored. Following administration of dopamine, urine flow in oliguric or anuric patients may increase to normal levels.

For administration, the contents of one ampule (5 ml containing 200 mg) are transferred to either a 250-ml or 500-ml bottle of one of the following: 1) sodium chloride injection, U.S.P.; 2) dextrose 5% injection, U.S.P.; 3) dextrose 5% and sodium chloride 0.9% injection, U.S.P.; 4) 5% dextrose in 0.45% sodium chloride solution; 5) dextrose 5% in lactated Ringer's solution; 6) sodium lactate (one-sixth molar) injection, U.S.P., or 7) lactated Ringer's injection, U.S.P. These dilutions yield a final concentration of 800 mcg/ml of dopamine in 250 ml or 400 mcg/ml in 500 ml. Solutions are stable for a minimum of 24 hours after dilution in the aforementioned solutions. Dopamine is not compatible with alkaline diluent solutions.

After dilution, dopamine is administered intravenously, utilizing an IV drip chamber to control the rate of flow in drops/minute. Each patient should be individually titrated to the desired hemodynamic and/or renal response. The optimum dosage rate for the desired increase in systolic blood pressure may require rapid administration after which the rate is reduced. Administration at rates greater than 50 mcg/kg/min can be used in emergencies.

Careful monitoring of the cardiac output, blood pressure, and urine flow are necessary when dopamine is given. Adverse reactions include ectopic beats, aberrant conduction, tachycardia, bradycardia, widened QRS complex, azotemia, hypotension, and vasoconstriction. Nausea and vomiting may occur along with dyspnea.

Use of dopamine with cyclopropane or halogenated hydrocarbon anesthetics is contraindicated since they increase cardiac autonomic irritability and may sensitize the myocardium to the action of catecholamines. Dopamine should not be used in patients with pheochromocytoma, or with uncorrected tachyarrhythmias or ventricular fibrillation. Its use should be avoided in pregnant animals.

Diluted dopamine should be infused intravenously, since injection into tissues may cause necrosis and slough. If extravasation occurs, the ischemic area should be infiltrated as soon as possible with 10 to 15 ml of saline solution containing 5 to 10 mg of phentolamine, an adrenergic blocking agent.

Since the duration of action of dopamine is short, no remedial measures are usually necessary in case of accidental overdosage. Phentolamine can be used if the patient's condition does not stabilize.

Levarterenol Bitartrate, U.S.P. (*l*-arterenol; *l*-norepinephrine; *l*-noradrenalin; Levophed)

Levarterenol has both alpha- and beta-adrenergic properties, the alpha predominating. It is the principal pressor amine found in postganglionic adrenergic nerves. The bitartrate is a white, water-soluble powder. On exposure to air and light, it tends to darken and should be discarded. Levarterenol bitartrate is a water-soluble salt of the levorotatory isomer of arterenol. The latter is the unmethylated precursor of epinephrine.

Levarterenol has a marked vasopressor action, slowing the pulse rate and producing little effect on cardiac output. The vasopressor action is due to generalized vasoconstriction; this characteristic is used clinically in treatment of hypotension due to surgery, hemorrhage, anesthetic agents, or tranquilizers. It does not increase the circulating blood volume and therefore is not a substitute for administration of whole blood or plasma expanders. Rather, it is an adjunct to treatment of these conditions. Levarterenol should be used cautiously with cyclopropane, chloroform, or other anesthetic agents that sensitize the heart, because of the possibility of producing ventricular fibrillation.

The inactivation and excretion of levarterenol and epinephrine are similar. Small quantities are excreted in the urine.

Because of its vasoconstrictor property, levarterenol may produce necrosis and slough when injected into tissues.

According to Stowe (1965), an average dose of levarterenol bitartrate is 0.01 to 0.02 μg/kg/min, using a dilution of 2 μg/ml in 5% dextrose. The duration of infusion is determined by return of blood pressure to a normal level. Patients should be "weaned" from levarterenol infusions since sudden withdrawal may cause hypotension. Withdrawal should take place over a period of several hours.

Dilution of levarterenol for infusion should be in 5% dextrose to protect against loss of potency by oxidation. The infusion fluid is prepared by diluting 4 ml of 0.2% levarterenol bitartrate solution (equivalent to 0.1% of base) in 1000 ml of 5% dextrose. Saline should not be used for this purpose because oxidation occurs with saline solutions.

Epinephrine Hydrochloride, U.S.P. (Adrenalin)

Epinephrine hydrochloride is a white, crystalline, odorless powder consisting of hormone formed by the adrenal medulla (Fig. 4–16). It is produced commercially by either synthesis or extraction from the adrenal glands of animals. A 1:1000 aqueous solution of epinephrine is used clinically. It oxidizes upon exposure to air and light, first to a pink color and then to a reddish brown. For this reason, it is protected by packaging in brown bottles.

Epinephrine is ineffective when given orally. Solutions may be injected intramuscularly, subcutaneously and, in emergencies, intravenously or intracardially. Intravenous injections produce a rapid and marked effect. The intramuscular dose necessary to produce a comparable response is 25 to 50 times greater. For this reason, intravenous and intracardial epinephrine should be used with caution. Epinephrine in the tissues is oxidized by amine and phenol oxidases and by the cytochrome system. The end products appear to be melanin pigments (Blaschko et al., 1937). A small amount of unoxidized epinephrine is conjugated with sulfuric acid and excreted in the urine.

Injection of epinephrine produces a quick rise in both systolic and diastolic blood pressure. This effect is mainly caused by arteriolar constriction, but is augmented by cardiac acceleration, increased myocardial contraction, and contraction of the spleen. The initial constrictor effect is caused by epinephrine stimulating the myoneural junction of blood vessels. A second rise in blood pressure may occur owing to stimulation of the vasoconstrictor center; thus, on a recording, two peaks or rises may be seen. After the rises, a fall below normal occurs followed by a return to the initial level. Subsequent intravenous injections of equal quantities of epinephrine cause progressively smaller pressor effects in the dog.

The vascular response to epinephrine varies depending upon the body location. Vessels of the abdominal viscera, including those of the kidneys, are constricted. On the other hand, the arterioles of the skeletal muscles are usually dilated. This can be explained on the basis of Cannon's "Emergency Theory," which states that the effect of epinephrine is to supply blood to those organs most needed during an emergency.

Epinephrine should not be used in the treatment of hypotension caused by phenothiazine tranquilizers. The latter produce alpha blockade and, if epinephrine is administered, "epinephrine reversal" may follow. The alpha (vasoconstrictor) effects of epinephrine are blocked leaving the beta (vasodilatory) effects unopposed. Fatal shock due to extreme vasodilatation may follow.

Epinephrine is a powerful cardiac stimulant, acting directly on the β_1 receptors, and producing increased force of contraction, shortening of systole, and increased output. It stimulates the cardiac accelerator nerve causing an increased heart rate. It is thought to cause the potassium current within Purkinje's fibers to fall more rapidly, thus speeding depolarization of the cell membrane (Hauswirth et al., 1968). Increased blood pressure produces stimulation of the caroticoaortic pressor receptive mechanism which, in turn, stimulates the vagus nerve to depress the heart. The heart rate is thus slowed even as the blood pressure reaches its maximum.

The stimulating action of epinephrine on the myocardium is used in combating cardiac arrest. In this situation, 0.5 to 1.0 ml of 1:10,000 epinephrine is injected intravenously, following which the heart is massaged to force epinephrine-containing blood into the coronary vessels. Holmes et al. (1980) have shown that epinephrine is more effective in maintaining cerebral and coronary blood flows during cardiopulmonary resuscitation than are phenylephrine and isoproterenol (Table 20–4). Although intracardial injection has often been employed successfully, it has no advantage over the intravenous route and may damage the heart.

Epinephrine may also be detrimental to the myocardium, a high concentration producing cardiac dilatation and ventricular fibrillation. Epinephrine-induced ventricular fibrillation is seen particularly with chloroform, cyclopropane, and halothane. These anesthetics sensitize the myocardium to the stimulant action of the drug. Under these conditions, a dose of epinephrine that normally has no cardiac effect will induce fibrillation. Acepromazine has a protective effect against epinephrine-induced arrhythmias and ventricular fibrillation in thiamylal-halothane anesthetized dogs (see Chap. 8).

Epinephrine is sometimes used for its direct effect upon the blood vessels. Mixed with local anesthetic agents, a solution of 1:100,000 produces local vasoconstriction, preventing toxic reactions and prolonging the action of the agent. A 1:10,000 or 1:20,000 solution is sometimes sprayed on mucous membranes or injected locally to prevent hemorrhage during surgical procedures. Systemic toxicity can result from extensive absorption of epinephrine when used for this purpose. Use of epinephrine with halothane anesthesia is contraindicated.

Epinephrine has no direct effect upon respiration and should not be used as a respiratory analeptic. If blood pressure response to epinephrine is appreciable, an inverse respiratory response occurs. Respirations are decreased during the period of increased blood pressure and then increased as the blood pressure falls. This response is probably due to blood pressure changes in the carotid sinus and aortic arch.

Epinephrine has little effect on other body organs or functions; the gastrointestinal tract is inhibited, the pupil of the eye is dilated, and the basal metabolic rate is accelerated. Epinephrine causes glycogenolysis, hypergly-

TABLE 20–4. Drug Effects During Cardiopulmonary Resuscitation

	Cardiac Output (ml/min)	*Cerebral Blood Flow (ml/min)*	*Coronary Blood Flow (ml/min)*	*Kidney Blood Flow (ml/min)*
Saline	392	37	25	44
Epinephrine	319	54	79	4
Phenylephrine	255	29	26	16
Isoproterenol	475	28	15	29

(From Holmes, H.R., Babbs, C.F., Voorhees, W.D., Tracker, W.A., and DeGaravilla, B.: Influence of Adrenergic Drugs upon Vital Organ Perfusion During CPR. Crit. Care Med., 8:137, 1980).

cemia, and transient glycosuria; this action potentiates barbiturate anesthesia. In the cat, epinephrine stimulates salivary flow, which is thick and viscid.

In excessive doses, epinephrine causes tachycardia, palpitation, high blood pressure, dyspnea, pupillary dilatation, vertigo, rapid collapse, and death. The latter occurs from acute cardiac dilatation, pulmonary edema, and ventricular fibrillation. When injected subcutaneously or intramuscularly in dogs, 0.5 to 1.0 ml of 1:1000 epinephrine may produce edematous swelling followed by necrosis at the site of injection.

Only symptomatic treatment is used in epinephrine poisoning. Because of its rapid metabolism by enzymes within the body, the effects are transient.

Recommended subcutaneous or intramuscular doses of a 1:1000 solution of epinephrine hydrochloide are 4 to 8 ml in adult cattle and horses and 1 to 3 ml in sheep and swine; 1 to 5 ml of a 1:10,000 solution is recommended in dogs and cats.

Intravenously, one-fifth to one-half of the aforementioned dose as a 1:10,000 solution is recommended (Stowe, 1965).

Amphetamine Sulfate, U.S.P. (Benzadrine Sulfate, N.N.R.)

Amphetamine is a racemic mixture of d, l, and dl-beta forms of the drug. The dextrorotatory form is known as *Dextro-Amphetamine, U.S.P.* (Dexedrine Sulfate).

Amphetamine is classified both as a sympathomimetic amine and as a respiratory analeptic. It releases norepinephrine from adrenergic terminals. Possessing both alpha- and beta-adrenergic properties, it produces an elevation of blood pressure due to peripheral vasoconstriction, stimulates the heart muscle, relaxes the bronchial and intestinal muscles, and dilates the pupil. As a respiratory analeptic, it stimulates the cerebrospinal axis, particularly the brain stem and cortex. It is a potent stimulant of the medullary respiratory center, thus relieving central depression caused by anesthetics. A marked increase in rate and depth of respiration results from its central stimulating action. Large doses of amphetamine have been shown to increase oxygen consumption markedly in experimental animals. With repeated doses, tachyphylaxis occurs.

Gunn (1939) showed that amphetamine produced uterine contraction in all animals examined, including nonpregnant cats. Mydriasis is also produced.

Amphetamine is destroyed in the body by deamination and excretion of the unchanged portion in the urine. Amine oxidase has little effect on this compound.

Amphetamine is available in 5.0% solution. Craige (1943) reported that 5 mg/kg of amphetamine sulfate intravenously is the MLD in normal unanesthetized dogs. The optimum dose for anesthetized, critically depressed dogs is 4.0 to 4.5 mg/kg intravenously. Doses of less than 1 mg/kg are ineffective in this situation, whereas larger doses are superfluous and may be fatal. Dogs dying from large doses have severe hemorrhagic gastroenteritis on necropsy.

When amphetamine was given to dogs anesthetized with pentobarbital sodium (28.5 mg/kg), 1 of 10 dogs died following injection of 11 mg/kg, and the LD_{50} appeared to be in excess of 44 mg/kg.

The usual dose of amphetamine for large animals is 0.2 to 0.7 mg/kg given intramuscularly or intravenously.

Amphetamine is a Schedule II drug under federal regulations, and for the reason its use in veterinary medicine is decreasing.

Metaraminol Bitartrate (Aramine)

Metaraminol is a potent vasopressor with prolonged duration of action. It liberates norepinephrine and is itself taken up by adrenergic neurones and the heart. Its actions, therefore, are almost identical to those of norepinephrine. It is available in solution containing 10 mg/ml. The dose for dogs is 0.05 to 0.20 mg/kg intravenously or 0.5 to 1.0 mg/kg intramuscularly.

Following injection in hypotensive dogs, there is a rapid rise in blood pressure due to peripheral vasoconstriction. An increase in cardiac output and coronary blood flow also occurs, caused by amplified myocardial contractility (Sarnoff et al., 1954). In dogs with hemorrhagic hypotension, a significant increase in survival has been noted by Sarnoff and Kaufman (1954).

The central nervous system is not stimulated as with some other sympathomimetic amines, and there is a slight tendency to prolong barbiturate narcosis. Respiration is either unaffected or is moderately slowed following injection.

There is little evidence of tachyphylaxis. Following administration of epinephrine and some other sympathomimetic amines, secondary vasodilation occurs. This is not observed with metaraminol.

Injection may be made intravenously, intramuscularly, or subcutaneously. The onset of action is approximately 1 minute, 10 minutes, and 20 minutes respectively and lasts for 20 minutes to 1 hour. Metaraminol does not appear to cause cardiac arrhythmias, but its use with cyclopropane and halogenated inhalant agents is not recommended.

BETA-ADRENERGIC AGENTS

Mephentermine Sulfate, U.S.P. (Wyamine)

Mephentermine acts both directly and by release of endogenous norepinephrine. It produces a betamimetic effect with increased cardiac output and heart rate. Goldberg et al. (1953), in comparing sympathomimetic drugs, found that it had prominent inotropic and chronotropic actions on the dog heart, apparently due to release of endogenous norepinephrine in the heart itself.

Mephentermine, when given intravenously, produces an effect for 30 to 50 minutes; on intramuscular injection, it lasts up to 4 hours. Repeated intravenous injections in dogs produce tachyphylaxis, apparently caused by norepinephrine depletion in the heart.

Mephentermine is marketed in sterile vials containing 1 or 10 ml (15 mg/ml) for parenteral administration. The intravenous dose for dogs is 0.3 mg/kg.

Isoproterenol Hydrochloride, U.S.P. (Isuprel)

Isoproterenol hydrochloride is a potent beta-adrenergic agent with virtually no alpha-adrenergic property. It is used as a cardiac stimulant in anesthesiology and in the treatment of shock and bronchospasm. In dogs, the toxic dose of isoproterenol is approximately 1000 times the therapeutic dose.

Isoproterenol is supplied as a 1:5000 solution for parenteral use. It contains 0.2 mg/ml of isoproterenol hydrochloride, 0.12 mg of lactic acid, 1.8 mg of sodium lactate, 7 mg of sodium chloride, not more than 1 mg of sodium bisulphite as preservative, and the pH is adjusted with hydrochloric acid. It is sold in ampules of 1 and 5 ml.

It has been shown by Starzecki et al. (1968) that isoproterenol markedly increases the survival of dogs subjected to endotoxin shock. This is attributed to increased cardiac output with decreased peripheral, renal, and mesenteric resistance resulting in an increased perfusion of tissues (see Tables 20–2, 20–3). Renal output is increased markedly by this drug. It has been used to increase cardiac output and to improve tissue perfusion in the horse by slow IV drip (0.2 to 0.4 mg in 1000 ml of lactated Ringer's solution) (Riebold et al., 1982).

Isoproterenol (1:5000) is diluted in 5% dextrose solution (5 ml in 500 ml) for administration to patients in shock. The mixture is infused at a rate of 0.25 to 2.5 ml/min. Higher concentrations of drug can be used where the total amount of fluid administered should be controlled.

Isoproterenol should not be used in cardiopulmonary resuscitation because it shunts blood away from vital organs (Holmes et al., 1980).

Isoproterenol has been shown to be a potent bronchodilating agent, even in doses that have little effect on the cardiovascular system (Cohen et al., 1949). In contrast to epinephrine, it may be used in patients anesthetized with cyclopropane. For treatment of bronchospasm during anesthesia, isoproterenol is given intravenously in an initial dose of 0.01 mg (0.5 ml of a 1:50,000 solution, repeated as necessary). The 1:50,000 solution is prepared by diluting 1 ml of a 1:5000 solution with sterile saline. Halmagyi et al. (1964) have shown that isoproterenol given to sheep anesthetized intravenously with thiopental at the rate of 0.33 μg/kg/min increased lung compliance approximately 50%.

Dobutamine Hydrochloride (Dobutrex)

Dobutamine is a synthetic catecholamine which, in comparison to the naturally occurring catecholamines and isoproterenol, appears to be more cardioselective. It is a direct-acting inotropic agent with primary activity on the β_1-receptors of the heart, while producing comparatively mild chronotropic or arrhythmogenic effects. Dobutamine has weak action on the α- and β_2-adrenergic receptors resulting in mild hypertension. Because it does not cause release of endogenous norepinephrine as does dopamine, it avoids the undesirable effects of norepinephrine and eliminates possible loss of potency in patients with depleted norepinephrine.

Dobutamine is indicated for parenteral administration in short-term treatment of cardiac decompensation due to depressed contractility as might result from cardiac surgical procedures or organic heart disease. In patients with atrial fibrillation and rapid ventricular response, a digitalis preparation should be used prior to instituting therapy with dobutamine.

In experiments with dogs anesthetized with halothane, dobutamine, dopamine, and isoproterenol were administered for 5-minute periods in successively increasing doses (Holloway and Frederickson, 1974). Dobutamine produced no obvious extremes in cardiac output, heart rate, stroke volume, arterial pressure, or total peripheral resistance. Isoproterenol caused excessive tachycardia, and high doses of dopamine caused hypertension. Dopamine caused serious arrhythmias and death more than twice as frequently when these drugs were administered in large inotropically equivalent doses. Dopamine and dobutamine were compared in vagotomized dogs anesthetized with pentobarbital (Robie and Goldberg, 1975). Both agents increased myocardial contractility, but dobutamine had a greater effect on cardiac output. Infusions of dopamine greater than 5 mcg/kg/min increased mean aortic pressure, whereas dobutamine raised the systolic pressure slightly without altering mean aortic pressure. Dopamine infusions up to 10 mcg/kg/min increased renal and mesenteric blood flow and decreased vascular resistance; in contrast, dobutamine had negligible effects on renal and mesenteric blood flows but produced dose-related increases in femoral blood flow.

Hinds and Hawthorne (1975) compared cardiac dynamics with constant infusions of dobutamine and isoproterenol in conscious dogs. With increasing doses of dobutamine, linear increases were significant in all measured indices of myocardial contractility, such as T/P_{40}, mean velocity of left ventricular fiber shortening, ejection fraction, and stroke work. When dobutamine was infused in doses of 5 to 20 μg/kg/min, these changes occurred without changes in end-diastolic volume, mean aortic pressure, or heart rate. Isoproterenol also caused linear changes, but in doses of 0.02 to 0.10 μg/kg/min. It produced a significantly higher heart rate than dobutamine. Cardiac minute work (heart rate times stroke work) was increased by both drugs. With infusions of isoproterenol, however, the amount of cardiac work was significantly limited because of increases in heart rate, whereas with dobutamine, cardiac minute work increased to a higher level because of changes in myocardial contractility without changes in heart rate.

Tuttle and Mills (1975) found that dobutamine had an inotropic efficacy as great as that of epinephrine, owing to its direct action on β_1 cardiac receptors. Unlike epinephrine, dobutamine had slight effect on α and β_2 vascular receptors. In ischemic dog hearts, dobutamine did not cause significant arrhythmic activity, whereas dopamine, norepinephrine, and isoproterenol caused severe ectopic activity. In dogs with induced low cardiac contractility, low cardiac output, and hypotension, dobutamine produced dose-related increases in cardiac contractility and output, restoring arterial blood pressure, and reducing total peripheral resistance slightly. In contrast, isoproterenol failed to restore blood pressure and had only a meager effect on cardiac contractility and output. It caused extreme tachycardia and lowered peripheral resistance more than did dobutamine. Norepinephrine did not increase cardiac contractility or output as much as dobutamine and excessively elevated peripheral resistance and arterial blood pressure.

The short half-life of dobutamine (1 to 2 minutes) is due to rapid tissue uptake. It is metabolized in the tissues, and the metabolites reenter the systemic circulation. During continuous intravenous infusion in dogs, a steady-state level of dobutamine is reached in 8 to 10 minutes. During continuous IV infusion, the combined biliary and urinary excretion rates approach the infusion rates 3 to 4 hours after infusion is started. Forty-eight hours after dobutamine administration, 67% is excreted in urine and 20% in feces (Murphy et al., 1976).

Dobutamine is supplied in 20-ml rubber-stoppered vials containing 250 mg of sterile powder. Hydrochloric acid is used to adjust the pH to between 2.5 and 5.5. The powder is constituted with sterile water for injection or 5% dextrose injection. Diluent (10 ml) is added to the vial, which contains 250 mg of dobutamine. It may be stored under refrigeration for 48 hours or at room temperature for 6 hours. Reconstituted dobutamine is further diluted in 5% dextrose injection, 0.9% sodium chloride injection, or sodium lactate injection. Dilute solutions should be used within 24 hours. Solutions may exhibit a pink color caused by slight oxidation of the drug; it indicates no significant loss of potency. The rate of administration and duration of therapy must be adjusted to the patient's response as determined by heart rate, presence of ectopic activity, blood pressure, urine flow and, where possible, measurement of cardiac output. The usual rate of infusion ranges from 2.5 to 10 mcg/kg/min, with rates up to 40 mcg/kg/min occasionally being required to produce the desired effect. In case of overdosage, the rate of administration is temporarily discontinued. Because the duration of action is short, usually no remedial measures are necessary.

According to Kittleson (1980), dobutamine is preferable to all other sympathomimetics for cardiac support because of its negligible effects on heart rate, blood pressure, and dysrhythmogenesis.

ALPHALYTIC AGENTS

Phentolamine Mesylate (Regitine)

Phentolamine is a potent alphalytic agent of relatively short duration. In dogs, it lowers arterial blood pressure and peripheral vascular resistance, while increasing venous return (Bradley, 1965).

Phentolamine is available in ampules containing 5 mg of phentolamine mesylate and 5 mg of lactose in lyophilized form. It is reconstituted with sterile water. The dose for dogs is 1 to 3 mg administered intramuscularly or *very slowly* intravenously. Fluids must be given concurrently to prevent severe hypotension.

It has been used in man for diagnosis and treatment of pheochromocytoma and in the treatment of shock. It is uniformly hypotensive in dogs, cats, rabbits, rats, and guinea pigs (Meier et al., 1949).

Phenoxybenzamine Hydrochloride (Dibenzyline, Dibenyline)

Phenoxybenzamine is an alpha-adrenergic blocking agent used for treatment of hypertension and the diagnosis of pheochromocytoma in man. By producing and maintaining "chemical sympathectomy," this agent causes peripheral blood flow to be increased while systemic blood pressure is decreased. It has no effect on the parasympathetic system. In treatment of shock, it is used to prevent acute arterial vasoconstriction and thus to increase organ perfusion.

Phenoxybenzamine is given slowly by intravenous infusion. Extravascular administration should be avoided since the solution may cause tissue damage. The onset of action is slow, requiring approximately 30 minutes. The intravenous dose is 0.25 to 2 mg/kg diluted in 250 to 500 ml of 5% dextrose or 0.9% sodium chloride solution. The response is persistent, lasting approximately 24 hours.

Phenoxybenzamine hydrochloride solution for injection contains 50 mg of phenoxybenzamine hydrochloride, 48.5% v/v absolute alcohol, 0.5% v/v hydrochloric acid, and propylene glycol q.s.ad. 1.0 ml.

In treatment of acute hypotension caused by phenoxybenzamine, the usual pressor agents are not effective. Epinephrine is contraindicated since it may produce a further fall in blood pressure caused by "epinephrine reversal." Levarterenol may be administered intravenously since its effect may not be completely blocked.

Phenothiazine Tranquilizers

The phenothiazine tranquilizers are alphalytic. They are described in Chapter 8.

BETALYTIC AGENTS

Propranolol Hydrochloride (Inderal)

Propranolol hydrochloride is a beta-adrenergic blocking agent that reduces the chronotropic and inotropic actions of sympathetic stimulation on the heart. It thus prevents cardiac overactivity produced by fear, pain, vagolytic drugs, anesthesia, surgical trauma, respiratory acidosis, and either exogenous or endogenous catecholamines (Johnstone, 1966). It is used in anesthesia for treatment of cardiac arrhythmias and fibrillation. It has a half-life of approximately 40 to 60 minutes when given intravenously.

Beta-adrenergic blockade with propranolol produces a fall in heart rate, a reduction in cardiac output, a reduction in resting stroke volume, reduced oxygen consumption, and an increase in left ventricular end-diastolic pressure. Following administration, the effects of beta-adrenergic stimulation are blocked for up to 4 hours. Propranolol has been shown to block the release of plasma-free fatty acids produced by administration of catecholamines.

In pentobarbital- or chloralose-anesthetized dogs, intravenous injection of propranolol reduces heart rate, cardiac contractile force, arterial blood pressure, and aortic blood flow due to decrease in cardiac output. Propranolol has been shown to block the chronotropic and inotropic actions of isoproterenol, epinephrine, and norepinephine and to block stellate ganglion stimulation. It does not affect the response to phenylephrine.

Williams and Sekiya (1963) and Erlij and Mendez (1964) found that beta blockade prevented the ventricular arrhythmias produced by cardiac glycosides in isolated guinea pig hearts and anesthetized dogs. Benfey and Varma (1966), studying propranolol in guinea pigs, concluded that it possesses an antifibrillatory property that may not be directly related to its beta-receptor blocking activity. Lucchesi et al. (1967) showed that propranolol was effective in reversing or preventing several types of experimentally induced cardiac arrhythmias in dogs. Lucchesi and Iwami (1968) demonstrated that pretreatment with 0.5 mg/kg intravenously protected dogs against halothane-epinephrine-induced ventricular tachycardia and ventricular fibrillation.

In subacute toxicity studies, propranolol has been given to dogs intravenously at the rate of 7.5 mg/kg without ill effects. Studies of blood levels on long-term oral administration indicate there is no accumulation in the blood with oral doses as high as 60 mg/kg daily.

During halothane anesthesia, tachyarrhythmias may arise with carbon dioxide accumulation, surgical stimulation, or catecholamine administration. These may be treated by intravenous administration of propranolol. However, it may cause cardiac collapse in dogs anesthetized with ether or chloroform (Rouse, 1966). When combined atropine and propranolol are administered, the heart is essentially denervated and its rate becomes the intrinsic rate of the S-A node (Jose, 1966).

Propranolol also protects the heart from the positive intropic and chronotropic effects of excessive levels of catecholamines as occur in pheochromocytoma. Alpha-adrenergic blocking agents (phenoxybenzamine and phentolamine) reduce the risk of excessive hypertension from this tumor before and during surgery, but do not prevent excessive cardiac stimulation by catecholamines. Alpha-receptor blockers should always be used with propranolol since antagonism of the dilator (beta) action of epinephrine on peripheral vessels may leave the constrictor (alpha) action unopposed and cause a serious rise in blood pressure.

The intravenous dose is up to 0.2 mg/kg administered with ECG and central venous pressure monitoring. The rate of administration should not exceed 1 mg (1 ml) per minute. Once an alteration in rhythm is recorded, no further drug should be given until the full effect is observed. If bradycardia occurs, atropine should be administered intravenously. If central venous pressure rises inordinately, administration should be stopped unless the patient is first digitalized (Winnie, 1968).

Propranolol is supplied in 1-ml ampules each containing 1 mg of drug in sterile water. The pH is adjusted with citric acid.

CARDIAC GLYCOSIDES

The cardiac glycosides (digitoxin, digoxin, and ouabain) produce an increase in the force of ventricular contraction in both normal and failing hearts. Cardiac output is increased, and the effects of heart failure, such as pulmonary and peripheral edema, are reversed (Fig. 20–11). Increased cardiac output reflexly slows heart rate by reducing the high adrenergic tone associated with heart failure.

Digitalization slows the rate by decreasing conduction velocity in cardiac muscle and the atrioventricular conduction system. Furthermore, it enhances vagal slowing of the sinoatrial (SA) node. These effects slow ventricular response to supraventricular tachycardia, such as atrial flutter and fibrillation. In the failing heart, digitalis decreases intraventricular volume and filling pressure, and thus produces a net reduction in myocardial oxygen consumption.

Glycosides appear to inhibit cell membrane Na^+-K^+ ATPase. Inhibition causes an intracellular accumulation of Na^+ that exchanges by means of an electroneutral carrier system with Ca^{++} localized superficially on the outer surface of the cell membrane (Fig. 20–12). The result is an increased efflux of Na^+ and an increased inward movement of Ca^{++} into the cell to activate myofilaments.

Deutsch and Dalen (1969) have pointed out that, in the absence of overt cardiac failure, atrial flutter, or fibrillation, administration of cardiac glycosides in preparation of the patient for anesthesia is controversial. They recommended preanesthetic digitalization in man 1) to decrease the incidence of heart failure due to the stress of anesthesia and surgery, and 2) to lower the incidence of intra- and postoperative arrhythmias (Table 20–5). However, since cardiac glycosides have a low therapeutic index and the possibility of toxicity exists, it is probably wise to use these drugs only for established indications (Atlee and Rusy, 1981).

From a clinical standpoint, digoxin is the only glycoside of importance; digitoxin and ouabain are seldom used. Digoxin therapy is indicated in the long-term treatment of cardiogenic shock. For immediate therapy, dobutamine or dopamine should be given by continuous infusion.

Cardiac glycosides are listed in Table 20–6. Signs of digitalization in the failing heart are: 1) slowing of the heart to near normal rate, e.g., from 150 to 70 beats per minute; 2) reduction

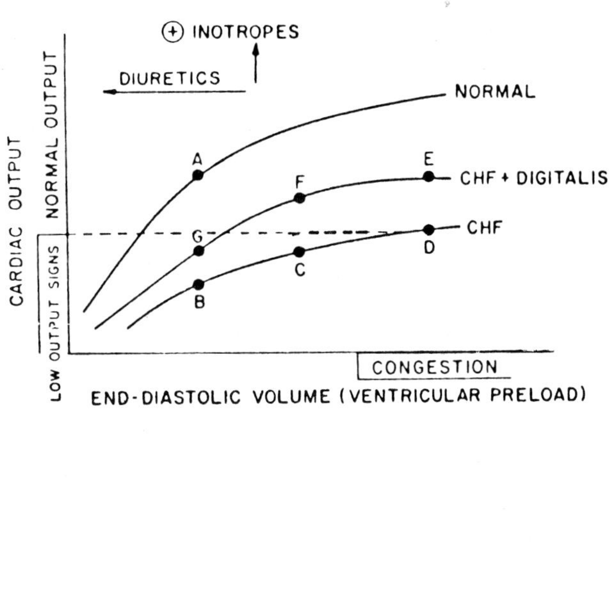

Figure 20–11. Ventricular function curves in congestive heart failure. The effect of blood volume (end-diastolic volume) on cardiac output is shown. As ventricular preload increases, cardiac output is augmented. Normal hearts function near point A. With heart failure (B), the ventricular function curve shifts down and to the right. Compensatory mechanisms retain fluid and salt, maintaining cardiac output at the expense of congestive signs (D). The administration of a diuretic relieves edema (C) but results in low output signs (e.g., azotemia). Administration of digitalis shifts the ventricular function curve up and to the left (E). Diuretic therapy now relieves edema, and cardiac output is adequate (F). Excessive diuretic therapy still can be hazardous (G). CHF = congestive heart failure. (From Bonagura, J.D.: The Clinical Pharmacology of Cardiovascular Drugs. Scientific Proceedings of the Am. Anim. Hosp. Assoc., 1981. Adapted from Bonagura, J.: Acute Heart Failure. In *Current Veterinary Therapy VII*. Edited by R.W. Kirk. W.B. Saunders, Philadelphia, 1980.)

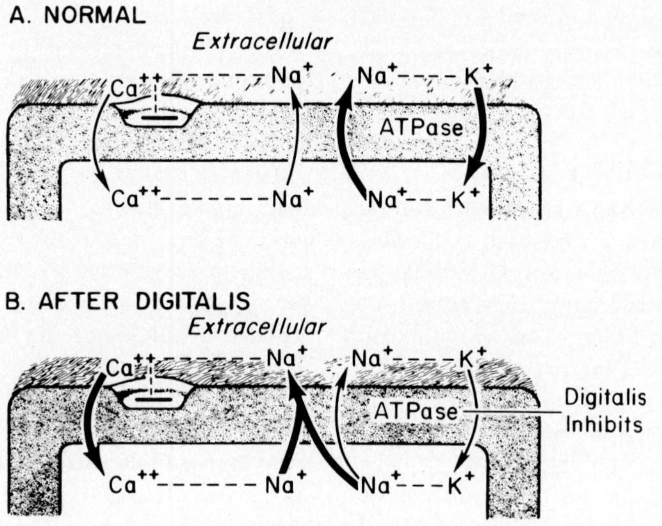

Figure 20–12. Schematic representation of the proposed mechanism for the inotropic action of cardiac glycosides. Inhibition of Na^+–K^+ ATPase ("sodium pump") by digitalis results in increased intracellular concentrations of sodium available for exchange with calcium. The heavy arrows designate the dominant pathway of ion exchange during normal conditions *(A)* and after inhibition by digitalis of Na^+–K^+ ATPase *(B)*. (From Parker, J.L., and Adams, R.H.: Drugs and the Heart Muscle. J.A.V.M.A., 171:78, 1977.)

in central venous pressure; 3) electrocardiographic changes, such as increased PR interval and depression of ST segment; 4) lessening of pulmonary congestion; and 5) diuresis.

The therapeutic index for cardiac glycosides is quite low; therefore, the effect of anesthetics on toxicity is important in digitalized patients that must be anesthetized. It has been shown that epidural and systemic lidocaine lower toxicity, whereas pentobarbital has no effect and cyclopropane increases it. The relative potency of anesthetics in converting ouabain-induced ventricular tachycardia to sinus rhythm is, in order of descending effectiveness: diethyl ether, methoxyflurane, enflurane, isoflurane, and pentobarbital (Ivankovich et al., 1976).

The LD_{50} of ouabain is significantly increased by ketamine and fentanyl-droperidol. The effect of the latter is attributed to the droperidol component, since fentanyl alone has no effect (Ivankovitch et al., 1975).

The most serious signs of digitalis intoxication are arrhythmias. Varying degrees of heart block, premature ventricular contractions, ventricular tachycardia, and fibrillation may result. Hypokalemia due to diuretics or administration of calcium are common causes in digitalized

TABLE 20–5. Recommendations for Preoperative Digitalization

I. ESTABLISHED INDICATIONS
    - Overt heart failure
    - Atrial fibrillation or flutter

II. PROPHYLACTIC DIGITALIZATION
    - To prevent intra-or postoperative heart failure
        - Past history of heart failure even though now well-compensated
        - Cardiac enlargement disclosed by chest roentgenogram
        - ECG evidence of left or right ventricular hypertrophy
    - To prevent or to control postoperative arrhythmias
        - History of documented episodes of atrial fibrillation or flutter
        - All patients undergoing cardiac surgery
        - Aged patients undergoing pulmonary surgery
        - Patients with aortic or mitral stenosis (with or without cardiac enlargement)

(Adapted from Deutsch, S., and Dalen, J.E.: Indications for Prophylactic Digitalization. Anesthesiology, 30:648, 1969.)

TABLE 20–6. Doses of Cardiac Glycosides

Product	Dog	Cat	Horse	Cow
Digoxin (Lanoxin)	Rapid IV digitalization, 0.01 to 0.02 mg/kg; administer one-half dose and follow incrementally with remaining half during next 8 hrs	Rapid IV digitalization, 0.01 mg/kg; administer as for dog	IV loading dose 14 μg/kg divided into thirds and given over 1- to 2-hr intervals; IV maintenance 7 μg/kg/day	Rapid IV digitalization, 0.88 mg/100 kg; administer as for dog
	Oral maintenance, 0.01 to 0.02 mg/kg divided bid	Oral maintenance, 0.007 to 0.01 mg/kg divided bid	Oral loading dose 70 μg/kg; oral maintenance 35 μg/kg/day	Oral therapy not effective due to degradation in rumen
Digitoxin	Rapid IV digitalization 0.01 to 0.03 mg/kg; administer one-half dose and follow incrementally with remaining half during next 8 hrs	—	—	—
	Oral maintenance, 0.06 to 0.1 mg/kg divided bid or tid	—	Oral digitalizing dose, 3.3 to 6.6 mg/kg; administer in 6 divided doses; oral maintenance, approximately one-eighth to one-fifth of digitalizing dose	Oral therapy not effective due to degradation in rumen
Ouabain (G-Strophanthin)	Rapid IV digitalization, 0.022 to 0.033 mg/kg; administer one-half dose and follow in 2 hrs with other half incrementally	—	Rapid IV digitalization, 1.32 to 2.2 mg/100 kg; administer as for dog	Same as horse

patients. Phenytoin is an almost specific treatment for digitalis-induced ventricular arrhythmias. Potassium chloride is specific for hypokalemia-induced digitalis toxicity.

Digoxin (Lanoxin, Cardoxin)

Digoxin is available for injection in 2-ml ampules containing 0.5 mg. The biological half-life is 20 to 38 hours in the dog (Bonagura, 1981) and 23.1 hours in the horse (Button et al., 1980). Cats have a lower tolerance to digoxin (Bonagura, 1981). For intravenous digitalization, one-half the dose should be given immediately. The remaining half should be given in increments during the next 8 hours, based on the patient's status and ECG. For long-term therapy, the patient can be switched to oral digoxin or digitoxin.

Ouabain is considered obsolete for intravenous digitalization.

TABLE 20–7. Classification of Antiarrhythmic Drugs

Group	Agent
I	Quinidine Procainamide Disopyramide
II	Lidocaine Phenytoin Mexiletine* Tocainide*
III	Propranolol Metoprolol
IV	Bretylium
V	Verapamil* Nifedipine*

*Not currently available for routine clinical use.

(From Federman, J., and Vlietstra, R.E.: Series on Pharmacology in Practice. 2. Antiarrhythmic Drug Therapy. Mayo Clin. Proc., 54:531, 1979.)

ANTIARRHYTHMIC AGENTS

Antiarrhythmic drugs are of dual importance in anesthesiology because 1) their use in emergencies may be life-saving, and 2) patients to be anesthetized may already be receiving these drugs. Antiarrhythmic drugs have been classified into five groups (Federman and Vlietstra, 1979) (Table 20–7). Of these, the most important in veterinary use are quinidine, procainamide, lidocaine, phenytoin, propranolol, and bretylium. While not listed, acepromazine is also a potent antiarrhythmic agent (see Chap. 8).

Group I. These drugs act by depressing Na^+ conductance. They slow the action potential upstroke in phase 0, thus slowing conduction velocity, and prolonging the action potential and refractoriness. Automaticity is decreased by decreasing the slope of phase 4 depolarization.

They are effective in supraventricular and ventricular arrhythmias that are due to either an automatic focus or a reentry circuit (Fig. 20–13). With reentry arrhythmias, they increase the refractoriness of one or more components of the circuit. Atrioventricular node conduction, His bundle conduction, and intraventricular conduction are suppressed. The P-R interval, QRS duration, H-V interval, and Q-T interval are prolonged. Complete heart block may result, and suppression of lower pacemakers may cause asystole. Because some drugs in this group also manifest an atropine-like effect, which tends to counter the direct action on atrioventricular node conduction, the net effect may be to accelerate atrioventricular conduction.

Group II. These drugs have little influence on the conduction velocity of normal myocardium. A selective decrease in conduction in ischemic myocardium has been shown with both lidocaine and phenytoin. Thus, their action in

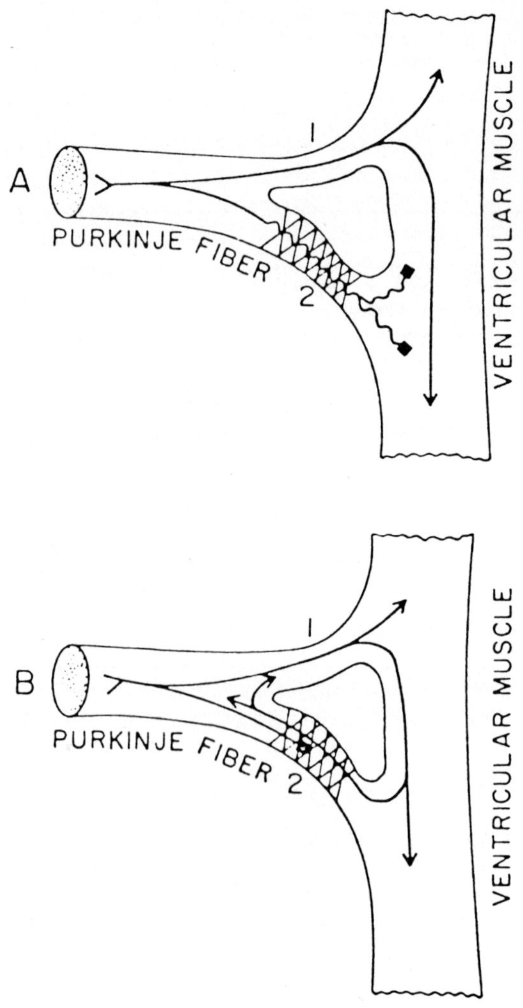

Figure 20–13. Schematic representation of branching Purkinje fiber terminating on a ventricular muscle fiber; model for reentry of excitation. Reentry is prevented in Panel A, but permitted in Panel B. In Panels A and B, the impulse arriving from above conducts normally through branch 1 and excites the ventricular muscle fiber. The impulse in branch 2, however, fails to conduct normally. This may happen when the fibers are subject to hypoxia, stretch, catecholamines, digitalis excess, electrolyte imbalances or, possibly, anesthetics. In Panel A, the impulse *propagates slowly* through branch 2 to excite the ventricular fiber, which is now refractory following previous excitation by the impulse conducted through branch 1. In Panel A, reentry is not possible because the impulse traveling through branch 1 cannot be conducted antidromically through branch 2, and the impulse traveling orthodromically and slowly through branch 2 cannot excite the ventricular fiber. Reentry of excitation is possible in Panel B where the orthodromically conducted impulse is *blocked* in branch 2. The impulse conducted through branch 1 excites the ventricular fiber and returns antidromically through branch 2, which is no longer absolutely refractory. The impulse traveling back through branch 2 excites the more proximal portions of the Purkinje fiber and returns via branch 1 to reexcite the ventricular fiber resulting in a return extrasystole. If the reentry circuit is maintained, a series of extrasystoles or tachycardia results. Reentry is abolished if another impulse from above reaches branch 1 before the return extrasystole coming back up branch 2. Whereas the reentrant circuit involves the ventricular muscle-Purkinje fiber junction, the potential for reentry exists anywhere in the heart. (From Atlee, J.L., III: Antiarrhythmic Agents. In *Drug Interactions in Anesthesia.* Edited by N.T. Smith, R.D. Miller, and A.N. Corbascio. Lea & Febiger, Philadelphia, 1981).

reentry ventricular arrhythmias associated with myocardial infarction is to increase the conduction block in the reentry loop. Lidocaine has little effect on atrial tissue and is relatively ineffective against supraventricular arrhythmias.

Group III. These drugs have group I and group II effects, plus the ability to produce beta-adrenergic blockade. They are effective in supraventricular and ventricular arrhythmias. In high doses they may occasionally cause atrioventricular nodal block and may suppress lower pacemaker foci, with resulting asystole. They have little effect on the H-V interval.

Group IV. Originally, the antiarrhythmic actions of bretylium were thought to be related to its effects on the adrenergic neuron. More recent work indicates that its antiarrhythmic properties may be due to its quaternary ammonium structure. It has been shown to reduce the disparity in duration of action potential between normal and ischemic zones.

Group V. This group acts by blocking the slow inward channels that carry Ca^{++} and Na^{+} ions. These drugs act in both supraventricular and ventricular arrhythmias and in hearts resistant to group I, II, and III drugs.

Use of antiarrhythmic drugs requires continuous ECG monitoring during anesthetic induction, maintenance, and recovery. Three of these drugs (quinidine, phenytoin, lidocaine) increase the threshold shock strength needed for ventricular defibrillation in dogs (Babbs et al., 1979). This may present a problem since fibrillation may occur after these drugs, particularly lidocaine, are given. In contrast, bretylium tosylate reduces the defibrillation threshold by as much as 16% for energy and 31% for current (Tacker et al., 1980).

Quinidine Gluconate or Sulfate, U.S.P.

Quinidine causes depression of myocardial contractility and excitability and slows the velocity of cardiac conduction. It prolongs the myocardial refractory period. Peripheral arteries are dilated, and the blood pressure is reduced. Quinidine also possesses anticholinergic and antivagal effects.

Quinidine has been used in humans for years in treatment of atrial and ventricular arrhythmias. It often converts atrial fibrillation in man to normal sinus rhythm; however, it has not proved as successful in animals. The dose for the dog is shown in Table 20–8. In emergency situations, it has largely been supplanted by other drugs such as propranolol.

Quinidine gluconate is available in 10-ml vials containing 80 mg/ml for intravenous use. Quinidine sulfate tablets contain 200 mg; gluconate tablets contain 330 mg.

Quinidine has been shown to cause digitalis toxicity (Leahey et al., 1978).

Procainamide Hydrochloride (Pronestyl)

Procainamide has been used for over two decades in control of atrial and ventricular arrhythmias. When it is given orally, the mean biological half-life is only 3.5 hours. The primary route of elimination is via the kidneys.

Procainamide depresses excitability and slows conduction in atria and ventricles. High doses prolong the QRS complex and P-R and Q-T intervals. Antivagal and anticholinergic effects of the drug may increase the heart rate.

Procainamide hydrochloride is available in 10-ml vials containing 100 or 500 mg/ml and in 250- and 500-mg capsules. The dose for the dog is shown in Table 20–8. When given intravenously, procainamide causes hypotension because of sympathetic ganglionic blockade; therefore, it is best given orally. It is a good replacement for intravenous lidocaine (Bonagura, 1981).

The major metabolite of procainamide is N-acetyl procainamide (Napa), which is approximately equal in potency to its parent compound, but is eliminated more slowly by the kidneys. Thus, the potential for dangerous levels of Napa exist in patients with impaired renal function. For this reason, procainamide/Napa assays are utilized in man to ascertain therapeutic levels.

Lidocaine Hydrochloride Injection, U.S.P. (Xylocaine)

Lidocaine has been used extensively in treatment of ventricular arrhythmias that develop during anesthesia. It is *not* recommended for supraventricular arrhythmias. The dose is

TABLE 20–8. Antiarrhythmic Drugs

Drug	*Dose*	*Comments*
Digoxin	Rapid oral digitalization (dog): 0.02 to 0.06 mg/kg divided bid for one day	Does not convert atrial fibrillation to sinus rhythm, but slows ventricular response
	Rapid IV digitalization (dog): 0.01 to 0.02 mg/kg; administer ½ of calculated dose IV, wait 30 to 60 minutes and administer ¼ of dose; wait 30 to 60 minutes and administer remaining dose if necessary	
	Oral maintenance (dog): 0.01 to 0.02 mg/kg divided bid	
	Oral maintenance (cat): 0.007 to 0.015 mg/kg divided bid	
Digitoxin (dog)	Rapid IV digitalization: 0.01 to 0.03 mg/kg; administer as per digoxin	
	Oral maintenance: 0.06 to 0.1 mg/kg divided bid to tid	
Propranolol	0.04 to 0.6 mg/kg (IV)*	Administer cautiously in heart failure
	(Cat): 2.5 to 10 mg tid (oral)	Maintenance dose; initial low dose is increased to effect
	(Dog): 0.2 to 0.3 mg/kg tid (oral)	Initial oral dose; increase dose daily to effect
	(Dog): 5 to 50 mg tid (oral)	Daily maintenance dose
Lidocaine	(Dog): 2 to 6 mg/kg (IV)	Administer bolus over 2 to 3 minutes
	(Dog): 25 to 80 μg/kg/minute†	Constant-rate infusion‡
	(Cat): 0.25 to 0.75 mg/kg (IV)	Administer slowly to avoid neuroexcitability and hypotension
Procainamide	(Dog): 6 mg/kg qid (IV, IM)	Beware of hypotension
	(Dog): 10 to 40 μg/kg/minute (IV)	Constant-rate infusion
	(Dog): 12 to 20 mg/kg qid (oral)	Adverse effects: emesis, diarrhea, hypotension, ↑ $Q\text{-}T_c$ interval
Quinidine sulfate or gluconate	(Dog): 6 to 16 mg/kg tid to qid (IM, oral)	Adverse effects: same as procainamide
Diphenylhydantoin	(Dog): 50 to 100 mg (IV)	Administer very slowly
	(Dog): 8 to 15 mg/kg tid (oral)	For digitalis-induced dysrhythmias

*1 mg = 0.001 g
†1 μg = 0.001 mg

‡Formula for constant-rate infusion: $\left(\frac{\text{infusion dose in mg}}{\frac{\text{kg}}{\text{min}}} \times \text{body weight in kg} \right) (360 \text{ min}) = \text{total dosage in mg given for a 6-hr period}$

(From Bonagura, J.D.: The Clinical Pharmacology of Cardiovascular Drugs. Scientific Proc., Am. Anim. Hosp. Assoc., 1981.)

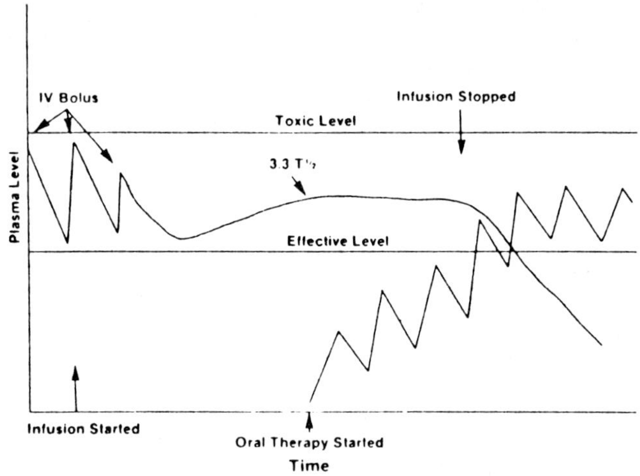

Figure 20–14. Initial therapy of acute ventricular arrhythmias includes an IV bolus of lidocaine or procainamide. If effective, a constant IV infusion is begun, and supplementary boluses are given until steady-state drug levels are attained (approximately 3.3 half-lives). Supplementary doses are smaller than the initial bolus. Following stabilization of the cardiac rhythm, oral replacement therapy can be initiated, if required. Oral therapy is given for one or two days; then the infusion rate is halved and, finally, it is discontinued. Maintenance oral antiarrhythmic therapy is administered. (From Bonagura, J.D.: The Clinical Pharmacology of Cardiovascular Drugs. Scientific Proceedings of the Am. Anim. Hosp. Assoc., 1981.)

shown in Table 20–8. Clinically used doses have little effect on myocardial contractility or blood pressure. Blood levels decline rapidly after a single bolus injection; therefore, constant infusion is required to maintain a therapeutic blood level (Fig. 20–14). When ventricular extrasystoles are detected on the ECG monitor, a lidocaine bolus (2 to 6 mg/kg) should immediately be given intravenously followed by a continuous infusion. In emergencies, where venous access is difficult or impossible, lidocaine may be injected into the pulmonary tree via endotracheal catheter and is rapidly absorbed.

Intravenous lidocaine boluses (total 11 mg/kg) interspersed with thiopental injections have been used to prevent arrhythmias on induction of anesthesia by Rawlings and Kolata (1983). They advocated this technique for use especially in patients with cardiopulmonary disease.

Use of lidocaine as a local anesthetic is described in Chapter 15.

Phenytoin Sodium (Diphenylhydantoin, Dilantin)

Phenytoin has been used in treating various arrhythmias in humans. In man, it is almost specific treatment for those that are digitalis-induced. The intravenous dose is 5 mg/kg, and up to 15 mg/kg may be given. Use of this drug in veterinary medicine is not well documented. The dose for the dog is given in Table 20–9. The serum half-life of phenytoin is increased in dogs under pentobarbital anesthesia (Sanders et al., 1979). Phenytoin has been shown to have teratogenic effects in mice and humans (Millicovsky and Johnston, 1981).

Bretylium Tosylate (Bretylol)

Bretylium tosylate accumulates in sympathetic ganglia and postganglionic adrenergic neurons, inhibiting norepinephrine release by depressing adrenergic nerve terminal excitability. It suppresses ventricular arrhythmias and fibrillation, while lowering the defibrillation threshold (Tacker et al., 1980).

Bretylium produces a chemical sympathectomy-like state resembling surgical sympathectomy. Catecholamine stores are not depleted, but catecholamine effects on the myocardium and on peripheral vascular resistance may be seen shortly after administration, because it causes an early release of norepinephrine from adrenergic postganglionic nerve terminals. Subsequently, bretylium blocks the release of norepinephrine in response to neuronal stimulation. Peripheral adrenergic blockage causes orthostatic hypotension in humans, but has less effect on supine blood pressure. The relationship of adrenergic blockade to antifibrillatory and antiarrhythmic actions is not clear (Bigger and Jaffe, 1971; Hammermeister et al., 1972; Cardinal and Sasyniuk, 1978).

Bretylium is indicated in the treatment of life-threatening ventricular arrhythmias that have not responded to lidocaine. There are no contraindications to its use in ventricular fibrillation or in refractory ventricular arrhythmias. Suppression of ventricular fibrillation is rapid, usually occurring within minutes following intravenous administration (Holder et al., 1977). Suppression of ventricular tachycardia and other ventricular arrhythmias occurs more slowly, usually 20 minutes to 2 hours after administration (Bernstein and Koch-Weser, 1972).

Because of the initial release of norepinephrine from adrenergic postganglionic nerve terminals, transient hypertension or increased frequency of premature ventricular contractions and other arrhythmias may occur. This initial release of norepinephrine may aggravate digitalis toxicity. Bretylium should be used only if the arrhythmia is not caused by digitalis toxicity, and other antiarrhythmic drugs are not effective.

Bretylium tosylate is available in 10-ml ampules containing 500 mg. It should be diluted for intravenous use with 4 parts of Dextrose Injection, U.S.P. or Sodium Chloride Injection, U.S.P. Rapid intravenous injection may produce nausea and vomiting; therefore, diluted solution should be infused over a period of at least 8 minutes. When one is treating ventricular fibrillation, 5 mg/kg of bretylium should be given intravenously as rapidly as possible, and may be given without dilution.

Bretylium should be administered with constant electrocardiographic monitoring. Since there is a delay in onset of action, it should not be considered or used as a replacement for rapid-acting antiarrhythmic agents. Clinical use of bretylium is for short term only. If ventricular fibrillation persists, the dosage may be increased to 10 mg/kg and repeated at 15- to 30-minute intervals, until a dose of not more than 30 mg/kg has been given.

Bretylium is eliminated intact by the kidneys, approximately 70 to 80% being excreted in the urine during the first 24 hours, with an additional 10% over the next 3 days. Estimates of the half-life have varied from 5 to 10 hours. Since bretylium is excreted principally by the kidneys, the dosage should be reduced in patients with impaired renal function.

ANTIHYPERTHERMIC AGENTS

Several agents have been used in prevention and treatment of malignant hyperthermia. Among these are procainamide, phenytoin, acepromazine, and dantrolene.

Dantrolene Sodium (Dantrium)

Dantrolene sodium is available as a slightly soluble oral powder and a sterile lyophilized formulation for intravenous use. Unlike other muscle relaxants, it acts directly upon skeletal muscle. It is believed to act upon excitation-contraction coupling, raising the rheobase by decreasing the release of calcium from the sarcoplasmic reticulum (Morgan and Bryant, 1977). It affects neither neuromuscular transmission nor the electrical properties of skeletal muscle membranes (Bianchine, 1980). Dantrolene has been found effective for the prevention and treatment of porcine malignant hyperthermia. Although doses of 1 to 10 mg/kg IV have been used, Flewellen and Nelson (1980) have reported the 95% effective prophylactic and therapeutic dose to be 3.5 mg/kg. Dantrolene has also been recommended for treatment of malignant hyperthermia in man and other species. In the horse, a dose of 500 mg orally has been used (Riebold et al., 1982). Absorption of dantrolene from the gastrointestinal tract is slow; it is slowly metabolized by the liver and excreted via the urine. It is currently used in man for alleviation of skeletal muscle spasticity but, when used for long periods (e.g., 60 days), has a potential to cause hepatotoxicity (Bianchine, 1980).

THE ADRENOCORTICAL STEROIDS

Adrenocortical steroids assist in regulating the volume and composition of body fluids and support essential cellular metabolism, thus maintaining homeostasis in the body. They are of three types: 1) glucocorticoids, which cause gluconeogenesis, eosinopenia, hyperglycemia, sodium retention, edema, and potassium loss (cortisone, hydrocortisone, and their derivatives); 2) mineralocorticoids, which principally affect electrolyte and water metabolism (aldosterone, corticosterone, and desoxycorticosterone); and 3) androgenic corticoids (adrenosterone).

Pharmacologically, all glucocorticoids produce the same actions. These include gluconeogenesis, hyperglycemia, glycosuria, and a negative nitrogen balance. Sodium is retained by the kidneys, and potassium is excreted. When large amounts of potassium are excreted, diuresis occurs. Excessive therapy may produce sodium retention with edema, hypochloremia, hypocalcemia, hypokalemia, and metabolic alkalosis. This condition can be corrected by concurrent administration of potassium. When given during the last trimester of pregnancy, corticosteroids may induce premature parturition, followed by dystocia, fetal death, retained placenta, and metritis. Prolonged therapy with corticosteroids should be avoided since this produces atrophy of the adrenal cortex with elimination of calcium, phosphorus, and nitrogen, which in turn produces osteoporosis and occasional fractures. Furthermore, animals that have been on continuous corticoid therapy require an increased amount during periods of stress, such as anesthesia and surgery.

Glucocorticoids stabilize cell membranes and reduce the inflammatory response to tissue insult. Vascularization and fibroblastic activity with formation of granulation tissue and intercellular ground substance are inhibited. This action slows wound healing and should be considered if these drugs are administered to surgical patients. Exacerbation of latent infections may also occur.

The glucocorticoids are absorbed readily from the gastrointestinal tract. For continuous therapy, however, they must be administered three or four times during a 24-hour period in order to obtain sustained hormonal effect. Metabolites of glucocorticoids are eliminated through the kidneys in conjugation with glucuronic and sulfuric acids.

In periods of acute stress, the normal output of cortical hormone may need to be multiplied 10 times or more. If the pituitary-adrenal axis is incapable of meeting this demand, falling blood pressure, increase in pulse rate, hemoconcentration, coma, and eventual death will occur (Fig. 20–15).

Cortical hormone is involved in maintenance of capillary tone which, in turn, is important to homeostasis. With excessive catecholamine activity, the intercellular matrix between myofibers of the vascular musculature becomes damaged. Administration of corticosteroids will reestablish its patency. Corticosteroids have also been shown to increase erythrocyte 2,3-DGP content and concentration, and P_{50} values. Increased arterial-venous oxygen difference, found in adrenalectomized dogs, is reduced (Thompson et al., 1977).

In shock, an intravenous preparation, such as hydrocortisone sodium succinate, prednisolone sodium succinate or phosphate, or dexamethasone phosphate, will restore vascular sensitivity to vasopressors (Fig. 20–16).

The efficacy of corticosteroids in shock is controversial, but their use continues. Bowen (1980) has listed the possible beneficial effects:

1. Enhancement of endothelial integrity, particularly of capillaries.

2. Interference with degranulation of polymorphonuclear leukocytes, presumably by stabilization of lysosomal membranes. Breakdown of lysosomes releases acid hydrolases (e.g., cathepsins), which promote formation of myocardial depressant factor (MDF) through plasma proteolysis. Lysosomal enzymes are more active in acidosis, as is usually the situation in shock. MDF weakens the force of cardiac contraction through a direct effect on the myocardium and constricts the splanchnic vasculature, enhancing release of lysosomal enzymes with formation of additional MDF. It depresses the activity of fixed macrophages of the reticuloendothelial system, which are necessary for clearance and inactivation of MDF and lysosomal enzymes.

3. Production of a small dose-dependent vasodilating effect. Alpha-blocking agents are more effective in producing vasodilation in shock.

4. Protection against activation of the coagulation pathways. High-dosage corticosteroids exert a marked anticoagulant effect.

5. Inhibition of complement activation by endotoxin, a process that mediates many of the adverse effects caused by endotoxin.

6. Reduction of elevated antidiuretic hormone levels toward normal, thus enhancing kidney function.

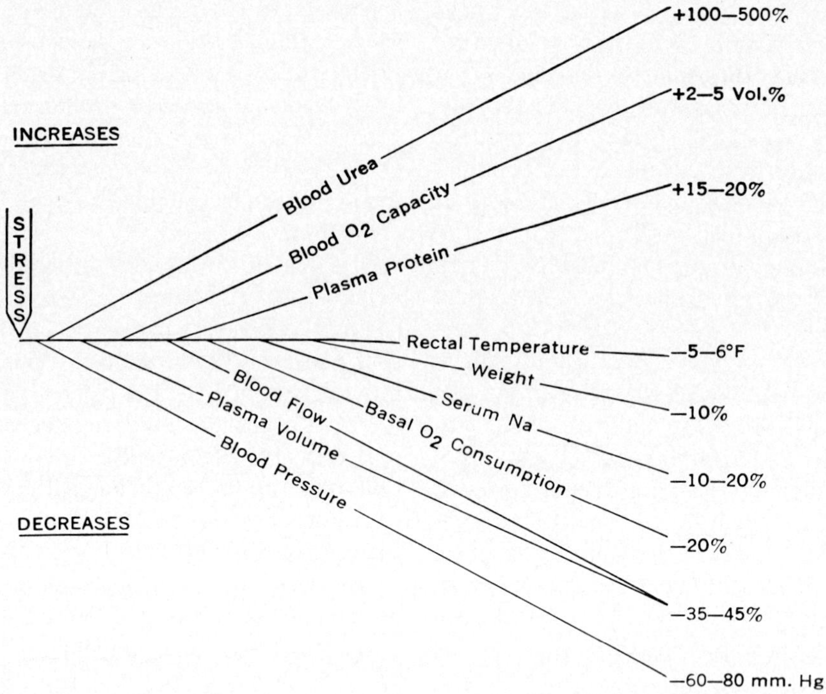

Figure 20–15. Symptoms of stress with cortical insufficiency. (Courtesy of Dr. K.B. Haas, The Upjohn Company, Kalamazoo, Michigan.)

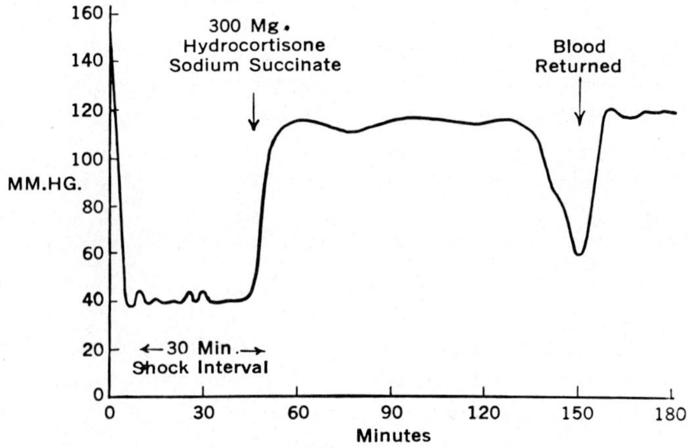

Figure 20–16. Effect of intravenous hydrocortisone sodium succinate on the blood pressure of a dog subjected to experimental hemorrhagic shock. (From Connolly, J.E., Bruns, D.L., and Stofer, R.C.: The Use of Intravenous Hydrocortisone in Hemorrhagic Shock. Surg. Forum, 9:17, 1958.)

7. Reduction of edema in the central nervous system (CNS trauma).

Of the several forms of shock, endotoxin shock is the only one for which almost universal agreement exists that corticosteroids are valuable. Here they stop the continued production of endotoxin. In other types of shock, corticosteroids are probably useful, but primary attention should be placed on other forms of shock therapy.

The dose of hydrocortisone sodium succinate for small animals is up to 50 mg/kg, depending upon the condition. In hypotensive shock, an average of 200 mg is required to elevate blood pressure to 90 mm Hg.

The dose of prednisolone sodium succinate for small animals is up to 40 mg/kg. For maintenance, one-half the initial dose may be given at intervals of 4, 8, and 12 hours afterward as deemed necessary. Prednisolone sodium succinate (0.3 to 0.5 mg/lb IV) may be used in the horse.

The intravenous dose of dexamethasone sodium phosphate in shock is 4 to 6 mg/kg of base, followed by continuous perfusion or intramuscular injections of the drug. The plasma half-life is 200 minutes (Davis, 1976).

Repeated doses of glucocorticoids are important and are usually required in shock. An intramuscular injection can be given for prolonged therapy at the same time the first injection is made intravenously.

CARDIAC DEFIBRILLATOR AND ARREST KIT

Many brands of defibrillators are available commercially, and their use has become widespread in veterinary practice.

Although it is possible to make a simple alternating current (AC) defibrillator (Booth et al., 1958), operator safety and thermal damage to the patient's heart should be considered before such an undertaking. Even commercially made AC defibrillators present hazards to the operator and patient that are objectionable. In addition, AC defibrillators are not as efficient as direct current defibrillators. For these reasons, the DC defibrillator is now standard.

Safety for the operator of a defibrillator should be considered because high voltages are used with both direct (internal) and indirect (external) defibrillation. Ventricular fibrillation may be induced in the operator by a weak or short burst of alternating current. With a single pulse discharge from a capacitor (direct current), fibrillation can occur only during the ventricular vulnerable period. This corresponds with the rising T-wave of the ECG (Fig. 20–17) and is only about one-sixth of the duration of the cardiac cycle.

McFarlane et al. (1967) found that when DC delivered from a capacitor was used, the optimum time constant for defibrillation of the canine heart was 1.0 millisecond. Wada (1969) has stated that the defibrillation threshold for the dog is 8 to 32 watt-seconds (700 to 1400 volts), which releases practically no harmful high energy.

Tacker et al. (1968), applying trans-chest capacitor-discharge defibrillation in dogs (12 to 16.5 kg), found that approximately 28 watt-seconds were required from a 29 μf capacitor charged to 1,400 volts. As the duration of discharge was decreased, the energy requirement increased. With high-energy, high-current, short-duration capacitor discharge, cardiac damage resulted, and the heart was unable to recover function.

Peak current value to defibrillate canine hearts by transventricular capacitor discharge is 0.82 A/kg of body weight or 89.5 mA/g of heart. This dose plus two standard deviations (1.42 A/kg) is suggested to be the 100% success level for defibrillation in normal canine hearts (Armayor, 1979).

Body hypothermia significantly lowers transventricular defibrillation thresholds 4.1%/°C for current and up to 5.9%/°C for energy (Arrendondo et al., 1980).

Witzel et al. (1966) successfully defibrillated two calves weighing 100 and 150 kg, but were unable to defibrillate the ventricles of a 200-kg calf despite application of up to 2710 watt-seconds directly to the heart. Witzel et al. (1968) directly defibrillated the heart of a 140-kg pony with 60 Hz AC for 0.05 second at voltages of 500 and 600, thus delivering 250 and 360 watt-

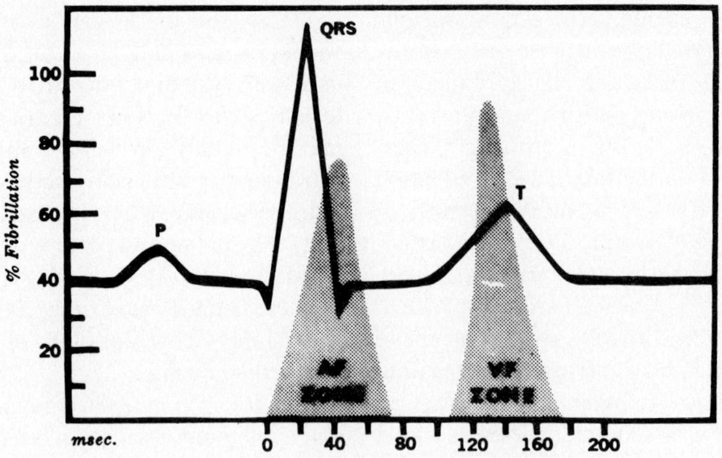

Figure 20–17. Fibrillation danger zones charted on the electrocardiogram. Shaded triangles represent zones where electroshock is most likely to produce atrial fibrillation (AF) or ventricular fibrillation (VF). (From Lown, B., Amarasingham, R., Neuman, J., and Berkovits, B.V.: The Use of Synchronized Direct Current Countershock in the Treatment of Cardiac Arrhythmias. J. Clin. Invest., 41:1381, 1962.)

seconds at 10 and 12 amperes. Larger equine hearts could not be defibrillated with this equipment, despite delivery of larger amounts of electrical energy. By extrapolation, they determined that horses weighing 450 to 500 kg would require an energy level of approximately 3 million watt-seconds.

For a defibrillator to be of value, it must be kept in a convenient location, and saline for moistening the electrodes should be stored with it.

Because, in addition to the defibrillator, several drugs are necessary in cardiopulmonary resuscitation (CPR), an arrest kit containing all necessary supplies should be kept in readiness in the operating room. It should include:

Atropine sulphate injection
Bretylium tosylate
Calcium gluconate or chloride, 10%
Dantrolene hydrochloride
Digoxin, injectable
Disposable syringes (5, 10, and 50 ml)
Dobutamine hydrochloride
Dopamine hydrochloride
Doxapram hydrochloride
Endotracheal tubes with adapters
Epinephrine hydrochloride, 1:10,000
Hypodermic needles
Instruments for thoracotomy
Intravenous fluids (normal saline or Ringer's lactate solution)
Intravenous fluid administration sets
Intravenous catheters and CVP catheter
Lidocaine hydrochloride, 2%
Manual resuscitator bag
Methoxamine
Naloxone hydrochloride
Potassium chloride, 2%
Prednisolone sodium succinate or dexamethasone sodium phosphate, injectable
Propranolol hydrochloride
Sodium bicarbonate, 7.5% and/or tromethamine

Calcium Chloride

The calcium ion increases contractility of the heart muscle and prolongs systole. When the heart is dilated and flaccid, it enhances cardiac muscle tone and irritability.

Following massage, if the heart is flabby and ventricular standstill exists, 0.5 to 3 ml of 10% calcium chloride or calcium gluconate should be injected intravenously and massage continued. In the horse, 1 ml/20 lb of 10% solution is used intravenously; alternatively, calcium borogluconate may be used.

Use of calcium in CPR has been criticized by Redding et al. (1983), who believe that it may prevent cerebral reperfusion following successful circulatory resuscitation. This occurrence reduces the chance of ultimate survival or increases the probability of serious neurologic sequelae.

Potassium Chloride

Ventricular fibrillation can be stopped by intravenous or intraventricular injection of 50 mg/kg of 5% potassium chloride. This effect is due to cardiac relaxation and inhibition produced by the potassium ion. In the absence of a defibrillator, this technique coupled with massage may prove life-saving. However, it is not as effective as electrical defibrillation and should be used only as an adjunct. See Chapter 13 for other cardioplegic solutions.

ANALEPTICS

Drugs that stimulate the respiratory center and produce an increased respiratory exchange are termed *respiratory analeptics*. Among these are doxapram hydrochloride (Dopram), pentylenetetrazol (Metrazol), methetharimide (Mikedimide), amphetamine (Benzedrine), and carbon dioxide. All but the latter produce an "arousal" effect characterized by a return toward consciousness of the patient. During the period of stimulation, which is short, animals may arouse enough to bump and bruise themselves severely or even have convulsions. In recent years, several investigators have stated that analeptics are contraindicated for respiratory depression produced by barbiturates. Following stimulation for a brief period, the respiratory center becomes more depressed than it was prior to administration of the analeptic agent. Current belief is that artificial ventilation until the barbiturate is detoxified is the most effective means of management.

Doxapram Hydrochloride (Dopram-V)

Doxapram hydrochloride, a pyrrolidone, is marketed as a clear colorless 2% aqueous solution with a pH of 3.5 to 5.0. It contains 0.5% chlorobutanol as a preservative. Because of its pH, it is incompatible with barbiturates, but it can be mixed in 5 or 10% dextrose or normal saline.

Doxapram may be given by any route. In emergencies, intravenous injection produces response in 10 to 30 seconds. In dogs, the dose for respiratory stimulation is 1 mg/kg, while the "arousal" dose is 5 mg/kg. In horses, the dose is 0.25 mg/lb. There is a wide margin of safety. The intravenous LD_{50} is 75 mg/kg. In conscious cats, the ratio of convulsive dose to respiratory stimulatory dose is 70:1 (Funderburk and Alphin, 1962). The response in dogs is more marked than in some other species. Cats do not show as marked a respiratory response, whereas rats do not show arousal.

Studies with dogs indicate that doxapram is the most effective agent when compared with other analeptics or combinations of analeptic agents (Klemm, 1966*a*). Polak and Plum (1964) found doxapram superior to methetharimide when compared in cats. Jensen and Klemm (1967) found doxapram effectively increased ventilation in dogs anesthetized with morphine-atropine-pentobarbital, promazine-pentobarbital, and atropine-fentanyl-droperidol-pentobarbital. The best responses were obtained in dogs given either promazine or atropine-fentanyl-droperidol as preanesthetics. Cats receiving pentobarbital alone had consistent increases in rate and depth of breathing. When second injections of doxapram were given to dogs and cats, they were effective but not to the same degree as initially.

Doxapram produces a striking and sustained hyperventilation with increased blood pressure in doses far below the convulsive dose. The action is primarily on the brain stem, producing increased tidal volume and respiratory rate, although it also produces a lesser stimulation of the aortic and carotid chemoreceptors (Kato and Buckley, 1964). Larger doses stimulate the cortex and spinal cord producing arousal effects. It does not produce convulsions in barbiturate-anesthetized animals.

In pentobarbital-anesthetized dogs, 2 mg/kg of doxapram increased respiratory minute volume by 200% at one minute after injection (Klemm, 1966*a*), whereas 4 mg/kg increased it 540% (Klemm, 1966*b*). Soma and Kenny (1967) measured a variety of parameters in pentobarbital-anesthetized dogs given doxapram at the rate of 2 and 4 mg/kg. With 2 mg/kg, there was an immediate increase in respiratory rate averaging 388% of the preinjection value within the first minute. The rate subsequently declined to a plateau that remained above control levels.

There was a maximal increase of 19% in the tidal volume within the first minute, followed by a rapid decline to below control levels. Because the rate increased, the minute volume remained above control levels despite the decline in tidal volume. After injection of 2 mg/kg of doxapram, blood pH values increased and P_{CO_2} values decreased. The P_{O_2} values increased after respiratory stimulation reflecting improved alveolar ventilation (Fig. 20–18).

Blood pressure increases, primarily because of stimulation of brain stem vasomotor areas, and is mediated through the sympathoadrenal system. Spinal section at C_2 abolishes the pressor effect. Intravenous infusion produces a marked increase in total blood and urinary catecholamines. In dogs, Soma and Kenny (1967) found a mean increase of 29% in systolic and diastolic blood pressures within one minute. Heart rate also increased but more slowly, a mean increase of 22% occurring within 4 minutes. After injection of 4 mg/kg, a transient hypotension occurred followed by an increase above control levels. This hypotension did not occur after injection of 2 mg/kg.

Changes in EEG patterns after intravenous doxapram were not observed in dogs under deep pentobarbital or moderate thiopental anesthesia (Soma and Kenny, 1967).

Use of doxapram in horses after anesthesia with chloral hydrate, chloral and magnesium sulfate, and pentobarbital has been reported by Short et al. (1970). Respiratory rate and volume were increased while arousal time was materially shortened. Riebold et al. (1982) have recommended 0.25 mg/lb IV in the horse.

Doxapram is primarily metabolized in the body with small amounts eliminated unchanged in the urine. When the drug is tagged with radioactive carbon, 38% of the radioactive material is found in the feces after 72 hours.

Winnie and Collins (1965) have described the

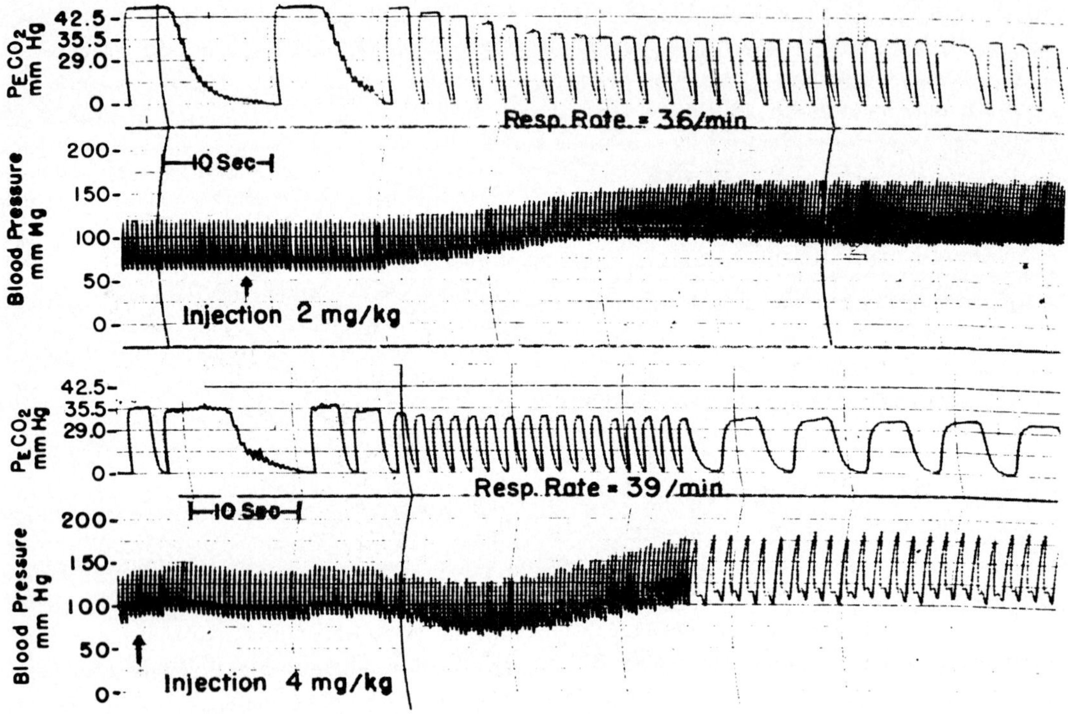

Figure 20–18. A transient decrease in blood pressure occurs when 4 mg of doxapram per kilogram of body weight is administered intravenously (bottom). This decrease before the increase in blood pressure does not occur when smaller doses are given (top). The reduction in expired carbon dioxide tension (P_{CO_2}) occurs rapidly in both instances and in parallel with the change in ventilation. (From Soma, L.R., and Kenny, R.: Respiratory, Cardiovascular, Metabolic, and Electroencephalographic Effects of Doxapram Hydrochloride in the Dog. Am. J. Vet. Res., 28:191, 1967.)

"doxapram test" for differential diagnosis of apnea in man following the use of general anesthesia and muscle relaxants (see Chap. 14). This test is used to differentiate between apnea due to *central depression* or *peripheral neuromuscular blockade*.

Doxapram may be contraindicated following xylazine sedation in the dog (see Chap. 8).

Pentylenetetrazol, U.S.P. (Metrazol, Leptazol) and Methetharimide (Mikedimide, Megimide)

Because doxapram has proved to be more effective, these two agents are seldom used today. For information concerning them, the reader is referred to the previous edition of this text.

Amphetamine and carbon dioxide are discussed elsewhere in this text.

THE NARCOTIC ANTAGONISTS

Since the discovery of opiate receptors in the CNS, much has been learned about the competitive actions of narcotic agonists and antagonists. The ratio of agonist to antagonist activity determines the net effect of a given agent. The following narcotic "antagonists" vary in their effects because of differences in this ratio.

Nalorphine Hydrochloride (Nalline) and Levallorphan Tartrate (Lorfan)

Nalorphine and levallorphan are synthetic congeners of morphine and are classified as agonist-antagonists. Respiratory depression caused by narcotics is reversed. Their effect is specific for narcotics, and they are not effective in respiratory depression due to barbiturates, anesthetics, or other agents. *They should not be used as general analeptics.*

When these drugs are given intravenously to dogs deeply sedated with morphine, the initial effects are observed within 15 seconds after injection (Aronson and Gans, 1959*a*). A deep inspiration is followed by change in the panting type of respiration, seen with morphine, to breathing with a greater tidal volume and slower rate. After 90 seconds, almost all signs of morphine hypnosis disappear. The same changes are seen with these drugs if given following other narcotics. When they are injected into pentobarbital-anesthetized dogs that have not received preanesthetic narcotics, a moderate depression of ventilation and a small but transient fall in blood pressure are observed.

When dogs anesthetized with pentobarbital are given morphine or meperidine intravenously followed by nalorphine, a rapid increase in ventilation, decrease in arterial carbon dixode content, and a return of blood pressure toward normal levels occur without substantially altering the plane of anesthesia.

Nalorphine or levallorphan given without prior administration of a narcotic will produce central nervous depression. The antagonism of these drugs for the narcotics is a competitive inhibition.

One milligram of nalorphine is recommended for every 10 mg of morphine or 20 mg of meperidine used preanesthetically. One milligram of levallorphan is recommended for every 50 mg of morphine or 100 mg of meperidine. Since levallorphan and nalorphine are themselves depressant drugs, the total amount given in a 4-hour period should not exceed 5 mg of levallorphan or 25 mg of nalorphine for a 25-pound dog. When one is treating neonatal respiratory depression produced by narcotic analgesics, the dose of either drug should be approximately one-fifteenth to one-twentieth of the adult dose. Good results have been reported by Kirk (1961) when narcotic-depressed newborn pups were injected in the umbilical vessels with 0.1 ml of nalorphine (0.5 mg).

Aronson and Gans (1959*b*) have stated that administration of levallorphan or nalorphine in pentobarbital-anesthetized dogs depressed by narcotic analgesics permits resumption of adequate respiration without altering the level of anesthesia. In addition, narcotic analgesics may be given during prolonged surgery as supplemental anesthesia, respiratory depression being prevented or overcome by the use of these antagonists.

Naloxone Hydrochloride (Narcan)

Naloxone hydrochloride is the N-allyl derivative of a potent narcotic analgesic, oxymorphone. Because it has no agonist properties, it does not produce analgesia or respiratory depression when used alone. Naloxone reverses the effects of its parent compound, oxymorphone, and other narcotics such as morphine, meperidine, and fentanyl. The LD_{50} of naloxone in dogs is 500 mg/kg. It is 13 times more potent than nalorphine and 3 times more potent than levallorphan in counteracting narcotic-induced respiratory depression in rabbits and narcosis in rats. The half-life of antagonistic action is 12 to 40 minutes. For this reason, patients should be closely watched following narcotic reversal.

In dogs, 3 mg/kg of naloxone intravenously caused no change in cardiovascular dynamics (Schweichel et al., 1979). When naloxone was given after fentanyl administration, total peripheral resistance decreased rapidly, and stroke volume index and cardiac index increased. These changes were believed to be caused by fentanyl reversal. The authors commented that these changes might be unwanted in patients with cardiac disease.

When naloxone (10 mg/kg) was given to endotoxin-shocked rats, mean arterial and pulse pressures returned to control values. Further studies demonstrated the same effect in rats and dogs subjected to hemorrhagic shock and in rats with traumatized spinal cords. Holaday and Faden (1978, 1981; Faden and Holaday, 1981) have hypothesized from these experiments that pituitary endorphins are released in shock, and act upon opiate receptors in the brain to depress cardiovascular function. The mechanism of naloxone action is to block their toxic cardiovascular effects.

The role of naloxone and endorphins in acute cerebral ischemia has been investigated by Hosobuchi et al. (1982). They found that experimentally induced stroke could be reversed by naloxone, which suggests its use following ischemic accidents during anesthesia.

When naloxone is administered with oxymorphone, the respiratory depression produced by the latter is eliminated, but the analgesic effect remains. According to Palminteri (1966), the best results in cats and dogs are obtained with a mixture of 0.02 to 0.03 mg of naloxone to 1.5 mg of oxymorphone.

Naloxone may be administered intravenously in the umbilical vein of puppies delivered under anesthesia employing a narcotic. The dose is 0.1 mg for the average puppy of approximately 10 oz.

Naloxone hydrochloride has been found to be a specific antagonist for pentazocine (Kallos and Smith, 1968), and will reverse the effects of d-propoxyphene. Naloxone will significantly reduce the duration of anesthesia and LD_{50} of pentobarbital or methohexital in rats (Fürst et al., 1977).

Cyprenorphine (M-285) and Diprenorphine (M-5050)

Cyprenorphine is a potent narcotic antagonist with an action similar to that of nalorphine. Its potency is up to 35 times that of nalorphine, with a duration of action 2 to 3 times as long. In game animals, a satisfactory and rapid reversal of etorphine (M-99) is usually produced by administration of 2.5 times the amount of etorphine given.

Diprenorphine is similar chemically and in potency to cyprenorphine. No analgesic, cardiac, respiratory, or central nervous system action has been reported. Its use as an antagonist for combined etorphine and methotrimeprazine in the dog has been reported by Alford and Wozniak (1970). A dose four times that of the etorphine administered was found to be most favorable. Because of its few side effects, diprenorphine is supplanting cyprenorphine in clinical use.

OTHER ANTAGONISTS

Recently, considerable attention has been given to 4-aminopyridine (4-AP) and yohimbine as antagonists for a wide variety of drugs used in anesthesia.

4-AP partially reverses nondepolarizing types of neuromuscular and ganglionic blockade. In addition, it partially antagonizes xylazine depression in cattle and dogs, ketamine anesthesia in cats, and barbiturate anesthesia in dogs and cats. These actions are believed to be due to enhanced release of acetylcholine and other neurotransmitters from prejunctional nerve endings. Combined with naloxone, it reverses the neuroleptanalgesia of droperidol-fentanyl (Booth et al., 1982).

Yohimbine blocks central a_2-adrenoreceptors (Hsu, 1981). It partially antagonizes barbiturates, ketamine, xylazine, benzodiazepines, and phenothiazines. It may also influence cholinergic, dopaminergic, serotonergic, and GABA receptors. In mice and chickens, 1 mg/kg of yohimbine abolishes the effect of xylazine.

When 4-AP and yohimbine are combined, they are capable of rapidly reversing the effects of ketamine anesthesia in cats, xylazine sedation in cattle, xylazine-acepromazine sedation in dogs, and xylazine-pentobarbital anesthesia in dogs (Kitzman et al., 1982; Cronin et al., 1983; Hatch et al., 1983).

Although 4-AP and yohimbine are not currently available commercially for animal use, it appears that they will be soon.

REFERENCES

Aberg, M., Hedner, U., and Bergentz, S.E.: Effect of Dextran on Factor VIII (Antihemophilic Factor) and Platelet Function. Ann. Surg., 189:243, 1979.

Alford, B.T., and Wozniak, L.A.: Neuroleptanalgesia in the Dog and Reversal by an Antagonist. J.A.V.M.A., 156:208, 1970.

Armayor, M.R., Savino, G., Valentinuzzi, M.E., Clavi, O.E., Monzon, J.E., and Arredondo, M.T.: Ventricular Defibrillation Thresholds with Capacitor Discharge. Med. Biol. Eng. Comput., 17:435, 1979.

Aronson, A.L., and Gans, J.H.: The Narcotic Analgesics and Their Antagonists as Adjuncts to Barbiturate Anesthesia. I. Physiological and Pharmacological Considerations. Am. J. Vet. Res., 20:909, 1959*a*.

Aronson, A.L., and Gans, J.H.: The Narcotic Analgesics and Their Antagonists as Adjuncts to Barbiturate Anesthesia. II. Clinical Applications. J.A.V.M.A., 134:459, 1959*b*.

Arrendondo, M.T., Armayor, M.R., Clavin, O.E., Valentinuzzi, M.E., and Scida, E.E.: Effect of Body Hypothermia on Transventricular Simple-Capacitor-Discharge Defibrillation Thresholds. Am. Physiol. Soc., H675, 1980.

Atlee, J.L., III, and Rusy, B.F.: Digitalis. In *Drug Interactions in Anesthesia*. Edited by N.T. Smith, R.D. Miller, and A.N. Corbascio. Lea & Febiger, Philadelphia, 1981.

Auer, L., Bell, K., and Coates, S.: Blood Transfusion Reactions in the Cat. J.A.V.M.A., 180:729, 1982.

Babbs, C.F., Yim, G.K.W., Whistler, S.J., Tacker, W.A., and Geddes, L.A.: Elevation of Ventricular Defibrillation Threshold in Dogs by Antiarrhythmic Drugs. Am. Heart J., 98:345, 1979.

Benfey, B.F., and Varma, D.R.: Antisympathomimetic and Antifibrillatory Effects of Pronethalol and Propranolol. Br. J. Pharmacol., 26:3, 1966.

Bernstein, J.G., and Koch-Weser, J.: Effectiveness of Bretylium Tosylate Against Refractory Ventricular Arrhythmias. Circulation, 45:1024, 1972.

Biachine, J.R.: Drugs for Parkinson's Disease; Centrally Acting Muscle Relaxants. In *The Pharmacological Basis of Therapeutics,* 6th ed. Macmillan Publishing Co., Inc., New York, 1980.

Bigger, J.T., and Jaffe, C.C.: The Effect of Bretylium Tosylate on the Electrophysiologic Properties of Ventricular Muscle and Purkinje Fibers. Am. J. Cardiol., 27:82, 1971.

Bishop, R.L., and Weisfeldt, M.L.: Sodium Bicarbonate Administration During Cardiac Arrest. J.A.M.A., 235:506, 1976.

Blaschko, H., Richter, D., and Schlossmann, H.: The Oxidation of Adrenaline and Other Amines. Biochem. J., 31:2187, 1937.

Bonagura, J.D.: The Clinical Pharmacology of Cardiovascular Drugs. Proc. 48th Mtg. A.A.H.A., 1981.

Booth, N.H., Hatch, R.C., and Crawford, L.M.: Reversal of the Neuroleptanalgesic Effect of Droperidol-Fentanyl in the Dog by 4-Aminopyridine and Naloxone. Am. J. Vet. Res., 43:1227, 1982.

Booth, N.H., Will, D.H., Moss, L.C., and Swenson, M.J.: An Electrical Apparatus and Its Application in Defibrillating the Heart of the Dog. J.A.V.M.A., 132:117, 1958.

Bowen, J.M.: Are Corticosteroids Useful in Shock Therapy? J.A.V.M.A., 177:453, 1980.

Bradley, E.C.: Results with Phentolamine (Regitine) in the Treatment of Selected Patients with Shock. Calif. Med., 103:314, 1965.

Breznock, E.M., and Strack, D.: Blood Volume of Non-Splenectomized and Splenectomized Cats before and after Acute Hemorrhage. Am. J. Vet. Res., 43:1811, 1983.

Brill, I.C., Krueger, J.D., and McCawley, E.L.: Restoration of Sinus Rhythm in Experimental and Clinical Ventricular Arrhythmias by Methoxamine Hydrochloride. Am. J. Cardiol., 3:307, 1959.

Button, C., Gross, D.R., Johnston, J.T., and Yakatan, G.J.: Digoxin Pharmacokinetics, Bioavailability, Efficacy, and Dosage Regimens in the Horse. Am. J. Vet. Res., 41:1388, 1980.

Cardinal, R., and Sasyniuk, B.I.: Electrophysiological Effects of Bretylium Tosylate on Subendocardial Purkinje Fibers from Infarcted Canine Hearts. J. Pharmacol. Exp. Ther., 204:159, 1978.

Clark, C.H., and Woodley, C.H.: A Comparison of Blood Volumes as Measured by Rose Bengal, T-1824 (Evans Blue), Radiochromium-Tagged Erythrocytes, and a Combination of the Latter Two. Am. J. Vet. Res., 20:1067, 1959.

Cohen, E.N., Van Bergen, F.V., and Knight, R.T.: Bronchodilation under Anesthesia with 1(3,4-Dihydroxyphenyl) 2 Isopropyl Aminoethanol Hydrochloride: A Comparative Study (Preliminary Report). Anesthesiology, 10:451, 1949.

Cotter, S.: Blood Transfusion Reactions in Cats. J.A.V.M.A., 181:5, 1982.

Craige, A.H., Jr.: Amphetamine in Veterinary Practice: Special Reference to Dosage. J.A.V.M.A., 103:28, 1943.

Cronin, M.F., Booth, N.H., Hatch, R.C., and Brown, J.:

Acepromazine-Xylazine Combination in Dogs: Antagonism with 4-Aminopyridine and Yohimbine. Am. J. Vet. Res., 44:2037, 1983.

Cullison, R.F.: Toxicosis in Cats from Use of Benzyl Alcohol in Lactated Ringer's Solution. J.A.V.M.A., 182:61, 1983.

Darby, T.D., and Anderson, S.J.: Tolerance and Toxicity of THAM. Ann. Anesth., Franc., 7:585, 1966.

Davis, L.E.: Pharmacology of Adrenocorticosteroids. Clinical Pharmacology Newsletter. Colorado State University, 2:6, 1976.

De Beer, E.J., Wnuck, A.L., Fanelli, R.V., Norton, S., and Ellis, C.H.: The Restoration of Arterial Pressure from Various Hypotensive States by Methoxamine. Arch. Int. Pharmacodyn., 104:487, 1956.

DeBoer, A.: Body Fluid Compartment Changes Following Large Volume Hemodilution. Arch. Surg., 98:602, 1969.

Deutsch, S., and Dalen, J.D.: Indications for Prophylactic Digitalization. Anesthesiology, 30:648, 1969.

Dinerstein, R.J., Vannice, J., Henderson, R.C., Roth, L.J., Goldberg, L.I., and Hoffman, P.C.: Histofluorescence Techniques Provide Evidence for Dopamine-Containing Neuronal Elements in Canine Kidney. Science, 205:497, 1979.

Effron, M.B., Guarnieri, T., Frederiksen, J.W., Greene, H.L., and Weisfeldt, M.L.: Effect of Tris (Hydroxymethyl) Aminomethane on Ischemic Myocardium. Am. J. Physiol., 235:H167, 1978.

Erlij, D., and Mendez, R.: The Modification of Digitalis Intoxication by Excluding Adrenergic Influences on the Heart. J. Pharm. Exp. Ther., 144:97, 1964.

Faden, A.I., and Holaday, J.W.: A Role for Endorphins in the Pathophysiology of Spinal Cord Injury. In *Neurosecretion and Brain Peptides*. Edited by J.B. Martin, S. Reichlin, and K.L. Bick. Raven Press, New York, 1981.

Federman, J., and Vlietstra, R.E.: Antiarrhythmic Drug Therapy. Mayo Clin. Proc., 45:531, 1979.

Firt, P., and Hejhal, L.: Treatment of Severe Haemorrhage. Lancet, 273:1132, 1957.

Flewellen, E.H., and Nelson, T.E.: Dantrolene Dose Response in Malignant Hyperthermia-Susceptible (MHS) Swine: Method to Obtain Prophylaxis and Therapeusis. Anesthesiology, 52:303, 1980.

Funderburk, W.H., and Alphin, R.S.: Electrical Changes in the CNS Produced by a New Respiratory Stimulant, AHR-619. Fed. Proc., 21:324, 1962.

Fürst, Z., Foldes, F.F., and Knoll, J.: The Influence of Naloxone on Barbiturate Anesthesia and Toxicity in the Rat. Life Sci., 20:921, 1977.

Gibson, G.E., Shimada, M., and Blass, J.P.: Protection by Tris (Hydroxymethyl)-Aminomethane against Behavioral and Neurochemical Effects of Hypoxia. Biochem. Pharmacol., 28:747, 1979.

Glogar, D.H., Kloner, R.A., Muller, J., DeBoer, L.W.V., and Braunwald, E.: Fluorocarbons Reduce Myocardial Ischemic Damage after Coronary Occlusion. Science, 211:1439, 1981.

Goldberg, L.I., Cotten, M. deV., Darby, T.D., and Howell, E.V.: Comparative Heart Contractile Force Effects of Equipressor Doses of Several Sympathomimetic Amines. J. Pharmacol. Exp. Ther., 108:177, 1953.

Gunn, J.A.: The Pharmacological Actions and Therapeutic Uses of Some Compounds Related to Adrenalin: Lecture I. Br. Med. J., 2:155, 1939. Lecture II. Ibid. 2:214, 1939.

Halmagyi, D.F.J., Colebatch, H.J.H., Starzecki, B., and Horner, G.J.: Pulmonary Alveolar-Vascular Reflex. J. Appl. Physiol., 19:105, 1964.

Hammermeister, K.E., Boerth, R.C., and Warbasse, J.R.: The Comparative Inotropic Effects of Six Clinically Used Antiarrhythmic Agents. Am. Heart J., 84:643, 1972.

Hatch, R.C., Booth, N.H., Clark, J.D., Crawford, L.M., Jr., Kitzman, J.V., and Wallner, B.: Antagonism of Xylazine Sedation in Dogs by 4-Aminopyridine and Yohimbine. Am. J. Vet. Res., 43:1009, 1983.

Hauswirth, O., Noble, D., and Tsien, R.W.: Adrenaline: Mechanism of Action on the Pacemaker Potential in Cardiac Purkinje Fibers. Science, 162:916, 1968.

Hayes, A., Mastrota, F., Mooney, S., and Hurvitz, A.: Safety of Transfusing Blood in Cats. J.A.V.M.A., 181:4, 1982.

Hinds, J.E., and Hawthorne, E.W.: Comparative Cardiac Dynamic Effects of Dobutamine and Isoproterenol in Conscious Instrumented Dogs. Am. J. Cardiol., 36:894, 1975.

Holaday, J.W., and Faden, A.I.: Naloxone Reversal of Endotoxin Hypotension Suggests Role of Endorphins in Shock. Nature, 275:450, 1978.

Holaday, J.W., and Faden, A.I.: Naloxone Reverses the Pathophysiology of Shock Through an Antagonism of Endorphin Systems. In *Neurosecretion and Brain Peptides*. Edited by J.B. Martin, S. Reichlin, and K.L. Bick. Raven Press, New York, 1981.

Holder, D.A., Sniderman, A.D., Fraser, G., and Fallen, E.L.: Experience with Bretylium Tosylate by a Hospital Cardiac Arrest Team. Circulation, 55:541, 1977.

Holloway, G.A., Jr., and Frederickson, E.L.: Dobutamine, a New Beta Agonist. Anesth. Analg., 53:616, 1974.

Holmes, H.R., Babbs, C.F., Voorhees, W.D., Tacker, W.A., and DeGaravilla, B.: Influence of Adrenergic Drugs Upon Vital Organ Perfusion During CPR. Crit. Care Med., 8:137, 1980.

Hosobuchi, Y., Baskin, D.S., and Woo, S.K.: Reversal of Induced Ischemia Neurological Deficit in Gerbils by the Opiate Antagonist Naloxone. Science, 215:69, 1982.

Howard, J.M., Ebert, R.V., Bloom, W.L., and Sloan, M.H.: The Present Status of Dextran as a Plasma Expander. Am. J. Surg., 97:593, 1959.

Howland, W.S., and Schweizer, O.: Physiologic Compensation for Storage Lesion of Bank Blood. Anesth. Analg., 44:8, 1965.

Hsu, W.H.: Xylazine-Induced Depression and Its Antagonism by Alpha Adrenergic Blocking Agents. J. Pharmacol. Exp. Ther., 218:188, 1981.

Ivanokovich, A.D., El-Etr, A.A., Janeczko, G.F., and Maronic, J.A.: The Effects of Ketamine and of Innovar® Anesthesia on Digitalis Tolerance in Dogs. Anesth. Analg., 54:106, 1975.

Ivankovich, A.D., Miletich, D.J., Grossman, R.K., Albrecht, R.F., El-Etr, A.A., and Cairoli, V.J.: The Effect of Enflurane, Isoflurane, Fluroxene, Methoxyflurane and Diethyl Ether Anesthesia on Ouabain Tolerance in the Dog. Anesth. Analg., 55:360, 1976.

Jensen, E.C., and Klemm, W.R.: Clinical Evaluation of the Analeptic Doxapram, in Dogs and Cats. J.A.V.M.A., 150:516, 1967.

Johnstone, M.: Propranolol (Inderal) During Halothane Anaesthesia. Br. J. Anaesth., 38:516, 1966.

Jones, E.W., and Brock, W.E.: Unpublished Data. Oklahoma State University, Stillwater, 1960.

Jose, A.D.: The Effect of Combined Sympathetic and Parasympathetic Blockade on Heart Rate and Cardiac Function in Man. Am. J. Cardiol., 18:476, 1966.

Kahn, R.C., Jascott, D., Carlon, G.C., Schweizer, O., Howland, W.S., and Goldiner, P.L.: Massive Blood Replacement: Correlation of Ionized Calcium, Citrate, and Hydrogen Ion Concentration. Anesth. Analg., 58:274, 1979.

Kallos, T., and Smith, T.C.: Naloxone Reversal of Pentazocine-Induced Respiratory Depression. J.A.M.A., 204:932, 1968.

Kaneko, J.J.: *Clinical Biochemistry of Domestic Animals*. Academic Press, New York, 1980.

Kanter, G.S.: Effect of Massive Sodium Bicarbonate Infusion on Renal Function. Technical Documentary Report No. SAM-TDR-63-15. U.S.A.F. School of Aerospace Medicine, Brooks Air Force Base, Texas, 1963.

Kato, H., and Buckley, J.P.: Possible Sites of Action of the Respiratory Stimulant Effect of Doxapram Hydrochloride. J. Pharmacol. Exp. Ther., 144:260, 1964.

Kirk, R.W.: Personal Communication. Cornell University, Ithaca, New York, 1961.

Kittleson, M.D.: Dobutamine. J.A.V.M.A., 177:642, 1980.

Kitzman, J.V., Booth, N.H., Hatch, R.C., and Wallner, B.: Antagonism of Xylazine Sedation by 4-Aminopyridine and Yohimbine in Cattle. Am. J. Vet. Res., 43:2165, 1982.

Klemm, W.R.: Evaluation of Effectiveness of Doxapram and Various Analeptic Combinations in Dogs. J.A.V.M.A., 148:894, 1966*a*.

Klemm, W.R.: Physiologic Responses to Equivalent Doses of Doxapram and Various Analeptic Combinations in Acute Barbiturate Narcosis in Dogs. Toxicol. Appl. Pharmacol., 8:505, 1966*b*.

Lahti, R.E., Brill, I.C., and McCawley, E.L.: The Effect of Methoxamine Hydrochloride (Vasoxyl) on Cardiac Rhythm. J. Pharmacol. Ther., 115:268, 1955.

Lapin, R., Friedman, A.E., Levine, E.M., Hutchins, H.L., Malhotra, V., Daniel, D., and Barasch, S.: The Preoperative Use of Fluosol-DA 20% in Major Abdominal Surgery. J. Abd. Surg., 22:15, 1980.

Lazrove, S., Waxman, K., Shippy, C., and Shoemaker, W.C.: Hemodynamic, Blood Volume, and Oxygen Transport Responses to Albumin and Hydroxyethyl Starch Infusions in Critically Ill Postoperative Patients. Crit. Care Med., 8:302, 1980.

Leahey, E.B., Jr., Reiffel, J.A., Drusin, R.E., Heisenbuttel, R.H., Lovejoy, W.P., and Bigger, J.T.: Interaction Between Quinidine and Digoxin. J.A.M.A., 240:533, 1978.

Lee, W.H., Rubin, J.W., and Huggins, M.P.: Clinical Evaluation of Priming Solutions for Pump Oxygenator Perfusion. Ann. Thorac. Surg., 19:529, 1975.

Livesay, J.J., Follette, D.M., Fey, K.H., Nelson, R.L., DeLand, E.C., Barnard, R.J., and Buckberg, G.D.: Optimizing Myocardial Supply/Demand Balance with α-Adrenergic Drugs during Cardiopulmonary Resuscitation. J. Thorac. Cardiovasc. Surg., 76:244, 1978.

Lucchesi, B.R., and Iwami, T.: The Antiarrhythmic Properties of ICI 46037, A Quaternary Analog of Propranolol. J. Pharmacol. Exp. Ther., 162:49, 1968.

Lucchesi, B.R., Whitsitt, L.S., and Stickney, J.L.: Antiarrhythmic Effects of Beta-Adrenergic Blocking Agents. Ann. N.Y. Acad. Sci., 139:940, 1967.

Malm, J.R., Manger, W.N., Sullivan, S.F., Papper, E.M., and Nahas, G.G.: The Effect of Acidosis on Sympatho-adrenal Stimulation. J.A.M.A., 197:161, 1966.

Marshall, B.E., Wurzel, H.A., Neufeld, G.R., Aukburg, S.J., Ewing, B.C., Fried, R.J., and Barnes, C.: Effects of Fenwal 4C2423 Transfusion Microfilter on Microaggregates and Other Constituents of Stored Blood. Transfusion, 18:38, 1978.

McFarlane, J., Geddes, L.A., Maddus, J.S., and Hoff, H.E.: Threshold Energy for Defibrillation of the Canine Ventricle. Cardiovasc. Res. Cent. Bull, 6:58, 1967.

McNamara, J.J., Burran, E.L., Larson, E., Omiya, G., Suehiro, G.P., and Yamase, H.: Effect of Debris in Stored Blood on Pulmonary Microvasculature. Ann. Thorac. Surg., 14:133, 1972.

Meier, R., Yonkman, F.F., Craver, B.N., and Gross, F.: 17083 P. A New Imidazoline Derivative with Marked Adrenolytic Properties. Proc. Soc. Exp. Biol. Med., 71:70, 1949.

Mettar, J.A., Weil, M.H., Shubin, H., and Stein, L.: Cardiac Arrest in the Critically Ill. II. Hyperosmolar States Following Cardiac Arrest. Am. J. Med., 56:162, 1974.

Millicovsky, G., and Johnston, M.C.: Maternal Hyperoxia Greatly Reduces the Incidence of Phenytoin-Induced Cleft Lip and Palate in A/J Mice. Science, 212:671, 1981.

Mishler, J.M., and Durr, H.K.: Macroamylasaemia Following the Infusion of Low Molecular Weight-Hydroxyethyl Starch in Man. Eur. Surg. Res., 11:217, 1979.

Mishler, J.M., Nicora, R.W., Yoshatake, T., Oishi, K., Kawasake, T., and Shimizu, K.: Hemodilution with Hydroxyethyl Starch During Cardiopulmonary Bypass: Review of a Multi-Institutional Study. Amsect, 7:140, 1975.

Morgan, K.G., and Bryant, S.H.: The Mechanism of Action of Dantrolene Sodium. J. Pharmacol. Exp. Ther., 201:138, 1977.

Moss, G.: Fluid Distribution in Prevention of Hypovolemic Shock. Arch. Surg., 98:281, 1969.

Munoz, E., Raciti, A., Dove, D.B., Stahl, W.M., and Guercio, L.R.M.: Effect of Hydroxyethyl Starch Versus Albumin on Hemodynamic and Respiratory Function in Patients in Shock. Crit. Care Med., 8:255, 1980.

Murphy, P.J., Williams, T.L., and Kau, D.L.: Disposition of Dobutamine in the Dog. J. Pharmacol. Exp. Ther., 199:423, 1976.

Nahas, G.G.: The Clinical Pharmacology of THAM (Tris (Hydroxymethyl)-Aminomethane). Clin. Pharmacol. Ther., 4:784, 1963.

Nahas, G.G.: Use of an Organic Carbon Dioxide Buffer *in vivo*. Science, 129:782, 1959.

Ohyanagi, M.D., Toshima, M.D., Sekita, M., Okamoto, M., Itoh, T., Mitsuno, T., Naito, R., Suyama, T., and Yokoyama, K.: Clinical Studies of Perfluorochemical Whole Blood Substitutes: Safety of Fluosol-DA (20%) in Normal Human Volunteers. Clin. Ther., 2:306, 1979.

Palminteri, A.: Clinical Appraisal of the Narcotic Antagonist N-Allylnoroxymorphone. J.A.V.M.A., 148:1396, 1966.

Polak, A., and Plum, F.: Comparison of New Analeptics in Barbiturate-Poisoned Animals. J. Pharmacol. Exp. Ther., 145:27, 1964.

Rawlings, C.A., and Kolata, R.J.: Cardiopulmonary Effects of Thiopental/Lidocaine Combination during Anesthetic Induction in the Dog. Am. J. Vet. Res., 44:144, 1983.

Redding, J.S., Haynes, R.R., and Thomas, J.D.: Drug Therapy in Resuscitation from Electromechanical Dissociation. Crit. Care Med., 11:681, 1983.

Reid, P.R., and Thompson, W.L.: The Clinical Use of Dopamine in the Treatment of Shock. Johns Hopkins Med. J., 137:276, 1975.

Riebold, T.W., Goble, D.O., and Geiser, D.R.: *Large Animal Anesthesia, Principles and Techniques*. The Iowa State Press, Ames, 1982.

Ring, J., and Messmer, K.: Incidence and Severity of Anaphylactoid Reactions to Colloid Volume Substitutes. Lancet, 1:466, 1977.

Robie, N.W., Goetter, W.E., and Goldberg, L.I.: Systemic and Renal Hemodynamic Effects of Dopamine and Prostaglandin A Alone and in Combination. Blood Vessels, 11:86, 1974.

Robie, N.W., and Goldberg, L.I.: Comparative Systemic and Regional Hemodynamic Effects of Dopamine and Dobutamine. Am. Heart J., 90:340, 1975.

Rock, G., and Wise, P.: Plasma Expansion During Granulocyte Procurement: Cumulative Effects of Hydroxyethyl Starch. Blood, 53:1156, 1979.

Rouse, W.: Cardiac Effects of Propranolol During Anesthesia in Dogs. Am. J. Cardiol., 18:406, 1966.

Rumbaugh, G.E., Carlson, G.P., and Harrold, D.: Clinicopathologic Effects of Rapid Infusion of 5% Sodium Bicarbonate in 5% Dextrose in the Horse. J.A.V.M.A., 1783:267, 1981.

Rush, B.F., Richardson, J.D., Bosomworth, P., and Eiseman, B.: Limitations of Blood Replacement with Electrolyte Solutions. Arch. Surg., 98:49, 1969.

Sanders, J.E., Yeary, R.A., Powers, J.D., and DeWet, P.: Relationships Between Serum and Brain Concentrations of Phenytoin in the Dog. Am. J. Vet. Res., 40:473, 1979.

Sarnoff, S.J., Case, R.B., Berglund, E., and Sarnoff, L.C.: Ventricular Function. V. The Circulatory Effects of Aramine; Mechanism of Action of "Vasopressor" Drugs in Cardiogenic Shock. Circulation, 10:84, 1954.

Sarnoff, S.J., and Kaufman, H.E.: Effect of Aramine on the Survival of Dogs Subjected to Hemorrhagic Hypotension. Circ. Res., 2:420, 1954.

Schalm, O.W.: *Veterinary Hematology,* 2nd ed. Lea & Febiger, Philadelphia, 1965.

Schweichel, E., Schmidt, D., Schneider, E., and Brüchner, J.B.: Circulatory Pattern and Duration of Action of Naloxone in Dogs with and without Opioid Pretreatment. Acta Anaesthesiol. Scand., 23:336, 1979.

Short, C.E., Cloyd, G.D., and Ward, J.W.: The Use of Doxapram Hydrochloride with Intravenous Anesthetics in Horses. Part I. Vet. Med./Small Anim. Clin., 65:157, 1970.

Smith, J.E., Mahaffey, E., and Board, P.: A New Storage Medium for Canine Blood. J.A.V.M.A., 172:701, 1978.

Soma, L.R., and Kenny, R.: Respiratory, Cardiovascular, Metabolic, and Electroencephalographic Effects of Doxapram Hydrochloride in the Dog. Am. J. Vet. Res., 28:191, 1967.

Starzecki, B., Reddin, J.L., and Spink, W.W.: Effect of Isoproterenol on Survival in Canine Endotoxin Shock. Ann. Surg., 167:35, 1968.

Stormont, C.J.: Blood Groups in Animals. J.A.V.M.A., 181:1120, 1982.

Stowe, C.M.: Adrenergic Drugs. In *Veterinary Pharmacology and Therapeutics,* 3rd ed. Edited by L.M. Jones. Iowa State University Press, Ames, 1965.

Tacker, W.A., Havens, W.W., and Geddes, L.A.: Minimum Duration of Capacitor Discharge Current for Indirect Ventricular Defibrillation in the Dog. Cardiovasc. Res. Cent. Bull., 7:12, 1968.

Tacker, W.A., Niebauer, M.J., Babbs, C.F., Combs, W.J., Hahn, B.M., Barker, M.A., Seipel, J.F., Bourland, J.D., and Geddes, L.A.: The Effect of Newer Antiarrhythmic Drugs on Defibrillation Threshold. Crit. Care Med., 8:177, 1980.

Thompson, F.N., Armstrong, K., Kreuz, S.S., and Cornelius, L.N.: Effect of Adrenalectomy in the Dog on Blood Gas Tensions and Oxygen Content. Am. J. Vet. Res., 38:235, 1977.

Trinkle, J.K., Rush, B.F., and Eiseman, B.: Metabolism of Lactate Following Major Blood Loss. Surgery, 63:782, 1968.

Tucker, W.K., Rackstein, A.D., and Munson, E.S.: Comparison of Arrhythmic Doses of Adrenaline, Metaraminol, Ephedrine, and Phenylephrine during Isoflurane and Halothane Anesthesia in Dogs. Br. J. Anaesth., 46:392, 1974.

Tuttle, R.R., and Mills, J.: Development of a New Catecholamine to Selectively Increase Cardiac Contractility. Circ. Res., 36:185, 1975.

Van den Berg, C.J., and Pineda, A.A.: Plasma Exchange in the Treatment of Acute Renal Failure Due to Low Molecular-Weight Dextran. Mayo Clin. Proc., 55:387, 1980.

Wada, J.: Cardiac Defibrillation. In *Cardiac Arrest and Resuscitation,* 3rd ed. Edited by H.E. Stephenson, Jr. C.V. Mosby Co., St. Louis, 1969.

Walter, A.K.Y.: Blood Microfiltration. Anaesthesia, 33:35, 1978.

Webb, W.R., Lemmer, R.A., and Elman, R.: Absorption Rates, Electrolyte and Volume Changes Following Subcutaneous and Intraperitoneal Injections of Solutions Containing Salt, Glucose, and Amino Acids. Surg. Gynecol. Obstet., 91:265, 1950.

Williams, E.M., and Sekiya, A.: Prevention of Arrhythmias Due to Cardiac Glycosides by Block of Sympathetic B-receptors. Lancet, 1:420, 1963.

Wingfield, W.E.: Personal communication. Colorado State University, Fort Collins, Colorado, 1984.

Winnie, A.P.: Arrhythmia Beta Blockade Catecholamines. Division of Anesthesiology, Cook County Hospital, and The Hektoen Institute of Medical Research, Cook County Hospital, Chicago, 1968.

Winnie, A.P., and Collins, V.J.: The Doxapram Test: A New Technique for the Differential Diagnosis of Apnea. Anesthesiology, 26:265, 1965.

Witzel, D.A., Geddes, L.A., Hoff, H.E., and McFarlane, J.: Electrical Defibrillation of the Equine Heart. Am. J. Vet. Res., 29:1279, 1968.

Witzel, D., Geddes, L.A., and McFarlane, J.: Electrical

Ventricular Defibrillation in the Calf. Southwest. Vet., 20:25, 1966.
Wong, D.W., Mishkin, F.S., and Tanaka, T.T.: The Effects of Bicarbonate on Blood Coagulation. J.A.V.M.A., 244:61, 1980.
Zenoble, R.D., and Stone, E.A.: Autotransfusion in the Dog. J.A.V.M.A., 172:1411, 1978.
Zontine, W.J., and Donovan, M.L.: Effect of Hypodermoclysis with Dextrose in Dogs. Am. J. Vet. Res., 30: 605, 1969.

CHAPTER 21

Anesthetic Complications and Emergencies

Despite all precautionary measures, anesthetic emergencies occasionally develop. It has been stated (Anonymous, 1950), "Although certain surgical procedures may be classified as 'minor operations' we need wider recognition of the fact that there is no such thing as a 'minor anesthetic'. . . . It is during . . . 'minor' procedures that the anesthetic accident often occurs." By scrupulous care, many emergencies can be avoided; by prior preparation and training, emergencies can usually be brought to a successful conclusion for the patient.

RESPIRATORY SYSTEM

Signs indicative of abnormal respiration include the following: 1) apnea (respiratory arrest), 2) hypopnea (hypoventilation), 3) irregular and slow breathing, 4) tracheal tug, apneustic breathing, and gasping, 5) hyperpnea (hyperventilation), and 6) tachypnea (accelerated respiratory rate). Since these signs often reflect hypoxia and/or hypercapnia, which predispose the heart to arrest, immediate correction with maintenance of efficient oxygenation and elimination of carbon dioxide are essential (see Chap. 6). Serial blood gas determinations and/or end tidal gas analyses will show the degree of respiratory insufficiency, and will indicate the efficacy of therapy.

Apnea

Apnea may result from 1) respiratory obstruction, 2) depression of the respiratory center by cardiac arrest or by general anesthetics, sedatives, and narcotics, 3) the use of muscle relaxants, 4) hyperventilation with concomitant hypocapnia and suppression of the stretch receptors, 5) reflex stimulation, especially during light anesthesia (surgical stimulation, irritation of celiac plexus, irritation of upper respiratory tract), and 6) depression of the chemoreceptors by high oxygen tensions following hypoxia.

Should apnea occur, administration of anesthetic should cease, the presence of effective heart action and a patent airway should be assured, and effective ventilation should be maintained until the cause can be corrected. When mechanical ventilation has induced hyperventilation apnea, it may be necessary to administer air or air and oxygen via a nonrebreathing technique or to hypoventilate the patient until spontaneous respiration recurs (see Chap. 7). If respiratory analeptics are administered, it is important to appreciate that their action is usually short-lived, and respiratory arrest or ineffective ventilation may recur (see Chap. 20).

Hypopnea, Irregular and Slow Breathing

Respirations that are shallow, irregular, or slow are usually indicative of ineffective ventilation, with impaired oxygenation and carbon dioxide elimination. If ventilation is ineffective, respirations should be assisted, even when oxygen is being administered. Control is most effective if end-tidal or blood gases are monitored. Hypoventilation is more likely to occur in patients in which abdominal pressure is increased by distension, restraint, or obesity. Slow breathing may result from sedatives and narcotics and is associated with shallow breathing (hypopnea) during the deeper planes of gas anesthesia, barbiturate anesthesia, myoneural block, and overdosage of narcotics and sedatives. Although ineffective ventilation is usually more severe in the deeper planes of anesthesia, it may occur at all levels, and even presents a problem during induction, especially if a rapid injection technique has been employed. In such instances, transient apnea may even occur. This should not cause alarm unless cyanosis develops, for respirations usually resume as carbon dioxide tensions increase. Hypoventilation with irregular breathing (rate and depth) is a common occurrence during thiobarbiturate induction in the horse. Intubation, administration of oxygen, and controlled breathing are necessary when this persists. Specific antagonists are indicated when available.

Tracheal Tug, Apneustic Breathing, and Gasping

Other respiratory patterns occur that are further indications of depressed respiratory function. In deep anesthesia or during the use of muscle relaxants, a jerky type of inspiration, including posterior movement of the larynx and trachea, may occur. It is associated with intercostal and diaphragmatic paralysis. A series of slow deep inspirations, in which inflation is held for a brief period followed with exhalation by elastic recoil (apneustic breathing), may also occur during anesthesia that is too deep. This pattern of breathing arises in deep barbiturate and chloral hydrate anesthesia in the horse.

Prior to ultimate respiratory arrest, especially that resulting from cardiac arrest, a few deep gasping respirations may occur.

Hyperpnea and Tachypnea

An increase in the depth and rate of breathing results from surgical stimulation during anesthesia that is too light, from hypoxia, and from hypercapnia. It is essential under such circumstances to confirm the presence of a patent airway, a supply of oxygen, and effective carbon dioxide absorption. Respiratory obstruction will be indicated by respiratory effort that is disproportionate to the resulting chest excursions. Tachypnea may also be observed in dogs, cats, horses, and cattle during halothane anesthesia, especially when high concentrations are used. The tachypnea may be overcome by a small intravenous dose of meperidine.

Respiratory Obstruction

Obstruction to breathing is indicated by inadequate tidal exchange, evidenced by reduced excursion of the reservoir bag or weakness of the breathing sounds. If the obstruction is partial, breathing is noisy. Contrasting with the reduced tidal exchange, the respiratory effort is increased. There is increased diaphragmatic action with resulting excessive abdominal movement; there is use of the accessory respiratory muscles, and the increased inspiratory subatmospheric intrathoracic pressure may be sufficient to cause partial collapse of the thoracic wall. During anesthesia, especially deep anesthesia, these responses to airway obstruction are markedly suppressed and may go unobserved.

As a result of obstruction, the exchange of oxygen, carbon dioxide, and inhalant anesthetic (if used) is curtailed, with consequent hypoxia, hypercapnia, and delayed induction of or recovery from inhalation anesthesia. The respiratory effort causes increased work of breathing, and the negative pressure during inspiration may cause pulmonary edema.

Obstruction of the airway can occur from many causes. Unfavorable positioning of the patient during anesthesia may produce partial or complete obstruction. Other causes of nasopharyngeal obstruction are occlusion of the mouth and external nares by draping material, accumulation of mucus, saliva, blood clots, or vomitus in the pharynx, and posterior displacement of the base of the tongue with obstruction of the laryngeal orifice. The head should therefore be extended, the tongue pulled out, the nasopharynx freed of mucus, saliva, or exudate, and the nose and mouth cleared of draping materials. In brachycephalic dogs, elongation of the soft palate and eversion of the lateral ventricles may cause obstruction. Intubation is mandatory in such patients. Obstruction by the soft palate may occur in the horse and is a common cause of stertorous breathing during anesthesia of this species. Respiratory obstruction also results from laryngospasm and bronchospasm (see the following section).

Obstruction to breathing can result from faulty anesthetic apparatus. Prior to use, the supply of gases should be checked and the operation of valves examined by briefly exhaling into and inhaling from the circuit. Partial obstruction may also be caused by an insufficient gas flow with collapse of the reservoir bag.

The endotracheal tube is a common cause of obstruction. It may be partially or completely occluded with mucus, blood, or exudate, kinked, too small, or obstructed by overinflation of the cuff.

Laryngeal and Bronchial Spasm

Spasms of the larynx and/or bronchi may develop in any species, but are seen most commonly in cats, sheep, goats, swine, and rabbits given high concentrations of inhalation anesthetics or one of the thiobarbiturates.

Rex (1966) has shown that laryngospasm can be induced in the cat by inhalation of either halothane (6 to 8%) or ether (10 to 20%). The vocal cord adductor muscles were those stimulated. The sites of stimulation producing laryngospasm included not only the larynx but also the cervical trachea and lower respiratory tract. The contractions could be reduced by spraying the anterior larynx with lidocaine (2%), and abolished by cutting the internal branches of the superior laryngeal nerves.

Rosen (1960) has pointed out the dual origin of vagal fibers that arise in both the pons and medulla. Atropine, which blocks only postganglionic cholinergic nerve endings, not the myoneural junction of striated muscle, is of no value in therapeutic doses for treatment of laryngospasm. The efficacious results reported by Burstein and Rovenstine (1938) in cats were at extremely high dose levels and were probably due to central depressant effects.

Spasms usually occur in lightly anesthetized animals from stimulation of the respiratory tract (intubation attempts, inhalation of concentrated anesthetic vapors); they may also result from stimuli arising at the site of operation. The result is coughing and a high-pitched inspiratory sound accompanied by some degree of cyanosis. Hall (1959) has suggested intravenous meperidine in this situation for its spasmolytic action. Oxygen should be administered by mask or oral or nasopharyngeal tube until such time as the laryngospasms are relaxed by induction of deeper anesthesia or by the use of a muscle relaxant. An endotracheal catheter is then inserted. Forcible intubation through a closed glottis may cause trauma with subsequent edema; therefore, intubation should be done gently. Spasm can be prevented by the topical application of 4% lidocaine to the larynx, by intubation only after laryngeal reflexes are obtunded, by use of a muscle relaxant, or by intravenous administration of 2% lidocaine.

Bronchial or bronchiolar spasms result, likewise, from inadequate suppression of reflexes and are associated with stimulation by secretions, anesthetic vapor, intubation, especially when the carina is stimulated, and operative procedures. The syndrome is characterized by wheezing, coughing, gasping, inadequate ventilation, and even cyanosis. Although it occurs in most species, it is most common in ruminants. Management should include respiratory support, meperidine, intravenous lidocaine, or isoproterenol.

Pulmonary Ventilation—Blood Flow Inequality

When pulmonary ventilation and blood flow are uneven, the lung exchanges gases less efficiently, arterial oxygen tensions are likely to fall, and carbon dioxide tensions increase (see Chap. 6). Hypoxemia without hypercapnia after abdominal surgery in man has been attributed to regional ventilation-perfusion inequality in the lungs and to shunting of pulmonary capillary blood through unventilated areas of alveolar collapse (Cullen, 1967). In anesthetized horses in lateral recumbency, Gillespie et al. (1969) have reported large differences between alveolar and arterial oxygen tensions.

In addition to atelectasis secondary to hypoventilation and recumbency, ventilation-perfusion inequalities during or following anesthesia may result from pneumothorax, intrapleural effusion and hemorrhage, abdominal distension, and aspiration and accumulation of blood, secretions, and stomach contents. Regardless of the cause, it should be corrected if possible, and the resulting atelectasis overcome by increased inflation of the lungs.

When pulmonary embolism occurs, the alveoli affected are not perfused and therefore constitute increased dead space. This complication occasionally results from jugular phlebitis induced by such irritants as chloral hydrate, or in swine from venipuncture of the anterior vena cava. Treatment includes oxygen therapy, sedation, and anticoagulants.

Aspiration of Chest Following Thoracic Surgery

Any form of pneumothorax leads to hypoventilation (see Chap. 6). For this reason, following thoracic surgery the chest should be continuously aspirated. This will 1) remove any residual air and correct atelectasis; 2) remove any fluid or blood remaining in the pleural cavity after chest closure; and 3) indicate if hemorrhage is inadvertently occurring into the pleural cavity.

A catheter is inserted through a stab wound adjacent to the thoracotomy wound and connected to a suction device (Fig. 21–1). Generally, prolonged aspiration is unnecessary, the tube being removed from the chest as the animal shows signs of awakening. The Heimlich valve can be used in lieu of a 2- or 3-bottle chest drainage system in both anesthetized and awake, unrestrained animals (Heimlich, 1966; Sauer, 1969).

CARDIOVASCULAR SYSTEM

Shock

Shock is a general term implying the occurrence of prostration or stupor accompanied by decreased arterial blood pressure.

Physiologically, shock may be defined as a condition in which there is inadequate tissue perfusion resulting in cellular hypoxia (Baue, 1968). *It is a failure of blood flow, not of blood pressure.* Four general types of shock may be recognized by the surgeon and anesthesiologist. *Hypovolemic shock* is due to loss of whole blood, plasma, and body fluids. It may be caused by trauma, hemorrhage, burns, intestinal obstruction, dehydration, and hypoproteinemia. *Septic (endotoxic) shock* is caused by infection, usually with gram-negative organisms, though any terminal infection may be the cause. *Cardiogenic shock* results from deficiency in the myocardial ability to pump blood. Regardless of initiating cause, as the shock process develops, less distinction can be made between these types. For example, in fulminating hemorrhagic shock, myocardial function is always impaired and bacterial invasion develops. It must be recognized that anesthesia modifies the response of the patient to these phenomena.

Neurogenic shock is caused by complete transection of the spinal cord or by other phenomena that produce peripheral vasodilatation with hypotension and simulate this effect. High spinal

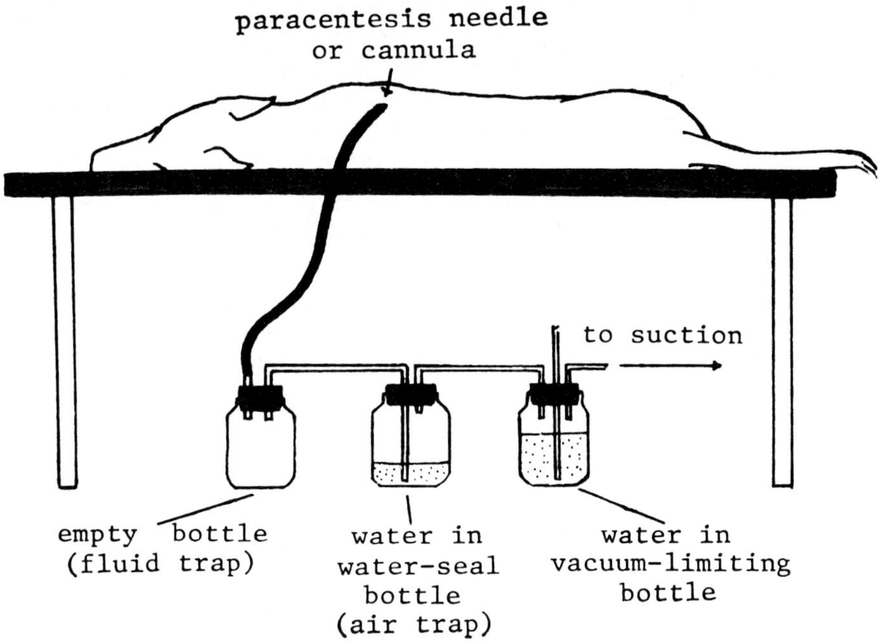

Figure 21–1. Aspiration of chest. The 3rd bottle (the vacuum-limiting bottle) can be omitted when an electrically driven suction device with a variable air bleed is used. If the water-seal bottle is more than 80 cm below the table, the water cannot be aspirated into the chest by even the most violent respiratory movements. (From Hall, L.W.: Better Management for Trauma in the Dog. Mod. Vet. Pract., 48:43, 1967.)

anesthesia is a modality that may cause this to occur. As pointed out by Hermreck and Thal (1968), use of the term *shock* for this condition is misleading since it bears little relationship to other forms of shock and is treated differently, at least initially. Pure neurogenic shock can be treated successfully with any of the alpha- or mixed alpha- and beta-adrenergic agents.

Once shock starts, the sequence of events is much the same regardless of cause. An understanding of these changes is essential to rational therapy. The changes are time-related and vary, depending upon the severity of the inciting cause.

Some physiologic compensations, especially increased sympathetic activity, take place to protect the animal. Among these are arterial and splenic constriction, increased cardiac rate, and selective distribution of the available blood supply. The vital organs are favored over the non-vital ones, causing superficial pallor, skin coldness, and weakened pulse. The most important organs are the central nervous system, heart, liver, and kidneys, the first being the most sensitive to decrease in blood flow. During shock, the organism makes every effort to supply blood to the central nervous system and survives as long as this is adequately maintained. On the other hand, if compensation is not adequate, shock will progress to the irreversible stage, resulting in death of the patient.

Low blood flows stimulate release of ACTH, antidiuretic hormone, renin-angiotensin, 17-hydroxycorticosteroid, aldosterone, and catecholamines. Arterial and venous vasoconstriction are produced, with a rise in peripheral vascular resistance and pooling of blood in the venous capacitance system. This is reflected in a low central venous pressure. If shock persists or is accentuated, the compensatory vasoconstriction breaks down. The accumulation of metabolic products, especially lactic acid, in the tissues promotes relaxation of the precapillary sphincters, which are susceptible to changes in pH. The constrictors on the venous side of the capillary bed, however, remain constricted, pooling of blood in the capillary bed is accentuated, and the stagnant phase of shock ensues. There is red cell agglutination and thrombosis, loss of fluid into the interstitial space, and a diffuse, often only transient, clotting of blood within the microcirculation (disseminated intravascular coagulation—DIC). For DIC to occur, there must not only be slow or stagnant capillary flow, but also a thromboplastic agent in the blood. A small amount of hemolysis is all that is necessary (Hardway, 1980). The combination of hemorrhage and hemolysis in traumatic shock produces the requirements for DIC to occur. Lysis of clots may result in embolism with tissue necrosis, compromise of the reticuloendothelial system, and inability to clear endotoxins normally entering the body from the gut. Owing to congestion and edema, right-to-left pulmonary shunting develops and may reach a peak of 80%. In fact, ventilatory failure is a major cause of death from shock in human patients. At necropsy, the lung is wet, heavy, and liver-like (''shock lung''). Histologically, congestion, hemorrhage, edema, alveolar obliteration, and hyaline membranes are observed.

Stagnation of sludged blood in dilated capillaries also reduces venous return to the heart, which must perform at a higher level of activity with reduced coronary circulation (Fig. 21–2). Decreased cardiac output further increases tissue, including myocardial, hypoxia and permeability of capillaries. A point is reached at which hypoxic capillaries become permanently damaged and irreversibly permeable to plasma colloids. This state characterizes irreversible shock. When it is reached, the capillary bed never again is able to retain blood or plasma transfused into the vascular system.

In shock, renal function is progressively diminished owing to constriction of the renal vessels with decreased blood flow to the kidneys. A blood pressure of at least 70 mm Hg is required for kidney function. The blood colloids have an osmotic pressure of 30 mm Hg, and a

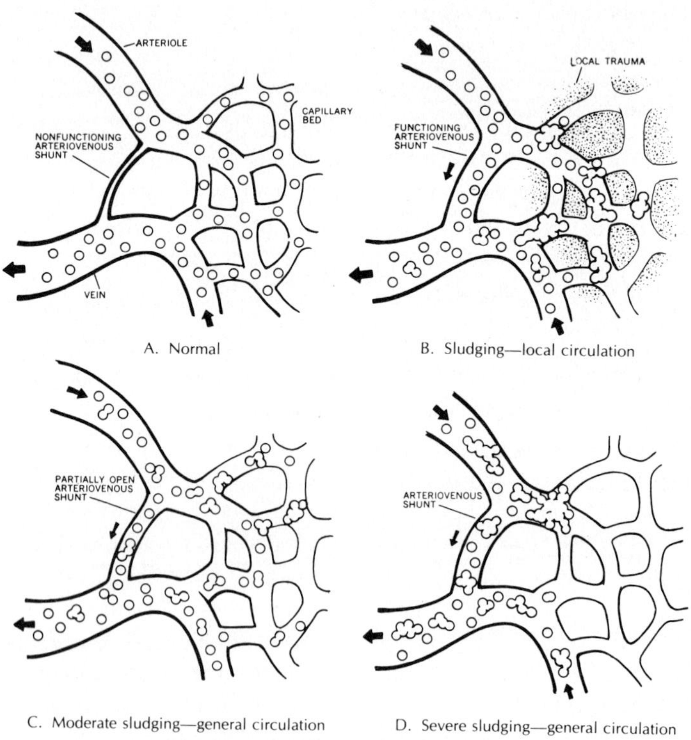

Figure 21–2. Progressive stages of blood sludging in the microcirculation. (Adapted from Bigelow, W.G.: Canad. J. Surg., 7: 237, 1964.) (From Rheomacrodex (Dextran 40): Flow Improver in Cardiopulmonary Bypass. Pharmacia Laboratories, Inc., Piscataway, N.J. 1967.)

pressure of 30 to 40 mm Hg is required to overcome resistance of the kidney tubule and remainder of the urinary tract. Thus, a prolonged fall in blood pressure results in complete loss of function with subsequent tubular necrosis.

Approximately 80% of the blood supply to the liver comes via the portal vein and 20% through the hepatic artery. Numerous workers have shown that interruption of the arterial blood supply to the liver causes rapid death in dogs owing to liver necrosis. If these dogs are treated with antibiotics just prior to ligation, most will survive. Death is caused by inability of the liver, deprived of oxygen, to cope with normal clostridial saprophytes that are constantly present in this organ. Only a little arterial blood is sufficient to prevent liver necrosis. Following hemorrhagic shock, there is disruption of hepatic lysosomes with release of hydrolytic lysosomal enzymes. An increase in arterial blood flow to the liver reduces liver damage and thereby mortality. Antibiotic therapy, to check bacterial proliferation, is also effective.

Invasive infection of the intestinal mucosa occurs from the normal bacterial flora of the intestine along with overgrowth of saprophytic clostridial bacteria in the liver. A causal relation between these lesions and regional hypotension has been demonstrated in cats (Haglund et al., 1976). Intracellular edema develops with mitochondrial changes and increased levels of lysosomal hydrolase enzymes. Lysosomal protease has a direct negative inotropic effect in some species. Endotoxins released from bacteria are no longer degraded by the reticuloendothelial system in the liver and splanchnic region owing to the marked decrease in hepatic and splanchnic blood flow. These endotoxins are thus disseminated widely and cause release of vasoactive agents (Al-Kaisi et al., 1977), and excessive and prolonged sympathetic nervous stimulation of the blood vessels with eventual loss of vascular tone (Fine, 1967).

Endotoxin binds to various blood cellular elements that sequester in the microcirculation of the lungs, liver, and spleen. Serotonin, histamine, lysosomal enzymes, and other factors are released. The terminal complement series is activated when there is an increase in epinephrine

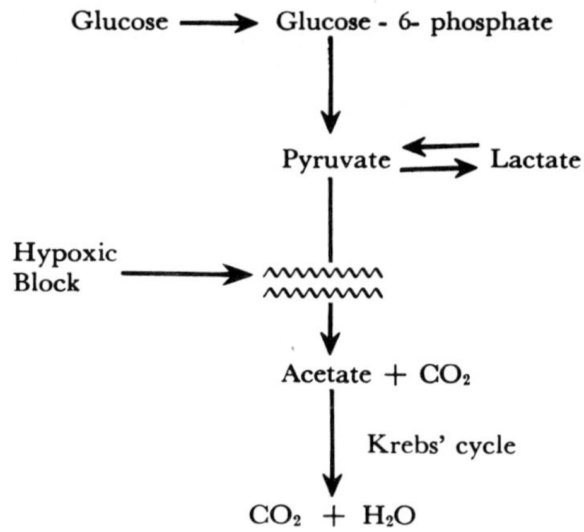

Figure 21–3. Formation of lactic acid (lactate) due to hypoxia. Note that the reaction is reversible and follows the law of mass action.

and norepinephrine. Kinins, prostaglandins, pyrogen, interferon, pancreatic myocardial depressant factor (MDF), and glucocorticoid-antagonizing factor are all increased in the systemic circulation (Burrows, 1981). It has been suggested that prostaglandins released because of endotoxin have significant vasoconstrictor and bronchoconstrictor activity (Al-Kaisi et al., 1977). In studies of experimental endotoxic shock, Faden and Holaday (1980) found that pituitary endorphins are also pathophysiologic factors and that the use of opiate antagonists may be of therapeutic benefit. In the horse, an animal sensitive to shock and especially endotoxin, treatment with flunixin meglumine, an antiprostaglandin, has been shown to alleviate experimental endotoxic shock (Bottoms et al., 1981).

Certain metabolic changes accompany the development of shock. Increase in blood lactic acid indicates cellular hypoxia. In hypoxia, aerobic oxidation of pyruvic acid is blocked, and it is converted to lactic acid (Fig. 21–3). The accumulation of lactic acid accounts, in part, for the progressive acidosis in shock (Broder and Weil, 1964). Functional impairment of cellular metabolism is followed by permanent cellular damage. Serum enzymes reflecting cellular damage are, therefore, elevated (e.g., GOT, GPT, and LDH). The severity of oxygen deprivation and the differential sensitiv-

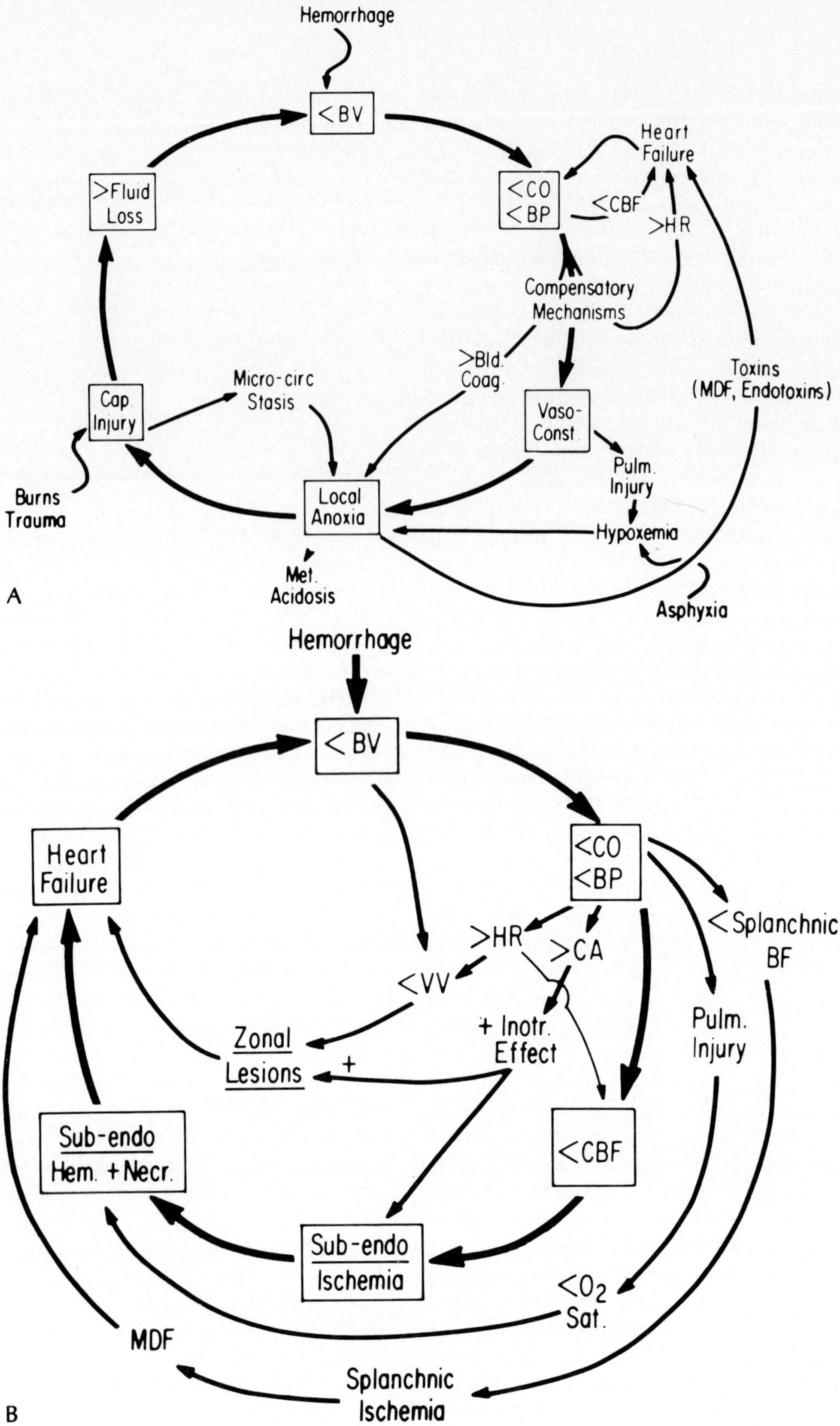
Hemorrhage
< BV
>Fluid Loss
< CO < BP
Heart Failure
< CBF
> HR
Compensatory Mechanisms
> Bld. Coag.
Toxins (MDF, Endotoxins)
Vaso-Const.
Micro-circ Stasis
Cap. Injury
Burns Trauma
Local Anoxia
Pulm. Injury
Hypoxemia
Met. Acidosis
Asphyxia
A
Hemorrhage
< BV
Heart Failure
< CO < BP
> HR
> CA
< Splanchnic BF
< VV
+ Inotr. Effect
Zonal Lesions
+
Pulm. Injury
Sub-endo Hem. + Necr.
< CBF
Sub-endo Ischemia
< O2 Sat.
MDF
Splanchnic Ischemia
B

ity of tissues to oxygen lack are immediate determinants of survival. Measurement of excess lactate provides a means of assessing oxygen debt. In pentobarbital-anesthetized dogs subjected to hemorrhagic shock, a blood lactic acid level over 40 mg/dl is a grave prognostic sign and over 50 mg/dl is fatal (Swan and Nelson, 1969).

Cellular hypoxia causes decreased aerobic oxidation of glucose through the Krebs' cycle and increased anaerobic glycolysis through the Embden-Meyerhof pathway. After a certain period its rate of glycolysis begins to decline, owing to progressive acidosis, which appears to inhibit the process at the phosphofructokinase step (Markov et al., 1981). Because anaerobic glycolysis is less efficient, the amount of energy available to the tissues is reduced. Hepatic glycogen breakdown causes early hypoglycemia and eventual hyperkalemia and glycogen depletion. Tissue adenosine triphosphate (ATP) decreases. Both pyruvate and lactate increase, with lactate increasing most. Acid metabolites produce metabolic acidosis and, as the alkali reserve of the body is diminished, the blood pH may fall below 7.0. Malm et al. (1966) have shown that acidosis per se is a significant stimulus to catecholamine release and to hypotension.

Increased breakdown of protein in the peripheral tissues and reduced amino-acid metabolism due to hepatic hypoxia cause increased plasma nonprotein nitrogen. This increase is exacerbated by reduced renal function and is generally proportional to the severity of shock. There is also loss of sodium and an increase in potassium of the blood. Coagulability of the blood is decreased. Hemoconcentration produces a rise in the hematocrit, which may serve as a rough measurement of the degree of shock, since it is an indirect method of measuring capillary permeability.

Clinically, shock is characterized by paleness of the skin and mucous membranes from diminished circulation to these organs. Decreased oxygenation due to reduced circulation results in cyanosis. In an effort to compensate for diminished cardiac output, the heart rate increases. The pulse is fast and weak because of decreased circulating blood volume. If arterial blood pressure determinations are made, the reading will be less than 90 mm Hg. In the surgical field, lowered blood pressure and stagnation result in diminished bleeding, darkened blood, and cyanosis of the tissues. The blood viscosity is increased. As the heart becomes progressively more hypoxic, bradycardia develops.

In an attempt to increase oxygenation of the blood, respirations are accelerated. Shallow respirations indicate pulmonary edema caused by increased capillary permeability. Restlessness, depression, weakness, and prostration become evident in unanesthesized animals. The body temperature falls and extremities become cold. There is increased thirst, which may be accompanied by vomiting, dryness of the mucous membranes, and diarrhea. As functional activity gradually ebbs, the animal, if unanesthetized, becomes comatose due to progressive uncompensated circulatory failure. This indicates the irreversibility of the shock mechanism. Terminally, the pupils become widely dilated. Some of the mechanisms by which shock becomes irreversible are illustrated in Figure 21–4*A*, *B*.

In clinical practice, shock is occasionally seen on induction of anesthesia in animals that were normal, insofar as could be determined. This is due to the anesthetic agent and is probably a combination of anesthetic toxicity, reduced respiratory exchange, and reduction in blood pres-

Figure 21–4. *A*, Some of the vicious cycles of shock. Abbreviations: *Bld Coag*, blood coagulability; *BP*, systemic blood pressure; *BV*, effective blood volume; *Cap*, capillary; *CBF*, coronary blood flow; *CO*, cardiac output; *HR*, heart rate; *MDF*, myocardial depressant factor; *Met*, metabolic; *Const*, constriction; and *Pulm*, pulmonary; < = decrease and > = increase. *B*, Factors contributing to heart failure in shock. *BF*, blood flow; *CA*, catecholamines; *Hem*, hemorrhage; *Inotr*, inotropic; *Necr*, necrosis; *Sat*, saturation; *Sub-endo*, subendocardial; and *VV*, ventricular volume. (From Hackel, D.B., Ratliff, N.B., and Mikat, E.: The Heart in Shock. Circ. Res., 35:805, 1974. By permission of the American Heart Association, Inc.)

sure owing to loss of muscle tone with decreased venous return to the heart.

During surgery at least four factors may cause development of shock: 1) prenaesthetic and anesthetic effects, 2) hemorrhage, 3) manipulation of the viscera or rough handling of tissues in general, and 4) cooling of the abdominal cavity and its contents. According to Dukes (1947), a reduction of 40 to 50% in the blood volume of an unanesthetized dog results in severe shock. Hay and Webb (1951) found that the amount of blood loss necessary to produce irreversibility varies widely. Experimentally, it varied from 18 to 73% of the blood volume in dogs. Shock can be produced by trauma, such as compression or contusion of tissues, or manipulation of the intestine or other abdominal viscera. It has also been produced in dogs by cooling the abdominal cavity and its contents with water at 15° C for 2 to 2½ hours. The effects of cooling should, for this reason, be considered in prolonged abdominal surgery.

Treatment of Shock

The onset of shock is subtle and may go unnoticed for some time. For this reason, the wise course of action is to start a prophylactic intravenous drip of buffered Ringer's lactate solution or saline-dextrose whenever there is a significant potential for subsequent shock. In addition, hypotension should be avoided by minimizing hemorrhage and excessive anesthetic depth. The flow of fluid should be adjusted so that it more than replaces blood loss. If brisk hemorrhage occurs, the flow should be immediately increased proportionally. The circulating blood volume is thus maintained in the face of hemorrhage, and access to the venous system is ensured in the event drugs need to be quickly administered. Routine adherence to this principle will many times prevent the necessity for more heroic measures later.

In the event of shock, anesthesia should not be induced, except in extreme emergency, until the animal has been resuscitated. It is essential to correct metabolic acidosis with sodium bicarbonate and to provide fluid replacement prior to the use of vasodilator drugs. If possible, a balanced anesthetic regimen should be used and phenothiazine-derivative tranquilizers avoided. Ketamine, diazepam, narcotics with nitrous oxide-oxygen and, if needed, a muscle relaxant, are anesthetic drugs deserving consideration. Alternatively, conduction anesthesia may be utilized. Survival rate in hemorrhagic shock of rats has been shown to be significantly higher with ketamine anesthesia in contrast to pentobarbital sodium, halothane, and fluroxene (Longnecker and Sturgill, 1976). Halothane or methoxyflurane should be used with care because of possible potentiation of hypotension. Increased right-to-left intrapulmonic shunting and decreased functional residual capacity in shock necessitate reexpansion of atelectatic alveoli by volume-controlled ventilation with continuous positive airway pressure (CPAP) (Kirby, 1973).

Once shock has become apparent, the *first step* in its treatment is to provide adequate ventilation. In many instances, the patient will be anesthetized and intubated, so that all that is necessary is to assure an adequate minute volume and to supply supplemental oxygen. In instances when long-term ventilation therapy is needed in conscious patients, a tracheostomy may be performed. Regardless of the method used, adequate oxygenation and carbon dioxide elimination must be maintained. It should be reemphasized that it is possible for a patient to be well oxygenated and still have carbon dioxide retention and respiratory acidosis. Measurement of arterial blood gases and pH is important to determine the degree of CO_2 retention with acidosis, which contributes to shock.

The *second step* must be directed toward achieving an adequate circulating blood volume. Circulatory function can be roughly estimated by exerting pressure on the mucous membranes of the mouth, and thus determining capillary refill time (Table 21–1). Because estimation of blood loss is at best inaccurate without sophisticated equipment and because replacement of blood loss may not provide an adequate circulating blood volume, central venous pressure (CVP) monitoring is currently considered to be an effective determinant of adequate fluid replacement. In normal animals, CVP usually ranges from 3 to 7.5 cm of water. In recumbent large animals, it is generally

TABLE 21–1. Evaluation of Capillary Refill Time

Color	CRT	Interpretation
Bright pink	1 sec or less	Normal to high cardiac output
Brick red	1 sec or less	Vasodilation; normal to low cardiac output
		Low arterial blood pressure and cardiac output
Pale blue	1 to 3 sec	Possible venule dilation and/or reflux of venous blood into the capillary bed

(From Whittick, W.G.: Normal Canine Models. In *Veterinary Critical Care*. Edited by F.P. Sattler, R.P. Knowles, and W.G. Whittick. Lea & Febiger, Philadelphia, 1981.)

higher. In man, a rule of thumb is to transfuse until either the blood pressure or the CVP rises. If the blood pressure rises first, a volume deficit exists; if the CVP rises first, a cardiac deficit exists. In shock, a CVP of 0 to 5 cm of water is an indication to give fluids rapidly; from 6 to 12 cm, fluids are probably needed, but at a slower rate based upon the patient's condition; above 15 cm, fluids are contraindicated.

For blood volume expansion, the most effective fluid for immediate use is buffered Ringer's lactate solution, which can be given in quantities as much as 8 times greater than the amount of blood actually lost (Moss, 1969). The use of buffered Ringer's lactate solution *prior* to administration of whole blood is more effective in improving cardiac output and oxygen consumption in dogs with shock than treatment with blood alone. An hematocrit of less than 30% is an indication for administration of whole blood. Often in acute blood loss, it is necessary to use multiple simultaneous infusions to provide rapid and adequate replacement. Use of pumping devices may be necessary (see Fig. 20–3).

Since a significant decrease in functional extracellular fluid volume occurs in shock, use of a volume expander alone may not be adequate (Kirby, 1973). Excessive amounts of lactated Ringer's solution may cause pulmonary edema unless sufficient intravascular osmotic pressure is maintained. Plasma, or substitutes thereof, are recommended until the hematocrit falls below 30% or until coagulopathies occur. These may be overcome by the use of plasma (Buchanan, 1977). Brasmer (1979) emphasizes that the volume of fluid necessary for replacement far exceeds the blood lost. In dogs, a loading dose of 90 ml/kg is recommended. It is not unusual to find that 200 ml/kg is required in dogs to produce evidence of normal perfusion.

Because the circulating blood volume in cats is small (~56 ml/kg or 4% of body weight), fluids should be administered judiciously to prevent overloading. This is particularly true in cats with cardiac, renal, or hepatic disease (Breznock and Strack, 1983).

Despite the simplicity and value of CVP monitoring, it only provides an indication of right heart competence. A good index of the functional competence of the left heart can be obtained by monitoring pulmonary wedge pressure with a Swan-Ganz catheter. Fluid load may be evaluated as with the CVP. Keeping the pulmonary wedge pressure below 10 to 12 mm Hg prevents pulmonary edema. Incorporation of a thermistor wire in the Swan-Ganz catheter permits determination of blood temperature and thereby cardiac output by thermal dilution.

The *third step* in shock therapy is to assure the patency of the pumping mechanism, namely, the heart. In shock, cardiac reserve decreases, and the heart eventually fails. As it does so, tissue perfusion deteriorates, further contributing to the patient's demise. Deterioration of the heart is signaled by a high or rising CVP and/or pulmonary wedge pressure without obvious clinical improvement of the patient. A strong pulse wave, good capillary perfusion, and a normal CVP are indicative of a relatively high cardiac output. Monitoring of arterial pressure, CVP, and vital signs is desirable. In critical cases, pulmonary wedge and cardiac output measurements are advantageous. An intravenous drip of dobutamine or isoproterenol increases heart rate and cardiac output and, at the same time, lowers peripheral vascular resistance. Digitalization should be considered where long-term therapy is needed.

The *fourth step* is to provide other supportive treatment. Sodium bicarbonate or tromethamine should be given intravenously to compensate for acidosis. Corticosteroids are indicated, especially when endotoxin absorption is anticipated, where adrenal insufficiency is suspected, or where shock is prolonged. Broad-spectrum antibiotics should also be given, intravenously if possible, to protect the animal against facultative pathogens and their toxins. Tetracyclines are contraindicated in the horse because of the propensity for colitis.

Kolata (1980) has found that measurement of the skin temperature between the third and fourth phalanges of the hindlimb in dogs is a useful reflection of limb blood flow and, indirectly, reflects the severity of shock. In normal dogs, the difference between toe web and rectal temperatures is 1 to 5°F. In shock the difference exceeds 10°F. Web temperatures can be taken with either a glass thermometer (scale 70° to 110°F) or an electronic one. The bulb of the thermometer is placed (or taped) against the skin between the toes.

Hypothermia has been shown to have a protective action in shock. Extensive peripheral vasodilation induced by application of external heat may accentuate the volume deficit. For this reason, vigorous attempts to warm the patient should be avoided, and the patient should never be made hyperthermic.

Markov et al. (1981) have attempted to restore glycolysis by administration of fructose-1, 6-diphosphate. This therapy appeared to be of potential benefit in irreversible hemorrhagic shock. In endotoxic shock, Faden and Holaday (1980) have found intravenous and intracerebroventricular naloxone to be beneficial in rodent and canine models (see Chap. 20).

Cardiac Arrhythmias

Normal sinus rhythm in various species usually falls within the following range: horse, 28 to 40 per minute; cow, 40 to 80; small ruminant, 70 to 80; pig, 60 to 80; dog, 60 to 160; and cat, 110 to 200. Arrhythmias are classified as those arising above the atrioventricular (A-V) node, at the node, and below the node. They include sinus tachycardia, bradycardia, atrial tachycardia (atrial fibrillation, atrial flutter, and paroxysmal atrial fibrillation), atrial bradycardia, ectopic atrial and nodal beats, nodal tachycardia, atrioventricular dissociation, nodal bradycardia, ventricular ectopic (premature) beats, ventricular tachycardia, and ventricular fibrillation. Conduction disturbances comprise first-, second-, and third-degree heart block, right and left bundle branch block, and Wolff-Parkinson-White syndrome. Figures 21–5, 21–6, and 21–7 illustrate methods for differential diagnosis of arrhythmias.

Clement (1978) has described the relevance, classification, and diagnosis of cardiac arrhythmias as they relate to anesthesia. They are common during general and regional anesthesia and surgery, and are most frequent during induction and intubation. *Arrhythmias usually precede cardiac arrest,* and the causes of each are closely related. Cardiac arrhythmias may be the only sign of cardiovascular disease, and may be either the cause or the effect of progressive myocardial dysfunction. They may occur in the normal heart and be of little significance, or may severely impair the function of the heart which is already compromised. Atrial contractions are especially important when there is obstruction between the atrium and ventricle, when the ventricle requires extra pressure for adequate distension, or when the ventricle is suddenly stressed by increased arterial resistance. Abnormalities of atrial contraction are, therefore, of greater significance under such circumstances. Abnormal slowing of the heart is hazardous if the heart is unable to compensate fully by increased filling and stroke volume, or if there is aortic incompetence or stenosis. In tachycardia, there may be lack of time for diastolic filling in normal hearts and in cases of mitral stenosis; there is also an increase in tension-time index and myocardial oxygen consumption, and an adverse effect in ventricular hypertrophy.

Cessation of the heartbeat is often preceded by cardiac arrhythmias induced by factors that cause or predispose to arrest.

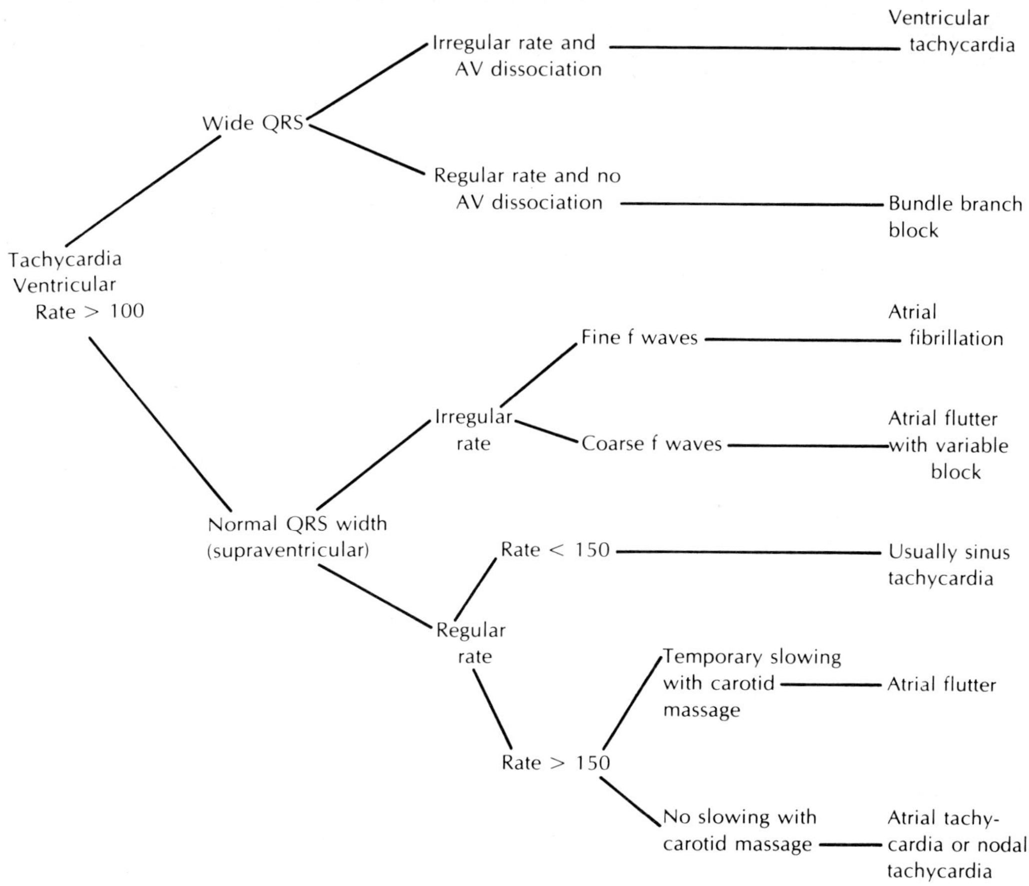

Figure 21–5. Differential diagnosis of ventricular tachycardia. (From Whittick, W.G.: Normal Canine Models. In *Veterinary Critical Care*. Edited by F.P. Sattler, R.P. Knowles, and W.G. Whittick. Lea & Febiger, Philadelphia, 1981.)

It has been known for at least 50 years that irregularities in the heartbeat are associated with the vagus nerve. The efferent vagal fibers are preganglionic and end in peripheral ganglia located in the atria. Postganglionic fibers innervate the S-A and A-V nodes along with the atrial muscle and A-V bundle. A constant cardioinhibitory tone is maintained by the vagus. Although much was made of vagovagal reflexes in older publications, these were often incriminated without adequate evidence. In the well-ventilated animal, the effects of vagal stimulation are minimal. They are, however, marked in association with hypercapnia, hypoxia, asphyxia, or electrolyte imbalance (Condon, 1962; Erlanger, 1962; Katz and Bigger, 1970).

More recently, it has become apparent that reflex cardiac arrhythmias during anesthesia may be initiated by various combinations of sympathetic and parasympathetic stimulation and/or inhibition (Katz and Bigger, 1970). A relative or absolute increase in parasympathetic tone induces bradycardia, hypotension, and cardiac arrhythmias; similarly, relative or actual increased sympathetic tone may cause tachycardia, hypertension, and arrhythmias (see Fig. 8–1).

Reflex arrhythmias may be triggered by stimulation of the pharynx and trachea, by traction on intrathoracic and abdominal structures, by manipulation of the eye, and by stimulation of the carotid sinus. Such arrhythmias occur especially during endotracheal intubation, but are transient and usually insignificant in the well-

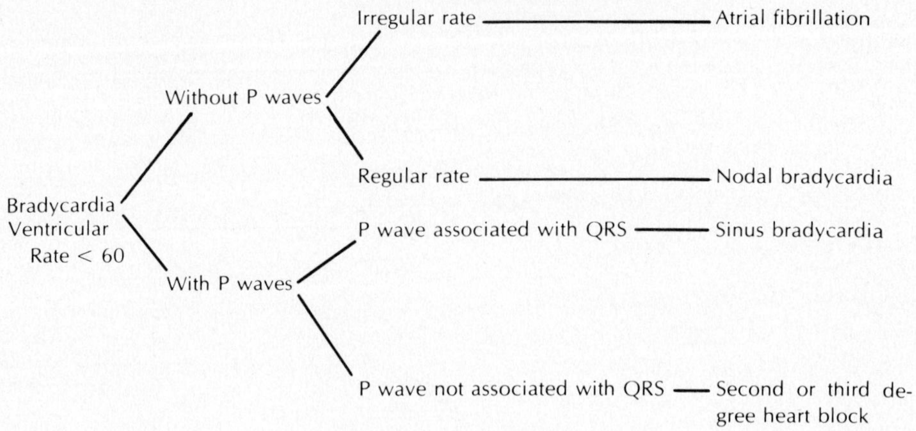

Figure 21–6. Differential diagnosis of ventricular bradycardia. (From Whittick. W.G.: Normal Canine Models. In *Veterinary Critical Care*. Edited by F.P. Sattler, R.P. Knowles, and W.G. Whittick. Lea & Febiger, Philadelphia, 1981.)

ventilated patient. Their etiology remains uncertain; some workers have implicated a vagovagal mechanism (Reid and Brace, 1940; DeVault et al., 1960). Whatever the mechanism, the central nervous system is important in the production and maintenance of many cardiac arrhythmias. In support of this, certain neurodepressant drugs (e.g., chlordiazepoxide, chlorpromazine, acepromazine, pentobarbital, and diazepam) have antiarrhythmic properties. Muir et al. (1975*a*) concluded that intravenous diazepam (1 mg/kg) was effective in reducing ventricular ectopic activity in dogs.

The occurrence of cardiac arrhythmias during anesthesia varies considerably with the anesthetic agent. In 1913, Levy showed that ventricular fibrillation could be produced in cats under chloroform anesthesia by allowing the animals to struggle during induction, by administering chloroform intermittently, or by increasing the chloroform concentration suddenly. Arrhythmias commonly occur also under cyclopropane and trichlorethylene anesthesia. They are more likely to occur during the administration of excessive concentrations. Halothane, methoxyflurane, and fluroxene are less likely to cause arrhythmias, while they are rarely induced by diethyl ether and nitrous oxide (Katz and Bigger, 1970). Cardiac arrhythmias commonly occur during thiobarbiturate anesthesia. They have been reported in 68 to 80% of dogs anesthetized with thiamylal sodium, and in 40%

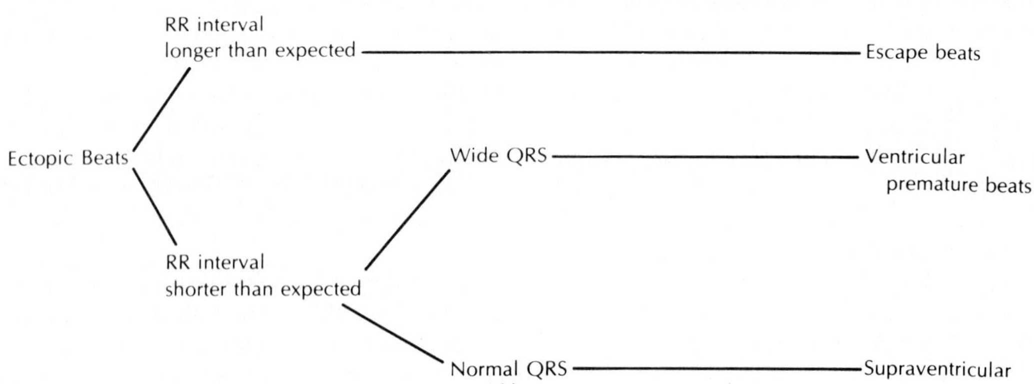

Figure 21–7. Differential diagnosis of ectopic beats. (From Whittick, W.G.: Normal Canine Models. In *Veterinary Critical Care*. Edited by F.P. Sattler, R.P. Knowles, and W.G. Whittick. Lea & Febiger, Philadelphia, 1981.)

of those anesthetized with thiopental sodium. These arrhythmias are mostly benign; bigeminal rhythm is especially common (Wiersig et al., 1974).

It is well established that cardiac arrhythmias commonly occur during anesthesia when defective ventilation causes hypercapnia and/or hypoxia. The threshold arterial P_{CO_2} necessary to produce cardiac arrhythmias in cyclopropane anesthesia has been reported to range from 44 to 107 mm Hg (Lurie et al., 1958; Price et al., 1958). This threshold was inversely proportional to the cyclopropane concentration. A similar relationship has been reported between arterial P_{CO_2} tensions and halothane concentrations (Black et al., 1959).

It appears that respiratory acidosis during anesthesia stimulates central vasomotor areas, thereby increasing sympathetic outflow and catecholamine release (Katz and Bigger, 1970). Hypoxia similarly leads to release of catecholamines and cardiac arrhythmias. The mechanisms involved remain uncertain. Adrenals, peripheral chemoreceptors, central vasomotor centers, and direct effects upon the cardiac muscle have been implicated.

Cullen and Eger (1970) demonstrated that the cardiorespiratory response to moderate hypoxia (P_{O_2} 45 mm Hg) persisted to deep levels of halothane anesthesia in dogs. Cardiorespiratory responses were further stimulated by severe hypoxia (P_{O_2} 30 mm Hg) at light planes of halothane anesthesia in the dog, but were depressed with consequent respiratory and/or cardiac arrest at 1 to 1.5% end-tidal halothane concentrations.

Katz and Epstein (1968) have reviewed the interaction of anesthetics and adrenergic drugs in relation to cardiac arrhythmia. Although sufficiently large doses of catecholamines, such as epinephrine, norepinephrine, and isoproterenol, cause arrhythmias in the unanesthetized patient, induction of anesthesia with thiobarbiturates, halogenated hydrocarbons, or cyclopropane reduces the dose of catecholamine necessary to induce such arrhythmias. Inhalant anesthetics predisposing to catecholamine-induced arrhythmias, listed in order of decreasing sensitizing ability in the dog, are trichloroethylene, ethyl chloride, cyclopropane, halothane, chloroform, methoxyflurane, and fluroxene. Likewise, small intravenous doses of epinephrine induce ventricular arrhythmias in dogs during thiamylal anesthesia (Muir et al., 1975*b*). This arrhythmogenic effect is exacerbated by premedication with xylazine and is prevented by prior use of acepromazine in thiamylal and halothane anesthesia (Muir et al., 1975*c*). Adrenergic agents incriminated include epinephrine, norepinephrine, metaraminol, epinine, kephrine, cobefrin, and dopamine. Ephedrine, propadrine, benzedrine, paredrine, synephrine, phenylephrine, methoxamine, and mephentermine rarely induce arrhythmias. Anesthetic-adrenergic cardiac arrhythmias are induced by beta-adrenergic stimulation and are facilitated by increased heart rate and arterial pressure and by release of potassium (Katz and Bigger, 1970).

Since normal function of the cardiac cell depends on cyclic movement of ions across its cell membrane, it is not surprising that variation in the concentrations of these ions causes arrhythmias. Hypokalemia may cause supraventricular or ventricular ectopic beats or rhythms, ST depression, decreased amplitude of the T-wave, and accentuation of the toxic effects of digitalis (Katz and Bigger, 1970). Hyperkalemia, on the other hand, may cause sinus bradycardia, A-V block, asystole, ventricular tachycardia, and fibrillation. The electrocardiogram in hyperkalemia has peaked T-waves and shortening of the QT interval. The effects of potassium are in general opposed by those of calcium, which causes increased contractility, prolongation of systole, shortening of diastole, and eventual arrest in systole.

Use of succinylcholine during anesthesia is also a common cause of arrhythmias and accentuates the arrhythmogenicity of epinephrine during halothane anesthesia (Tucker and Munson, 1975). Bradycardia, sinus arrest, and supraventricular and ventricular arrhythmias have been reported in man, cats, dogs, and monkeys (Katz and Bigger, 1970). In the horse, tachycardia, arterial hypertension, and cardiac arrhythmias have been reported (Hall, 1971). Katz and Bigger (1970) conclude that the cardiovascular actions of succinylcholine result from ganglionic stimulation. When one is considering the effect of succinylcholine, it is important to recall that this drug may cause hyperkalemia in patients with severe trauma, spinal cord injuries, and regional paralysis. Arrhythmias also commonly occur as a result of the administration of xylazine, and premature ventricular beats are commonly encountered in dogs after administration of morphine-like drugs (Green, 1979).

When reviewing cardiac arrhythmias during anesthesia and operation, Katz and Bigger (1970) have indicated:

1. Arrhythmias occur frequently even in well-managed patients, in which case they rarely require treatment.

2. Because arrhythmias may result from faulty anesthetic techniques, their occurrence requires immediate evaluation of the techniques in use.

3. Slow supraventricular rhythms (atrial rhythm, A-V junctional rhythm, and wandering pacemaker) are benign and do not require treatment; ventricular arrhythmias should be regarded as serious.

4. Most arrhythmias result from imbalances of the autonomic nervous system, namely sympathetic or parasympathetic dominance.

5. Arrhythmias may result not only from changes occurring within the heart itself, but also from primary changes in the central nervous system or the periphery.

The increasing propensity for serious arrhythmias with progressive hypoxia, hypercapnia, and anesthetic depth necessitates the maintenance of optimal gaseous exchange and the use of no greater anesthetic depth than necessary. Consideration of the appropriate anesthetic regimen, of fluid, and of thermal homeostasis is also essential.

Direct observations and use of monitoring equipment alert the anesthesiologist to the presence of such dangerous situations. Ventricular arrhythmias should always be considered serious and treated appropriately. Bradycardia should be treated with intravenous atropine, tachycardia with an intravenous beta blocker such as propranolol, and ventricular ectopic beats with intravenous lidocaine. If the latter do not respond to lidocaine, bretylium should be used (see Chap. 20). A rising CVP indicates that the heart is not pumping all venous blood returned to it and should be treated with isoproterenol or dobutamine.

History of Cardiac Arrest and Resuscitation

In the sixteenth century, Vesalius made three great discoveries that initiated the study of cardiac arrest and resuscitation. He developed a method for endotracheal intubation and artificial respiration, described ventricular fibrillation, and made the first attempt to resuscitate a nonbeating heart. He also noticed that hypoxia predisposed to ventricular fibrillation.

William Harvey, in the seventeenth century, was next to record attempts at cardiac resuscitation. He was the first to use manual manipulation as a resuscitative technique.

Moritz Schliff, a professor of physiology at Florence, Italy, is credited with laying the basis for future work on cardiac arrest and resuscitation by his experimentation with dogs in the 1870s. He was able, by cardiac massage and endotracheal insufflation, to reestablish the heart beat in dogs up to 11½ minutes after it had stopped.

In 1900, J. Prus in Lemberg, Germany described studies in cardiac resuscitation of dogs. Artificial respiration and cardiac massage were used. In 16 of 21 killed with chloroform, the heart action was restored.

Batelli introduced the electrical defibrillator in 1900, but it was not until 1947 that the first successful defibrillation of a human heart was reported.

Since 1900 many cases of human cardiac resuscitation have been recorded, and there is a wealth of literature on this subject. A cardiac arrest registry has been established at the University of Missouri, School of Medicine, and physicians the world over are invited to cooperate in recording cases. Some interesting information has been compiled through this procedure. The incidence of cardiac arrest in man is approximately 1 in every 2125 operations. The incidence in males is higher than in females, the ratio being 1.5:1. Twenty-one percent of arrests occur in persons in the age group from birth to 10 years of age. The greatest number happen in the operating room, 14.2% developing outside in a series of 1710 cases. Of the 1710 recorded cases, only 11.3% evidenced ventricular fibrillation.

Nagel (1970) has indicated that the current era in cardiopulmonary resuscitation was introduced around 1958 with advances in the techniques of resuscitation by expired air, external defibrillation, and closed-chest cardiac massage. These developments provided the necessary components for successful cardiopulmonary resuscitation, namely: 1) establishment of an airway; 2) positive pressure ventilation of the lungs; 3) artificial circulation of the blood; and 4) restoration of a normal heartbeat (including defibrillation and supportive drug therapy).

Causes of Cardiac Arrest

Causes of cardiac arrest during anesthesia are generally considered to include one or more of the following factors:

1. Hypoxia caused by ineffective pulmonary ventilation, inadequate supply of oxygen, and impaired organ perfusion (anemia, shock, right-to-left circulatory shunts).
2. Hypercapnia (hypercarbia) caused by inadequate pulmonary ventilation or depletion of the carbon dioxide absorbent.
3. Hypocapnia that occurs suddenly after hypercapnia (Brown and Miller, 1952).
4. Electrolyte changes, especially hyperkalemia, which may cause asystolic arrest or ventricular fibrillation. High concentrations of serum potassium result from hypoxia, hypercapnia, extensive tissue breakdown, administration of succinylcholine, especially in paretic patients, and transfusion of stored blood.
5. Circulating catecholamines. The potential of these drugs to induce arrhythmias is enhanced by the halogenated hydrocarbons, cyclopropane, and thiobarbiturates.
6. Anesthetic drugs directly depress the myocardium or increase the excitability of the ventricular muscle; as the dose increases, they cause respiratory depression and arterial hypotension with resulting hypercapnia and hypoxia.
7. Cardiac disease may predispose to arrest during anesthesia because of low cardiac output with inability to compensate for decreased peripheral resistance. It may be associated with a hypoxic heart which is susceptible to ventricular fibrillation.
8. Electrocution is an increasing hazard with the common use of monitoring equipment; alternating currents are more likely to be fatal at lower voltages than are direct currents.

Diagnosis of Cardiac Arrest

Since, at normal body temperatures, permanent brain damage results if cardiac arrest remains untreated for longer than 4 minutes, prompt diagnosis and treatment are essential. Fifteen seconds after cessation of cerebral blood flow, the brain's oxygen stores are totally depleted. In 5 minutes, glucose and glycogen stores are used up and even anaerobic glycolysis ceases. All energy-dependent reactions stop. One of the latter is the plasma-membrane sodium pump, with the consequence of increased intracellular sodium and cellular edema. Changes of this type continue for an hour or so, after which time necrosis becomes evident (Safar, 1981). Diagnosis of cardiac arrest is based on absence of breathing, absence of a pulse, dilatation of the pupils, and on certain ancillary signs (Nagel, 1970).

Absence of Breathing. In the absence of blood flow to the respiratory centers, respiratory arrest results. This may be preceded by a few gasps during the first minute or so of arrest. Since respiratory failure frequently precedes cardiac arrest, *immediate recognition and artificial ventilation* will often prevent ventricular fibrillation. The clinician should therefore check first for the absence of breathing.

Absence of Pulse. Although the peripheral pulse may be imperceptible in shock, the carotid and femoral pulse may be palpable in those species in which they can be detected. If no pulse can be detected, the blood pressure is markedly suppressed or absent, and the heart is no longer an effective pump. In small species or in neonates, palpation of the heartbeat is often more suitable.

Dilatation of the Pupils. The pupils dilate widely immediately after cessation of the heartbeat. They constrict once again if effective cardiac massage is immediately instigated. It is important to recall that the pupils may be dilated by drugs such as atropine and that the intensely constricted pupil, such as occurs after morphine administration, may not immediately dilate when arrest occurs.

General Appearance. The mucous membranes and nonpigmented skin are cyanotic, and there is no sign of circulation. The latter may be detected by compression of buccal mucous membranes or the ventral surface of the tongue. During surgery, the habit of observing the color of the tissues and blood, the degree of bleeding, and the pulsation of local vessels should be acquired.

Absence of Heart Sounds. Auscultation to search for heart sounds is to be condemned. If, however, heart action is being monitored with the aid of an esophageal stethoscope, auscultation will provide a useful means for detection of ineffective pumping or arrest. In dogs, Swann and Brucer (1951) have pointed out that all heart sounds cease at a systolic pressure of 50 mm Hg and therefore, if no sounds are heard, circulation has probably failed.

Electrocardiogram. Determination and accurate interpretation of electrical activity at the time of cardiac arrest are essential because the patterns of electrical activity are not always the same. The arrhythmias occurring with cardiac arrest are ventricular fibrillation, asystole, and electromechanical dissociation. Ventricular fibrillation is characterized by totally uncoordinated electrical activity, asystole by absence of electrical activity, and electromechanical dissociation by relatively normal electrical pattern, but with absence of a pulse. Ventricular fibrillation is usually preceded by premature ventricular contractions (PVCs) and/or ventricular tachycardia. Asystole is usually preceded by widening of the PR interval, heartblock, and/or severe bradycardia. Electromechanical dissociation may occur during resuscitative procedures or as a primary event (Sladen, 1976).

Electroencephalogram. Electroencephalographic monitoring, on the other hand, provides an excellent means of determining cessation of circulation. Within about 20 seconds after total anoxia of the brain, alpha, beta, and gamma waves are absent (see Figs. 19–19, 24–1). Thus, cerebral anoxia may be noted before electrocardiographic tracings show cessation of electrical activity in the heart.

Central Venous Pressure. If central venous pressure is being monitored, this increases abruptly and may exceed 15 or even 20 cm H_2O in dogs.

Treatment of Cardiac Arrest

Cardiac arrest can be successfully corrected, provided it is recognized immediately and the appropriate steps speedily accomplished. Delay in diagnosis and institution of resuscitation will invariably be fatal. Delay in diagnosis is responsible for approximately 85% of the failures to resuscitate successfully. The best rule of thumb is that if there is no palpable apex beat or evidence of pulse pressure, and both have disappeared suddenly, then cardiac arrest has occurred. Patients seldom survive a delay of more than 4 minutes before artificial circulation is maintained by massage. The greatest time lapse usually is between arrest and diagnosis. This period is often spent by the anesthesiologist in searching for a stethoscope, in injecting ineffective stimulants, in searching for an endotracheal catheter, in looking for the instruments necessary for thoracotomy, or in seeking a consultant. The person who should treat cardiac arrest is that person immediately available. It must be kept constantly in mind that *cardiac arrest is a 3-minute emergency* necessitating the immediate supply of adequate oxygen to and removal of carbon dioxide from the brain. Once these vital basic functions have been reestablished, efforts to restore normal rhythmic cardiac contractions can be taken more leisurely. The only exception is the patient currently being monitored. Arrhythmias with functional cardiac arrest are detected immediately, and primary resuscitative therapy can be initiated before the complications of serious hypoxia and acidosis occur.

When cardiac arrest is suspected, the cardiopulmonary resuscitation (CPR) procedure is as follows:

1. Airway and Ventilation. Administration of anesthetic should be discontinued and the presence of a patent airway should be established. If necessary, obstruction due to mucus,

TABLE 21–2. Effect of Varying External Cardiac Compression (ECC) Rates on Carotid Flow during Resuscitation

	Carotid Flow (ml/min)			
Dog	*ECC 48*	*ECC 60*	*ECC 72*	*ECC 120*
1	10	16	20	28
2	12	14	16	25
3	5	5	7	12
4	0	9	14	14
Mean	7 ± 4	11 ± 4	14 ± 4	20 ± 7

(From Harris, L.C., Kirimli, B., and Safar, P.: Ventilation-Cardiac Compression Rates and Ratios in Cardiopulmonary Resuscitation. Anesthesiology, 28:806, 1967.)

stomach contents, or soft tissues should be corrected. Unless an endotracheal catheter is immediately at hand or an anesthetic machine is already in use, time should not be wasted intubating the small animal at this time. Instead, its lungs should be inflated as fully as possible by cupping the hands about the muzzle and blowing into them. This procedure should be repeated several times to ensure that there is chest excursion with each ventilation. If this is not possible, manual compression of the chest is of some temporary value. In larger animals, intubation and some form of mechanical ventilation (bag or ventilator) are necessary immediately.

2. Cardiac Compression. If the heart beat is absent or ineffective, the chest should be compressed over the heart at 70 to 100 times per minute in dogs and cats. From a practical viewpoint, a rate of 70 to 80 per minute is maximal for one operator for a long period. Harris et al. (1967) reported that when ventricular fibrillation was induced in 8- to 12-kg mongrel dogs, there was a consistent increase in the carotid flow with increasing rates of external cardiac compression (ECC) from 7 ± 4 ml/min at a rate of 48 to 20 ± 7 ml at a rate of 120/min (Table 21–2). However, there was no statistically significant increase in carotid flow when the rate of cardiac compression was increased from 72 to 120/min. When studying regional blood flow during cardiopulmonary resuscitation in dogs, Voorhees et al. (1980) found that in comparison with flow during normal sinus rhythm, the ratio for cerebral blood flow was 90%, for coronary 35%, for renal 15%, and for spleen and small intestine 33%. More recently it has been reported that blood flow results not only from cardiac compression (cardiac pump mechanism), but also from thoracic compression (thoracic pump mechanism) (Babbs, 1980) (Fig. 21–8).

The lungs should be inflated between every fifth or sixth cardiac compression. Harris et al. (1967) indicated that lung inflations interposed between sternal compressions were superior to simultaneous inflation of the lung and compression of the heart (Table 21–3). These authors reported that whenever possible the lung should be inflated once and the heart compressed for 4 to 5 times. If only one operator was on hand, a sequence of 3 inflations and 15 cardiac compressions was preferred. Cardiac output has been shown to remain constant despite changes in ventilation pressures from 10 to 50 cm of H_2O (Babbs et al., 1980). The advent of high-frequency ventilation offers the potential for independent ventilation and cardiac compression procedures. Methods for cardiac compression in larger animals have yet to be developed. In dogs, several techniques have been employed:

a. Ott (1962) positioned dogs in dorsal recumbency and applied pressure to the sternum. By this technique, carotid blood flows have averaged 12% and aortic blood pressures 31% of control values (Redding and Cozine, 1961).

b. Swann and Brucer (1951) placed dogs on their sides and, with a hand on either side of the chest, compressed the heart 100 times per minute.

c. Burnap (1970) placed the dog on its back, interlocked the fingers of each hand, placed the joined hands over the sternum, and compressed each side of the chest with the heels of the hands.

d. Automatic sternal compression with a Beck-Rand sternal compression machine has been used by other workers (Harris et al., 1967; Safar and Harris, 1963).

e. More recently accepted techniques in small animals have been reported by Ross and Breznock (1981) (Fig. 21–9).

In horses and cattle in lateral recumbency, pressure can be applied with one foot or, preferably, immediate emergency thoracotomy per-

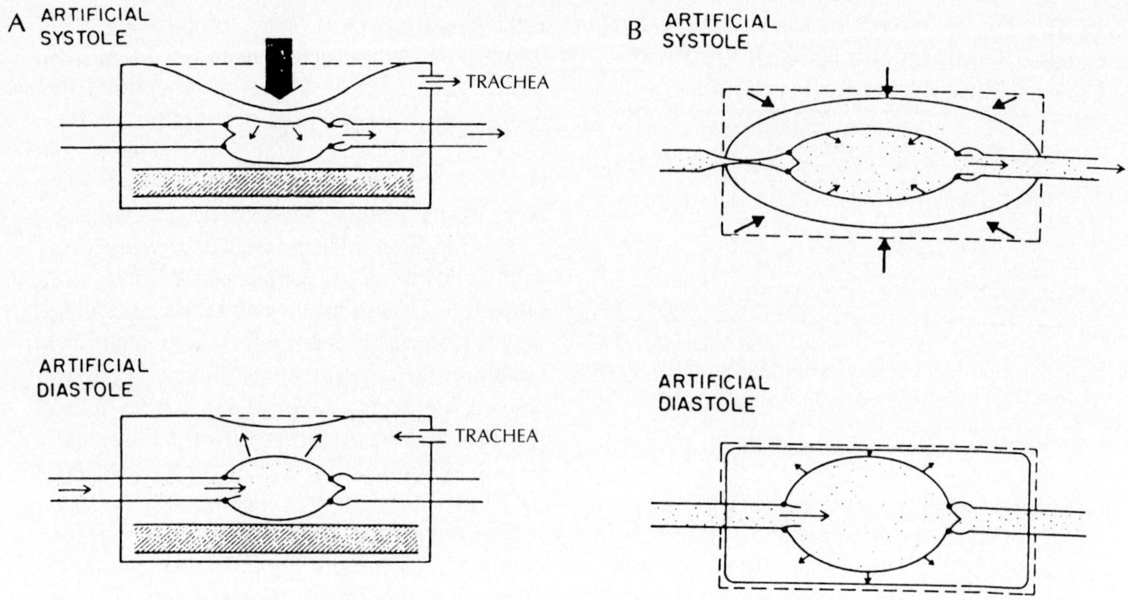

Figure 21–8. *A*, Cardiac pump mechanism for generating blood flow during CPR. During artificial systole, central chest compression squeezes the heart against the spine, forcing blood out. Air is vented from the thorax via the trachea *(top left)*. During artificial diastole, chest resiliency creates negative pressure for filling. The site of application of force *(broad arrow)* is critical. For simplicity only one pumping chamber is shown. *B*, The thoracic pump mechanism for generation of blood flow during CPR. During artificial systole, thoracic compression or cough generates intrathoracic pressure which is vented by arterial outflow to peripheral tissues. During artificial diastole, release of intrathoracic pressure allows for filling. Site of application of force is not important. (From Babbs, C.F.: New Versus Old Theories of Blood Flow During CPR. Crit. Care Med., 8:191, 1980.)

TABLE 21–3. Arterial Oxygen Saturation and pH During Cardiopulmonary Resuscitation

	Oxygen Saturation%		*pH*	
Dog	*Interposed**	*Simultaneous†*	*Interposed*	*Simultaneous*
	A. Three Minutes Resuscitation			
1	98	92	7.54	7.48
2	89	77	7.32	7.19
3	90	82	7.54	7.38
4	97	95	7.31	7.32
5	99	82	7.62	7.30
Mean	94.5 ± 4.7	85.5 ± 7.4	7.46 ± 0.14	7.33 ± 0.11
	B. Eighteen Minutes Resuscitation			
1	99	55	7.13	7.05
2	89	80	7.15	7.45
3	87	54	7.41	7.48
4	85	62	7.23	7.10
5	99	85	7.53	7.29
Mean	91.8 ± 6.7	67.2 ± 14.5	7.29 ± 0.17	7.45 ± 0.08

*Interposed = lung inflation interposed between cardiac compressions.
†Simultaneous = lung inflation simultaneous with cardiac compression.

(From Harris, L.C., Kirimli, B., and Safar, P.: Ventilation-Cardiac Compression Rates and Ratios in Cardiopulmonary Resuscitation. Anesthesiology, 28:806, 1967.)

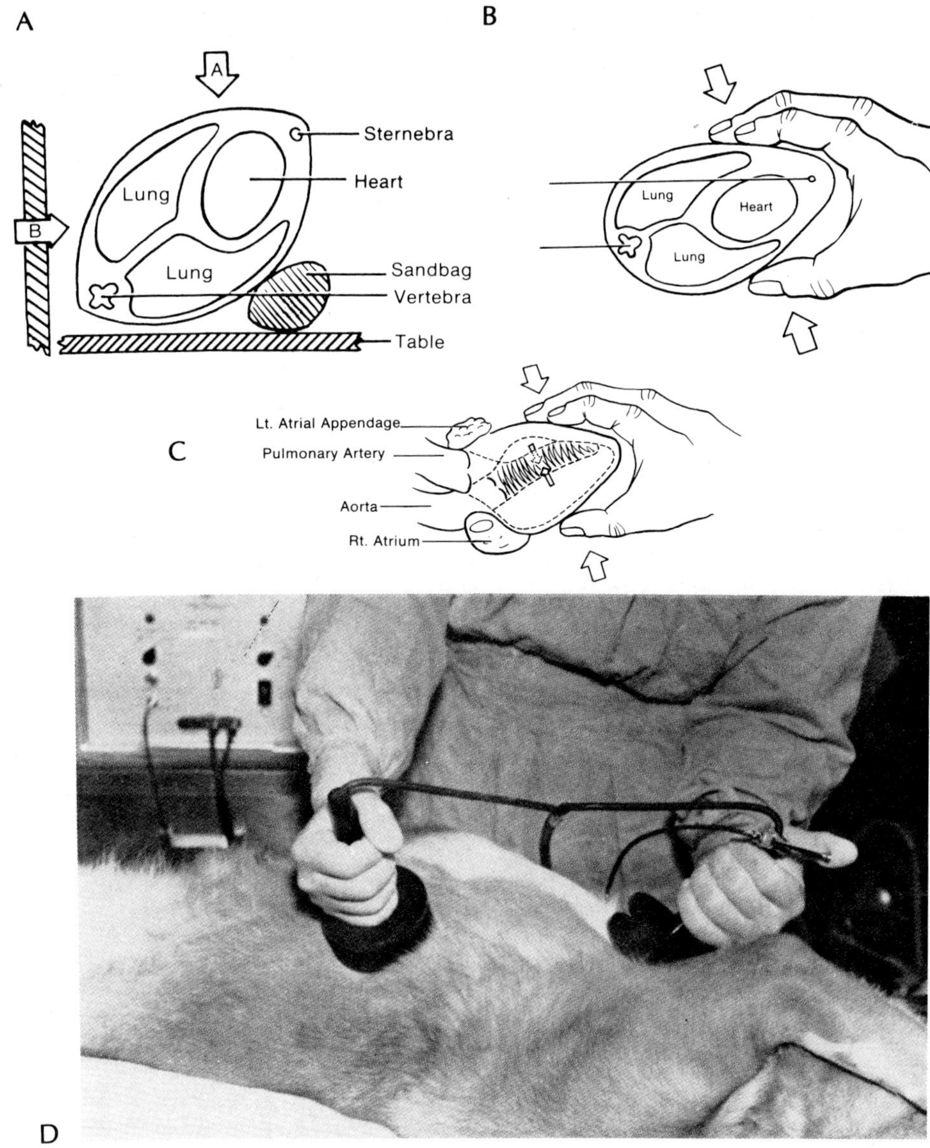

Figure 21–9. *A*, Diagram illustrating the technique of external cardiac compression in most animals (5 to 60 kg in body weight). Rhythmic downward force A is applied with the heel of the hand to the left lateral thorax (80 times per minute) in the area of the costochondral junction at the level of the sixth rib. The patient is stabilized by force B, which may be a wall or other object, another person, or the resuscitator's other hand. *B*, Diagram illustrating the technique of external cardiac compression in small animals (less than 5 kg in body weight). The fingers and thumb of one hand are used to compress the right and left hemithorax at the costochondral junction at the level of the sixth rib. The compression rate in smaller animals should approach 120/min. *C*, Diagram illustrating a technique of internal cardiac compression in small animals. The palmar surfaces of the fingers and thumb of one hand are used to compress the ventricular free walls toward the interventricular septum. *D*, Placement of external defibrillator electrodes over the manubrium and on the left precordial region. (*A*, *B*, and C from Ross, J.N., and Breznock, E.M.: Resuscitation. In *Veterinary Critical Care*. Edited by F.P. Sattler, R.P. Knowles, and W.G. Whittick. Lea & Febiger, Philadelphia, 1981. *D* from Ott, B.S.: Closed Chest Cardiac Resuscitation. Small Anim. Clin., 2:572, 1962.)

formed and internal cardiac compression initiated. External cardiac compression (20 compressions/min) has been found to be successful in ponies (Frauenfelder et al., 1981). Whatever the external technique employed, the pressure should be applied firmly over the heart just dorsal to the costochondral junction and released fully between each compression to allow expansion of the chest and filling of the heart. Should the chest be open, direct compression of the heart between the thumb and fingers can be performed (Fig. 21–9). In larger animals it may be necessary, as in adult man, to compress the heart between both hands (Brooks, 1967).

When comparing closed and open cardiac compression in dogs, Redding and Cozine (1961) found little difference between the circulation induced. Elam (1968) indicated, however, that in man the skilled operator can improve cardiac output by open-chest cardiac compression. In the closed-chest technique, severe trauma, such as fractured ribs, mediastinal hemorrhage, and liver lacerations, may result when maximal force is used to obtain the highest possible pressure. Open-chest cardiac compression has the added advantage of visual diagnosis of ventricular fibrillation, visual assessment of reestablished cardiac function, and direct injection of drugs into the heart chambers. It also provides better cardiac output in animals weighing over 50 kg (Ross and Breznock, 1981). Cerebral circulation may be improved by simultaneous compression of the thoracic aorta. Disadvantages include pulmonary collapse, the need for rib retractors, the added time required, the possibility of inadvertent atrial rupture, and the danger of postresuscitation infection.

Whatever the technique employed, effectiveness is best judged by detection of a carotid or femoral pulse. A femoral pulse can be palpated if the blood pressure is greater than 60 mm Hg (Ott, 1962). Effective cardiac compression and pulmonary ventilation are judged by constriction of the pupils. Cardiac compression and ventilation should be continued with an absolute minimum of interruption until rhythmic cardiac and respiratory action are restored.

3. Intubation. As soon as effective ventilation and circulation have been reestablished by means of exhaled air ventilation and closed-chest compression, the trachea should be intubated if this has not already been done. Intubation should be accomplished rapidly, in less than 30 seconds.

4. Mechanical Ventilation. Although mechanical ventilation may have been performed previously with the aid of a mask, an endotracheal tube with inflated cuff is preferred. The complications of gastric inflation and aspiration of regurgitated stomach contents are thus avoided. Suitable equipment for mechanical ventilation includes anesthetic machines, self-inflating bags with nonrebreathing valves, and automatic ventilators. It is important to appreciate that concurrent pulmonary inflation and cardiac compression may cause pressures that will induce alveolar rupture, and that pressure-cycled ventilators are ineffective during chest compression. The rapid compression of the chest triggers the cycling mechanism of the respirator, and the response is similar to that encountered during respiratory obstruction.

5. Drug Therapy. *Epinephrine*. Epinephrine (0.5 to 3 ml of 1:10,000) should be administered intravenously into the jugular vein or via an indwelling intravenous catheter. Although many inject directly into the heart, this has little or no advantage over injection into larger veins and may damage the heart. Epinephrine improves cerebral and coronary blood flow, intracardiac conduction, pacemaker activity, and myocardial tone, and is appropriate for asystolic arrest. In ventricular fibrillation, it coarsens fine fibrillatory action and improves the chances of successful defibrillation. Recommendations have been made for immediate empirical intravenous or intracardiac injection of epinephrine for the aforementioned reasons (Clark, 1977). If there is doubt that arrest has occurred in animals under halogenated hydrocarbon anesthesia, it should be avoided owing to its propensity to cause ventricular fibrillation. Profibrillatory effects of epinephrine are reduced by prior administration of lidocaine. Isoproterenol may be used to maintain cardiac rate and to enhance cardiac output once arrest is overcome. It may, however, cause excessive tachycardia. Metaraminol may be more beneficial since it increases cardiac contractility without increasing rate or peripheral resistance excessively. Dopamine and glucagon have also received consideration (Clark, 1977).

Methoxamine. The use of epinephrine, which has both α- and β-adrenergic activity, in CPR has been challenged by Redding et al. (1983). They state that methoxamine, a pure α-adrenergic agonist, is more effective because it does not produce subendocardial vasoconstriction as does epinephrine. In 10 dogs asphyxiated until asystole developed, they restored spontaneous respiration in all with injections of methoxamine. These authors believe that methoxamine is the drug of choice during resuscitation from cardiac arrest, regardless of the ECG pattern.

Sodium Bicarbonate. Five percent sodium bicarbonate should be administered intravenously (1.0 mEq/kg over a 10-minute period) to combat acidosis and to improve the action of the epinephrine. Both sodium bicarbonate and epinephrine should be administered within 2 minutes of initial arrest (Elam, 1968). Since the degree of acidosis varies markedly, it has been suggested that the initial dose of sodium bicarbonate should be related to the duration of cardiac arrest (Gilston, 1965) according to the formula:

$$\text{Dose of bicarbonate in mEq} = \frac{\text{wt of patient in kg}}{5} \times \frac{\text{duration of arrest in min}}{2}$$

Jones (1972) also recommends intravenous injection of corticosteroid immediately after injection of sodium bicarbonate, to supplement potentially exhausted adrenal output and to stabilize lysosomal membranes. Its capacity to ameliorate brain damage, however, is unsubstantiated (Safar, 1981). Tromethamine may be used as an alternative to sodium bicarbonate. It is a stronger base and penetrates the cell more readily than sodium bicarbonate. When it was compared in dogs, no significant differences were noted between these two drugs (Minuck and Sharma, 1977).

Calcium Chloride. Intravenous administration to the dog of 0.5 to 3 ml of 10% calcium chloride (10 mg/kg) or calcium gluconate (10 to 20 ml of 10% solution every 10 minutes for an average dog) improves myocardial tone. Twenty to 40 ml of calcium borogluconate (20% solution) has been recommended for intravenous administration to the horse (Goldstein et al., 1981).

Lidocaine. Lidocaine, 2 to 6 mg/kg in dogs, may be injected intravenously to reduce myocardial irritability and thereby to increase the threshold to fibrillation.

6. Defibrillation. The occurrence of ventricular fibrillation is recognized only by monitoring the electrocardiograph (Fig. 21–10) or by direct observation of the heart with the pericardial sac open. For successful defibrillation, it is essential that the heart be in optimal condition. The tone of the heart should first be improved by compression for several minutes, thereby providing the best possible myocardial oxygenation; acidosis should be reversed, and epinephrine recently administered. Improved myocardial condition is reflected by its color and tone and by replacement of fine almost invisible fibrillations with coarse fibrillations that appear on the electrocardiograph as vigorous (1 millivolt) potentials.

Defibrillation is accomplished by passage of an electrical current through the heart, thereby causing all myocardial fibers to have their refractory period simultaneously. A normal beat may then occur spontaneously or may require tactile stimulation with the finger or manual compression. The defibrillating countershock is, depending on condition, applied externally to the closed chest or internally directly to the heart. For external defibrillation, electrode paste or saline-soaked pads are applied to either side of the chest over the heart. The electrodes are then firmly pressed on these areas (see Fig. 21–9*D*), and a shock is administered. Geddes et al. (1974) have reported that there is a body weight to electrical shock strength relationship. In the duration range of 3 to 10 ms, the electrical dose was nearly 1 A/kg of body weight. Others

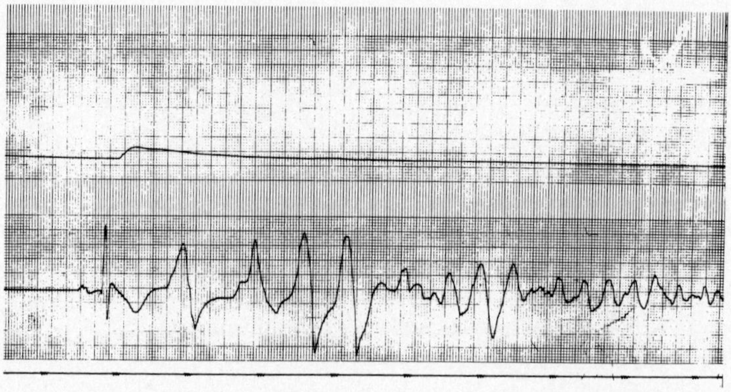

Figure 21–10. Onset of cardiac fibrillation. Top trace is blood pressure; lower trace is the electrocardiogram. One relatively normal QRS complex is shown at extreme left along with a pulse wave. As fibrillation develops, pulse waves no longer occur.

have questioned such a direct relationship, because of the possible influence of such factors as hypoxemia, drug therapy, acid-base and electrolyte status, and duration of arrest. Energy requirements for successful countershock are directly proportional to the duration of fibrillation (Yakaitis et al., 1980). Higher energies than necessary may decrease the success of defibrillation, possibly because of the production of secondary arrhythmias (Jones and Jones, 1980).

Myocardial lesions and/or death have occurred in dogs given suprathreshold shock (3.2 to 10.6 A/kg) transthoracically. The severity of damage was increased by decreasing the electrode size, by applying it directly to the heart, and by reducing the time interval between shocks (Van Vleet et al., 1977). Should defibrillation be unsuccessful, it is repeated after additional efforts to improve the condition of the heart, by compression, ventilation, and administration of epinephrine, calcium, and bicarbonate. Newer antiarrhythmic drugs (bretylium, clofilium) significantly decrease the defibrillation threshold and have been shown to produce chemical defibrillation in the absence of defibrillator countershock (Tacker et al., 1980). In any case, if ventricular fibrillations are "fine," they should be converted to "coarse" by intravenous injection of epinephrine. This facilitates defibrillation.

Once heart action is reinitiated, blood pressure and coronary circulation may be enhanced by administration of norepinephrine, and a lidocaine infusion may help prevent recurring fibrillation. Further measures, as outlined under Treatment of Shock, should be undertaken to support the patient until it has clearly recovered. The treatment of cardiac arrest is summarized in Figure 21–11.

NERVOUS SYSTEM

Cerebral Edema

It is an old axiom in anesthesiology that, "If the lips are blue, the brain is too!" Hypoxia of the brain leads to cerebral edema. Successful CPR may still produce an unsuccessful end result, due to fulminating brain edema with neuronal necrosis, leaving a vegetative patient. Coma, irregular stertorous respiration, tachycardia, sweating, muscular twitching, nystagmus, fully dilated pupils, blindness, and continuous pacing may be observed. Postresuscitation efforts should be directed at preventing this disaster.

Because the skull is inelastic, increases in intracranial volume initiate elevations in intracranial pressure (ICP). Initial increases can be compensated by reduction in cerebrospinal fluid volume. However, elevated intracranial pressure eventually leads to a reduction in cerebral perfusion pressure (CPP = arterial blood pressure − intracranial pressure). This result produces a fall in cerebral blood flow (CBF) with accumulation of acid metabolites, cerebral

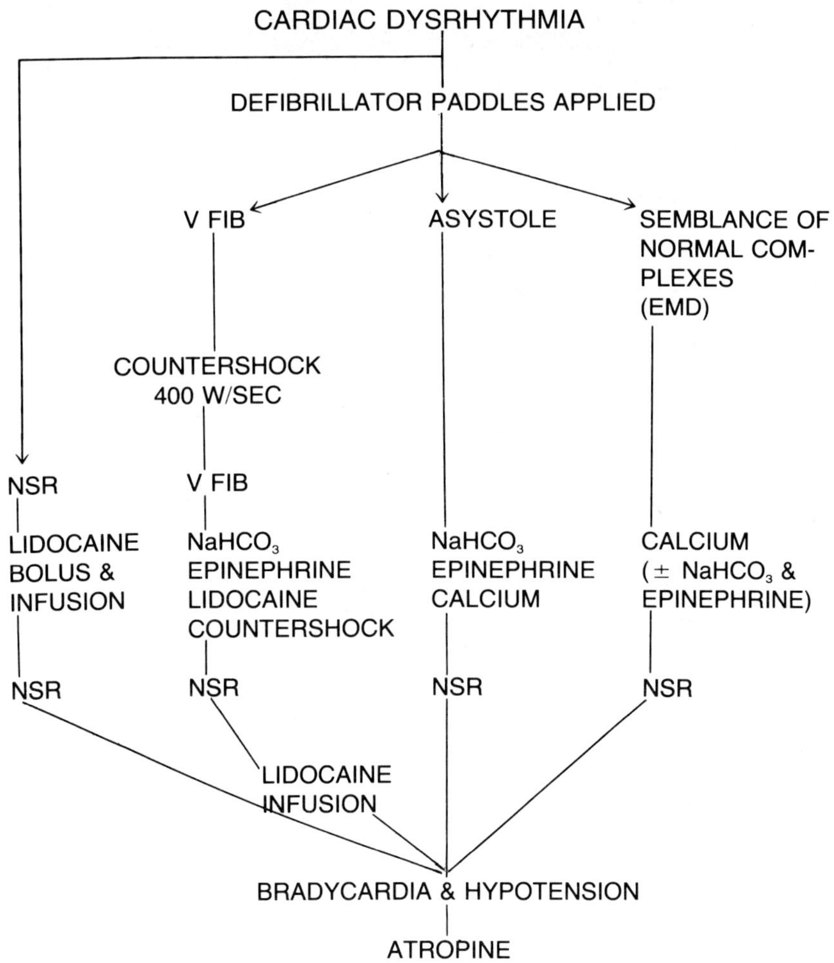

Figure 21–11. Drug treatment of cardiac dysrhythmias associated with absence of cardiac output. All drugs, alone or in combination, may have to be repeated. External or internal cardiac massage must be maintained except with normal sinus rhythm (NSR). V FIB, ventricular fibrillation; EMD, electromechanical dissociation. (Adapted from Sladen, A.: Pharmacologic Management of Cardiopulmonary Resuscitation. Refresher Courses in Anesthesiology, 4:113, 1976.)

edema, and inability of the autoregulatory mechanism to regulate brain blood flow. Thus a vicious cycle begins in which increased blood flow causes increased ICP, which in turn causes cerebral edema with neurologic damage as the end result (Fig. 21–12).

Ideally in this situation, ICP is monitored continuously with a ventricular cannula or a subarachnoid screw. Hyperventilation should be maintained to lower P_{CO_2} and thus reduce cerebral blood flow. Postarrest systemic normotension or even slight hypertension is essential, for even mild hypotension has been shown to be deleterious (Safar, 1981). Traditional treatments have included diuretics to increase blood osmotic pressure, such as mannitol (1.5 g/kg IV, administered over one hour) and furosemide (5 mg/kg IV). Corticosteroids, such as dexamethasone (2 to 4 mg/kg IV), have also been used routinely (see Chap. 20). Barbiturates, such as thiopental and pentobarbital, have been given to lower CPP with conflicting results (Steen et al., 1979; Ventureyra and Ivan, 1979; Marshall et al., 1979). Sodium nitroprusside is contraindicated (Clubb et al., 1980), as is hypothermia (see Chap. 13).

Ketamine, halothane, methoxyflurane, and enflurane are contraindicated as anesthetics be-

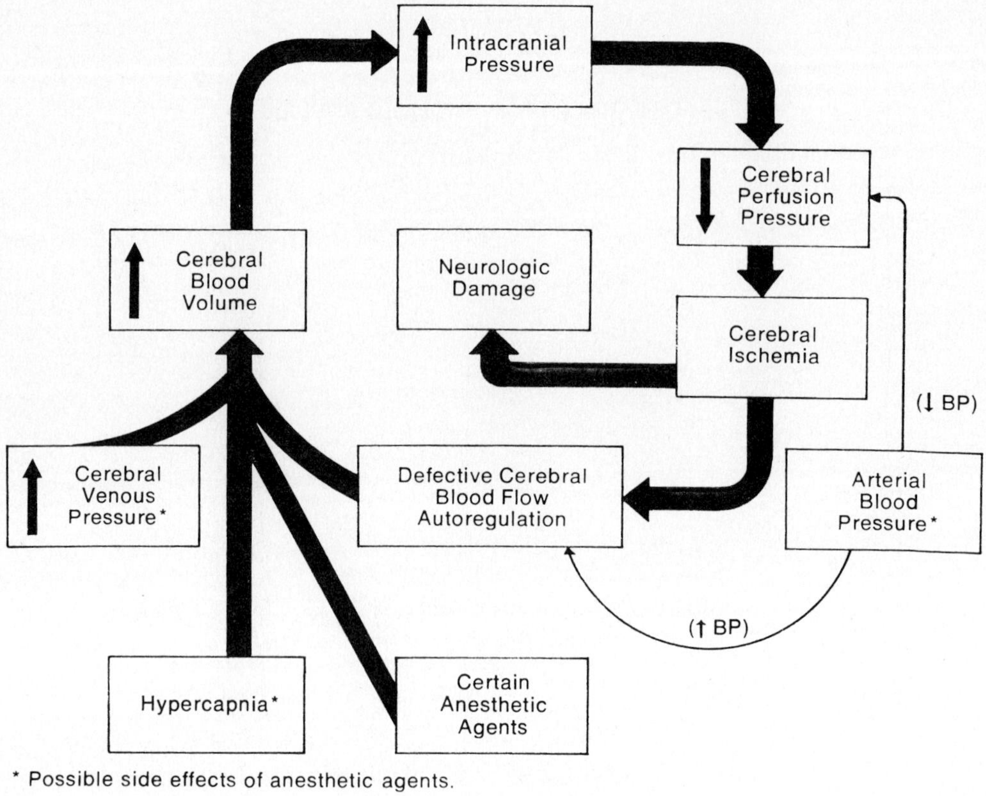

Figure 21–12. The vicious cycle of increased intracranial pressure. (From Shapiro, H.M., Wyte, S.R., and Barton, M.D.: Increased Intracranial Pressure: Physiology and Pharmacology. Scientific Exhibit, Annual Meeting, American Society of Anesthesiologists, San Francisco, 1973.)

cause they raise ICP. Thiopental, fentanyl-droperidol, and etomidate may be the anesthetics of choice in cerebral edema. Lidocaine (1.5 mg/kg IV) has been found as effective in preventing neurologic deficits as thiopental, without the cardiovascular depression (Bedford et al., 1980). Naloxone has been used successfully in treating localized cerebral edema and may prove effective in brain edema from any cause (Hosobuchi, 1982).

The aforementioned principles apply also to anesthesia of patients with cranial trauma.

REGURGITATION AND VOMITION

Regurgitation is the *passive* discharge of stomach contents into the pharynx, whereas vomiting is the *active* discharge. Vomition during induction is not uncommon in dogs, cats, and primates. Regurgitation may occur in dogs, cats, and other small animals during anesthesia, despite adequate preanesthetic preparation. Relaxation of the cardia allows gastric contents to flow up the esophagus if the animal is positioned in dorsal recumbency, or if there is manipulation of abdominal viscera. Often the flow of material from the mouth is the only evidence that this has occurred. Gastric juice is brown and contains dark flocculent material. Although regurgitation in small animals under anesthesia is usually not as serious as vomition, immediate steps should be taken to remove regurgitated material as outlined in this section. Pooling of gastric juice in the esophagus over a long period leads to esophagitis and possibly formation of stricture (Grier, 1975). Gastric secretions may be reduced by premedication with glycopyrrolate or cimetidine.

Silent (inapparent) regurgitation has been reported in 7.8% of 900 human patients under general anesthesia. Of those regurgitating, 8.6% aspirated the vomitus (Blitt et al., 1970).

In ruminants, regurgitation under anesthesia is common despite preanesthetic starvation and medication. Pressure on the rumen produced by recumbency along with relaxation of the cardia are the probable causes. The regurgitated material may be copious and will contain a considerable amount of feed. In a study of 110 cases of halothane anesthesia of cattle, Weaver (1971) reported that tympany was not a problem, but regurgitation occurred in 16% of cases. Regurgitation was most frequent in stage 3 anesthesia. In 2 of 3 cases in which it occurred prior to intubation, the result was fatal. Although not significant, regurgitation was more common in intra-abdominal operations, in animals in lateral recumbency, and during the first hour of anesthesia. There was no relationship to preoperative restriction of food and water.

The hazards of regurgitation and subsequent aspiration in the ruminant can be minimized by the following procedures:

1. Intubation should be performed as soon as possible. Fortunately, with the exception of the goat, laryngospasm is not common, and an endotracheal tube can be inserted when anesthesia is light. Intubation is facilitated by use of a topical anesthetic to suppress laryngeal and tracheal reflexes.

2. While recumbent, the ruminant should be positioned to minimize regurgitation and aspiration. Sternal recumbency with the head down is preferred. When this is not possible, the chest should preferably be higher than both the abdomen and the head.

3. Accumulation of gas with associated excessive intra-abdominal pressure should be avoided by the routine use of a stomach tube.

If regurgitation occurs, drainage from the pharynx should be assured by elevation of the poll region and by suction.

Occasionally, it is necessary to anesthetize animals without preanesthetic preparation, and vomiting may occur on induction or during anesthesia. In man, occlusion of the esophagus by back pressure on the cricoid has been recommended (Sellick's maneuver). Usually vomition is preceded by several abortive retching movements that are easily recognized having once been observed. Immediate treatment is necessary to prevent unfavorable sequelae and even fatality from this event. As soon as retching movements occur, the operating table should be tilted so that the patient is positioned with its head down, and 100% oxygen should be given either through the mouth or with a nasal catheter. The pharynx should be cleared of vomitus manually and with suction, if available, and the larynx and bronchial tree should be cleaned by direct laryngoscopy and bronchoscopy. An endotracheal catheter should be inserted, the cuff inflated to prevent further aspiration in the event vomiting again occurs, and oxygen administration continued.

Aspiration Pneumonitis

Aspiration pneumonitis has been studied experimentally in rabbits (Bannister et al., 1961), cats (Lewinski, 1965), and dogs (Hamelberg and Bosomworth, 1964; Exarhos et al., 1965). When gastric juice is introduced into the trachea of dogs, the immediate effects are apnea, cyanosis, tachypnea, hypotension, and bronchospasm (Table 21–4). Pulmonary edema, patchy atelectasis, hemorrhagic areas, and frank necrosis subsequently develop in the lungs, the severity depending upon the amount and pH of the fluid. Aspiration of large quantities of gastric juice (4 ml/kg) with a pH of 1.1 inevitably causes death. Aspiration of stomach contents may also cause hypoxia due to laryngospasm and cardiac inhibition from reflexes originating in the bronchi.

Experimentally it has been shown that aspirated gastric juice containing no ingesta is rapidly dispersed throughout the lung, making attempts to remove it by irrigation virtually worthless. Nevertheless, bronchial lavage has been recommended. Repeated saline aliquots are used until washings are clear.

Hydrocortisone solution intratracheally has been shown to be more effective than irrigation with either saline or 1.3% sodium bicarbonate solution.

Antibiotics have no direct effect on the inflammatory process, but are probably indicated for secondary complications.

TABLE 21–4. Circulatory Responses to Aspiration of Gastric Juice

	Control	*Postaspiration 2 minutes*	*Postaspiration 15 minutes*
Mean arterial pressure	106 mm Hg	71 mm Hg	91 mm Hg
Pulmonary systolic arterial pressure	21 mm Hg	27 mm Hg	31 mm Hg
Femoral arterial oxygen saturation	98%	79%	56%
Femoral arterial pH	7.45	7.22	7.12

Five dogs subjected to aspiration of gastric juice (pH 1.10), 4 ml per kg of body weight.

(From Hamelberg, W., and Bosomworth, P.P.: Aspiration Pneumonitis: Experimental Studies and Clinical Observations. Anesth. Analg., 43:673, 1964.)

Specific drug therapy is indicated to support the patient and to prevent inflammation and infection in the respiratory tract. This therapy should include:

1. A corticosteroid intratracheally and intravenously, followed by intramuscular injections for the next 2 to 3 days. Nonsteroidal anti-inflammatory drugs may be used alternatively or concurrently. Steroid therapy has not been found effective in fresh-water drowning or aspiration pneumonitis due to hydrochloric acid (Calderwood et al., 1975).
2. A broad-spectrum antibiotic either intravenously or intramuscularly.
3. Continued administration of 100% oxygen through a nasal catheter, in an oxygen chamber, or with a tracheostomy and ventilator to maintain adequate oxygenation. Ventilation with PEEP at an optimal level (greatest improvement in PaO_2 with least depression of cardiac output) is desirable.
4. Aminophyline (0.05 to 0.2 g for dogs) intravenously or in suppositories twice daily for 2 or 3 days for its bronchodilating effect.
5. Expectorant cough mixtures to produce thin bronchial secretions that may aid in removal of vomitus not removed by manual cleaning.
6. Inhalation of a detergent aerosol that may aid in prevention of atelectasis.

AIR EMBOLISM

Little information exists concerning air embolism in animals, except for instances in which it has been experimentally produced and in a reported fatality associated with canine pneumocystography (Ackerman et al., 1972).

In man, air embolism may cause death due to hypoxia and cardiac arrest or to cerebral damage. Common causes of air embolism are: 1) open heart surgery, 2) operations involving the large veins, and 3) diagnostic air injections.

Worman and Seidel (1966) were unable to produce a standard cerebral lesion in dogs by injection of 0.75 ml/kg of air into the carotid artery, though some deaths due to cardiac arrest and some cerebral lesions resulted. Pate and Birdsong (1964) found an "all or none" effect in cats. All cats receiving 3.0 ml/kg of air in the carotid artery survived, whereas all receiving 3.5 ml/kg or more died with convulsions and respiratory arrest. At necropsy, the right heart was filled with foam, and death was attributed to loss of effective circulation.

Air infused at a constant rate for one hour into the jugular vein of dogs caused transient hypotension, elevated central venous pressure, and a fall in arterial oxygen tension (Wycoff and Cann, 1966). When a lethal amount of air (0.69 ml/kg/min) was infused, a characteristic cardiac murmur and heart failure developed, with a marked rise in CVP and a fall in blood pressure. When studying the slow intravenous infusion of air (0.12 to 2.20 ml/kg/min) in dogs, Adornato et al. (1978) encountered an elevated CVP and hypotension. They also reported an abrupt increase in pulmonary arterial pressure and a progressive decrease in peripheral resistance. An early electrocardiographic change was peaking of the P waves. Later there was depression of the S-T segment. Changes in heart sounds were only detected after significant cardiovascular decompensation had occurred.

The possibility that serious or fatal air embolism can be produced, particularly by the venipuncture techniques commonly employed in large animals, should be considered. Gabel (1970) has reported that 1 L of air produces splashing heart sounds in horses, and 4 L may be fatal. He cautioned against leaving open needles or catheters in the jugular vein of the horse.

If a murmur is heard, the following steps should be taken (Wycoff and Cann, 1966): 1) control air entry into vein; 2) place patient on left side; 3) aspirate air in the heart; and 4) perform external cardiac massage.

ANESTHETIC RESPONSES AND OVERDOSE

An *excessive* normal response to the usual dose of a drug is termed *hypersensitivity.* An *unusual* and *abnormal* response to the usual dose of a drug is termed *idiosyncrasy.* These two terms have been used many times to explain anesthetic deaths that actually were caused by a total disregard for basic principles, such as failure to assure a proper airway.

Anesthetic overdose may be either *relative* or *absolute*. A relative overdose occurs when an animal develops complications from administration of the normal calculated dose. An absolute overdose occurs when more than the correct calculated dose is administered.

When anesthetic overdose is suspected, the obvious first procedure is to stop administration. Although overdose of inhalation anesthetics can and does occur, additional discussion of this phenomenon is not needed because of the inherent ease with which these anesthetics can be removed from the body by controlled ventilation. The barbiturates, however, present a different problem.

Anaphylactoid Reactions

Many drugs used during anesthesia release histamine; these include morphine, meperidine, tubocurarine, succinylcholine, hexamethonium, gallamine, phenothiazine derivatives, atropine, basic antibiotics, adriamycin and similar antibiotics, dextran and polyvinyl pyrrolidone, radiopaque substances, and shortacting intravenous anesthetics, especially steroids. Sensitivity (histaminoid) reactions have been reported to occur commonly in cats as a result of steroid (alphaxalone/alphadalone) anesthesia. Reactions included hyperemia or edema of the ears, forepaws, and face with mild progressive hypotension (Dodman, 1980). The mechanism of histamine release is uncertain, but is similar to that induced by IgE and antigen in a typical allergic reaction. Release of endogenous histamine in the heart leads to severe cardiac dysfunction with arrhythmias, prolongation of cardiac conduction, and cardiac arrest. In studies with tubocurarine, the response appeared to be dose-related. Reactions were more readily provoked with bolus injections than with slow infusions. Histamine release was blocked by high levels of circulating glucose and epinephrine, and enhanced by hypoglycemia, cholinergic agents, and low circulating levels of epinephrine (Beaven, 1981).

Drug Interactions

Animals requiring anesthesia have frequently already received several drugs. Interaction of these with anesthetic drugs may have dangerous consequences. Interactions may occur as a result of physical or chemical incompatibility, such as the precipitation resulting from mixing thiopental with pancuronium or meperidine. Common beneficial interactions at the site of absorption are the slowing effect of epinephrine upon the uptake of local anesthetics, and the influence of nitrous oxide on the absorption of other inhalants (second gas effect, see Chap. 10). Drug distribution may be affected by competition for protein-binding sites (see Chaps. 2, 12). Drugs may also compete for common binding sites, such as those of the myoneural junction for which tubocurarine and acetylcholine vie. Antibiotics, especially those of the aminoglycoside group, may enhance neuromuscular blockade of muscle relaxants or cause respiratory depression, probably by binding calcium at the neuromuscular junction and by interfering with the release of acetylcholine (Cullen and Miller,

1979). Respiratory depression may also occur during recovery from anesthesia owing to administration of such antibiotics. It is likely that aminoglycoside antibiotics, by altering Ca^{++}-dependent functions, interact synergistically with anesthetics to accentuate cardiovascular depression (Adams et al., 1976). Drug interactions may also alter excretion; narcotics, for instance, depress respiration and thereby the excretion of inhalant anesthetics.

Anesthesia-Associated Hepatitis and Nephropathy

Despite the linkage of halothane to postanesthetic hepatitis in man, clinical cases have not been reported in veterinary patients (Benson and Brock, 1980). The syndrome is probably associated with excessive dosage, decreased hepatic blood flow and/or hypoxia, defective hepatic enzymes, and possibly genetic predisposition (see Chap. 2). Similar hepatotoxicity has been observed in some laboratory animals (rats, mice, guinea pigs, and mink), especially when repeated exposures were given (Greenham and Ware, 1979; Benson and Brock, 1980). The latter authors indicate that because the syndrome occurs in man and certain laboratory animals, it is possible that such a syndrome exists in veterinary patients. They indicate, however, that preexisting hepatic disease is not a contraindication for the use of halothane. It should be noted that a hepatitis syndrome has also been associated with methoxyflurane anesthesia in man.

Despite the occurrence of methoxyflurane-related nephropathy in man, this condition has not been observed in veterinary patients, although transient polyuria and polydypsia have been noted in dogs (Benson and Brock, 1980). The syndrome is characterized as a nephrogenic diabetes insipidus resulting from renal tubular damage. An identical condition, the intensity of which is dose-related, has been reported as a consequence of methoxyflurane administration to rats. It appears to be caused by inorganic fluoride released during metabolism of the anesthetic. The condition is aggravated by obesity, by prolonged methoxyflurane administration, and by concurrent administration of nephrotoxic drugs, especially tetracycline and gentamicin. Repeated methoxyflurane administration has been associated with hepatorenal failure in one dog. Initial exposure of two horses to methoxyflurane was complicated by hepatic necrosis, and several equine and bovine cases complicated by postanesthetic jaundice have been observed (Benson and Brock, 1980). These authors also caution that veterinarians chronically exposed to trace concentrations of halothane and/or methoxyflurane may be at higher risk than the general population when they themselves undergo anesthesia.

Barbiturate Overdose

Overdose of barbiturates is not uncommon in small animals, particularly when repeated doses are administered, since even the ultrashort-acting agents are cumulative (Fig. 12–8). The incidence of prolonged anesthesia is discussed in Chapter 23 and tabulated in Table 23–13.

Self-induced barbiturate overdose occurs commonly in man and, for this reason, has been studied extensively in animals and man. As described in Chapter 12, the blood pH dictates the degree of dissociation of a barbiturate in blood and its subsequent ability to penetrate cell walls.

In barbiturate overdose, a vicious cycle sets in. Respiration is depressed, respiratory acidosis develops, and additional barbiturate enters the brain cells, further depressing the respiratory and cardiac centers.

To correct the cycle, the following procedure should be used:

1. Hyperventilate to reduce CO_2 and to increase the blood pH, thus producing more dissociated or ionized barbiturate.
2. Give sodium bicarbonate or tromethamine intravenously to increase pH and to cause ionization of the barbiturate. The dose used depends upon the degree of acidosis as measured by arterial blood pH and/or base deficit.
3. Maintain tissue perfusion by alpha-adrenergic blockade with a phenothiazine tranquilizer, phentolamine, or dibenzyline to prevent anaerobic metabolism with lactic acid formation. Central venous pressure should be monitored concurrently.

4. Maintain blood volume and urine output by administration of fluids and diuretics.

a. Administer saline solution intravenously. Dextrose or lactate solutions should not be used because of the possible "glucose effect" (see Chap. 12).

b. Administer 10% mannitol (2.5 g/kg intravenously).

c. Administer furosemide (2 mg/lb) intravenously or intramuscularly, repeated every 6 hours. It is important to recall that thiazide diuretics predispose to hypokalemia and an increased propensity for arrhythmias.

5. Maintain normal body temperature, and turn frequently to prevent hypostatic congestion of the lungs.

Other methods of removing barbiturates from the patient that have been tried include peritoneal dialysis (Berman and Vogelsang, 1964; Bourne, 1964), hemodialysis with an artificial kidney (Schreiner, 1958), and hemoperfusion with ion-exchange resins (Nealon et al., 1966) or activated charcoal. When hemodialysis and hemoperfusion were compared in dogs given large doses of barbiturates, hemoperfusion proved superior (Medd et al., 1973).

While 4-aminopyridine and yohimbine have been shown to be partial antagonists of pentobarbital, they are not currently available commercially.

Treatment of barbiturate slough is discussed in Chapter 12.

TEMPERATURE MANAGEMENT

During general anesthesia, body temperature regulation is abolished. The temperature regulating center no longer functions normally, and the animal is unable to shiver. In addition, several anesthetics reduce peripheral vasoconstrictor tone, thereby facilitating heat exchange with the environment (Stephen, 1970). Anesthetized animals thus tend to become poikilothermic, and temperatures of 35 to 33°C have been recorded in cats and dogs anesthetized with barbiturates and/or inhalant anesthetics (Hartsfield, 1979*a*). A relatively large surface in relation to body mass, such as in newborn and young animals, encourages heat exchange with the environment. Heat loss is also promoted by the use of nonrebreathing techniques, by surgical exposure of the tissues and body cavities, and by intravenous administration of cool fluids. Although reduction of the basal metabolic rate concomitant with body temperature may be an advantage during anesthesia, requirements for chemical anesthetics are reduced as body temperature falls, and the patient may be slow to recover and have depressed reflexes postoperatively (Stephen, 1970). The halothane or methoxyflurane requirement for anesthesia drops 5% for each degree centigrade less than 37° C. Together with increasing depth, reduced capacity of the liver to detoxify drugs may delay recovery if injectable agents have also been used. In addition, the condition is further complicated by a potential for cardiac dysrhythmias, decreased circulating blood volume, hemoconcentration, bradycardia, and depressed cardiac output. These complications are most likely if the temperature falls below 32° C for an extended period (Hartsfield, 1979*a*).

Morris and Wilkey (1970) have recommended that the operating room for surgery of man should be maintained between 21 and 23.9° C (70 to 75° F), and that esophageal or nasopharyngeal temperatures should always be monitored during major surgical procedures. In rooms cooler than 21° C, the body temperatures of patients were less than 36° C 45 minutes after induction and declined at a mean rate of 0.3° C per hour during the next 2 to 3 hours. Demands on the respiratory and circulatory systems from the spontaneous hypothermia and from attempts to restore normothermia postoperatively by shivering may be hazardous, if pulmonary and cardiovascular disease exists (Goldberg and Roe, 1966). In human patients having a fall in temperature, oxygen consumption increased as much as 80%. This increase coincided with the onset of shivering.

Animals should, therefore, be kept warm during anesthesia and the ensuing recovery period. The operating room temperature should be at least 70° F, intravenous fluids should be warmed, and a pad should be placed between a metal table and the animal. Animals emerging from anesthesia should likewise be kept warm.

Blankets, heat lamps, heating pads, and warm water (temperature 40.5° C) circulating blankets are satisfactory. It must, however, be remembered that these animals cannot escape excessive heat and may be burned or even killed by the injudicious use of heating pads or other warming devices. Burns have not been reported with water blankets although, for safety, a cotton drape between the patient and blanket is recommended (Hartsfield, 1979*b*).

Since thermoregulation is impaired during anesthesia, the potential for hyperthermia should be considered, especially in large animals that may be anesthetized in an environmental temperature greater than that of their body. Heat dissipation is impaired by obesity, heavy hair coats, high humidity, and respiratory embarrassment. Tolerance to heat in animals varies significantly among the various species. Maximal rectal temperatures tolerated for a brief period have been shown to vary from 43.4° C in the rabbit and cat to 41.7° C in the dog (Wallin, 1977). Hyperthermia is characterized by panting, tachycardia, red mucous membranes, warm skin, and an elevated or rising temperature. As the syndrome progresses, hemoconcentration, hypovolemia, disseminated intravascular coagulation, cardiac dysrhythmias, decreased urine volume, acidosis, hyperkalemia, coma, and respiratory arrest all may occur (Hartsfield, 1979*b*). Even when animals are removed from the heat source, delayed death may occur in 1 to 20 hours (Wallin, 1977). Causes of hyperthermia relative to anesthesia include preanesthetic stress, misuse of external heat, excitement and struggling during recovery, pyrogens, CNS lesions, and malignant hyperthermia. Excitement, excessive restraint, and struggling during induction or recovery, especially in animals having difficulty in dissipating heat, all contribute to possible hyperthermia. Premedication and suitable environment will usually prevent such a problem. During recovery, cold water circulating blankets, cold water baths, and use of an antiprostaglandin (e.g., flunixin meglumine) with both analgesic and antipyretic effects are helpful. It is important to recall that environmental temperature is of utmost importance in the determination of drug effects; there is a critical environmental temperature above which some drugs produce a rise of body temperature and below which they produce a decline (Wallin, 1977). The effect of temperature on the action of drugs has been extensively reviewed by Weibe (1973). Indiscriminate inadequately supervised use of external heat during anesthesia or anesthetic recovery may easily produce hyperthermia, especially in neonates, well-insulated animals, and febrile animals. This problem can be avoided by temperature monitoring and removal of the heat source if the rectal temperature exceeds the normal value.

Lesions in the anterior hypothalamus may impair thermoregulation. These may develop during anesthesia as a result of fat embolism, low cerebral oxygen tensions, and trauma (surgical or accidental) to the cranial or anterior spinal cord regions (Hartsfield, 1979*a,b*).

MALIGNANT HYPERTHERMIA

In 1960, a syndrome in which uncontrolled hyperpyrexia developed rapidly in anesthetized humans was described. Subsequently, it was reported to occur in swine (Jones et al., 1970). With increasing recognition of malignant hyperthermia (MH) in man and recognition of a similar, if not identical, syndrome in swine, numerous studies were undertaken to clarify the pathogenesis, to identify susceptible patients, and to develop effective prophylactic and therapeutic procedures.

This inherited syndrome has been reviewed by Hartsfield (1979*b*), Gronert (1980), and Hall et al. (1980). In susceptible animals, MH is triggered by potent volatile anesthetics, succinylcholine, decamethonium, environmental stress (exercise, heat, anoxia), and excitement. Triggering in the absence of anesthetic agents has been proved primarily in swine, although there is significant presumptive evidence that factors other than anesthetic agents are implicated in man. Parasympatholytic and sympathomimetic drugs, cardiac glycosides, and calcium salts may exacerbate the syndrome, whereas phenothiazine tranquilizers may suppress the response. Amide local anesthetics may also induce MH, although it has not been possible to confirm this in swine susceptible to MH. The mode of inheritance is uncertain, and its determination has possibly been complicated by variation in the ease by which it may be triggered. In swine the inheritance may vary from breed to breed; it is, however, thought to be an autosomal recessive characteristic and may be linked to certain blood types. Anesthetic-induced and, in some instances, stress-induced MH has also been reported in the horse, cat, dog, deer, birds, and wild animals during capture (see the following section on Capture Myopathy).

With the onset of MH, skeletal muscle suddenly increases oxygen consumption and lactate production with greater heat production, hyperpyrexia, respiratory and metabolic acidosis, muscle rigidity, sympathetic stimulation, and increased cellular permeability. Initial increases in serum magnesium, phosphorus, calcium, and potassium are followed by a fall in potassium and calcium, and by myoglobinuria. The syndrome probably results from an inability to control calcium concentrations in muscle fibers and may involve a generalized cellular or subcellular membrane permeability. Diagnosis is based upon the rapid change in temperature and acid-base status, and the common occurrence of muscle rigidity. Susceptibility can be predicted by in vitro response of muscle biopsy specimens to halothane, caffeine, potassium, and succinylcholine. History of occurrence in related animals and significant elevation of plasma CPK are important indicators of potential susceptibility. Specific treatment may be accomplished by administration of dantrolene sodium (see Chap. 20) while muscle perfusion still persists. Dantrolene suppresses calcium release within the muscle without influencing calcium uptake. The minimal effective dose in swine is 3.5 to 5 mg/kg intravenously; it may also be used prophylactically in potentially susceptible animals. Other treatment includes immediate termination of anesthetic administration, intravenous administration of procaine (if dantrolene is unavailable), corticosteroids, hyperventilation, 2 to 4 mEq/kg of sodium bicarbonate by rapid intravenous injection, and aggressive body cooling with the aid of ice, cold fluids, and gastric or peritoneal lavage. Cardiac arrhythmias usually require control, and adequate urine flow should be maintained. Suggested anesthetic agents for known susceptible patients include thiopental, opiates, droperidol, pancuronium, nitrous oxide, along with preoperative dantrolene.

CAPTURE MYOPATHY

Capture myopathy is a syndrome that may develop in wild animals following acute stress. The subject has been reviewed by Spraker (1982), who describes four forms: peracute death syndrome, acute death syndrome, ataxic myoglobinuric syndrome, and ruptured muscle syndrome. The pathogenesis of all four syndromes appears to involve the same factors, namely, fear, stimulation of the pituitary-adrenal and sympathetic systems, and severe muscular exertion. The interplay of these factors seems to determine the severity of the disease. Capture myopathy has been reported in a variety of wild quadrupeds and primates, including those that are free-ranging or confined.

Fear stimulates an outpouring of epinephrine and corticosteroids from the adrenal gland, and norepinephrine from the sympathetic nerve endings. With prolonged or excessive stimulation, these responses become exhausted, resulting in decreased tissue perfusion, tissue hypoxia, and capillary stagnation. Shock, vascular collapse, and cellular necrosis develop. Intracellular potassium entering the general circulation may cause ventricular fibrillation (peracute death syndrome). Prolonged muscular exertion, accompanied by excessive heat production, leads to anaerobic metabolism and buildup of lactate in skeletal muscles with acidosis, cellular death, and subsequent death of the animal due to shock (acute death syndrome).

Ataxic myoglobinuric syndrome is observed hours to several days after capture. The clinical signs include ataxia, torticollis, and myoglobinuria, with elevated serum GOT, CPK, LDH, and BUN levels. Clinical signs may vary from mild to severe, with recovery or death of the animal. Skeletal muscle lesions are characterized by rhabdomyolysis; kidney lesions include dilated tubules, myoglobin casts within the tubules, and tubular nephrosis.

If the animal recovers, it may still have varying degrees of muscle necrosis and tubular nephrosis resulting from renal hypoxia and, possibly, from toxic myoglobinemia. If the muscular necrosis is in weight-bearing muscles, movement of the animal may cause the muscle to rupture (ruptured muscle syndrome). This commonly is manifested as a marked drop in the hindquarters and hyperflexion of the hock. At necropsy, the gross lesions consist of massive subcutaneous hemorrhages and multifocal pale soft lesions in the muscles of the limbs, neck, and diaphragm.

Several treatments have been used with varying success. Among these are corticosteroids, vitamins, antibiotics, sodium bicarbonate, intravenous electrolyte solutions, selenium, and cooling with water. The relationship of capture myopathy and malignant hyperthermia has not been elucidated. However, it appears that dantrolene (see Chap. 20) might be efficacious in treatment of this syndrome, as it is in treatment of malignant hyperthermia.

PHYSICAL INJURIES AND COMPLICATIONS

Large animals, especially horses, are subject to temporary or even permanent loss of sensory and/or motor nerve function, during or subsequent to anesthesia. The injury may result from stretching, tension, pressure paralysis, or direct trauma. It is therefore essential to avoid unnecessary traction, abduction, or stretching of the limbs, especially during anesthesia when muscles are well relaxed. Superficial nerves should be protected by bandaging, padding (2 to 4 inches thick), and padded halters or hoods. The use of protective pads, cushions, inflated inner tubes, or water beds beneath recumbent animals is mandatory, and the period of recumbency should be reduced to a minimum.

Nerves commonly affected are the radial, peroneal, and facial. Paralysis of the radial nerve usually occurs as a result of body pressure on the nerve as it crosses the musculospiral groove of the humerus. Pressure upon the brachial plexus may also be a cause. During recumbency, compression of the brachial artery with subsequent ischemia of foreleg muscles may also cause radial paralysis. In this instance, lameness develops several hours after recovery from anesthesia (Riebold et al., 1982). Usually radial paralysis lasts 1 to 3 days.

Prophylaxis necessitates adequate use of padding and other protective devices, and extension of the down front leg so that the thorax lies over the belly of the triceps muscle rather than on the humerus itself. Therapy includes protective bandaging and padding, and steroidal and/or nonsteroidal anti-inflammatory agents, diuretics, and hydrotherapy.

Peroneal paralysis is also usually temporary, lasting 1 to 3 days, and results from pressure of the body on the down rear leg or from excessive posterior extension of the pelvic limb. This syndrome has also been observed in dogs placed head-down on a tilted table with hindlimbs extended over the upper table edge and fastened underneath. Prophylaxis requires the use of body padding and normal positioning of the legs during anesthesia.

Facial nerve paralysis is usually caused by direct trauma or improper padding. Auriculopalpebral paralysis also occurs in the dog as a result of injury during anesthesia. Prevention requires use of pads, padded halters, or hoods, and care to avoid accidental trauma. Therapy likewise requires the use of anti-inflammatory agents. Because of prolonged recumbency or inadequate padding, areas of edema or ultimately of local tissue necrosis and sloughing may occur from lying on a hard surface or operating table. These problems can be overcome by adequate padding, such as afforded by a water bed, and by minimizing the duration of recumbency.

Other miscellaneous injuries encountered in the large animal, especially during induction and recovery, include rupture of a vertebral artery as a result of falling head first (Riebold et al., 1982), rupture of the stomach or large bowel, rupture of an aneurysm, hematomas, wound disruption, ocular injuries, and fractures of the skull, vertebrae, and long bones. Ducharme et al. (1983) reported that 5.11% of 181 equine colic cases developed long bone fractures during the recovery period, despite use of a padded stall.

Following the recumbency of anesthesia, the horse may develop postanesthetic myopathy. The triceps is most commonly affected, although the quadriceps, extensors of the pelvic limb, gluteals, and masseters may be involved, and a generalized myopathy may also occur (White, 1982). Some believe thoroughbreds may be more susceptible than standardbreds, whereas others report that the syndrome more commonly occurs in males, in horses undergoing strenuous training (Waldron-Mease and Rosenberg, 1979), or in heavily muscled horses, especially draft horses (Riebold et al., 1982).

The condition is associated with prolonged recumbency (generally greater than 2 hours) during anesthesia. Lack of adequate padding of the affected areas, arterial hypotension, and hypoxia contribute to the disorder, which is thought to result from muscle ischemia. A compartmental syndrome (local muscle ischemia within a closed osteofascial compartment) resulting from trauma, exercise, ischemia or drug overdose has been recognized in man and has been produced experimentally in the dog. Intracompartmental muscle pressures recorded from forelimbs during prolonged recumbency of the anesthetized horse suggest that equine postanesthetic lameness is a similar syndrome (Lindsay et al., 1980). Others have related postoperative lumbar or generalized muscle rigidity with pain to malignant hyperthermia, based upon in vitro exposure of muscle biopsy specimens to halothane and caffeine (Waldron-Mease and Rosenberg, 1979).

Postanesthetic myopathy may occur during recovery from anesthesia or up to several hours thereafter. It is characterized by weakness of the affected muscle groups. If the triceps is affected, the elbow is dropped, whereas the fetlock is knuckled when there is extensive damage of the hindlimb. Affected muscles may be flaccid or hot, swollen, hard, and painful; muscle tremors or fasciculations frequently occur. Pain may be manifested by anxiety, sweating, and colic. Generalized myopathy may also occur. Serum CPK levels greater than 300 IU are indicative of muscle damage, and levels greater than 1000 IU are indicative of generalized muscle disease. Myoglobinuria and hypocalcemia are also observed (White, 1982), although others have not been able to detect changes in serum calcium (Lindsay et al., 1980).

Once muscle damage has occurred, treatment is symptomatic and comprises rest, administration of steroidal and/or nonsteroidal anti-inflammatory drugs, plus fluid and electrolyte therapy to maintain hydration, urine flow, and acid-base balance. Muscle relaxants, such as dantrolene sodium (4 mg/kg) or guaifenesin, may help relieve pain and muscle rigidity.

Prevention necessitates limitation of the duration of recumbency to 2 hours or less, use of minimal anesthetic depth, avoidance of arterial hypotension, assurance of adequate oxygenation, use of adequate padding (4 inches thick), and proper positioning of the limbs. If, in lateral recumbency, the lower forelimb is extended and the upper one is parallel with the lower or is elevated, muscle pressure has been found acceptable (White, 1982). Dorsal recumbency also necessitates thorough padding and even positioning, without leaning.

Injuries in small animals are less common, but do occur, particularly in the recovery period. Wound disruption, hematomas, broken teeth, tongue and ocular injuries, and fractures are most common. Drowning in water pans can occur unless they are removed. Violent movements during recovery should always be controlled with tranquilizers and/or narcotics. Padding should be provided to protect the patient from possible trauma. For further information on aftercare, see Chapter 22.

MISCELLANEOUS ANESTHETIC MISHAPS

A study of human factors and preventable mishaps at a human hospital revealed that 82% of these involved human error. Breathing circuit connections, inadvertent changes in gas flows, and drug syringe errors were frequent problems. Although overt equipment failures comprised only 14% of preventable mishaps, equipment design contributed to human error in many instances, as did inadequate experience and lack of familiarity with equipment and/or the surgical procedure. The most frequent incidents in order of frequency were breathing circuit disconnection, inadvertent gas flow change, syringe swap, gas supply problem, intravenous apparatus disconnection, laryngoscope malfunction, premature extubation, breathing circuit connection error, hypovolemia, and tracheal airway device position changes (Cooper et al., 1978) (see also Tables 23–9, 23–15, 23–16).

It is well recognized in man and animals that excessive inflation of endotracheal tube cuffs causes mucosal ischemia and tracheal injury. Latex cuffs have been shown to exert highest mucosal pressures and silicone cuffs the lowest. Stiff cuffs impair mucosal blood flow more than compliant cuffs, which are therefore preferred (Dobrin and Canfield, 1977; Pedersoli and Krista, 1979).

With the virtual cessation of use of explosive anesthetics, this hazard has been reduced significantly. Should explosive mixtures be used, full precautions are essential (see Chap. 11).

Complications with injectable agents include perivascular accidents, inadvertent intra-arterial injection, and penile prolapse (in the horse). Although every effort should be made to prevent perivascular accidents, when they occur they should be treated by injection of procaine and saline into the area to dilute the effect (see Chap. 12). Occasionally, inadvertent intracarotid injection may be made in the horse. Convulsions frequently result, and a muscle relaxant or a general anesthetic may be required (Riebold et al., 1982).

Phenothiazine tranquilizers, with or without narcotics, cause reversible prolapse of the equine penis. Occasionally the prolapse is associated with permanent prolapse and/or erection and consequent trauma. One survey has indicated the occurrence of 11 cases of persistent prolapse; 3 occurred in young colts receiving acepromazine, and the remaining 8 in animals given acepromazine and etorphine, with diprenorphine for recovery. The use of xylazine is preferred over acepromazine for breeding stallions. Should the condition occur, prompt treatment by manual compression or a compression bandage is indicated (Gering, 1981).

TEMPERAMENT CHANGES CAUSED BY ANESTHETIC AGENTS

Unfortunately, an occasional animal may exhibit transient or permanent changes in temperament following administration of preanesthetic and/or anesthetic agents. This change most frequently occurs with tranquilizers, but may occur with other drugs, and is observed in both small and large animals. Most reports are anecdotal; however, one of the authors has experienced this phenomenon in his own animals. Obviously, it is in the veterinarian's best interest to use minimal restraint and to be selective in the choice of drugs employed, since at least one lawsuit has occurred following alleged mishandling and emotional trauma to the animal (Hannah, 1977).

INJURIES TO PERSONNEL

In addition to the injuries that may occur to animal patients, the anesthesiologist, technician, or other assisting personnel may be subjected to injury. Particularly with large animals, the risk of being struck, kicked, bitten, or squeezed is always present. Smaller patients frequently scratch, claw, or bite.

Another source of danger lies in the use of extremely potent pharmacologic agents (Haigh and Haigh, 1980). These drugs may be inadvertently injected into humans in a veterinary hospital or "in the field." In at least one instance, this has caused the death of a veterinarian (Anonymous, 1976). Ketamine, etorphine, fentanyl, carfentanil, xylazine, nicotine, and succinylcholine are probably the dangerous agents most frequently used. Needless to say, extreme precautions should be taken to protect personnel from accidental injection or from ocular, oral, or even skin exposure. Antagonists, if available, should always be at hand during use of these drugs, along with equipment for cardiopulmonary resuscitation.

Waste anesthetic gases are also toxic for personnel and are discussed in Chapter 11.

REFERENCES

Ackerman, N., Wingfield, W.E., and Corley, E.A.: Fatal Air Embolism Associated with Pneumourethrography and Pneumocystography in a Dog. J.A.V.M.A., 160:1616, 1972.

Adams, H.R., Teske, R.H., and Mercer, H.D.: Anesthetic-Antibiotic Interrelationships. J.A.V.M.A., 168:409, 1976.

Adornato, D.C., Gildenberg, P.L., Ferrario, C.M., Smart, J., and Frost, E.A.M.: Pathophysiology of Intravenous Air Embolism in Dogs. Anesthesiology, 49:120, 1978.

Aitken, M.M., and Sanford, J.: Correspondence: Immobilon: Reactions to VPC Decision. Vet Rec., 99:35, 1976.

Al-Kaisi, N., Parratt, J.R., Siddigui, H.H., and Zeitlin, I.J.: Feline Endotoxin Shock: Effects of Methylprednisolone on Kininogen-Depletion, on the Pulmonary Circulation and on Survival. Br. J. Pharmacol., 60:471, 1977.

Anonymous: Inquest—Veterinary Surgeon's Immobilon Death "Accidental." Vet. Rec., 98:414, 1976.

Anonymous: The Prevention of Anesthetic Accidents. Lederle Bulletin Newsletter, July, 1950.

Babbs, C.F.: New Versus Old Theories of Blood Flow During CPR. Crit. Care Med., 8:191, 1980.

Babbs, C.F., Voorhees, W.D., Fitzgerald, K.R., Holmes, H.R., and Geddes, L.E.: Influence of Interposed Ventilation Pressure upon Artificial Cardiac Output During Cardiopulmonary Resuscitation in Dogs. Crit. Care Med., 8:127, 1980.

Bannister, W.K., Sattilaro, A.J., and Otis, R.D.: Therapeutic Aspects of Aspiration Pneumonitis in Experimental Animals. Anesthesiology, 22:440, 1961.

Baue, A.E.: Recent Developments in the Study and Treatment of Shock. Surg. Gynecol. Obstet., 127:849, 1968.

Beaven, M.A.: Editorial Views: Anaphylactoid Reactions to Anesthetic Drugs. Anesthesiology, 55:3, 1981.

Bedford, R.F., Persing, J.A., Pobereskin, L., and Butler, A.: Lidocaine or Thiopental for Rapid Control of Intracranial Hypertension? Anesth. Analg., 59:435, 1980.

Benson, C.J., and Brock, K.A.: Halothane-Associated Hepatitis and Methoxyflurane-Related Nephropathy: A Review. J. Vet. Pharmacol. Ther., 3:187, 1980.

Berman, L.B., and Vogelsang, P.: Removal Rates for Barbiturates Using Two Types of Peritoneal Dialysis. N. Engl. J. Med., 270:77, 1964.

Black, G.W., Linde, H.W., Dripps, R.D., and Price, H.L.: Circulatory Changes Accompanying Respiratory Acidosis during Halothane (Fluothane) Anesthesia in Man. Br. J. Anaesth., 31:238, 1959.

Blitt, C.D., Gutman, H.L., Cohen, D.D., Weisman, H., and Dillon, J.B.: "Silent" Regurgitation and Aspiration during General Anesthesia. Anesth. Analg., 49:707, 1970.

Bottoms, G.D., Fessler, J.F., Roesel, O.F., Moore, A.B., and Frauenfelder, H.C.: Endotoxin-Induced Hemodynamic Changes in Ponies: Effects of Flunixin Meglumine. Am. J. Vet. Res., 42:1514, 1981.

Bourne, C.W.: The Effect of Albumin on the Extraction of Barbiturate by Peritoneal Dialysis. Invest. Urol., 2:107, 1964.

Brasmer, T.H.: Fluid Therapy in Shock. J.A.V.M.A., 174:475, 1979.

Breznock, E.M., and Strack, D.: Blood Volume of Non-Splenectomized and Splenectomized Cats before and after Acute Hemorrhage. Am. J. Vet. Res., 43:1811, 1983.

Broder, G., and Weil, M.H.: Excess Lactate: An Index of Reversibility of Shock in Human Patients. Science, 143:1457, 1964.

Brooks, D.K.: *Resuscitation*. Edward Arnold, Ltd., London, 1967.

Brown, E.B., Jr., and Miller, F.L.: Ventricular Fibrillation Following a Rapid Fall in Alveolar Carbon Dioxide Concentration. Am. J. Physiol., 169:56, 1952.

Buchanan, E.C.: Blood and Blood Substitutes for Treating Hemorrhagic Shock. Am. J. Hosp. Pharmacol., 34:631, 1977.

Burnap, T.K.: Personal communication. Harvard School of Medicine, Boston, Massachusetts, 1970.

Burrows, G.E.: Endotoxaemia in the Horse. Review Article. Equine Vet. J., 13:89, 1981.

Burstein, C.L., and Rovenstine, E.A.: Respiratory Action of Some Shorter Acting Barbituric Acid Derivatives. J. Pharmacol. Exp. Ther., 63:43, 1938.

Calderwood, H.W., Modell, J.H., and Ruiz, B.C.: The Ineffectiveness of Steroid Therapy for Treatment of Fresh-Water Near-Drowning. Anesthesiology, 43:642, 1975.

Clark, D.R.: Recognition and Treatment of Cardiac Emergencies. J.A.V.M.A., 171:98, 1977.

Clement, A.J.: Anaesthesia and Cardiac Disease. In *A Practice of Anaesthesia*, 4th ed. Edited by H.C. Churchill-Davidson. W.B. Saunders Co., Philadelphia, 1978.

Clubb, R.J., Maxwell, R.E., and Chou, S.N.: Experimental Brain Injury in the Dog. The Pharmacological Effects of Pentobarbital and Sodium Nitroprusside. J. Neurosurg., 52:189, 1980.

Condon, R.E.: Pathophysiologic Mechanisms in Cardiac Arrest. Surg. Gynecol. Obstet., 114:8, 1962.

Cooper, J.B., Newbower, R.S., Lang, C.D., and McPeek, B.: Preventable Anesthesia Mishaps: Study of Human Factors. Anesthesiology, 49:399, 1978.

Cullen, B.F., and Miller, M.G.: Drug Interactions and Anesthesia: A Review. Anesth. Analg., 58:413, 1979.

Cullen, D.J., and Eger. E.I.: The Effects of Halothane on Respiratory and Cardiovascular Responses to Hypoxia in Dogs. Anesthesiology, 33:487, 1970.

Cullen, S.C.: *The Year Book of Anesthesia*. Year Book Medical Publishers, Inc., Chicago, 1967.

DeVault, M., Greifenstein, F.E., and Harris, I.C., Jr.: Circulatory Responses to Endotracheal Intubation in Light General Anesthesia: The Effect of Atropine and Phentolamine. Anesthesiology, 21:360, 1960.

Dobrin, P., and Canfield, T.: Cuffed Endotracheal Tubes: Mucosal Pressures and Tracheal Wall Blood Flow. Am. J. Surg., 133:562, 1977.

Dodman, N.H.: Complications of Saffan Anaesthesia in Cats. Vet. Rec., 107:481, 1980.

Ducharme, N.G., Hackett, R.P., Ducharme, G.R., and Long, S.: Surgical Treatment of Colic. Results in 181 Horses. Vet. Surg., 12:206, 1983.

Dukes, H.H.: *The Physiology of Domestic Animals*, 6th ed. Comstock Publishing Co., Ithaca, New York, 1947.

Elam, J.O.: Treatment of Cardiac Arrest. Lecture No. 142, Annual Refresher Course Lectures. Am. Soc. Anesth., Washington, D.C., 1968.

Erlanger, H.: Cardiac Arrhythmias in Relationship to Anesthesia: Past and Present Concepts. Am. J. Med. Sci., 243:651, 1962.

Exarhos, N.D., Logan, W.D., Abbott, O.A., and Hatcher,

C.R.: The Importance of pH and Volume in Tracheobronchial Aspiration. Dis. Chest, 17:167, 1965.

Faden, A.I., and Holaday, J.W.: Experimental Endotoxin Shock: The Pathophysiologic Function of Endorphins and Treatment with Opiate Antagonists. J. Infect. Dis., 142:229, 1980.

Fine, J.: Defense Mechanisms in Massive Injury. 17th Gaines Vet. Symp., October, 1967.

Frauenfelder, H.C., Fessler, J.F., Latshaw, H.S., Moore, A.B., and Bottoms, G.D.: External Cardiovascular Resuscitation of the Anesthetized Pony. J.A.V.M.A., 179:673, 1981.

Gabel, A.: Air Embolism. J.A.V.M.A., 156:283, 1970.

Geddes, L.A., Tacker, W.A., Rosborough, J.P., Moore, A.G., and Cabler, P.S.: Electrical Dose for Ventricular Defibrillation of Large and Small Animals Using Precordial Electrodes. J. Clin. Invest., 53:310, 1974.

Gering, E.L.: Priapism and ACP in the Horse. Vet. Rec., 109:64, 1981.

Gillespie, J.R., Tyler, W.S., and Hall, L.W.: Cardiopulmonary Dysfunction in Anesthetized, Laterally Recumbent Horses. Am. J. Vet. Res., 30:61, 1969.

Gilston, A.: Clinical and Biochemical Aspects of Cardiac Resuscitation. Lancet, 2:1039, 1965.

Goldberg, M.J., and Roe, C.F.: Temperature Changes During Anesthesia and Operations. Arch. Surg., 93:365, 1966.

Goldstein, M.A., Schwark, W.S., Short, C.E., and White, K.K.: Cardiopulmonary Resuscitation in the Horse. Cornell Vet., 71:225, 1981.

Green, C.J.: *Animal Anaesthesia*. Laboratory Animals Ltd., London, 1979.

Greenham, L.W., and Ware, G.C.: Mustelid Anaesthesia and Halothane Hepatitis. Vet. Rec., 105:104, 1979.

Grier, R.L.: Esophageal Disease as a Result of Improper Patient Positioning. Arch. A.C.V.S., 4:4, 1975.

Gronert, G.A.: Malignant Hyperthermia. Anesthesiology, 53:395, 1980.

Haglund, U., Abe, T., Ahrén, C., Braide, I., and Lundgren, O.: The Intestinal Mucosal Lesions in Shock. II. The Relationship Between the Mucosal Lesions and the Cardiovascular Derangement Following Regional Shock. Eur. Surg. Res., 8:448, 1976.

Haigh, J.C., and Haigh, J.M.: Immobilizing Drug Emergencies in Humans. Vet. Human Toxicol., 22: 94, 1980.

Hall, G.M., Lucke, J.N., and Lister, D.: Malignant Hyperthermia—Pearls out of Swine? Br. J. Anaesth., 52:165, 1980.

Hall, L.W.: Accidents and Emergencies in Anesthesia. Mod. Vet. Pract., 40:28, 1959.

Hall, L.W.: *Wright's Veterinary Anaesthesia and Analgesia,* 7th ed. Baillière, Tindall & Cassell, London, 1971.

Hamelberg, W., and Bosomworth, P.P.: Aspiration Pneumonitis. Experimental Studies and Clinical Observations. Anesth. Analg., 43:669, 1964.

Hannah, H.W.: Temperament Changes Due to Treatment. J.A.V.M.A., 170:693, 1977.

Hardway, R.M., III.: Mechanism of Traumatic Shock. Surg. Gynecol. Obstet., 151:65, 1980.

Harris, L.C., Kirimli, B., and Safar, P.: Ventilation-Cardiac Compression Rates and Ratios in Cardiopulmonary Resuscitation. Anesthesiology, 28:806, 1967.

Hartsfield, S.M.: Body Temperature Variations Associated with General Anesthesia. A Review Part I: Hyperthermia. Southwestern Vet., 32:95, 1979*a*.

Hartsfield, S.M.: Body Temperature Variations Associated with General Anesthesia. A Review Part II: Hyperthermia. Southwestern Vet., 32:179, 1979*b*.

Hay, E.B., and Webb, J.K.: The Effect of Increased Arterial Blood Flow to the Liver on the Mortality Rate Following Hemorrhagic Shock. Surgery, 29:826, 1951.

Heimlich, H.J.: Drainage of the Pleural Cavity. GP, 33:86, 1966.

Hermreck, A.S., and Thal, A.P.: The Adrenergic Drugs and Their Use in Shock Therapy. Curr. Prob. Surg., July, 1968.

Hosobuchi, Y., Baskin, D.S., and Woo, S.K.: Reversal of Induced Ischemia Neurological Deficit in Gerbils by the Opiate Antagonist Naloxone. Science, 215:69, 1982.

Jones, E.M.: Personal communication. Oklahoma State University, Stillwater, 1972.

Jones, E.W., Burnap, T.K., Nelson, T.E., Anderson, I.L., and Kerr, D.D.: Preliminary Studies on Fulminant Hyperpyrexia in a Family of Swine. Proc., Am. Soc. Anesth. Meeting, New York, 1970.

Jones, J.L., and Jones, R.E.: Postshock Arrhythmias—A Possible Cause of Unsuccessful Defibrillation. Crit. Care Med., 8:167, 1980.

Katz, R.L., and Bigger, J.T., Jr.: Cardiac Arrhythmias during Anesthesia and Operation. Anesthesiology, 33:193, 1970.

Katz, R.L., and Epstein, R.A.: The Interaction of Anesthetic Agents and Adrenergic Drugs to Produce Cardiac Arrhythmias. Anesthesiology, 29:763, 1968.

Kirby, R.R.: Pathophysiology and Treatment of Shock. Regional Refresher Courses in Anesthesiology, I:69, 1973.

Kolata, R.J.: The Clinical Management of Circulatory Shock Based on Pathophysiological Patterns. Compend. Cont. Ed. Pract. Vet., 2:314, 1980.

Lewinski, A.: Evaluation of Methods Employed in the Treatment of the Chemical Pneumonitis of Aspiration. Anesthesiology, 26:37, 1965.

Lindsay, W.A., McDanell, W., and Bignell, W.: Equine Postanesthetic Forelimb Lameness: Intracompartmental Muscle Pressure Changes and Biochemical Patterns. Am. J. Vet. Res., 41:1919, 1980.

Longnecker, D.E., and Sturgill, B.C.: Influence of Anesthetic Agent on Survival Following Hemorrhage. Anesthesiology, 45:516, 1976.

Lurie, A.A., Jones, R.E., Linde, H.W., Price, M.L., Dripps, R.D., and Price, H.L.: Cyclopropane Anesthesia: Cardiac Rate and Rhythm during Steady Levels of Cyclopropane Anesthesia at Elevated and Normal End-Expiratory Carbon Dioxide Tensions. Anesthesiology, 19:457, 1958.

Malm, J.R., Manger, W.M., Sullivan, S.F., Papper, E.M., and Nahas, G.G.: The Effect of Acidosis on Sympathoadrenal Stimulation. J.A.M.A., 197:161, 1966.

Markov, A.K., Oglethorpe, N., Young, D.B., and Hellems, H.K.: Irreversible Hemorrhagic Shock. Treatment and Cardiac Pathophysiology. Circ. Shock, 8:9, 1981.

Marshall, L.F., Smith, R.W., and Shapiro, H.M.: The Outcome with Aggressive Treatment in Severe Head Injuries. Part II: Acute and Chronic Barbiturate Administration in the Management of Head Injury. J. Neurosurg., 50:26, 1979.

Medd, R.K., Widdop, B., Braithwaite, R.A., Rees, A.J., and Goulding, R.: Comparison of Haemoperfusion and Haemodialysis in the Therapy of Barbiturate Intoxication in Dogs. Arch. Toxicol., 31:163, 1973.

Minuck, M., and Sharma, G.P.: Comparison of THAM and Sodium Bicarbonate in Resuscitation of the Heart After Ventricular Fibrillation in Dogs. Anesth. Analg., 56:38, 1977.

Morris, R.H., and Wilkey, B.R.: The Effects of Ambient Temperature on Patient Temperature During Surgery Not Involving Body Cavities. Anesthesiology, 32:102, 1970.

Moss, G.: Fluid Distribution in Prevention of Hypovolemic Shock. Arch. Surg., 98:281, 1969.

Muir, W.W., III, Werner, L.L., and Hamlin, R.L.: Antiarrhythmic Effects of Diazepam During Coronary Artery Occlusion in Dogs. Am. J. Vet. Res., 36:1203, 1975a.

Muir, W.W., III, Werner, L.L., and Hamlin, R.L.: Arrhythmias in Dogs Associated with Epinephrine and Thiamylal Anesthesia. Am. J. Vet. Res., 36:1291, 1975*b*.

Muir, W.W., III, Werner, L.L., and Hamlin, R.L.: Effects of Xylazine and Acetylpromazine upon Induced Ventricular Fibrillation in Dogs Anesthetized with Thiamylal and Halothane. Am. J. Vet. Res., 36:1300, 1975*c*.

Nagel, E.: Cardiopulmonary Resuscitation. Lecture No. 112, Annual Refresher Course Lectures. Am. Soc. Anesth., New York, 1970.

Nealon, T.F., Sugerman, H., Shea, W., and Fleeger, E.: An Extracorporeal Device to Treat Barbiturate Poisoning. J.A.M.A., 197:158, 1966.

Ott, B.S.: Closed Chest Cardiac Resuscitation. Small Anim. Clin., 2:572, 1962.

Pate, J.W., and Birdsong, S.: Carotid Air Embolism. Arch. Surg., 89:685, 1964.

Pedersoli, W.M., and Krista, L.M.: Alterations in Tracheal Epithelium in Dogs Due to Endotracheal Intubation. Vet. Anesth., 6:34, 1979.

Price, H.L., Lurie, A.A., Jones, R.E., Price, M.L., and Linde, H.W.: Cyclopropane Anesthesia: Epinephrine and Norepinephrine in Initiation of Ventricular Arrhythmias by Carbon Dioxide Inhalation. Anesthesiology, 19:619, 1958.

Redding, J.S., and Cozine, R.A.: A Comparison of Open-Chest and Closed-Chest Cardiac Massage in Dogs. Anesthesiology, 22:280, 1961.

Redding, J.S., Haynes, R.R., and Thomas, J.D.: Drug Therapy in Resuscitation from Electromechanical Dissociation. Crit. Care Med., 11:681, 1983.

Reid, L.C., and Brace, D.E.: Imitation of Respiratory Tract and Its Reflex Effect on Heart Rate. Surg. Gynecol. Obstet., 70:157, 1940.

Rex, M.A.E.: Stimulation of Laryngospasm in the Cat by Volatile Anaesthetics. Br. J. Anaesth., 38:569, 1966.

Rosen, M.: Atropine in the Treatment of Laryngeal Spasm. Br. J. Anaesth., 32:190, 1960.

Riebold, T.W., Goble, D.O., and Geiser, D.R.: *Large Animal Anesthesia: Principles and Techniques*. The Iowa State Univesity Press, Ames, 1982.

Ross, J.N., and Breznock, E.M.: Resuscitation. In *Veterinary Critical Care*. Edited by F.P. Sattler, R.P. Knowles, and W.G. Whittick. Lea & Febiger, Philadelphia, 1981.

Safar, P.: Dynamics of Brain Resuscitation After Ischemic Anoxia. Hosp. Pract., 16:67, 1981.

Safar, P., and Harris, L.C.: The Beck-Rand External Cardiac Compression Machine. Anesthesiology, 24:586, 1963.

Sauer, B.W.: Valve Drainage of the Pleural Cavity of the Dog. J.A.V.M.A., 155:1997, 1969.

Schreiner, G.E.: The Role of Hemodialysis (Artificial Kidney) in Acute Poisoning. Arch. Intern. Med., 102:896, 1958.

Sladen, A.: Pharmacologic Management of Cardiopulmonary Resuscitation. Regional Refresher Courses in Anesthesiology, 4:113, 1976.

Spraker, T.R.: An Overview of the Pathophysiology of Capture Myopathy and Related Conditions that Occur at the Time of Capture of Wild Animals. Proc. N. Am. Symp.: Chemical Immobilization of Wildlife. Milwaukee, April, 1982.

Steen, P.A., Milde, J.H., and Michenfelder, J.D.: No Barbiturate Protection in a Dog Model of Complete Cerebral Ischemia. Ann. Neurol., 5:343, 1979.

Stephen, C.R.: Temperature Management—Problems and Solutions Outline. Annual Refresher Course Lectures, Am. Soc. Anesth., New York, 1970.

Swan, H., and Nelson, A.W.: Personal communication. Colorado State University, Fort Collins, 1969.

Swann, H.G., and Brucer, M.: The Sequence of Circulatory, Respiratory and Cerebral Failure During the Process of Death: Its Relation to Resuscitability. Texas Reports Biol. Med., 9:180, 1951.

Tacker, W.A., Niebauer, M.J., Babbs, C.F., Combs, W.J., Hahn, B.M., Barker, M.A., Seipel, J.F., Bourland, J.D., and Geddes, L.A.: The Effect of Newer Antiarrhythmic Drugs on Defibrillation Threshold. Crit. Care Med., 8:177, 1980.

Tucker, W.K., and Munson, E.S.: Effects of Succinylcholine and d-Tubocurarine on Epinephrine-Induced Arrhythmias During Halothane Anesthesia in Dogs. Anesthesiology, 42:41, 1975.

Van Vleet, J.F., Tacker, W.A., Jr., Geddes, L.A., and Ferrans, V.J.: Acute Cardiac Wave-Form Defibrillator. Am. J. Vet. Res., 38:617, 1977.

Ventureyra, E.C.G., and Ivan, L.P.: Brain Resuscitation. Can. J. Neurol. Sci., 6:71, 1979.

Voorhees, W.D., Babbs, C.F., and Tacker, W.A.: Regional Blood Flow During Cardiopulmonary Resuscitation in Dogs. Crit. Care Med., 8:134, 1980.

Waldron-Mease, E., and Rosenberg, H.: Post-Anesthetic Myositis in the Horse Associated with In Vitro Malignant Hyperthermia Susceptibility. Vet. Sci. Communications, 3:45, 1979.

Wallin, R.F.: Quest Discussion—Thermoregulatory Defect in Rats During Anesthesia. Anesth. Analg., 56:14, 1977.

Weaver, A.D.: Complications in Halothane Anaesthesia of Cattle. Zbl. Vet. Med. A, 18:409, 1971.

Weibe, W.H.: The Effect of Temperature on the Action of Drugs. Ann. Rev. Pharmacol., 13:409, 1973.

White, N.A., II: Postanesthetic Recumbency Myopathy in Horses: Cont. Ed. Pract. Vet. Large Anim. Suppl., 4:44, 1982.

Wiersig, D.O., Davis, R.H., Jr., and Szabuniewicz, M.: Prevention of Induced Fibrillation in Dogs Anesthetized with Ultrashort Acting Barbiturates and Halothane. J.A.V.M.A., 163:341, 1974.

Worman, L.W., and Seidel, B.: Treatment of Cerebral Air Embolism in the Dog. Am. J. Surg., 111:820, 1966.

Wycoff, C.C., and Cann, J.E.: Experimental Pulmonary Air Embolism in Dogs. Calif. Med., 105:361, 1966.

Yakaitis, R.W., Ewy, G.A., Oho, C.W., Taren, D.L., and Moon, T.E.: Influence of Time and Therapy on Ventricular Defibrillation in Dogs. Crit. Care Med., 8:157, 1980.

CHAPTER 22

Aftercare

Small Animals

Large Animals

Although in most instances recovery from anesthesia is uneventful, the patient should be kept under observation during the recovery period to prevent untoward sequelae. In animal hospitals and laboratory animal facilities, it is wise to have a recovery room for this purpose, since all the necessary equipment, drugs, and materials can be kept in one place, and it is less difficult to observe several animals. In some instances, the "prep" room may also serve as the recovery room; alternatively, recovery and intensive care functions may be combined. Such facilities should be conveniently located for nursing staff.

SMALL ANIMALS

Following removal from the operating room, the animal should be placed in its cage in lateral recumbency. While the animal remains unconscious or immobile, monitoring deemed necessary in the operating room should be continued. In any case, vital signs should be recorded at 15-minute intervals until the animal regains consciousness. Continued supervision is especially important until extubation and the return of coughing and swallowing reflexes. A blanket, pad, or even newspaper, should be placed under and over the patient to conserve body heat. In very small or newborn animals, the ambient temperature should approximate body temperature. Incubators designed for babies are helpful in maintaining body temperature and are used routinely in many laboratories where birds, rodents, and primates are anesthetized. In newborn pigs, an environmental temperature of 90° F has been found desirable (Landy, 1961). Otherwise, shivering occurs with increased oxygen and energy requirements, and hypoglycemia may result. During recovery, birds should be housed at 100° F, mice, hamsters, and small primates at 95° F, rats, guinea pigs, and rabbits at 90° F, and cats, dogs, and similar carnivores at 77 to 86° F (Green, 1979). Depending upon environmental temperatures, heat lamps, heating pads, or warm water blankets may be required (see Temperature Management in Chap. 21). If fluid therapy is used, fluids should be warmed to body temperature.

During recovery, the tongue should be pulled forward to preclude its blocking the pharynx. In brachycephalic breeds or in animals in which respiratory function is compromised, an endotracheal tube should remain in place until upper airway reflexes and jaw movements return. In such animals, sternal recumbency, if practical, is preferred. Care is necessary to assure freedom of the airway from blankets or paper. The water pan should always be removed from the cage to prevent accidental drowning, in the event the semiconscious patient should place its nose and mouth or endotracheal catheter in the container. As soon as the animal regains the righting reflex, the water pan should be returned to the cage and the animal encouraged to drink a small quantity. Food may be offered as soon as the patient can stand.

Predisposition to postoperative respiratory failure may result from continuing drug-induced respiratory depression, postextubation spasm or glottic edema, other respiratory obstructions, diffusion hypoxia (see Chap. 10), mechanical splinting associated with pain and/or dressings, and from persistent hypoventilation and/or atelectasis during anesthesia. Careful evaluation of respiration during the immediate postanesthetic period is therefore essential. If hypoventilation is identified, predisposing causes should be corrected if possible and, if necessary, supportive respiratory therapy should be initiated. Since postoperative hypotension may also occur as a result of a persistent drug effect, hemorrhage, and inadequate volume, adequacy of cardiovascular function should also be carefully and frequently evaluated.

Under no circumstances should an anesthetized animal be placed in the same cage with a conscious one, since the former cannot protect itself. Cannibalism has been known to occur, particularly where the anesthetized patient had an open wound!

When preanesthetic sedation has not been used, animals may thrash and struggle, bruising themselves severely and even breaking teeth during the recovery period. Coursing breeds, such as greyhounds, Russian wolfhounds, and Afghans, are particularly prone to this phenomenon. Judicious use of tranquilizers or narcotics in small doses will quiet animals in this condition. Plastic-covered sponge rubber mats or other suitable pads in recovery cages will also afford protection.

Following administration of pentobarbital, an occasional animal will have an extremely prolonged recovery period (see Chaps. 12 and 21; Table 23–13). Cats are more prone to this than dogs, sometimes sleeping as long as 72 hours before arousing. Special attention must be given these animals to prevent hypostatic congestion and subsequent pneumonia. They should, of course, be kept warm and turned frequently. In addition, prophylactic antibiotic therapy should be given, and a protective ophthalmic ointment instilled in the eyes to prevent corneal drying. Intravenous electrolyte solutions in moderate amounts prevent dehydration. If barbiturates have been used, dextrose or lactate solutions should be avoided because of their reanesthetizing potential.

Constrictive bandaging of the head or throat must be avoided because of the danger of asphyxiation. Occasionally cats that have been tightly bandaged around the abdomen show evidence of posterior paralysis on recovery. This condition is apparently caused by circulatory obstruction to the hindquarters. Removal of the bandage quickly restores them to normal.

Once the patient has regained righting reflexes, further postanesthetic care will be dictated by the animal's condition and the procedure for which anesthesia was administered.

It is unwise to send anesthetized animals home, since owners are generally unable to cope with any unusual situation that may arise. In addition, they may become alarmed by the signs of approaching consciousness and may demand service unnecessarily during the night or other inconvenient hours.

LARGE ANIMALS

Like the small animal, the large animal should be removed to a recovery room (stall). The room should be padded to minimize injury during emergence from the anesthetic and recovery of righting reflexes. Availability of oxygen and suction is essential. If a padded floor and pads are not available and it is necessary to use bedding material such as straw, this should be covered with a tarpaulin so that it is kept clear of the external nares or end of the endotracheal tube and the eyes. Use of pads beneath the head and limbs is essential (see Physical Injuries and Complications, Chap. 21). In the horse especially, protection of bony prominences from abrasion is essential. It is an excellent practice to bandage and pad all limbs prior to anesthesia and to keep these in place until recovery is complete. The head of the horse is especially subject to trauma during recovery with resulting abrasions, edema, and even facial paralysis. It should, therefore, be protected with a pad or a padded hood. Halters or headstalls should be used only while necessary and should be padded.

Whenever possible, the horse should be allowed to lie quietly in a darkened environment and should be neither restrained nor disturbed. The possibility of emergence struggling and of attempts to stand before coordination is fully recovered is thus less likely. If an endotracheal tube has been used, it should remain in situ until the return of upper airway and jaw reflexes necessitates its removal. As with the small animal, food and water should be removed from the stall until recovery is complete. If straw or other bedding material is used, the animal should be observed to prevent it from eating this. When eye reflexes have fully returned, and nystagmus and pupillary dilatation are absent, the horse is usually able to stand. While the animal is attempting to rise, a steady influence exerted by the handlers in holding up the head and in upward traction on the tail may be helpful.

Some horses, despite preanesthetic sedation, struggle during recovery from anesthesia. Restraint is therefore necessary. In such instances, hobbles and restraining ropes may be used to hold the head and neck down and in extension, or a tranquilizer or guaifenesin may be administered. Control by medication is preferable, although recovery may be prolonged with large doses. Small amounts of xylazine (~ 100 mg) have proved useful in alleviating pain and calming recovery without unduly lengthening it. Some veterinarians routinely restrain the horse either on the operating table or by ropes and hobbles until they judge the animal is able to stand. Such a practice predisposes to struggling and injuries.

When recovery rooms are not available, it may be necessary to permit recovery in the operating room. Operating rooms having a padded floor, or padded floor with table that lowers to floor level, are suitable. Restraint on the operating table until recovery is complete is undesirable, especially for the horse; struggling is likely and abrasions and nerve injuries are common. Rupture of the colon has been attributed to such restraint in several instances. If a cart is available to transport the animal, a grassy plot is a desirable location for recovery.

Ruminants are handled in a manner similar to that used for horses. Struggling and resulting trauma are usually not problems. Instead, it is necessary to minimize possible regurgitation and aspiration of rumen contents, and ruminal tympany. The endotracheal tube with cuff inflated should, therefore, remain in position as long as possible. Use of a speculum to prevent damage to or constriction of the tube is helpful. During recovery, the ruminant should be placed in sternal recumbency. If the flexed limbs are abducted slightly, it is usually possible to prop the animal in this position. Padded bolsters, other supports, or even bales of hay can be used to assist in maintaining this position. The head should be down and extended and the end of the endotracheal tube unobstructed. When anterior epidural anesthesia has been used, the hind legs should be hobbled to a degree sufficient to prevent abduction until muscle control is regained.

The recovering large animal should be protected from temperature extremes. In the absence of heating or air conditioning, blankets, heaters, or fans may be necessary. If an outside recovery area is used, the animal should be shaded from direct sunlight in hot weather and blanketed in cold weather. When recovery is prolonged, the animal should be turned frequently and warmed fluids should be administered intravenously.

As with the small animal, vital signs should be continually and routinely monitored until return of coughing, swallowing, and righting reflexes.

REFERENCES

Green, C.J.: *Animal Anaesthesia*. Laboratory Animals Ltd., London, 1979.

Landy, J.J.: The Use of Large Germfree Animals in Medical Research. J.A.M.A., 178:1084, 1961.

CHAPTER 23

Statistics and Records

REASONS FOR KEEPING RECORDS

Death of a patient from any cause is always unpleasant, but a fatality from anesthesia is even more so because it is obviously induced by the anesthesiologist. One will occasionally hear a veterinarian state that he has never lost an animal from anesthesia. This is conceivably true, though highly unlikely if a sizable number of animals have been anesthetized. Obviously, the criteria for anesthetic mortality in this instance must be defined. It is human nature to forget the disagreeable and to excuse a fatality by blaming it on something over which the anesthesiologist has no control.

As long as anesthetics are administered, the hazard of death can never be eliminated completely; it can, however, be minimized, particularly if one is willing to investigate and to learn from mistakes. Once an anesthetic fatality has occurred, the preceding events should be reviewed, and a necropsy should be performed to piece together its pathogenesis and etiology. Armed with this information, the anesthesiologist can then take steps to prevent a recurrence of this tragedy.

Unfortunately, there is little recorded information concerning mortality in animals anesthetized in clinical practice. This is because 1) busy practitioners do not have time to collect the necessary data, 2) there is no economic gain to be derived from such collection, and 3) there is lack of interest on the part of individuals best able to obtain these data. Clinics of veterinary schools in the United States are just beginning to have valid information on this subject.

DATA COLLECTION

To obtain meaningful data concerning anesthesia, certain information must be collected and definite criteria established. A record must be made for each animal anesthetized, with the owner's name and the case number written on it. Among the items that should be recorded are:

1. species, breed, age, sex, weight, and physical status of the animal;
2. surgical procedure or other reason for anesthesia;
3. preanesthetic agents given;
4. anesthetic agents used and method of administration;
5. person administering anesthesia (veterinarian, technician, student, lay personnel);
6. duration of anesthesia;
7. supportive measures; and
8. difficulties encountered and methods of correction.

Tabulation of these data will give not only extensive information on anesthesia, but also the incidence of surgical diseases in various species, age groups, and breeds.

Obviously, moribund patients are not good anesthetic risks, and if a single agent is used to anesthetize them, the mortality rate for this agent may appear to be disproportionately high.

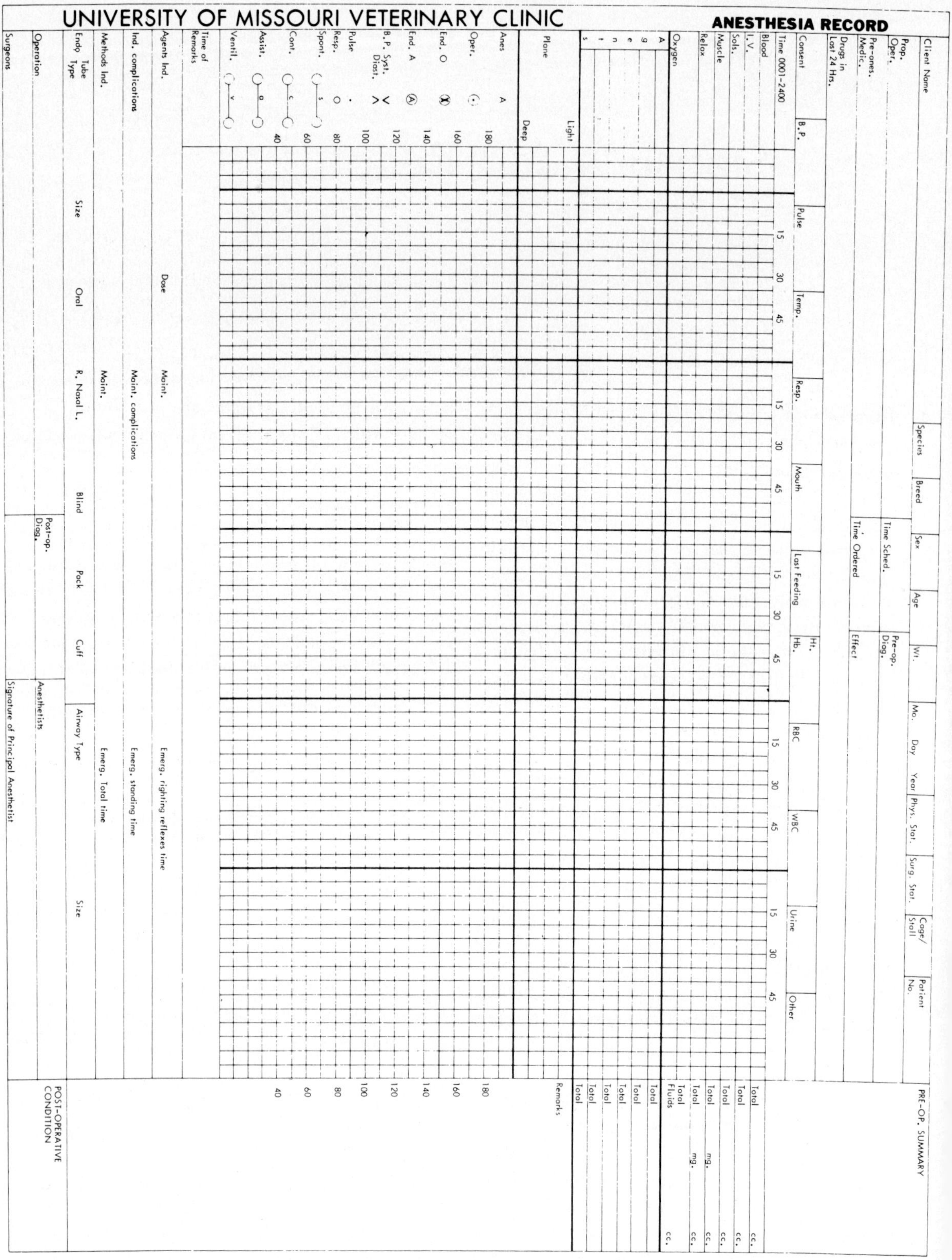

Figure 23–1. Anesthetic record used at the University of Missouri Veterinary Clinic.

Category			
	Morph.	Innovar	Barb.
PRE-MED.	Dem.	Atrop.	
	I.M.	I.V.	
	Rectal	Oral	
	Satis.	Inadeq.	Excess
RELAX	d-T-C	Succin.	Over Dose
	Flax.		Antidote
VASO-CONST.	Epinep.	Nor-ep.	Other
I.V. THERAP.	Blood	Plasma	Dextran
	Packed Cells	Albumin	
	5 % Gluc. & H_2O	Gluc./Sal.	Saline
	Ringers	Lactate	
PHYSICAL STATUS	1. Good	2. Fair	
	3. Poor	4. Bad	
	5. Emergency (Good)		
	6. Emergency (Bad)		
	7. Moribund		
PRE-OP. THERAP.	Digit.	Antihypert	Endocr.
	Barbit.	Narcot.	Blood
	Fluids	Vasoconst.	
AGE OF PATIENT	- 1 mo.	- 6 mo.	- 1
	- 2	- 3	- 4
	- 5	- 6	- 7
	- 10	-15	+ 15
WEIGHT OF PATIENT	- 5	- 10	- 25
	- 50	- 100	- 250
	- 500	- 1000	+ 1000
HEAD & NECK	Nasal	Eye	Dental
	Plastic	Ear	Neck
	Superficial	Intracranial	
THORAX	Cardiac	Great Vessels	Lung
	Mediast.	Intrapleural	Thor. Cage
	Thor. Superfic.		
UPPER ABDOMEN	Stom. & Duoden.	Colon	Pancreas
	Spleen	Rumen	Liver
	Renal	Retro-perit.	Other
LOWER ABD.	Bowel		U.G. Ops.
	Preg. Ops.	Gyn. Ops.	Other
ABD. WALL	Inguin.	Lumbar	Abdomen Super.
	Extra-perit.		
PERIN.	Perin. U.G.	Perin Gyn.	Perin. Obs.
	Anorectal	Other	
EXTRE.	Column	Cord	Spine
	Bone	Upper	Joint
	Soft	Lower	Foot
POSITION	Supine	Prone	Trendel.
	L. Lat.	R. Lat.	Flexed
	Head up	Head down	
	Heparin	Protomine	Klot
pH	Na bicarbonate		Na lactate
VASO. PRESS	Neo-Syn.	I.V.	Isuprel
	Drip.	Levophed	
DEATH	Prevent.	Non-prevent	Pt. Disease
	Anes.	Surg.	Complic.

PRE-OP. SUMMARY

POST-OP. SUMMARY

PREV. ANES. COMPLICATIONS

RESP.	11. Pneu. 12. Hemorrhage 13. Bronch. 14. Trach. 15. Laryng. 16. Empyema
	17. Emphysema 18. Foreign body.
CARDIO VASC.	19. Cong. H.D. 20. R.H.D. 21. Arterioscle. 22. Hypertens. 23. Hypotens.
	24. Failure 25. Arrhyth. 26. Pulm. Edema 27. Other
NEUROL.	28. Br. Tu. 29. Cd. Tu. 30. Lues 31. Epilep. 32. Paral.
	33. Irrat 34. Other
G.I.	35. Int. Obst. 36. Perf. Vis. 37. Periton. 38. Ileus 39. Carcinoma
	40. Emesis 41. Other
G.U.	42. Cystit. 43. Pyel. 44. Nephrit. 45. Anuria 46. Hemat. 47. Album. 48. Glucos.
	49. Acetone 50. Other
METABOL.	51. Diab. 52. Obese 53. Acid 54. Alkal. 55. Dehydration 56. Other
HEMATOL.	57. Anemia 58. Hypovol. 59. Polycyth. 60. Leuco. 61. Leucopenia 62. Other
NO. COMP.	63. No. Pre-op. 64. No. Post-op. 65. Neither 66. Death 67. Autopsy

Category	Method	Ind.	Main	Emer.	Sup-ple
GENERAL METHODS	O.D.				
	NRB				
	Mask				
	Semi-closed				
	Circle				
	To & Fro				
	Insuff.				
	I.V.				
	I.M.				
	Rectal				
	Other				

Category	Agent	Ind.	Main	Emer.	Supp.
GENERAL AGENTS	Ether				
	C_HCl_3				
	Elect.				
	Nitrous Oxide				
	Chloral				
	Surital				
	Pentothal				
	Other Barb.				
	Metafane				
	Fluothane				

Category			
ENDO.	L. Nasal	R. Nasal	Oral
	Cuff	Pack	₮ Cuff or Pack
	Blind	Under Mask	

Category	
IND. COMPLIC.	Excitability
	Cardiac arrest
	Respiratory arrest
	Brady cardia
	Tachy cardia
	Over dosage
	Under dosage
ANES. COMPLIC.	Cardiac arrest
	Respiratory arrest
	Brady cardia
	Tachy cardia
	Other arrhyth.
	Hypertension
	Hypotension
	Inst. muscle relax.
	Pain
	Alkalosis
	Acidosis
	Hypoxia
EMER. COMPLIC.	Excitement
	Convulsions
	Paralysis
	Vomiting
	Cynosis
	Laryngeal spasm
	Laryngeal edema
	Pulmonary edema
	Hemorrhage

Category			
STIM.	Mike.	Ritalin	Amph.
	Dopram	I.V.	
CARD. CONT.	$CaCl_2$	Ca Glu	Digit.
	Pronestyl	Xylo.	Epinep.
	I.V.		

Figure 23–1 ***Continued.***

TABLE 23–1. ASA Classification of Physical Status

1. A normal healthy patient.
2. A patient with a mild systemic disease.
3. A patient with a severe systemic disease.
4. A patient with severe systemic disease that is a constant threat to life.
5. A moribund patient not expected to survive 24 hours with or without operation.

In the event of emergency operation, precede the number with an E.

When one is discussing anesthetic mortality, therefore, it is necessary to categorize the physical status of the patient. The American Society of Anesthesiologists (ASA) has developed a five-division classification (Table 23–1).

It should be emphasized that physical status, anesthetic risk, and operative risk are entirely different. To determine anesthetic risk, many factors must be considered, including the degree of skill of the anesthetist, the anesthetic to be employed, and the physical status of the patient. To determine operative risk, the foregoing must be appraised and, in addition, the operation to be performed and the skill of the surgeon must also be taken into consideration.

For man, it is considered absolutely necessary that each step of anesthetic administration be recorded along with the patient's response. Commonly, the pulse, blood pressure, and respiratory rate are monitored at 5-minute intervals and charted. Trends in these parameters thus become apparent before the patient's condition deteriorates seriously, so that remedial steps may be taken. This type of recording has been introduced in veterinary anesthesia, principally in university hospitals (Fig. 23–1).

Marginal punched cards have also been used. The holes along the margins are coded according to the information to be recorded (Schwabe and Davis, 1954). The face of each card may have the code printed on it, or a master code card may be used and the other cards punched using it as the key.

Combinations utilizing the principles of both systems have been used for man. Where large numbers of animals are anesthetized, marginal punched cards become cumbersome to manage during data retrieval. For this reason, computerization of records has been adopted in large institutions and is gradually becoming more widespread.

SURVEY OF ANESTHESIAS AT COLORADO STATE UNIVERSITY (1955–1957)

During the years 1955 through 1957* records were kept of all small animal anesthesias at the Colorado State University Veterinary Hospital, using marginal punched cards (Lumb, 1963). Results of 2912 anesthetic periods in dogs and cats, using a wide variety of preanesthetics and general anesthetics, are summarized in Tables 23–2 through 23–13.

An anesthetic death was defined as *any death occurring from the time of induction until the righting reflex returned, regardless of cause.*

The mean age of both dogs and cats dying under anesthesia was slightly higher than the mean age for each species (Tables 23–4 and 23–5). Mortality in spayed females of both species was higher than in intact animals of either sex (Table 23–6). This finding suggests that physiologic changes produced by spaying may have an adverse affect on the animal's ability to withstand the stress of anesthesia and surgery. On the other hand, the mean age of all spayed animals (4.465 years) was considerably higher than the mean age of the group.

By breed, the highest mortality was in the cocker spaniel, which at this time was probably the most common purebred seen at the clinic (Table 23–7). Only two brachycephalic dogs died: a bulldog and a pekingese.

Table 23–8 lists the relationship of physical status to deaths. As expected, the mortality rate increased sharply as physical status deteriorated. There were various reasons for poor physical status (Table 23–9). In some instances, anesthesia was administered and surgery performed as a last resort on animals that otherwise would have died within hours. The percent mortality in all categories of physical status was higher in cats than dogs indicating a species intolerance to the anesthetics used.

*Except summer months.

TABLE 23–2. Physical Status and Percent Mortality of 2406 Dogs Anesthetized with Various Agents (Colorado State University, 1955–1957)

	*Status I**			*Status II**			*Status III**			*Status IV**			*All Categories*		
Agent(s)	*Total*	*Died***	*% Mortality†*	*Total*	*Died***	*% Mortality†*	*Total*	*Died***	*% Mortality†*	*Total*	*Died***	*% Mortality†*	*Total*	*Died***	*% Mortality†*
Pentobarbital	939	5	0.532	384	6	1.562	62	0	0.0	16	2	12.50	1401	13	0.928
Thiamylal	118	0	0.0	361	0	0.0	64	0	0.0	8	2	25.0	551	2	0.363
Thiopental	—	–	—	1	0	0.0	—	–	—	—	–	—	1	0	0.0
Combuthal‖	3	0	0.0	5	0	0.0	1	1	100.0	—	–	—	9	1	11.111
Pentobarbital-thiamylal	11	0	0.0	14	0	0.0	1	0	0.0	2	1	50.0	28	1	3.571
Ether (S)‡	—	–	—	1	0	0.0	—	–	—	—	–	—	1	0	0.0
Ether (C)§	1	0	0.0	4	0	0.0	1	0	0.0	—	–	—	6	0	0.0
Ether (S & C)	—	–	—	—	–	—	1	0	0.0	1	1	100.0	2	1	50.0
Pentobarbital-ether (S)	9	0	0.0	3	0	0.0	1	0	0.0	—	–	—	13	0	0.0
Pentobarbital-ether (C)	4	0	0.0	9	0	0.0	1	0	0.0	2	0	0.0	16	0	0.0
Thiamylal-ether (C)	55	1	1.818	113	1	0.885	40	1	2.50	24	5	20.833	232	8	3.448
Combuthal-ether (C)	1	0	0.0	—	–	—	—	–	—	—	–	—	1	0	0.0
Thiopental-ether (C)	—	–	—	2	0	0.0	—	–	—	—	–	—	2	0	0.0
Pentobarbital-thiamylal-ether (C)	1	0	0.0	—	–	—	—	–	—	—	–	—	1	0	0.0
Halothane (C)	—	–	—	—	–	—	1	0	0.0	—	–	—	1	0	0.0
Pentobarbital-halothane (C)	1	0	0.0	2	0	0.0	—	–	—	1	0	0.0	4	0	0.0
Thiamylal-halothane (C)	39	1	2.564	65	0	0.0	24	0	0.0	6	0	0.0	134	1	0.746
Thiopental-halothane (C)	—	–	—	—	–	—	1	0	0.0	—	–	—	1	0	0.0
Combuthal-halothane (C)	2	0	0.0	—	–	—	—	–	—	—	–	—	2	0	0.0
Totals	1184	7	0.591	964	7	0.726	198	2	1.010	60	11	18.333	2406	27	1.122

*For Physical Status see Table 23–8.
**Includes all animals dying for any reason between induction of anesthesia and return of righting reflex.

$$\dagger\text{Percent mortality} = \frac{\text{Number dead}}{\text{Number anesthetized}}$$

‡S = Administered by semiopen drop method.
§C = Administered in a closed system with carbon dioxide absorption by soda lime.
‖ = Mixture of thiopental (75%) and pentobarbital (25%).

TABLE 23–3. Physical Status and Percent Mortality of 506 Cats Anesthetized with Various Agents (Colorado State University, 1955–1957)

	Status I*			Status II*			Status III*			Status IV*			All Categories		
Agent(s)	*Total*	*Died*	*% Mortality†*	*Total*	*Died**	*% Mortality†*	*Total*	*Died***	*% Mortality†*	*Total*	*Died***	*% Mortality†*	*Total*	*Died***	*% Mortality†*
Pentobarbital	234	3	1.282	37	1	2.702	10	1	10.0	1	0	0.0	282	5	1.773
Thiamylal	114	0	0.0	44	0	0.0	15	0	0.0	2	1	50.0	175	1	0.571
Thiopental	1	0	0.0	—	–	—	—	–	—	—	–	—	1	0	0.0
Combuthal‖	2	0	0.0	1	0	0.0	—	–	—	—	–	—	3	0	0.0
Pentobarbital-thiamylal	2	0	0.0	1	0	0.0	1	0	0.0	—	–	—	4	0	0.0
Ether (C)§	—	–	—	—	–	—	2	0	0.0	4	1	25.0	6	1	16.667
Pentobarbital-ether (C)	1	0	0.0	—	–	—	—	–	—	—	–	—	1	0	0.0
Pentobarbital-ether (S)‡	5	1	20.0	1	0	0.0	—	–	—	—	–	—	6	1	16.667
Thiamylal-ether (C)	—	–	—	—	–	—	—	–	—	1	1	100.0	1	1	100.0
Thiamylal-ether (S)	—	–	—	1	0	0.0	—	–	—	—	–	—	1	0	0.0
Thiamylal-cyclopropane (C)	—	–	—	—	–	—	—	–	—	1	0	0.0	1	0	0.0
Ethyl chloride (S)	1	0	0.0	—	–	—	2	0	0.0	—	–	—	3	0	0.0
Trichloroethylene (S)	17	0	0.0	5	0	0.0	—	–	—	—	–	—	22	0	0.0
Totals	377	4	1.061	90	1	1.111	30	1	3.333	9	3	33.333	506	9	1.778

*For Physical Status see Table 23–8.

**Includes all animals dying for any reason between induction of anesthesia and return of righting reflex.

$$\dagger\text{Percent mortality} = \frac{\text{Number dead}}{\text{Number anesthetized}}$$

‡S = Administered by semiopen drop method.

§C = Administered in a closed system with carbon dioxide absorption by soda lime.

‖ = Mixture of thiopental (75%) and pentobarbital (25%).

TABLE 23–4. Mean Age and Sex of Dogs and Cats Anesthetized at Colorado State University (1955–1957)

Species	*Total Anesthetized*	*Mean Age**	*Sex*			
			M	*CM†*	*F*	*SF‡*
Canine	2406	2.798	967	38	1103	298
Feline	506	1.818	201	33	250	22
Canine and Feline	2912	2.308	1168	71	1353	320

*Of animals with known age. Animals less than 1 year figured as 7 months.
†CM = Castrated male.
‡SF = Spayed female.

TABLE 23–5. Age of Animals Dying Under Anesthesia (Colorado State University, 1955–1957)

Canine		*Feline*	
Age in Years	*Number*	*Age in Years*	*Number*
<1	1	<1	2
1	6	1	1
2	5	2	1
3	2	3	2
4	2	9	1
5	1	Unknown	2
6	2		
7	3		
Unknown	5		
Mean Age* 3.122 Years		Mean Age* 2.738 Years	

*Of animals with known age. Animals less than 1 year figured as 7 months.

A high mortality in healthy animals was associated with ovariohysterectomy. Four cats and four dogs died during or following this operation. All eight were anesthetized and operated upon by students. Three of these animals died of hemoperitoneum with associated cardiovascular collapse.

Some deaths occurred from poor judgment on the part of the anesthesiologist. Examples include administration of morphine, pentobarbital, or pentobarbital-thiamylal to animals in physical status IV (Table 23–10). A more serious error was injection of a gross overdose of pentobarbital. Six animals received glucose, which may have deepened barbiturate anesthesia in the presence of shock. One death occurred because of ineptitude in placement of an endotracheal catheter.

Cardiac massage was performed in four dogs. Two of these resumed function but died after 8 and 14 hours, respectively.

Approximately two-thirds of the fatalities occurred after surgery was completed and the animal was presumably recovering (Table 23–11). Of the 36 animals that died, 7 were found dead without previous knowledge of complication. Continuous surveillance of these animals was not maintained. Closer postoperative observation would probably have saved some of these.

Two cats given pentobarbital remained anesthetized for 24 and 36 hours and succumbed despite resuscitative measures.

Complications requiring some type of cor-

TABLE 23–6. Sex of Animals Dying Under Anesthesia Compared to Total Anesthetized (Colorado State University, 1955–1957)

	Sex	*Deaths*	*Total Anesthetized*	*Percent Mortality*	*Ratio*
Canine	Male	11	967	1.137	1:87.9
	Castrated male	0	38	—	—
	Female	11	1103	0.997	1:100
	Spayed female	5	298	1.678	1:59.6
Feline	Male	2	201	0.995	1:100
	Castrated male	0	33	—	—
	Female	5	250	2.00	1:50
	Spayed female	2	22	9.09	1:11

TABLE 23–7. Breed of Animals Dying Under Anesthesia (Colorado State University, 1955–1957)

Dogs		*Cats*	
Breed	*Number*	*Breed*	*Number*
Mixed breed	13	Domestic	9
Cocker spaniel	4		
Chihuahua	2		
Dachshund	2		
Bulldog	1		
Chesapeake retriever	1		
English cocker spaniel	1		
Greyhound	1		
Labrador retriever	1		
Pekingese	1		

rective measure arose in 5.46% of animals anesthetized with a general anesthetic. Hypopnea and respiratory arrest were most common and occurred with a variety of anesthetic agents (Table 23–12). Shock and hemorrhage were encountered less frequently, occurring in 18 dogs and 3 cats.

Several animals remained anesthetized for prolonged periods and eventually aroused (Table 23–13). The susceptibility of cats to pentobarbital, and even thiamylal, was evident; 4.6% of all cats receiving pentobarbital were anesthetized 14 hours or more, whereas only 0.57% of the dogs were so affected. When thiamylal was used in cats, 1.14% were anesthetized 15 hours or longer.

Violent excitement on recovery was seen in 8 dogs, 4 greyhounds and 4 of mixed breeding. These quieted on administration of meperidine.

Other miscellaneous complications included one case of hyperpnea, due to exhaustion of soda lime during thiamylal-ether anesthesia, and one instance of mechanical failure of an anesthetic machine.

Reflex contraction of the diaphragm synchronous with the heartbeat developed in a dog following a hypoxic episode (Brown and Lumb, 1958). This was successfully treated by intravenous administration of 1 ml of 50% calcium gluconate.

Nonfatal cardiac arrest occurred in one dog and one cat. Direct cardiac massage was successful in the dog, but it was blind and ataxic thereafter. The cat was treated with external massage and intracardial epinephrine and completely recovered.

TABLE 23–8. Relationship of Physical Status to Anesthetic Deaths (Colorado State University, 1955–1957)

	*Physical Status**	*Deaths*	*Total Anesthetized*	*Percent Mortality*	*Ratio*
Canine	I	7	1184	0.591	1:169
	II	7	964	0.726	1:138
	III	2	198	1.010	1:99
	IV	11	60	18.333	1:5.4
Feline	I	4	377	1.061	1:94
	II	1	90	1.111	1:90
	III	1	30	3.333	1:30
	IV	3	9	33.333	1:3

	**Physical Status*	*Possible Examples of This Category*
I	Healthy No discernible disease	Animals entered for ovariohysterectomy, ear trim, caudectomy
II	Preexisting disease No discernible systemic symptoms	Skin tumor, fracture without shock, uncomplicated hernia, localized infection, compensated cardiac disease
III	Preexisting disease Mild systemic symptoms	Low fever, slight dehydration, slight anemia, slight cachexia
IV	Preexisting disease Severe systemic symptoms	Uremia, toxemia, severe shock, severe dehydration, anemia, cardiac decompensation, emaciation, high fever; includes all moribund animals.

TABLE 23–9. Analysis of Anesthetic Deaths in 36 Dogs and Cats (Colorado State University, 1955–1957)

A. CANINE

Anesthetic Agent	*P.S.**	*Sex*	*Age (Yr)*	*Breed*	*Reason for Anesthesia*	*Reason for Physical Status*	*Reason for Death, if Known*
Pentobarbital	I	F	2	Lab. ret.	Ovariohysterectomy	Healthy	Hemoperitoneum
		F	Unknown	Mixed	Ovariohysterectomy	Healthy	Hemoperitoneum
		F	1	Mixed	Ovariohysterectomy	Healthy	Respiratory failure followed by cardiac failure; cardiac massage unsuccessful
		F	7	C. spaniel	Ovariohysterectomy	Healthy	Gross overdose of anesthetic
		M	Unknown	Mixed	Liver biopsy	Healthy	Undetermined; died during night
	II	Sp F	2	Mixed	Excision of nasal tumor	Nasal tumor	Died on induction; thoracotomy and cardiac massage, died 14 hrs later
		Sp F	2	Chihuahua	Umbilical herniorraphy	Umbilical hernia	Undetermined; found dead 13 hrs postinduction
		M	Unknown	Bulldog	Entropion operation	Entropion	Died before surgery; endotracheal catheter in esophagus; cardiac massage unsuccessful
		M	2	Mixed	To perform cerebral angiogram	Anesthetized previous day with pentobarbital and not fully recovered	Died after both carotid arteries injected with Diodrast
		M	1	Mixed	Prostatectomy	Suppurating wound on thorax	Respiratory arrest during operation
		M	Unknown	Mixed	Castration	Distemper, without systemic symptoms	Undetermined, died during night
	IV	F	4	Pekingese	Lumbar myelogram	Ruptured intervertebral disc with systemic infection, urinary retention	Died 3 hrs following myelogram
		F	<1	Mixed	To control convulsions	Distemper with encephalitis	Died 1 hr postinduction
Thiamylal	IV	F	3	C. spaniel	Débridement and suturing of severe skin laceration	Severe skin laceration with hemorrhage, shock, internal injuries	Respiratory failure during operation, shock, internal hemorrhage
		F	1	Mixed	Ligation of hepatic artery	Systolic murmur, ascites	Cardiac failure

(Continued on p. 620.)

TABLE 23–9. Analysis of Anesthetic Deaths in 36 Dogs and Cats (Colorado State University, 1955–1957) *(Continued)*

A. CANINE

Anesthetic Agent	*P.S.**	*Sex*	*Age (Yr)*	*Breed*	*Reason for Anesthesia*	*Reason for Physical Status*	*Reason for Death, if Known*
Thiamylal-ether	*I*	*M*	*7*	*Mixed*	*Esophagogastrectomy*	*Healthy*	*Surgical shock*
(Closed system)	*II*	*Sp F*	*1*	*Mixed*	*Diaphragmatic herniorrhaphy*	*Had recent surgery*	*Hemothorax and shock*
	III	*F*	*1*	*Chihuahua*	*Cesarean section*	*Dystocia, dehydrated, thin*	*Shock from intrauterine hemorrhage*
	IV	*M*	*2*	*C. spaniel*	*Diaphragmatic herniorrhaphy*	*Diaphragmatic hernia with severe dyspnea*	*Died from shock during operation*
		M	*6*	*English c. spaniel*	*Herniorrhaphy and partial splenectomy*	*Traumatic ventral hernia*	*Shock*
		M	*7*	*C. spaniel*	*Thoracotomy*	*Debilitated, weak, temperature 104° F*	*Undetermined; died during night*
	IV	Sp F	7	Dachshund	Exploratory celiotomy	Nephritis	Died on induction; toxemia and shock
		Sp. F	4	Mixed	Intestinal anastomosis	Peritonitis from perforated intestine; vomiting, dehydration; temperature 100.4° F	Shock, toxemia
Thiamylal-halothane (Closed system)	I	F	1	Mixed	Ovariohysterectomy	Healthy	Died during induction of halothane; probably gross overdose; cardiac massage, died 8 hrs later
Combuthal†	III	M	5	Dachshund	Excision of intervertebral disc	Ruptured intervertebral disc	Respiratory arrest
Pentobarbital-thiamylal	IV	M	6	Chesapeake	Liver biopsy	Generalized neoplastic disease	Undetermined; died during night
Ether (Open and closed system)	IV	F	3	Greyhound	Ovariohysterectomy	Dystocia with metritis, toxemia, temperature 106° F; macerated fetuses	Toxemia; died on induction

B. FELINE

Pentobarbital	I	Sp F	7	Domestic	Splenectomy	Healthy	Found dead following morning
		F	1	Domestic	Ovariohysterectomy	Healthy	Hemoperitoneum
		F	<1	Domestic	Ovariohysterectomy	Healthy	Undetermined; found dead 9 hrs postoperatively
	II	F	3	Domestic	Ovariohysterectomy	Thin but otherwise asymptomatic	Died 36 hrs following induction without arousing
	III	Sp F	7	Domestic	Splenectomy	Off feed, dehydrated, infected skin wound, temperature 101.8° F	Died 24 hrs following induction without arousing
Pentobarbital-ether (Open)	I	F	2	Domestic	Ovariohysterectomy	Healthy	Pentobarbital anesthesia lightened so ether administered by mask; respirations and heartbeat ceased
Ether (Closed system)	IV	M	9	Domestic	Excision of ampulla of Vater, with reimplantation into duodenum	Cachectic, jaundiced, dyspnea	Surgical shock; common bile duct occluded at duodenum
Thiamylal	IV	M	<1	Domestic	Catheterization of urethra	Urinary retention, uremia, depression	Respiratory arrest; bladder ruptured on induction
Thiamylal-ether (Closed system)	IV	F	3	Domestic	Pulmonary lobectomy	Emaciated, dehydrated, temperature 102.8° F; pulmonary abscess diagnosed radiographically	Airway occluded by pus from abscess

*P.S. = Physical Status (see Table 23–8).
† = Mixture of thiopental (75%) and pentobarbital (25%).

TABLE 23–10. Preanesthetic and Anesthetic Agents Used in Fatalities (Colorado State University, 1955–1957)

A. CANINE

Preanesthetic(s)	*Anesthetic(s)*	*P.S.**	*Fatalities*
Atropine	Thiamylal-ether (C†)	I	1
		III	1
		IV	2
	Ether (S‡ and C)	IV	1
Morphine-Atropine	Pentobarbital	I	5
		II	6
		IV	2
	Pentobarbital-thiamylal	IV	1
	Combuthal§	III	1
	Thiamylal-ether	II	1
		IV	2
	Thiamylal	I	1
		IV	1
None	Thiamylal	IV	1
	Thiamylal-ether	IV	1
B. FELINE			
Atropine	Pentobarbital	I	1
	Thiamylal-ether (C)	IV	1
None	Pentobarbital	I	2
		II	1
		III	1
	Pentobarbital-ether	I	1
	Ether	IV	1
	Thiamylal	IV	1

*P.S. = Physical Status (see footnote Table 23–8).
†C = Closed system with carbon dioxide absorption by soda lime.
‡S = Semiopen.
§ = Mixture of thiopental (75%) and pentobarbital (25%).

TABLE 23–11. Time of Death (Colorado State University, 1955–1957)

Species	*Before Surgery*	*During Surgery*	*After Surgery*
Canine (27 deaths)	6	6	15
Feline (9 deaths)	0	2	7

TABLE 23–12. Hypopnea and Respiratory Arrest (Colorado State University, 1955–1957)

	Hypopnea		*Respiratory Arrest*	
Agent	*Canine*	*Feline*	*Canine*	*Feline*
Pentobarbital	32	1	22	1
Thiamylal	2	2	8	—
Thiamylal-ether	—	—	3	—
Thiamylal-halothane	—	—	5	—

TABLE 23–13. Prolonged Anesthesia (Colorado State University, 1955–1957)

Duration of Anesthesia in Hours	*Pentobarbital*		*Thiamylal*	*Thiamylal-Pentobarbital*
	Canine	*Feline*	*Feline*	*Canine*
14	3	2	—	—
15	—	—	1	—
16	1	2	—	—
17	—	4	—	—
18	1	2	1	—
19	2	—	—	—
22	—	1	—	—
24	—	1	—	—
30	1	—	—	—
31	—	—	—	1
72	—	1	—	—
Totals	8	13	2	1

SURVEY OF ANESTHESIAS AT COLORADO STATE UNIVERSITY (1979–1981)

A more recent survey of anesthesia in dogs, cats, and horses has been made by Perkins et al. (1982) at Colorado State University. They anesthetized 9968 animals of these species between 1979 and 1981, with an overall mortality rate of 0.53% (Table 23–14).

Surprisingly, of the 32 dogs and cats that died, one-half were in ASA physical status I or II (Tables 23–1; 23–15). No breed predisposition to fatality was observed in dogs; 18 breeds were represented in 27 deaths. Only one dog was brachycephalic. Deaths in dogs were attributed to a variety of problems. Overdosage of anesthetic(s) was a common cause of death. Failure to add oxygen to nitrous oxide produced hypoxic deaths in two dogs and one cat. Mechanical problems with endotracheal tubes contributed to two deaths. Hypothermia occurred in some cases. Hypoventilation and cardiovascular collapse were the most common causes.

The lowest mortality rate (0.25%) was in cats, which compares favorably with the data of Lumb (1963) where the rate was 1.78%. The improvement can be attributed to several factors, including abandonment of pentobarbital and/or ether, use of newer agents and techniques, and improvement in supervision and training of student anesthetists. The 5 cats that died were all of the domestic breed and were given various preanesthetic and anesthetic agents.

The highest mortality rate was in horses (1.18%), attesting to the difficulty of anesthetizing and maintaining homeostasis in such a large species. Many of these animals were in acute condition from colic before being anesthetized (Table 23–16). On the other hand, two died from human error in the use of N_2O and

TABLE 23–14. Summary of Anesthetic Fatalities in Dogs, Cats, and Horses at Colorado State University (1979–1981)

	Anesthesias				*Anesthetic Fatalities*			
Year	*Canine*	*Feline*	*Equine*	*Total*	*Canine*	*Feline*	*Equine*	*Total*
1979	1,757	588	442	2,787	12	3	6	21
1980	2,097	605	609	3,311	7	1	6	14
1981	2,406	737	727	3,870	8	1	9	18
Total	6,260	1,930	1,778	9,968	27	5	21	53
Percent Mortality					0.43	0.25	1.18	0.53

(From Perkins, D., Heath, R.B., and Lumb, W.V.: Unpublished data. Colorado State University, Fort Collins, 1982.)

TABLE 23–15. Analysis of Anesthetic Deaths in 32 Dogs and Cats at Colorado State University (1979–1981)

*Sex**	*Age*	*Breed*	*Reason for Anesthesia*	*Physical Status† and Reason*	*Preanesthetic and Anesthetic Agents Used*	*Reason for Death*
Dogs, 1979						
s/F	10 yrs	Scottie	Rectal pull through for stricture due to previous surgery for tumor removal	II, Decreased potassium level	Atropine, oxymorphone, halothane-N_2O	O.d.‡ halothane, K^+ in drip, PCVs, arrest; no response to CPR
F	2 mos	German shepherd	Vascular ring anomaly	II, Decreased cardiac function	Atropine, oxymorphone, methoxyflurane-N_2O	Bradycardia, isoproterenol, fibrillation; no response to CPR
M	10 yrs	Chihuahua	Diaphragmatic hernia	II, Dyspnea	Atropine, oxymorphone, acepromazine, methoxyflurane	Hypothermia—off table at 96° F, died 6 hrs later in ICU
M	2 yrs	Samoyed	Pulmonic stenosis	III, Right heart enlargement, grade III systolic murmur	Atropine, oxymorphone, acepromazine, methoxyflurane	Poor monitoring—o.d. halothane
M	3 yrs	Beagle	Open heart surgery (Epstein anomaly)	IV, Epstein anomaly	Atropine, oxymorphone, acepromazine, methoxyflurane	Bypass machine not heparinized properly, blood clotted, fibrillated
s/F	6 yrs	Saint Bernard	Amputation	II, Osteosarcoma	Atropine, fentanyl, droperidol, halothane	O.d. halothane
M	5 mos	Afghan	Wound repair	II, Post-trauma	Atropine, fentanyl, halothane, methoxyflurane	Both halothane and methoxyflurane inadvertently used, o.d.
M	8 yrs	Dachshund	Cervical slotting	III, Cardiac valvular insufficiency	Atropine, diazepam, ketamine, methoxyflurane	Right heart failure
F	2 mos	Cocker spaniel	Patent ductus arteriosus	IV, Patent ductus arteriosus	Atropine, halothane then methoxyflurane	Acute hemorrhage from surgical error
F	9 yrs	Golden Labrador	Cesarean section	II, Emphysematous fetus	Atropine, mepivacaine epidural	Hypotension, hypoventilation
F	3 yrs	Pomeranian	Fractured ulna repair	II, Recent traumatic fracture	Atropine, oxymorphone, acepromazine, halothane-N_2O	Turned on N_2O without O_2
M	1 yr	Irish setter	Salivary mucocele	II, Salivary mucocele	Atropine, oxymorphone, acepromazine, methoxyflurane-N_2O	Possibly vagal stimulation

Dogs, 1980						
M	2 mos	Australian shepherd	Patent ductus arteriosus	III, Patent ductus arteriosus	Atropine, acepromazine, halothane (mask) then methoxyflurane	O.d. or endotracheal tube too long
M	9 yrs	Poodle	Exploratory laparotomy	E III, Elevated liver enzymes	Atropine, acepromazine, halothane (mask), methoxyflurane-N_2O	Circulatory collapse-brain death
F	3 yrs	Malamute	Thoracotomy	III, Pericarditis-coccidioidomycosis, pleural effusion	Atropine, acepromazine, thiopental, methoxyflurane	Hypoxia due to hypoventilation
M	3 yrs	Irish setter	Gastrotomy repair	IV, Peritonitis, septicemia	Atropine, acepromazine, oxymorphone, methoxyflurane	Septicemic shock
M	11 yrs	Mix	Skull roentgenogram	II, Senility	Atropine, acepromazine, thiopental, methoxyflurane	Respiratory then cardiac arrest
M	6 yrs	Malamute	Repair anastomosis	E IV, Peritonitis	Atropine, acepromazine, thiopental, methoxyflurane	Septicemic shock
M	1 yr	Cocker	Castration	I, Healthy	Atropine, acepromazine, thiopental, methoxyflurane	Turned on N_2O without O_2
Dogs, 1981						
M	21 mos	West Highland terrier	Repair of ventricular septal defect	III, Ventricular septal defect	Atropine, acepromazine, oxymorphone, methoxyflurane, then hypothermia on pump for cardiopulmonary bypass	Hypotension and hypothermia
F	3 mos	Bulldog	Angiogram	III, VSD, right heart enlargement, congestive heart failure	Atropine, acepromazine, thiopental, methoxyflurane	Hypoventilation, circulatory collapse, bradycardia, o.d.
						Insufficient cardiac contractility, electrical activity continued while there was no functional pulse and respiratory arrest
M	6 yrs	German shepherd	Whole body hyperthermia treatment for cancer	IV, Mammary adenocarcinoma with metastasis to lungs	Atropine, thiopental, methoxyflurane	Pulmonary edema, respiratory and cardiac collapse
F	6 mos	German shepherd	Reduction of cervical spine	II, Post-trauma	Atropine, thiopental, methoxyflurane-N_2O	Electromechanical dissociation of heart

(Continued on p. 626.)

TABLE 23–15. Analysis of Anesthetic Deaths in 32 Dogs and Cats at Colorado State University (1979–1981) *(Continued)*

*Sex**	*Age*	*Breed*	*Reason for Anesthesia*	*Physical Status† and Reason*	*Preanesthetic and Anesthetic Agents Used*	*Reason for Death*
M	2 mos	Irish setter	Thoracotomy	II, Persistent right aortic arch, megaesophagus	Atropine, acepromazine, oxymorphone, methoxyflurane-N_2O	Respiratory arrest immediately after surgery; possible pneumothorax or mucus plugging ET tube
M	3 mos	Newfoundland	Thoracotomy	II, Patent ductus arteriosus (PDA)	Atropine, acepromazine, oxymorphone, methoxyflurane	Surgical tear in PDA, hypovolemia
F	4 yrs	Irish setter	Thoracotomy	III, Lung torsion	Atropine, oxymorphone, halothane	Cardiac arrest following PCVs and fibrillation
M	9 yrs	Borzoi	Laryngotomy-tracheostomy	IV, Cancerous larynx, poor nutritional state, age	Halothane (mask), methoxyflurane	Vagal stimulation-bradycardia, then cardiac arrest
Cats, 1979						
M	2 yrs	Domestic	Declaw	I, Healthy	Atropine, acepromazine, ketamine	Positional hypoxia
s/F	6 yrs	Domestic	Ear ablation	II, Chronic otitis externa	Atropine, halothane (mask), methoxyflurane	O.d. methoxyflurane
c/M	4 yrs	Domestic	Perineal urethrostomy	II, Cystitis	Atropine, xylazine, halothane-N_2O	Turned on N_2O without O_2 Brain damage—died 24 hours later
Cats, 1980						
F	6 mos	Domestic	Ovariohysterectomy-onychectomy	II, Preoperative tachycardia	Atropine, acepromazine, ketamine, halothane	O.d.—ruptured lung during CPR
Cats, 1981						
F	2 yrs	Domestic	Repair fractured femur	III, Traumatic fracture	Atropine, acepromazine, ketamine, halothane-N_2O	Emboli in pulmonary artery

*c/M = castrated male; s/F = spayed female.
†ASA classification, see Table 23-1.
‡ O.d. = overdose.

(From Perkins, D., Heath, R.B., and Lumb, W.V.: Unpublished data, Colorado State University, Fort Collins, 1982.)

TABLE 23–16. Analysis of Anesthetic Deaths in 21 Horses at Colorado State University (1979–1981)

Sex*	Age	Breed	Reason for Anesthesia	Physical Status† and Reason	Preanesthetic and Anesthetic Agents Used	Reason for Death
Horses, 1979						
M	1 yr	Quarter	Abdominal exploration	IV, Colic, severe shock	Guaifenesin and thiamylal	Toxic shock
F	9 yr	Appaloosa	Abdominal exploration	III, Postparturient colic for 48 hours	Xylazine, ketamine, halothane	Tachycardia for 20 minutes postinduction, then cardiac arrest
c/M	7 yr	Quarter	Abdominal exploration	III, Colic, shock	Xylazine, ketamine, halothane	Cardiac arrest
M	7 yr	Quarter	Abdominal exploration	IV, Colic, severe shock	Xylazine, chloral hydrate, ketamine, halothane	Toxic shock
c/M	10 yr	Quarter	Abdominal exploration	IV, Colic, severe shock	Xylazine, ketamine, halothane	Toxic shock
c/M	5 yr	Quarter	Abdominal exploration	V, Colic, severe shock (Preoperative heart rate 100, PCV 65%, cyanotic)	Xylazine, ketamine	Toxic shock
M	8 yr	Mixed breed	Abdominal exploration	E III, Colic	Xylazine, ketamine, halothane	Inadequate perfusion, arrhythmia, and fibrillation
Horses, 1980						
F	6 mos	Mixed breed	Repair of fractured olecranon	II, Trauma, fracture	Xylazine, halothane-N_2O	O.d.‡ halothane
c/M	11 yr	Arabian	Abdominal exploration	III, Shock	Xylazine, ketamine, halothane	O.d., toxic animal
M	6 mos	Quarter	Repair of fractured nasal bones	II, Trauma, compound fracture of nasal bones	Xylazine, ketamine	Hemorrhage into lungs, could not oxygenate
F	1½ yr	Quarter	Laminectomy	I, Elective (research horse)	Xylazine, guaifenesin, ketamine, halothane	Cardiac arrest
M	7 yr	Thoroughbred	Penis reconstruction	II, Penile laceration, previous anesthesia with severe myopathy	Xylazine, guaifenesin, thiamylal, halothane	Fractured both femurs on recovery, lacerated femoral artery and bled out, hypovolemic shock

(Continued on p. 628.)

TABLE 23–16. Analysis of Anesthetic Deaths in 21 Horses at Colorado State University (1979–1981) *(Continued)*

*Sex**	*Age*	*Breed*	*Reason for Anesthesia*	*Physical Status† and Reason*	*Preanesthetic and Anesthetic Agents Used*	*Reason for Death*
Horses, 1981						
F	4 yr	Thoroughbred	Dorsal laminectomy	II, "Wobbler"	Xylazine, ketamine, halothane-N_2O	O.d.
M	1 mo	Thoroughbred	Exploratory laparotomy	E III, Shock	Halothane	O.d.
F	5 yr	Quarter	Fractured ulna	II, Recent trauma	Xylazine, ketamine, halothane	O.d.
F	13 yr	Quarter	Ovariectomy	I, Elective	Xylazine, guaifenesin, thiamylal, halothane	Cardiac and renal disease on necropsy
F	1 mo	Quarter	Abdominal exploratory	IV, Ruptured bladder	Halothane	Toxic shock following ruptured bladder
M	3 yr	Quarter	Tattoo cornea	I, Elective	Acepromazine, xylazine, guaifenesin, thiamylal, halothane-N_2O	N_2O given instead of O_2
F	3 yr	Arabian	Laparotomy	E IV, Colic	Xylazine, ketamine, halothane	Toxic shock
F	4 yr	Thoroughbred	Dorsal laminectomy	II, "Wobbler"	Xylazine, ketamine, halothane-N_2O	Unknown
F	6 yr	Quarter	Ovariectomy	I, Elective	Xylazine, ketamine, halothane	N_2 given instead of O_2

*c/M = castrated male.
†ASA classification, see Table 23–1.
‡O.d. = overdose.

(From Perkins, D., Heath, R.B., and Lumb, W.V.: Unpublished data, Colorado State University, Fort Collins, 1982.)

TABLE 23–17. Claims Involving Anesthesia, Surgery, and Medicine Presented to the AVMA Professional Liability Insurance Trust, 1976–1982

Species	Total No. of Claims	Claims Involving: Anesthesia (%)	Surgery (%)	Medicine (%)
Horses	542	13.8	41.7	44.5
Cattle	436	3.9	44.2	51.8
Dogs	1225	13.1	42.5	44.4
Cats	216	6.5	45.8	47.7

(Courtesy of Dinsmore, J.R.: AVMA Professional Liability Insurance Trust, Chicago, Illinois, 1983.)

N_2 instead of O_2. Four animals were in physical status I, and were anesthetized for elective surgery.

Data on anesthesia in cattle are not as available, probably because local, regional, and epidural techniques are commonly used with this species. Bowen and Seidel (1976), performing ova transplants at Colorado State University, had three anesthetic deaths in over 1000 cases of halothane anesthesia. As they pointed out, this operation can be performed under optimal circumstances, since it is elective.

SURVEY OF ANESTHESIAS IN HORSES AT NORWEGIAN COLLEGE OF VETERINARY MEDICINE

Tevik (1983) conducted a retrospective study of fatalities in horses undergoing anesthesia and surgery at the Norwegian College of Veterinary Medicine from 1965 to 1981. Of 1216 horses, 33 did not survive. Twenty-seven of these were given halothane-N_2O, the remainder received sedatives only. Anesthesia alone was considered to be the cause of death in 10 horses (0.8%). Eight of the 33 (24.2%) died from postanesthetic rhabdomyolysis.

INSURANCE CLAIMS INVOLVING ANESTHESIA

Table 23–17 lists claims presented to the American Veterinary Medical Association Professional Liability Insurance Trust from 1976 through 1982 for anesthetic, surgical, and medical losses.

For additional data on anesthetic administration in animals, the reader is referred to the previous edition of this text.

REFERENCES

Bowen, J.M., and Seidel, S.: Anesthesia in the Cow. Vet. Anesth., 3:100, 1976.

Brown, J.D., and Lumb, W.V.: Tracheal Obstruction in a Dog. J.A.V.M.A., 132:521, 1958.

Heath, R.B.: Personal communication. Colorado State University, Fort Collins, 1970.

Lumb, W.V.: *Small Animal Anesthesia.* Lea & Febiger, Philadelphia, 1963.

Perkins, D., Heath, R.B., and Lumb, W.V.: Unpublished data. Colorado State University, Fort Collins, 1982.

Schwabe, C.W., and Davis, L.R.: Marginal Punched Cards in Veterinary Research. Am. J. Vet. Res., 15:634, 1954.

Tevik, A.: The Role of Anesthesia in Surgical Mortality in Horses. Nord. Vet. Med., 35:175, 1983.

CHAPTER 24

Euthanasia*

INTRODUCTION

Euthanasia is the act of inducing painless death, specifically painlessness for the animal being subjected to euthanasia. The distress that human beings may experience when observing euthanasia or death in any form is an emotional response dependent on the functionally complex and highly developed human brain. Kinship of human beings with higher animals, however distant, serves to transfer the unpleasantness associated with death of human beings to death of other animals. Such human distress occurs even though the observer experiences no physical pain. This distress may be minimized by perfection of the technique of euthanasia.

The sensation of pain is initiated by damage to or intense stimulation of almost any part of the body. In tissues, pain receptors react to substances released when tissue is damaged. Substances such as histamine, angiotonin, serotonin, prostaglandins, bradykinin, adenosine triphosphate, and H^+ and K^+ ions are released from tissues and modulate or stimulate pain receptors (Breazile 1971; Guyton, 1976; Swenson, 1977).

Pain perception in animals other than man has been discussed by Breazile and Kitchell (1969). Recognition of pain by an animal depends on impulses from pain receptors traversing pain pathways leading to the thalamus and cerebral cortex. For pain to be experienced, the cerebral cortex and subcortical structures must be functional. An unconscious animal does not experience pain because the cerebral cortex is not functioning. If the cerebral cortex is rendered nonfunctional by any means such as hypoxia,

*The major portion of this chapter is the Report of the American Veterinary Medical Association Panel on Euthanasia. This Report was published in the J.A.V.M.A., 173:59, 1978. Panel members were:

L.E. McDonald, DVM, PhD *(Chairman)*, College of Veterinary Medicine, University of Georgia, Athens, GA 30602
N.H. Booth, DVM, PhD, College of Veterinary Medicine, University of Georgia, Athens, GA 30602
W.V. Lumb, DVM, PhD, College of Veterinary Medicine and Biomedical Sciences, Colorado State University, Fort Collins, CO 80523
R.W. Redding, DVM, PhD, School of Veterinary Medicine, Auburn University, Auburn, AL 36830
D.C. Sawyer, DVM, PhD, College of Veterinary Medicine, Michigan State University, East Lansing, MI 48824
Lois Stevenson, Science Writer and Columnist, 49 Rock Rd West, Green Brook, NJ 08812
W.M. Wass, DVM, PhD, College of Veterinary Medicine, Iowa State University, Ames, IA 50011

depression by drugs, electric shock, or concussion, pain is not experienced.

In an unconscious animal, stimuli that evoke pain will elicit reflex responses manifested by motor movement. For this reason, purposeful or nonpurposeful movements of an animal are not reliable indicators of cerebral pain reception. Conversely, an animal can experience pain, even though no body movements occur in response to painful stimuli, if the animal is given muscle paralyzing agents such as curare, succinylcholine, gallamine, pancuronium, nicotine, or decamethonium. These muscle paralyzing agents do not depress the cerebral cortex or thalamus.

As with other procedures applied to animals, euthanasia commonly requires some physical control over the animal. The degree of control needed is variable. Important factors in determining the magnitude and kind of restraint are species or breed of animal, whether wild or domesticated, presence or absence of painful injury or disease, method of euthanasia, and degree of excitement. Suitable control is vital for satisfactory performance of euthanasia to minimize intensity and duration of pain in animals involved, to assure safety of the person performing euthanasia and, frequently, to protect other animals and people in the immediate environment.

Selection of the method of euthanasia in any given situation is dependent on the species of animal involved, available means of control of the animal, skill of personnel, numbers of animals, economic factors, and other considerations.

BEHAVIORIAL CONSIDERATIONS

The behavioral and physiologic responses to noxious stimulation include distress vocalization, struggling and attempts to escape, defensive-redirected aggression, and immobility or "freezing." Other responses include salivation, urination, defecation, evacuation of anal glands, pupillary dilation, tachycardia, sweating, and reflex contractions of skeletal muscles causing shivering, tremors, or other muscular spasms.

In very young animals, autonomic and reflexive reactions are evident, although overt behavioral reactions may differ. With maturation, there is gradual development of pain perception.

The need to reduce fear and apprehension must be considered in determining the method of euthanasia to be employed. Reactions of an animal, such as distress vocalizations, fearful behavior, and release of certain odors, may cause anxiety and apprehension in other animals present. Gentle restraint, careful handling, and talking during administration of euthanasia agents are often effective in calming an animal. However, these methods may not be effective with wild animals or animals that are injured or sick. Where capture or restraint may cause pain, injury, or anxiety to the animal or danger to the operator, the use of tranquilizing or immobilizing drugs may be necessary.

MODES OF ACTION OF EUTHANATIZING AGENTS

Euthanatizing agents terminate life by three basic mechanisms: 1) hypoxia, direct or indirect; 2) direct depression of neurons vital for life function; and 3) physical damage or concussion of brain tissue (Table 24–1).

Agents that produce death by direct or indirect hypoxia (depriving tissues of oxygen) have different sites of action and different times of onset of unconsciousness. With some agents, unconsciousness occurs prior to cessation of motor activity (muscle movement). Thus, even if animals demonstrate muscular contractions, they are not perceiving pain. The uninformed observer may find this difficult to accept when muscle contractions are observed. Conversely, muscle relaxants produce a flaccid muscular paralysis so that the animal is conscious until death eventually occurs from hypoxia and hypercarbia due to paralysis of respiratory muscles. To the uninformed observer, the animal appears relaxed with no visible evidence that it actually is in a state of panic and can feel pain. Outwardly this would appear to be an ideal form of euthanisia, but it is not. Agents that do not produce unconsciousness prior to death are in the curariform group: curare, succinylcholine, gallamine, nicotine, magnesium salts, pancuronium,

TABLE 24–1. Mode of Action of Euthanatizing Agents

	Site of Action	*Classification*	*Comments*
1. HYPOXIC AGENTS			
Carbon monoxide	Carbon monoxide combines with hemoglobin of RBC preventing combination with oxygen	Histotoxic hypoxia	Unconsciousness occurs rapidly; motor activity persists after unconsciousness
Hydrogen cyanide gas	Depression of oxygen transport at tissue level; no O_2 available in tissues	Histotoxic hypoxia	Unconsciousness occurs rapidly; motor activity persists after unconsciousness
Curariform drugs: curare, succinylcholine, gallamine, decamethonium	Paralysis of respiratory muscles; oxygen not available to blood	Hypoxic hypoxia and hypercarbia	Unconsciousness develops slowly, preceded by anxiety and fear; no motor activity
Rapid decompression	Reduced partial pressure of oxygen available to blood	Hypoxic hypoxia	Unconsciousness occurs rapidly; motor activity persists after unconsciousness
Nitrogen inhalation	Reduced partial pressure of oxygen available to blood	Hypoxic hypoxia	Unconsciousness occurs rapidly; motor activity persists after unconsciousness
Electrocution when current does not pass through brain	Spastic paralysis of respiratory muscles and ventricular fibrillation; oxygen not available to blood in lungs	Hypoxic hypoxia	Unconsciousness develops slowly, occurring after violent muscle spasms
2. DIRECT NEURON-DEPRESSING AGENTS			
Anesthetic gases: ether, chloroform, methoxyflurane, halothane, nitrous oxide, and enflurane	Direct depression of cerebral cortex and subcortical structures and vital centers	Ultimate cause of death is hypoxia; respiration ceases due to depression of vital centers	Unconsciousness occurs first; no anxiety or pain; possible involuntary motor activity after unconsciousness; no motor activity after brief period
Carbon dioxide	Direct depression of cerebral cortex and subcortical structures and vital centers; direct depression of heart muscle	Ultimate cause of death is hypoxia; respiration ceases due to depression of vital centers	Unconsciousness occurs first; usually no motor activity
Barbituric acid derivatives	Direct depression of cerebral cortex and subcortical structures and vital centers; direct depression of heart muscle	Ultimate cause of death is hypoxia; respiration ceases due to depression of vital centers	Unconsciousness reached rapidly; no anxiety; no excitement period; no motor activity; best to administer by intravenous (IV) or intracardiac (IC) administration
Chloral hydrate and chloral hydrate combinations	Direct depression of cerebral cortex and subcortical structures and vital centers; direct depression of heart muscle	Ultimate cause of death is hypoxia; respiration ceases due to depression of vital centers	Transient anxiety, unconsciousness occurs rapidly; no motor activity
T-61	Direct depression of cerebral cortex and subcortical structures and vital centers; direct depression of heart muscle	Ultimate cause of death is hypoxia; respiration ceases due to depression of vital centers and muscle paralysis	Transient anxiety and struggling may occur before unconsciousness when given too rapidly; tissue damage may occur if not given IV or at recommended dosage; best given IV or IC
3. PHYSICAL AGENTS			
Electrocution through brain	Direct depression of brain	Ultimate cause of death is hypoxia; respiration ceases due to depression of vital centers	Violent muscle contractions occur at same time as unconsciousness
Gunshot or captive-bolt into brain	Direct concussion of brain tissue	Ultimate cause of death is hypoxia; respiration ceases due to depression of vital centers	Instant unconsciousness; motor activity may occur after unconsciousness
Microwave irradiation	Direct inactivation of brain enzymes	Ultimate cause of death is hypoxia; respiration ceases due to depression of vital centers	Currently used only in small laboratory animals; further study needed

and decamethonium. In addition, strychnine and potassium salts do not induce unconsciousness before death. Use of any of these agents alone for euthanasia is absolutely condemned.

The second group of euthanatizing agents (Tables 24–1, 24–2) directly affects nervous tissue. All these agents depress nerve cells of the brain first, blocking apprehension and pain perception, with unconsciousness following.

Some of these agents ''release'' muscle control during the first stage of anesthesia, resulting in an ''excitement or delirium phase,'' during which there may be vocalization and some muscle contraction (Lumb, 1974). Although these appear to be purposeful, they are not. The ultimate cause of death is hypoxia caused by direct depression of respiratory centers.

With the third group (Table 24–1), direct electrical flow through the brain, concussion, or physical damage to the brain produces instant unconsciousness (Warrington, 1974). Muscular activity may follow unconsciousness. When electrocution is properly used, muscular contraction occurs concomitantly with loss of consciousness; with the other methods in this group, muscular contraction may occur. Although this may be unpleasant to the observer, the animal is not suffering.

Electroencephalograms (brain waves) and other physiologic variables of dogs often are employed to measure characteristics of many euthanatizing agents (Fig. 24–1*A* to *D*).

CRITERIA FOR JUDGING METHODS OF EUTHANASIA

Several criteria were used in evaluating methods of euthanasia: 1) ability to produce death without causing pain; 2) time required to produce loss of consciousness; 3) time required to produce death; 4) reliability; 5) safety of personnel; 6) potential for minimizing undesirable psychologic stress; 7) compatibility with requirement and purpose; 8) emotional effect upon observers or operators; 9) economic feasibility; 10) compatibility with histopathologic evaluation; and 11) drug availability and abuse potential.

INHALANT AGENTS

Occupational exposure to inhalation anesthetics constitutes a health hazard. The National Institute of Occupational Safety and Health has recognized as primary health concerns an increase in both spontaneous abortion and congenital abnormalities in offspring of personnel exposed to trace amounts of inhalation anesthetic agents (DHEW, 1977). In addition, other potential health problems indicate that exposure levels for volatile liquid anesthetics (ether, halothane, methoxyflurane, ethrane, and chloroform) must be less than 2 ppm and for nitrous oxide must be less than 50 ppm. Moreover, chloroform is an hepatotoxin and a suspected carcinogen and should be avoided or used with extreme caution. When these agents are used, effective procedures must be employed to protect personnel from anesthetic vapors.

Inhalant Anesthetics: Ether, Chloroform, Halothane, Methoxyflurane, Enflurane, Cyclopropane, and Nitrous Oxide

The inhalant anesthetics, primarily ether, chloroform, halothane, and methoxyflurane, have been used for euthanasia of many species (Booth, 1977*b*). A newer agent, enflurane, has been seldom used. With these agents, the animal ordinarily is placed in a closed receptacle containing cotton or gauze soaked with the anesthetic (American Humane Association, 1969; Universities Federation for Animal Welfare, 1968; Sawyer, 1976). Vapors are inhaled until respiration ceases and death ensues (Table 24–2). Humane considerations dictate that the animal not contact the liquid anesthetic. In addition, air or oxygen must be available to the animal during the initial induction period (American Humane Association, 1969; Universities Federation for Animal Welfare, 1968).

Other inhalation anesthetics are seldom used for euthanasia because of low potency, high cost, or danger. Cyclopropanc, a gas, is highly flammable and explosive (Lumb and Jones, 1973). It requires special equipment for administration. Nitrous oxide, a compressed gas, may be used alone to produce mild analgesia, anesthesia, and death by hypoxia. Nitrous oxide is

TABLE 24–2. Efficacy of Inhalant Anesthetics for Euthanasia

Agent	Safety for Personnel	Ease of Performance	Rapidity	Economic Considerations	Tissue Changes	Efficacy	Species Suitability	Remarks
Ether	Flammable and explosive	Easily performed with closed container or chamber	Slow onset of anesthesia	Relatively inexpensive	Slight changes may occur in parenchymatous organs	Highly effective provided subject is sufficiently exposed	Suitable for cats and young dogs, birds, rodents, and other small species	Acceptable
							Administration to larger animals requires specialized equipment and training; onset is slow; vapors are irritating	Not acceptable
Chloroform	Nonflammable and nonexplosive; chronic exposure of animals or personnel is dangerous because of potential liver or kidney damage	Easily performed with closed container or chamber; can be administered to large animals by means of a mask	Rapid onset of anesthesia	Inexpensive	Extensive changes may occur in parenchymatous organs	Highly effective provided subject is sufficiently exposed	Suitable for cats and young dogs, birds, rodents, and other small species	Acceptable
							Useful in large animals in emergency situations	Not acceptable, except in emergencies
Halothane*	Nonflammable and nonexplosive; chronic exposure of animals or personnel to vapor may be hazardous	Easily performed with closed container or chamber; can be administered to large animals by means of a mask	Rapid onset of anesthesia	Expensive	May occur in parenchymatous organs	Highly effective provided subject is sufficiently exposed	Suitable for cats and young dogs, birds, rodents, and other small species	Acceptable
							Useful in large animals in emergency situations	Not acceptable, except in emergencies
Methoxyflurane†	Nonflammable and nonexplosive under normal environmental conditions; chronic exposure of animals or personnel to vapor may be hazardous	Slow with closed container or chamber; may be difficult to obtain necessary vapor concentration; can be administered to large animals by means of a mask	Slow onset of anesthesia	Expensive	May occur in parenchymatous organs	Highly effective provided subject is sufficiently exposed	Suitable for cats and young dogs, birds, rodents, and other small species	Acceptable
							Administration to large animals requires specialized equipment and training; slow onset	Not acceptable
Nitrous oxide	Nonflammable and nonexplosive but will support combustion; chronic exposure of animals or personnel to gas may be hazardous	Easily performed with closed container or chamber	Rapid onset in 100% concentration	Relatively expensive	Hypoxic lesions may occur	Highly effective provided subject is sufficiently exposed	Suitable for cats, small dogs, birds, rodents, and other small species	Acceptable
							Not recommended alone for larger animals	Use in large animals requires supplementation with other agents
Enflurane‡	Nonflammable and nonexplosive; chronic exposure of animals or personnel to vapors may be harmful	Easily performed with closed container or chamber; can be administered to large animals by means of a mask	Rapid onset of anesthesia	Expensive	May occur in parenchymatous organs, particularly kidneys	Highly effective provided subject is sufficiently exposed; deep anesthesia may be accompanied by motor activity (twitching)	Suitable for cats and young dogs, birds, rodents, and other small species	Acceptable, but not recommended because of motor activity in deep plane of anesthesia
							Useful in large animals in emergency situations	Not acceptable, except in emergencies

*Fluothane, Ayerst Laboratories, New York, NY; Halocarbon, Halocarbon Laboratories, Hackensack, NJ.
†Metofane, Pitman-Moore, Inc, Washington Crossing, NJ; Penthrane, Abbott Laboratories, Chicago, Ill.
‡Ethrane, Ohio Medical Products, Division of Airco, Inc., Madison, Wis.

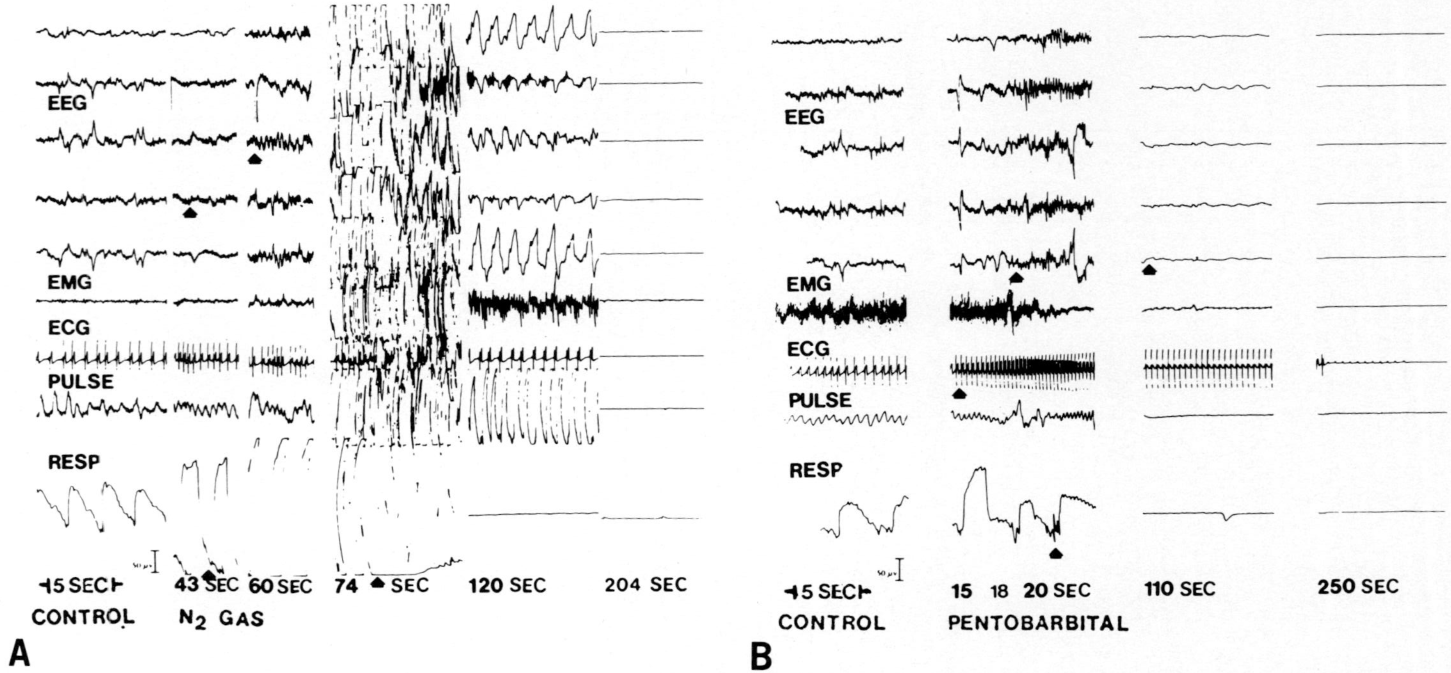

Figure 24–1. Recordings of physiologic activity of dogs undergoing euthanasia. Recordings of the electroencephalogram (EEG), (5 top lines); electromyogram (EMG), electrocardiogram (ECG), pulse (using a photoelectric pulse transducer on the ear), and respiration (RESP) made with a strain gauge differential airflow transducer with the input from a 12-gauge needle in the tracheal lumen. The needle was inserted between two tracheal cartilage rings. The recording polygraph was a Grass (Grass Instrument Co., Quincy, Mass.) Model 6 Electroencephalograph with two channels of DC amplifier. The paper speed was 6 mm/sec. (See time base on recordings.) The standardization for the EEG was 50 μv/cm. (See standardization on recordings.) The time interval from onset of injection or inhalation of the euthanasia agent is indicated on the bottom of each tracing in seconds for each demonstrated change indicated by arrows on tracing.

A, Use of 100% nitrogen gas inhalation administered by placing the animal's head in a 3 L flexible, clear plastic container with an ingoing and outgoing port. The nitrogen gas was introduced at rapid flow of 10 L/minute for 1 minute to exhaust the air in the container. The flow was then reduced to maintain a constant positive pressure inside. The plastic container assured a 100% nitrogen concentration. In 43 seconds, there was medium-voltage fast activity in the EEG indicating apprehension, ECG and pulse activity were increased, and heart rate suggested response to apprehension. At 60 seconds, there were higher voltage slow waves of EEG indicating unconsciousness. At 74 seconds, generalized convulsions occurred. At 120 seconds, there was postictal slowing of the EEG and EMG response was active, pulse waves were extremely high, there were ECG abnormal wave forms, and respiration ceased. At 43 seconds and 60 seconds, there was marked increase in depth of respiratory effort. At 74 seconds, both the depth and rate of respiratory effort were extreme. The EEG was flat at 130 seconds, and cardiac activity ceased at 204 seconds.

B, Use of pentobarbital sodium intravenously via the cephalic vein. The dose was 66.0 mg/kg (30 mg/lb) administered rapidly as a bolus. In 15 seconds, there was rapid fall in blood pressure as indicated by marked reflex increase in pulse rate and ECG rate increase. At 18 seconds, unconsciousness occurred as indicated by EEG medium-voltage slow waves. Arrow on respiration (RESP) recording indicates onset of apnea at 20 seconds. At 110 seconds, the EEG tracing was almost flat, indicating complete lack of brain function. At 250 seconds, ECG activity was no longer detectable, and EEG became completely flat, indicating brain death.

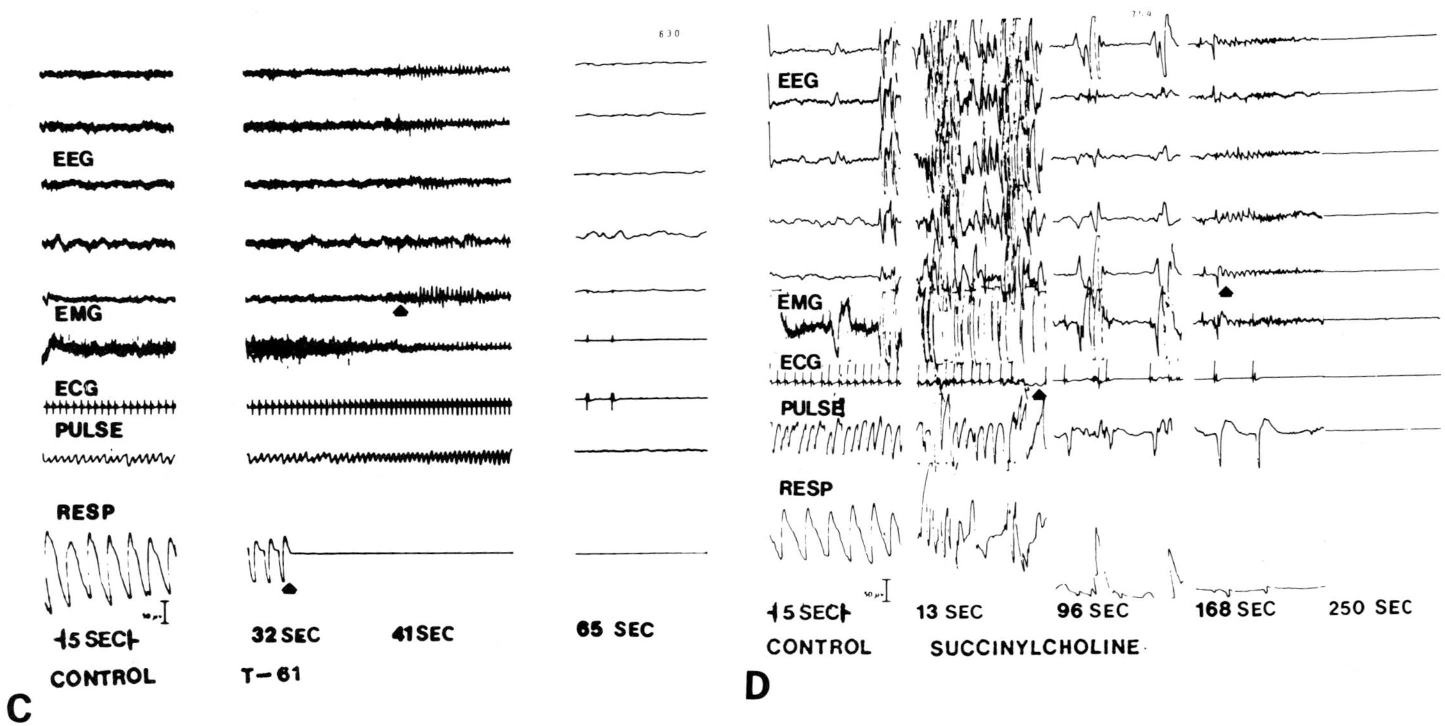

Figure 24–1 ***Continued.*** *C,* Use of T-61 euthanasia solution intravenously via the cephalic vein. The dose was 0.3 ml/kg (0.14 ml/lb) administered at two-thirds the total dose at a rate of 1 ml/5 sec. The remaining third was administered rapidly. In 32 seconds, respiratory movements ceased. At 41 seconds, there were EEG high-voltage slow waves of unconsciousness. At 65 seconds, cardiac activity terminated and EEG became flat, indicating complete lack of brain function.

D, Use of succinylcholine chloride intravenously via the cephalic vein. The dose was 1.0 mg/kg (0.45 mg/lb) administered rapidly as a bolus. In 13 seconds, the high-voltage EMG and EEG fast activity indicated severe apprehension, fear, panic, possibly pain, and respiratory irregularity. At 96 seconds, EEG indicated that consciousness was still present, ECG indicated irregular cardiac activity, and respiratory tracing indicated respiratory efforts persisted. At 168 seconds, EEG contained medium-voltage slow waves suggestive of true unconsciousness. Cardiac activity and pulse were still present. At 250 seconds, EEG tracing became flat and cardiac activity ceased.

nonflammable and nonexplosive, but will support combustion.

Advantages. 1) The inhalant anesthetics are particularly valuable in euthanasia of birds, rodents, and cats, and in young dogs when venipuncture may prove difficult. 2) Chloroform, halothane, enflurane, methoxyflurane, and nitrous oxide are nonflammable and nonexplosive under ordinary environmental conditions.

Disadvantages. 1) Struggling and anxiety may be manifested by the animal during the induction stage of anesthesia before unconsciousness develops. These states are provoked initially by irritating vapors of the anesthetics and subsequently by their excitant effects on the central nervous system. 2) Ether cannot be used near an open flame because it is flammable and explosive. Chloroform is not explosive but can be hazardous when used in the presence of flame because phosgene gas may form. 3) Exposure to these agents can be injurious to personnel and other animals. 4) Halothane, methoxyflurane, nitrous oxide, and enflurane are relatively expensive.

Recommendations. Under certain circumstances, ether, chloroform, halothane, enflurane, methoxyflurane, and nitrous oxide administered by inhalation are useful for euthanasia of small animals such as birds, rodents, cats, and young dogs. These agents are not recommended for general use in larger animals because of their cost and difficulty in administration. In emergency situations, chloroform, halothane, or enflurane may be administered to large animals.

Nitrogen (N_2)

Nitrogen, a colorless, odorless gas, constitutes 78% of the normal atmospheric air. It is inert, nonflammable, and nonexplosive.

Euthanasia is accomplished by placing the animal in a closed container into which pure N_2 is introduced at a rapid flow rate. Nitrogen displaces atmospheric oxygen in the container, thus producing hypoxic death. Commercially available N_2 equipment for euthanasia consists of closed chambers for containing animals in the N_2 gas, an oxygen monitor to determine that N_2 concentration is adequate and has displaced the atmospheric oxygen (1.5% O_2 or less in 45 to 50 seconds), and a timer to insure adequate exposure to the gas. The system is operated at normal atmospheric pressure. Because N_2 mixes with room air when the chamber is opened, there is minimal danger to personnel provided adequate ventilation is supplied.

Dogs became unconscious within 76 seconds when N_2 was flushed into an enclosure to reach a final concentration of 98.5% in 45 to 60 seconds. An isoelectric (flat) EEG was reached at a mean of 80 seconds with zero arterial blood pressure achieved in an average of 204 seconds. Prior to unconsciousness, respiratory activity increased in all dogs. Herin et al. (1978) concluded that this method produced death without pain. Following unconsciousness, yelping, gasping, convulsions, and muscular tremors occurred in some dogs. At the end of a 5-minute exposure period, all dogs were dead. These results are similar to those for rabbits (Noell and Chinn, 1949) and for a single dog as shown in Figure 24–1*A*.

Glass et al. (1944) showed that newborn dogs, rabbits, and guinea pigs can survive a N_2 atmosphere much longer than adults of these species. Newborn dogs and rabbits survived 31 minutes and guinea pigs 6 minutes, whereas adult dogs and guinea pigs survived 3 minutes and adult rabbits 1½ minutes. Nitrogen has been used for euthanasia of mink (Vinter, 1957).

Advantages. Nitrogen gas is highly effective, N_2 gas is readily available, and hazards to the operator are minimal.

Disadvantages. 1) It is not esthetically acceptable to observers because of unpleasant responses in the unconscious animal. 2) Very young animals are not rapidly euthanatized. 3) Equipment or operator malfunctions may occur. 4) Rapid N_2 flow may produce a noise that may frighten animals. 5) The chamber may be overcrowded, causing undesirable animal behavior. 6) In some areas the use of N_2 for euthanasia has been prohibited by law.

Recommendations. Nitrogen is considered an effective agent for euthanasia provided that the equipment is properly constructed, correctly maintained, and proficiently operated, and that no animals under 4 months of age are subjected to this method. Personnel using N_2 must be instructed thoroughly in its use and must understand its hazards and limitations. An exhaust or ventilatory system is essential to insure against exposure of personnel to high concentrations of N_2.

Hydrogen Cyanide Gas

Hydrogen cyanide gas is one of the most rapidly acting poisons (Swineyard, 1975). The maximum allowable concentration for occupational exposure in industry is 10 ppm for 8 hours of exposure.

Hydrogen cyanide gas for euthanasia is produced by placing pellets of sodium cyanide in sulfuric acid, thus producing the gas. An airtight chamber is required to protect the operator and to confine the gas to the chamber.

Cyanide reacts readily with the ferric ion of cytochrome oxidase in cell mitochondria to form cytochrome oxidase-cyanide complex. A cytoxic hypoxia occurs.

There is no evidence to suggest that the effects of cyanide are painful (Sanford, 1976). Cyanide promotes intense respiratory stimulation and may cause excitement, which may result in distressing respiratory sounds before death. In addition, cyanide possesses a pungent and rather unpleasant smell and, because of its highly toxic properties, it is probably best avoided. The United Kingdom allows destruction of rabbits, foxes, and badgers in dens by cyanide gas generated when cyanide powder comes into contact with moisture (Scott, 1976).

Advantages. Hydrogen cyanide gas induces rapid death, and it can be used under field conditions where other agents are impractical.

Disadvantages. 1) The animal manifests violent convulsive seizures and opisthotonos prior to death. 2) The responses are disagreeable to most observers. 3) The gas is exceedingly irritating to the respiratory mucosa. 4) There is extreme danger to the operator from the highly toxic gas.

Recommendations. Although the effect of hydrogen cyanide gas is rapid, reliable, and irreversible, it endangers the operator, and the manner of death is esthetically objectionable (Austin, 1973). Other methods of euthanasia are preferable.

Carbon Monoxide (CO)

Carbon monoxide combines with hemoglobin to form carboxyhemoglobin. This blocks the uptake of oxygen by the erythrocytes, leading to fatal hypoxemia.

Common sources of CO are domestic and industrial furnaces and gasoline engines. It may be produced chemically by mixing sodium formate and sulfuric acid. Three methods have practical application to mass euthanasia of animals: 1) chemical interaction of sodium formate and sulfuric acid, 2) exhaust fumes from engines combusting petroleum, and 3) commercially compressed CO gas in cylinders.

Haldane (1895) concluded that clinical signs caused by CO depend on the extent to which hemoglobin has been saturated with CO. Thus, CO is a cumulative poison. Distinct signs are not produced by CO until the concentration is 0.05% in air, and acute signs do not occur until the concentration is approximately 0.2%. In man, exposure to 0.32% and 0.45% of CO for one hour will produce unconsciousness and death, respectively (Bloom, 1972).

Carding (1968) used sodium formate and sulfuric acid to generate CO for euthanasia and found a marked reduction in the average time of collapse and death in dogs exposed to increasing concentrations from 2 to 3% CO in air.

In a report by Ramsey and Eilmann (1932), guinea pigs collapsed in 40 seconds to 2 minutes, and death occurred within 5¾ minutes in a chamber concentration of 8% CO.

For euthanasia of mink (Vinter, 1957) and chinchillas, CO was used. These animals collapsed in 1 minute, breathing ceased in 2 minutes, and then were considered dead when the heart stopped beating in approximately 5 to 7 minutes.

Blood et al. (1972) reported excellent results in producing CO euthanasia in cats and dogs. Several chamber concentrations were tested, and they concluded that a 6% CO concentration gave fastest results. No advantage was observed by increasing the CO concentration.

Carbon monoxide in gasoline engine exhaust

piped into an enclosed chamber reaches levels above 8% quickly; saturation of hemoglobin to the 70% level occurs more rapidly than with concentrations lower than the optimal 6%. Use of cylinder gas allows rapid attainment of optimal chamber concentration.

Carbon monoxide produced by a gasoline engine was compared with cylinder CO for effectiveness and cost of euthanasia (Moreland, 1974). Differences in effectiveness were negligible, but operational costs were less for the gasoline engine method.

In production of CO by combustion, oxides of nitrogen and hydrocarbons, oxygenates of hydrocarbons, and heat must be controlled to prevent discomfort to the animal. This may be done by passing exhaust gases through a water chamber and a metal gauze filter with a cloth screen. The water chamber cools the gas, removes some carbon particles, and entraps the oxides of nitrogen and hydrocarbons and oxygenates of hydrocarbons. The cloth filter further removes carbon particles, allowing relatively clean nonirritating CO gas to enter the chamber. Carbon monoxide is generated in greater quantities when the fuel-to-air ratio is high; therefore, an idling engine running on a rich mixture produces the largest percentage of CO in the exhaust gas. In all cases, CO must be considered extremely hazardous for personnel because its presence is difficult to detect and because it is highly toxic. An exhaust or ventilatory system is essential to prevent accidental exposure of human beings.

Advantages. 1) Carbon monoxide fumes produce rapid and painless death. 2) Hypoxemia produced by CO is insidious so that the animal is completely unaware of it. 3) Unconsciousness occurs without pain or appreciable discomfort.

Disadvantages. 1) Safeguards must be observed to prevent discomfort to animals and hazard to personnel. 2) During chemical generation through the use of sodium formate and sulfuric acid, irritating vapors of sulfuric acid must be filtered out by passing the generated CO through a solution of 10% sodium hydroxide. 3) Exhaust gas must be filtered and cooled.

Recommendations. Carbon monoxide used for individual or mass euthanasia is acceptable for small animals, including dogs and cats, provided the following precautions are carefully observed:

1. Personnel using CO must be instructed thoroughly in its use and must understand the hazards and limitations.
2. The CO generator and chamber must be located in a well-ventilated environment, preferably out-of-doors.
3. The chamber must be equipped with internal lighting and viewports that allow direct visual surveillance of collapse and death of animals.
4. The gas generation process should be adequate to achieve a CO concentration throughout the chamber of at least 5% within no more than 20 minutes after animals are placed in the chamber.
5. If chemical generation through the use of sodium formate and sulfuric acid is used, the generated CO must have the irritating acid vapors filtered out by passing it through a 10% solution of sodium hydroxide.
6. If CO generation is by combustion of gasoline in an engine, the engine must be operating efficiently and only at idling speed with a rich fuel-air mixture; prior to entry into the chamber, the exhaust gas must be cooled to less than 125° F (51.7° C); the chamber must be equipped with accurate temperature gauges monitored by attendants to assure that internal temperature of the chamber does not exceed 110° F (41.3° C); and the exhaust gas must be passed through water and cloth filtration processes to remove irritants and carbon particles before entering the chamber.
7. Exhaust gas piped into a chamber on a cruising vehicle is not acceptable.

Carbon Dioxide

Room air contains 0.04% CO_2. Pure CO_2 is heavier than air and nearly odorless. Inhalation of CO_2 in concentrations of 7.5% elevates the pain threshold, and higher concentrations of CO_2 have a rapid anesthetic effect (Klemm, 1964; Leake and Waters, 1929; Mattsson et al., 1972; Woodbury et al., 1958).

Inhalation of 60% CO_2 results in loss of consciousness within 45 seconds and arrest of respiration within 5 minutes (Glen and Scott, 1973). The marked depressant action of CO_2 has been utilized effectively in group euthanasia of small laboratory animals such as mice, rats, guinea pigs, chickens, and rabbits (Breazile and Kitchell, 1969; Kline et al., 1963; Kotula et al., 1961; Stone et al., 1961), and for humane slaughter of swine for human food (Dodman, 1977). According to Croft (1967), animals do not detect the presence of CO_2 immediately, and the depressant action of the gas takes place almost unnoticed.

Leake and Waters (1929) reported the experimental use of CO_2 as an anesthetic agent in the dog. They observed that concentrations of 30 to 40% CO_2 with oxygen produced anesthesia within 1 to 2 minutes, usually without struggling, vomiting, or retching. The combination of 40% CO_2 and approximately 3% CO has been used experimentally by Carding (1968) for euthanasia of dogs. Carbon dioxide has been used for euthanasia of cats (Universities Federation for Animal Welfare, 1976–1977; Hall, 1972; McArthur, 1976). A CO_2 cabinet has been designed for cats and for small laboratory animals (McArthur, 1976).

Carbon dioxide euthanasia does not distort cellular architecture (Feldman and Gupta, 1976).

Advantages. 1) Carbon dioxide may be purchased in cylinders or in a solid state as "dry ice." 2) CO_2 is inexpensive, nonflammable, nonexplosive, and presents minimal hazard to the operator when used with properly designed equipment. 3) CO_2 does not result in accumulation of tissue residues in food-producing animals.

Disadvantages. Because CO_2 is heavier than air, incomplete filling of a chamber may permit a climbing animal to avoid exposure and to survive.

Recommendations. Rapid depressant and anesthetic qualities of CO_2 have been well established in small laboratory animals, and in cats and young dogs. Chambers should be designed to enable cleaning and removal of dead animals with minimum loss of CO_2. Compressed CO_2 gas in cylinders is preferred over dry ice. If dry ice is used, it should not come in contact with animals because discomfort from freezing or chilling will occur. Carbon dioxide euthanasia is recommended for small laboratory animals, dogs under 3 weeks old, and cats.

NONINHALANT PHARMACOLOGIC AGENTS

The noninhalant agents that can be used to produce euthanasia are widely diverse in chemical composition (Hatch, 1977; Lumb, 1974). Although death can be produced by administering these drugs via many routes (intravenous, intracardiac, intraperitoneal, intrathecal, intramuscular, intrathoracic, subcutaneous, and oral), intravenous administration is preferred because the effect is fastest and most reliable. Intrapulmonic injections should be avoided in situations where intravenous injection is feasible because intrapulmonically administered agents may irritate delicate lung tissue.

Oral, rectal, and intraperitoneal routes of administration are inadvisable for euthanasia because of slowness of onset, wide range in lethal doses, and possible irritant effect of drugs on tissue. With some drugs, an hour or more may elapse from time of administration to observation of maximal drug effect. Some drugs, such as chloral hydrate and T-61, are irritating when given intraperitoneally and produce definite signs of abdominal pain. Others may produce tissue changes depending on dose and route of administration (Feldman and Gupta, 1976; Sawyer et al., 1978).

Intracardiac injection is objectionable because crying and struggling may follow improper administration. Skill is required to penetrate the heart of an animal with one thrust of a hypodermic needle especially if the animal is not easily controlled. Intracardiac injection of drugs is not recommended for euthanasia, except in small, depressed, or comatose animals. Intrathecal use of drugs in unanesthetized animals is not recommended because of the difficulty in puncturing the cisterna magna without producing pain and struggling.

If the animal to be subjected to euthanasia is excitable or vicious, use of analgesics, tranquilizers, narcotics, ketamine, xylazine, or other depressants is recommended before administration of the euthanatizing agent.

Barbituric Acid Derivatives

Barbiturates depress the entire central nervous system, but quantitatively, various areas are affected differently. Within seconds of intravenous administration, unconsciousness is induced, which progresses to deep anesthesia (Fig. 24–1*B*). Breathing stops from depression of the respiratory center, and cessation of heart action quickly follows. Direct action on the medulla accounts for respiratory depression when high doses are given. Several barbiturates are acceptable, but pentobarbital sodium is most commonly used for euthanasia.

Advantages. A primary advantage of barbiturates is speed of action. This effect is dependent not only on the dose, but also on concentration and rate of injection. The barbiturates give smooth induction of euthanasia, minimal discomfort to the animal during injection, and a favorable impression on the observer because the animal dies quietly (Fig. 24–1*B*).

Disadvantages. 1) Intravenous injection is necessary for best results, necessitating trained personnel. 2) Each animal must be individually restrained. 3) Current federal drug regulations require strict accounting for the barbiturates and, by necessity, these must be used under the supervision of personnel registered with the US Drug Enforcement Agency.

Recommendations. The advantages of using barbiturates for euthanasia in small animals far outweigh the disadvantages The intravenous injection of a barbituric acid derivative is the preferred method for euthanasia of individual dogs, cats, and other small animals. Some animals, because of nervousness or viciousness, should be quieted by prior administration of a tranquilizer or sedative.

T-61*

T-61 is an injectable nonbarbiturate, nonnarcotic mixture of three drugs used to induce euthanasia. These drugs provide a combination of general anesthetic, curariform, and local anesthetic actions. Death results from severe CNS depression, hypoxia, and circulatory collapse. T-61 has been used in Germany since 1962 and became available in the United States soon thereafter (Eikmeier, 1962; Kuepper, 1964; Lumb et al., 1978; Quin, 1963). Because it is not currently listed as a controlled substance under federal drug regulations, it has gained popularity in recent years.

A comparative study of T-61 and pentobarbital (at 57.1 mg/kg of body weight) indicated that either agent induced euthanasia smoothly and without undesirable reactions (Lumb et al., 1978). The dogs given T-61 received two-thirds of the total dose (0.3 ml/kg of body weight) at a rate of 0.2 ml/sec with the last one-third given at 1.2 ml/sec. With both pentobarbital and T-61, the EEG changed from a normal awake pattern to one of low frequency and increased amplitude for approximately 5 seconds followed quickly by electrical silence. The dogs treated with pentobarbital required 12 seconds longer for the occurrence of electrical silence. With both agents, alterations in ECG developed immediately, and arterial pressure dropped to zero. Results of this study indicate that painless death is produced by pentobarbital or T-61 (Figs. 24–1*B*, *C*).

Advantages. T-61 may be used in mammalian species including dogs (Lumb et al., 1978), cats, horses, laboratory animals, and birds. The terminal gasp (Fowler and Foster, 1970) that may accompany pentobarbital euthanasia is not evident with T-61.

Disadvantages. 1) Intravenous injection is recommended for T-61; therefore, it has most of the same limitations as barbiturate derivatives. T-61 may be given intracardially. 2) T-61 is not approved for use in animals intended for human consumption. 3) Except in the horse, if T-61 is injected at a rapid rate, the animal may appear to experience pain or discomfort immediately prior to becoming unconscious. 4) If larger than recommended doses are given, pulmonary edema and other tissue lesions may be produced. This is an important consideration

*Each milliliter contains: 200 mg of N-[2—(m-methoxyphenyl)—2-ethyl-butyl-(1)]—gamma-hydroxybutyramide, 50 mg of 4,4′-methylene-bis (cyclohexyl-trimethyl-ammonium iodide), and 5 mg of tetracaine hydrochloride, with 0.6 ml dimethylformamide in distilled water.

when tissues are required for histopathologic examination following euthanasia.

Recommendations. If barbiturates cannot be used, T-61 appears to be a suitable substitute. T-61 must be administered in recommended dosages and at proper injection rates.

Chloral Hydrate

Chloral hydrate depresses the cerebrum slowly so that restraint during induction may create a problem in some animals. A fatal dose causes death by progressive depression of the respiratory center. Death may be preceded by gasping, muscle spasm, and whining or crying.

Recommendation. Chloral hydrate is not recommended for euthanasia of dogs, cats, and other small animals because the associated signs may be severe and are esthetically objectionable.

Combination of Chloral Hydrate, Magnesium Sulfate, and Sodium Pentobarbital

This combination has been used for anesthesia of large animals and may be administered in overdosage for euthanasia (Lumb and Jones, 1973).

Recommendation. This mixture is an acceptable large animal euthanatizing agent when administered intravenously.

Strychnine

Strychnine increases the excitability of the CNS, leaving the animal conscious and excessively responsive to stimuli. Strychnine produces violent convulsions and associated contraction of skeletal muscles that are painful (Franz, 1975).

Recommendation. Strychnine is absolutely condemned for euthanasia.

Magnesium Sulfate ($MgSO_4$)

Magnesium ions act at myoneural junctions, but exert little if any direct depressant or analgesic effect on the CNS. Dosages of $MgSO_4$ previously recommended for euthanasia have been shown to cause complete neuromuscular block and death due to asphyxia (Bowen et al., 1970).

Recommendation. Magnesium salts must not be used alone for euthanasia because of the lack of analgesic or anesthetic effect.

Nicotine

Nicotine is an alkaloid obtained from several species of tobacco. It is an odorless, clear liquid, soluble in water. Lethal doses can be absorbed through mucous membranes and intact skin, making its use dangerous for personnel.

Nicotine has been used extensively in the past in capture equipment for immobilizing wild game and feral and domestic dogs. Because of the high mortality rate, other drugs have replaced it.

Nicotine is an agent with curariform activity. It produces a short period of stimulation followed by paralysis of autonomic ganglia.

When injected in sufficient quantity, nicotine produces a muscle relaxant effect, with paralysis of the respiratory muscles and, subsequently, asphyxic death. Salivation, vomiting, defecation, and convulsions commonly occur prior to death.

Recommendation. Because nicotine is an extremely dangerous drug for personnel and induces serious side effects prior to death, it is absolutely condemned for euthanasia.

Curariform Drugs

Drugs such as curare, succinylcholine, pancuronium, guaifenesin, and other neuromuscular blocking agents produce death by immobilizing the respiratory muscles, causing fatal suffocation. There is no depressant action on the brain (Fig. 24–1*D*). Human patients given these drugs have described periods of full consciousness accompanied by complete muscular immobility and intense anxiety (Lumb and Jones, 1973).

Hicks and Bailey (1978) administered massive doses of succinylcholine to dogs and observed changes in ECG, EEG, and respiratory responses. They found initial bradycardia with elevated arterial blood pressure; as the myocardium failed, tachycardia was followed by a fall in arterial pressure. The EEG indicated no loss of consciousness as the normal awake wave form progressed to an activated EEG. The EEG activity continued long after cessation of respiration (> 7 min) before becoming isoelectric. Urination, salivation, and defecation commonly occurred along with muscular fasciculations. Asphyxial struggling was sometimes accompanied by violent fasciculations and head movements. These authors concluded that dogs given succinylcholine are conscious for prolonged intervals before dying of respiratory and cardiac arrest, and for this reason it should not be given as the sole agent for euthanasia.

Recommendations. Where standard methods of restraint are impractical, impossible, or dangerous, or where manual capture and restraint may cause pain and injury through struggling and anxiety, the use of immobilizing drugs is justified. Because the immobilized animal is fully conscious and subject to death by suffocation, euthanasia by captive-bolt, electrocution, or other methods must be accomplished immediately. Curariform drugs alone are not to be used for euthanasia.

Other Parenteral Preparations

Several injectable agents are currently available for immobilizing domestic and feral animals. Drugs such as ketamine HCl and xylazine are used for immobilization, analgesia, and anesthesia. The effect occurs within minutes following intramuscular injection, making these drugs useful for restraint. Currently, these agents are not included as controlled substances by federal drug regulations. Narcotics also may be used for sedation and analgesia, but detailed records must be kept and their use properly supervised by a licensed professional registered with the US Drug Enforcement Agency. Although it is possible to cause death with high doses of these drugs, such use would be impractical and may produce convulsions before death.

PHYSICAL METHODS

Electrocution

Electrocution as a form of euthanasia has been employed for years (British Veterinary Association, 1974; Carding, 1977; Croft, 1976; Croft and Hume, 1956; Croft, 1953; Croft, 1959; Hatch, 1977; Loftsgard et al., 1972; Roberts, 1974; Roberts, 1954; Swan, 1970; Warrington, 1974; WHO, 1962). Elaborate devices have been used for dogs and cats, such as closed wooden cabinets with separated front and rear metal floor sections serving as electrodes, or with a full metal floor plus a metal collar and chain serving as electrodes.

Experiments in dogs have shown the necessity of directing the electrical current through the brain in order to produce instant stunning with loss of consciousness. In the dog, when the electricity passes between front and rear limbs or neck and feet, it causes the heart to fibrillate promptly, but does not produce unconsciousness by action on the brain. The animal does not lose consciousness until affected by cerebral anoxia, which occurs a minimum of 12 seconds after cardiac fibrillation is induced by the electrical shock. These data dictate against use of the older-style euthanasia cabinets that direct current through the heart and not directly through the brain. An apparatus that applies electrodes to opposite sides of the head, or in another way directs electrical current immediately through the brain, is necessary to induce unconsciousness instantly. This effect should be followed promptly by electrically induced fibrillation of the heart.

Disadvantages. 1) Electrocution is not a useful method for mass euthanasia because so much time is required with each animal. 2) It is not a useful method for a vicious, intractable animal. 3) Violent extension and stiffening of the legs, head, and neck occur. 4) Electrocution is esthetically objectionable. 5) In small animals, electrocution may not result in death because ventricular fibrillation and circulatory collapse do not always persist after cessation of current flow. 6) It is hazardous to personnel.

Recommendations. Electrocution is humane only if special skills and equipment are employed to assure passage of sufficient current through the brain to produce unconsciousness followed by electrically induced fibrillation of the heart.

Gunshot and Captive-Bolt Pistol

Under some circumstances, gunshot may be the only practical method of euthanasia. It should be performed by a trained marksman utilizing a rifle or pistol appropriate for the situation. The projectile should be accurately placed to enter the brain, causing instant unconsciousness (Anis, 1976; Carding, 1977).

The captive-bolt pistol is more appropriate when there is effective restraint of the animal (Anis, 1976). This pistol utilizes a blank cartridge as propellant. When it is applied to the forehead, it fires a bolt through the skull, penetrating the brain. Since the bolt remains attached to the gun, the hazard of ricochet is eliminated.

Advantages. Euthanasia is instant and, under field conditions, gunshot may be the only effective method available.

Disadvantages. 1) It is dangerous to personnel; 2) it is esthetically unpleasant; 3) under field conditions it may be difficult to hit the brain; and 4) the method is not suitable where brain examination must be conducted after death.

Recommendations. Use of a captive-bolt pistol in restrained animals is recommended. Where restraint cannot be effectively accomplished, gunshot is an acceptable method of euthanasia.

Rapid Decompression (Hypoxia)

Brain function and consciousness are highly dependent on an adequate oxygen (O_2) supply. Hypoxia is a deficiency of O_2 available to the tissues (Van Liere, 1942; Van Liere and Stickney, 1963). Aircraft pilots flying at high altitude and exposed to a low O_2 environment frequently experience euphoria, followed by depression of the CNS. Hypoxia may be so acute that loss of consciousness occurs rapidly without any prior warning (Busby et al., 1976*a,b*). Unconsciousness occurs within 10 seconds in dogs exposed to simulated pressure altitudes between 50,000 and 55,000 feet (equivalent to 68.8 mm of Hg), whether breathing air or 100% oxygen (Bancroft and Dunn, 1965). Properly designed and maintained chambers operate at these pressures.

The relationships among unconsciousness, absence of pain, and involuntary muscular activity have been reviewed earlier in this report. Humane (the animal) and esthetic (the observer) considerations are often in conflict. Bancroft and Dunn (1965) listed some of the body responses during decompression after loss of consciousness and pain perception, as follows. Respirations become deep and rapid for several seconds. Marked abdominal distension occurs immediately, owing to expansion of gases present in the gastrointestinal tract. The animal collapses in about 8 seconds. Mild convulsions generally occur in 10 to 12 seconds and last for several seconds. Decerebrate rigidity also may occur (Edelmann and Hitchcock, 1952). Following a convulsive seizure, the animal is quiescent except for occasional respiratory gasps. Usually lacrimation, salivation, and urination occur. Intravascular gas bubbles are not produced at 55,000 feet or below (Kemph and Hitchcock, 1952).

The literature on rapid decompression as a means of producing hypoxia and its use in euthanasia was reviewed by Booth (1978). Although there are differences of opinion, evidence supported by EEG recordings indicates that hypoxia rapidly induces unconsciousness in both animals and human beings subjected to high altitude simulated by the use of decompression chambers.

Advantages. When properly used, decompression euthanasia is efficient, humane, and safe for personnel.

Disadvantages. Some cities and states have passed legislation banning the use of decompression euthanasia. The method has fallen into disrepute because of: 1) improper design, operation, maintenance, and functioning of equipment; 2) accidental recompression with recovery of the animal followed again by decompression before death; 3) bloating, bleeding, vomiting, convulsions, urination, and defecation in the unconscious animal, which are esthetically unpleasant; 4) possible overcrowding of the chamber; 5) the increased tolerance of immature animals (under 4 months old) to hypoxia and the long periods of decompression required before respiration ceases; 6) respiratory or middle ear infections, or both, that may cause pain from unequalized pressure; and 7) failure to understand the mechanisms of action of hypoxia and its effects on animals.

Recommendations. Rapid decompression is a satisfactory procedure for euthanasia, provided the equipment is properly constructed, correctly maintained, and proficiently operated. Because many difficulties have arisen in using decompression and because there is a general lack of understanding of how hypoxia affects animals, other methods of euthanasia are preferable.

Other Physical Methods

If a blow of sufficient force and accuracy is delivered to the skull of an animal, immediate unconsciousness results. Death should then be assured by thoracotomy, exsanguination, or other means. Because this procedure is esthetically offensive, it is not recommended when more suitable techniques are available.

Disarticulation of skull and cervical vertebrae is a method of producing euthanasia in mice and poultry. Guillotine devices have been used for decapitating smaller laboratory animals, especially rats. Although this procedure may be esthetically offensive, it is rapid, inexpensive, and when properly done, produces instant death.

Microwave irradiation of the brain has been reported as a procedure for killing small rodents (Jones et al., 1974; Schmidt et al., 1971; Stavinoha et al., 1973). The animal is restrained in a plastic holder, and a metal wave guide is utilized so that most of the energy from the magnetron is delivered to the head region. Internal heating of the brain causes inactivation of endogenous tissue enzymes and immediate unconsciousness. Death occurs in 2 to 4 seconds and is painless.

Methods such as drowning or exsanguination without producing prior unconsciousness can be painful, unreliable, productive of fear or apprehension in the animals, and dangerous to personnel performing euthanasia. These methods are not recommended.

PRECAUTIONS REGARDING FOOD ANIMALS

In euthanasia of animals intended for human food, agents cannot be used that lead to tissue residues, unless approved by the US Food and Drug Administration (Booth, 1977*a*). Carbon dioxide is the only chemical currently used in euthanasia of animals for human food (primarily swine) that does not lead to tissue residues.

ADDENDUM

Since 1978, at least two agents, different than those previously described, have become available for euthanasia (Lumb and Moreland, 1982). One of these is isoflurane, a volatile liquid inhalant anesthetic with characteristics similar to those of halothane (see Chap. 10). It should be administered for euthanasia in the same manner as described for halothane and with the same precautions. The other agent is a mixture of pentobarbital and phenytoin.* The phenytoin is claimed to speed cardiac collapse and CNS depression. In addition, it reduces the possibility of drug abuse and, for this reason, the mixture is placed in Class III by the Drug Enforcement Agency.

REFERENCES

American Humane Association: Chloroform Box, Construction and Use. American Humane Assoc., Denver, 1969.

Anis, G.W.: Euthanasia of Domesticated Animals by Shooting. In *Humane Destruction of Unwanted Animals*. The Universities Federation for Animal Welfare, Potters Bar, Herts, England, 1976.

Austin, F.H.: Chemical Agents for Use in the Humane Destruction of Horses. Ir. Vet. J., 27:45, 1973.

Bancroft, R.W. and Dunn, J.E., II: Experimental Animal Decompressions to a Near Vacuum Environment. Aerospace Med., 36:720, 1965.

Blood, D.C., Johnston, D.E., and Blackwood, J.D.: Carbon Monoxide Euthanasia. A Report to the Committee of the Victorian Division of the Royal Society for Prevention of Cruelty to Animals. (Information provided for the 1972 Report of the AVMA Panel on Euthanasia.)

Bloom J.D.: Some Considerations in Establishing Divers' Breathing Gas Purity Standards for Carbon Monoxide. Aerospace Med., 43:633, 1972.

Booth, N.H.: Drug and Chemical Residues in the Edible Tissues of Animals. In *Veterinary Pharmacology and Therapeutics*, 4th ed. Edited by L.M. Jones, N.H. Booth, and L.E. McDonald. Iowa State University Press, Ames, 1977*a*.

Booth, N.H.: Effect of Rapid Decompression and Associated Hypoxic Phenomena in Euthanasia of Animals: A Review. J.A.V.M.A., 173:308, 1978.

Booth N.H.: Inhalant Anesthetics. In *Veterinary Pharmacology and Therapeutics*, 4th ed. Edited by L.M. Jones,

*See Appendix A for manufacturer.

N.H. Booth, and L.E. McDonald. Iowa State University Press. Ames, 1977*b*.

Bowen, J.M., Blackman, D.M., and Heavner, J.E.: Effect of Magnesium Ions on Neuromuscular Transmission in the Horse, Steer, and Dog. J.A.V.M.A., 157:164, 1970.

Breazile, J.E.: *Textbook of Veterinary Physiology.* Philadelphia, Lea & Febiger, 1971.

Breazile, J.E., and Kitchell, R.L.: Euthanasia for Laboratory Animals. Fed. Proc., 28:1577, 1969.

British Veterinary Association: Electrical Euthanasia of Dogs. Vet. Rec., 95:239, 1974.

Busby, D.E., Higgins, E.A., and Funkhouser, G.E.: Effect of Physical Activity of Airline Flight Attendants on their Time of Useful Consciousness in a Rapid Decompression. Aviat. Space Environ. Med., 47:117, 1976*a*.

Busby, D.E., Higgins, E.A., and Funkhouser, G.E.: Protection of Airline Flight Attendants from Hypoxia Following Rapid Decompression. Aviat. Space Environ. Med., 47:942, 1976*b*.

Carding, A.H.: Mass Euthanasia of Dogs with Carbon Monoxide and/or Carbon Dioxide. Preliminary Trials. J. Small Anim. Pract., 9:245, 1968.

Carding, T.: Euthanasia of Dogs and Cats. Animal Regulation Studies, 1:5, 1977.

Croft, P.G.: Anaesthesia and Euthanasia. In *UFAW Handbook on the Care and Management of Laboratory Animals,* 3rd ed. Williams & Wilkins, Baltimore, 1967.

Croft, P.G.: Electrical Euthanasia of Unwanted Dogs. In *Humane Destruction of Unwanted Animals.* The Universities Federation for Animal Welfare, Potters Bar, Herts, England, 1976.

Croft, P.G., and Hume, C.W.: Electric Stunning of Sheep. Vet. Rec., 68:318, 1956.

Croft, P.G.: Electric Stunning and Electrocution of Small Animals. Vet. Rec., 65:259, 1953.

Croft, P.G.: Euthanasia. In *Veterinary Annual.* Edited by W.A. Pool. John Wright and Sons Ltd., Bristol, 1959.

DHEW: Occupational Exposure to Waste Anesthetic Gases and Vapors. DHEW (NIOSH) No. 77–140, Washington, DC, March 1977.

Dodman, N.H.: Observations on the Use of the Wernberg Dip-lift Carbon Dioxide Apparatus for Pre-Slaughter Anaesthesia of Pigs. Br. Vet. J., 133:71, 1977.

Edelmann, A., and Hitchcock, F.A.: Observations on Dogs Exposed to an Ambient Pressure of 30 Mm Hg. J. Appl. Physiol., 4:807, 1952.

Eikmeier, H.: Experiences with a New Preparation for Painless Destruction of Small Animals (T-61). Die Blauen Hefte Tieraerztl., 5:22, 1962.

Feldman, D.B., and Gupta, B.N.: Histopathologic Changes in Laboratory Animals Resulting from Various Methods of Euthanasia. Lab. Anim. Sci., 26:218, 1976.

Fowler, N.G. and Foster, S.J.: The Last Gasp. Vet. Rec., 86:145, 1970.

Franz, D.N.: Central Nervous System Stimulants. In *The Pharmacological Basis of Therapeutics,* 5th ed. Edited by L.S. Goodman, and A. Gilman. Macmillan Publishing Co. Inc., New York, 1975.

Glass, H.G., Snyder, F.F., and Webster, E.: The Rate of Decline in Resistance to Anoxia of Rabbits, Dogs, and Guinea Pigs from the Onset of Viability to Adult Life. Am. J. Physiol., 140:609, 1944.

Glen, J.B., and Scott, W.N.: Carbon Dioxide Euthanasia of Cats. Br. Vet. J., 129:471, 1973.

Guyton, A.C.: *Textbook of Medical Physiology,* 5th ed. W.B. Saunders Co., Philadelphia, 1976.

Haldane, J.: The Action of Carbonic Oxide in Man. J. Physiol., 18:430, 1895.

Hall, L.W.: The Anaesthesia and Euthanasia of Neonatal and Juvenile Dogs and Cats. Vet. Rec., 90:303, 1972.

Hatch, R.C.: Euthanizing Agents. In *Veterinary Pharmacology and Therapeutics.* Edited by L.M. Jones, N.H. Booth, and L.E. McDonald. Iowa State University Press, Ames, 1977.

Herin, R.A., Hall, P., and Fitch, J.W.: Nitrogen Inhalation as a Method of Euthanasia in Dogs. Am. J. Vet. Res., 39:989, 1978.

Hicks, T. and Bailey, E.M., Jr.: Succinylcholine Chloride as an Euthanatizing Agent in Dogs. Am. J. Vet. Res., 39:1195, 1978.

Jones, D.J., Medina, M.A., Ross, D.H., and Stavinoha, W.B.: Rate of Inactivation of Adenyl Cyclase and Phosphodiesterase: Determinants of Brain Cyclic AMP. Life Sci., 14:1577, 1974.

Kemph, J.P., and Hitchcock, F.A.: Changes in Blood and Circulation of Dogs Following Explosive Decompression to Low Barometric Pressures. Am. J. Physiol., 168:592, 1952.

Klemm, W.R.: Carbon Dioxide Anesthesia in Cats. Am. J. Vet. Res., 25:1201, 1964.

Kline, B.E., Peckman, V., and Hesit, H.E.: Some Aids in Handling Large Numbers of Mice. Lab. Anim. Care, 13:84, 1963.

Kotula, A.W., Drewniak, E.E., and Davis, L.L.: Experimentation with In-line Carbon Dioxide Immobilization of Chickens Prior to Slaughter. Poult. Sci., 40:213, 1961.

Kuepper, G.: T-61 Used in Large Animals. Die Blauen Hefte Tieraeztl., 8:32, 1964.

Leake, C.D., and Waters, R.M.: The Anesthetic Properties of Carbon Dioxide. Current Researches in Anesthesiology and Analgesia (Cleve), 8:17, 1929.

Loftsgard, G., Braathen, S., and Helgobostd, A.: Electrical Stunning of Mink. Vet. Rec., 91:132, 1972.

Lumb, W.V., and Jones, E.: *Veterinary Anesthesia.* Lea & Febiger, Philadelphia, 1973.

Lumb, W.V.: Euthanasia by Noninhalant Pharmacologic Agents. J.A.V.M.A., 165:851, 1974.

Lumb, W.V., Doshi, K., and Scott, R.I.: A Comparative Study of T-61 and Pentobarbital for Euthanasia of Dogs. J.A.V.M.A., 172:149, 1978.

Lumb, W.V., and Moreland, A.F.: Chemical Methods for Euthanasia. Lab. Anim., 11:29, 1982.

Mattsson, J.L., Stinson, J.M., and Clark, C.S.: Electroencephalographic Power-Spectral Changes Coincident with Onset of Carbon Dioxide Narcosis in Rhesus Monkey. Am. J. Vet. Res., 33:2043, 1972.

McArthur, J.A.: Carbon Dioxide Euthanasia of Small Animals (Including Cats). In *Humane Destruction of Unwanted Animals.* The Universities Federation for Animal Welfare, Potters Bar, Herts, England, 1976.

Moreland, A.F.: Carbon Monoxide Euthanasia of Dogs: Chamber Concentrations and Comparative Effects of Automobile Engine Exhaust and Carbon Monoxide from a Cylinder. J.A.V.M.A., 165:853, 1974.

Noell, W.K. and Chinn, H.I.: Time Course of Failure of

the Visual Pathway in Rabbits During Anoxia. Fed. Proc., 8:119, 1949.

Quin, A.H.: Observations on a New Euthanasia Agent for Small Animals. Vet. Med., 58:494, 1963.

Ramsey, T.L. and Eilmann, H.J.: Carbon Monoxide Acute and Chronic Poisoning and Experimental Studies. J. Lab. Clin. Med., 17:415, 1932.

Roberts, T.D.M.: Correspondence Electrocution Cabinets. Vet. Rec., 95:241, 1974.

Roberts, T.D.M.: Cortical Activity in Electrocuted Dogs. Vet. Rec., 66:561, 1954.

Sanford, J.: Euthanasia of Domesticated Animals by Injection of Drugs. In *Humane Destruction of Unwanted Animals*. The Universities Federation of Animal Welfare, Potters Bar, Herts, England, 1976.

Sawyer, D.C.: Comparative Effects of Halothane. Gaines Dog Res. Prog., 1976.

Sawyer, D.C., Wallin, R.F., and Port, C.: Michigan State University, E. Lansing, Unpublished data. 1978.

Schmidt, M.J., Schmidt, D.E., and Robinson, G.A.: Cyclic Adenosine Monophosphate in Brain Areas: Microwave Irradiation as a Means of Tissue Fixation. Science, 173:1142, 1971.

Scott, W.N.: The Use of Poisons in Animal Destruction. In *Humane Destruction of Unwanted Animals*. The Universities Federation of Animal Welfare, Potters Bar, Herts, England, 1976.

Stavinoha, W.B., Weintraub, S.T., and Modak, A.T.: The Use of Microwave Heating to Inactivate Cholinesterase in the Rat Brain Prior to Analysis for Acetylcholine. J. Neurochem., 20:361, 1973.

Stone, W.S., Amiraian, K., Duell, C., and Schadeer, C.: Carbon Dioxide Anesthetization of Guinea Pigs to Increase Yields of Blood and Serum. Proc. Anim. Care Panel, 11:299, 1961.

Swan, J.F.C.: Effectiveness of Electrical Stunning. Vet. Rec., 86:212, 1970.

Swenson, M.J.: *Duke's Physiology of Domestic Animals*, 9th ed. Cornell University Press, Ithaca, N.Y., 1977.

Swineyard, E.A.: Noxious Gases and Vapors. In *The Pharmacological Basis of Therapeutics*, 5th ed. Edited by L.S. Goodman, and A. Gilman. Macmillan Publishing Co. Inc., 1975.

Universities Federation for Animal Welfare: *Humane Killing of Unwanted Animals*, 2nd ed. The Universities Federation for Animal Welfare, Potters Bar, Herts, England, 1968.

Universities Federation for Animal Welfare: Euthanasia (Carbon Dioxide). In *Report and Accounts*. The Universities Federation for Animal Welfare, Potters Bar, Herts, England, 1976–1977.

Van Liere, E.J.: *Anoxia, Its Effect on the Body*. University of Chicago Press, Chicago, 1942.

Van Liere, E.J. and Stickney, J.C.: *Hypoxia*. University of Chicago Press, Chicago, 1963.

Vinter, F.J.: *The Humane Killing of Mink*. The Universities Federation for Animal Welfare, London, 1957.

Warrington, R.: Electrical Stunning, A Review of Literature. Vet. Bull., 44:617, 1974.

WHO Joint FAO/WHO Expert Committee on Meat Hygiene. Second Report. World Health Org. Tech. Rep. Ser., 241, 1962.

Woodbury, D.M., Rollins, L.T., Gardner, M.D., Hirschi, W.L., Hogan, J.R., Rollison, M.L., Tanner, G.S., and Brodie, D.A.: Effects of Carbon Dioxide on Brain Excitability and Electrolytes. Am. J. Physiol., 192:79, 1958.

Appendix A

Sources for Drugs and Equipment* Described in the Text

DRUGS

Generic Name	*Trade Name*	*Manufacturer†*
Acepromazine maleate	Acepromazine	9
Adrenocorticosteroids		
Prednisolone Na succinate	Solu-Delta Cortef	57
Dexamethasone	Azium	51
Althesin	Saffan	29
Aminophylline		22
4-Aminopyridine	4-AP	52
Apomorphine hydrochloride		36
Atropine sulfate		25
Azaperone	Stresnil	32
Bretylium tosylate	Bretylol	6
Bupivacaine hydrochloride	Marcaine	59
Butacaine sulfate	Butyn	1
Butorphanol tartrate	Torbutrol	13
Calcium chloride solution		22
Carbon dioxide		40, 47
Carfentanil	R33799	32
Chloral hydrate (See also Pentobarbital sodium)		38
α-Chloralose		24, 46
Chlorobutanol	Chloretone	24
Chloroform		38
Chloroprocaine hydrochloride	Nesacaine	8
Chlorpromazine hydrochloride		22
Cocaine hydrochloride		36
Cyclopropane		40
Cyprenorphine hydrochloride	M-285	32
Dantrolene sodium	Dantrium	39
Dextran	Macrodex (Dextran 70)	44
	Rheomacrodex (Dextran 40)	44
Diazepam	Valium	50
Dibucaine hydrochloride	Nupercaine	16
Digoxin	Lanoxin	58
Diprenorphine hydrochloride	M50–50	32, 35
Dobutamine hydrochloride	Dobutrex	36
Dopamine hydrochloride	Inotropin	6
Doxapram hydrochloride	Dopram-V	49
Droperidol		32
Dyclonine hydrochloride	Dyclone	8
Edrophonium chloride	Tensilon	50
Enflurane	Ethrane	40
Epinephrine hydrochloride	Adrenalin	22
Ether		54
Ethyl chloride		27
Ethylisobutrazine	Diquel	33
Ethylene		40

*Inclusion of a drug or item of equipment on this list does not imply endorsement of the product by the authors and is for informational purposes only.

†The numbers in this column are keys to the names and addresses of manufacturers appearing on pages 651–653.

DRUGS

Generic Name	*Trade Name*	*Manufacturer*†
Etidocaine hydrochloride	Duranest	8
Etomidate	Amidate	1
Etorphine hydrochloride	M-99	32, 35
Etorphine–Acepromazine	Immobilon-LA	48
Etorphine–Methotrimeprazine	Immobilon-SA	48
Fentanyl citrate		32, 45
Fentanyl citrate–Droperidol	Innovar-Vet	45
Furosemide	Lasix	31
Gallamine triethiodide	Flaxedil	4
Glycopyrrolate	Robinul-V	49
Guaifenesin	Gecolate	55
	Glycodex	14
Halothane	Fluothane	9, 30
Heparin sodium		37, 49
Hetastarch	Hespan	3
Hexylcaine hydrochloride	Cyclaine	38
Hyaluronidase	Wydase	60
Isoflurane	Forane	40
Isoproterenol hydrochloride	Isuprel	22
Ketamine hydrochloride	Vetalar	42
	Ketaset	13
Lactated Ringer's solution		1
Levallorphan tartrate	Lorfan	50
Levarterenol bitartrate	Levophed	12
Levorphanol tartrate	Levo-Dromoran	50
Lidocaine hydrochloride	Xylocaine	8
Mannitol		5
Meperidine hydrochloride	Demerol	22
Mephentermine sulfate	Wyamine	60
Mepivacaine hydrochloride	Carbocaine	12
Metaraminol bitartrate	Aramine	38
Methadone hydrochloride	Dolophine	36
Methocel		21
Methohexital sodium	Brevital	36
Methotrimeprazine hydrochloride		48
Methoxamine hydrochloride	Vasoxyl	58
Methoxyflurane	Metofane	45
	Penthrane	1
Methoxymol		32
Methylpentynol		24
Metocurine iodide	Metubine	36
Metomidate hydrochloride	Hypnodil	32
Morphine sulfate		36
Nalorphine hydrochloride	Nalline	38
Naloxone hydrochloride	Narcan	23
Neostigmine methylsulfate	Prostigmine	50
Nitrous oxide		40, 47
Oxymorphone hydrochloride	Numorphan	23
Pancuronium bromide	Pavulon	41
Paraldehyde		38
Pentazocine lactate	Talwin-V	59
Pentobarbital sodium	Nembutal	1
	Bulk Powder (for euthanasia solution)	26
Pentobarbital sodium, chloral hydrate, and magnesium sulfate		25
Pentobarbital sodium and phenytoin	Beuthanasia-D Special (for euthanasia)	14
Perfluorochemical emulsion	Fluosol-DA	2
Phenobarbital sodium		36

†The numbers are keys to the names and addresses of manufacturers appearing on pages 651–653.

DRUGS

Generic Name	Trade Name	Manufacturer†
Phenoxybenzamine hydrochloride	Dibenzyline	53
2-Phenoxyethanol		24
Phentolamine mesylate	Regitine	16
Phenylephrine hydrochloride	Neo-Synephrine	59
Phenytoin sodium	Dilantin	22
Piperacetazine	Psymod	45
Piperocaine hydrochloride	Metycaine	36
Potassium chloride solution		1
Pralidoxime chloride	Protopam	9
Prilocaine hydrochloride	Citanest	8
Procainamide	Pronestyl	54
Procaine hydrochloride	Novocaine	59
Promazine hydrochloride		60
Proparacaine hydrochloride	Ophthaine	54
Propiopromazine hydrochloride	Tranvet	20
Propoxate hydrochloride	R7464	32
Propranolol hydrochloride	Inderal	9
Protamine sulfate		36
Pyridostigmine	Regonol	41
Quinadine gluconate		36
Quinaldine sulfate	Quinate	17, 24
Sodium bicarbonate		1
Sodium nitroprusside	Nipride	50
4-Styrlpyridine	4-Stilbazole	24
Succinylcholine chloride	Anectine	58
	Sucostrin	54
Tetracaine hydrochloride	Pontocaine	12
	Cetacaine (spray)	15
Thiambutene hydrochloride	Themalon	28
Thiamylal sodium	Biotal	11
Thiopental sodium	Pentothal	1
Tricaine methanesulfonate	MS-222	17, 24
Trichloroethylene	Trilene	40
Triflupromazine hydrochloride	Vetame	54
Trimethaphan	Arfonad	50
Tromethamine	THAM	1
Tubocurarine chloride		54
T-61		31
Urethan	Urethane	38
Xylazine hydrochloride	Rompun	10
Yohimbine		52

†The numbers are keys to the names and addresses of manufacturers appearing on pages 651–653.

DRUG MANUFACTURERS

1. Abbott Laboratories
   Abbott Park Dept 342
   North Chicago
   IL 60064
2. Alpha Therapeutic Corporation
   5555 Valley Boulevard
   Los Angeles, CA 90032
3. American Critical Care
   1600 Waukegan Road
   McGaw Park, IL 60085
4. American Cyanamid Company
   PO Box 400
   Princeton, NJ 08540
5. American Quinine
   Hospital Division of Natcon Chemical Company, Inc.
   1 Fairchild Court
   Plainview, NY 11803
6. Arnar-Stone Laboratories, Inc.
   McGaw Park, IL 60085
7. Arnold-Nasco Ltd.
   58 Dawson Road
   Guelph, Ontario
   Canada N1H 6P9
8. Astra Pharmaceutical Products
   7 Neoponset Street
   Worcester
   MA 01606

DRUG MANUFACTURERS

9. Ayerst Laboratories
685 3rd Avenue
New York, NY 10017
10. Bayvet Division
Miles Laboratories, Inc.
PO Box 390
Shawnee, KS 66201
11. Bio-Ceutic Laboratories, Inc.
PO Box 999
St. Joseph, MO 64502
12. Breon Laboratories, Inc.
Subsidiary of Sterling Drug, Inc.
90 Park Avenue
New York, NY 10016
13. Bristol Laboratories
Veterinary Products
Division of Bristol-Myers Company
Syracuse, NY 13201
14. Burns-Biotec Laboratories, Inc.
8536 K Street
Omaha, NB 68127
15. Cetylite Industries, Inc.
9051 River Road
Pennsauken, NJ 08110
16. Ciba Pharmaceutical Company
556 Morris Avenue
Summit, NJ 07901
17. Crescent Research Chemicals, Inc.
5301 North 37th Place
Paradise Valley, AZ 85253
18. Cutter Laboratories
Fourth and Parker Streets
Berkeley, CA 94710
19. Deseret Medical, Inc.
9450 South State Street
Sandy, UT 84070
20. Diamond Laboratories
2538 Southeast 43rd Street
PO Box 863
Des Moines, IA 50304
21. Dow Corning Corporation
Midland, MI 48640
22. Elkins-Sinn, Inc.
Subsidiary of A.H. Robins
2 Esterbrook Lane
Cherry Hill, NJ 08034
23. Endo Laboratories, Inc.
1000 Stewart Avenue
Garden City, NY 11530
24. Fisher Scientific Company
711 Forbes Avenue
Pittsburgh, PA 15219
25. Fort Dodge Laboratories
800 5th Street, N.W.
Fort Dodge, IA 50501
26. Ganes Chemical Works
1114 Avenue of the Americas
New York, NY 10036
27. Gebauer Chemical Company
9410 St. Catherine Avenue
Cleveland, OH 44104
28. W. Gimber & Sons, Ltd.
Veterinary Division
10./2 Queens Road
Peckham, London, S. E. 15
England
29. Glaxo Laboratories Ltd.,
Greenford
Middlesex, England UB6 OHE
30. Halocarbon Pharmaceutical Company
PO Box 833
Hackensack, NJ 07601
31. Hoechst-Roussel Pharmaceuticals, Inc.
Route 202-206 North
Somerville, NJ 08876
32. Janssen Pharmaceutica
Turnhoutsebaan 30
2340 Beerse
Belgium
33. Jensen-Salsbery Laboratories, Inc.
520 West 21st Street
Kansas City, MO 64141
34. Lederle Laboratories
Division of American Cyanamid Company
One Cyanamid Plaza
Wayne, NJ 07470
35. Lemmon Company
PO Box 1729
Rockville, MD 20850
36. Lilly, Eli and Company
640 East McCarty Street
Indianapolis, IN 42685
37. Med-Tech, Inc.
Elkan Estates
PO Box 338
Elwood, KS 66024
38. Merck & Company
126 East Lincoln Avenue
PO Box 2000
Rahway, NJ 07065
39. Norwich-Eaton Pharmaceuticals
PO Box 191
Norwich, NY 13815
40. Ohio Medical Products
PO Box 1319
3030 Airco Drive
Madison, WI 53701
41. Organon, Inc.
375 Mount Pleasant Avenue
West Orange, NJ 07052
42. Parke-Davis
Division of Warner Lambert Company
201 Tabor Road
Morris Plains, NJ 07950
43. Pfizer, Charles, & Company, Inc.
235 East 42nd Street
New York, NY 10017
44. Pharmacia Laboratories
Division of Pharmacia, Inc.
800 Centennial Avenue
Piscataway, NJ 08854
45. Pitman-Moore Company
PO Box 344
Washington Crossing, NJ 08560

Drug Manufacturers

46. Prolabo
    12 Rue Pelee
    Paris 11, France
47. Puritan Bennett Corporation
    10800 Pflumm Road
    Lenexa, KS 66215
48. Reckett and Colman Pharmaceuticals
    Dansom Lane
    Kingston-upon-Hull
    England HU8 7DS
49. Robins, A.H., Company
    1407 Cummings Drive
    Richmond, VA 23261–6609
50. Roche Laboratories
    Division of Hoffmann-La Roche Inc.
    340 Kingsland Road
    Nutley, NJ 07110
51. Schering Corporation
    Bloomfield, NJ 07003
52. Sigma Chemical Company
    PO Box 14508
    St. Louis, MO 63178
53. Smith Kline & French Laboratories
    1500 Spring Garden Street
    Philadelphia, PA 19101
54. Squibb Pharmaceutical Company
    E.R. Squibb and Sons, Inc.
    PO Box 4000
    Princeton, NJ 08540
55. Summit Hill Laboratories
    PO Box 1
    Avalon, NJ 08202
56. Travenol Laboratories, Inc.
    Morton Grove, IL 60053
57. Upjohn Company (The)
    7000 Portage Road
    Kalamazoo, MI 49001
58. Wellcome Veterinary Division
    Burroughs-Wellcome Company
    3030 Cornwallis Road
    Research Triangle Park, NC 27709
59. Winthrop Laboratories
    90 Park Avenue
    New York, NY 10016
60. Wyeth Laboratories
    PO Box 8299
    Philadelphia, PA 19101

Equipment

Description or Trade Name	*Manufacturer†*
Anesthesia carts	14
Anesthesia chambers	59
Anesthesia machines	12, 25, 29, 41, 42
Anesthetic gas analyzers for operating rooms	24
Animal control equipment (syringe guns, poles, blowguns, snares)	26, 36, 45, 57, 67, 69
Animal restrainers/positioners	3, 29, 53
Baralyme	15
Bayer's wedge	5
Blood filters, warming systems, banking and administration equipment	1, 23
Blood gas analyzers (oxygen, carbon dioxide, pH)	18, 33, 50
Blood pressure monitors (indirect, Doppler)	1, 35, 43
Blood pressure transducers and recorders (see also cardiac output)	1, 9, 19, 30, 47, 55
Blood volume monitor	44
Carbon dioxide monitors	1, 8, 42
Cardiac monitors and/or defibrillators	1, 10, 19, 30, 47, 63
Cardiac output equipment	20, 28, 30
Central venous pressure (CVP) monitor	7, 23
Drinkwater mouth gag	7
Electrocardiograph	8, 13, 30
Electroencephalograph	8, 30
Endotracheal catheters	
small animal	15, 39, 40, 41, 42, 49
large animal	25, 39
Esophageal stethoscope	41, 42
Euthanasia equipment	
captive bolt pistol	37
chambers	26, 60, 64
microwave	56
Heating/cooling pads and blankets	3, 16, 27, 63, 67
Humidifiers	12, 42
Incubators	1, 42, 59
Intravenous fluid administration sets, manifolds, flow regulators, and catheters	1, 7, 17, 23, 55
Laryngoscopes	
small animal	25, 41, 42, 49
large animal	25
Masks	12, 41, 42, 49
Microsyringes	61
Nerve stimulators	48, 65
Oncometers	33
Operating tables	
small animal	29, 53
large animal	54, 66
human	2
Oxygen blenders	12, 15, 25, 41, 42, 49
Oxygen chambers and cages	1, 15, 49, 59
Oxygen monitors	1, 11, 42
Oxygen regulators	15, 25, 41, 42, 49
Oxygenators (for heart-lung bypass)	9, 17
Pneumotachograph	32
Pressurized intravenous infusion equipment	6, 22, 23, 55
Pumps (for heart-lung bypass)	52
Rebreathing bags	15, 41, 42, 49
Reelite (for electric clippers)	4
Respiration monitors	10, 12, 42, 46, 63
Respirators/ventilators	1, 12, 41, 42, 49
Resuscitators	12, 31, 38, 42
Soda lime	42
Squeeze cages	51
Suction equipment	1, 55
Thermometers (thermistor)	58, 68
Tracheostomy tube (emergency airway)	34
Vaporizers	12, 15, 42, 49
Vetaspirator	62, 65

*The numbers on this column are keys to the names and addresses of manufacturers appearing on pages 654–655.

Equipment Manufacturers

1. Air Shields, Inc.
   330 Jacksonville Road
   Hatboro, PA 19040
2. Amsco Division
   American Sterilizer Company
   Erie, PA 16512
3. Ancare Corporation
   PO Box 354
   Manhasset, NY 11030
4. Appleton Electric Company
   Chicago, IL 60600
5. Arnold-Nasco Ltd.
   58 Dawson Road
   Guelph, Ontario
   Canada N14 6P9
6. Auto-Syringe, Inc.
   Londonderry Turnpike
   Hooksett, NH 03104
7. Bard-Parker
   Division of Becton, Dickinson and Company
   2 Bridgewater Lane
   Lincoln Park, NJ 07035
8. Beckman Instruments Company
   1548 South State College
   Anaheim, CA 92806
9. Bentley Laboratories, Inc.
   17502 Armstrong Avenue
   Irvine, CA 92714
10. Bickford, A.M., Inc.
    1581 Hubbard Road
    East Aurora, NY 14052
11. BioMarine Industries
    45 Great Valley Center
    Malvern, PA 19355
12. Bird Products/3M
    225-5S 3M Center
    St. Paul, MN 55144
13. Birtcher Corporation (The)
    4371 Valley Blvd.
    Los Angeles, CA 90032
14. Blue Bell Bio-Medical
    532 Township Line Road
    Blue Bell, PA 19422
15. Chemetron Medical Division
    Allied Health Products, Inc.
    1720 Sublette
    St. Louis, MO 63110
16. Cincinnati Sub-Zero Products, Inc.
    2612 Gilbert Avenue
    Cincinnati, OH 45206
17. Cobe Laboratories, Inc.
    11010 West 12th Avenue
    Lakewood, CO 80215
18. Corning Scientific Instruments
    Medfield, MA 02052
19. Datascope Corporation
    580 Winters Avenue
    Paramus, NJ 07652
20. Edwards Laboratories
    PO Box 11150
    Santa Ana, CA 92711
21. Euthanair Company
    13644 Camilla Street
    Whittier, CA 90601
22. Extracorporeal Medical Specialties, Inc.
    Ross and Royal Roads
    King of Prussia, PA 19406
23. Fenwal Laboratories
    Division of Travenol Laboratories
    Deerfield, IL 60015
24. Foxboro Analytical
    140 Water Street
    PO Box 5449
    South Norwalk, CT 06856
25. Fraser Harlake, Inc.
    145 Mid County Drive
    Orchard Park, NY 14127
26. Gerwig Manufacturing Company
    PO Box 679
    Ashland, OH 44805
27. Gorman-Rupp Industries Division
    American Hospital Supply Corporation
    Bellville, OH 44813
28. Gould Inc.
    Measurement Systems Division
    2230 Statham Boulevard
    Oxnard, CA 93030
29. Harvard Apparatus Company, Inc.
    22 Pleasant Street
    South Natick, MA 01760
30. Hewlett-Packard
    Medical Electronics Division
    175 Wyman Street
    Waltham, MA 02254
31. Hudson Oxygen Therapy Sales Company,
    Wadsworth, OH 44281
32. Instrumentation Associates, Inc.
    17 West 60th Street
    New York, NY 10017
33. Instrumentation Laboratory Inc.
    113 Hartwell Avenue
    Lexington, MA 02173
34. International Medical Devices, Inc.
    PO Box 408
    Canoga Park, CA 91303
35. IVAC Corporation
    10300 Campus Point Drive
    San Diego, CA 92121-1579
36. Ketch-All Company
    2537 University Avenue
    San Diego, CA 92104
37. Koch Supplies, Inc.
    1411 West 29th
    Kansas City, MO 64108
38. Laerdal Medical Corporation
    1 Labriola Court
    Armonk, NY 10504
39. Lane Manufacturing, Inc.
    5560 East Pacific Place
    Denver, CO 80222
40. Link Sales Company
    2426 South 73rd Street
    Milwaukee, WI 53219
41. North American Dräger
    148B Quarry Road
    Telford, PA 18969
42. Ohio Medical Products
    PO Box 1319
    3030 Airco Drive
    Madison, WI 53701

EQUIPMENT MANUFACTURERS

43. Parks Medical Electronics, Inc.
PO Box BB
Beaverton, OR 97075
44. Particle Data, Inc.
PO Box 265
Elmhurst, IL 60126
45. Paxarms Limited
PO Box 317
Timaru, New Zealand
46. Perkin-Elmer Medical Instruments
2771 North Garey Avenue
Pomona, CA 91767
47. Physio-Control Corporation
11811 Willows Road
Redmond, WA 98052
48. Professional Instruments Company
PO Box 38245
Houston, TX 77238-8245
49. Puritan Bennett Corporation
10800 Pflumm Road
Lenexa, KS 66215
50. Radiometer America, Inc.
81 Sharon Drive
Cleveland, OH 41145
51. Research Equipment Company
3904 North Texas Avenue
Bryan, TX 77806
52. Sarns, Inc.
6200 Jackson Road
PO Box 1247
Ann Arbor, MI 48106
53. Schroer Manufacturing Company
2217 Campbell
Kansas City, MO 64108
54. Shank's Machine Company, Inc.
1704 East 18th Street
Sterling, IL 61081
55. Sorenson Research Company
4455 Atherton Drive
PO Box 15588
Salt Lake City, UT 84115
56. Stoelting Company
1350 South Kostner Avenue
Chicago, IL 60623
57. Telonics
1300 West University Drive
Mesa AZ 85201
58. Temptronix
19782 MacArthur Boulevard
Suite 300
Irvine, CA 92714
59. TEN/SV Care
PO Box YY
Incline, NV 89450
60. Thermocare, Inc.
PO Drawer YY
Incline Village, NV 89450
61. Unimetrics
1853 Raymond Avenue
Anaheim, CA 92801
62. Veterinarian Specialties, Inc.
Cedar Rapids, IA 52406
63. Vetko
4931 Northpark Drive
Colorado Springs, CO 80907
64. Walz & Krenzer, Inc.
22 Flint Street
Rochester, NY 14608
65. Wellcome Animal Health, Inc.
520 West 21st Street
Kansas City, MO 64108
66. Westwood Enterprise
PO Box 112
Ovando, MT 59854
67. Wysong Medical Corporation
4925 North Jefferson Avenue
Midland, MI 48640
68. Yellow Springs Instrument, Co., Inc.
PO Box 279
Yellow Springs, OH 45387
69. Zulu Arms of Omaha
10315 Wright Street
Omaha, NB 68124

Appendix B

Standard Values and Equivalents*

METRIC WEIGHTS

1 gram (1 g)	=	weight of 1 cc water at 4° C
1000 g	=	1 kilogram (kg)
0.1 g	=	1 decigram (dg)
0.01 g	=	1 centigram (cg)
0.001 g	=	1 milligram (mg)
0.001 mg	=	1 microgram (μg)

METRIC VOLUMES

1 liter (L)	=	1 cubic decimeter or 1000 cubic centimeters (cc)
0.001 liter	=	1 milliliter (ml)

SOLUTION EQUIVALENTS

1 part in	10	=	10.00 %	(1 ml contains 100 mg)
1 part in	50	=	2.00 %	(1 ml contains 20 mg)
1 part in	100	=	1.00 %	(1 ml contains 10 mg)
1 part in	200	=	0.50 %	(1 ml contains 5 mg)
1 part in	500	=	0.20 %	(1 ml contains 2 mg)
1 part in	1,000	=	0.10 %	(1 ml contains 1 mg)
1 part in	1,500	=	0.066%	(1 ml contains 0.66 mg)
1 part in	2,600	=	0.038%	(1 ml contains 0.38 mg)
1 part in	5,000	=	0.02 %	(1 ml contains 0.20 mg)
1 part in	50,000	=	0.002%	(1 ml contains 0.02 mg)

The number of milligrams in 1 milliliter of any solution of known percentage strength is obtained by moving the decimal one place to the right.

APOTHECARIES' OR TROY WEIGHT

(Used in Prescriptions)

1 pound (lb)	=	12 ounces	=	5,760 grains
1 ounce (℥)	=	8 drams	=	480 grains
1 dram (ʒ)	=	60 grains		

Apothecaries' Volume

1 pint (O)	=	16 fluid ounces		
1 fluid ounce (fl. ℥)	=	8 fluid dram	=	480 minims (min)
1 fluid dram (fl. ʒ)	=	60 minims		

*Systeme International (SI) units and conversions are shown later in this appendix.

AVOIRDUPOIS OR IMPERIAL WEIGHT

(Used in commerce in the United States and in the British Pharmacopeia)

Grain	=	same as Troy grain		
Ounce (oz)	=			437.5 grains
Pound (lb)	=	16 oz	=	7000 grains
Ton	=	2000 lb		

IMPERIAL VOLUME

				Apothecaries' System
Minims (min)	=			0.96 ♏
Fluidrachm (fl dr)	=	60 min	=	0.96 fl ʒ
Fluidounce (fl oz)	=	8 drachms	=	0.96 fl ℥
Pint (O)	=	20 fluidounces	=	1.2 O
Gallon (C)	=	8 pints	=	1.2 C

APPROXIMATE EQUIVALENT WEIGHTS

1 kilogram	=	2.2 Avoirdupois or Imperial pounds
1 kilogram	=	2.6 Apothecary or Troy pounds
1 gram	=	15 (15.4) grains
1 milligram	=	1/60 (1/64) grain
1 ounce	=	30 grams
(Avoirdupois or Imperial	=	28.350 grams)
(Apothecary or Troy	=	31.1035 grams)
1 dram	=	4 grams
1 grain	=	60 milligrams

APPROXIMATE VOLUMES

1 liter	=	1 quart
1 milliliter or cubic centimeter	=	15 minims
1 pint	=	500 cubic centimeters
1 fluid ounce	=	30 cubic centimeters
(Imperial	=	28.412 cubic centimeters)
(Apothecary	=	29.574 cubic centimeters)
1 fluid dram	=	4 cubic centimeters

EQUIVALENTS OF CENTIGRADE AND FAHRENHEIT THERMOMETRIC SCALES

Centigrade Degree	*Fahrenheit Degree*	*Centigrade Degree*	*Fahrenheit Degree*
−17	+ 1.4	14	57.2
−16	3.2	15	59.0
−15	5.0	16	60.8
−14	6.8	17	62.6
−13	8.6	18	64.4
−12	10.4	19	66.2
−11	12.2	20	68.0
−10	14.0	21	69.8
− 9	15.8	22	71.6
− 8	17.6	23	73.4
− 7	19.4	24	75.2
− 6	21.2	25	77.0
− 5	23.0	26	78.8
− 4	24.8	27	80.6
− 3	26.6	28	82.4
− 2	28.4	29	84.2
− 1	30.2	30	86.0
0	32.0	31	87.8
+ 1	33.8	32	89.6
2	35.6	33	91.4
3	37.4	34	93.2
4	39.2	35	95.0
5	41.0	36	96.8
6	42.8	37	98.6
7	44.6	38	100.4
8	46.4	39	102.2
9	48.2	40	104.0
10	50.0	41	105.8
11	51.8	42	107.6
12	53.6	43	109.4
13	55.4	44	111.2
		45	113.0

GAS DENSITIES

(Wt of Unit Vol)

22.4 liters of any gas are equal to its molecular weight in grams at a pressure of 760 mm of mercury and 0° C

MOLECULAR WEIGHTS

Ethylene	=	28 g
Air	=	29 g
Oxygen	=	32 g
Cyclopropane	=	42 g
Nitrous oxide	=	44 g
Carbon dioxide	=	44 g
Ether	=	74 g
Chloroform	=	119 g

(From A.M.A.: *Fundamentals of Anesthesia,* 3rd ed. W. B. Saunders Co., Philadelphia, 1954.)

Special Symbols*

— Dash above any symbol indicates a *mean* value.
· Dot above any symbol indicates a *time derivative*.

FOR GASES

Primary Symbols (Large Capital Letters)			*Examples*		
V	=	gas volume	VA	=	volume of alveolar gas
$\dot{V}$	=	gas volume/unit time	$\dot{V}O_2$	=	O_2 consumption/min
P	=	gas pressure	PAO_2	=	alveolar O_2 pressure
$\bar{P}$	=	mean gas pressure	PCO_2	=	mean capillary O_2 pressure
F	=	fractional concentration in dry gas phase	FIO_2	=	fractional concentration of O_2 in inspired gas
f	=	respiratory frequency (breaths/unit time)			
D	=	diffusing capacity	DO_2	=	diffusing capacity for (O_2 (ml O_2/min/mm/Hg)
R	=	respiratory exchange ratio	R	=	$\dot{V}CO_2/\dot{V}O_2$

Secondary Symbols (Small Capital Letters)			*Examples*		
I	=	inspired gas	FICO_2	=	fractional concentration of CO_2 in inspired gas
E	=	expired gas	VE	=	volume of expired gas
A	=	alveolar gas	$\dot{V}$A	=	alveolar ventilation/min
T	=	tidal gas	VT	=	tidal volume
D	=	dead space gas	VD	=	volume of dead space gas
B	=	barometric	PB	=	barometric pressure
STPD	=	0° C, 760 mm Hg, dry			
BTPS	=	body temperature and pressure saturated with water vapor			
ATPS	=	ambient temperature and pressure saturated with water vapor			

*From THE LUNG by Julius H. Comroe, Jr., et al. (based on report in Fed. Proc., 9:602–605, 1950). Copyright © 1962 (Second Edition) Year Book Medical Publishers. Used with permission.

For Blood

Primary Symbols (Large Capital Letters)		Examples	
Q	= volume of blood	Qc	= volume of blood in pulmonary capillaries
$\dot{Q}$	= volume flow of blood/unit time	$\dot{Q}$c	= blood flow through pulmonary capillaries/min
C	= concentration of gas in blood	Ca_{O_2}	= ml O_2 in 100 ml arterial blood
S	= % saturation of Hb with O_2 or CO	Sv_{CO_2}	= saturation of Hb with O_2 in mixed venous blood

Secondary Symbols (small letters)		Examples	
a	= arterial blood	Pa_{CO_2}	= partial pressure of CO_2 in arterial blood
v	= venous blood	Pv_{O_2}	= partial pressure of O_2 in mixed venous blood
c	= capillary blood	Pc_{CO}	= partial pressure of CO in pulmonry capillary blood

For Lung Volumes

VC	= Vital Capacity	= maximal volume that can be expired after maximal inspiration
IC	= Inspiratory Capacity	= maximal volume that can be inspired from resting expiratory level
IRV	= Inspiratory Reserve Volume	= maximal volume that can be inspired from end-tidal inspiration
ERV	= Expiratory Reserve Volume	= maximal volume that can be expired from resting expiratory level
FRC	= Functional Residual Capacity	= volume of gas in lungs at resting expiratory level
RV	= Residual Volume	= volume of gas in lungs at end of maximal expiration
TLC	= Total Lung Capacity	= volume of gas in lungs at end of maximal inspiration

SYSTEME INTERNATIONAL*

The following information on SI units and factors for conversion between SI and older conventional units is provided for the convenience of readers and authors.

BASIC SI UNITS

Physical Quantity	*Name*	*Symbol*
Length	Meter	m
Mass	Kilogram	kg
Time	Second*	s
Electric current	Ampere	A
Thermodynamic temperature	Kelvin	K
Luminous intensity	Candela	cd
Amount of substance	Mole	mol

*Minute (min), hour (h), and day (d) will remain in use although they are not official SI units.

PREFIXES FOR SI UNITS

Factor	*Name*	*Symbol*	*Factor*	*Name*	*Symbol*
10^{18}	Exa	E	10^{-18}	Atto-	a
10^{15}	Peta	P	10^{-15}	Femto	f
10^{12}	Tera-	T	10^{-12}	Pico-	p
10^{9}	Giga-	G	10^{-9}	Nano-	n
10^{6}	Mega-	M	10^{-6}	Micro-	μ
10^{3}	Kilo-	k	10^{-3}	Milli-	m
10^{2}	Hecto-	h	10^{-2}	Centi-	c
10^{1}	Deca-	da	10^{-1}	Deci-	d

DERIVED SI UNITS

Quantity	*SI Unit*	*Symbol*	*Expression in Terms of SI Base Units or Derived Units*
Frequency	Hertz	Hz	1 Hz = 1 cycle/s (1 s^{-1})
Force	Newton	N	1 N = 1 kg·m/s^2 (1 kg·mPs^{-2})
Work, energy, quantity of heat	Joule	J	1 J = 1 N·m
Power	Watt	W	1 W = 1 J/s (1 J·s^{-1})
Quantity of electricity	Coulomb	C	1 C = 1 A·s
Electric potential, potential difference, tension, electromotive force	Volt	V	1 V = 1 W/A (1 W·A^{-1})
Electric capacitance	Farad	F	1 F = 1 A·s/V (1 A·s·V^{-1})
Electric resistance	Ohm	Ω	1 Ω = 1 V/A (1 V·A^{-1})
Flux of magnetic induction, magnetic flux	Weber	Wb	1 Wb = 1 V·s
Magnetic flux density, magnetic induction	Tesla	T	1 T = 1 Wb/m^2 (1 Wb·m^{-2})
Inductance	Henry	H	1 H = 1 V·s/A (1 V·s·A^{-1})
Pressure	Pascal	Pa	1 Pa = 1 N/m^2 (1 N·m^{-2}) = 1 kg/m·s^2 (1 kg·m^{-1}· s^{-2})

The liter (10^{-3} m^3 = dm^3), though not official, will remain in use as a unit of volume as also will the dyne (dyn) as a unit of force (1 dyn = 10^{-5} N).

*Reprints of these tables are available on request from The Canadian Anaesthetists' Society Journal, 178 St. George Street, Toronto, Canada, M5R 2M7.

SI Unit	Old Unit	Conversion Factors Old to SI (exact)	SI to Old (approx.)
kPa	mm Hg*	0.133	7.5
kPa	1 standard atmosphere† (approx: 1 Bar)	101.3	0.01
kPa	cmH_2O	0.0981	10
kPa	lbs/sq in	6.89	0.145

*e.g., systolic BP of 120 mm Hg = 16 kPa and diastolic BP of 80 mm Hg = 11 kPa
† = 760 mm Hg

BLOOD CHEMISTRY. UNITS AND CONVERSION FACTORS

Measurement	SI Unit	Old Unit	Conversion Factors Old to SI (exact)	SI to Old (approx.)
Blood				
Acid-Base				
P_{CO_2}	kPa	mm Hg	0.133	7.5
P_{O_2}	kPa	mm Hg	0.133	7.5
Standard bicarbonate	mmol/liter	mEq/liter	Numerically equivalent	
Base excess	mmol/liter	mEq/liter	Numerically equivalent	
Glucose	mmol/liter	mg/100 ml	0.0555	18
Plasma				
Sodium	mmol/liter	mEq/liter	Numerically equivalent	
Potassium	mmol/liter	mEq/liter	Numerically equivalent	
Magnesium	mmol/liter	mEq/liter	0.5	2
Chloride	mmol/liter	mEq/liter	Numerically equivalent	
Phosphate (inorganic)	mmol/liter	mEq/liter	0.323	3.0
Creatinine	μmol/liter	mg/100 ml	88.4	0.01
Urea	mmol/liter	mg/100 ml	0.166	6.0
Serum				
Calcium	mmol/liter	mg/100 ml	0.25	4.0
Iron	μmol/liter	μg/100 mol	0.179	5.6
Bilirubin	μmol/liter	mg/100 ml	17.1	0.06
Cholesterol	mmol/liter	mg/100 ml	0.0259	39
Total proteins	g/liter	g/100 ml	10.0	0.1
Albumin	g/liter	g/100 ml	10.0	0.1
Globulin	g/liter	g/100 ml	10.0	0.1

BIOCHEMICAL CONTENT OF OTHER BODY FUIDS

Measurement	SI Unit	Old Unit	Conversion Factors Old to SI (exact)	SI to Old (approx.)
Urine				
Calcium	mmol/24 h	mg/24 h	0.025	40
Creatinine	mmol/24 h	mg/24 h	0.00884	113
Potassium	mmol/liter	mEq/liter	Numerically equivalent	
Sodium	mmol/liter	mEq/liter	Numerically equivalent	
Cerebrospinal fluid				
Protein	g/liter	mg/100 ml	0.01	100
Glucose	mmol/liter	mg/100 ml	0.0555	18

HEMATOLOGY

Measurement	SI Unit	Old Unit	Conversion Factors: Old to SI	Conversion Factors: SI to Old
Hemoglobin (Hb)	g/dl	g/100 ml	Numerically equivalent	
Packed cell volume	No unit*	Percent	0.01	100
Mean cell Hb conc.	g/dl	Percent	Numerically equivalent	
Mean cell Hb	pg	$\mu\mu g$	Numerically equivalent	
Red cell count	Cells/liter	Cells/mm^3	10^6	10^{-6}
White cell count	Cells/liter	Cells/mm^3	10^6	10^{-6}
Reticulocytes	Percent	Percent	Numerically equivalent	
Platelets	Cells/liter	Cells/mm^3	10^6	10^{-6}

*Expressed as decimal fraction, e.g., normal adult male value 0.40 to 0.54.

PH AND NMOL/LITER OF H^+ ACTIVITY

pH	nmol/liter
6.80	158
6.90	126
7.00	100
7.10	79
7.20	63
7.25	56
7.30	50
7.35	45
7.40	40
7.45	36
7.50	32
7.55	28
7.60	25
7.70	20

CATHETER COMPARISON SCALE
FOR DAVOL & MAGILL (A.CHAS.KING CO.LTD.) CATHETERS

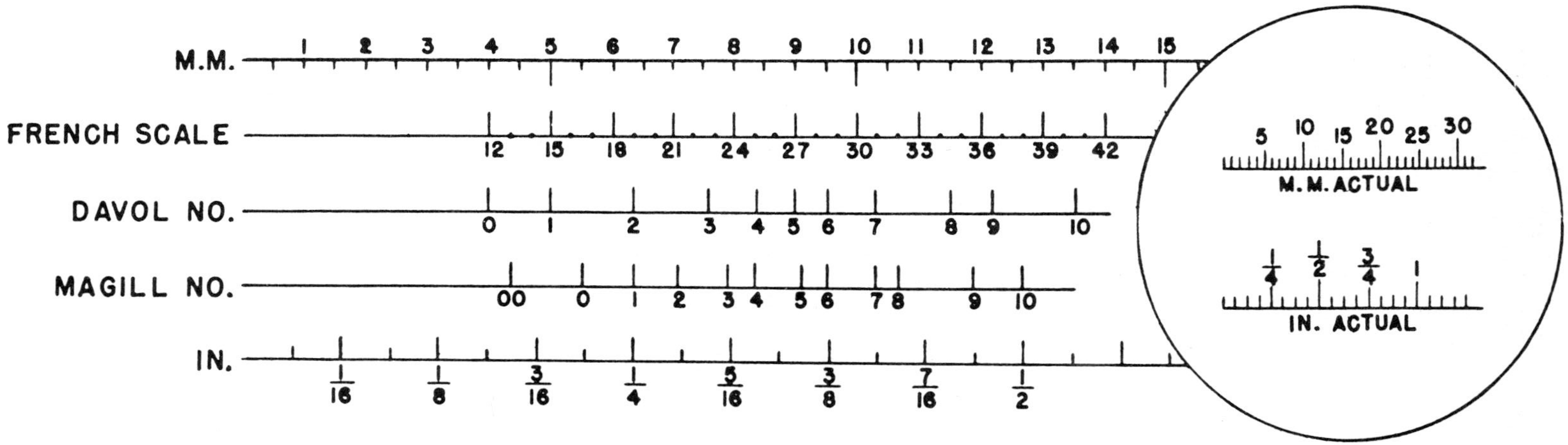

To compare catheter sizes, place a rule on one of the calibrations and check along the edge for the corresponding figures. The scale is enlarged eight times for easy reading. An actual-size scale is shown in the circle if measurements are required. (Courtesy of The British Oxygen Co., Ltd., London.) For an approximate conversion from French scale to internal diameter in millimeters, the French value can be divided by four.

Appendix C

Euthanasia Solution

Pentobarbital sodium, powder	259.2 g
Ethyl alcohol, 95%	400.0 ml
Sodium hydroxide solution, 10%	80.0 ml
Hot water q.s.	2000.0 ml

Give 1 ml/5 lb intravenously, more if necessary.

Index

Numbers in *italics* refer to figures; numbers followed by "t" refer to tables.